Trauma Team Dynamics

Lawrence Marshall Gillman • Sandy Widder
Editors

Trauma Team Dynamics

A Trauma Crisis Resource Management Manual

Second Edition 2025

Springer

Editors
Lawrence Marshall Gillman
University of Manitoba
Winnipeg, MB, Canada

Sandy Widder
University of Alberta
Edmonton, AB, Canada

ISBN 978-3-031-86311-0 ISBN 978-3-031-86312-7 (eBook)
https://doi.org/10.1007/978-3-031-86312-7

This Springer imprint is published by the registered company Springer Nature Switzerland AG
The registered company address is: Gewerbestrasse 11, 6330 Cham, Switzerland

To our families, friends, and colleagues. None of this would be possible without you.

—Lawrence M. Gillman

Foreword

Trauma, an enduring global challenge, continues to claim countless lives and inflict immeasurable suffering. While significant progress has been made in trauma care, with a proliferation of worldwide training programs and the establishment of trauma systems in various nations, the pivotal aspect of how trauma providers collaborate and care for critically injured patients remains paramount.

Trauma resuscitation, which is inherently multidisciplinary and perpetually high-stakes, hinges on the effectiveness of teamwork, communication, and coordination. Care of the multiply inured trauma patient is ever changing and the ability to accurately diagnose as well as provide care to these patients is profoundly influenced by the collaborative efforts of the trauma team. It is indisputable that seamless cooperation among healthcare professionals can markedly enhance the quality of trauma resuscitation, directly impacting patient outcomes.

The exceptional compilation of chapters in this second edition of "Trauma Team Dynamics" builds upon the foundations laid by its predecessor, and it brings fresh perspectives, insights, and expertise to the field of trauma resuscitation. The distinguished editors, recognized as international leaders in their respective domains, have meticulously assembled a diverse ensemble of acclaimed authors.

This collective effort culminates in what can be unequivocally hailed as a quintessential textbook on trauma team dynamics. What sets this textbook and its associated course, STARTT (Standardized Trauma and Resuscitation Team Training), apart is its unique focus on what has traditionally been described as nontechnical skills. These skills, however, are absolutely essential for effectively coordinating and communicating with the diverse array of trauma providers, which includes, but is not limited to, emergency medical providers, nurses, respiratory therapists, emergency department technicians, emergency room physicians, traumatologists, and a host of different surgeons.

"Trauma Team Dynamics" and the associated STARTT course provide the essential groundwork for facilitating and enhancing trauma team dynamics, giving healthcare professionals the tools and insights necessary to excel in their roles. This second edition will serve as an invaluable resource for healthcare providers, educators, and students alike, offering guidance and inspiration as they navigate the complex landscape of trauma care. I believe that the wisdom contained within these pages will foster an environment where every trauma resuscitation team can truly excel, ultimately saving more lives and mitigating the impact of this relentless global epidemic.

Departments of Surgery and Medicine
Schulich School of Medicine and Dentistry
Western University
London, ON, Canada

Neil G. Parry

Preface: Trauma as a Team Sport

The American College of Surgeons Advanced Trauma Life Support (ATLS®) Course has revolutionized trauma care by offering a standardized, reproducible, and universal approach to trauma patient management. ATLS® however focuses on management by a solo practitioner, which is rarely the case in modern trauma care. The introduction of a trauma team, no matter how small, brings with it new challenges and dynamics. To date no text (including the ATLS® manual) has addressed the unique dynamics created by a multidisciplinary trauma team and strategies to optimize them.

Further, morbidity and mortality reviews reveal that the majority of medical errors are nontechnical in nature, stemming from faulty decision-making, asynchronous information gathering, lack of situational awareness, and ineffective communication and team leadership. Reviews of accidents from other high-risk industries, including the airline industry, have had similar findings. This led NASA (National Aeronautics and Space Administration) and the airline industry to develop crew (now crisis) resource management (CRM) training. Medicine has begun adapting this training especially within the realms of anesthesia and critical care. Trauma surgery has been slower to utilize this work however simulation based training is increasing in popularity. These team-based training strategies address "nontechnical" skills to counteract human error and improve team and patient safety.

CRM is integral to the way that we manage ourselves, team members, and patients during emergency situations. It is essentially the ability to translate knowledge of what needs to be done into effective actions during a crisis situation. There are numerous publications on trauma diagnosis, management, and treatment of injuries, but little literature exists on communication within the trauma resuscitation, and how communication can be utilized to improve teamwork and crisis management, and potentially improve patient resuscitation outcomes.

This book is in no way meant to replace ATLS® training, but instead build on ATLS® principles and highlight how they can be applied by a multi-disciplinary trauma team. This textbook represents a unique standalone reference for others trying to teach or learn these Trauma Team Dynamics. Authored by an international group with a broad expertise in trauma, critical care, emergency medicine, nursing, respiratory therapy, and pre-hospital care (including NASA and United States military affiliated experts), we feel it forms a comprehensive, multidisciplinary manual for all trauma team members including pre- and out-of-hospital personnel, emergency and critical care physicians, trauma surgeons, nurses, and respiratory therapists, as well as their respective trainees.

Part I highlights the history of CRM including its beginnings with NASA and the airline industry, and its evolution to other high-risk industries including medicine. It goes on to introduce us to the guiding tenants of CRM and how they can be applied practically in a trauma setting. These concepts continue to be woven throughout the text as we highlight the importance of CRM principles while following the trauma patient from the scene, through prehospital care and transport, to the trauma bay and finally to definitive care.

In Part II we discover the structure of the modern trauma team, including pre-hospital personnel, highlighting the roles of the various trauma team members and design of the typical trauma bay. We also briefly explore the logistics of trauma system design and important quality control issues.

Part III begins with a review of ATLS® and resuscitation principles and then offers a practical and comprehensive approach to damage control resuscitation not seen in other texts. It goes on to discuss the complexities of trauma decision-making and ends with a practical highlight of common trauma bay procedures.

Part IV stresses certain challenges in the trauma management of specific patient populations including the pregnant patient, the head injured patient as well as the patient with multiple medical comorbidities and the elderly.

In Part V we discuss conventional and point of care imaging in the trauma patient including an in-depth look at basic and advanced trauma ultrasound, and new emerging techniques.

Part VI takes trauma to the battlefield, the mountain-top and beyond with discussions on tactical and battlefield medicine, trauma in austere environments and even space. In the course of this discussion we emphasize the unique challenges of chemical, biological, and nuclear injuries and how these affect both the patient and the trauma team.

Finally, crisis resource management skills are best taught through a crisis simulation curriculum and therefore Part VII offers practical tips and guidance on CRM curriculum design, debriefing, and evaluation.

It is our sincere hope that this text serves as a catalyst to improve communication in the trauma bay, improve multidisciplinary training of team members, and ultimately improve patient care. Trauma truly is a Team Sport and its time to finally teach it as such.

Winnipeg, MB, Canada Lawrence M. Gillman

Contents

Part I

Trauma Team Preparation

A Culture of Safety: Evolution of the S.T.A.R.T.T. Course

1

Lawrence Marshall Gillman, J. Damian Paton-Gay, Paul T. Engels, and Sandy Widder

The Simulated Trauma and Resuscitation Team Training (S.T.A.R.T.T.) Course is a multidisciplinary trauma team training course designed to teach non-technical (crisis resource management) skills to all trauma team members involved in the care of the multi-injured patient, including prehospital personnel (emergency medical technicians and paramedics), nurses, respiratory therapists, physician assistants, nurse practitioners, emergency physicians, anaesthetists and surgeons.

History

The S.T.A.R.T.T. course evolved from humble beginnings. The course foundation was initially devised in 2010 by two keen staff surgeons (LG and SW) who had completed their Trauma/Critical Care training and realized there was a need for optimizing trauma team dynamics during resuscitations. With the burgeoning national Royal College Acute Critical Events Simulation (ACES) course (now under the auspices of the Canadian Critical Care Society) [1] and monthly local crisis simulations, critical care training had embraced Crisis Resource Management (CRM) principles; however, trauma and surgical training was lagging behind. The course was started at their local institutions in Edmonton and Winnipeg as a way to improve general surgery resident trauma training specifically focussing on non-technical skills training. The success of this concept locally quickly led to the educational expansion to a national platform, but prior to implementation, the foundations needed to be established.

A needs analysis of general surgery program directors across the country was undertaken. The response rate was 64.7% (11 of 17). Only a minority of programs had CRM training and trauma simulation as part of their local curricula. The vast majority saw value in this training, however, and supported the creation of a national curriculum and training program [2].

This led to the formation of the S.T.A.R.T.T. course committee and a discussion about the format, content and curriculum of the initial pilot course. It quickly became clear that training residents in isolation would do little to improve the actual functioning of the full trauma team. While many CRM training programs included non-physician team members in their simulations, most were confederates whose roles were to support resident learning but not necessarily act as learners. This prompted us to expand the planned S.T.A.R.T.T. course to a multidisciplinary model where all participants enter each simulation blindly and are treated as equal participants. Not only was the premise to enhance team trust, but also to reflect the reality of the unpredictable nature of trauma, highlighting team dynamics that were not previously apparent. The inaugural S.T.A.R.T.T. course was held in conjunction with the Canadian Surgery Forum in Calgary on September 12, 2012. Twenty general surgery residents (PGY 1–6), five practicing nurses and four respiratory therapists participated in the course supported by eleven instructors. These participants represented eight universities from six different Canadian provinces, with all the respiratory therapists and nurses from local hospitals. The course was overwhelmingly well received with 97.5% of participants rating the course as "good" or "excellent" and 97.5% recom-

L. Marshall Gillman (✉)
Departments of Surgery Section of General Surgery, University of Manitoba, Winnipeg, MB, Canada

Internal Medicine Section of Critical Care, University of Manitoba, Winnipeg, MB, Canada
e-mail: Lawrence.Gillman@umanitoba.ca

J. D. Paton-Gay · S. Widder
Department of Surgery, University of Alberta, Edmonton, AB, Canada
e-mail: patongay@ualberta.ca

P. T. Engels
Departments of Surgery and Critical Care Medicine, McMaster University, Hamilton, ON, Canada
e-mail: engelsp@mcmaster.ca

L. Marshall Gillman, S. Widder (eds.), *Trauma Team Dynamics*, https://doi.org/10.1007/978-3-031-86312-7_1

mending it to others. On pre- and post-course testing, all groups also showed a significant improvement in attitudes towards CRM principles specifically within the domains of teamwork and safety climate [2].

While the bulk of the feedback was positive, there were constructive criticisms as well. Most importantly, even though the non-physician participants were told they were equal participants, some felt the simulation cases, and debriefs were still physician-centric, and they did not truly feel like true participants and team members. Over the ensuing courses, extensive work was done to overhaul the scenarios, including obtaining input from non-physician stakeholders. Learning objectives and tasks were created for each participating discipline and unique scenario designs were created, including distance simulations and staggered entry scenarios in order to engage non-physician participants and improve the experience for all. Not only did these changes accomplish these goals, they broadened the learning objectives and added important layers to the debriefs [3]. These will be discussed in more detail later in the chapter on Multidisciplinary Simulation Design.

One of the most well received and beneficial changes we made was to our instructor assignments. As is common with simulation courses, we initially had instructors assigned to each simulation scenario and the participants rotated as a team from scenario to scenario. While this allowed instructors to become familiar with their stations the participants felt they were receiving significant repetition in the content of the debrief from scenario to scenario. We therefore made a change, assigning one of our senior instructors, termed a "team coach" or "team navigator", to spend the day with each team. Other instructors were assigned to individual simulation stations. This had multiple immediate benefits. First, it allowed a single instructor to get to know the group for the duration of the day. The coach was tasked with leading all the debriefs and therefore could build on lessons learned from the previous scenario while helping their team focus on areas of weakness or new areas in subsequent scenarios. It also built rapport between the debriefer and the team members, and ensured a culture of safety so that the debriefer could understand personalities, unique team dynamics, and bring out comments from all team members. We also ensured that our team coaches had received formal debriefing training to ensure they were skilled to control the room and the post simulation debrief maintaining a balanced discussion that identified and closed performance gaps.

As the course content developed, two distinct versions of the course emerged. The first was the standard course, involving physicians, respiratory therapists, nurses and physician assistants. The second was an expanded course incorporating pre-hospital personnel as part of the participating groups. This addition was extremely well received as it not only incorporated mass casualty management and transport issues, it also added an additional layer of communication and handover. The format brought together two distinct groups of practitioners (hospital and prehospital personnel) that frequently interact and work together but rarely, if ever, train together [4].

In 2017, we introduced the surgical cut suit, otherwise known as "Human Worn Partial Task Surgical Simulators" (Strategic Operations, Inc.), as a routine component of the course. This one-piece zip-up suit is worn by standardized patients and takes the place of classic mannequin-based simulation. The cut suit allows for procedures including cricothyroidotomy, chest tube insertion, laparotomy and even ED thoracotomy to be performed directly (and safely) on a live, talking actor, enhancing both conceptual and physical realism. This addition was similarly met with overwhelming support, as more than 70% of participants reported the suits as an essential part of the course and more than 90% reported the suits as valuable to the course and an improvement in course realism [5].

Documented Outcomes

To date, we have held 17 courses in major trauma centres across Canada and an international course in Melbourne, Australia. We have trained over 300 trauma providers and have more than 50 trained instructors. We held our first French language course in Quebec City. The challenge of running a communication course for francophone participants coached by predominantly anglophone faculty was a welcome and rewarding learning experience for the course leadership [6].

The ideal venue for S.T.A.R.T.T. courses remains an area of debate. The majority of S.T.A.R.T.T. courses to date have been held at large national and international meetings. However, we have also run a number of local courses, notably in Winnipeg and Montreal, involving local trauma teams. Running smaller local courses has the advantage of training teams that work together on a regular basis, improving the camaraderie and non-technical skills of established teams while fostering further local work and innovation. On the opposite side, holding courses at larger national and international meetings brings together participants (and experts) from multiple centres, each offering their own local flavour and expertise with the ability for participants to return to their own centres with new shared knowledge. The reality is that there is no perfect model. Using local courses to reinvigorate the culture of safety and ongoing quality improvement at the site level, while using larger national courses to share information and maintain a cohesive trauma community are likely both worthwhile endeavours.

Future Direction

With the COVID-19 pandemic, the S.T.A.R.T.T. course reached a crossroads. The feasibility of a large-scale, in-person, training curriculum was unclear in that challenging environment. Thankfully it seems we have weathered the pandemic and restarting larger courses at national and international meetings seems possible again. However, the COVID pandemic has allowed us to consider other shifts in philosophy for the S.T.A.R.T.T. course. As with all challenges, there is an opportunity for innovation. We are currently looking at hybrid models using virtual platforms to offer simulation over distance and training local trauma teams from multiple institutions simultaneously [7]. This may allow us to share knowledge across the national and international communities, while allowing local teams to hone their responses within the culture and environment of their home facilities. With technological development, other potential avenues of pursuit may include courses held in virtual reality environments, allowing for participants across vast distances to simulate together in a virtual classroom.

Regardless of how S.T.A.R.T.T. evolves to meet this new challenge, the need for continual training and updating of our trauma practitioners remains. After all, trauma care is the ultimate high-performance team sport, and no team gets better without dedicated practice.

Key Points

- A trauma crisis resource management team training course adds important skills not currently available elsewhere.
- The structure and venue of this course will need to continue to evolve as this training becomes more widely available and ubiquitous.

References

1. Canadian Critical Care Society. About National Acute Critical Event Simulation (N-ACES). https://www.canadiancriticalcare.org/N-ACES. Accessed 9 Nov 2022.
2. Ziesmann MT, Widder S, Park J, Kortbeek JB, Brindley P, Hameed M, et al. S.T.A.R.T.T.: development of a national, multidisciplinary trauma crisis resource management curriculum-results from the pilot course. J Trauma Acute Care Surg. 2013;75:753–8. https://doi.org/10.1097/TA.0b013e3182a925df.
3. Gillman LM, Brindley P, Paton-Gay JD, Engels PT, Park J, Vergis A, et al. Simulated Trauma and Resuscitation Team Training course-evolution of a multidisciplinary trauma crisis resource management simulation course. Am J Surg. 2016;212:188–1e3. https://doi.org/10.1016/j.amjsurg.2015.07.024.
4. Gillman LM, Martin D, Engels PT, Brindley P, Widder S. French C. S.T.A.R.T.T. plus: addition of prehospital personnel to a national multidisciplinary crisis resource management trauma team training course. Can J Surg. 2015;58:010915–5.
5. Johnson GGRJ, Brindley PG, Gillman LM. Fidelity in surgical simulation: further lessons from the S.T.A.R.T.T. course. Can J Surg. 2020;63:E161–3. https://doi.org/10.1503/cjs.017818.
6. Trauma Simulation in Bilingual Canada. Insurmountable barrier or unexpected strength? Insights from the first bilingual S.T.A.R.T.T. course. Can J Surg. 2016;59:80–2. https://doi.org/10.1503/cjs.014115.
7. Johnson GGRJ, Beaumont J, Paton-Gay JD, Widder S, Gillman LM. Multidisciplinary, multisite trauma team training during COVID-19: lessons from the first virtual E-S.T.A.R.T.T. course. Can J Surg. 2021;64(6):E609–12. https://doi.org/10.1503/cjs.009921.

The Genesis of Crew Resource Management: The NASA Experience

2

David J. Alexander

Humble Beginnings

The *National Aeronautics and Space Administration* (NASA) has been intimately involved with the process of Crew Resource Management (CRM) and one of the early innovators of the systematic procedures to eliminate human error in the cockpit. The first effort was the development of the aviation checklist. This was due to the crash of the Boeing Model 229 aircraft on October 30th, 1935. The Boeing Model 229 was an extremely complex aircraft for the time. It had many revolutionary design elements incorporated. The pilot, who had never flown the Model 229, had neglected to release the elevator lock prior to takeoff. The Boeing chief test pilot aboard the aircraft, Leslie Tower, realized the error once airborne. He attempted to release the lock but was too late to save the doomed aircraft. The design was in serious jeopardy after the crash. The press had labeled the aircraft as too complex to fly. Army Air Corps officers pleaded to proceed with the project and eventually 12 aircraft were delivered to the 2nd Bombardment Wing at Langley Airfield in Virginia. It was emphasized to the pilots that any further accidents would result in the cancellation of further orders. The pilots came together and developed four checklists. These were the Take-off, Flight, Pre-landing, and After Landing checklists. They eventually proved that the Model 229 was not "too much aircraft for a man to fly"; it had systems more complex than any one man's memory. These checklists were the assurance that no item was forgotten. These 12 aircraft went on to safely fly 1.8 million miles without a serious accident. The Model 229 went on to be developed as the B-17. It was one of the workhorse bombers of World War II and helped to destroy Nazi Germany's war industries. The checklist was then integrated into subsequent Air Corps aircraft and the civilian airline industry.

Human error as a cause for an accident was placed in the public eye again on the night of December 29th, 1972. An Eastern Airlines Lockheed L-1011, Flight 401 would be a sentinel event in safety. Flight 401 was en route from JFK Airport, New York, to Miami International Airport. The Lockheed L-1011 had rolled out of the factory only four months previously. This particular flight carried 163 passengers and 13 crewmembers. The journey was routine up until 11:32 pm. The aircraft was on approach to Miami International, and the landing gear was lowered. The landing gear indicator was not illuminated, indicating the gear was not down and locked. The landing gear was cycled again, and the illuminator still did not light. The light on the indicator was burned out, and the cockpit crew began replacing the bulb. The crew discontinued the approach and began a circling pattern to work on this problem. The second officer was sent into the lower avionics bay to view through a small window and confirm the gear was down. The aircraft autopilot was activated to maintain 2000 ft. During this time, the pilot accidently leaned against the yoke (control column) and changed the modes on the autopilot from altitude hold to CWS (Control Wheel Steering—in which the pilot controlled the pitch of that aircraft). This forward pressure also started the aircraft to descend. After descending 250 ft, a C-cord alarm was sounded in the cockpit. This alarm was designed to alert the crew that they had descended from their assigned altitude. The frustrated, fatigued crew who were concentrating only on the burned out light did not notice the alarm. The engineer was not on the flight deck as well and could not have heard the alarm from the avionics bay. The plane was over the Everglades at night, and therefore, there was no ground references to indicate the plane had descended. In fifty seconds, the aircraft was now down to 1000 ft. The co-pilot then initiated a 180 degree turn to maintain a holding pattern and noticed the discrepancy in altitude. This triggered the following conversation .

Co-pilot: We did something to the altitude.
Pilot: What?
Co-pilot: We're still at 2000 ft, right?
Pilot: Hey—what's happening here?

D. J. Alexander (✉)
Johnson Space Center, Houston, TX, USA
e-mail: david.j.alexander@nasa.gov

L. Marshall Gillman, S. Widder (eds.), *Trauma Team Dynamics*, https://doi.org/10.1007/978-3-031-86312-7_2

Ten seconds later, the aircraft impacted the Everglades. This resulted in the deaths of 101 persons and was the first accident of a wide-bodied airliner. At that time, it was the second deadliest single aircraft disaster in the United States [1–4].

Another accident around this same time period highlighted human error in the cockpit. United Airlines Flight 173 (UAL 173) was making its final approach to Portland International Airport after a routine flight on December 28, 1978 [5]. The aircraft ran out of fuel and crashed into a residential area, killing eight passengers and two crew members and seriously injuring 23 others. While circling, the first officer and flight engineer told the pilot that the plane was running low on fuel. The pilot ignored the warnings of his junior officers. These and other accidents aroused the interest publically in accidents due to human error.

In all of the cases, the aircrafts were mechanically sound; the crews were experienced and technically competent. The system at the time simply did not catch mistakes in time to prevent these fatal errors. In 1978, the Military Inspector General determined that poor crew interactions were a major factor in aircraft accidents. NASA then led the way to change the aviation community to prevent these accidents from occurring. In 1979, NASA conducted the *Resource Management on the Flightdeck* workshop at the Ames Research Center [6, 7]. NASA had for many years been conducting research into human factors and performance in aviation since the early 1970s at the Ames Research Center. In 1973, interviews with aircrews were conducted, and this highlighted the lack of training for airline Captains in leadership. H.P. Ruffel-Smith (1979) conducted a 747 simulator-based study on human behavior [8]. He found that in both routine and emergency simulations, the better the cockpit resources were utilized and using effective crew communications, the better the performance in the cockpit. Several other studies suggested that incorporating "Crew Resource Management" into routine flight operations training would greatly aid in preventing these accidents. During the workshop, it was soon discovered that 60–80% of aviation accidents were the result of human error. Clearly the aviation industry had to change. After another NASA/Federal Aviation Administration (FAA) workshop conducted in January 1981, the FAA began incorporating a CRM platform into its regulatory program. United Airlines was the first to add CRM into its training syllabus in 1981.

A New Paradigm Is Born

Crew Resource Management does not focus on technical aptitude or skills. CRM focuses on cognitive and interpersonal communication needed to organize a complex aviation environment. Cognitive skills focus on situational awareness, planning, and decision-making. Situational awareness provides an organized way to recognize salient factors and conditions that affect the safe operation of the aircraft. Planning takes the decision construction process across all phases of the flight. This also incorporates subordinate input into the decision formation process but still maintains a hierarchical structure with the Captain retaining authority and responsibility for the flight. Interpersonal skills concentrate on communications and team building. Essential to CRM is communication. Research has proven that good communication not only transfers accurate information but helps to build a unified understanding of the problems at hand. It helps everyone to build a mental model of the environment and enhances situational awareness. Team building incorporates the entire crew's skills and experience, resulting in the combined efforts far exceeding the capability of one individual. Emotional climate and stress management skills are also taught in CRM training. Research showed that the creation of a positive tone on the flight deck enhanced the cognitive and interpersonal proficiencies of the crew. Stress management in the cockpit can be managed by an organizational culture that efficiently assigns tasks and establishes priorities. This also incorporates the empowerment of subordinates by training them in the skills that will enable them to take on additional responsibility when the circumstances demand it.

The airlines embraced CRM training as well as the military. NASA took these concepts and incorporated them into the shuttle training program. One aspect of CRM was simulation training in the management of complex contingency operations that occur in spaceflight. These had been incorporated into the NASA culture since the earliest phases of spaceflight. From Mercury through today's International Space Station training, simulators have been a mainstay of spaceflight practice. NASA has also learned hard lessons from its failures. The Challenger accident highlighted several lapses in the NASA "Safety Culture" that contributed to the disaster. The investigation highlighted NASA's and Morton Thiokol's failure to respond to the design flaw of the O-rings in the Solid Rocket boosters. Rather than redesign the joint, it was defined as an acceptable flight risk. This was the "Normalization of Deviancy" or the violation of standards of practice repeatedly such that they actually become routine over time. This occurs by errors, lapses, or mistakes that go unattended, unappreciated, or unresolved for an extended period of time. The report also impugned the decision to launch. It cited numerous failures in communication that resulted in a decision to launch 51-L. The decision was based on "incomplete and sometimes misleading information, a conflict between engineering data and management judgments, and a NASA management structure that permitted internal flight safety problems to bypass key Shuttle managers" [9] .

Attention once again focused on the attitude of NASA management toward safety issues in 2003, after the Space Shuttle *Columbia* loss. The Columbia Accident Investigation Board (CAIB) deduced that NASA had not incorporated the lessons of *Challenger*. One highlight was that the agency had not set up a truly independent office for safety oversight. The CAIB concluded that in this area, "NASA's response to the Rogers Commission did not meet the Commission's intent" [10]. The CAIB believed that "the causes of the institutional failure responsible for *Challenger* have not been fixed" [10]. They declared that the same "flawed decision making process" that had culminated in the *Challenger* accident was at fault for *Columbia*'s destruction. The *Challenger* and *Columbia* accidents are now used as case studies in how several concepts in CRM broke down. The lessons for NASA were breakdowns in communication, lapses in group decision making and most importantly, revealed the dangers of groupthink (in which the desire for conformity or amity in a group results in a deviant or flawed decision-making conclusion).

NASA continues to improve the CRM process. The shuttle crews incorporated CRM directly into their training. These Shuttle Transportation System (STS) crews underwent numerous case simulations of normal and emergent situations. These incorporated the lessons learned from aviation and the shuttle accidents. These were incorporated into CRM for the entire shuttle operational teams. The crews were together for several years prior to launching. This included not only the mission's onboard crewmembers, but the Mission Control Teams dedicated to the particular missions. Numerous crew bonding activities to promote communication and team building were incorporated in to training regimens. Events such as the National Environmental Leadership School (NOLS) classes to teach leadership became important in astronaut training. These sessions incorporate leadership curriculum, outdoor ethics, and wilderness skills to help develop good leadership and communication. NASA management also undergoes CRM training to produce a true safety culture. These lessons are still integral to the International Space Station training and the future mission culture of NASA.

Medicine has also learned from these experiences in aviation. Helmreich and Schafer proposed using the NASA-inspired Crew Resource Management from the airline industry in operating rooms [11]. Subsequent to that in 1999, Sexton et al. compared flight crew interactions with operating room staff. This extensive multiyear study showed a remarkable difference in the attitudes about teamwork. The surgical staff showed that the surgical attendings and residents reported high levels of teamwork, but the ancillary staff (anesthesiology attendings, residents, nurses, and OR nurses) reported exceptionally low levels of teamwork. A significant amount of attending surgeons preferred the use of steep hierarchies (with junior team members being limited in questioning the decisions and actions of a superior). This was in stark contrast to the airline crews, instilled with the Crew Resource Management styles, who 94% preferred the flat hierarchies (in which junior members are encouraged to voice concerns about the senior members choices and decisions) [12]. The study also revealed the attitudes toward fatigue. A vast majority of the surgical staff agreed with the statement "Even when fatigued, I perform effectively during critical times." In stark contrast, only 26% of the flight crews agreed with that statement [12]. In 2000, a landmark report from the Institutes of Medicine (IOM) was released that sparked a large amount of public debate. The report "To Err Is Human: Building a Safer Health System" examined medical errors in healthcare systems. The report cited results from Colorado and Utah that up to 44,000 people died due to medical errors. It then went on to refer to one New York study, which indicated that up to 98,000 died due to errors in the medical system [12]. The report then concluded emphatically "healthcare is a decade or more behind other high-risk industries in its attention to ensuring basic safety." These lead to public outcries which subsequently lead to President Bill Clinton executing an executive order to require federal departments to develop safer practices in healthcare [13]. This lead to the Joint Commission on Accreditation for Healthcare Organizations (JCAHO) to support aviation teamwork applications in training programs for hospitals [14, 15].

The Sexton study and several other papers around that time triggered numerous changes to training programs, which incorporated aviation-inspired Crew Resource Management. Critical areas such as the Emergency Departments, Operating Suites, and Labor/Delivery were identified as those areas that could benefit from CRM training [16–18]. Anesthesiology incidents that were related to human error were proclaimed to be as high as 65–70% [15]. This prompted the VA Palo Alto Healthcare System and Stanford University to develop the Anesthesia Crisis Resource Management (ACRM) system based on CRM [16, 19]. The Army Research Laboratory and Dynamics Research Corporation developed the MedTeams behavior-based teamwork system. This drove military-based aviation experience into the Emergency Medicine training [18]. This system was expanded into labor and delivery units. The system eventually drove specific training and assessment tools incorporated into the Emergency Team Coordination Course. Similar to aviation CRM, the entire philosophy was centered on avoiding errors, ensnaring errors when they occurred, and mitigating all the consequences of decisions and actions that may have been taken in error. Peer monitoring is critical in all the medical CRM approaches. This insures maintaining adequate situational awareness during essential dynamic medical procedures. This then aids in incorporating good practices into procedures and improving training programs.

There is much debate currently on the effectiveness of CRM in medicine. Like aviation, it is difficult to show direct correlations to improvements in safety. Studies are challenging to design and very few studies to date incorporate a control group. Subjective and anecdotal data do suggest that aviation-based CRM in medicine is an improvement in the culture. and training previously offered [16, 17, 19]. Aviation has the advantage of 20 years of CRM training and experience. The improvements in performance for pilots have been shown in yearly evaluations, actual flight performance evaluations, and simulator training. The NASA/University of Texas Line/LOS Checklist (LINE/LOS Checklist) rating scales for critical crew performance during different phases of flight has shown improvements [20–23]. Again, NASA helped lead the way for safety improvement and evaluation. Analogous studies need to be performed in medicine.

Shifts in the culture of medicine to shift from centering only on technical expertise to include the facilitation of human interactions will take time. This effort is only now getting started. Crew resource management is a new paradigm in a centuries-old institution. This book marks a first step in introducing CRM to the trauma bay.

Key Points

- NASA has been intimately involved in aviation safety since the 1970s.
- Several airline accidents gained public attention when very experienced crews became distracted and initiated a series of errors that led to major accidents.
- Ground-breaking studies on human performance by NASA Ames Laboratories led to the NASA/FAA workshop in January 1981 to recommend Crew Resource Management (CRM) be incorporated into aviation safety.
- CRM focuses on cognitive and interpersonal communication needed to organize a complex aviation environment.
- NASA incorporated CRM into its safety culture, followed closely by the US Military and the major airlines.
- Reducing human error in the skies and in hospitals are noble endeavors.

References

1. Eastern airlines flight 401. [Internet]. [cited December 30, 2013]. Available from: https://sites.google.com/site/eastern401/
2. Kilroy K. Special report: Eastern airlines flight 401. [Internet]. AirDisaster.com. 1997 [updated 2013; cited December 30, 2013]. Available from: http://www.airdisaster.com/special/special-ea401.shtml
3. Eastern airlines flight 401 tribute group: The heritage of CRM. [Internet]. [updated February 2010; cited December 30, 2013]. http://www.ealflt401.blogspot.com
4. National Transportation Safety Board. Washington, DC: Aircraft accident report: Eastern Airlines Inc., L-1011 N310EA, Miami Fla, December 29, 1972, NTSB AAR-73-14
5. National Transportation Safety Board. Washington DC: Aircraft accident report: United Airlines, Inc., McDonnell-Douglass, DC-8-61, N8082U, Portland Oregon, December 28, 1978, NTSB-AAR-79-7
6. Cooper GE, White MD, Lauber JK. Resource management on the flightdeck: proceedings of a NASA/Industry Workshop, NASA Conference Publication No. CP-2120. Moffett Field: NASA – Ames Research Center; 1980.
7. Lauber JK. Cockpit resource management: background and overview. In: Orlady HW, Foushee HC, editors. Cockpit resource management training: proceedings of the NASA/MAC workshop, NASA Conference Publication No. 2455. Moffett Field: NASA – Ames Research Center.
8. Ruffel Smith HP. A simulator study of the interaction of pilot workload with errors, vigilance, and Decisions NASA Technical Memoraridum 78482. SMC-8. 1978;12:867–75.
9. Rogers Commission (June 6, 1986). Report of the presidential commission on the space shuttle challenger accident. Chapter V: The contributing cause of the accident
10. Columbia Accident Investigation Board. Report of Columbia accident investigation board. 2003;I(Chapter 7):178.
11. Helmreich RL, Schaefer HG. Team performance in the operating room. In: Bogner MS, editor. Human error in medicine. Hillside: Laurence Erlbaum; 1998.
12. Sexton JB, Thomas EJ, Helmreich RL. Error, stress, and the teamwork in medicine and aviation: cross sectional surveys. BMJ. 2000;320:745–9.
13. Altman DE, Clancy C, Blendon RJ. Improving patient safety – five years after the IOM report. N Engl J Med. 2004;351(20):2041–3.
14. O'Leary D. Patient safety: "instilling hospitals with a culture of continuous improvement". Testimony Before the Senate Committee on Governmental Affairs. JCAHO; 2003.
15. Sundar E, Sundar S, Pawlowski J, Blum R, Feinstein D, Pratt. Crew resource management and team training. Anesth Clin. 2007;25:283–300.
16. Howard SK, Gaba DM, Fish KJ, Yang G, Sarnquist FH. Anesthesia crisis resource management training: teaching anesthesiologists to handle critical incidents. Aviat Space Environ Med. 1992;63:763–70.
17. Halamek LP, Kaegi DM, Gaba DM, Sowb YA, Smith BC, Smith BE, et al. Time for a new paradigm in pediatric medical education: teaching neonatal resuscitation in a simulated delivery room environment. Pediatrics. 2000;106:E45.

18. Risser DT, Rice MM, Salisbury ML, Simon R, Jay GD, Berns SD. The potential for improved teamwork to reduce medical errors in the emergency department. The MedTeams Research Consortium. Ann Emerg Med. 1999;34:373–83.
19. Gaba DM, Howard SK, Fish KJ, Yasser SA. Simulation-based training in Anesthesia Crisis Resource Management (ACRM): a decade of experience. In: Simulation & gaming, vol. 32. Sage.
20. Gaba DM, Howard SK, Flanagan B, Smith BE, Fish KJ, Botney R. Assessment of clinical performance during simulated crises using both technical and behavioral ratings. Anesthesiology. 1998;89:8–18.
21. Barker JM, Clothier CC, Woody JR, McKinney EH Jr, Brown JL. Crew resource management: a simulator study comparing fixed versus formed aircrews. Aviat Space Environ Med. 1996;67:3–7.
22. Wiegmann DA, Shappell SA. Human error and crew resource management failures in Naval aviation mishaps: a review of U.S. Naval Safety Center Data, 1990–96. Aviat Space Environ Med. 1999;70:1147–51.
23. Helmreich RL, Wilhelm JA, Gregorich SE, Chidester TR. Preliminary results from the evaluation of cockpit resource management training: performance ratings of flight crews. Aviat Space Environ Med. 1990;61:576–9.

3 Evidence Supporting Crisis Resource Management Training

Christopher Hicks

Introduction

Error is ubiquitous in trauma care, occurring in as many as 100% of trauma resuscitations [1]. The trauma room represents a perfect storm for adverse outcomes; multiple team members of various backgrounds and training levels, holding different and often competing patient care priorities, must interact in the face of diagnostic uncertainty, high patient acuity and extreme time pressures to rapidly diagnose and manage multiple potentially life-threatening injuries.

Prior work has established a taxonomy of common errors that occur during the care of the trauma patient, which are known to have a detrimental effect on patient outcomes [2, 3]. The majority of these errors are non-technical in nature, stemming from faulty decision-making, asynchronous information gathering, lack of situational awareness and ineffective communication and team leadership.

Accordingly, there is a need to develop team-based training strategies that address these non-technical skills as a specific strategy to counteract medical error and improve patient safety. Simulation-based team-training has its origins in high-risk industries, such as civilian and military aviation, and has been used effectively in health to train teams in surgery, critical care and emergency medicine, improving patient safety and decreasing error rates [4–6]. Team training is not a "one-size" intervention, and training applications need to be adapted and developed to suit domain-specific needs [6–8].

C. Hicks (✉)
St. Michael's Hospital, University of Toronto, Toronto, ON, Canada

Li Ka Shing Knowledge Institute, University of Toronto, Toronto, ON, Canada

Emergency Medicine, Division of Emergency Medicine, University of Toronto, Toronto, ON, Canada

Department of Medicine, University of Toronto, Toronto, ON, Canada

The Case for CRM: Origins of Team Training in Aviation

Aviation may be classified as a high-hazard industry: the safety of flight crew and, in the case of commercial aviation, passengers depends on the precise execution of multiple high-risk manoeuvres coordinated by a team of skilled pilots and technicians. Over the past several decades, the commercial aviation industry has garnered wide recognition for its safety record, taking its place among military and nuclear operations as an example of a high-reliability organization (HRO). HROs are organizations that exist in hazardous environments where errors carry high consequences, yet the error rate is extremely low [9].

Prior to the 1980s, training of civilian and military pilots focused almost exclusively on the technical aspects of flight [10]. Prompted by a series of high-profile, high-fatality airline incidents, the aviation and aerospace industries began to take a critical look at why planes crashed. An example is the Tenerife disaster in 1977, where two fully loaded jumbo jets (KLM Flight 4805 and Pan Am Flight 1736) collided on the runway of a small Canary Island airport during a failed take-off manoeuvre, killing 583 passengers and crewmembers—the most fatal disaster in aviation history. A large international panel of experts were involved in the crash investigation, which implicated errors in communication, rushed and incomplete procedure and failure to challenge the decision-making of senior KLM Captain van Zanten when it was obvious to crew members that his actions were hasty and ill-informed [11].

In 1976, the National Aviation and Space Agency (NASA) began collecting data on all aviation mishaps via the Aviation Safety and Reporting System (ASRS). Designed in close cooperation with the aviation industry, the ASRS was a voluntary reporting system created to assist in the analysis of aviation catastrophes and near misses [12]. Early reports from the ASRS implicated human error as the root cause of 60–80% of all aviation incidents [13]. The US General Accounting Office reported that a lack of team coordination,

L. Marshall Gillman, S. Widder (eds.), *Trauma Team Dynamics*, https://doi.org/10.1007/978-3-031-86312-7_3

failure to assign tasks and lack of effective leadership and supervision were a contributing cause in nearly half of fatal accidents between 1983 and 1985 [14]. In 1984, Billings and Reynard published a review of seven years of data and over 35,000 reports in the ASRS in an attempt to better understand and classify the nature of consequential cockpit errors. The majority of events could be attributed to either human or system factors: at the system level, over 70% of reported incidents involved faulty information transfer [12]. Although information quality was typically not the culprit, failure to effectively communicate key data to the personnel responsible for tactical decision-making frequently led to erroneous decisions with dire consequences. Reported human factor error included failure of flight crews to effectively manage resources, plan for contingencies, question authority and request clarification [12]. Whether or not human error resulted in a consequential accident depended largely on the environment in which the error occurred—as an example, the authors point out that an altitude error is more likely to result in an accident when the plane is close to the ground. Furthermore, errors were found to be more consequential if they occurred during periods of high workload or non-routine operations [12]. In contrast, technical problems including aircraft malfunction and equipment failures were comparatively rare, and in general had a less significant impact on aircraft accidents. Billings concluded:

> The disease or disorder called "human error" causes half of the preventable deaths in both civil and military flying personnel. It is the largest single cause of premature mortality in this population. This disorder needs to be attacked as aggressively and effectively as we have attacked the physiological and medical disorders responsible for the remainder of preventable deaths [12].

The development of pilot training programs targeting human factors can be traced back to a 1980 NASA workshop entitled *Resource Management on the Flightdeck* [15]. Research presented at this conference explored the human and team behaviours most frequently implicated in air crashes. Key targets of cockpit team performance included interpersonal communication, decision-making and leadership [16]. The term "Cockpit Resource Management" (CRM) was created to refer to non-technical (i.e. human resource) cockpit team training that focused on these specific aspects of human and team behaviour [17]. CRM training was touted as an important tool to reduce the incidence of consequential aviation mishaps occurring as a result of human error.

Following the NASA workshop, and in response to recommendations made in the wake of the Tenerife investigation, aviation and aerospace moved quickly to develop CRM-based team training programs tailored to suit specific industry needs. Since that time, CRM training has undergone a significant evolution as it became integrated into the fabric of aviation safety culture and cockpit training. First-generation CRM programs mainly used seminar and table-top exercises to engender elements of effective managerial style and professional behaviour in the cockpit. More recent iterations have cut a broader and more inclusive swath, using realistic flight simulators to address human factor training in the context of simulated missions [16]. Third and fourth generations saw simulation-based Line-Oriented Flight Training (LOFT) become a required component of pilot training and expanded its scope to include flight technicians, attendants and mechanics in an attempt to engender common attitudes towards safety across disciplines [16]. Although each generation has had demonstrated successes in influencing flight crew's attitudes towards human factors, LOFT training has had the most robust impact on achieving buy-in from participants by producing demonstrable changes in behaviours observed during formal Line Operational Evaluations (LOE) of crews in full mission simulation [17]. The Federal Aviation Administration (FAA) currently requires airlines to provide CRM and LOFT training for all flight crews, while still allowing for carriers to maintain a degree of flexibility in training under the Advanced Qualifications Program (AQP) [1, 18].

A common thread spanning generations of CRM training is the notion that its primary goal should be to reduce the incidence of consequential human error through focused instruction on effective communication, leadership, resource utilization, problem solving and situational awareness. Helmreich, Merritt and Wilhelm have argued that even when these specific behaviours are being taught, the link between human factors training and error management needs to be explicitly drawn, such that CRM is regarded as a series of countermeasures with three lines of defense: the avoidance, capturing and mitigation of error and its consequences [16]. In this framework, error is regarded as "ubiquitous and inevitable", and instruction is re-focused on the natural limitations of human ability, the nature of cognitive errors and the effects of stress, fatigue and work overload on team performance during both routine and crisis situations.

Proponents of CRM have pointed to a gradual but distinct decrease in airline incidents and fatalities occurring as a result of human error over the past 25 years as evidence of the effectiveness of formal team training to improve safety in aviation. However, aviation incidents are extremely rare events, and drawing specific conclusions about the impact of training in the accident rate per million flights is problematic [16]. Proposed surrogates have included direct observation crew attitudes and behaviours using formal LOE protocols. Regardless, in the absence of a criterion standard for evaluating performance, it is not possible to say with certainty that CRM training, rather than advances in technology or "smarter planes", can account for the bulk of safety improvements. Nevertheless, based on the strong face validity of CRM principles, the majority of aviation crews believe that CRM training has had a significant impact on flight safety [19].

In 2001, Salas, Burke, Bowers and Wilson published a review of 58 reports of CRM training in search of evidence for its effectiveness in preventing consequential error in commercial and military aviation [13]. Drawing extensively from the framework for evaluating training programs developed by Kirkpatrick [20], Salas and colleagues argue that while there is reasonable evidence that aviators enjoy CRM training and learn about CRM as a result of LOFT and other programs, evidence of a demonstrable impact on outcomes measured in terms of organizational outcomes is nearly non-existent. Although simulation-based LOFT and LOE do generally demonstrate that CRM training has an impact on behaviour, the link between improved cockpit dynamics in a simulated environment and safety outcomes in the real world remains by and large theoretical. The most powerful reports are those that assess the impact of CRM training on multiple levels and include higher levels of evidence (i.e. influences behaviours and outcomes) in their analysis—not surprisingly, there is a paucity of such multilevel reports in the literature, yet these studies generally offer the most compelling evidence that CRM training can have a broad impact on attitudes, knowledge, behaviour and outcomes [13].

Overall, the weight of evidence suggests that CRM training programs do offer something of value in promoting safety and human factors in aviation, and there is a general belief that human factors training does contribute to "safety in the skies". However, as Salas and colleagues point out, larger and more rigorous multilevel studies are needed in order to accurately assess the impact of team training on aviation safety.

CRM in Medicine: Principles, Limitations and Frontiers

Although the Institute of Medicine's condemning report on the consequences of medical error was published in 1999, medicine and in particular anaesthesiology had been investigating ways to adopt elements of aviation team training as a tool to combat error in the operating room (OR) for more than a decade before the report was released. Several investigations into the causes of OR catastrophes have confirmed that at least half of critical incidents are caused by human error [21, 22]. In the late 1980s, David Gaba, Steven Howard and a team of researchers at the VA Palo Alto Health Care System at Stanford University began to experiment with the use of high-fidelity human patient simulators as a tool to teach aviation-style team training to OR staff [4]. The result was Anesthesia Crisis Resource Management (ACRM), a simulation-based instructional paradigm for OR staff that focused on teaching principles derived from aviation CRM; leadership, problem-solving, situational awareness, communication skills and resource management are still at the forefront of present day ACRM protocols [23].

ACRM places participants in a realistic OR environment, complete with monitors, alarms, scrubs, drapes and actors playing OR team members—the "patient" is a full-sized computer-operated human mannequin capable of reproducing realistic physiologic responses to procedural (i.e. intubation) or pharmacological interventions (i.e. induction of general anaesthesia). A skilled simulation technician, who observes the scenario and programmes responses from an adjacent room, controls mannequin responses. Gaba and his group developed and utilized the CASE (Comprehensive Anaesthesia Simulation Environment) simulation system, created specifically for the purpose of investigating human performance, to faithfully reproduce a wide variety of OR crises, observe participant behaviour and provide instruction via focused debriefings using videotaped recordings of the crisis event as a stimulus for discussion with a skilled facilitator [24]. In many centres, anaesthesia staff, residents, nurses and even medical undergraduates now participate in ACRM training using high-fidelity simulation [24–26]. ACRM instruction and evaluation principles have been adopted for a multitude of disciplines across medicine, from radiology to critical care and emergency medicine [27–30]. Although these applications differ in structure and design, the basic elements of CRM training are similar:

1. Leadership: An effective leader stands back and manages the team, avoids authority gradients by listening to and accepting input from the team and demonstrates prompt and firm decision making.
2. Situational Awareness: Maintaining a "big picture" perspective—avoiding fixation error by actively re-assessing and re-evaluating the situation.
3. Communication: Closed-loop communication (i.e. give an order/confirm its receipt/confirm its execution).
4. Resource Utilization: Mobilizing key human and equipment resources, asking for help.
5. Problem Solving: Demonstrating an organized approach, thinking "outside the box" and rapidly implementing solutions.
6. Team-Based Behaviours: Mutual support, adaptability, role clarity, cross-checking.

Effective ACRM training programs are based on three crucial tenants, as endorsed by Gaba: knowledge (understanding key team training principles), practice (the ability to use the simulator to safely practice team training skills again and again without threat of harm to patients) and recurrence (the need to repeat CRM training over time to combat skills decay) [31].

CRM is not a one-size-fits-all intervention—effective team training strategies need to be adapted to suit the operational, knowledge, cultural and skills-based environment unique to each medical discipline [6]. To that end, many disciplines outside of anaesthesia have made initial strides towards the development of targeted team training interventions, including emergency medicine, critical care and more recently trauma [32–36].

Human Factors in Trauma Care

What evidence is there that CRM training has had an impact on patient safety in trauma? As is the case in aviation, the answer is not easily arrived at. Numerous studies are available demonstrating the impact of CRM-type training on knowledge and attitudes of healthcare professionals. Simulation-based CRM training paired with focused debriefing has been shown to be effective at improving team communication, [37] fostering positive attitudes towards team training [19, 34, 35] and enhancing team performance in a simulated environment [32, 34]. To date, there is a paucity of evidence to support the notion that CRM training has an impact on patient safety and outcomes [38–40]. In 2010, Capella et al. [41] were able to demonstrate that structured trauma team training based on TeamSTEPPS [42] human patient simulation led to significant decreases in time from arrival to computerized tomography scanner, endotracheal intubation and operating room were significantly decreased.

While there is a clear need to evaluate the impact of team training on patient-centred outcomes, the cumulative evidence to date along with the strong face validity supports the continued pursuit of structured, high-quality human factors training as a mechanism to promote patient safety and reduce consequential error in the trauma bay.

Key Points

1. Crisis resource management (CRM) training consists of a training program to improve leadership, situational awareness, communication, resource utilization, problem solving and team-based behaviours.
2. While it is difficult to establish a clear link between CRM training and patient outcomes, it has strong face validity and has been proven effective at improving team communication, fostering positive attitudes towards team training and enhancing team performance in a simulated environment.

References

1. Clarke J, Spejewski B, Getner A. An objective analysis of process errors in trauma resuscitations. Acad Emerg Med. 2000;7:1272–7.
2. Gruen R, Jurkovich GJ, McIntyre LK, Foy HM, Maier RV. Patterns of errors contributing to trauma mortality. Ann Surg. 2006;244:371–80.
3. Sarcevic A. Understanding teamwork in high-risk domains through analysis of errors. Boston: CHI; 2009.
4. Gaba D, Howard S, Fish K. Simulation-based training in anesthesia crisis resource management (ACRM): a decade of experience. Simul Gaming. 2001;32:175–93.
5. Morey J, Simon R, Jay G, Wears R, Salisbury M, Dukes K. Error reduction and performance improvement in the Emergency Department through formal teamwork training: evaluation results of the MedTeams Project. Health Serv Res. 2002;37:373–83.
6. Hicks C, Kiss A, Bandiera G, Denny C. Crisis Resources for Emergency Workers (CREW), Phase II: results from a pilot study and simulation-based crisis resource management course for emergency medicine residents. Can J Emerg Med. 2012;14(6):354–62.
7. Burke C, Salas E, Wilson-Donnelly K, Priest H. How to turn a team of experts into an exert medical team: guidance from the aviation and military communities. Qual Saf Health Care. 2004;13:96–104.
8. Hicks C, Bandiera G, Denny C. Building a crisis resource management course for emergency medicine, Phase 1: results from an interdisciplinary needs assessment survey. Acad Emerg Med. 2008;15:1136–43.
9. Baker D, Day R, Salas E. Teamwork as an essential component of high-reliability organizations. Health Serv Res. 2006;41:1576–98.
10. Helmreich R. On error management: lessons from aviation. Br Med J. 2000;320:781–5.
11. Tenerife Disaster. 2008. http://en.wikipedia.org/wiki/Tenerife_disaster. Accessed 6 May 2008.
12. Billings C, Reynard W. Human factors in aircraft incidents: results of a 7-year study. Aviat Space Environ Med. 1984;55:960–5.
13. Salas E, Burke S, Bowers C, Wilson K. Team training in the skies: does crew resource management (CRM) training work? Hum Factors. 2001;43:641–74.
14. Human Factors. FAA's guidance and oversight of pilot crew resource management training can be improved. Washington, DC: U.S. General Accounting Office.
15. Cooper G, White M, Lauber J. Resource management on the flightdeck: proceedings of a NASA/indurstry workshop (NASA CP-2120). Moffet Field: NASA-Ames Research Center: Academic; 1980.
16. Helmreich R, Merritt A, Wilhelm J. The evolution of crew resource management training in commerical aviation. Int J Aviat Psychol. 1999;9:19–32.
17. Helmreich R, Foushee H. Why crew resource management? Empiric and theoretical bases of human factors training in aviation. In: Weiner E, Kanki B, Helmreich R, editors. Cockpit resource management. San Diego: Academic; 1993. p. 3–45.
18. Birnbach R, Longridge T. The regulatory perspective. In: Weiner E, Kanki B, Helmreich R, editors. Cockpit resource management. San Diego: Academic; 1993. p. 263–82.
19. Grogan E, Styles R, France D, Speroff T. The impact of aviation-based teamwork training on the attitudes of health care professionals. J Am Coll Surg. 2004;199:843–8.
20. Kirkpatrick D. Evaluation of training. In: Craig R, editor. Training and development handbook: a guide to human resources development. New York: McGraw-Hill; 1976. p. 18.1-.27.

21. Cooper J, Newbowser R, Kitz R. An analysis of major errors and equipment failures in anesthesia management: considerations for prevention and detection. Anesthesiology. 1984;60:34–42.
22. Gaba D. Dynamic decision-making in anesthesiology: cognitive models and training approaches. In: Evans D, Patel V, editors. Advanced models of cognition for medical training and practice. Berlin: Springer; 2004. p. 123–47.
23. Howard S, Gaba D, Fish K, Yang G, Sarnquist F. Anesthesia crisis resource management training: teaching anesthesiologists to handle critical incidents. Aviat Space Environ Med. 1992;63:763–70.
24. Blum R, Raemer D, Carroll J, Sunder N, Feinstein D, Cooper J. Crisis resource management training for an anesthesia faculty: a new approach to continuing education. Med Educ. 2004;38:45–55.
25. O'Donnell J, Fletcher J, Dixon B, Palmer L. Planning and implementing an anesthesia crisis resource management course for student nurse anesthetists. CRNA. 1998;9:50–8.
26. Flanagan B, Nestel D, Joseph M. Making patient safety the focus: crisis resource management in the undergraduate curriculum. Med Educ. 2004;38:56–66.
27. Sica G, Barron D, Blum R, Frenna T, Raemer D. Computerized realistic simulation: a teaching module for crisis management in radiology. AJR. 1999;172:301–4.
28. Kim J, Neilipovitz D, Cardinal P, Chiu M, Clinch J. A pilot study using high-fidelity simulation to formally evaluate performance in the resuscitation of critically ill patients: The University of Ottawa Critical Care Medicine, High-Fidelity Simulation, And Crisis Resource Management I Study. Crit Care Med. 2006;34:2167–74.
29. Reznek M, Smith-Coggins R, Howard S, et al. Emergency Medicine Crisis Resource Management (EMCRM): pilot study of a simulation-based crisis management course for emergency medicine. Acad Emerg Med. 2003;10:386–9.
30. Shapiro M, Morey J, Small S, et al. Simulation based teamwork training for emergency department staff: does it improve clinical team performance when added to an existing didactic teamwork curriculum? Qual Saf Health Care. 2004;13:417–21.
31. Hunt E, Shilkofski N, Stavroudis T, Nelson K. Simulation: translation to improved team performance. Anesthesiol Clin. 2007;25:301–19.
32. Hicks C, Kiss A, Bandiera G, Denny C. Crisis Resources for Emergecny Workers (CREW II): results of a pilot study and simulation-based crisis resource management course for emergency medicine residents. Can J Emerg Med. 2012;14:354–62.
33. Brindley PG, Reynolds SF. Improving verbal communication in critical care medicine. J Crit Care. 2011;26:155–9.
34. Knudson MM, Khaw L, Bullard K, et al. Trauma training in simulation: translating skills from SIM time to real time. J Trauma Acute Care Surg. 2008;64:255–64.
35. Ziesmann MT, Widder S, Park J, Kortbeek JB, Brindley P, Hameed M, et al. S.T.A.R.T.T.: development of a national, multidisciplinary trauma crisis resource management curriculum-results from the pilot course. J Trauma Acute Care Surg. 2013;75(5):753–8.
36. Domouras AG, Keshet I, Nathens AB, Ahmen N, Hicks C. Trauma Non-Technical Training (TNT-2): the development, piloting and multilevel assessment of a simulation-based, interprofessional curriculum for team-based trauma resuscitation. Can J Surg. 2014;57(5):354–5.
37. Blum R, Raemer D, Carroll J, Dufrense R, Cooper J. A method for measuring the effectiveness of simulation-based team training for improving communication skills. Anesthes Analges. 2005;100:1375–80.
38. Doumouras AG, Keshet I, Nathens AB, Ahmen N, Hicks C. A crisis of faith? A review of simulation in teaching team-based crisis management skills to surgical trainees. J Surg Educ. 2012.
39. Shear TD, Greenberg SB, Tokarczyk A. Does training with human patient simulation translate to improved patient safety and outcome? Curr Opin Anesthesiol. 2013;26(2):159–63.
40. Petrosoniak A, Hicks C. Beyond crisis resource management: new frontiers in human factors training for acute care medicine. Curr Opin Anesthesiol. 2013;26(6):699–706.
41. Capella J, Smith S, Philp A, et al. Teamwork training improves the clinical care of trauma patients. J Surg Educ. 2010;67(6):439–43.
42. TeamSTEPPS. http://teamstepps.ahrq.gov/

Trauma Team Development: Leadership and Collaboration

4

Brent Hunter and K. Dean Gubler

Introduction

Effective leadership is a common theme found throughout the professional world. Spanning from military to finance and ranging from healthcare to sports, the search for effective leadership is ubiquitous. What is effective leadership? Are leaders born or created? To reference Winston Churchill, "the price of greatness is responsibility". For our purposes, the concept of leadership is crucial for the trauma team. The trauma team leader is not only a leader in the context of medical care for the critically injured, but also in the context of professional development, adherence to policy, and interprofessional collaboration. Regardless of context or specific situation, the trauma team leader must always be a leader.

The 1995–1996 Chicago Bulls are widely recognized as one of the greatest basketball teams ever assembled. They finished the season with an astonishing 72 wins and 10 losses, a record that persisted for over 20 years. The Bull's success is largely attributed to Michael Jordan, universally known as the apex of NBA basketball prowess. Evaluation of the team, however, reveals that it takes more than a single superstar to be extraordinary. Coaches, administration, staff, athletic directors, team physicians, and other role players are all critical components that allowed this team to become one of the greatest. What made this team extraordinary? The answer lies in the dynamics, the interplay between players.

In the world of trauma, the goal is to be a high-performance team like the Bulls. It does not take a team full of All-star caliber players, but it does take a team with impeccable dynamics, interplay, unified behavior, and execution. It takes a team that understands one another's roles, promotes each other's strengths, and recognizes the inherent strength of a leader.

Severe traumatic injury is a unique and complex clinical event. It represents the initiation of an interdisciplinary and multidimensional path of medical and surgical intervention. While duration, context, and outcomes vary, the necessity of multispecialty care is ubiquitous. Pre-hospital personnel, nurses, technicians, and multiple providers are all needed in the initial moments of care for the critically injured. Without an orchestrated leadership model, this scenario can easily devolve into chaos with preventable morbidity and mortality.

The acute care of the critically ill and injured is predisposed to a highly emotionally charged environment with uncertain outcomes. The uncertainty of appropriate responses to clinical challenges, individual roles, and outcomes creates the potential for patient care to degrade into chaos. Avoidance of the potential chaos requires a corradiated team response under skilled leadership. The purpose of this chapter is to explore problem solving and decision making in the context of trauma team dynamics.

Modern Trauma: A Collaborative History

The beginnings of modern trauma teams are deeply rooted in the soils of caring for injured military personnel. The first trauma manual was a product of the American Civil war and the Abraham Lincoln administration. The principles conceived during that time served as the foundation for rapid medical advancement during World War II and even as a model for the modern trauma system [1].

Further advances in rapid casualty evacuation, rapid triage, and definitive care came during the Korean and Vietnam wars. David B Hoyt, former Executive director of the American College of Surgeons, highlighted the collaboration between military and civilian systems saying "Collaboration between civilian and military health systems started at least

B. Hunter
Mountain View Emergency Medicine GME, Los Angeles, CA, USA
e-mail: brent.hunter@hcahealthcare.com

K. Dean Gubler (✉)
Rocky Vista University, Englewood, CO, USA
e-mail: dgubler@rvu.edu

L. Marshall Gillman, S. Widder (eds.), *Trauma Team Dynamics*, https://doi.org/10.1007/978-3-031-86312-7_4

100 years ago. These partnerships helped advance care both during peacetime and during times of conflict."

Further collaboration between military and civilian partners saw the initiation and development of Emergency Medical Services (EMS), establishment of trauma algorithms, quantifiable research on reduction in trauma morbidity, and standardization and verification of trauma care. The continued partnership has led to what is known as the Joint Trauma System. This system prompted the military trauma system to incorporate civilian-led practices in battlefield trauma. Notable highlights of this program include advancement in bleeding control, forward surgical care, use of whole blood products for resuscitation, and new insights into management of traumatic brain injury [2, 3], important topics discussed in this book.

Defining Trauma Designation and Verification

Trauma centers are distinguished by two separate classification systems: designation and verification. Designation refers to the resources available at each location and is the deciding factor on the breadth and depth of trauma that can be managed at that location. Designations follow a five-tier system and are regulated by local governments. Level I is the most comprehensive and can provide complete care. Level V provides initial evaluation and stabilization and initiates transfer to the next appropriate level of care. Each level has specific criteria mandates that will include specialties represented, ancillary care, and other resources [4].

Verification is the supervisory branch that grants "accreditation" and substantiates the facility's ability to hold a specific designation. In the United States, verification is provided by the American College of Surgeons Committee on Trauma (COT) and/or by local state governments. As noted on the COT website, "The designation of trauma facilities is a geopolitical process by which empowered entities, government or otherwise, are authorized to designate. The ACS does not designate trauma centers; instead, it verifies the presence of the resources listed in *Resources for Optimal Care of the Injured Patient*" [5].

The Trauma Team

Utilizing the NBA sports analogy, it is important to identify how we define "team." In basketball, there are typically 15 players, but only 5 on the court at a time. This provides several available players and depth at each of the five playing positions. The same is true for trauma care. Depending on the severity of the trauma and the specific designation of the facility, the trauma team can be modified to meet the needs of the situation. A smaller team can be utilized for a prehospital environment or a larger, more robust, team for care that takes place in an operating room environment under the leadership of a fellowship trained trauma surgeon. The primary resuscitation team is supported by physicians and surgeons of all specialties along with their respective supporting technical and administrative staff. All designated trauma care facilities require continued support from the pre-hospital community, administration, and facilities. These entities provide organization, dedicated resources, as well as planning and operational policy development.

While context will dictate situational specifics, a generic trauma team may be composed of a trauma team leader, primary physician, airway team (anesthesia/emergency room physician/respiratory therapist), trauma nurse(s), radiology technician, recorder, laboratory and blood bank technicians, chaplain, and social services. Each component of the trauma team must be technically proficient in their respective fields, but also able to understand the dynamics of the team. The unique roles of the trauma team members are discussed further in Chaps. 21 and 22.

Consider the analogy of some orchestral ensembles: Under direction of the conductor, orchestral members combine individual technical expertise with non-technical cohesiveness. It is a harmonious union of mastery and compliance.

In a marvelous display of ability, members of these organizations emphasize the beauty of unified effort. The ebb and flow of music requires a give and take from the musicians. Forte at times, followed by pianissimo at others. The ability to know when to be at the forefront is just as important as the ability to know when not to be. As we examine the intricacies of the interplay between instruments, we can learn more about the importance of contrast in trauma care.

Trauma Team Leadership

The inherent stress associated with the care of the critically injured demands that the trauma team performs at consistently high levels. Efficiency, preparation, poise, and level of performance are all directly proportional to the quality of the team's leadership. The trauma team leader is responsible for their team's preparation, training, and performance. They alone carry the trust and obligation for operations carried out during their tenure. These individuals must embody the principles of personal responsibility, accountability, decisiveness, and composure.

Similar to military commanders, trauma team leaders are not intended to be the technical experts, nor do they participate in the specific tasks of trauma care. Their responsibility is to oversee, anticipate, plan, execute, and adapt. Military leadership models employ several tiers of ancillary staff and executive officers. It is this auxiliary staff that are responsible for filtering and relaying accurate information so that decisions can be made. Data about resources, policy, unit morale, operational capability, and site mission are all incorporated and analyzed into a congruent information feed that allows the Commander to observe, orient, decide, and act (OODA).

Similarly, the trauma team leader does not participate in specifics such as intravenous access, airway management, or performing physical exams. Those duties are delegated to other team members. The trauma team leader designates and directs the management of the injured, relying on team members to provide real-time, accurate information. This affords the team lead the ability to maintain a global picture of medical and surgical management and the agility to constantly evaluate new information.

Considering the position and responsibility of the trauma team lead, it is crucial to understand that the trauma team leader is the focal point for decision making and management of the injured patient. Good leaders value their team's input and consider their specific perspectives; however, the team leader must apply individual perspectives into the global context of comprehensive trauma management.

Crisis Resource Management

Crisis resource management represents principles used for the efficiency and quality of trauma evaluation and management [6, 7]. These principles are intended to help unify the trauma team's goals, streamline actions, and increase coordination to an evolving event. The principles of CRM can for ease be separated into two categories: decision-making and team management [8].

Decision-making	Team management
Use all available information	Early recognition of needed resources
Allocate attention wisely	Designated leadership
Mobilize resources	Established role clarity and task delegation
Use cognitive aids	Effective communication
Pattern anticipation	Situational awareness and a shared mental model

It is important to highlight that the roles and responsibilities of trauma team leadership do not occur exclusively within the confines of direct medical care. It does not start when the patient arrives nor does it end with discharge. Trauma team leadership is an ongoing, continuous process that encourages and promotes coherence between all supporting aspects of care. To promote optimal trauma team dynamics, trauma team leaders are also engaged in activities that support their trauma teams. Examples include team debriefing, simulation and communication training, policy development, prehospital/EMS coordination, transfer protocols, disaster preparedness, and administrative processes. These additional responsibilities represent an extension of CRM principles.

Engagement in these activities is a fundamental part of trauma care and represents an inherent part of the team leader's role. Effective leaders understand that purposeful CRM is essential to their team's ability to perform at high levels. Its employment promotes synergistic, highly effective trauma teams by providing them with the necessary resources, training, policy, and guidance.

Observe, Orient, Decide, Act OODA Loop

The OODA loop is a decision-making process that, like trauma structure, shares historical ties to the military. John Boyd, an American fighter pilot in the Korean war, developed the concept to direct combat operations. The process, with various refinements, is now utilized in multiple industries and sectors. OODA refers to the four actions:

Orient
Observe
Decide
Act

The OODA loop is not a single event, but a series of multiple feedback mechanisms that influence our thought, perceptions, forward thinking, and actions. It is a representation for receiving, processing, and acting on information as it arrives. Its applicability to the trauma setting is ideal, as medical intervention often happens without complete information or context. Because of this information gap, a mental model that allows for flexibility is advantageous.

Observe

Utilizing the analogy of aerial combat, we can highlight the importance of orienting ourselves. When Boyd devised this concept, he was concerned with the combat environment. Air speed, arsenal, opponent's resources, and location are all crucial pieces of information. In the trauma setting, this orientation is equally as important. Mechanism of injury, vitals, environment, and resources factor into the management of the patient.

Not only is the information important, but considering the source, integrity, and validity of that information is essential. In a common team building exercise (and child's game) known as broken telephone, information is initiated at one end of a line and then subsequently whispered to the last person. Often, the information at the end of the line scarcely resembles the original information. The same is true, and significantly more important for this discussion.

Clear, concise, accurate information needs to be relayed through multiple sources. It needs to remain unadulterated and precise. Problems in conveyance can arise anywhere in the management of trauma including faulty medical devices, communications equipment disturbances, interpersonal miscommunication, and so forth. Once information is received it needs to be processed and communicated to the trauma team by the team leader in a precise and concise manner. This communication allows for transparency and clarity around the care plan. It allows team members to stay involved and promotes collaboration and creative thinking. It allows team members to employ their own OODA loop.

Orient

Once an individual has received information, it is necessary to process the information and organize it based on relevancy. Essentially, the information needs to be filtered. In the inundation of input, look for the data that helps you to formulate a course of action. Again, the analogy of aerial combat. The color of the sky is probably not as important as airspeed, altitude, or enemy location. All of that information is available, but which is most beneficial? It may be helpful to ask some clarifying questions.

What am I missing?
What are the trends?
What else do I need to make a decision?

In addition to filtering information, it is important to know that the orientation step of the OODA loop is the most subjective. During the observe phase, obtaining information is paramount. This is an objective endeavor. How we perceive information, however, varies wildly. In a study comparing surgeons, non-trauma to trauma, there were eight categories that were identified as "educational dilemmas" [9]. The areas of concern were:

1. Thinking physiologically
2. Damage control surgery
3. Priorities and time management
4. Impact of environment
5. Managing limited resources
6. Lack of general medical skills
7. Different cultural behavior
8. Ethical issues

Several of these categories are the result of past experiences. Our personal experiences, in large part, shape how we filter and eventually apply information. Because of this, the orient step is the point in the OODA loop where personal biases can cloud judgement and undermine our team efforts.

Boyd said:

> The second O, orientation—as the repository of our genetic heritage, cultural tradition, and previous experiences—is the most important part of the O-O-D-A loop since it shapes the way we observe, the way we decide, the way we act [10].

Because of the multidisciplinary aspect of trauma care, there is the pitfall and high likelihood of multiple opinions and miscommunications occurring at this point. Situations can become complex when multiple perspectives are derived from the same objective information.

Consider, for example, hemodynamics. The average blood pressure for a newborn is 64/41 and 95/58 in a 2-year-old. For a practicing pediatrician, these numbers would be appropriate. In the trauma patient, however, these numbers would be alarming and may be indicative of poor prognosis. Context, background, perspective, and training all become potential points of division and can undermine team dynamics.

To mitigate inefficiencies and bolster effectiveness during this stage, simulation scenarios in conjunction with team building exercises are often employed. However, it is still important to realize the potential for inadequacies.

Decide and Act

When the information has been processed and filtered, the next step of the OODA loop is to decide and act. Decisions need to weigh the anticipated result with the associated risks. This balance should help guide the course of care. To assist with this, specific algorithms can become effective. These specific models will outline a step-by-step guide for the course of treatment. Some examples that include CPR (cardiopulmonary resuscitation), ATLS (Advanced Trauma Life Support), ACLS (Advanced Cardiac Life Support), PALS (Pediatric Advance Life Support), institution specific protocols, etc.

Once a decision has been made, the team lead must communicate that decision to the team and to delegate responsibilities. The team lead's responsibility is continual, just like the OODA model, and comprises synthesizing the information, devising a plan of action, and motivating the team to follow through.

It is important to recognize that the OODA loop does not stop at this point. The stages that have been described occur frequently and often through the entire process and are consistently re-examined as new and pertinent information arrives. Modification of the management of the critically injured should be anticipated and embraced as more information becomes available and care progresses. It is important for the team lead to evaluate the effectiveness of the clinical evaluation and clinical interventions as more information becomes available. Further decisions and actions depend this ability to be flexible and responsive to new information.

Conclusion

Not every team is great. There can be problems with management, teamwork, logistics, resources, or communication. Extraordinary teams possess not only technical competence, but members also have the emotional maturity to know when to lead and follow. They know how to communicate, how to relay reliable information, and know that ultimate decision making is the responsibility of the team leader.

In support of their team, the team leader recognizes and employs effectively CRM. This responsibility is crucial to team success and is an inherent part of the team leader's role. By managing resources, promoting development, providing guidance, and employing policy the trauma team leader enables their team to perform at high levels and as a cohesive unit. This synergistic unity promotes open communication, information sharing, and flexibility during acute medical care. The OODA loop is a continuous cycle that can only be effective when the trauma team shares information openly and freely. Engaging in active CRM and the OODA loop utilization, trauma teams can be what patients and their families deserve.

References

1. Part 1: A brief history of trauma systems. American College of Surgeons. https://www.facs.org/quality-programs/trauma/tqp/systems-programs/trauma-series/part-i. Accessed 22 Dec 2020.
2. Part 2: Why the U.S. trauma system needs a robust civilian-military partnership. American College of Surgeons. https://www.facs.org/quality-programs/trauma/tqp/systems-programs/trauma-series/part-ii. Accessed 22 Dec 2020.
3. Part 3: Sixty-year military-civilian partnership serves as a model for the national trauma system. American College of Surgeons. https://www.facs.org/quality-programs/trauma/tqp/systems-programs/trauma-series/part-iii. Accessed 22 Dec 2020.
4. Trauma Center Levels Explained. American Trauma Society. https://www.amtrauma.org/page/TraumaLevels. Accessed 22 Dec 2020.
5. Trauma Centers. American College of Surgeons. https://www.facs.org/search/trauma-centers. Accessed 22 Dec 2020.
6. Joshi N. Crisis Resource Management. ALiEM. http://www.aliem.com/crisis-resource-management/. Published 12 Nov 2016. Accessed 22 Dec 2020.
7. Gaba DM. Crisis resource management and teamwork training in anaesthesia. Br J Anaesth. 2010;105(1):3–6. https://doi.org/10.1093/bja/aeq124.
8. Burden A. High-fidelity simulation education and crisis resource management. Clinical Key. https://www-clinicalkey-com.proxy.rvu.edu/. Published 1 Dec 2020. Accessed 22 Dec 2020.
9. Sonesson L, Boffard K, Lundberg L, Rydmark M, Karlgren K. Decision-making in management of the complex trauma patient: changing the mindset of the non-trauma surgeon. World J Surg. 2018;42(8):2392. https://search-ebscohost-com.proxy.rvu.edu/login.aspx?direct=true&db=edb&AN=130602864&site=eds-live&scope=site. Accessed 22 Dec 2020
10. Boyd J. Organic design for command and control. Address presented at the: May 1987. http://publiclibrariesonline.org/2018/05/observation-orientation-decision-action-applying-the-ooda-loop-concept-to-libraries/. Accessed 22 Dec 2020.

5 Improving Human Factors, Teamwork, and Communication in Trauma Care

Peter G. Brindley and Jocelyn M. Slemko

Introduction: Why Does Teamwork Matter?

The real problem of humanity is the following: we have paleolithic emotions; medieval institutions; and god-like technology.
E. O. Wilson. Biologist

Talent wins games, but teamwork, and intelligence wins championships
Michael Jordan. Basketball God

Introduction

While accepting that aviation will never be exactly the same as trauma medicine, even the greatest cynic should accept that other high-stakes, high-reliability industries still offer numerous oven-ready ideas. Hence, this chapter will cover aviation's crew resource management and how it dovetails with medicine's crisis resource management. We hope to offer a concise primer, while evergreening a topic (CRM) that needs to be further developed, and even more widely understood. Regardless, the best trauma team members will welcome practical insights and reminders, no matter the source or repetition. Excellence does not happen by accident. It starts with the humility to (over)learn from others and a commitment to constant self-reflection and iterative improvement.

The literature has now made it abundantly clear that inadequate teamwork and inadequate communication are among the most common reasons for preventable error in both aviation and acute care medicine [1–6]. The debate is over, and now the issue is how to operationalize what we already know. For example, in trauma care, there is an increasing acceptance of the importance of simulation training, and the need to deliberately address human factors and team dynamics, but we need to go further [1, 2].

Table 5.1 Practical strategies to improve team work in a medical crisis

Team factor	Recommendation
Climate and culture	More "we," less "me" Mutual respect; calm and decisive Hierarchy still has a role "What" is right, not "who" is right
Establish structure	Assign roles Assign responsibilities Establish 3 priorities Communicate throughout
Shared mental model	Ensure all on 'same page' Invite input when possible Share the priorities; update prn Set the emotions of the team
Cross monitor	Monitor performance Monitor workload Flatten hierarchy Encourage feedback
Maintain resilience	Routine practice sessions Request feedback Encourage debrief Provide time for casual interaction

Our medical profession is overdue in terms of embracing a culture of safety and self-reflection and peer-review. We have also yet to accept how much can be achieved from the aggregation of marginal gains and empowering all members of the healthcare team, not just senior administrators. Even if medicine does not equal aviation, the latter offers translatable strategies regarding how to promote a "science of reducing complexity," "science of team performance," and a "science of safety" (See summary Tables 5.1 and 5.2).

As has been outlined in numerous medical lectures, the largest aviation disaster occurred in 1977 when flights KLM 4805 and Pan Am 1736 collided. Five hundred and eighty-three died. Investigators concluded that not only was the accident wholly preventable, but that a major cause was because the crews had "failed to take the time to become a team." [1] In a similar vein, evidence shows that fewer planes

P. G. Brindley (✉) · J. M. Slemko
Department of Critical Care Medicine, University of Alberta Hospital, Edmonton, AB, Canada
e-mail: Peter.Brindley@albertahealthservices.ca; Jocelyn.slemko@albertahealthservices.ca

L. Marshall Gillman, S. Widder (eds.), *Trauma Team Dynamics*, https://doi.org/10.1007/978-3-031-86312-7_5

Table 5.2 Practical strategies to improve verbal communication in a medical crisis

Perform regular simulation exercises
Practice active-listening
Model "transmitter-oriented language"
Ban "mitigating language"
Cite names; be **C**lear/concise; **C**lose the loop (3 **C**'s of Communication)
Structure communication using "SBAR" and "repeat-backs"
"Call out" when significant changes occur
Practice "escalating assertiveness"
Avoid "somebody"/"anybody" comments
Respect communication "sterility"; control interruptions

crash when the co-pilot is flying [7]. There are many reasons why, but part of it is because, firstly, the senior pilot is unafraid to speak up, and, secondly, because the subordinate is now actively involved [7]. In other words, an ad hoc team is formed, and that team has larger mental and physical capacity than previously existed. Evidence suggests the same for acute care medicine [2]. In short, trauma training needs more "we" and less "me" [2].

Our profession has been slower than aviation to realize that team skills are not innate and therefore cannot be left to chance or intuition. In addition, these are non-technical skills, require novel approaches, and must be practiced. This is why simulation is not a luxury but rather a part of core business. As will be outlined, team skills encompass effective communication; adaptability; compensatory behavior; mutual monitoring and the ability to give and receive feedback [2]. In short, modern trauma care is as much about "team-dexterity" and "verbal dexterity" (see below) as it is about traditional factual knowledge or procedural skill.

Another readily applicable aviation example is the 1935 crash of the B17 bomber during a test flight; when it was lamented that "the modern plane is just too much for one man to fly." [1]. Similarly, the complexity of trauma-care makes the modern patient simply too much for one clinician to manage. After all, the modern critical care unit patient has been estimated to require approximately 180 steps per-patient per-day [1]. Regardless of the exact number, clearly such complexity exceeds even the most capable individual. Therefore, it is not hyperbolic to argue that without effective teamwork, high-quality trauma care is largely impossible. In short, trauma care truly is a team sport [2].

What Does It Take to Create a Team?

Teamwork, which can be defined as "cooperative efforts to achieve a common goal," is more than just subordinates doing as the leader tells them [2]. Instead, it is about maximizing the mental and physical problem-solving capabilities, such that the sum exceeds the parts [2]. Additionally, task demands (rescuing the patient) and social demands (running the team) have to work in parallel [2, 8]. In other words, there is a difference between taskwork (getting finite things done) and teamwork (nurturing a group of people so that they can achieve many things). We need to turn individuals into team players, or else the team fails, and the patient pays the price. Individual team members will not share their abilities unless they feel safe to do so [2]. This does not mean that we no longer need a leader and leadership: it means that we cannot create the teams that we want unless we create the culture that we need [8].

Team Culture: Not Just Leaders; Followers Too

Most people accept that culture matters, but unfortunately, "culture" is rarely defined or measured. As such, "culture change" seems to be little more than a buzzword than an overdue imperative. This chapter does not allow for an in-depth discussion, but the work of Dutch Psychologist, Geert Hofstede, offers a good starting point [9]. His group outlined six indices of culture, which include: Power Distance Index (i.e., how the powerful and less powerful accept their status); Individualism (i.e., loyalty versus everyone for themselves); Masculinity vs Femininity (i.e., money-focus; self-centeredness); Uncertainty Avoidance (i.e., comfort with uncertainty; reliance on rules vs style); Long-Term Orientation (i.e. persistence, and the importance of shame), and Indulgence vs Restraint (i.e., individual freedom vs societal norms).

Culture is a complex whole that encompasses the knowledge, beliefs, customs, and habits of a group, not just the habits and beliefs of an individual. Group culture has a powerful influence upon behaviors, attitudes, and action. Medicine has had a laudable culture that emphasizes patient ownership and self-reliance. The downside is that this can promote the individual agenda over team cohesion. Similarly, traditionally, we have also assumed that success results from individual efforts (and failure from individual shortcomings), ignoring the contributions of all team members and the environment. Accordingly, remedies have previously focused on individual competence or blame. It's time to update.

A thriving, effective medical culture requires commitment to hard work over years rather than the typical trauma timescale, namely hours or even less. We must ensure that empathy is cultivated and shared, and workplace complacency (or toxicity) is not tolerated. Buzzwords aside, we really do need to create and nourish a safe work environment. Teams absolutely still need structure and hierarchy, but the skill is to simultaneously ensure that we leverage everybody's knowledge and skills [10]. It is important to understanding that those actively talking (i.e., resuscitating by voice) are no more important than those actively listening [10]. Team leaders may be largely responsible for setting the dynamic, but, importantly, we all own and affect culture.

Skilled leadership improves team performance, satisfaction, and efficiency [11]. However, just like culture, the definition of a good leader is difficult. An effective leader knows when to be hands-on (explicit leadership) and when to step back and delegate (implicit leadership) [10]. Leadership requires skill and experience and cannot always be intuited. Leaders must simultaneously earn the team's trust, present an acceptable shared mental model, centralize information flow, coordinate tasks, and overcome emotions (their own and others') [12]. Through managing and monitoring the overall situation, they accept disproportionate responsibility (i.e., including when they are not at fault). They step up and get their hands dirty when required. Leaders also teach, mentor, and model a standard for the whole team [11]. This is why hierarchy matters—you earn the right to lead; it isn't just awarded on day one. It is also why leadership is difficult and followers should help leaders and forgive occasional failings. Leadership traits and skills are discussed further in Chap. 20.

Much of the medical literature focusses on the qualities of an effective leader, but there is a paucity of discussion on what makes an excellent follower. To date, there are 60 publications on leadership for every one publication on followership [13]. Self-identifying as a "follower" (i.e., a relative subordinate) is still associated with significant stigma, even though 85% of healthcare workers are better understood to be followers, and the system simply could not function without them. Once again, these skills should be taught and highly valued. In short, followership is an advanced and impressive skill.

Effective followers have capacity to step up when required and do not take it personally when they need to step back. They are able to self-manage and use their emotional intelligence to size up when and what they should contribute [10].

Members of the trauma team oscillate between assuming leadership and followership roles. Therefore, one should simply talk about high functioning team members, who, in turn, are those dexterous enough to adapt to *what* (rather than *who*) is right. Effective leaders and followers also cross monitor, meaning that while they manage themselves, they also remain vigilant to the needs of others. Every good trauma team member has a "sixth sense," where you size up a situation and decide to step up or step back, depending on what will best serve the patient and team.

Resuscitations often require sub-teams, while each team member maintains a global perspective and sub-teams divide up the work and can thereby narrow their focus—to minimize task overload and maximize cognitive offload [14]. Examples include an airway team or vascular access team. The goal is to divide the resuscitation into manageable chunks and enable the leader to maintain a more supervisory role, or "thousand-foot view." [14] In nature, there are two types of attentiveness. System-1 is a focused spotlight gaze, such as when a predator focuses on only what truly matters, namely catching prey. System-2 involves scanning from stimulus to stimulus. In nature, the potential prey must avoid fixating on one spot and instead adjust their attention constantly in order to avoid being eaten [11].

The most common team failings (and therefore the areas on which to focus our resources and energies) are the inability to assign roles and responsibilities; to hold team members to account; to advocate a position or a corrective action; to use check-backs (i.e., "closed-loop communication"); to seek usable information (as opposed to just "data"); to prioritize tasks; and to cross-monitor other team members [2]. In short, it should be clear why a team of experts is not the same as an expert team [2].

Teamwork: Good and Bad

Teamwork is probably the best way to mitigate task-overload and fixation errors. However, not all teamwork is inherently good. As a result, psychology also offers useful cautionary tales for the modern trauma team. Zimbardo's infamous Stanford Prison experiment (which had graduate students assume the roles of prisoners and prison guards) demonstrates how easily we can be made to assume roles even when not beneficial. Even though supposedly play-acting, the students quickly formed into two teams, with one becoming excessively unruly (the prisoners) and the other excessively sadistic (the guards). In a similar vein, Stanley Milgram's work (where he was able to get people to administer electric shocks to others) further demonstrates our propensity toward blind obedience [15]. Solomon Asch's experiments (where he could get experts to give incorrect answers just by having other confederates answer incorrectly beforehand) show how easily we can be made to do things that we know are wrong. Importantly, in Asch's experiments there was no overt coercion, merely the power of embarrassment and social conformity [15].

The apparent irrationality of modern humans and their blind spots is tough for some professionals to accept [8]. However, humans have evolved as social beings and are therefore highly susceptible to social pressures [2, 8]. Regardless, it should not be surprising that we resort to behaviors that have worked well for most of our evolutionary past, especially during crises [8]. Moreover, we all have biases, and while we may be adept at seeing them in others, we are less likely to see them in ourselves. Regardless, good team leaders know to capitalize on the best of our primitive crisis behavior and mitigate against innate shortcomings. For example, good leaders can capitalize on our propensity to obedience during a crisis. At the same time, good team leaders realize that too much hierarchy will suppress the team's larger cognitive capacity [8].

Insightful team leaders should know that once a majority of team members have formed an opinion, they usually stick with it despite contradictory information [2]. This is done subconsciously to reduce a sense of isolation and "cognitive dissonance" (the discomfort that humans have with holding two or more contradictory ideas simultaneously) [15]. As a result, a good team leader will deliberately and routinely challenge assumptions (why are you so certain this is hemorrhagic shock?). Similarly, "group think" means that teams may follow the majority opinion rather than the rational argument ("if we all agree then we can't be wrong") [2, 15]. As a result, the effective team leader will force the team to seek out contradictory information ("I still want to see that ECG before we take this patient to the operating room"). Interestingly, teams can also amplify individual behavior. For example, groups tend toward greater risk if an individual's initial tendency was to be risky and toward more caution if individuals were risk averse [2, 15]. Team behavior can (and must) be managed and is a key leadership skill that can be taught.

Team Leadership 101: The Shared Mental Model

Leadership includes providing structure to chaos, and organization where previously there was none [8]. A key strategy is the "shared mental model" (a common understanding, or, in colloquial terms, a sense that everyone is "on the same page") [2]. This helps to form a task-focused (rather than power-focused or ego-focused) team as well as a structure that prioritizes duties, manages information, establishes roles, stabilizes emotions, and can build confidence [2]. If time allows, then the team leader should invite members to suggest a mental model ("what do you think?, what should we do?"). After all, diverse inputs can provide the team with a more comprehensive view [2, 8]. However, under time pressure, the leader has to rapidly establish a reasonable mental model that members will support ("I believe its hemorrhagic shock, unless I'm missing something please do the following") [3]. Studies have shown that the best situational awareness and the shortest reaction time come from practice and prior exposure [8]. In this way, simulation is a great way to develop team "reflexes" and for leaders to learn the power of the "shared mental model."

The greater the overlap in shared mental models, the more likely that team members will predict, adapt, and coordinate—even if dealing with stress or novelty [2]. It is also essential to regularly update the shared mental model ("okay, the airway is secured; our next priority is…") and to ensure that it still makes sense as new knowledge comes to light ("I now have an ECG that shows ST elevation—please listen up because things have changed"). Task assignment is usually specified by profession (e.g., anesthetists intubate and surgeons operate) [2]. Therefore, this does not usually need to be negotiated in the mental model. However, if there is confusion (i.e., both the anesthetist and surgeon could insert central lines), then the good leader predicts that it may cause confusion and hence that it needs to be explicitly stated ("Dr Smith, you intubate, Dr Jones you do lines"). In short, the mental model must be clear, proactive, flexible, and shared.

Say What You Mean and Mean What You Say

Mounting evidence shows that ineffective communication during an acute medical crisis is one of the commonest reasons for preventable medical error and preventable death [3, 7, 16]. This should not be a surprise, after all we have long known that poor cockpit communication—especially between junior and senior crew—is one of the commonest reasons why mechanically-sound planes crash [3, 7, 16]. It is also time to understand that our "verbal dexterity" is every bit as important as factual knowledge or procedural dexterity during a crisis [3]. Most of what follows is not native to medicine. It is, however, highly translatable to our reality.

Many shortfalls in communication can be summarized using the following pithy quote by Rall and Gaba: "**Meant is not said; said is not heard; heard is not understood; understood is not done.**" [17]. However, it is also important not to oversimplify something as complex as communication. For example, communication is far more than just talking. Communication aids task execution; enables information exchange, and helps (or hinders) relationship building [2]. Communication is also more than just what is said. It also includes how it is said and how it is understood [2]. As a result, non-verbal communication (which includes posture, facial expressions, gestures, and eye contact), as well as para-verbal communication (which includes pacing, tone, volume, and emphasis), is at least as important as verbal communication [2, 16]. This is especially true when there is incongruence between the words used and the facial expression or the tone [15]. As a result, while this section will present several practical verbal techniques (again borrowed from aviation and adapted to medicine), we are only scratching the surface. Readers are strongly encouraged to read more and to realize that expertise in acute trauma means expertise in all facets of crisis communication [2, 3, 16].

Flight investigators made a priority of flattening the authority gradient. [7] One way to do so is to mandate more "horizontal communication" [7, 16]. This means that all members of the team are authorized—in fact they are obligated—to speak up, and to do so clearly, regardless of rank [7]. Moreover, aviation has mandated "transmitter orientated" communication (where it is the speaker's responsibility to be understood) rather than "receiver orientated" communication (where it is the listeners responsibility to unravel what was meant) [7]. However, making communication more deliberate means that we also promote active listening [2]. This requires that we confirm understanding and demand clarification, regardless of seniority or embarrassment. [2, 4, 5] All team members take responsibility for how messages are delivered, received, understood, and carried out [2, 3, 8, 16].

Crisis Communication 101

A common feature following aviation crashes is black-box silence during minutes prior to a crash. [3, 7] Similarly, ask most nurses about the last bad resuscitation they witnessed, and it is likely notable for the same thing: silence despite chaos. Therefore, team members need to be taught strategies regarding how to speak up [3, 7, 16]. Physicians may not speak due to stress or uncertainty, or simply because they do not have the usable lines [18]. For example, instead of silence, we can teach the leader standardized verbal responses. An example would be: "we still have no pulse… what am I missing?" Another would be: "I am unclear what happened before we arrived; who can summarize?" [3]. Other team members need verbal strategies to become part of the trauma team rapidly. An example could be "I am from General Surgery; is there any job that needs doing?" Just as teamwork does not come naturally, neither does crisis communication. Again, simulation is an ideal tool. It enables us to discover what works and to master what are, after all, lifesaving skills.

The military and aviation have long used the **SBAR** acronym (Situations, Background, Assessment, Recommendation) in order to provide a recognizable structure to communication [3, 19]. While it may seem overly formal—especially when team members are either familiar with each other or if the problem is routine—it can offer a very useful construct for junior staff and for unfamiliar situations [19]. A simple example could be: Situation: "this is Dr X, I need your help right away"; Background: "he's a 35 year old with a splenic injury"; Assessment: "he is still hypotensive despite four units of blood." Recommendation: "You should review him now regarding need for surgery."

In addition to getting aviators to speak up, they are also taught how to be acknowledged and how to be taken seriously. Therefore, they learn how to use levels or grades of assertiveness [2, 3, 7, 16, 18, 20–22]. For example, Robert Besco's iconic four-step P.A.C.E communication progresses as follows: Probing, Alerting, Challenging, and finally Emergency [22]. Other constructs include up to six steps. Regardless, the intention is to offer strategies from least to most direct. For example, this includes the "hint" (e.g., "should things look like this?"); "preference" (e.g., "I would suggest…"); "query" (e.g., "what do you think?"); "shared suggestion" (e.g., "you and I could"); "statement" (e.g., "we need to") and "command" (e.g., "do this now!"). Of note, those actively listening should also pick up on the escalating urgency and react accordingly. It is worth re-emphasizing that leaders understand that crisis communication is as much about listening as talking.

Without instruction, junior team members may only hint and, if ignored, fail to escalate their assertiveness further [7]. On the other extreme, without instruction, senior team members may rely too heavily upon blunt "commands." [7]. This style is certainly unequivocal and is needed when team members have repeatedly failed to appreciate the seriousness of a situation. However, it can destroy the team structure if routinely used as the initial, or the only, communication style [7]. With the same purpose in mind, aviation also teaches a five-step model of advocacy and confirmation [18]. The following includes aviation examples and medical corollaries: Attention Getter ("Captain/Doctor"), State Your Concern ("We're low on fuel/the patient is hypotensive"), State the Problem as You See It ("I don't think we can land/I think we need to operate now"), State a Solution ("Let's re-route to a closer airport/I'll book the OR theatre"), Obtain Agreement ("Okay, Captain/Doctor?") [18].

Applying the "C's of communication" mean that we must **cite** names (to avoid diffusion of responsibility); that we must be **clear** and **concise** (to avoid confusion); and most importantly, that we must **close-the-loop** (to confirm that it has been done) [3–5, 16, 18]. This means that we reinforce our instructions by demanding verbal feedback. For example, we tell a specific person to intubate but also to tell us when it is done (or to tell us the end tidal CO_2). This also means we do not just ask for two units of blood but rather "Nurse, give two units of blood…and tell me the blood pressure when it is in" or "Jim, poke for an arterial blood gas… and bring the result back to me." In other words, there are many ways to "close the loop," but as a strategy it confirms that the instruction was heard, understood, and done. A potential additional C includes **crowd control**. This means ensuring that there are enough people present ("we do not have someone who can do a surgical airway, go and get me Dr X"), or that we have the right people present ("please tell me your role"), or that we do not have too many people present ("thank you for responding, but we need to clear out all but the following people…").

Another strategy is the "call out." [18]. This means that we alert the team whenever there are important changes ("he's starting to go back into ventricular fibrillation") [18].

Similarly, the "step back method" means we verbally force a "time-out." This compels the team to reassess their assumptions ("stop chest compressions, we need to know if we're still in asystole"). The "repeat back method" [18] provides a safety check by repeating an order to confirm mutual understanding ("so was that one full milligram of epinephrine?"). The "read back method" [18] means we confirm a verbal order before processing it ("okay, so first you want two units of packed cells, then repeat a hemoglobin, then call you if it has not increased").

While team members must be encouraged to speak up, they need to be taught how to make those inputs task-focused and appropriately timed. If not, it can further exacerbate the cacophony and chaos [2, 8]. Non-helpful interruptions are considered such a safety hazard in aviation that they are now addressed in this industry's standard operating procedures. The "Sterile Cockpit Rule" means that no non-operational talk is allowed during critical phases such as taxi, take-off, or landing [16, 23, 24]. Of note, it applies to all those in the cockpit to enforce it, not just those currently talking. [16, 23, 24] We understand the need for microbiologic sterility in surgery, so why not "communication sterility."

The Sterile Cockpit Rule [23, 24] can be readily adapted to medical practitioners during resuscitation [3, 8]. In less-critical situations, we should confirm if others are able to focus their attention ("I want your opinion, do you have two full minutes?") [3]. In more critical situations, we can demand attention ("I need you to stop that conversation and focus on this critically ill trauma patient"). A great example comes from the everyday operating room: the anesthetist is in his or her critical phase during induction and awakening. Therefore, the surgeon must avoid unnecessary noise or distraction. Once the operation is underway, the surgeon is now in his or her critical phase even if the anesthetist no longer is. It is now just as important for the anesthetist to avoid unnecessary interruptions or disturbances of the surgeon. In other words, all members are responsible for creating the right environment so that the right team communication can be leveraged to benefit the patient [3, 16].

Ambiguous or non-committal speech (aka "mitigating speech") is common prior to airline crashes, as well as during medical crises [7]. This is why, during crises, we must replace comments like "perhaps we need a surgeon," or "we should think about operating," with "get me a surgeon" and "we need to go to the operating theatre now." Junior members (or those that feel "unsafe" in their role) may mitigate speech to show deference when embarrassed or if unsure [2, 3]. Interestingly, if time permits, then "mitigating language" can be harmless and may aid team building ("if you get a moment could you help me with this patient?"). However, if the wrong communication tool is used during a crisis, it can be no less dangerous than the wrong surgical instrument. It is about being as dexterous with your communication as with your hands.

Over-cautious language is inappropriate during crises, just as overly strident language can be inappropriate at less critical times. Crisis communication should still be polite but must be unambiguous ("Jessica, your next job is to intubate, do it now, please"). Communication must also be addressed to a specific person to avoid diffusion of responsibility [2, 4, 5]. This is why comments like "could someone" and "does anybody" are inappropriate even if they are polite [2]. However, just as we need to control communication during a crisis, we need to loosen the reigns once it has abated. As a result, at other times we also need to promote more free-flowing communication. This is essential for debriefing, conflict management, and stress relief. In other words, communication is also essential to keep the team resilient ahead of the next crisis [2].

Conclusion

Despite a culture that typically trumps the individual, modern medicine (and especially acute care medicine) demands teamwork and team communication. In addition, it requires team leaders and followers who understand the basics of human psychology, and how this can be utilized to the patient's benefit. Practitioners, educators, and administrators should agree that teamwork must not be assumed or left to chance. Instead, teamwork should be deliberately taught, routinely practiced, and reliably funded. We also need to adapt, and then to freely share, the best strategies learned from other high-stakes professions but also from each other. The question is whether we have the requisite humility, insight, common sense, and culture to evolve.

Key Points

- Non-technical skills likely have the greatest impact upon patient safety and outcome.
- We must make a "science of reducing complexity"—fortunately practical strategies can be taught.
- Teamwork is key to reducing chaos and complexity.
- Communication is the key leadership skill.
- Good teamwork (and communication and followership) cannot (and need not) be left to chance.

References

1. Gawande A. The checklist. In: Gawande A, editor. The checklist manifesto. New York: Henry Holt and Company; 2009. p. 32–48.
2. St Pierre M, Hofinger G, Buerschaper C. Crisis management in acute care settings: human factors and team psychology in a high stakes environment. New York: Springer; 2008.
3. Brindley PG, Reynolds SF. Improving verbal communication in critical care medicine. J Crit Care. 2011;26:155–9.
4. Gaba DM, Fish KJ, Howard SK. Crisis management in anesthesiology. New York: Churchill Livingstone; 1994.
5. Gaba DM. Dynamic decision-making in anesthesiology: cognitive models and training approaches. In: Evans DA, Patel VI, editors. Advanced models of cognition for medical training and practice. Berlin: Springer-Verlag; 1992. p. 123–47.
6. Aron D, Headrick L. Educating physicians prepared to improve care and safety is no accident: it requires a systematic approach. Qual Saf Health Care. 2002;11:168–73.
7. Gladwell M. The ethnic theory of plane crashes. In: Gladwell M, editor. Outliers. New York: Little, Brown and Company; 2008. p. 177–223.
8. Ripley A. The unthinkable: who survives when disaster strikes – and why. New York: Crown Publishers; 2008.
9. Hofstede G. Attitudes, values and organizational culture: disentangling the concepts. Organ Stud. 1998;19(3):477–92.
10. Gillman LM, Brindley PG, Blaivas M, Widder S, Karakitsos D. Trauma team dynamics. J Crit Care. 2016;32:218–21.
11. Gillman LM, Widder S, Blaivas M, Karakitsos D. Trauma team dynamics. 1st ed. Springer; 2016.
12. Brindley PG, Reynolds SF. Improving verbal communication in critical care medicine. J Crit Care 2011;26(2):155–159. Available from: https://doi.org/10.1016/j.jcrc.2011.03.004
13. Leung C, Lucas A, Brindley P, Anderson S, Park J, Vergis A, et al. Followership: a review of the literature in healthcare and beyond. J Crit Care 2018;46:99–104. Available from: https://doi.org/10.1016/j.jcrc.2018.05.001
14. Hicks C, Petrosoniak A. The human factor: optimizing trauma team performance in dynamic clinical environments. Emerg Med Clin North Am. 2018;36(1):1–17.
15. Heffernan M. Willful blindness: why We ignore the obvious at our peril. Canada: Doubleday/Random House; 2011.
16. Cyna AM, Andrew MI, Tan SGM SGM, Smith AF. Handbook of communication in anaesthesia and critical care. A practical guide to exploring the art. Oxford University Press; 2010.
17. http://www.skygod.com/quotes/cliches.html. Accessed Aug 2012
18. Dunn EJ, Mills PD, Neily J, Crittenden MD, Carmack AL, Bagian JP. Medical team training: applying crew resource management in the veterans health administration. Jt Comm J Qual Patient Saf. 2007;33(6):317–25.
19. SBAR Institute for Healthcare Improvement. SBAR Technique for Communication: a situational briefing model. Available at: http://www.ihi.org/IHI/Topics/PatientSafety/SafetyGeneral/Tools/SBARTechniqueforCommunicationASituationalBriefingModel.htm. Accessed Aug 2012
20. Leonard M, Graham S, Bonacum D. The human factor: the critical importance of effective communication in providing safe care. Qual Saf Health Care. 2004;13(suppl):i85–90.
21. Fischer U, Orasanu J. Cultural diversity and crew communication. 1999. Available at http://www.lcc.gatech.edu/~fischer/AIAA99.pdf. Accessed Aug 2012
22. Besco RO. To intervene or not to intervene? The copilots 'catch 22': Developing flight crew survival skills through the use of 'P.A.C.E'. 1994. Available at http://www.crm-devel.org/resources/paper/PACE.PDF. Accessed Aug 2012.
23. Airbus flight operations briefing notes. Human performance: managing interruptions and distractions. Available at: http://www.skybrary.aero/bookshelf/books/176.pdf. Accessed 15 May 2012.
24. The Sterile Cockpit Rule Aviation Safety Reporting System (ASRS). 1993. Available at: http://asrs.arc.nasa.gov/publications/directline/dl4_sterile.htm. Accessed Aug 2012.

6 Introduction to Leadership: Self-Awareness and Self-Management

David Kolthoff and Sandy Widder

Trauma resuscitations are a time of chaos, high emotions, and multiple moving parts within the system. A trauma leader needs to guide and act as an emotional compass keeping the team working in synergy and goal focussed. They cannot rely on a single and linear style but need multiple tools in their leadership toolbox to utilize based on the situation and emotional temperature of the team. This chapter will provide the first steps to building an accountable, authentic, and grounded leader and bring greater success to your team.

Background

Trauma can be an environment of chaos. As such, meaningful leadership skills are required to deliver timely care and to optimize outcomes. Resuscitating the trauma patients can be demanding due to the concomitant stress of rescuing unstable multi-injured patients and directing the needs of the multidisciplinary team. Therefore, a leader must first lead themselves before they can effectively lead the team to success. Leadership is the most essential nontechnical skill for a trauma team to be successful [1]. Furthermore, effective leadership reinforces a culture of collaboration and teamwork within the trauma team [2].

A growing body of literature suggests that training focused on leadership, team building, and team training is greatly related to increased team coalition and improved success with outcomes. Thomas et al. studied pediatric residents undertaking a common neonatal resuscitation program but provided deliberate team training to only half. This single intervention was associated with increased information sharing, inquiry, assertion, vigilance, and workload management. Other studies have similarly concluded that leadership and team structure improve team performance [3–6]. Accordingly, courses such as Advanced Life Support and Pediatric Advanced Life Support courses supplied by the American Heart Association that historically were focused on factual knowledge now included modules in leadership and teamwork [7].

D. Kolthoff (✉)
Alberta Health Services, Edmonton, AB, Canada
e-mail: David.kolthoff@albertahealthservices.ca

S. Widder
University of Alberta, Edmonton, AB, Canada
e-mail: sandy.widder2@albertahealthservices.ca

Leadership Styles

Despite the multiple styles of leadership available within literature and the web, they can be grouped into three categories: empowering, directive or commanding, and passive. In 1939, psychologist Kurt Lewin led one of the most influential leadership studies. Lewin studied school children and placed them in three groups with an authoritarian (commanding), democratic (empowering), and laissez-faire (passive) leader (See Table 6.1). Lewin found three distinct groups of behaviors based on the group the children were placed in. The children were less creative in the authoritarian/commanding group due to the top-down approach, where the leader is typically the most knowledgeable with little input from the team or group. Lewin found the children in the democratic group to be more empowered and creative, with greater quality with their contributions but less productive than the authoritarian group. The laissez-faire leader was found to be passive, less productive, and creative than the other two groups but also created more demands on the leader. They also showed an inability to work independently and also demonstrated little cooperation with each other.

Subsequently, multiple studies have identified leadership styles and dissected them further into more detail. Goleman divided leadership into two distinct categories: resonant and dissonant. He further dissected these two categories into greater detailed styles: resonant styles-visionary, coaching, affiliative, and democratic. Dissonant styles- pacesetting and commanding. The resonant styles create inspiration, creativity, and motivation where the dissonant styles share the same

L. Marshall Gillman, S. Widder (eds.), *Trauma Team Dynamics*, https://doi.org/10.1007/978-3-031-86312-7_6

Table 6.1 Leadership styles

Empowering	Commanding
Motivates and inspires Coaching and mentoring Creates emotional bonds Reinforces participation and collaboration Reinforces communication Nourishes a learning environment	Top-down approach "Do what I tell you" "Do as I do now" Demands immediate compliance Minimal to no input from team Transactional (punish or reward)

characteristics of Lewin's autocratic style with a top-down approach that is needed at times but should be used with caution.

During a trauma resuscitation, there is a time and place for the leader to use multiple styles, exercising situational awareness, social awareness, and emotional intelligence. In 2005, Yun, Faraj, and Sims studied leadership within trauma resuscitations and found the style of leadership was dependent on the trauma complexity. A commanding or dissonant style was more effective with high severities and an inexperienced team. Dealing with lower severities and a highly experienced team, a resonant style was recommended. The authors also supported Goleman's approach describing how an empowering and resonant leader provided greater learning opportunities versus a commanding approach. The use of multiple leadership styles contingent on the situation was the greatest significant finding within this study as described by the authors.

The leader in any group has been the one who others look for clarity and direction during chaos and uncertainty or appreciation when things are going well. The leader is the emotional guide or compass for the group. Guiding the emotions of a group can be fleeting and open to interpretation but is vital in achieving outcomes within a highly emotionally charged team such as a trauma team.

Building the Foundation of Leadership

The evolution of a great leader and building effective leadership skills is similar to learning any new technical or social skill, and a foundation needs to be firmly built and reinforced. An effective leader needs to first lead themselves before they can lead others. This skill requires an abundance of self-reflection and self-awareness. These attributes are also the foundation of emotional intelligence (EI). Daniel Goleman popularized EI in the mid-1990s where Goleman described EI as "how leaders handle themselves and their relationships." [3] A leader who exercises self-awareness is then able to self-manage, create social awareness, and furthermore manage relationships based on empathy.

Fundamentals of Emotional Intelligence

Self-Awareness

Self-awareness is the knowing of one's emotions, values, strengths but also limitations [3]. They are typically honest with themselves and are neither self-critical nor naïve but demonstrate a state of realism. Self-awareness mandates continuous self-reflection either planned or impromptu. Without effective self-awareness, we leave ourselves vulnerable to being sidetracked to other stimuli, emotions, and leading void of direction and purpose. Self-awareness is our rudder or emotional compass and enables the leader to guide the group to success.

Effective self-awareness enables the leader to know their strengths and limitations and avoid blind spots [6]. When things are going well, it is easy for leaders to default upon their strengths and collaborate, motivate others, and engage the team. Unfortunately, when leaders are not aware of their limits, they do not always realize opportunities for improvement, and more importantly, that they themselves may be leading the team astray. When the leader is uncomfortable, they may default to an autocratic/commanding leadership style that can deteriorate the confidence and dynamics of the trauma team.

Resources to aid with reflection and self-awareness could be the use of a diary, meditation, or just setting out quiet moments in your day to reflect. Some of these skills are discussed further in the chapter on Mindfulness. Even taking a pause during and reflecting on the current situation as too what is going well and what could go better.

Self-Management

Once there is clarity surrounding your emotions and your purpose from reflection and self-awareness, the next step in the process of EI is self-management. We need to know our emotions before we can manage our response to them. In many ways, this is self-control and is much easier when we are dealing with positive, happy emotions, but dealing with negative emotions such as frustration and anger with a lapse of self-management can be disastrous and lead to poor outcomes. As healthcare providers and front-line leaders, we are typically attuned to managing our emotional response to stimuli around us. This is especially true when dealing with patients and family members during difficult times, but at times we are subjected to an emotional hijack.

Emotional hijack, or amygdala hijack, is when we act upon our emotions without that subconscious pause. It's bypassing the neuro-circuitry that links our emotions with intellect. The prefrontal area of the brain is the "command center" and collects and analyzes all information from different areas [8].

During a resuscitation when emotions are high, and the room is filled with multiple distracting stimuli, an emotional hijack is quite possible and could lead to suboptimal outcomes versus keeping those impulses in check. Emotional hijack could cause a leader to demonstrate unprofessional behaviours such as an emotional outburst, offensive language, or blatant nonverbal, and facial expressions. The emotional intelligent leader exercising effective self-management would pause and reflect "the patient is hypotensive, we have two large bore IV's infusing boluses now, the team is working well." Furthermore, utilizing effective self-management and avoiding emotional hijack have a contagion effect. It is leading by example and modelling for others in the team. "Leading by example is much more effective than leading by command." [9]

Social Awareness

Simply put, social awareness is the ability of an emotional intelligent leader to empathize. Being aware of the emotions of team members around you. Being aware of facial expressions, posture, and verbal tone allows more information to fine tune within the prefrontal command centre. Furthermore, an emotionally intelligent leader who exercises social awareness is much more effective at messaging to team members. Being attuned to the emotions of the team, the leader can effectively guide the team and potentially deescalate if needed. Messaging is much more clear and authentic due the leader being attuned to the emotions of the group.

Despite empathy being the core competence of social awareness, the emotionally intelligent, empathetic leader isn't attempting to please everyone. Exercising empathy within the team isn't sacrificing your own emotions and adopting other's emotions. Neither is it creating a kumbaya moment, but an empathic leader makes decisions by taking other's emotions into consideration. Empathetic leaders tap into the groups emotions and guide them through difficult times. They are seen as approachable and create a psychologically safe environment: flourishing learning, motivation, and teamwork.

Relationship Management

As we further build the foundation of an emotionally intelligent leader who is self-aware, which enables them to self-manage and express empathy, the leader can optimally manage relationships. Typically, the term leadership is described as motivating and inspiring others. This may be why management of relationships is the most perceptible trait in leadership. Relationship management enables the leader to guide emotions, manage conflict, and collaborate effectively within the team based on being attuned and authentic with their emotions, and values. When the leader is dishonest and deceitful and attempts to manipulate, typically members' social awareness picks up these dissonant cues and a mistrust for leader may evolve. If this were to happen, a team can be divided, and the dynamics significantly altered. These relationships may be irreparable.

Trauma resuscitation is a time where emotions can run high, there is a sense of urgency in the form of (hopefully) controlled chaos with multiple moving parts of a system with the goal of patient survival. With a diverse range in experience and skills, collaboration is key, and trust is ultimately the foundation of collaboration. The EI leader who effectively manages relationship among their team fosters cooperation and communication and influences the members to achieve high performance. A leader without the trust of his team will struggle with the relationships between themselves and the teammates and endure extreme difficulties accomplishing tasks (Table 6.2).

Table 6.2 Fundamentals of emotional intelligence

EI component	Definition	Attributes	Example
Self-awareness	Knowing of one's emotions, values, strengths, limitations, values, and goals	Self-assessment Self-confidence Realistic Honest about themselves	The trauma team leader knows they overstimulated during the onset of a trauma resuscitation but attempts to self-soothe and deescalate themselves
Self-management	Controlling and self-regulating one's emotions and impulses	Self-soothing Avoiding emotional hijack Clarity Optimistic	During the resuscitation there is difficulty with the team establishing IV access. The leader resists the urge to scream. Instead, the leader calmly asks for other solutions to the team
Social awareness	The ability to empathize and be aware of the team members emotions around you	Empathetic Aware of the emotions of team members Messaging is authentic and clear	The leader reads the room and emotions are high which is causing some issues with the dynamics of the team. The leader then takes a moment to pause and summarize with their team and ask for any suggestions to cultivate empathy and collaboration
Relationship management	Managing the relationships around to guide emotions, manage conflict and enable collaboration within the team	Guides emotions, manages conflict and collaboration within the team Fundamental in building trust in teams	Subspecialist is attempting to give input regarding the case but feels reluctant. The leader encourages input and validates that input from other members of the trauma team and subspecialties included in that case

Validation

Summarizing this brief journey into leadership theories and styles, it is important to mention validation and recognition within the team. This is especially true within the task and emotion-saturated environment of a trauma resuscitation. Recognition is an emotional currency, and your trauma team needs this to replenish their emotional bank. Otherwise, team members may feel taken for granted and ultimately a climate of depreciation which over time will reinforce a poor team culture and likely poor patient outcomes. Utilizing authentic, personalized recognition validates team members to strive for greatness and creates a culture of community, creativity, and learning.

Putting It All Together

Leadership as well as any skill demands ongoing education, practice, and reflection to assess accomplishments, needs, and areas for improvement. There is an abundance of information available surrounding leadership, and within this chapter, we attempted to condense the content to either initiate a strong foundation or enhance the leadership skills already learned. The foundation to effective leadership is building and leading one's self before you can lead others.

Reviewing the various leadership styles, there are empowering styles that resonate or create resonance within the group. This fosters collaboration, communication, creativity, and trust within the group. A culture of learning and community is also nurtured, enabling members to learn among themselves but also mirror the attributes from the leader. On the other side of the leadership coin, we have the commanding and dissonant styles, which establish a top-down approach and inhibit input from members of the team. Finally, the passive style which wasn't described in great detail due to the fact it has little relevance within the trauma team. Every style of leadership despite being resonant or dissonant is effective and applicable but is contingent on the situation. A leader who is grounded within emotional intelligence can utilize these various styles dependent on the data they are receiving from the team. Social awareness yields data in form of verbalizations and tone, facial expressions, and body posture. The leader can then interpret this data and dip into their "toolbox" of leadership styles to use the most appropriate approach to reap success. Therefore, leadership is not a "cookie cutter" approach because one style will not always work, and if the leader utilizes a linear approach to leadership and disregards the incoming data from the group, it will create mistrust and dyssynchrony within the team. A high-fidelity team with multiple working parts, such as a trauma team, needs trust to enhance collaboration and optimize processes and outcomes.

Key Points

- Leadership skills and training can lead to increased team coalition during times of chaos and potentially affect outcomes.
- Many leadership styles exist, but the two ends of the spectrum are empowering and commanding styles.
- Leadership styles can vary depending on the situation, team members, and sense of urgency.
- Self awareness and management of self are key emotional intelligence pillars to become a great leader.

References

1. Hjortdahl M, Ringen A, Naess AC. Leadership is the essential non technical skill in the trauma team–results of a qualitative study. Scand J Trauma Rescue Emerg Med. 2009;17:49.
2. Cole E, Crichton N. The culture of trauma team in relation to human factors. J Clinical Nursing. 2006;15:1257–66. https://doi.org/10.1111/j.1365-2702.2006.01566.x.
3. Thomas EJ, Taggart B, Crandell S, Lasky RE, Williams AL, Love LJ, et al. Teaching teamwork during Neonatal Resuscitation Program: a randomized trial. J Perinatol. 2007;27:409–14.
4. Sakran JV, Finneman B, Maxwell C, Sonnad SS, Sarani B, Pascaul J, et al. Trauma leadership: does perception drive reality? J Surg Educ. 2012;69(2):236–40.
5. Driscoll P, Vincent C. Organizing an efficient trauma team. Injury. 1992;23:107–10.
6. Xiao Y, Seagull F, Mackenzie C, Klein K. Adaptive leadership in trauma resuscitation teams: a grounded theory approach to video analysis. Cognit Technol Work. 2004;6:6158–64.
7. ATLS Subcommittee, American College of Surgeons' Committee on Trauma, International ATLS Working Group. Advanced trauma life support (ATLS(R)): the ninth edition. J Trauma Acute Care Surg. 2013;74(5):1363–6. [PubMed] [Google Scholar]
8. Goleman D, Boyatzis R, McKee A. Primal leadership: learning to lead with emotional intelligence. Boston, MA: HBR Review Press; 2004. p. 6.
9. Kouzes JM, Posner BZ. The leadership challenge: how to make extraordinary things happen in organizations. 5th ed. San Francisco: Jossey-Bass; 2012. p. 17. Ford K, Menchine M, Burner E, Arora S, Inaba K, Demetriades D, Yersin B. Leadership and teamwork in trauma and resuscitation. West J Emerg Med. 2016;17(5):549–56. https://doi.org/10.5811/westjem.2016.7.29812. Epub 2016 Aug 22. PMID: 27625718; PMCID: PMC5017838; Yun S, Faraj S, Sims HP Jr. Contingent leadership and effectiveness of trauma resuscitation teams. J Appl Psychol. 2005;90(6):1288–96. https://doi.org/10.1037/0021-9010.90.6.1288. PMID: 16316282; Goleman D. Working with emotional intelligence. New York: Bantam Books. 1998

Followership

7

Jacqueline Beaumont and Lawrence Marshall Gillman

Intro

> In many ways, great followership is harder than leadership. It has more dangers and fewer rewards, and it must routinely be exercised with much more subtlety. But great followership has never been more important. —Warren Bennis

Followership has only recently become a more common topic of literature as it relates to teamwork and functioning in complex systems. Most research has historically focused on the leadership role, particularly as it relates to a more hierarchical teamwork design [1]. As the emphasis decreases regarding hierarchical leadership, it has become increasingly important to understand the role of followership, especially within the health system, where group interaction and participation are vital [2].

Followership can be difficult to define, but as described by Leung et al., it is the processes by which people follow, who they follow, and how much engagement and influence they exert [3]. Robert Kelley in his writing of the "Art of Followership" described the most well-known theory of followership [4]. He described five basic styles: passive, conformist, alienated, pragmatist, and effective [4]. He placed these styles on two continuums: participation, which can range from passive to active; and thinking, which runs from dependent to independent. He used a 2 × 2 table to describe this phenomenon where pragmatic style is at the center and the other styles are arranged according to where they fall on the continuum [5]. These styles are described in more detail later in the chapter.

Followership is beginning to become recognized as an important skill for healthcare teams and one that should be taught and discussed with just as much vigor as leadership [6]. Many of the qualities of good followership reflect those of good leadership; as a result, individuals who develop strong followership skills are more likely to translate into better leaders [7]. Certain followership styles in healthcare may also lead to improved job satisfaction and patient satisfaction [8]. The purpose of this chapter is to familiarize the reader with the concept of followership, why it is important, and what may define a good or bad follower. As you progress through this chapter, we encourage the reader to reflect on one's own experience with these roles, and how we can understand and improve these dynamics in our own environment.

The History of Followership

In the early and mid-twentieth century, there was an attempt to distinguish between the leader and follower in such a way to make them two "different species." [9] There was a change of view when Edwin Hollander, in the late-twentieth century, spoke to the critical role of the follower for the leader. He stated "… leadership is a process that involves followership. Followers are crucial because they either give leaders their support or withhold it." [9] In 1975, George Graen formulated the Vertical Dyad Linkage hypothesis [9]. This hypothesis described the relationship between a leader and followers as "links" including an "in-group" and an "out-group" of followers that are connected to the leader in a single direction [9]. This idea turned into the Leader-Member Exchange theory that described a multi-directional relationship between leaders and followers. This relationship yielded mutual support, respect, loyalty, and greater autonomy within a team, allowing improved performance and job satisfaction [8, 10]. Full-range leadership model then followed which identified both transactional and transformational behaviors. Briefly transactional leadership utilizes punishments and rewards to motivate followers and works well to ensure that basic tasks are done reliably, while transformational leadership focuses on inspiring followers by obtaining buy-in, focusing on vision and modelling expected behaviors. This mode encouraged the empowerment and influence of followers, inspiring

J. Beaumont (✉) · L. Marshall Gillman
Department of Surgery, University of Manitoba, Winnipeg, MB, Canada
e-mail: umbeaum2@myumanitoba.ca

L. Marshall Gillman, S. Widder (eds.), *Trauma Team Dynamics*, https://doi.org/10.1007/978-3-031-86312-7_7

them to perform beyond their perceived capabilities [11]. This cooperation, empowerment, and mutual support between followers and leaders is still encouraged in present day team environments [8].

What Is Followership

Three independent ideas on followership styles have been published in the last few decades and will be discussed in this section. It was Robert Kelley, in 1988, who first developed a theory that focused exclusively on followers [10]. He described five basic styles of followership based on a 2 × 2 matrix that compared the follower's engagement, and their independent/critical thinking [12]. This is visualized in Fig. 7.1. These followership styles can be applied to any team work environment including healthcare. The following were described:

1. Passive followers are those that do not take initiative or think critically and are sometimes thought of as "sheep." They look to the leader for directions and motivation.
2. Conformists are also sometimes referred to as "yes people." They are often engaged and motivated and fulfill their tasks with energy, but rely on the leader to direct the next steps.
3. Alienated followers are those that think independently but have a negative energy and low motivation to accomplish tasks. These individuals are smart but do not put their energy toward constructive solutions for the team.
4. Pragmatic followers think and act independently but are reluctant to cause conflict. They tend to "sit on the fence" to see which way something is headed before determining whether to get on board.
5. The effective/"star" followers think for themselves, are motivated, and have the capacity to recognize errors and speak up when necessary. These individuals often move fluidly between roles of follower and leader and are the most effective type of follower style.

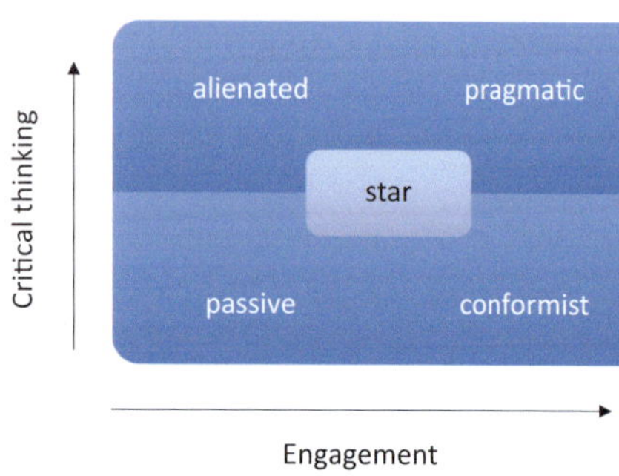

Fig. 7.1 Robert Kelley's followership styles matrix

A second model by Ira Chaleff, in 2008, focused on followership in the workplace and a framework to developing these skills [13]. He described the power that followers exhibit and distinguished that power as courage, therefore calling his model "Courageous Follower model," with five dimensions, as listed as follows:

1. The courage to support the leader
2. The courage to assume responsibility for a common goal
3. The courage to constructively challenge the leader's behaviors and opinions
4. The courage to participate in any transformation needed
5. The courage to take a moral stand when warranted to prevent abuse

With these dimensions, Chaleff differentiated four styles of followership based on the degree of courage the follower displayed to support or challenge the leader [13].

1. The resource style of followership exhibits low support and low challenge toward the leader. This follower may not support the leader but also doesn't openly challenge them.
2. The individualist style represents low support and high challenge. This follower will speak up but often takes an opposing position to the leader.
3. The implementer style demonstrates high support and low challenge. These followers will typically follow the leader blindly, without questions.
4. The partner style is characterized by high support and high challenge, assuming full responsibility for their actions and acting accordingly.

Chaleff's model emphasizes courage in limiting toxic leaders, and encouraging followers to be more effective.

A third model published in 2008 by Barbara Kellerman described five followership styles based on a continuum of low engagement to the committed follower [13].

1. Isolates are completely detached and do not know or care about their leaders.
2. The bystanders observe and do not participate.
3. Participant followers are more engaged, and they either favor their leaders and organizations or are clearly opposed.
4. Activists feel strongly and act accordingly.
5. Diehards are deeply devoted to their leaders, and their followership defines who they are and determines what they do.

Kellerman's model focuses on the level of engagement a follower has; the more engaged they are the more influence they have on the system.

Despite Kelley's model being the most well-known, it is important to note that each author agrees that there are different styles of followership, and there is a difference between effective and ineffective followership. As well, followers can and should influence their leaders [13]. Since these models were published, followership literature has continued to explore how followers contribute to leadership and organizational performance. The concept of shared-leadership has been highlighted, with increasing attention given to followers and the importance of follower-leader communication and cooperation [8, 14, 15].

Why Is Followership Important?

These followership models can be a useful framework when considering what makes an effective team, whether one is in a leadership or a followership role. The hospital is a highly complex organization, and each role in the system involves both leadership and followership components. At times, individuals may be followers, and other times, they may lead [8]. Follower and leader cooperation is crucial in order to deliver accurate, efficient, and safe patient care [8]. Since followers hold great importance within healthcare, studies have examined the relationship between followership style and job satisfaction. One study identified that followers who are actively engaged have much higher job satisfaction than those who are not [16]. Other studies have suggested that ineffective leader-follower exchange among other high stressors in healthcare environments increases burnout [17]. They also demonstrated that some followership styles, such as "exemplary" and "pragmatist" styles, were associated with less burnout [17]. In the business industry where these concepts have been most studied, it appears the most successful organizations have high numbers of "star followers" or "effective" followers who are able to think and act independently and have the courage to speak up when necessary [12]. In the medical community this concept is much less studied, however, "star followers" are likely to thrive in this environment as well. In the end, these styles are likely dynamic, and the ideal mix of followership styles that make up an organization depend on the leader and the task to be accomplished, but each style plays an important role within the organization [12].

When considering the importance of followers to speak up when required, a few strategies have been described that can help guide how one can advocate for patients in a respectful and assertive manner [18]. These strategies are discussed below and include: The effective followership algorithm, the two challenge rule, "CUS," and the "CHAT" pneumonic [18, 19]. These strategies are important in healthcare as the presence of hierarchy between team members has contributed to significant communication breakdowns and adverse patient outcomes [18]. When hierarchies are present, team members may fail to challenge decisions made by leaders despite concerns about patient outcomes [18].

The effective followership algorithm model begins with the "3W's": "what I see," "what I'm concerned about," and "what I want." [18] This allows the follower a structure to providing their concerns and expectations to the leader. If this fails to engage the team leader, the next level in the model is the 4-Step Assertive Tool [18]. This tool starts with capturing the leader's attention, followed by stating that the follower is concerned for patient safety, then offering a proposed solution or course of action, and closing the interaction with a question allowing the leader to engage. The next level in the algorithm if the previous two methods have not been effective, is to engage the team and allow other followers to advocate for patient safety [18]. The next step would be to involve the chain of command, and offer concerns to higher levels of authority [18]. Finally, effective followers should be prepared to take action when verbal tools fail and threats to safety are imminent [18].

The two challenge rule may be utilized within other frameworks and suggests that the concern be stated at least two times to ensure that it has been heard [19].

The "CUS" model to voice one's concerns uses words similar to the 4-Step Assertive Tool to advocate concerns regarding patient safety [19]. For example:

C: "I'm concerned"
U: "I'm uncomfortable" or "this is Unsafe"
S: "this is a safety issue" or "I am scared"

Finally, the CHAT pneumonic is a communication tool for team members to model their concerns [19], it goes as follows:

C: Context of the concern
H: History/background
A: Assessment of problem
T: Tentative plan of action

Table 7.1 provides examples of how to apply each of these strategies to a clinical scenario that requires a follower to speak up to the team leader about a patient safety concern.

All these models give the follower language that make it clear the concerns are patient or safety focused and do not challenge the decision making of the leader. In the healthcare environment, focusing on the patient well-being is an excellent way to unite the team towards a common goal and hopefully are not seen as challenges to one's ego. Having this language readily available and practiced allows the follower a toolbox of techniques that they can pull from in a crisis situation.

Table 7.1 Clinical example: The physician has restarted a patient's anti-hypertensive medication despite the patient having low blood pressure in the hospital; the bedside nurse is concerned about causing hypotension with this medication

Strategy	Application
The effective followership algorithm	1. 3 W's: "I see that you have restarted patient X's blood pressure medication. I am concerned that this will cause significant hypotension in this patient. I want you to re-evaluate holding this medication." 2. 4 step assertive tool: "Dr. Y, I am concerned for patient X's safety, I think we should hold his BP[a] medication as his BP has been low, what do you think?" 3. Engage the team 4. Engage the chain of command 5. Take action: do not give the medication
The two challenge rule	1."I am concerned that giving patient X his BP medication will cause significant hypotension" 2."I am concerned that giving patient X his BP medication will cause significant hypotension, I think we should hold it"
The CUS model	1. "I am *C*oncerned that giving patient X his BP medication will cause significant hypotension" 2. "It is *U*nsafe to restart patient X's BP medication at this time" 3. "I am *S*cared that the patient will have significant hypotension if we give them their BP medication"
The CHAT model	1. Context: "We restarted patient X's home BP medication today." 2. History/background: "The patient has been having low BP for the last couple of days." 3. Assessment of problem: "I am concerned we will cause hypotension if we give this medication." 4. Tentative plan: "I think we should continue to hold this medication."

[a]*BP* blood pressure

Unfortunately, there appears to be a level of discourse in knowledge of the role of followership within medicine [20]. A study in the UK by Gordon et al. found that medical trainees understanding of leadership and followership was of individualistic behaviors and hierarchy, often influenced by the structures they work in.[20] These attitudes are likely established early in training, and as a result, there should be dedicated education on this topic. Fortunately, training in crisis resource management principles and regular simulation exercises have emphasized the importance of multidisciplinary training, team cooperation, open communication, and effective leader-follower dynamics.[7] This type of training should be encouraged among all centers, to improve young trainees understanding of effective team dynamics including leadership and followership.

Summary

It is becoming increasingly obvious that good followership is just as important as good leadership. Engaged and open dialogue between team members allows for improved performance outcomes, feelings of job satisfaction, and less burnout among the team [16, 17]. Until more development in our knowledge and understanding of followership, the best approach may be to identify, reflect, and promote the ideas of modern follower and leader dynamics. This may allow young trainees to analyze their own behavior and those around them to hopefully improve the way we engage with each other and the system.

Key Points

- Followership is just as important as leadership.
- Understanding followership can improve team dynamics, job satisfaction, and decrease burnout.
- Followership can teach us advocacy techniques and improve patient safety.

References

1. Rost JC. Followership: an outmoded concept. In: Riggio R, Chaleff I, Lipman-Blumen J, editors. The art of followership: how great followers create great leaders and organizations. San Francisco: Jossey-Bass; 2008. p. 53–64.
2. Morgan SC. Followers make the differences: hospital performance and job satisfaction in relation to followership style. Minneapolis: Capella University; 2014.
3. Leung C, et al. Followership: a review of the literature in healthcare and beyond. J Crit Care. 2018;46:99–104. https://doi.org/10.1016/j.jcrc.2018.05.001.
4. Miller L. Followership. J Perinat Neonatal Nurs. 2007;23:38.
5. Kelley RE. The power of followership: how to create leaders people want to follow, and followers who lead themselves. New York: Doubleday/Currency; 1992.
6. Phelps G, Loh E, Dickinson H, Bismark M. Followership: a critical shortfall in health leadership. Royal Australasian College of Physicians; 2016. https://doi.org/10.1111/imj.12990.
7. Brindley P, Lucas A, Gillman LM, Cardinal P. Leadership and Followership Skills in Acute Care Medicine. In: Optimizing crisis resource management to improve patient safety and team performance. A handbook for all acute care health professionals. 1st ed. Royal College of Physicians and Surgeons of Canada. Ontario: Canada; 2017. p. 47–57.

8. Morgan S. Followers make the difference: hospital performance and job satisfaction in relation to followership style. Capella University; 2014.
9. Hollander EP, Julian JW. Contemporary trends in the analysis of leadership processes. Psychol Bull. 1969;71:387–91, quoted in Goethals and Sorenson, 871.
10. Riggio R. Why followership? New Dir Stud Leadersh. 2020;2020(167):15–22. https://doi.org/10.1002/yd.20395. © 2020 Wiley Periodicals LLC.
11. Antonakis J, House RJ. The full-range leadership theory: the way forward. In: Transformational and charismatic leadership: the road ahead 10th anniversary edition (Monographs in leadership and management), vol. 5. Emerald Group Publishing Limited; 2013. p. 3–33. https://doi.org/10.1108/S1479-357120130000005006.
12. Klingensmith ME. Leadership and followership in surgical education. Am J Surg. 2017;213(2):207–11.
13. Suda L. In praise of followers. In: Paper presented at PMI® Global Congress 2013—North America. New Orleans, LA/Newtown Square, PA: Project Management Institute; 2013.
14. Kohles JC, Bligh MC, Carsten MK. A follower-centric approach to the vision integration process. Leadersh Q. 2012;23(3):476–87. https://doi.org/10.1016/j.leaqua.2011.12.002.
15. Carsten MK, Uhl-Bien M. Follower beliefs in the co-production of leadership: examining upward communication and the moderating role of context. Z Psychol. 2012;220(4):210–20. https://doi.org/10.1027/2151-2604/a000115.
16. Gatti P, Ghilieri C, Cortese C. Relationships between followers' behaviors and job satisfaction in a sample of nurses. PLoS One. 2017;12(10):e0185905. https://doi.org/10.1371/journal.pone.0185905.
17. Crawford J, Daniels M. Follow the leader: how does "followership" influence nurse burnout? Nurs Manag (Springhouse). 2014;45(8):30–7. https://doi.org/10.1097/01.NUMA.0000451999.41720.30.
18. Sculli G, Fore A, Sine D, Paull D, Tschannen D, Aebersold M, Seagull J, Bagian J. Effective followership: a standardized algorithm to resolve clinical conflicts and improve teamwork. J Healthc Risk Manag. 2015;35(1):21–30.
19. Team communication: speaking up. CMPA. www.cmpa-acpm.ca.
20. Gordon L, Rees C, Ker J, Cleland J. Dimensions, discourses and differences: trainees conceptualising health care leadership and followership. Med Educ. 2015;49:1248–62. https://doi.org/10.1111/medu.12832.

8 Situational Awareness and Human Performance in Trauma

Peter G. Brindley and Jocelyn M. Slemko

Introduction

> From error to error, one discovers the entire truth. (Sigmund Freud)

> The issue is not that you screwed up, Peter- it's how you're gonna make sure it doesn't happen again. (The author's Mum on several weary occasions)

The factors that determine outcome in a crisis are more non-technical (or social) than technological (or procedural). In other words, trauma outcome and performance have more to do with human behavior than with just factual-recall or manual-dexterity [1–10]. How we act in a crisis is complex, but it is often predictable. Our responses are more ancient than many people assume. Our behavior is more influenced by psychology than simple rationality, meaning that we are more psycho-logical than logical [2]. In other words, once you understand the psychological and social forces at work, the responses make more sense. This in no way excuses high error rates, it is merely the first step in implementing a solution.

The human brain is one of the most complex structures in the known universe, and humans are capable of compassion, ingenuity, and hard work. However, we still rely upon the same "brain hardware" as our hominid ancestors. In healthcare, we also still have to manage overstretched teams. We too-often work within inflexible institutions and alongside eye-watering complexes. We need to look for each marginal gain, especially as these can add up over time.

Under stress, we tend to resort to behaviors that served us evolutionarily. This means we should get to know our "oldest personalities" [2] and our typical habits during crisis, rather than the manicured ones "on show" during controlled daily life. It is also why we steer away from overly simplistic questions such as "why did you do that?" and strive to understand "why at the time did that seem like the right thing to do?"

If an engineer wants to know if something is "up to the job," he or she pressure tests each part of the system [2]. The same should apply to trauma practitioners, trauma teams and organizations. Our brains have evolved to do many remarkable things, but resuscitation is not one of them. Competence cannot be assumed, and situational awareness is not innate. Fortunately, both can be taught and honed and maintained, but it takes work.

As should become clear, our brains (and our teams) can also be "rewired," meaning that we can be nudged toward doing better or worse. This means that, our job, as traumatologists, includes not just treating one patient at a time but also affecting culture change at the team and system level. To borrow from high performance sports, "we also play how we practice." This is because preparation and practice influence how we react and perform under stress, and long well after the exercise. This chapter provides applicable insights. After all, as both opening quotes illustrate, errors may be inevitable and predictable, but the outcome is not, and nor is the future [2].

Situational Awareness

Situational awareness encompasses three steps: identify, synthesize, and predict. Each step builds upon the previous one [3, 7]. Accordingly, this discussion sequentially outlines how humans (especially those under stress) perceive (or fail to perceive) relevant cues, how we connect and amalgamate these cues into mental models, and how we anticipate what is likely to happen next [3, 4].

P. G. Brindley (✉)
Department of Critical Care Medicine, University of Alberta, Edmonton, AB, Canada

Dossetor Ethics Centre, University of Alberta, Edmonton, AB, Canada
e-mail: peter.brindley@albertahealthservices.ca

J. M. Slemko
Department of Critical Care Medicine, University of Alberta, Edmonton, AB, Canada

University of Alberta Hospital, Edmonton, AB, Canada
e-mail: Jocelyn.slemko@ahs.ca

L. Marshall Gillman, S. Widder (eds.), *Trauma Team Dynamics*, https://doi.org/10.1007/978-3-031-86312-7_8

Table 8.1 Human factors associated with situational awareness and performance

	Benefits	Risks
Perception		
Scanning attention	Sample many stimuli Avoid fixing on one stimulus	Stimulus overload Lack of prioritization
Focused attention	Prioritize Eliminate "unimportant" cues	Fixation error Miss "important" cues
Synthesis		
Cognitive modeling	Recognize patterns (heuristics) Reduce workload Predictable response	See patterns where they do not exist Premature closure/confirmation bias Resistant to new ideas
Projection		
Anticipation	Predict future events	Incorrect assumptions
Sharing	Increased resources (cognitive/physical)	Need to coordinate a team
Stress		
	Increased vigilance Enhanced physical performance	Exhaustion/overload Impaired complex thinking

Step-one in improving situational awareness—even before heading to the bedside or simulator—is to commit to "metacognition." In other words, we need to "think about thinking." More specifically, we need to examine how we problem-solve, under normal circumstances, under stress, and over the course of lengthy careers. This helps identify our relative cognitive strengths and weaknesses, and how we might improve individual and team performance (See Table 8.1) [5, 6]. It means a career-long commitment to iterative improvement. Without doing so, healthcare providers are more vulnerable, the team is less resilient, the system fails to evergreen, and the patient is more at risk [3–6]. In the face of the information overload, and given the high-stakes of acute care medicine, our ability to maintain situational awareness can be quite literally life-saving.

Situational Awareness: Level One

The first level of situational awareness involves the perception of stimuli: otherwise known as "cues" [3]. Importantly, this requires the individual to focus their attention [5]. However, we must also realize that by focusing "here" we risk missing "there." In other words, we have finite attention or "cognitive bandwidth."

Because of the avalanche of stimuli, we must make conscious and unconscious decisions about where to prioritize and what to ignore (or postpone). This can lead to fixation errors: where we focus our attention inappropriately and where we miss relevant cues. This is especially true during stress—when we tend to develop cognitive tunnel vision.

In moderation, tunnel vision is important. It lets us focus on what really matters (i.e., airway, breathing, and circulation) and eliminate what can wait (i.e., mildly abnormal blood work). In excess, we fixate inappropriately and miss what really matters (i.e., we commit a fixation error). Examples abound but could include the cardiologist who only looks for cues of myocardial ischemia and therefore misses sepsis or pulmonary embolus. It could be the internist who misses post-operative bleeding because he looks everywhere but under the dressing.

Other examples of fixation errors are outlined below, but readers are encouraged to think of their own examples. This should be easy as fixation errors appear to happen to practitioners of all specialties and levels. The difference appears to be that seasoned practitioners know (hopefully) where the most-deadly fixations usually occur and how to mitigate them quicker [5]. Additionally, seasoned practitioners have previously experienced fixation errors and have therefore adapted, both consciously and subconsciously. This should include ensuring appropriate checks, balances, fail-safes, and standard operating procedures. As well as having predictable standardized approaches, the true expert stays open to other's opinions and has reached the "awkward realization" that we humans are not omnipotent.

For those still unconvinced about our cognitive fallibility, an excellent book by Christopher Chabris and Daniel Simons reviews their famous psychological experiment (aka "the invisible gorilla") [8]. In brief, Simons produced a video where viewers are asked to simply count basketball passes between actors wearing white and black shirts. Given the complex things that most professions do in their daily jobs, this may seem elementary. However, regardless of seniority, typically only half are correct. This is because the others are distracted by an actor who walks into the video frame midway through. He is wearing a gorilla suit and spends 8 seconds pounding his chest.

Typically, viewers see either the gorilla or get the number of passes correct, but rarely both. What is equally insightful is when the video is replayed many viewers refuse to believe that there was ever a gorilla on the original (they assume the video must has been monkeyed with…groan).

In short, our attention is imperfect, but so is our insight. The excellent video demonstrates how we have blind spots in our vision (and in our judgment) such that we only see what we are primed to see. Our brains are prone to looking without seeing, but also to hearing without listening and to acting without truly thinking [8].

Situational Awareness: Level Two

The second level of situational awareness is synthesis, which in turn facilitates comprehension [3, 9]. In other words, we fuse disjointed pieces of data (e.g., chest pain; ECG changes; elevated troponin) into a recognizable model (i.e., the diagnosis of myocardial ischemia) [3, 9, 10].

By creating a cognitive model, our brains can accelerate both our understanding and our action. In other words, mental models provide shortcuts or "heuristics" [5, 9]. This in turn allows for pattern recognition. Ideally, recognition of a model (i.e., a diagnosis or clinical syndrome) is how prior classroom knowledge (pathophysiology, pharmacology) is retrieved and applied. Because of the importance of visual and emotional triggers in learning and behavior change, a better way to unlock and apply knowledge is often through situational exposure, such as immersion followed by reflection using realistic simulation and extensive clinical experience.

Mental models are also useful because they reduce the individual's cognitive workload (and maintain bandwidth). This can free up scarce mental resources for other demands. However, once again, we need to be aware that upsides come with potential downsides. Firstly, we may see patterns when they do not actually exist and are slow to recognize exceptions (i.e., we continue to rationalize a routine diagnosis by downplaying contradictory information). Secondly, all species conserve energy whenever possible. Pattern recognition and mental models make this easier. Unfortunately, subconsciously this means that we rationalize shortcuts and decreased effort. We need to be wary of our propensity to create overly simple models (so-called premature closure) when we actually need to continue the search for other explanations (e.g., the infection that fails to respond to antibiotics because it is an abscess that requires surgical drainage). We need to understand that in a crisis, vigilance and persistence are every bit as important as traditional "cleverness." Laziness can kill and tenacity can save. Expressed another way, we are often paid just to be present, engaged and patient-focused, not brilliant.

The other downside of our desire to reduce cognitive workload is that it can make us resistant to change. For example, the "Semmelweis effect" [11] is the reflex-like tendency to reject new evidence or knowledge because it conflicts with established norms, beliefs or paradigms (i.e., the "new" does not fit with our current mental model). This is named after Ignaz Semmelweis who discovered that neonatal mortality could be greatly decreased by hand washing. There is more to this story than a simplistic refusal of those with power and privilege to listen, but once we accept that few people want to change or believe that they could be the problem, it becomes easier to understand why others dismissed and mocked Semmelweis's ideas. Fast forward, and it explains why modern medicine continues to retard innovation.

Situational Awareness: Level Three

The third level of situation awareness involves "projection." This in turn allows the individual or team to respond proactively [6, 9, 10]. Once a mental model is created, assumptions can be shared, and this allows for anticipation and planning. For example, without even seeing a patient whom you know to have a severe head injury, you can predict that they may need airway control. Moreover, it is reasonable to assume that the patient may become hemodynamically unstable and hence will need to be where experienced staff and advanced monitoring are immediately available. In short, this patient will either need to be in an ICU, or near to one, regardless of the specifics of their case.

The need for anticipation and preparation is also why another high-stakes profession, namely the military, talks of the eight p's of crisis management: "proper prior planning and preparation prevents piss-poor performance." Expressed another way, "failing to prepare is akin to preparing to fail." Regardless, it should be clear why situational awareness is one of the prime ways for individuals to safeguard the deteriorating patient; another is to maximize collective awareness by optimizing the team.

Crisis management is a team sport [5]. Therefore, we need situational awareness at the team level, not just within the leader's head. Obviously, each individual has his or her own experience and limitations. However, they must also know enough about each other's skills and limitations in order to perform in a unified fashion. Therefore, each individual needs to hone their own situational awareness but also appreciate others'. Like a Venn diagram, individuals' situational awareness must overlap in order to function together as a team [1, 9].

The above should explain why we don't just silently perform a primary survey, we announce the findings. This way all members have an equal opportunity to achieve the first level of situational awareness. Subsequently, each team member can then focus on his or her specific area. For example, the anesthetist evaluates the patient's airway and chest regarding airway capture and ventilation. The surgeon also examines the chest, but for typical surgical interventions such as chest drains or central venous lines.

As each team member builds an individual awareness, they report their findings and plans back to the team leader. The team leader then integrates these individual models into a shared mental model that summarizes the patient's current state (level two of situational awareness) and predicts their trajectory (level 3 of situational awareness). In this way, the team's awareness amplifies each individual's awareness. A good team leader is one whose behavior encourages all team members to share pertinent information. His or her job is then to emphasize or deemphasize that information, make sense of it, and establish the next priority. In short, team performance is creative and even artistic. It is something we should take pride in cultivating.

Factors Affecting Awareness and Performance

Attention

During a crisis, the volume of stimuli will typically exceed even the most capable individual. In order to process information, the individual focuses attention on relevant stimuli [2, 5]. Attention is like a searchlight—highlighting things that the individual can then either perceive as a cue (important for the cognitive model) or background (irrelevant at this time).

As the complexity of a situation increases, the number of possible cues requiring attention also increases. Unfortunately, like the diameter of the searchlight's beam, our attention is limited. This can cause selection bias either because our attention is misdirected (toward irrelevant stimuli) or simply insufficient (not enough cues are collected) [5, 12].

Fortunately, we can mitigate our innate selection bias. There are two main types of attention in nature, and both can be applied in acute care medicine. Firstly, there is the scanning vigilance typified by prey (where focus is routinely refocused from one area to the next) [13]. By constantly redirecting our attention and sampling different inputs, we reduce the likelihood of selection bias (and fixation errors) [3, 5, 12]. For example, during trauma resuscitation, we scan the trauma bay looking for cues that suggest patient distress. Just like lifeguards who scan the beach, we avoid looking at just one spot.

When danger strikes, we need the second type of attention typified by the focused gaze of a predator [13] (or exemplified by the life-guard ignoring others as he focuses on someone in possible distress). This is where non-essential stimuli are minimized and tunnel-vision takes over [5]. This second technique avoids wasting attention. However, as outlined, its potential downside is the fixation error and the illusion of centrality (that nothing outside of our immediate attention matters) [2, 5].

In civilian disasters, a common three-phase survival arc exists: denial, deliberation, and decision [2]. Preparation (whether through simulation or experience) decreases denial; means you have already done the work of deliberation, and means you have a cognitive roadmap for decisive action. This is part of why emergency drills save future lives. This is also why survival following plane evacuations is consistently higher for those that watched the in-flight safety video and confirmed their exit [2]. A related three-part model has been summarized by Leach et al.: just like other animals, we humans respond to crisis either through "fight, flight, or freeze" [14].

How our brains respond depends greatly upon complexity and familiarity. So-called "automatic responses" occur immediately because responses are embedded due to simplicity or repetition [4, 7]. For example, once the surgeon has begun to tie a knot, the actual tying consumes little of their attention. As such, attention is freed up [5]. "Simple decisions" (for example, which intravenous fluid to order) occur when there are a few possible responses available. Therefore, subconscious choosing usually takes a second or two. "Complex decisions" (e.g., being presented with a cluster of symptoms that you have never seen before) take longer because there is no appropriate response in your personal database. A response has to be created and this consumes additional precious time. Finally, there is the "inability to make decisions" where no behavioral schema exists, and no temporary schema can be created [14]. This typically causes stress, panic, or even paralysis [2].

Stress

Stress is a common word in modern life but can be difficult to define. It is usually understood to be a state of psychological or physical activation [2, 5]. Stress is also often uncomfortable because the need to act is seen as a threat and because there is a perceived imbalance between demands and resources. It is common to all high-risk professions but is also a personal experience [2, 3, 6]. In short, we perform a situational assessment and feel stressed if we feel threatened or unprepared or under-resourced.

Notably, in its original meaning, stress was not always negative: it simply described activity and arousal [2]. At low levels, stress stimulates attention, focus, and vigilance, and this can aid task completion [2, 3, 5, 9]. Interestingly, when faced with personal disaster, people appear to perform best with a mildly elevated heart rate (typically, 115–145 beats per minute) [2]. However, for every gift that adrenaline gives it takes one away.

Higher heart rates are associated with both exhaustion and impaired decision-making. In the battle to decide what to prioritize and what to neglect, our senses may become heightened, but stress hormones interfere with complex thinking [2]. Accordingly, soldiers are taught strategies such as "combat breathing techniques" (aka square breathing) to manage the undesirable physical effects of stress (breath in for four; hold for four; out for four) [2].

Similarly, soldiers train so often that the unfamiliar and stressful become familiar and automatic. In short, they aim to become overcompetent but not over confident. As outlined, under stress, our ability to see (and our judgment) shrinks such that we reduce periphery vision (and peripheral judgment). We can also get tunnel hearing where certain sounds are muted and others amplified [2]. As such, stress is closely associated with fixation errors [5].

A notorious fixation error occurred in 2005 in the UK [15, 16]. During anesthetic induction of an elective case, a mother of two, Ms. Elaine Bromiley, could not be intubated with an endotracheal tube. Multiple consultant anesthetists repeatedly attempted laryngoscopy. Each failed to sound the alarm or to move on to alternate strategies. Similarly, less senior members were concerned but failed to intervene.

Tragically, Ms. Bromiley—whose husband was a pilot and an expert in crisis management—died with severe anoxic brain injury. Similarly, in the trauma bay, physicians have been known to focus on the abnormal ECG, while the patient's oxygen saturation declines unnoticed. In other words, once we appreciate the basics of how we respond to crisis, our behavior makes more sense, and we are more likely to guard against it. Accordingly, we should speak less of medical errors as if they are unique and surprising, and more of predictable human errors but in an unforgiving high-stakes medical environment.

The inability to cognitively re-evaluate is also known as task myopia or task saturation [2, 5, 17]. Our tendency to fixate can be mitigated by stepping back, literally and figuratively. For example, the senior physician standing back from the action often surprises junior colleagues by his/her ability to pick up on peripheral things that they missed ("have you considered this possible diagnosis, guys?").

As outlined above, lifeguards (and also the police and military) are taught to scan to the full extent of their peripheral vision to avoid fixation. In the complex environments where even scanning techniques are insufficient, we can reduce stimuli into manageable pieces through task delegation. For example, commercial pilots assign one person to focus solely on flying the plane at all times, while other routine tasks (e.g., navigation or radio communication) are delegated. Within a medical team we can do similarly (e.g., "I am going to intubate. I won't be able to see the monitor—let me know when the vitals change").

As discussed, our brains function better when familiar with the problem. We feel more in control basically because we are, and because we can model and predict [2, 5]. In contrast, cognitive overload and the absence of a working model can lead to feeling out-of-control and out of rational responses. Therefore, we are more likely to resort to primitive reflexes such as panic (i.e., the hysterical airline passenger on a turbulent flight) or even paralysis (i.e., the passenger who refuses to leave a burning plane) [2]. Panic is actually not that common. This is worth empathizing as many organizations have been reluctant to perform disaster drills under the fallacious assumption that they will cause panic or lack of confidence [2].

Interestingly, paralysis may be an ancient evolutionary survival technique where the motionless prey looks dead and is therefore avoided by a predator. Regardless, it appears that every animal (including humans) has the instinct to shut down under extreme fear (e.g., the deer that freezes in the car headlights; the human that refuses to leave the burning building) [2]. We also tend to exhibit herd instincts in a crisis. This is probably why we are typically more obedient when disaster strikes [2]. This is why flight attendants are instructed to be firm with passengers during an evacuation, and why it is not automatically wrong if a doctor raises his or her voice. In the same way that an animal comes out of its daze after a loud noise (i.e., the slam of a car door), a human can be reoriented with unequivocal orders. In other words, if individuals have temporarily lost their situational awareness, then it is the team's responsibility to bring them back.

Conclusion

Crisis behavior requires an understanding of where our behaviors originated, how they can be mitigated, and why practice (i.e., crisis immunization) is our best defense. We need to expedite the mental model but then deliberately and repeatedly challenge it. Situational awareness means continually scanning the environment in order to minimize premature closure and selection bias. Each team member is responsible for forming and sharing the mental model. In addition, being the team leader means communicating that mental model, maintaining global awareness, and amplifying the team's situational awareness.

Without deliberate strategies, a small crisis can spiral into a runaway crisis. However, a vicious cycle can also be turned into a virtuous cycle. Strategies include (i) metacognition (being aware of our behavioral norms), (ii) mandating checks due to the likelihood of human error, and (iii) regular exposure (ideally through realistic simulation). Managing the medical crisis is a fascinating combination of science, art, psychology, and engineering. It need not be scary. In fact, it can be exhilarating, creative, and life affirming.

Key Notes

- Factors that determine outcome in a crisis are more social than technological.
- First level of situational awareness is the perception of stimuli (aka "cues").
- Second level requires synthesis with the goal of comprehension.
- Third level involves projection, anticipation, and planning.
- Our attention and response to stress can be improved upon by metacognition (being more aware of our behavioral norms) and through regular "crisis immunization."

References

1. Pruitt CM, Liebelt EL. Enhancing patient safety in the pediatric emergency department: teams, communication, and lessons from crew resource management. Pediatr Emerg Care. 2010;26(12):942–8.
2. Ripley A. The unthinkable: who survives when disaster strikes. New York: Three Rivers Press; 2008.
3. Endsley MR. Toward a theory of situation awareness in dynamic systems. Hum Factors. 1995;37(1):32–64.
4. Endsley MR. Theoretical underpinnings of situation awareness: a critical review. In: Situation awareness analysis and measurement. Mahwah: Lawrence Erlbaum Associates; 2000. p. 3–32.
5. St Pierre M, Hofinger G, Buerschaper C, Simon R. Crisis management in acute care settings. 2nd ed. New York: Springer; 2011.
6. Gaba DM, Howard SK, Small SD. Situation awareness in anesthesiology. Hum Factors. 1995;37(1):20–31.
7. Durso FT, Sethumadhavan A. Situation awareness: understanding dynamic environments. Hum Factors. 2008;50(3):442–8.
8. Chabris CF, Simons DJ. The invisible gorilla: and other ways our intuitions deceive us. New York: Crown Publishers, Random House; 2010.
9. Wickens CD. Situation awareness: review of Mica Endsley's 1995 articles on situation awareness theory and measurement. Hum Factors. 2008;50(3):397–403.
10. Stanton NA, Chambers PR, Piggott J. Review of situational awareness: concept, theory, and application. Saf Sci. 2001;39(39):189–204.
11. Semmelweis Reflex. Wikipedia. Available at: http://en.wikipedia.org/wiki/Semmelweis_reflex. Accessed Dec 2012.
12. Singh H. Understanding diagnostic errors in medicine: a lesson from aviation. Qual Saf Health Care. 2006;15(3):159–64.
13. Proctor RN, Schiebinger L. Agnotology: the making and unmaking of ignorance. Stanford: Stanford University Press; 2008.
14. Leach J. Why people "freeze" in an emergency: temporal and cognitive constraints on survival responses. Aviat Space Environ Med. 2004;75(6):539–42.
15. Martin Bromiley. Just a routine operation (You Tube). Available at: http://www.youtube.com/watch?v=JzlvgtPIof4. Accessed Dec 2012.
16. NHS Institute for Improvement and Innovation. Safer care: improving patient safety. Available at: http://www.institute.nhs.uk/safer_care/general/human_factors.html. Accessed Dec 2012.
17. Federal Aviation Authority. Pilot's handbook of aeronautical knowledge: aeronautical decision making. Available at: http://www.americanflyers.net/aviationlibrary/pilots_handbook/chapter_16.html. Accessed Dec 2012.

9 Handovers in Trauma

Michelle Au and Lawrence Marshall Gillman

Handover and Patient Safety

High-quality handovers are crucial to the safety of patients at all stages within their contact with the healthcare system. A handover is defined as the transfer of responsibility and accountability of care of a patient or groups of patients to another person, temporarily or permanently [1]. Information shared during handovers typically include the patient's identification, their condition, any changes in their clinical course, previous and current treatments, any complications and future management plans [1–6]. Miscommunication was identified to be the leading cause of sentinel events reported to the Joint Commission in the United States [7, 8]. A large proportion of preventable medical errors and adverse events are due to communication failures, and up to 80% of serious or preventable adverse events are due to miscommunication during handover [8]. Handovers require complex communication skills and clinical acumen to convey the priorities in a patient's care while balancing equally important details in a pressured, time-limited environment.

As many skills in medicine, a good handover develops over time. A lack of handover experience may result in the loss of important information and could potentially place the patient at higher risk for harm. Experience is an example of an individual factor that may affect the quality of the handover. In addition to experience, there must be education on how to perform a high-quality handover. Handovers are also affected by the environment in which it takes place. Handing over critically ill trauma patient in the resuscitation bay is significantly different than handing over a stable patient on the wards. The sense of urgency, patient complexity and a louder physical environment can make handing over more difficult. Figure 9.1 is a representation of the various factors that affect handovers.

In trauma scenarios, the complexity of handovers significantly increases. Handovers occur at multiple stages during a trauma patient's care (Fig. 9.2). Handovers can occur during the prehospital phase, the emergency department (ED) phase and the post-emergency department stage [9]. Pre-hospital handovers occur when the patient receives care from emergency medical services (EMS) responders and is transported directly to a trauma centre or may be transferred to a non-trauma healthcare centre before transported to a trauma centre. The emergency department phase consists of handover from the EMS responders to the emergency department team (physicians and nurses). During this handover, other teams including the trauma surgery team and other surgical services may be present. Further services may be consulted for management or transfer of care. If a patient requires surgical intervention, then handover occurs at multiple points: ED to the operating room (OR), OR to the post-anesthetic recovery unit (PACU), and the PACU to the ICU, a high-acuity bed, or to the ward. A trauma patient may have more than ten major handovers during their stay, not including the handovers that occur during shift changes. Each of these handovers are potential areas for patient harm due to issues with the continuity of care and miscommunication. In critically injured trauma patients, it has been found that 48% of patients had information discrepancy during their handover [10].

Currently, there is no universally agreed upon best practice for handovers. This is due to varying roles (paramedic, nurse, physician), specialties and subspecialties. Each profession may have different priorities and expectations during handover and may have varying levels of skills and knowledge. This chapter will aim to define the roles in a handover, the differences in handovers in varying environments, handover strategies and challenges that may be encountered.

M. Au · L. Marshall Gillman (✉)
University of Manitoba, Department of General Surgery, Winnipeg, MB, Canada
e-mail: aut@myumanitoba.ca; Lawrence.Gillman@umanitoba.ca

L. Marshall Gillman, S. Widder (eds.), *Trauma Team Dynamics*, https://doi.org/10.1007/978-3-031-86312-7_9

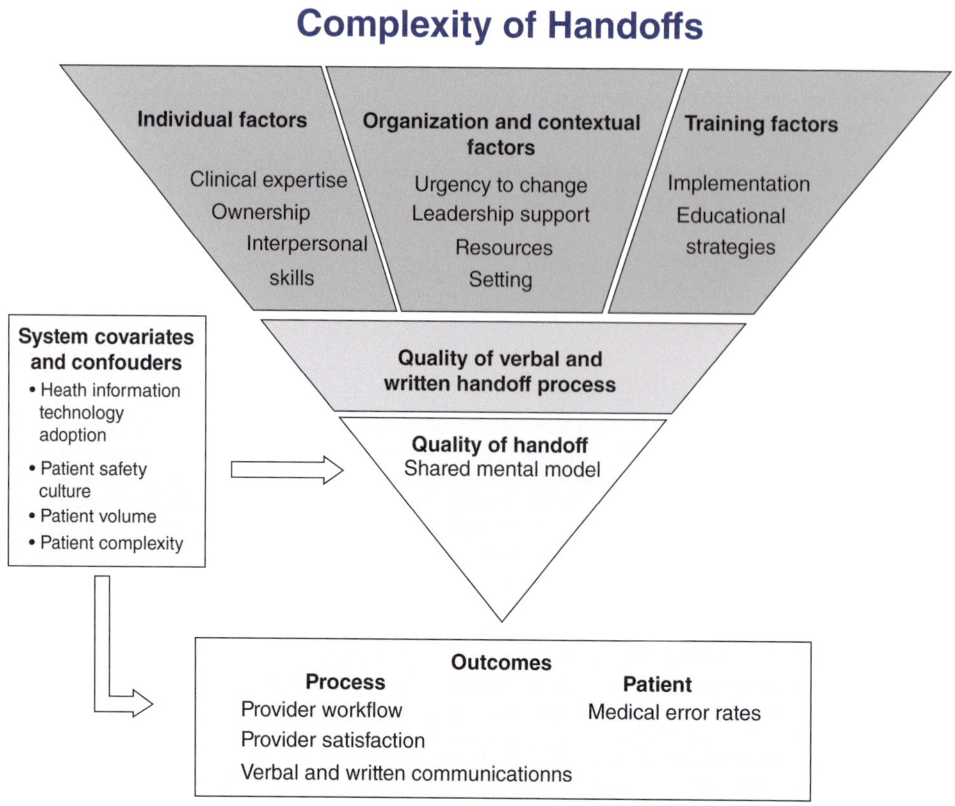

Fig. 9.1 Handoff complexity as portrayed by Starmer et al. [15]

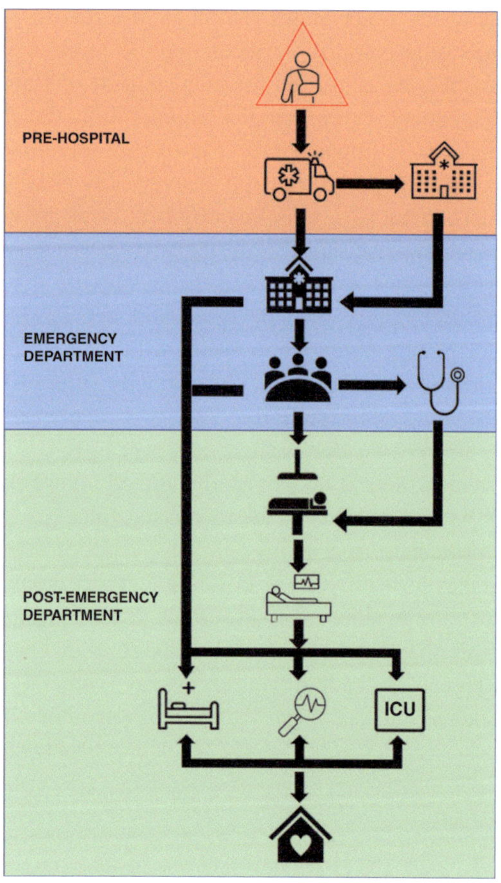

Fig. 9.2 A trauma patient's course through the healthcare system

Handover Foundations

> **Case 1: Tom**
> Tom is a 31-year-old male driver, previously healthy, who was T-boned by a semi-truck while driving home from work. The patient had fluctuating levels of consciousness at the scene and was hypotensive and hypoxic with the EMS responders. Upon arrival in the ED, he was intubated and resuscitated. There were decreased breath sounds to the right chest; as such, a right-sided chest tube was placed. The patient remained hypotensive despite ongoing fluid resuscitation. A massive transfusion protocol was activated. A FAST scan showed some fluid in the right upper quadrant. As such, the trauma surgery team took the patient for an emergency laparotomy.

In Case 1, numerous team members can be identified: EMS responders, ED physicians, ED nurses, respiratory therapist, trauma surgery team and the operating room staff. For this patient to managed efficiently and effectively, every team member must be on the same page. This is called a *Shared Mental Model*. A shared mental model is defined as "individually held knowledge structures that help team members function collaboratively in their environments"

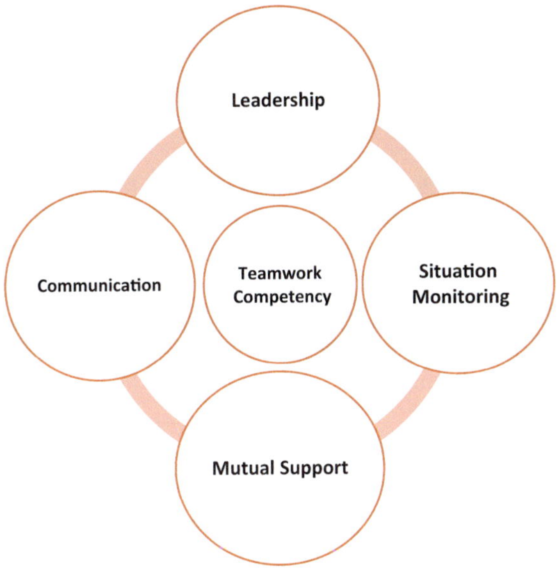

Fig. 9.3 TeamSTEPPS's 4 key areas in teamwork competency

[11]. In other words, the team operates in an environment where there is a shared understanding of the structure and roles of each member, thus making communication and coordination more effective.

The Agency for Healthcare Research and Quality's TeamSTEPPS program has been successfully implemented in healthcare settings to help train teams to achieve better communication [4]. TeamSTEPPS identifies four key areas in teamwork competency (Fig. 9.3).

Leadership Effective leadership ensures that roles are clearly identified, and expectations are clearly established. Task delegation is an important part of leadership to ensure appropriate use of resources.

Situation Monitoring Situation monitoring is defined as the assessment of a clinical situation by capturing behaviours and actions. Situation monitoring allows a team member to have situational awareness. When all team members share their situational awareness through communication, a shared mental model is developed.

Mutual Support Team members must be in a non-judgemental environment that allows each individual of the team to feel openly communicate their needs and thoughts. Each member understands that they all play an important role in the team and their input is valued.

Communication Information amongst all team members is shared accurately and efficiently. Communication is also standardized to minimize loss of key information. Team members should also use closed-loop communication to reduce the risk of misinterpretation. Closed-loop communication occurs when the receiver of the message confirms the points that were communicated, and the sender verifies the accuracy of the confirmation.

Using the TeamSTEPPS model for effective communication, we can extrapolate the features of a high-quality handover. A handover is successful when the people involved in the handover understands each other's roles, skills, and expectations, thus having a shared mental model. There must also be open communication, and the communication should be conducted in a standardized manner. When team members perceive handover as a team priority, handover will likely be more successful.

Other important factors that lead to better handovers include face-to-face communication. By handing over in person, the sender can emphasize the importance of key information while incorporating nuanced body language, and the receiver has opportunities to clarify and confirm the information. The receiver of information must be actively listening [12]. The 3 A's of active listening are Attitude, Attention, and Adjustment [13]. Listeners must be open-minded and non-reactive. Listeners must also be engaged and focused on the information being conveyed by the sender. An active listener is also flexible in their expectations and can ask for clarifications when needed.

Key Takeaways
- Using a shared mental model results in better handovers.
- Each team member needs to feel valued and comfortable to voice their thoughts.
- Receiving handover as an active listener is as important as the person giving handover.

Handover Challenges

Trauma presents a different level of complexity to handovers. The resuscitation bay is not necessarily the optimal environment for a good handover. Ideally, a good handover is done in an environment free of interruptions and distractions, with minimal external pressure such as time. Challenges to performing a good handover can be categorized into internal factors, external factors, and systemic factors (Fig. 9.4).

Team members each bring their own expectations, knowledge, experience, and communication styles. This is especially true during trauma handovers, as there are multiple different healthcare providers present with different professional backgrounds.

Individual factors Both the roles of a sender or receiver of information require categorizing, processing, and communicating accurate information. Factors such as fatigue and multitasking can result in cognitive overload. Fatigue may result in slower processing of information, confusion, impaired memory, inattention, and ultimately impaired communica-

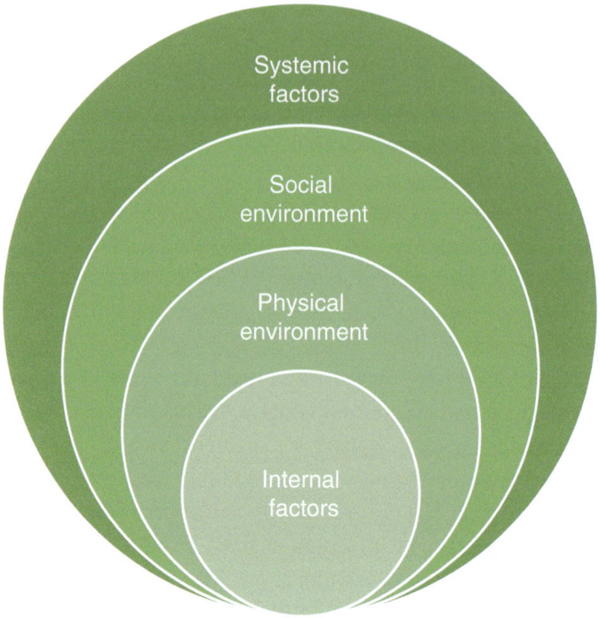

Fig. 9.4 Factors that can affect the quality of a handover

tion. Passive listening may also be a result of fatigue or inattention. Studies assessing information transfers and information degradation during handovers have shown that the most key piece of information was not conveyed in up to 60% of handovers, despite the perception from the sender that it was communicated. A study also found that only 56% of information during handover was accurately retained by the receiver [14].

Physical environment Whether it is in the resuscitation bay or on the wards, handovers are always strife with interruptions and distractions. These can include interruptions from the team asking for clarifications, loud noises in the environment such as beeping monitors and nearby conversations, or visual distractions such as people trying to complete tasks during handover (e.g. hooking up monitors or inserting IVs). Having a dedicated space that is large enough to accommodate the whole team is important for handover. The physical environment can increase the risk of the sender miscommunicating and decreased retention of information by the receiver.

Social environment There are always hierarchies within the healthcare system, which can either be clearly defined or unspoken. Attendings, physician trainees, students, interprofessional team members, and patients and their families all hold differing levels of power in a situation. This hierarchical difference can affect the way a person communicates based on how empowered the individual may feel to speak up or how comfortable they may be to ask questions. Ambiguous roles can also result in miscommunication during handover. Oftentimes, team members may not know the professional role of another interprofessional team member and their responsibilities. This may lead to different expectations about what key information needs to be communicated.

Systemic factors A person's ability to provide a high-quality handover is not only a result of their internal factors and external factors; it is also due to the training that they have received. Handover is a skill that needs to be taught, and medical institutions need to ensure that the training is provided. Additionally, the healthcare institution should adhere to a standardized format for handover. Furthermore, regular feedback on handover should be provided to the team members to ensure that education is ongoing.

Key Takeaways
- Multiple factors can result in poor handover.
- Ensure that handover is done in an environment that is non-judgemental, has minimal interruptions and physical distractions.
- Practice makes better—ensure that team members are trained in handover and consistently receive feedback during handover.

Handover Structure

There are several handover tools that have been used in the healthcare setting. Handover tools help reduce cognitive load by using a mnemonic and have been shown to significantly reduce medical errors. The specific handover tool used may be dependent on the environment that it is being used in (e.g. pre-hospital vs. the ward). The Joint Commission International (JCI) and the World Health Organization (WHO) have suggested the use of the SBAR tool. Other tools include I-PASS, SIGNOUT, ANTICipate, and IMIST-AMBO among many others (Table 9.1).

Regardless of the mnemonic used, there are key elements that should be included patient handovers. These include identification information (demographics), patient's stability and illness severity, their admission diagnosis, their medical history and code status, active issues, list of tasks needed to be completed, any anticipated issues and plans, and confirmation of key information by the receiver as part of engaging in closed loop communication.

Although there is no consensus on which mnemonic is better, certain mnemonics may be more appropriate depending on the complexity of the situation. Standardization of handover using mnemonics can result in a more efficient handover with improved relaying and retention of material and greater satisfaction for those involved in the handover.

Table 9.1 Handover mnemonics

SBAR	I-PASS	SIGNOUT	ANTICipate	IMIST-AMBO
Situation	Illness severity	Sick or DNR	Administrative data	Identification
Background information	Patient summary	Identifying data	New information (clinical update)	Mechanism/medical issue
Assessment and anticipated events	Action List	General hospital course	Tasks needed to be done	Injuries/information relevant to medical issue
Recommendations	Situation awareness and contingency planning	New events	Illness (stability)	Signs
	Synthesis	Overall clinical condition	Contingency plan/code status	Treatment and trends
		Upcoming possibilities and plan		Allergies
		Tasks to complete		Medications
				Background history
				Other information

Written Handover

In addition to verbal handovers, written handovers also significantly improve the quality of information transfer. Like mnemonics in verbal handovers, having a written handover document acts as a valuable cognitive aid, especially when there are multiple caregivers and multiple patients. Written documentation is the only source of information that is carried forward with the patient throughout their clinical course. Handover documents should be up to date and contain information in the same format as a verbal handover: demographic information, past medical history, medications, allergies, medical issues, pertinent information during their course in hospital, anticipated issues, and plans. By having an updated written document present during handover, clinical team members can focus on the details of issues and plans, rather than trying to remember demographic information. This improves the efficiency and accuracy of the information transferred in handover.

It is important to remember that written handover documents contain sensitive patient information and need to be handled and disposed of appropriately to maintain patient confidentiality. Team members must be aware of the Personal Health Information Act.

Key Takeaways

- A standardized method of handover should be adopted.
- Verbal and written handovers should be used concurrently to ensure efficient and accurate handovers.

Conclusion

Trauma patients are one of the most complex patients to provide handover for given the acute and dynamic nature of the situation, further augmented by the numerous settings that the patient can transition to (scene, trauma bay, operating room, ICU, ward). Trauma care is a team sport that requires a shared mental model with each team member playing a crucial role. A good handover between team members ensures that less avoidable medical errors are made, resulting in safer patient care.

References

1. Evans SM, Murray A, Patrick I, Fitzgerald M, Smith S, Cameron P. Clinical handover in the trauma setting: a qualitative study of paramedics and trauma team members. Qual Saf Health Care. 2010;19(6):e57.
2. Makkink AW, Stein COA, Bruijns SR, Gottschalk S. The variables perceived to be important during patient handover by South African prehospital care providers. Afr J Emerg Med. 2019;9(2):87–90.
3. Sujan M, Spurgeon P, Inada-Kim M, Rudd M, Fitton L, Horniblow S, et al. Clinical handover within the emergency care pathway and the potential risks of clinical handover failure (ECHO): primary research, Health services and delivery research, No. 2.5. Southampton: NIHR Journals Library; 2014. p. 1–144.
4. Bismilla Z, Wong B. Handover Toolkit: a resource to help teach, assess and implement a handover improvement program. Royal College of Physicians and Surgeons of Canada; 2018.
5. Fahim Yegane SA, Shahrami A, Hatamabadi HR, Hosseini-Zijoud S-MM, Yegane SAF, Shahrami A, et al. Clinical information transfer between EMS staff and emergency medicine assistants during handover of trauma patients. Prehosp Disaster Med. 2017;32(5):541–7.
6. Puzio TJ, Murphy PB, Virtanen P, Harvin JA, Hartwell JL. Handover practices in trauma and acute care surgery: a multicenter survey study. J Surg Res. 2020;254:191–6. Available from: https://doi.org/10.1016/j.jss.2020.04.023.
7. Joint Commission Centre for Transforming Healthcare. Joint Commission Centre for Transforming Healthcare releases targeted solutions tool for hand-off communications. 2012. Available from: https://www.jointcommission.org/-/media/deprecated-unorganized/imported-assets/tjc/system-folders/blogs/tst_hoc_persp.
8. Peer M, O'Regan NB, Evans B, Fowler A, Dubrowski A. Patient handover in emergency trauma situations. Cureus. 2020;12(8):e9544.

9. Merten H, Van Galen LS, Wagner C. Safe handover. BMJ. 2017;359:1–5. Available from: https://doi.org/10.1136/bmj.j4328.
10. Zakrison TL, Rosenbloom B, McFarlan A, Jovicic A, Soklaridis S, Allen C, et al. Lost information during the handover of critically injured trauma patients: a mixed-methods study. BMJ Qual Saf. 2016;25(12):929–36.
11. McComb S, Simpson V. The concept of shared mental models in healthcare collaboration. J Adv Nurs. 2014;70(7):1479–88.
12. Stelfox HT, Leigh JP, Dodek PM, Turgeon AF, Forster AJ, Lamontagne F, et al. A multi-center prospective cohort study of patient transfers from the intensive care unit to the hospital ward. Intensive Care Med. 2017;43(10):1485–94.
13. Jahromi VK, Tabatabaee SS, Abdar ZE, Rajabi M. Active listening: the key of successful communication in hospital managers. Electron Physician. 2016;8(3):2123–8. Available from: https://pubmed.ncbi.nlm.nih.gov/27123221.
14. Carter AJEE, Davis KA, Evans LV, Cone DC. Information loss in emergency medical services handover of trauma patients. Prehosp Emerg Care. 2009;13(3):280–5.
15. Starmer AJ, O'Toole JK, Rosenbluth G, et al. Development, implementation, and dissemination of the I-PASS handoff curriculum: a multisite educational intervention to improve patient handoffs. Acad Med. 2014;89(6):876–84.

Engaging Team Members

10

Mellissa Ward, Laura Morrison, Cheryl Ffrench, and Debrah Wirtzfeld

Activation of the trauma team brings together a complex assortment of individuals who need to come together under high anxiety and stress in a fast-paced environment. It is imperative that each person knows their role in caring for the trauma patient. Trauma Systems Management has advanced the knowledge of best practices to enhance survival and decrease morbidity. An important aspect of trauma team management is in engaging team members toward a common goal and keeping them focused on attaining these important objectives. Engaging team members should be considered as an important and strategic tactic for enhancing overall individual and team performance. This chapter will provide a cohesive and comprehensive approach to acquisition of skills to engage team members and enhance overall team performance.

How to Approach This Chapter

Successfully engaging team members is achieved through integrating new habits, purposefully relinquishing old habits, and a developing a different way of seeing things. As such, adoption of the ten principles of engaging team members will require persistence and a shift in mindset. Reading this chapter and being able to recite the important principles of engaging team members is not enough. Engagement can only be successfully achieved through repeated practice of the principles outlined in this chapter. Leaders need to communicate what they require from team members, understand what team members need from them, and be invested in the time and dedication it will require to reach peak performance.

The Difference Between a Group of Individuals and a Team

When a trauma code is activated, healthcare providers from different disciplines come together for a common purpose: to save a patient's life. It is this unifying goal that distinguishes these individuals as a *team*, rather than a *group*. A group is a collection of individuals gathered or classed together, while a team is a collection of individuals, each with independent yet complementary talents, who share a clear and common purpose [1]. The shared goal is distinct and specific to all team members. At any given time in the emergency department, there are groups of doctors, nurses, respiratory therapists, healthcare aides, lab and radiology technicians, orthopedic technicians, prehospital personnel, and more who are working in concert with one another, yet may have separate goals. These same individuals become a *team* in the moment a trauma code is activated. They are unified in the goal of resuscitating a trauma patient, and each member of the team has a distinct skillset which is essential for team success. Although the make-up of the trauma team can vary depending on the human resources available at the time, or at the site, they share the same common goal during the time the resuscitation is taking place.

Training and education of the trauma team have historically focused on task work — specifically responsibilities of each team member — with little emphasis on team development and management [2]. There is a pervasive belief that effective team dynamics will naturally develop in a healthcare setting. This mentality is not seen in other professional

M. Ward (✉)
Department of Surgery, University of Manitoba, Winnipeg, MB, Canada

L. Morrison
Department of Surgery, Cumming School of Medicine, University of Calgary, Calgary, AB, Canada
e-mail: laura.morrison1@ucalgary.ca

C. Ffrench
Department of Emergency Medicine, University of Manitoba, Winnipeg, MB, Canada

D. Wirtzfeld
Department of Surgery, Faculty of Medicine and Dentistry University of Alberta, Edmonton, AB, Canada

L. Marshall Gillman, S. Widder (eds.), *Trauma Team Dynamics*, https://doi.org/10.1007/978-3-031-86312-7_10

settings, which require the coordinated efforts of a team, such as software development companies [2]. These organizations place team training around engagement and communication front and center in order to ensure organizational goals are met and that teams succeed. The trauma team is a unique entity in that it can change from day-to-day or even from code to code in the same day. Each new team has to function at its full potential in order to meet the patient's needs. For this reason, every member who participates in a trauma code should be familiar with effective team dynamics. Effective teams have a designated leader; they trust their members to perform their designated roles, and they often oscillate from individual to team effort without direction [3, 4]. For example, the trauma team leader may rely on the anesthesiologist to simultaneously assess and manage the patient's airway without giving specific directions on how or what to do. At the same time, the lab technician may be preparing their supplies to draw blood from the patient while the radiology technician is positioning the patient for an x-ray. While tasks are being individually, yet simultaneously performed, the trauma team leader may then bring the team back to a unified moment in order to review the current findings and upcoming plan. The important skills of engaging team members toward a common goal are not inherent; they should be taught as a part of any trauma training.

What Do Leaders Require from Their Teams?

Ability to Meet Team Goals

Leaders, in the most general sense, want high levels of performance to achieve common goals. The overarching goal for the trauma team is to salvage the patient and preserve function [3]. There are a number of metrics used to measure achievement of these goals through trauma care processes and patient outcome measures. The most obvious patient outcome is mortality. Other metrics include complication rates, hospital readmissions, and length of stay. These metrics reflect not just the trauma team care but also care throughout their stay. Process measures can be more specific to the trauma team and include securing the airway in low GCS patients, reducing joint dislocation in under 1 hour, and transfer to ICU or surgery under 1 hour, where needed [3]. Together these outcome and process metrics form the basis of quality improvement programs [4]. Quality improvement will be discussed further in Chaps. 27 and 28.

Achieving quality patient care relies on an expert team with effective communication, efficient feedback, and team member cohesion. These non-technical skills are more difficult to measure directly during trauma resuscitation and patient care but are important markers of team function and are necessary to achieve a shared goal [5]. Team performance has been enhanced through video review of simulated resuscitations with established non-technical scoring systems [6]. Video-facilitated feedback is widely used in simulation and has been demonstrated to improve future performance [7]. Further, the use of video-recording resuscitations in the clinical setting allows for review of real-life team performance and may improve team clinical performance [8]. Time to critical interventions such as establishing a definitive airway, CT scanning, and transfer to the operating room are improved [9]. Simulation-based training leads to a reduction in resuscitation time and time to task completion. However, use of this tool has been limited, likely due to a combination of legal and ethical issues associated with the inability to obtain patient and provider consent in the setting of an acute trauma. Video review of trauma will be discussed further in Chap. 15.

Team Cohesion and Relationship Building

High-functioning teams focus not only on their deliverables or objectives but also on the team as an entity unto itself, which must be developed and fostered [10]. When there is strong group cohesion, there is a willingness to collaborate and share ideas and feedback. Strong cohesion is associated with both improved perceived team effectiveness and better patient outcomes [11]. Cohesion develops when there are shared goals, a shared commitment to accomplishing team tasks, and a belief that teammates are trustworthy [12]. Trauma teams can improve their communication, commitment, and ultimately teamwork through simulation [13, 14].

Important to team cohesion is psychological safety, a culture where all team members feel comfortable speaking up [15]. When team members feel safe speaking up, problems can be addressed, and the positive reinforcement helps maintain the safety and cohesion within the group. When working as a team, the result of any conversation or team interaction will build the relationship capital necessary to future team performance. These two aspects cannot happen in isolation, rather they must happen in parallel. Successful trauma teams epitomize this construct.

What Do Team Members Need from Their Leaders?

A Sense of Belonging

Diversity can be defined as the ways in which we are all different [16]. This definition does not attempt to define a specific dominant group as the norm and others as being a deviation from that. It defines all people as being important entities unto themselves with differences which make them unique. Inclusivity is how the voices and thoughts of the group are heard [16]. If diversity is the "what," inclusivity is the "how." An inclusive environment in turn fosters each individual's sense of belonging which is felt when an individual experiences that their social group identity is both connected with and accepted in an organization. Medicine and surgery have typically placed value on hierarchical systems in both educational pathways and the clinical practice environment. These types of leadership structures can introduce fear and anxiety in less empowered members of the team and lead to detrimental divisions in the group dynamic. More horizontal team structures, where every member of the team feels valued, have been found to improve performance. Furthermore, the best results stem from diverse teams; teams that include members with differing viewpoints and perspectives [17]. Acceptance of diverse views is strengthened by the degree of respect given to each perspective.

Respect

Respect is an offshoot of belonging that involves recognizing each member for their specific strengths and contributions. Specifically, it is operationalized when an individual experiences a "culture of civility and positive regard for diverse perspectives and ways of knowing" [16]. Not only does a member of the team feel that they are accepted, they also believe that their opinions and ideas are regarded with high value. When an individual is respected, a psychologically safe space is created for new ideas to be brought forward which have the capacity to improve team performance.

Due to the high stakes environment of a trauma resuscitation, presenting new ideas can be challenging. Hjortdal et al. conducted a series of interviews with trauma team members at four different hospitals to obtain a deeper understanding of the non-technical skills that are important to team members [18]. They found that maintaining the authority of leadership while providing constructive feedback or new ideas was essential to preserving team confidence. For example, feedback can be formulated as a question or a proposal: "What do you think about the patient's blood pressure?" In this way, the team member can feel safe to make a contribution while both being respected and respecting the leader.

Bidirectional and Open Communication

Critical to the success of any team, but distinctly important in a trauma setting, is the ability of the leader to communicate effectively. In the interview series by Hjortdal et al., participants indicated that they appreciated leaders with the ability to communicate distinctly and clearly [18]. The leader must have the capacity to analyze multiple sources of information (e.g., handover from the emergency transport team, information from the primary survey, inputs from the trauma team) and relay findings to the team in a calm, cool, and confident manner. The ability of the leader to radiate confidence in communication was highly regarded by team members, as it instilled confidence in the whole team. This circles back to the distinction of the trauma team as a *team* rather than a group. The leader needs to be in frequent communication with the members of the team because their role may be affected by ongoing developments. For example, if the leader finds the patient to have a pneumothorax, the anesthesiologist should be aware of a possible impending compromise to ventilation, the medical assistant can begin preparing a chest tube kit, and the radiology technician can start setting up for a post-procedural x-ray. Communication is vital to synchronizing the team's efforts to save the patient.

Opportunities for Continued Growth

The transient nature of a trauma team allows one to conceptualize each trauma team activation as a single project. Each trauma team activation should therefore culminate with a review of successes and failures [19]. This can be done in the form of an "after-action review" or a debrief. This stage is key to not only highlighting excellence but serves as a time to reflect on possible areas of learning to enhance future performance. In the Advanced Trauma Life Support Training model, the optimal time for the debrief is immediately after the patient is transferred to definitive care. Effective team behavior should be reinforced, and areas of excellence should be highlighted. For example, the trauma team leader might say, "I think we all did a great job minimizing extraneous noise in this code, let's keep that up next time." Furthermore, this is an opportunity to openly share opinions and discuss how the code went. General questions to consider include: What could we have done differently? What have we learned for next time? Are there any actions we need to take before our next trauma team activation? If a culture of psychological safety and respect has been adequately developed in the team environment, the flow of feedback can be multidirectional. The members will look for opportunities for continued growth, as will the team leader. Chapter 63 will discuss debriefing strategies further.

Resources

In order to sustain a culture of continued growth, team members should have access to a number of resources. Most notably, within a trauma team activation, the availability of adequately trained human resources is of utmost importance [20]. This includes an experienced trauma team leader and a full complement of team members, each with a clear understanding of their roles. In addition, physical resources to perform the resuscitation should be readily available and accessible. Petroniak et al. analyzed the traffic patterns of clinicians performing an emergency cricothyroidotomy during simulation and found that decreased travel was associated with a faster time-to-completion of the emergency procedure. Analysis of the simulation revealed that the clinician with the most efficient performance used a pre-prepared airway kit and delegated roles which included travelling to obtain more equipment. This is an example of effective use of resources in the trauma setting. Trauma bay design will be covered further in Chap. 24. Furthermore, all members who participate in trauma team activations should have the opportunity to engage in ongoing training which could include specialty seminars, simulation-based training, and video review [21].

The Four Stages of Competence

In the acquisition of skills and formation of new habits associated with the successful engagement of team members, one moves from unconscious incompetence through various stages until they finally arrive at a state of unconscious competence [22]. When someone initially takes on a new task, they are not aware they do not possess the skills, habits, and mindset required to be successful. This is the state of unconscious incompetence (Fig. 10.1). Over time and with repeated practice, they will eventually become aware they are incompetent and move into a state of conscious incompetence. With this awareness, and further practice, often associated with repeated failures and revisions, one moves into a state of conscious competence where skills and tools are practiced with intent. This requires conscious awareness and effort that newly acquired skills and habits need to be continuously practiced. One is consciously competent. Finally, one moves to a state of skillful performance without having to devote intentional energy and focus on their performance. This is the state of unconscious competence and the end goal of expertise.

The movement from unconscious incompetence to unconscious competence is not achieved solely by the acquisition of new skills and habits. It often requires that old ways of doing things need to be consciously forgotten. If your preferred approach in a trauma setting has been to assume the position of an expert to whom everyone else on the team defers, it will take effort to "get rid" of this old habit in addition to developing new habits which will more effectively support successful team engagement. This is often the place where the transition to new practices fail as people are willing to incorporate new skills but they are unable to give up their old way of doing things. This is why it is important to reflect on old habits and how they detract from the goal of engaging team members. Reversion to old habits should not be seen as a failure and a signal that one cannot change. It should be seen for just that—a reversion to an old, comfortable way of doing things. The goal is to move from a situation where time is spent in old habits and skills to one where time is dedicated to new habits and skills. It takes time for the brain to be rewired in this way as one moves through from unconscious incompetence to a final state of unconscious competence.

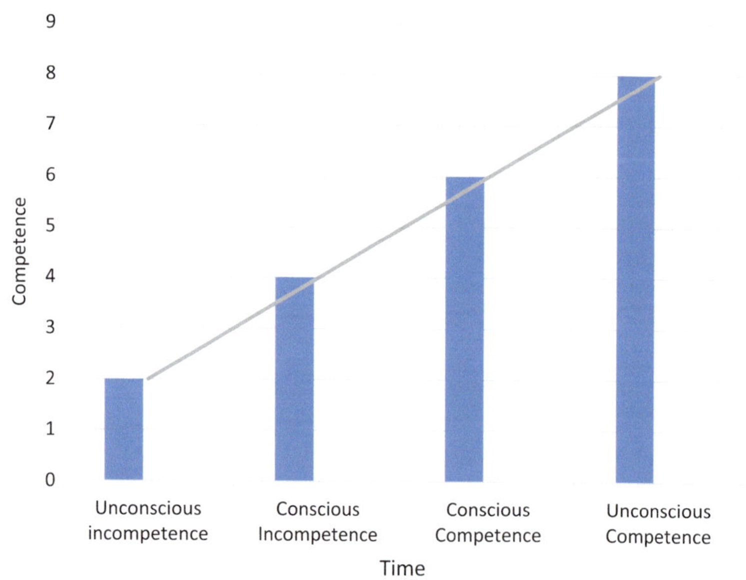

Fig. 10.1 Curtiss and Warren's four stages of competence model. (Modified from Curtiss and Warren [22, p. 89])

Ten Principles of Engaging Team Members

There are ten principles behind engaging team members. In moving from unconscious incompetence through to unconscious competence, leaders will need to make their teams aware that engaging the team is an important goal of the leader, as it should be for all team members. Open and frank discussion about how to best engage the team will enhance overall success.

1. Engage in Self-Reflection
Self-reflection can be undertaken as a series of conscious questions one asks themselves during the attainment of new skills. These questions include:

1. What happened during the trauma team activation and resuscitation?
2. What was the result or impact?
3. What was *the intended* result or impact?
4. Why did I handle it that way (especially when one reverts to old habits)?
5. How will I handle it in the future? What specific strategies will I employ?

An important aspect of reflection is to ask what internal or external aspects are continuing to support old habits. For example, if seeing yourself as the team leader with the expertise to which everyone must defer is part of how you see yourself, it will be important to recognize that this internal vision which supports old habits must be altered. In the moment, it will be important to remember that altering this vision will lead to enhanced benefits for the team, its individual members, and ultimately the patient.

2. Practice Active Listening
Active listening is a conscious activity whereby one focuses on correctly interpreting what the other person is saying. The distinction is found in hearing someone speak, but not understanding what is being said. This is a failure of listening, not of hearing. All of the principles involved in engaging team members can be tied back to active listening.

The components of active listening include the following [23]:

1. *Paying attention* by blocking out distractions and refraining from preparing a rebuttal while the other person is speaking,
2. *Showing you are listening* through open posture and eye contact
3. *Providing feedback* by paraphrasing and asking questions to clarify meaning
4. *Deferring judgement* by letting the other person finish what they are saying and responding in turn
5. *Responding appropriately* by showing respect and being open and honest in your responses

Active listening involves seeking to understand what the other person is saying over waiting until they finish so you can state your case. It is all about the other person.

3. Mentor Critical Thinking
To effectively engage their teams, leaders must ensure that all members feel valued. A leader's ability to mentor critical thinking and allow members to develop and showcase their strengths will significantly enhance engagement [24]. The concept of distributed leadership speaks to allowing all team members to lead where their strengths permit. This requires the leader to know their team members and be champions of inclusivity on the team. This will allow the team to expand the scope of their influence and limit the effect of their weaknesses on the successful completion of team objectives. It is the leader's responsibility to ensure that team members know their strengths in the team and that they are being supported to lead in these areas. For example, team members should have confidence in their own abilities and be able to identify when it is appropriate to act independently in pursuit of the team goal. Exemplary critical thinking includes identifying best evidence, addressing assumptions and biases, and critically appraising one's own leadership styles within the team.

4. Provide Constructive Feedback
Providing feedback is essential to team engagement. Feedback can be defined as specific information about the comparison between an individual's observed performance and a recognized and known standard [25]. Leaders should look for opportunities where feedback can be given, in the moment, and with the intent to improve the overall performance of the individual and enhance team performance. It should be encouraging, and if an error or mistake is made, the leader should seek to determine what led to the error and how things could be done differently next time. Feedback should be coached in "I" statements about what was observed and should recommend specific actionable behavior for improvement. For example, the leader might say, "I noticed you were standing behind everyone as you attempted to monitor the patient's vitals. I believe you were pushed aside because your name tag was not visible. Next time, ensure you speak up and that your name tag is visible. It will improve the function of the team." The feedback provided should promote specific aspects of performance to be maintained (if the behavior enhances team function) or redirect specific aspects performance in the future (if a change is nec-

essary to improve team performance). This type of feedback, known as directive feedback, is useful for small, simple corrections. For more complex tasks and decision-making inquiring about the person's frame of reference when making that choice can be more enlightening and help facilitate better discussion, engaging the team more effectively. This type of technique is termed advocacy inquiry and will be discussed further in Chap. 63. An example might be "I noticed you chose not to immediately intubate the patient on arrival. I was concerned that he might obstruct his airway and I wondered if this should be done immediately. How did you see your priorities at that moment?". It may be that the leader had a very rational thought process as to why that should be delayed and if not inquired properly may never come to light.

5. Adopt a Spirit of Servant Leadership

Servant leadership, popularized by Robert K. Greenleaf, is a style of leadership which *serves others first*. He first described servant leadership as the natural feeling that one wants to serve followed by a conscious choice to lead [26]. This distinction, which the leader is first a *servant* and then a *leader*, emphasizes the value of those being led. The leader's primary job is to foster, nurture, and nourish the team members to be the best they can be. Servant leaders work closely with the members of their team to recognize strengths and weaknesses and to facilitate continuous improvement. This individual relationship building ultimately serves to strengthen the team's function as a whole. When members of the trauma team are led by a servant leader, they recognize their importance within the team and will be motivated to perform at a high level. Servant leadership also necessitates that all voices are heard, communicated, and disseminated within the team [27]. A spirit of servant leadership essentially labels that the leader will focus on what the team needs: a sense of belonging, respect, open communication, opportunities for growth, and necessary resources to succeed.

6. Offer Continual Encouragement

Team members must receive encouragement in order to be motivated toward the goals or objectives of the team and as a means of developing team relationships and supporting cohesion among team members. Positive or re-enforcing encouragement promotes self-efficacy, which supports development of team relationships and cohesion among members [28]. Continual surveillance of the situation for opportunities to encourage successful performance will enhance the overall function of the team. Unlike feedback, encouragement does not necessarily need to be tagged to a specific aspect of performance, rather it supports overall performance. It should also be used to recognize team members' strengths and their necessary inclusion among those with whom the team interacts. In the trauma team setting, this may include recognition by the patient or the patient's family. Encouragement, like feedback, is time sensitive and should be given only where appropriate.

7. Engage in Successful Dialogue

Engaging in dialogue is an active process, which requires concentration through undivided attention, listening to body language, and avoiding distractions [29]. It is estimated that over 50% of the meaning of a conversation is conveyed through non-verbal communication or body language [24]. Think about what it might mean if someone rolls their eyes, looks or moves away, or crosses their arms during a conversation. More subtle aspects of body language might include certain gestures others make when they anxious or nervous, the speed or cadence of spoken language, or posture.

Dialogue is a way of communicating where the primary aim is to seek to understand the other person first—nothing more and certainly nothing less. This can best be achieved through active listening, which involves seeking clarification, asking questions to promote understanding, and paraphrasing [30]. It entails listening when one wants to speak, especially when they feel the need to aggressively defend their position though interrupting or speaking over others [31]. Holding a successful dialogue is the first element in resolving conflict effectively.

8. Resolve Conflict Effectively

The first step in resolving conflict effectively is in recognizing that a leader must know what each side wants and they must be willing to engage in a dialogue to establish common ground [32]. A leader will need to shift from caring about what they are saying, and in some situations interrupting to get their point across, to actively listening to understand what the other person is saying. Resolving conflict is coached in the ability to separate your interpretation of the events, your story, from the actual facts of the situation [33]. Team leaders must be able to get to a state of mutually agreeable goals and ultimately, and they must be invested in a good outcome for all parties. Often teams will have difficulty resolving conflict because they have not defined a mutually agreeable goal. In trying to develop ideas and strategies, there is an inability to come to a consensus. For example, if there are multiple people around the table and some of them are interested in furthering the ability of the team to function as a whole while others are interested in avoiding a lawsuit, it may be difficult to come up with strategies which will actually achieve both. It must be recognized that active listening and establishing a dialogue is paramount [32].

9. Set Realistic Expectations

The process of setting expectations is a dynamic and inclusive process [34]. Leaders must be willing to consult with other team members to ensure that expectations align with recognized personal strengths of team members and with the team's needs as a whole. There must be a common understanding of why certain expectations exist and how they align with the overall objectives of the team. Leaders should consider delegating the development of expectations to others, especially to those whom the expectations will apply. In the same way, responsibility for ensuring expectations are met should be a joint responsibility of leaders, those to whom the expectations apply, and the team as a whole as they seek to define where best to employ each member's strengths.

There may be situations in which expectations need to be achieved within a short time frame, and trauma teams are commonly in this position. In these situations, it is important that expectations of all members and the entire team are realistic and known in advance. We would not expect a very junior member of the team to support the airway without appropriate guidance and this should be clear to everyone on the team. Expectations should be set before the situation arises where they will need to be enacted. Unclear or unrealistic expectations will threaten the function of the team, engagement of team members, and ultimately patient outcomes.

10. Look for Opportunities
Self-reflection and actively listening, like other skills involved in engaging teams, require one to look for opportunities. They require conscious performance when one is in a space of unconscious incompetence and through to unconscious competence. These skills require time and effort when one is first seeking to practice them consistently. The propensity to fall back to bad habits will need to be specifically kept in check in strengthening these basic tenets, which are necessary for addressing the ten principles of engaging team members.

Engaging Virtual Teams

Engaging virtual teams is become increasingly more important during COVID-19. Although trauma teams may not engage virtually at the time of a trauma, some of the relationship building and simulation exercises may move to a virtual format. Leaders need to recognize that within the environment of virtual teams all processes must be simplified, clearly defined, and delegated appropriately [35]. It is the responsibility of the leader to set the parameters with clear direction and a shared mental model, including the roles to be taken on by team members in the virtual setting. When individuals understand their roles and other's contributions to the team, they are able to anticipate activities which can decrease the effort needed to coordinate the team.

For a virtual team to function equivalently to a face-to-face team requires more time and effort on the part of the leader [36]. This is challenging in a traditional hierarchical leadership model and can be supplemented with structural supports such as routines and reward systems as well as shared team leadership. This would include collaborative decision-making, where appropriate, and shared responsibility, both of which contribute to trust and group cohesion. Through frequent communication and shared responsibility, leaders can adapt and effectively engage with virtual teams. One of the ways of achieving this is through the development of a communication charter.

Develop a Communication Charter

One of the important challenges in virtual teams is the loss of informal communication, including access to non-verbal cues, meetings within meetings, and attention to emotional aspects of the environment, which normally function to establish trust through connectedness [37]. To overcome the loss of informal communication, leaders can create prompts and rules to guide discussion. A formal communication charter should be established which outlines how communication will take place in the virtual setting such that all voices are heard and timely discussions related to issues can be held [35]. A team charter can also help maintain a common understanding of group purpose, which is a marker of a healthy team [38].

Virtual Water Cooler

In-person meetings and interactions are inclusive of the opportunity for team members to interact and strengthen team relationships and support cohesion [35]. This is an aspect which has traditionally been missing from virtual interactions. An example of introducing the opportunity for informal interaction into the virtual team setting has been to establish a virtual water cooler [39]. Purposeful scheduling of white time as the start of a meeting can allow people to interact outside of the context of the meeting agenda. Allowing for informal break out rooms can strengthen this concept.

Together, a communication charter and virtual water cooler help to engage teams and create connectedness that forms the basis of team trust. Addressing the challenges of trust and informal communication help to create norms and cohesion, which are essential to effective team function [35].

The Role of Simulation in "Engaging Team Members" Skill Development

Overall enhancement of patient care in the trauma team setting can be achieved through the acquisition of effective team leadership skills, including engaging team members, in a simulation-based environment [40]. Simulation-based leadership development for trauma team leaders has been employed with emergency medicine residents with self-perceived improvements in pre-arrival brief and prioritization of tasks, both through enhanced communication and engagement of team members. These results were found to be maintained up to 24 months following the simulation training. Patient outcomes were not specifically evaluated.

Simulation can be used to define team member roles and allow communication around how to enhance efficiencies, enhance communication, and enhance empathy for the challenges of other members of the team [41]. For example, more junior members can be provided with information on the role they will play and what they need to focus on to be successful and proficient in that role. They can even be introduced to slightly more complex roles, both in terms of specific tasks and communication with other team members, and come to understand the impact they have on other team members and their roles. The simulation setting is particularly responsive to learner's needs and can help to develop a shared purpose of what it means to engage teams in communication and collaboration.

Simulated trauma situations can be used to specifically define the educational goals related to engaging team members [41]. Conflict can be built into the situation by "planting a mole" to evaluate and teach constructs related to the ten principles of engagement, including speaking up in the face of conflict and providing effective feedback. A mole or confederate is a member of the simulation team who is instructed to perform in a certain manner, without the knowledge of the rest of the team members, in order to ensure the team reaches a specific learning goal. The design of simulation scenarios and curricula can be found in Chaps. 61 and 62. Simulation is especially well suited to providing feedback in the moment around specific educational goals, with the opportunity to cement concepts through participation in an immediate second simulation following an effective debrief.

The debrief is an exceptionally important part of the simulation experience [42–45]. As such, those undertaking the debrief must be trained in how best to perform this part of the simulation. The debrief must be formative for learners and identify what went well, what areas must be improved upon, and how the learner can enhance their education to become more proficient. The debriefing process itself must be seen as a way to continue to engage members involved in the simulation experience. Importantly, those performing the debrief must be open to receiving feedback on their own debriefing techniques in order to enhance the experience for future learners. An introduction to basic debriefing techniques can be found in Chap. 63.

Conclusion

Engaging team members is of primary importance to optimal performance of the trauma team. Trauma teams are not static; each activation will result in a team whose membership is different from the last. As such, trauma team leaders must recognize that their members will be at different points in understanding their roles, interacting in teams, and responding under stress. The leadership skills involved in engaging team members can be acquired, with simulation-based scenarios followed by appropriate debriefing being paramount. Engagement of team members and ensuring appropriate team function are as important to limiting morbidity and mortality in the acute trauma setting as learning the ABCs of trauma.

References

1. Saltman DC, O'Dea NA, Farmer J, Veitch C, Rosen G, Kidd MR. Groups or teams in health care: finding the best fit. J Eval Clin Pract. 2001;13(1):55–60.
2. Hicks C, Petrosoniak A. The human factor: optimizing trauma team performance in dynamic clinical environments. Emerg Med Clin North Am. 2018;36(1):1–17.
3. Santana MJ, Stelfox HT, Asbridge M, Ball CG, Cameron P, Dyer D, et al. Development and evaluation of evidence-informed quality indicators for adult injury care. Ann Surg. 2014;259(1):186–92.
4. Truchon C, Moore L, Belcaid A, Clément J, Trudelle N, Ulysse MA, et al. Shaping quality through vision, structure, and monitoring of performance and quality indicators: impact story from the Quebec trauma network. Int J Technol Assess Health Care. 2017;33(4):415–9.
5. Briggs A, Raja AS, Joyce MF, Yule SJ, Jiang W, Lipsitz SR, et al. The role of nontechnical skills in simulated trauma resuscitation. J Surg Educ. 2015;72(4):732–9.
6. Hamilton NA, Kieninger AN, Woodhouse J, Freeman BD, Murray D, Klingensmith ME. Video review using a reliable evaluation metric improves team function in high-fidelity simulated trauma resuscitation. J Surg Educ. 2012;69(3):428–31.
7. Scherer LA, Chang MC, Meredith JW, Battistella FD. Videotape review leads to rapid and sustained learning. Am J Surg. 2003;185(6):516–20.
8. Brogaard L, Uldbjerg N. Filming for auditing of real-life emergency teams: a systematic review. BMJ Open Qual. 2019;8(4):588.
9. Noonan M, Olaussen A, Mathew J, Mitra B, Smit DV, Fitzgerald M. What is the clinical evidence supporting trauma team training (TTT): a systematic review and meta-analysis. Medicina. 2019;55(9):1–14.
10. Salas E, Estrada AX, Vessey WB. Team cohesion: advances in psychological theory, methods and practice. Bingley: Emerald Group Publishing Limited; 2015.
11. Lemieux-Charles L, McGuire WL. What do we know about health care team effectiveness? A review of the literature. Med Care Res Rev. 2006;63(3):263–300.
12. Michalisin M, Karau S, Tangpong C. Leadership's activation of team cohesion as a strategic asset: an empirical simulation. J Bus Strateg. 2007;24(1):1–26.
13. Miller D, Crandall C, Washington C, McLaughlin S. Improving teamwork and communication in trauma care through in situ simulations. Acad Emerg Med. 2012;19(5):608–12.
14. Shapiro MJ, Morey JC, Small SD, Langford V, Kaylor CJ, Jagminas L, et al. Simulation based teamwork training for emergency department staff: does it improve clinical team performance when added to an existing didactic teamwork curriculum? Qual Saf Health Care. 2004;13(6):417–21.
15. Manthous CA, Hollingshead AB. Team science and critical care. Am J Respir Crit Care Med. 2011;184(1):17–25.

16. West MA, Hwang S, Maier RV, Ahuja N, Angelos P, Bass B, et al. Ensuring equity, diversity, and inclusion in academic surgery: an American surgical association white paper. Ann Surg. 2018;268(3):403–7.
17. Hoogendoorn S, Oosterbeek H, Van Praag M. The impact of gender diversity on the performance of business teams: evidence from a field experiment. Manag Sci. 2013;59(7):1514–28.
18. Hjortdahl M, Ringen AH, Naess AC, Wisborg T. Leadership is the essential non-technical skill in the trauma team – results of a qualitative study. Scand J Trauma Resusc Emerg Med. 2009;17(1):1–9.
19. Committee on Trauma. Advanced trauma life support: student course manual. 10th ed. Chicago: The American College of Surgeons; 2018. p. 444.
20. Petrosoniak A, Almeida R, Pozzobon LD, Hicks C, Fan M, White K, et al. Tracking workflow during high-stakes resuscitation: the application of a novel clinician movement tracing tool during in situ trauma simulation. BMJ Simul Technol Enhanc Learn. 2019;5(2):78–84.
21. Tiel Groenestege-Kreb D, Van Maarseveen O, Leenen L. Trauma team. Br J Anaesth. 2014;113(2):258–65.
22. Curtiss PR, Warren PW. The dynamics of life skills coaching. Life skills series. Prince Albert: Training Research and Development Station, Department of Manpower and Immigration; 1974.
23. Active listening: hear what people really are saying. n.d. Retrieved from: https://www.mindtools.com/Commskll/ActiveListening.htm.
24. Coates DE, Bell MM. Connect with your team: mastering the top 10 communication skills. London: First Summit Publishing; 2020.
25. Van De Ridder JMM, Stokking KM, McGaghie WC, Ten Cate OTJ. What is feedback in clinical education? Med Educ. 2008;42:189–97. Retrieved from: https://onlinelibrary.wiley.com/doi/full/10.1111/j.1365-2923.2007.02973.x.
26. Greanleaf RK. The servant as leader. Westfield: The Greenleaf Center for Servant Leadership; 1970.
27. Savel RH, Munro CL. Servant leadership: the primacy of service. Am J Crit Care. 2017;26:97–9. Retrieved from: https://doi.org/10.4037/ajcc2017356.
28. Barbee J, Alexander M, Penman J, Dynlacht J. Twelve tips for clinical preceptors to deliver meaningful feedback. MedEdPublish. 2012;7(4):1–9.
29. Groysberg B, Slind M. Leadership is a conversation. Hard Bus Rev. 2012;90(6):76–84.
30. Daimler M. Listening is an overlooked leadership tool. Hard Bus Rev [Internet]. 2012 May 25. Retrieved from: https://hbr.org/2016/05/listening-is-an-overlooked-leadership-tool.
31. Carmichael SG. Everything you need to know about becoming a better listener. Hard Bus Rev [Internet]. 2015 Feb 6. Retrieved from: https://hbr.org/2015/02/everything-you-need-to-know-about-becoming-a-better-listener.
32. Patterson K, Grenny J, McMillan R, Switzler A. Explore others' paths. In: Crucial conversations: tools for talking when the stakes are high. 2nd ed. New York: McGraw-Hill; 2012. p. 155–76.
33. Patterson K, Grenny J, McMillan R, Switzler A. Putting it all together. In: Crucial conversations: tools for talking when the stakes are high. 2nd ed. New York: McGraw-Hill; 2012. p. 211–22.
34. Harter J, Adkins A. What great managers do to engage employees. Hard Bus Rev [Internet]. 2015 Apr 2. Retrieved from: https://hbr.org/2015/04/what-great-managers-do-to-engage-employees.
35. Hunsaker PL, Hunsaker JS. Virtual teams: a leader's guide. Team Perform Manag. 2008;14(1–2):86–101.
36. Hoch JE, Kozlowski SWJ. Leading virtual teams: hierarchical leadership, structural supports, and shared team leadership. J Appl Psychol. 2014;99(3):390–403.
37. Cowan LD. E-leadership: leading in a virtual environment – guiding principles for nurse leaders. Nurs Econ. 2014;32(6):312–22.
38. Cascio WF. Managing a virtual workplace. Acad Manag Exec. 2000;14:81.
39. Watkins M. Making virtual teams work: ten basic principles. Hard Bus Rev. 2013;1:1–6. Retrieved from: https://hbr.org/2013/06/making-virtual-teams-work-ten.
40. Rosenman ED, Vrablik MC, Brolliar SM, Chipman AK, Fernandez R. Targeted simulation-based leadership training for trauma team leaders. West J Emerg Med. 2019;20(3):520–6.
41. Aggarwal R, Mytton OT, Derbrew M, Hananel D, Heydenburg M, Issenberg B, et al. Training and simulation for patient safety. Qual Saf Health Care. 2010;19(Suppl 2):i34–43.
42. Sawyer T, Eppich W, Brett-Fleegler M, Grant V, Cheng A. More than one way to debrief: a critical review of healthcare simulation debriefing methods. Simul Healthc. 2016;11(3):209–17.
43. Eppich W, Cheng A. Promoting excellence and reflective learning in simulation (PEARLS): development and rationale for a blended approach to health care simulation debriefing. Simul Healthc. 2015;10(2):106–15.
44. Rudolph JW, Simon R, Rivard P, Dufresne RL, Raemer DB. Debriefing with good judgment: combining rigorous feedback with genuine inquiry. Anesthesiol Clin. 2007;45:361–76.
45. Rosen KR. The history of medical simulation. J Crit Care. 2008;23:157–66.

The Trouble with Teams: Practical Tools for Complex Trauma Team Dynamics

11

Christopher Hicks and Andrew Petrosoniak

None of us is as smart as all of us.

– Ken Blanchard

Anyone who has worked in the complex ecosystem of team-based trauma resuscitation can attest to the notion that effective teamwork is not intuitive, that a team of experts does not make an expert team and that to function as a cohesive inter-professional is a unique and specific skill set separate but not divorced from content or procedural knowledge. Exactly *what* that skill set looks like can be difficult to pinpoint: At any given time in a resuscitation, team members may be called upon to speak up, to keep quiet, to act, to remain hands off, to work together, to work independently, to work quickly or to slow things down. That the issue is complex does not mean that solutions have to be—in effect, good team behaviors can be scaffolded along a set of practical and tangible concepts, and then shaped by local, cultural and domain-specific understanding to create elite, high reliability, expert-level group performance.

Implicit Coordination

At the summit of our understanding of elite team performance is the concept of implicit coordination, or the ability to anticipate the needs of other team members in concert with carrying out your own role without an excess amount of chatter and cross-talking [1]. Effective teams tend to be surprisingly quiet, a concept that runs counter the Crisis Resource Management (CRM) principle of verbalizing thoughts or notion of "flying the patient"—a concept borrowed from aviation that describes the act of speaking aloud your thought process for the rest of the team members to hear [2]. Indeed, there is a time for speaking up, and a series of concepts to support doing so effectively (discussed subsequently), but the concept of implicit communication is nonetheless a cornerstone of expert team performance. Implicit coordination can be measured by way of an *anticipation ratio (AR)*, the frequency with which information is offered compared to the frequency with which it is requested [3]. The implication is that if team members are provided the information they need to carry out their roles without having to ask (AR > 1), the team is demonstrating implicit coordination by anticipating the needs of their fellow team members. This is important because it suggests that a team has a shared sense of situation awareness, current priorities, and anticipated next steps.

Implicit coordination is in turn predicated on the notion of *shared mental models*: the idea that all team members have a shared understanding of both team and task-based process for a given clinical scenario [4]. Experimental studies in combat aviation and military teams demonstrate that the degree to which team members share mental models is directly correlated with mission success [5]. This is particularly relevant in trauma resuscitation, where competing priorities can create confusion and interfere with one another, predisposing to consequential delays as well as errors of omission and commission. The concepts that follow are selected deliberately to facilitate the creation of shared, flexible, and accurate mental models for team-based trauma resuscitation, with the goal of building capacity for implicit coordination.

Psychological Safety and Emotional Contagion

In order to function cohesively under stressful, time-pressured conditions, team members need to be reassured that they have the permission to ask questions, admit mistakes, or challenge the team leader. The key to facilitating

The authors attest to having no relevant conflicts of interest to declare.

C. Hicks (✉) · A. Petrosoniak
St. Michael's Hospital, Li Ka Shing Knowledge Institute, Toronto, ON, Canada

Department of Medicine, University of Toronto, Toronto, ON, Canada
e-mail: christopher.hicks@unityhealth.to

L. Marshall Gillman, S. Widder (eds.), *Trauma Team Dynamics*, https://doi.org/10.1007/978-3-031-86312-7_11

positive social interactions within teams is establishing a sufficient sense of psychological safety: that is, that the team environment is safe for interpersonal risk-taking [6]. Psychological safety is correlated with improved safety behaviors like error reporting and promotes knowledge and power sharing, cogeneration and team learning [7].

Fostering psychological safety requires all team members, and perhaps most notably the team leader, to admit uncertainty, express doubt, seek input, and ask for help. Traditional models of team leadership that call upon the team leader to assume an all-seeing, all-knowing posture are counterproductive to establishing psychological safety and quite often call upon the team leader to compensate for these vulnerabilities by assuming an authoritative and at times authoritarian posture. Such negative emotional valence rapidly translates to the remainder of the team, a concept described by Soares and Lopes as *emotional contagion* [8]. Conversely, by openly embracing vulnerability and uncertainty when it exists, emotional contagion can be harnessed to generate more positive attitudes and behaviors, including voicing concern, cooperation, collaboration and mutual support. Creating a robust sense of psychological safety is the means by which the positive attributes of an inter-professional team may be brought to bear, cueing and facilitating the *transactive memory* of a diverse group of team members towards a common and shared goal [1]. Far from displaying weakness, team leaders who are willing to admit uncertainty and appreciate their limitations are generally regarded as better and more effective than those who do not.

Team leaders can foster psychological safety in several concrete ways. Seeking team input by asking "What am I missing?" sends a powerful message that the leader is willing to both admit uncertainty and seek input. Clearing cognitive dissonance by articulating ambiguity may also help realign mental models by provoking a conversation about next best steps: "The patient didn't respond as expected to a volume challenge, raising the possibility that other causes of shock might be in play; I seek your input on what our immediate next steps should be." Opportunities to build psychological safety are multiple and include the pre-primary survey (the Zero-Point Survey), during pre-briefings, and at set check-in or recap points that occur as the resuscitation progresses.

The Zero-Point Survey

In an organized resuscitation, the primary survey should be preceded by a series of steps to ensure self, team, and environmental preparation. Ideally, effective teams start preparing to resuscitate before patients arrive.

The Zero-Point Survey (ZPS) is a consensus-derived framework for organizing pre-primary survey discussions around self, team, and environmental preparation [9]. The ZPS is designed to create shared mental models and facilitate implicit coordination by direct team-based discussion and preparation prior to patient arrival, and is updated periodically once the resuscitation commences. The STEP-UP mnemonic is used to recall the elements of the ZPS (Fig. 11.1). Although diagrammed as a linear process, the interplay between elements of the ZPS (e.g., self and team) necessitates a back-and-forth reappraisal as the scenario progresses.

Prior to patient arrival, team members are prompted to examine and appraise their own sense of psychological preparedness, or *fitness to execute* via I'M SAFE (Illness, Medication, Stress, Alcohol, Fatigue, Eating/Elimination), with the implication that reversible incumbrancers to individual performance are identified and addressed, or partially mitigated before engaging in patient care. This is followed by a focused examination of roles, anticipated early priorities, and an environmental scan for equipment safety and logistics. Environmental preparation should occur well in advance, but in the immediacy of a pending resuscitation team members should at a minimum be made aware of the location of and anticipate the need for key equipment and planned pathways for patient and team member movement. Non-clinical personnel should be assigned specific roles to support clinical logistics, including equipment gathering, layout, and patient positioning.

A pre-primary survey facilitates the creation of robust shared mental models; a mental model is *shared* when that same cognitive representation is mutually understood and acknowledged between team members [5]. As a dynamic event progresses, the mental model needs to be periodically updated to incorporate new data and changing priorities. A structured Zero-Point Survey can help to clarify elements of

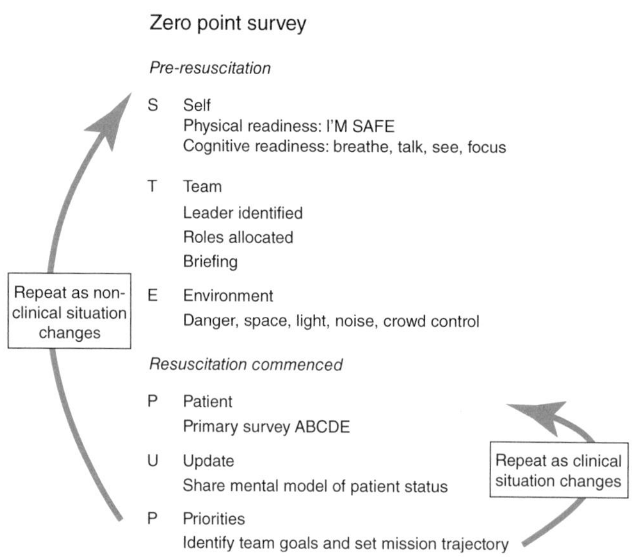

Fig. 11.1 Zero-Point Survey and the STEP-UP mnemonic

an ambiguous clinical event, allow for team input and challenge-response queries, and allow the team leaders to establish early goals and priorities.

The resuscitation environment can be hazardous for providers, and in many situations, team hazards are accepted as an unavoidable or unnoticed element of resuscitation practice. In many cases, a simple and focused environmental and equipment scan can help identify and mitigate latent safety hazards before they can inflict harm. This may include the provision of adequate lighting, positioning and spacing of procedure trays and carts in relation to the provider, positioning the stretcher centrally to ensure 360-degree patient access, and unencumbering monitoring wires and sterile equipment.

Once the patient arrives and the primary survey commences, adjustments to team structure, composition, and environment will invariably be required in response to dynamic patient needs. Assigning a *logistics and safety officer*—someone *other* than the clinical team leader—can assist with managing clinical logistics and optimizing the safe and efficient execution of clinical tasks. This is separate from clinical oversight and task prioritization and may include crowd and noise control, patient positioning, equipment logistics, safe movement of clinical personnel, and planning for patient egress. The importance of the safety officer has been highlighted in recent years by the need to monitor personal protective equipment protocols in light of emergent infectious diseases like COVID-19 [10].

Briefings and Checklists

Structured briefings can help create psychological safety by clarifying what is known, and by extension what remains unknown about a clinical scenario and provide an avenue for team members to ask questions and request clarification ahead of engaging in the hands-on work of the primary survey. Team-based pre-briefing—which takes place *prior to* patient arrival—is an effective way to establish *relational coordination* within an ad hoc team. Relational coordination theory refers to elements of teamwork that facilitate optimal functioning and are characteristic of high-performance organizations and teams and includes shared knowledge and goals that go beyond an individual's task-specific requirements, understanding how a team member's role integrates into the broader team framework, and establishing mutual respect as a means of facilitating psychological safety [11].

An ideal pre-briefing is rapid, team-based, and focused on immediate roles and priorities. At our trauma center, we use a four-question pre-brief in challenge-and-response format (Fig. 11.2). The intent is to quickly establish what is *known* (mechanism, injuries, clinical status, arrival time),

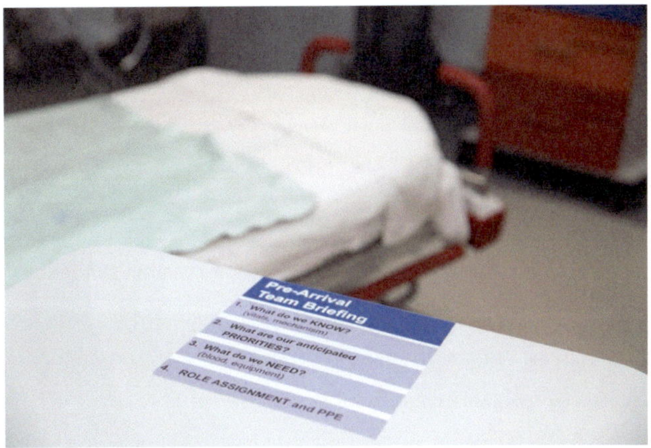

Fig. 11.2 The four-point trauma pre-brief: conducted in under a minute, led by the nurse co-lead, focusing on early and immediate priorities

discuss early anticipated *priorities* (blood, airway management, chest trauma), what is *needed* to address those priorities (massive hemorrhage protocol, difficult airway setup, finger thoracostomy cart), and *roles* (who will do what). Importantly, our pre-briefings are nurse-led, a modification that helps to establish our preferred nurse-physician co-lead trauma team model.

Transitions in care (patient hand-offs or sign-over) are high-risk periods in patient care. Standardized sign-over protocols can improve data transfer and ensure a smooth transition between care teams. This is of particular relevance to sign-over between pre-hospital and trauma teams, wherein the need for repetition is associated with degradation in both the quality and quantity of information transferred [12]. We emphasize a *hands-off, eyes-on* approach to sign-over, whereby team members refrain from engaging with the patient while sign-over takes place. The exception is when sign over and active resuscitation must take place concurrently; A balance between the two may include asking the prehospital team "Do you have any concerns that require our immediate attention before we proceed with sign-over?"

Checklists can help integrate safety behaviors into both standard and non-standard operations in situations where omissions are otherwise common, high stakes, or both. When used correctly, checklists can *force-function* elements of care that might otherwise be bypassed. The World Health Organization (WHO) has developed a trauma care checklist that we have modified according to identified local needs [13]. In our trauma center, we use the modified WHO checklist as a *pre-departure review* prior to egressing from the trauma bay to summarize key tasks, seek input from team members, and ensure adequate preparations have been made to facilitate patient movement (Fig. 11.3).

Pre-Departure Checklist

1. **Is there potential for further airway compromise?**
   If yes, has the airway been SECURED prior to departure?
2. **Have we reviewed Chest and Pelvis X-RAYS?**
3. **Is the patient in SHOCK? If YES, have we notified the TRAUMA SURGEON?**
4. **Are BLOOD products required or the MHP needed?**
   Indicators: > 4U blood products in 1hr *OR* ABC Score > 2 *OR* evidence of shock
5. **Have we controlled EXTERNAL bleeding?**
6. **Is Tranexamic Acid indicated?**
   If YES, administer 2 grams IV
7. **Have we recorded TEMPERATURE and treated hypothermia (T < 35°C)?**
8. **Have we considered ANALGESIA, antibiotics and tetanus?**
9. **Have we documented the NEUROVASCULAR status of all 4 limbs?**
10. **Is VASCULAR ACCESS adequated and functional?**
11. **Do we have all MEDICATIONS necessary for TRANSPORT?**
12. **Do we have the TRANSPORT MONITOR connected and functioning?**
13. **Have we updated the FAMILY?**
14. **Have we contacted the RECEIVING UNIT?**
15. **Are there ANY CONCERNS or ISSUES from any team member?**

Fig. 11.3 Our trauma pre-departure checklist

Language and Team Coordination

Verbal and non-verbal communication set the tone for how a team performs and responds, particularly when time pressures mount and opportunities for error and ambiguity are abundant. Issues with communication arise in virtually every critical event debriefing, and yet there is surprisingly little attention paid to known and effective techniques for effective crisis communication.

(i) *Mitigating language*. Mitigating phrases are the often-subconscious choice of language that downplays or minimizes the meaning of what is being said. This includes phrases like "Could we place a chest tube?" or "Could someone draw up medications for RSI?" which are better rephrased as the commands they are intended to be: "Please perform a right-sided finger thoracostomy," "Mark, draw up 100 mg of ketamine." Concise and direct should not be thought of as synonymous with impolite or offensive. Not knowing names and roles can at times present a barrier to direct and non-mitigating communication; the introduction of name and role identification stickers placed over top of personal protective equipment may in part help to address this.

(ii) *Resuscitation lexicon*. Yamada et al. have proposed the development of a lexicon of short words or phrases that succinctly communicate commands and requests, similar to what is used by cockpit crews [14]. Examples include confirm ("Confirm pre-hospital systolic blood pressure was 70 mmHg"), I say again ("I say again: carotid pulse is absent"), request ("Request update on volume status"), and read-back ("Please read back the total count of blood products given").

(iii) *Closed-loop communication*. Closed-loop communication has three steps—directing an order or request to a specific individual, and having that request verbally acknowledged as both received and completed successfully [15]. The third step is the most challenging, as complete is not synonymous with completed correctly. Effective closed-loop communication, therefore, requires cross-monitoring and mutual support amongst team members, with a particular emphasis recognizing when an action or intervention does not achieve the predicted result.

(iv) *Graded assertiveness*. The two-challenge rule is meant to counteract authority gradients and provide a structured means for expressing concern about a plan of action in a graded fashion [16]. The two-challenge C-U-S framework begins with directly stating a *concern* ("I am concerned about using paralytics for this difficult airway"). If the desired result is not obtained, the next step is for a team member to identify they are *uncomfortable* moving forward with the plan as outlined ("I am uncomfortable paralyzing this patient given the presence of severe airway trauma"). Finally, a *safety issue* is declared if the plan moves forward without adequate modification or retraction ("We must pause here as this is unsafe; I will ask another senior physician to assist us in finding a path forward").

Tactical Pauses, Sit-Reps and Snap Briefs

As the resuscitation progresses, the mental model needs to be updated in an equally concise fashion. Led by the team leader, a tactical pause is a break in case action in order to summarize, reflect, and set priorities for next stages in care. During a tactical pause, all non-essential clinical activity stops and all team members listen, reflect, and are asked to respond as needed. *10 in 10 snap briefs* involve 10-second updates provided by the team leader every 10 minutes and include a brief recap of the case, clinical events happening now, anticipated next steps and priorities, and role allocation or clarification (Table 11.1) [2].

Tactical pauses should go beyond one-way data transfer from leader to team but actively seek input from team mem-

Table 11.1 The 10-in-10 snap brief model

1. Recap on what has been achieved (or not) do far
2. What's happening now
3. Agree next most important steps
4. Prioritize next steps (with indicative timelines if possible e.g. we need to be ready to go scan in 10 minutes)
5. Allocate specific people/kit/resource to achieve next steps

bers. This pause in the action provides an opportunity for team members to speak up about questions, observations, or concerns, provided there is sufficient psychological safety for them to feel comfortable doing so.

Adaptive Coordination

Teams that participate in team training augmented with regular *pause and reassess* situation updates are better able to maintain flexible mental models, utilize more effective forms of communication, and are more resilient to the influence of acute stress on performance. *Adaptive coordination* refers to a team's ability to predict and modify their behavior in response to dynamic clinical and environmental cues—in other words, this is how mental models and transactive memory are operationalized [17]. Entin and Serfaty examined the performance and communication strategies of five-member naval officer teams during anti-air warfare exercises under a number of experimental training conditions [3]. Teams whose leader periodically provided situation-assessment updates—*sit reps*—to summarize priorities and current situation assessment demonstrated better teamwork and task completion and were more resilient to the effects of stress and task load. In fact, teams that were armed with the combination of team training and a pause and reassess framework that included periodic sit-reps were the only experimental group to maintain their performance in the face of increasing task burden, with task overload used as a proxy for acute stress. This phenomenon will be familiar to anyone who has participated in a trauma resuscitation involving multiple injuries or multiple casualties: as time pressure mounts and task demand is high, high-performing teams need to be armed with specific strategies to maintain performance as demands begin to outstrip resources. Tipping the stress appraisal from *threat* to *challenge* is a key facet of what adaptive coordination training seems to accomplish.

In Entin and Serfaty's study, teams using sit-reps shifted from explicit to implicit modes of communication—that is, team members shared information with team members more frequently and directly, without having been asked to do so. This observation is consistent with the ability to anticipate the needs of fellow team members—a key feature of expert team performance. Translated to clinical practice, adaptive team behaviors are facilitated by team leaders who periodically pause and reassess to openly share information, summarize data, voice specific findings, and seek team input and feedback.

Making It Happen

The drive toward implicit coordination and expert team performance requires focused practice in addition to understanding the theory. Interprofessional team training by way of in situ simulation—simulation training that takes place in the physical workspace itself—is a powerful tool to drive home key knowledge, skills, and attitudes relevant to team performance. Opportunities for in situ simulation abound, from building *living morbidity and mortality rounds* based on difficult prior cases, to *just in time* simulation focusing on a discreet and manageable element of team behaviors. In our trauma center, simulation has played a key role in shaping elements of trauma team culture, from designing the environment to integrating pre-briefings into standard operating procedures. And beyond simulation, debriefing after live clinical events allows for the identification and mitigation of safety hazards—team-based, environmental, and systemic—that would otherwise go unnoticed or uncorrected.

To be successful, teams must be situated in an organizational framework that supports the importance of team training. Teams don't exist in a bubble, and the complex interprofessional work of a trauma team is much more likely to succeed when organizations show overt and explicit support for team training [18]. In a system predicated on individual resilience, the onus is on organizational leadership to ensure top-down support to push the envelope of trauma team performance.

Key Notes

- Effective teamwork is not intuitive, as a team of experts does not make an expert team; instead, they rely on specific training and actions to create a high-performance trauma team.
- Elite trauma team performance employs a combination of actions and concepts, including implicit coordination, psychological safety, briefings and checklists, adaptive coordination, and effective language.
- Interprofessional team training by way of in situ simulation—simulation training that takes place in the physical workspace itself—is a powerful tool to drive home key knowledge, skills, and attitudes relevant to team performance.
- In a system predicated on individual resilience, the onus is on organizational leadership to ensure top-down support to push the envelope of trauma team performance.

References

1. Nawata K, Yamaguchi H, Aoshima M. Team implicit coordination based on transactive memory systems. Team Perform Manag. 2020;26(7/8):37–390.
2. Carley S. Five free strategies to improve your Resus Room 2018. St Emlyn's Blog. https://www.stemlynsblog.org/stemlynslive-five-free-strategies-to-improve-your-resuscitation-practice-st-emlyns/. Accessed 10 Sept 2022.
3. Entin EE, Serfaty D. Adaptive team coordination. Hum Factors. 1999;41(2):312–25.
4. Cannon-Bowers JA, Salas E, Converse S. Shared mental models in expert team decision making. In: Castellan Jr NJ, editor. Individual and group decision making: current issues. Hillsdale: Lawrence Erlbaum Associates, Inc; 1993. p. 221–46.
5. Mathieu J, Heffner TS, Goodwin GF, et al. The influence of shared mental models on team process and performance. J Appl Psychol. 2000;85(2):273–83.
6. Delizonna L. High-performing teams need psychological safety: here's how to create it. Harv Bus Rev. 2017. https://hbr.org/2017/08/high-performing-teams-need-psychological-safety-heres-how-to-create-it. Accessed 10 Sept 2022.
7. Kim S, Lee H, Connerton TP. How psychological safety affects team performance: mediating role of efficacy and learning behaviour. Front Psychol. 2020;11:1581.
8. Soares AE, Lopes MP. Social networks and psychological safety: a model of contagion. J Ind Eng Manag. 2014;7(5):950–1012.
9. Reid C, Brindley P, Hicks C, et al. Zero point survey: a multidisciplinary idea to STEP UP resuscitation effectiveness. Clin Exp Emerg Med. 2018;5(3):139–43.
10. Hicks C, Bridley P. COVID-19 miniRAGE with Hicks and Brindley. LITFL. 2020. https://litfl.com/covid-19-minirage-with-hicks-and-brindley/. Accessed 10 Sept 2022.
11. Purdy E, Alexander C, Shaw R, Brazil V. The team briefing: setting up relational coordination for your resuscitation. Clin Exp Emerg Med. 2022;7(1):1–4.
12. Sanjuan-Quiles A, Hernandez-Ramon MP, Julia-Sanchis R, et al. Handover of patients from prehospital emergency services to emergency departments. J Nurs Care Qual. 2019;34(2):169–74.
13. WHO Trauma Care Checklist. https://www.who.int/publications/i/item/trauma-care-checklist. Accessed 10 Sept 2022.
14. Yamada NK, Fuerch JH, Halamek LP. Impact of standardized communication techniques on errors during simulated neonatal resuscitation. Am J Perinatol. 2016;33:385–92.
15. Hargestam M, Lindkvist M, Brulin C, et al. Communication in interdisciplinary teams: exploring closed-loop communication during in situ trauma team training. BMJ Open. 2013;3:e003525.
16. Pocket Guide: TeamSTEPPS 2.0. 2013. https://www.ahrq.gov/teamstepps/instructor/essentials/pocketguide.html#:~:text=on%20next%20steps.-,Two%2DChallenge%20Rule,that%20it%20has%20been%20heard. Accessed 10 Sept 2022.
17. Burke S, Salas E, Pierce L. Understanding team adaptation: a conceptual analysis and model. J Appl Psychol. 2002;91(6):1189–207.
18. Driscoll PA, Vincent CA. Organizing an efficient trauma team. Injury. 1992;23(2):107–10.

Biological and Psychological Interactions of the Stress Response: How to Build Resilient Trauma Teams

12

Rebecca J. Ryznar, Christian Clodfelder, and Jeffrey Edwards

Biological Basis for the Human Stress Response

The human response to stress is a homeostatic mechanism in place to allow humans the ability to adapt to either real or perceived environmental stressors. The overall response to stressors is a complex balance of many organ systems. The modality, source, and duration of stressors produce a myriad of dynamic physiologic responses that can be both adaptive and maladaptive.

The discussion of the entire human physiologic response to stress is complex and beyond the scope of what is relevant to this text. However, a cursory understanding helps trauma teams appreciate and manage the response that they will inevitably face. The basic mechanisms of the human stress response will be discussed in an acute versus chronic context and by individual organ system.

SNS and HPA: Effectors of the Stress Response

The acute response to a stressor is an immediate, coordinated effort by the body to adapt to a changing environment. The primary mechanisms of initiating this response are the sympathetic nervous system (SNS)—colloquially known as the "fight-or-flight" response—and recruitment of the hypothalamic-pituitary-adrenal axis (HPA). Activation of both physiologic systems occur within seconds of real or perceived stress. The SNS and HPA axis provide elevated energy resources and upregulate metabolic processes to respond to changes in the environment. They also initiate long-term processes that eventually result in downregulation of potentially negative inflammatory responses.

The SNS is the nervous system's mechanism for responding to stressful stimuli. It is a collection of nerves that innervate tissues in the body and release primarily the catecholamines, norepinephrine and epinephrine, in order to cause changes in those tissues, which promote survival in dangerous situations. For example, the SNS activates the heart to pump harder and faster, it constricts blood vessels to organs so blood can be diverted away from digestive processes and toward the muscles for physical movement, and it dilates the pupils for enhanced awareness of surroundings. The SNS also activates the adrenal medulla, which can be viewed as a modified SNS nerve, except instead of innervating individual tissues it releases catecholamines into the blood stream, causing systemic sensitization to SNS tissue signals. All of these are highly useful when the organism is motivated to avoid danger, but it is also involved in responding to physiological stimuli that we encounter each day without realizing it, such as combatting a drop in blood pressure when we stand up from sitting [1].

The HPA plays an important role in the stress response as well, but while the SNS sends nerve signals to the adrenal cortex to release catecholamines, the HPA axis sends hormonal signals to activate the adrenal cortex to release cortisol. The key players of the HPA are the paraventricular nucleus (PVN) within the hypothalamus, the anterior pituitary gland, and the adrenal cortex. In response to stressors via the same mechanism as the SNS, the PVN synthesizes and releases corticotropin-releasing factor (CRF). CRF reaches the anterior pituitary gland via the hypophyseal portal system, causing the release of adrenocorticotropic hormone (ACTH) from corticotroph cells into systemic circulation [2]. When ACTH reaches the adrenal cortex, it stimulates the production and release of glucocorticoids into the blood. The glucocorticoid with the most relevance to human physiology is cortisol. Cortisol is a steroid hormone that interacts with glucocorticoid receptors in many tissues

R. J. Ryznar (✉)
Rocky Vista University, Englewood, CO, USA
e-mail: rryznar@rvu.edu

C. Clodfelder
University of Nebraska Medical Center, Omaha, NE, USA
e-mail: Christian.clodfelder@rvu.edu

J. Edwards
Swedish Family Medicine, Englewood, CO, USA
e-mail: Jeffrey.edwards@rvu.edu

L. Marshall Gillman, S. Widder (eds.), *Trauma Team Dynamics*, https://doi.org/10.1007/978-3-031-86312-7_12

of the human body. Cortisol stimulates gluconeogenesis, glycogenolysis, and lipolysis, which together increase the amount of glucose and fatty acids in the bloodstream for cells and tissues to utilize. Cortisol also upregulates catecholamine receptors in arterioles, increasing their sensitivity to epinephrine and norepinephrine and effectively raising arterial blood pressure. Cortisol also has potent immunosuppressive and anti-inflammatory effects [3, 4].

The first step in the stress response is sensing the stressful change in the environment. Physiologically, this is achieved by various sensors and receptors throughout the body. Those sensors transmit a signal to the central nervous system (CNS), at which point they are interpreted and reacted to. It is important to keep in mind that although there are many types of sensory input, the stress response system still reacts via the SNS and HPA axis, meaning different stressors have similar effects on the body.

A sudden loss of blood pressure is an example of a "physiological stress" for which the body has developed systems to control and maintain homeostasis. A sudden drop in blood pressure is detected by baroreceptors in the aortic arch and carotid sinus, and that information is communicated via general visceral afferent fibers to various nuclei within the brainstem. Through a series of neural reflex arcs, the SNS is activated and information is communicated via sympathetic nerve fibers to various effector organs through the release of neurotransmitters, classically epinephrine and norepinephrine. The end result is an increase in arterial blood pressure, heart rate, metabolic rate, and blood glucose concentration, thus alleviating the stress of low blood pressure. One of the effector organs is the adrenal medulla, which can be viewed as a modified SNS nerve that causes a massive systemic release of epinephrine and norepinephrine, rather than just releasing those catecholamines in a synaptic cleft. This dramatic increase in catecholamines allows for the entire body to respond to changes quickly and simultaneously [1]. All stressors follow this general pattern of detection, integration, and a corrective response to a real or perceived change is constant.

Pain is an example of a physiological stressor that we are able to perceive; it starts with the detection of painful stimuli, such as high temperature or chemical signs of cell damage, which results in the transmission of signals through afferent neurons. Some of these signals synapse in spinal reflex arcs, resulting in immediate withdrawal from a painful stimulus, such as a hot flame. Others continue up into the brain, where they are perceived as pain.

Psychological pain is a bit more complex, but it is important to note that psychological pain, often referred to as stress, can have very similar consequences as physiological stressors. The same effector mechanisms that regulate the body's response to physiological stressors control the response to psychological and emotional stressors, leading to increased blood pressure, decreased perfusion of vital organs, and shifting into a catabolic state.

The amygdala, a portion of the limbic system which functions in responding to emotion, fear, and anxiety, receives inputs from many of the sensory organs of the body. Stimuli that the body perceives as dangerous or harmful, such as visual and auditory perceptions, can activate the amygdala, which in turn activates the hypothalamus and other SNS nuclei within the brain. This results in the same downstream effects as described above. Although acute perception of stress is useful at times, such as the classic ancestral example of seeing a bear and needing to run, chronic activation of this psychological stress pathway can be quite toxic and lead to profound mental and physical health detriments.

The limbic system, more generally, is a subset of brain structures that are important in memory, behavior, and emotion. It is important to note that the limbic system is not considered to be the sole driver responsible for all of human emotion and behavior. Rather, it is one of many systems that contribute to the complex biologic concept of human emotion. Since the stress experienced by trauma teams is often mental, emotional, or psychological—a brief discussion about the basics of the limbic system is warranted. Within the cerebral cortex, the limbic structures include the limbic lobe, orbitofrontal cortex, entorhinal cortex, and piriform cortex. The hippocampus and fornix are also cortical structures that are considered a part of the limbic system. Other structures of the limbic system include the amygdala, septal nuclei, nucleus accumbens, the hypothalamus, anterior nuclei of the thalamus, and the mammillary bodies.

The hippocampus is involved in learning and memory, and the piriform cortex is necessary for processing olfactory information. As mentioned previously, the amygdala is one of the better understood structures within the limbic system, and its primary function is emotional response and decision-making [5]. Klüver–Bucy syndrome is a condition when a patient has bilateral destruction of the temporal lobe—which leads to destruction or damage of the amygdala. Initially investigated on experiments in monkeys, monkeys that suffer damage to the amygdala experience a complex constellation of symptoms. The monkeys lose their fear response and react to stimuli with lower than usual aggression. This results in a very tame, docile affect. The monkeys also experience hyperphagia, pica, and hyperorality. Hypersexuality and visual agnosia are also commonly described in Klüver–Bucy syndrome. The same condition has been described in human beings, with docility, dietary changes, and hyperorality being the most common findings [6].

Fear and aggression have long been thought of as the primary role of the amygdala. It also is known to play a more nuanced role in human emotional processing. There is a correlation between higher rates of mental disorders, such as anxiety and depression, with patients who have a deficit in certain cell types of the amygdala. These patients with decreased concentrations of amygdala granule cells also have lower emotional functioning compared to standard controls.

Now that we have covered the inciting events of the stress response, let's discuss the downstream effects of those signals. Understanding both the short- and long-term physiologic changes is particularly valuable to emergency personnel because recognizing and anticipating changes that occur during difficult, stressful, and traumatic situations can improve performance and recovery.

Acute Versus Chronic Stress

The acute response to stress is regulated by negative feedback loops from downstream products like cortisol, epinephrine, and norepinephrine, which act on the adrenal gland, hypothalamus, and anterior pituitary to suppress continued stimulation. Normally, this negative feedback keeps the stress response from over-activating and maintains homeostasis. Chronic stress, however, occurs when a stressful stimulus is maintained for long periods of time, such as in repeated exposures or failures in the negative feedback loop. Repeated exposure to stressors is viewed as a cumulative process. Repeated or prolonged exposures to stressors cause an HPA response and thus a cumulative increase in glucocorticoid burden, colloquially known as "too much cortisol." Data shows that the adrenal gland becomes both larger and more sensitive to ACTH with repeated exposure to ACTH. For example, there is literature demonstrating that surgical stress can result in long-term, continuous secretion of cortisol despite an absence of a corresponding increase in ACTH levels [7]. Additionally, immune effectors experience higher rates of apoptosis and involution after repeated exposure to ACTH, resulting in decreased immunological competence and increased susceptibility to infection and cancer. It is believed that the mechanism responsible for this increased sensitivity to ACTH is due to downregulation of glucocorticoid receptors in the hypothalamus and other brain regions that are necessary for negative feedback regulation [3].

It is well established that dysregulation of the HPA (hypothalamus-pituitary-adrenal) axis is part of the underlying pathophysiology of mental health disorders, indicating low resilience. Low resilience disorders include depression, anxiety, PTSD, and burn out [3]. The main determinants of HPA axis and SNS activity include genetics, early life experiences, and current life stress and other experiences [1]. Repeated stress influences immunity by stimulating cortisol and adrenaline secretion from the adrenal cortex and medulla, respectively. Stress also causes the release of noradrenaline from postganglionic sympathetic nerve terminals in blood vessels and lymphoid organs. Glucocorticoids in turn result in changes in the production of regulatory type 1 and type 2 cytokines (Th1 and Th2). Downstream of this process, glucocorticoids regulate physiological events and inhibit further HPA axis activation through intracellular receptors located in the brain and peripheral tissues [2]. More specifically, this results in suppression of pro-inflammatory cytokine secretion while promoting anti-inflammatory cytokine secretion [2]. Chronic stress is associated with up-regulation of pro-inflammatory cytokines and down-regulation of the anti-inflammatory cytokine pathways [3].

Stress and the Cardiovascular System

One of the most obvious and immediate effects of the human stress response is its influence on the cardiovascular system. SNS effects on the heart can be either chronotropic, inotropic, or dromotropic, all of which combine to increase cardiac output. Chronotropic refers to an increase in heart rate. Inotropic is an increase in contractility of the myocardium. Dromotropic is an increase in conduction velocity within the electrical conduction system of the heart. SNS activation and the action of catecholamines also have important effects on blood vessels. Alpha-1 receptors cause vasoconstriction, whereas Beta-2 receptor activation results in vasodilation. Due to a differential distribution of these receptors on different vascular beds, blood is shunted away from the viscera and toward the heart, lungs, brain, and skeletal muscles—with a net overall increase in systemic vascular resistance and blood pressure. Additionally, cortisol upregulates Alpha-1 receptors within vascular smooth muscle cells, increasing their sensitivity to circulating catecholamines.

The ANS and HPA axis also influence an important cardiac parameter referred to as heart rate variability (HRV). Specifically, HRV refers to the variation in the interval between heartbeats, specifically the RR interval. In general, decreased parasympathetic input or increased sympathetic input will reduce the HRV, while increased parasympathetic or decreased sympathetic input will increase the HRV [8].

In the literature describing HRV, HRV is divided into either low frequency (0.04–0.15 Hz) or high frequency (0.15–0.40 Hz)—with low frequency referring to low HRV and therefore more sympathetic activity, and high frequency referring to high HRV and therefore more parasympathetic activity. High-frequency HRV has been demonstrated to be very clearly correlated with PSNS activity, while the connection between lower HRV and SNS activity appears to be more complex. Knowing that different frequencies of HRV are associated with different levels of autonomic activity, it is often used as a rough measure for "stress" levels during exercise, simulation, or research. It is also often used as a parameter gauging the health or responsiveness of an individual's autonomic and cardiac function. Literature demonstrates that low HRV has been shown to be a predictor of poor outcomes and mortality after acute myocardial infarction [9]. Patients who are victims of sudden cardiac death have also been found to have lower frequency HRV compared to healthy controls. Additionally, patients who survive sudden cardiac death are shown to have depressed HRV levels [10]. Correlations between HRV and differing outcomes in other conditions such as heart failure, post-cardiac transplantation outcomes, diabetic kidney disease, and susceptibility to SIDS are also currently being explored.

It is understood that the vagus nerve is a central player in both the parasympathetic SNS and the HPA axis. The connection between the vagus nerve and both of these systems is bidirectional, providing both inputs and outputs that these systems use to regulate the human stress response. As mentioned earlier, the correlation between high-frequency HRV and PSNS activity is well described. Additionally, cortisol levels, high-frequency HRV, and direct vagus nerve tone have all been shown to be strongly linked. Isolated increases in cortisol have been shown to increase resting HRV [11]. The connection and interplay between all of these physiological variables and their effect on HRV makes it an excellent candidate for a general marker for stress levels. This could be used to monitor stress levels on trauma teams during real life scenarios, as well as a marker for the effectiveness of simulation and training.

The kidneys also play an intimate role in the body's hemodynamic and cardiovascular response to acute stressors. Activation of Beta-1 receptors in the kidneys lead to the release of renin, eventually leading to release of angiotensin II. Angiotensin II further increases sympathetic activity, causes the kidneys to retain electrolytes and fluid, increases aldosterone and ADH secretion, and directly causes vasoconstriction. All of these serve to further increase blood pressure [4].

Overall, the cardiovascular response to stressors is substantial. The acute response to stress within the cardiovascular system can manifest as tachycardia, palpitations, and hypertension. The increased workload on the heart can result in myocardial infarction, essentially the heart working harder than it can handle. Although rare, the stress placed on the heart can also transiently weaken the musculature of the heart to result in severe dysfunction, a condition known as Takotsubo cardiomyopathy. Takotsubo cardiomyopathy is still poorly understood but often mimics myocardial infarctions and presents with chest pain and hemodynamic instability, usually following extreme emotional or physical stress and a sudden surge of catecholamines and corticosteroids. Chronic stressful stimuli are also a well-described driver of cardiovascular disease. High blood pressures and high volumes cause endothelial cell damage and are the driving force behind atherosclerosis and vascular disease. These can lead to coronary vascular disease and increased risk of myocardial infarction, as well as microvasculopathies that can cause renal disease and retinopathy, perfusion deficits, and impaired function of many organ systems. Overall, hypertension is the most important preventable risk factor for premature death worldwide [9].

Stress and the Immune System

The immune system is significantly altered in both acute and chronic stress exposure. Whether or not these effects are proinflammatory or anti-inflammatory is variable depending on the modality of stress, duration, repeated exposure, and an individual's perception of stress. The effect of chronic stress on the function of the immune system is a major driver of morbidity and mortality, so understanding the sequelae of chronic stress is essential to maintaining health and resilience in those with high stress lifestyles and careers.

As is the case with the rest of the body, the immune system's response to stressors begins with the HPA and SNS response. These integrated neuroendocrine and autonomic responses kick off signaling pathways that enhance humoral immunity while suppressing cellular immunity. This switch in modalities is accomplished by stimulating Th12 cells and suppressing the function of Th1 and antigen presenting cells. It is hypothesized that this is an evolutionary response to the primary stressor of early humankind: infections. This shift effectively limits the detrimental effects of a non-specific, systemic immune reaction, while simultaneously enhancing a specific, localized reaction. The proinflammatory cytokines IL-1, TNFa, and IFNy are downregulated, while anti-inflammatory cytokines, IL-10, and TGFb are stimulated. (Local tissues that are damaged or inflamed can still attract proinflammatory cytokines via neutrophil recruitment.)

In contrast to this rapid response, long-term exposure to stressful stimuli is a well-described risk for developing infection, autoimmune disease, and malignancy. This increased incidence in disease is attributed to disruption in the homeostasis of defense mechanisms. Studies have shown that during acute stress, the concentration of CD16-rich NK cells increases—which potentiate antibody-dependent immunity, but chronic stress results in a decline in NK cytotoxic activity. Not only does the concentration of NKs decline with chronic stress, but also their responsiveness to cytokines. T-cells have also been shown to lose their proliferative response to mitogens, lectins, and activation of the T-cell receptor when exposed to chronic stress [10].

Cellular immunity isn't the only thing affected by exposure to chronic stress. Several studies have demonstrated that individuals suffering from chronic stress have a diminished antibody response to vaccines. It is thought that chronic activation of the HPA axis leads to persistent elevation of glucocorticoids, which interrupts the normal balance of the Th1/

Th2 response, thus hindering an appropriate response to vaccinations [11].

Failure to appropriately regulate the stress response in both the SNS and HPA system have been linked to a variety of different pathologies. Hypertension, autoimmune disease, immunosuppression, affective, and psychological disorders have all been described in relation to exposure to chronic stress. There are well-described diagnoses like major depressive disorder and PTSD that are directly related to stressful exposures. The connection of chronic stress exposure and human disease is still poorly understood and ongoing researching into prevention and therapy is of specific value to healthcare workers, first responders, military personnel, and other individuals regularly exposed to high-stress situations [10].

The physiology and biochemical pathways involved in the human stress response are complex and multifaceted. Not every signaling pathway or secondary messenger translates directly into the lived experience of an individual. First responders, medical workers, and other members of trauma teams need to be aware of the acute physical and behavioral changes that accompany the stress response in order to recognize it and respond appropriately. This is important in the acute setting to manage stress and be an effective operator in each situation, but also in the setting of chronic sense to maintain resilience, health, and long-term performance (Fig. 12.1).

Stress and Sleep

During daily life, many of the body's homeostatic mechanisms are maintained and regulated over a 24-hour period by circadian rhythms, the body's internal clock. Circadian rhythms are maintained both by a neurological "master-clock" within the hypothalamic suprachiasmatic nucleus as well as numerous autoregulatory peripheral feedback loops in most tissues. Through a complex process of gene transcription, protein production, and negative feedback loops on itself, the genes *CLOCK* and *BMAL1* are able to generate an internal 24-hour rhythm in the body, allowing for time-of-day-dependent maintenance and regulation of essential body systems. Disruption of these internal mechanisms can lead to suboptimal physiologic performance and response to stressors, thereby exacerbating the detrimental effects of acute and chronic stress. Literature shows that disruptions to the normal maintenance of homeostasis through circadian mechanisms can manifest as cardiovascular, immune, metabolic, and cognitive pathology. This is particularly important to recognize for trauma teams, first responders, and healthcare workers, who are often subject to chaotic schedules and sudden interruptions at any time of the day.

Cortisol plays an important role in the maintenance of the circadian rhythm, a physiologic pattern that promotes appropriate wakefulness and relaxation to optimize both performance and recovery. In humans, cortisol is secreted in an anticipatory fashion, peaking in the morning just before waking, followed by a steady decline until its lowest levels, which are maintained during sleep. This system primes the body for when it expects to be under the most stress, such as during waking hours, and promotes relaxation when it is time to sleep. Fluctuations in cortisol levels occur throughout the day based on stressors and external factors, but the overall pattern of peak levels in the day time and lowest at night is maintained solely by circadian mechanisms.

Cortisol levels are just one example of anticipatory homeostatic control based on circadian rhythms. Tissue sensitivity to glucocorticoids, adrenal response to catecholamines, temperature control, and even behavior and physical activity are all known to be dependent on the time of day.

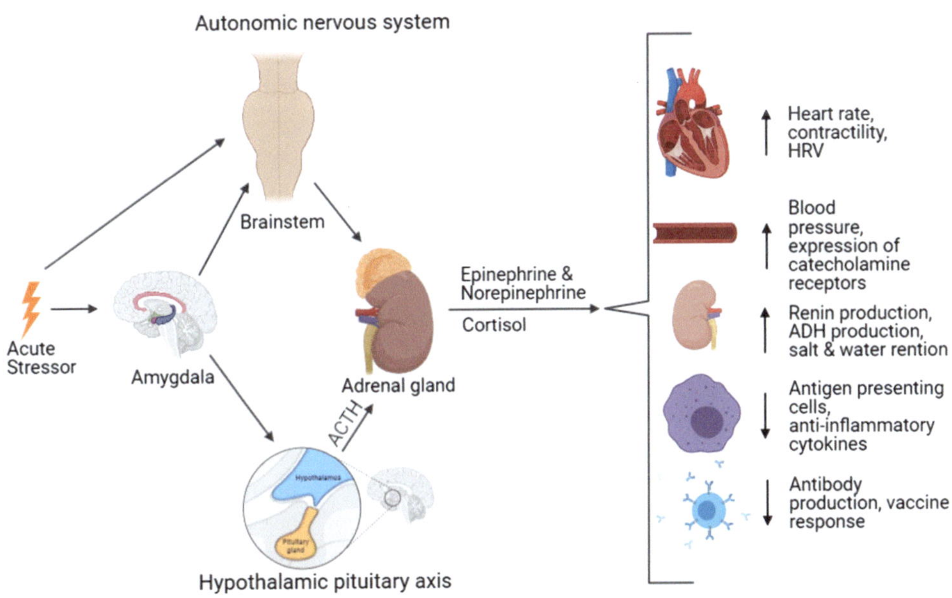

Fig. 12.1 Simplified schematic view of the human stress response and major downstream physiologic effects. (Figure made with BioRender)

It has long been understood that stress leads to elevated cortisol levels, and the negative health outcomes from stress are only due to consistently elevated cortisol. Literature is now showing that this is most likely an oversimplification. Losing synchronicity of cortisol levels with the inherent internal circadian rhythm has many poor health effects, even if average levels of cortisol are only minimally changed. In patients with primary hypocortisolism, the current treatment protocol is to administer steroids three times a day. Although peak levels of cortisol are achieved in the daytime, with low levels during sleep hours—the natural anticipatory rise in cortisol prior to awakening is absent. This shifts cortisol levels away from the natural cycle. These patients report increased morbidity and mortality from cardiovascular disease, malignancy, and infectious disease. They also often report fatigue and difficulty concentration. These patients are not exposed to chronically high levels of cortisol, but even just the disruption in the pulsatile release of cortisol produces symptoms analogous to chronic hypercortisolism. Synthetic glucocorticoids are one of the most widely used medications today. More than 75% of patients prescribed synthetic glucocorticoids report adverse side effects, even at low doses [1].

The chaotic schedules of trauma teams can affect more than just cortisol levels related to circadian disturbances. Sleep itself is an essential process. Sleep plays an important role in metabolism, immunity, brain function, and cardiovascular health. It is well understood that sub-optimal sleep has significant outcomes on health. Optimal sleep is defined by having sufficient duration, regularity, appropriate timing, and absence of disturbances. Maintaining all of these criteria is becoming increasingly difficult for trauma teams.

The downstream effects of sleep disruption include disruption of the circadian rhythm, which has previously been described to have dramatic implications with fluctuating cortisol levels. Additionally, sleep disruption increases the secretion of catecholamines, ACTH, and cortisol. It causes upregulation of proinflammatory cytokines such as IL-1, IL-6, and TNF. Sleep disturbance also has dramatic metabolic effects, including decreasing insulin sensitivity and disrupting the hormonal balance that controls appetite, leading to an increase in hunger. All of these effects cumulatively lead to a high risk of cardiovascular disease, type 2 diabetes, obesity, and cancer [12].

The health of trauma teams is obviously of utmost importance, but the safety of patients and overall efficacy of trauma teams is also hampered by fatigue and sleep disturbance. There are many studies that demonstrate how specific tasks, such as driving or tracking objects, are severely impaired in sleep-deprived subjects. In individual cases where fatigue or falling asleep has resulted in a poor patient outcome, these cases are generally viewed as isolated incidents. Currently, the general consensus within the healthcare industry is that fatigue or sleep deprivation of healthcare personnel is not associated with harm to patients. The current workplace culture of the healthcare industry, particularly emergency and trauma care, is that long hours and on-call time are necessary to provide enough exposure to trainees. Additionally, requiring continuous 24/7 coverage 365 days a year often requires long hours for those with the highest specialized training.

Other industries have been less hesitant to address to the potential harms of sleep-deprived workers. The aviation industry has very stringent, federally mandated rules to manage stress of pilots and other crewmembers. Additionally, when investigating accidents, the National Transportation Safety Board formally recognizes "fatigue" as a factor or cause in causing accidents [13]. Historically, aviation has a phenomenal safety record and is extremely safe for its customers. Further studies are necessary to see if the same strategies would have beneficial outcomes if applied to other fields related to trauma care.

It is clear that increases in overall concentrations of cortisol and other stress response molecules have implications for human health [1]. Their relation to times of day is also extremely important—particularly in the context of trauma teams. Understanding that the impact of stressful events can be potentiated when they occur outside of daytime hours has major implications for anyone who works unusual hours. Additionally, the direct effects of loss or disturbed sleep have dramatic consequences on the health and performance of trauma teams. Sleep hygiene, rotating schedules, mandatory rest/sleep times, and fatigue management may have greater implications in the health of trauma teams than previously anticipated.

Recognizing Chronic Versus Acute Stress

A simplified model for understanding how to discriminate between acute and chronic stress on human physiology has been described as "General Adaptation Syndrome." This term describes in general, the stress-induced physiologic changes through three separate stages: the alarm reaction stage, the resistance stage, and the exhaustion stage. The second two stages of this syndrome represent pathologic changes of prolonged exposure to stress, and it is important to recognize them as signs that chronic stress may be accumulating so that a response can be mounted.

The alarm response stage refers to the acute signs and symptoms in response to a stressor, as well as the "fight-or-flight" response. After resolution of the initial stressor, the body lowers catecholamine and cortisol levels, begins repairing any damage, and returns physiologic response to their resting levels (heart rate, blood pressure, etc.).

If the stressor continues to persist, the body's response will adapt to better cope with this chronic exposure to stress. Continued secretion of stress hormones will maintain the body's physiological stress mechanisms—this is called the resistance stage. Poor concentration, frustration, and irritability are common psychological consequences.

If the stressors still continue beyond this stage, the body will then begin to enter the exhaustion phase. This is where individuals will experience fatigue, depression, anxiety, burnout, and reduced tolerance to other stressors. Hypertension, immunosuppression, metabolic disturbances, and increased risks of malignancy are some of the physiologic consequences of the exhaustion stage [14].

One of the most effective ways to maintain resilience and avoid the long-term health consequences of stress can be avoidance of unnecessary exposure. Understanding the symptoms of each stage can help individuals recognize when they are experiencing a pathologic response to a prolonged stressor, prompting them to evaluate and change their behavior and exposures if necessary.

Psychological Basis for the Human Stress Response

While an understanding of the biological basis for the human stress response is certainly helpful, perhaps the most pragmatic lessons on this topic involve an analysis of the perceived experiences of people in their daily lives, which can be defined in psychological terms. The number of yearly articles on the psychology of trauma has increased exponentially over the last few decades, ramping up from dozens per year in the 1970s to hundreds and thousands by 2020. Clearly, this is a rising field of study, and it especially bears relevance in the medical community, which both treats trauma and is itself frequently a traumatic occupation.

Why We Care: Burnout

Burnout, a state of mental exhaustion, depersonalization, and decreased sense of personal accomplishment, is common among trauma team workers and can lead to impaired functioning and reduced happiness [15]. Factors leading to burnout include a physically and emotionally stressful work environment, risk of personal harm, low pay, and compounding sleep debt [16]. Burnout has been shown to have a negative effect on EMS worker performance and has been correlated with an increased number of sick days taken by those workers, as well as greater reported intention to leave the job [17, 18]. It is clearly a priority of trauma team leaders to address this issue.

Trauma and Its Lifelong Impacts: Brain Changes, Substance Abuse, Chronic Disease

The impact of psychological trauma on a person can begin very early, with adverse childhood experiences (ACEs) being correlated with both mental and physical health impacts [19]. Traumatic experiences in adulthood are also substantial, as professions such as first responders and trauma healthcare teams often undergo intensely stressful experiences and not uncommonly develop PTSD [20]. Although stress can be a valuable factor in human development, traumatic experiences can have lasting psychological and indeed neurobiological impacts, with pathologic brain morphology changes of PTSD overlapping with those of traumatic brain injuries [21].

ACEs have been correlated with decreases in prefrontal paralimbic gray matter volume (GMV) in the lower ventral, rostral and dorsolateral prefrontal, and insular cortical areas [22]. These morphological changes are not mere curiosity. In particular, the lowered insular GMV has been associated with a higher frequency of alcohol and cannabis use, which in turn has their own health consequences and professional risks [22]. Poor coping skills, such as self-blame, binge-eating, and substance abuse, have also been correlated with increased burnout [23]. It is easy to see that the combination of a stressful work environment with poor coping skills creates a vicious cycle, highlighting the need for stress management education and training.

Other consequences of chronic stress include an increased chronic disease burden. Occupational stress in first responders has been correlated with cardiovascular disease risk, including decreased cardiorespiratory fitness and sleep quality, as well as increased arterial stiffness [24]. These physical changes not only represent a risk of acute health events, but they also can affect work performance, decrease overall wellness through physical detriments that carry psychological consequences, and create a cycle of health-related stress and work-related stress that compounds on itself.

Bias in Studying PTSD: Variable Responses and Stigma

One of the more perplexing phenomena surrounding the human stress response is that people respond differently to comparable stressors, that some may develop PTSD while others apparently undergo only transient disruptions in their normal functioning [25]. We won't discuss the cultural, biological, or other sundry variables that lead to those individual responses because they are far too numerous and do not produce generalizable insight, and besides the risk of PTSD is high enough to warrant education regardless. However, this is an apt opportunity to point out that there is likely substantial bias underlying many studies in this area, although the slant of that bias is difficult to parse out; many people who cope do not seek treatment and are therefore not observed, and likewise, many who fail to cope also do not seek treatment or even exhibit external evidence of distress [26]. Another confounding variable is that there still exists significant stigma surrounding mental health, especially among professions with "cultures of toughness," such as in police forces, but also even in professions that are inherently educated in the biological and psychological ramifications of stress, such as the medical field, both of which have been shown to have higher rates of PTSD than the general population [26, 27]. In these cultures, it may be seen as "weak" to seek help because the individual is perceived as lacking self-sufficiency. That pervasive stigma is a primary reason why people who could benefit from mental health aid do not seek it, why it may go underreported even in anonymous surveys, and, practically speaking, why mental health education is so imperative.

Education Helps

It has been demonstrated that people with higher levels of education on mental illness, such as psychiatrists in comparison to medical students or non-healthcare workers, exhibit less mental health stigma and improved self-care [28]. This is why professional education on the human stress response and how to manage it are important, especially in the setting of stressful occupations: people who are more aware of mental health issues are empowered to take action or seek help by volition of that awareness. People with mental health education are also less likely to contribute to cultural stigma against seeking help, thereby affording others more chance to do so.

Practical Strategies for Alleviating Stress

Education is only one piece of the puzzle. Emerging research suggests that there are many practical strategies that can be employed in order to mitigate the effects of a stressful occupation and augment resilience in team members. Those strategies include individual approaches such as mindfulness, emotional regulation, and communication skills training; team approaches such as resiliency training and stress management workshops; as well as structural/organizational methods such as workload/schedule rotations, debriefing sessions, and focus groups [29]. Although genetics apparently do play a role in determining one's resilience, with some people being extremely predisposed to either developing PTSD or being hyper-resilient, these strategies have been shown to be effective for those in the window of opportunity that lies between those extremes [30]. These proven effective strategies have a wide range of benefits that may be tailored into approaches to suit team and individual goals (Table 12.1). The most recent literature reviews suggest that a bundled, multifaceted approached is best for achieving optimal results [29].

Mindfulness and mind-body practices, which train the individual to be cognizant of their physical and emotional states to better control those states, have been shown to have positive effects on PTSD symptoms, such as anxiety, depression, and intrusive memories [31]. Yoga, for example, has been highly studied, and implementing even a single session per week has been shown to reduce subjective stress and anxiety [32]. Improvements from yoga and mindfulness training have been shown to improve regulation of the sympathetic nervous system and the HPA axis, demonstrating improvements in physiological parameters such as blood pressure, heart rate, cortisol, and cytokine levels [33].

Table 12.1 Coping strategies and notable effects

Coping strategies	Effect
Mindfulness, mind-body practices	Decreased anxiety and depression Fewer intrusive memories
Yoga	Decreased subjective stress and anxiety Improved SNS and HPA axis regulation
General self-care (sleep, diet, exercise, social/spiritual activities)	Decreased burnout Particular benefit for newer team members
Reinforcement/reminders of coping strategies	Improved adherence to strategies Improved cooperation Decreased workplace stigma
Stress management workshops	Decreased burnout
Debriefing sessions	Improved resiliency Reduced compassion fatigue Fewer symptoms of PTSD
Shifts <12 hours, working <40 hours per week	Fewer adverse events
Fixed night shifts	Synchronization, improved performance Decreased job satisfaction Higher burnout rates

Note that not all effects are entirely positive

Self-care strategies, such as improving sleep hygiene, focusing on physical, spiritual, and social wellness, have demonstrated benefits particularly inexperienced trauma team members [34]. Coping styles that emphasize social integration and spiritual engagement, as well as specific strategies such as art therapy, have been correlated with decreased burnout rates [23, 35]. However, it is important for team leaders and members to appreciate that being informed on these strategies is not always ample for individuals to actually carry out these tasks, which admittedly can seem like additional work. It is therefore important to find ways to reinforce the importance of self-care on a regular basis, such as posting signs, encouraging healthy snacks, building a culture of support and civility, and organizing healthy group activities [36].

Team activities, such as stress management workshops, have also been proven effective, having been shown to decrease burnout measures in the medical field [37]. Debriefing sessions have also demonstrated efficacy, such as in improving resiliency and reducing compassion fatigue among emergency department staff [38]. While medical teams always strive to provide optimal care, mistakes do happen and result in not only patient harm, but also harm to care providers who are sometimes termed "second victims" of medical error [39]. In the setting of adverse events, Critical Incident Stress Debriefing (CISD) has been shown to reduce the risk of PTSD-like symptoms in emergency service personnel, although some reviews of the literature also demonstrate uncertainty this area [40, 41].

Structural strategies, such as organizing shift schedules to prevent burnout, are also important to consider. A 2016 literature review found that, although there is significant complexity in studying the effects of shift work, employees working shifts longer than 12 hours, working over 40 hours per week, and overly limiting break times are associated with adverse events [42]. Interestingly, an analysis of whether or not to implement rotating shifts does not provide clear recommendations; not surprisingly, working fixed night shifts results in lower job satisfaction, but working fixed night shifts also enables resynchronization to a sleep schedule, meaning it is up to leaders to appraise their team's situation and enact policy accordingly [42]. A 2017 review also found it difficult to make a conclusion on the impact of shift work due to multiple contextual and individual factors, but suffice to say that other studies have shown that shift irregularity and more frequent night shifts are correlated with higher burnout rates [43, 44].

With the realm of stress reduction being so complex, it is perhaps pertinent for teams and individuals to focus on only the most efficacious strategies with the highest amount of empirical evidence, while promoting an overall culture of valuing wellness. Fortunately, modern research techniques are becoming more and more suited to facilitating that goal.

Hyper-realistic Simulation Training

The field of self-care is vast and expanding with each year, but it is not always as efficient as would be suited to a professional environment. There are many pseudoscientific and even fantastical frameworks for self-care, some that may warrant expedient dismissal while others should be viewed with skeptical optimism. While most frameworks are anecdotally helpful to at least some individuals, when efficiency is a priority, they can actually represent a distraction from the pursuit of an effective strategy. With that in mind, one of the most promising methods for optimizing the psychological response to stressful scenarios is hyper-realistic simulation training. Simulation training has been shown to not only improve the subjective experience of individuals as well as physiologic, biochemical, and epigenetic parameters, but also to improve the quality of care during actual situations, including in the trauma team setting specifically [45].

The concept behind simulation training relies on an understanding of Inverted U Theory, which postulates that optimal performance is attained when there is a balance between pressure and stress. Pressure can be viewed as a positive motivator, whereas stress is translated into performance deficits. A person who has too little pressure to perform is unmotivated, but a person who has too much stress often experiences a decrease in performance. Stress can present as distracting thoughts, such as being worried about failure, or physical barriers to functioning, such as lack of sleep. Based on the evidence previously discussed that first responders and trauma teams have an abundance of stress, the goal of simulation training should be to acclimate team members to stressful scenarios so that real experiences are less intense. This allows team members to interpret situations more in terms of positive pressure and less in terms of negative stress on a cognitive level, and we can see the efficacy of simulation training by measuring biochemical markers of stress.

Development of a Stress Measurement Tool

One of the most difficult aspects of studying stress and creating mitigating strategies is the development of an accurate and precise screening tool for stress. Historically, these screening tools have been questionnaires that query an individual about their subjective experience in an effort to obtain quantifiable data. Although these tools have been validated clinically, the survey strategy presents several confounding variables.

One issue is the limitation of language; the meaning of words can be interpreted differently by different cultures, by different people within a culture, and even by the same people at different times. Finding effective ways to communicate is particularly difficult for surveys of feelings, and even more so when those feelings involve levels of conscious and unconscious understanding, such as they do in the setting of trauma.

Another issue is, again, stigma. People that live in a society or cultural niche where mental health is stigmatized may be hesitant to provide honest answers to questions about their own mental health. It is often beneficial to have mental health professionals administer surveys, which allows the use of counseling strategies to get more accurate information. Although clinically useful, that method also introduces a whole new level of bias.

One of the tools we have currently is the Brief Resilience Scale (BRS), which measures "resilience" and is a relatively strong predictor of mental health quality in the setting of traumatic experiences [46]. The BRS can help predict the effect of traumatic experiences such as ACEs on mental health, thereby allowing clinicians to make informed decisions on prognosis and treatment [47]. Another common tool that is popular in the primary care setting and which has been widely validated is the PHQ-9, a 9-item survey that stratifies patients into mild, moderate, and severe depression categories [48]. But even though tools like the BRS and PHQ-9 offer substantial clinical utility, there is still a clear impetus for more quantifiable and generalizable tools.

The next section will introduce new and upcoming research into biological markers of stress and mind wellness, or the ability to respond to stress. These methods are arguably more objective than survey screening tools and may serve as a bridge to further validate those methods as well as to explore new directions for research.

Resilience Is Individualized

Resilience is a key factor in determining the success of any trauma team dynamic. Resilience refers to the ability to bounce back, biologically and psychologically. This requires a combination of strong body and mind. For a trauma team to be resilient, the requirements are two-fold. Each individual member of the team must have developed resilience, and the team functioning in response to trauma must be resilient. Optimal team performance would fall under the optimum stress peak of the inverted U model of stress [54]. We are relying on individuals who have built their own resilience to stressful events by developing appropriate coping mechanisms and maintaining mental, emotional, physical health, and avoiding chronic social defeat and chronic substance abuse [49]. Resilience is critical for establishing a highly functional team that can handle stress appropriately without medical errors. The following sections highlight valuable points of understanding and improving resilience in a high-stress environment.

We know that HPA activity is quite individualized, resulting in cortisol levels and reactivity to stress that is highly variable depending upon the person. In order to avoid burnout or other disorders related to chronic stress, cortisol levels and stress reactivity must be regulated. Individuals with major depression, baseline cortisol concentrations appear to be increased; whereas, for bipolar disorder, cortisol concentrations are only increased in patients with a late age-of-onset. On the contrary, in patients with anxiety (generalized anxiety disorder, panic disorder), cortisol levels are decreased compared to healthy individuals. The same has been reported for posttraumatic stress disorder and individuals who have attempted suicide, where after an initial increase in cortisol release, the cortisol output decreases below baseline [57]. Both exaggerated/high and blunted/low stress reactivity of the HPA axis at baseline has been shown to correlate with mental health and disease outcomes. Interestingly, exaggerated stress reactivity at baseline predicted an increase in risk factors for cardiovascular disease and decreased telomere length at follow-up. In contrast, blunted stress reactivity predicted future increased adiposity and obesity, more depression, anxiety and PTSD symptoms, greater illness frequency, musculoskeletal pain and regulatory T-cell percentage, poorer cognitive ability, poorer self-reported health, and physical disability and lower bone mass [58]. Additionally, a pro-inflammatory state has been observed across many mental health disorders, including PTSD and individuals attempting suicide, including an increase in IL6 levels [59]. Altogether, it is clear that an imbalance in the concentration and reactivity of molecules that regulate the stress response is a hallmark of low resilience and poor coping. What can be done for individuals who struggle with low resilience?

Factors Contributing to Resilient Phenotypes

What determines an individual's resilience? Complex interactions between an individual's gene variants, his or her particular history of exposure to environmental stressors and an array of epigenetic changes that result in variable gene expression patterns, determine the degree of adaptability to novel challenges. The combination of genetics and epigenetics determines the function of the neural circuitry involved in stress responses whether they are acute, chronic, novel, or not (Fig. 12.2). Allelic variants in the following genes have been most tightly connected to resilient phenotypes: FKP5 (regulator of glucocorticoid sensitivity), CRHR1 (corticotropin releasing hormone receptor 1), SLC6A4 (human serotonin transporter), COMBT (regulator of dopamine and noradrenaline), NPY (Neuropeptide Y), and BDNF (brain-derived neurotrophic factor) [68]. Recent studies have begun to yield evidence of gene-gene and gene-environment interactions determining individual in stress responses. For example,

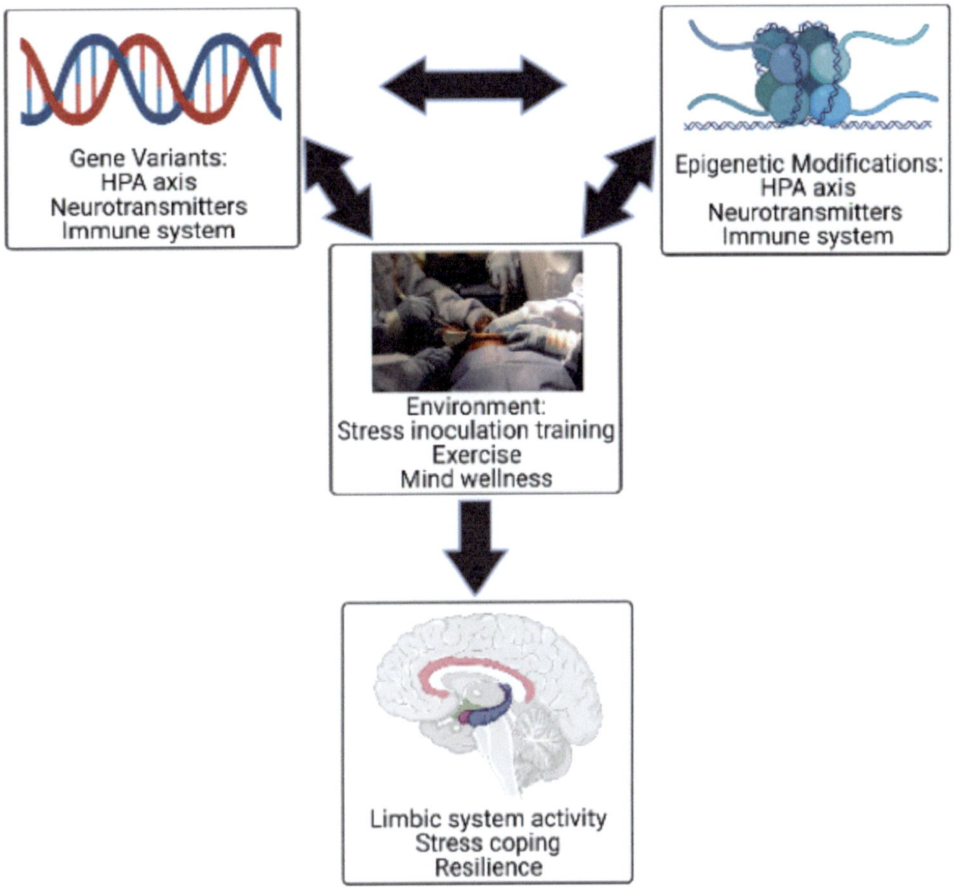

Fig. 12.2 Factors contributing to individualized resilience phenotypes. A combination of genetics, epigenetics, and environment all interplay to determine an individual's ability to cope with stress. (Figure made with BioRender)

interactions between 5-HTTLPR (region of SLC6A4), COMBT, and traumatic life events have been shown to affect the risk for depression and emotional reactivity to stressful stimuli. An additional example of gene-environment interactions determining resilience would be the observation that social support seems to mitigate the effects of the short allele of 5-HTTLPR, and the 5-HTTLPR and higher risk BDNF genotypes interact with stressful life events to result in higher risk for depression [67]. Lastly and most importantly, epigenetics contributes to individual resilience. Epigenetics refers to inheritance of biochemical information that is not encoded in the DNA sequence. This biochemical information in the form of modifications to histone tails and methylation to DNA causes stable changes in chromatin structure that underlies long-lasting alterations in gene expression. An additional form of an epigenetic mark includes non-coding RNA. Non-coding RNA typically functions to regulate gene expression though inhibition of mRNA translation, rather than altering chromatin structure directly. Genes that seem to be epigenetically modified in response to and regulating coping to traumatic stress fall under categories of players in the neural, endocrine, and immune pathways [68].

Epigenetic changes in genes regulating the HPA axis, specifically FKPB5 and NR3C1, are correlated with resilient phenotypes [79]. Key to note here is that the epigenome is different according to cell type and tissue, but studies are finding that alterations in the periphery can be indicative of epigenetic CNS dysregulation [67]. Studies have shown that DNA methylation of FKBP5 and NR3C1 in lymphocytes has been measured as predictors of psychotherapy outcome in combat veterans with PTSD. Results showed that increased NR3C1 DNA methylation measured pre-treatment did predict positive treatment outcome, although DNA methylation itself was not altered between pre- and post- treatment. On the other hand, FKBP5 DNA methylation pre-treatment did not predict treatment outcome but did decrease among those who responded to therapy. Among treatment-responders, FKBP5 mRNA expression was elevated, compared to non-responders. Also, as measured in peripheral blood, mononuclear cells in combat veterans with PTSD compared to combat veterans without PTSD. Methylation patterns at this location were also associated with three measures of functional GC activity. Results highlight that decreased NR3C1 methylation could either confer risk of PTSD development or be a result of PTSD development, and that epigenetic alteration of NR3C1 could functionally alter neuroendocrine system outputs [69, 70]. Both of these genes code for proteins that are key players in the stress response, so it is not surprising they are linked with susceptibility or protection to stress-related disorders.

Epigenetic variability contributing to resilience has also been detected in genes regulating the immune system. Activity of the HPA axis can result in changes to immune system components and overall inflammation. As mentioned in our earlier section of this chapter, glucocorticoids can serve an anti-inflammatory role and determine immune system responses in addition to regulating expression of various cytokines. These cytokines, in turn, can regulate functions of the central nervous system. A genome wide scale investigating epigenetic changes in peripheral blood cells of trauma exposed versus controls showed changes in genes regulating T-cell activation and immune networks [69]. Follow-up studies found differences in methylation patterns of IL6, IL8, IL17, IL18, and IFN-gamma based on traumatic stress exposure [70]. An additional study found differential DNA methylation in the IL-2A gene of highly traumatized individuals [71]. Lastly, miRNA expression of transcripts targeting immune system genes was observed to be dysregulated in individuals diagnosed with PTSD [72]. Overall, it is clear that epigenetic regulation of genes functioning in the immune system play a role in individual resilience patterns.

Variability of gene expression in the central nervous system undoubtedly contributes to individual resilient phenotypes. The challenge here is that unlike with the HPA and immune system networks where you can more accurately detect associated changes in related genes within the periphery, to definitively make conclusions about epigenetic changes in the CNS, one must detect these modifications in brain tissue. This is not a trivial task unless samples are collected post-mortem. Nevertheless, research investigations looking at epigenetic changes of CNS function related genes in the blood cells have been conducted and provide some insight into individual stress coping and resilience. One study has found that variable genotypes of the COMT gene correlate with methylation patterns and fear responses. More specifically, the MET/MET genotype of COMT showed an increase in promoter DNA methylation and also increased fear expression [73]. Additionally, a large-scale study analyzing epigenomes of first responders at the World Trade Center disaster, implicated differential methylation in genes associated with synaptic plasticity, oxytocin signaling, cholinergic synapse and inflammatory disease pathways.

Biological and Psychological Resilience Dynamics

Though both biological and psychological resiliencies are similarly defined as the "ability to bounce back," decline in the biological resilience with age could possibly coincide with the improvement in the psychological resilience in the same individuals. An accumulation of experienced trauma and chronic stress over time has been shown to speed up the aging process [78]. Even without experiencing trauma, resilience has been shown to decline with age. Specifically, there is a loss of resilience of neural architecture with aging, or a reduction in neuroplastic adaptation to stressful stimuli [75]. Other aging components that contribute to the decline in aging include depletion of body reserves with age such as HSCs (hematopoietic stem cells) losing the ability to self-renew and regenerate, slowdown of physiological processes and responses with age, and dysfunction and breakdown of cell repair and tissue cleaning, increasing allostatic load [76]. Fortunately, both trauma-induced aging and observed reduction in resilience as we age can be re-directed or even reversed with appropriate lifestyle choices and pharmacological interventions. Proposed practical anti-aging interventions to help reduce the rate of aging components and maintain or even improve resilience over time include caloric restriction and physical exercise. For example, BDNF may be a key feature of the depressive state, and elevation of BDNF by diverse treatments ranging from antidepressant drugs to regular physical activity may be a central feature of maintaining resilience over time. Some of the more cutting-edge techniques to slow down [80, 81] include stem cell therapy, mitochondrial transplantation, and a broad array of pharmacological interventions [76].

The beauty of epigenetics playing a major role in determination of resilience is the fact that it is dynamic. Individuals who are programmed epigenetically to have low resilience can be reprogrammed to have improved resilience. In some cases where genetically individuals may be at high risk for dysregulation of stress reactivity, epigenetics can help to bring the system back to balance. According to multiple studies conducted with animals and humans, it has been shown that there is a "window of epigenetic plasticity," or a duration of time during which appropriate lifestyle and occupational training can improve resilience, especially in individuals who are more genetically susceptible to negative effects of stress.

Many studies have provided insight into trends in stress responsiveness that can be used to predict susceptibility to poor stress coping skills and low resilience following future trauma. Tests are designed to measure HPA axis activity, such as cortisol, CRF, or ACTH. As mentioned in a previous section of this chapter, cortisol secretion follows along a circadian rhythm, and this rhythm has been found to change in patients experiencing stress. As a result, ACR (awakening cortisol response) can be used as a litmus test for both physiological and psychological wellness. Additionally, HPA axis or cortisol reactivity can also be utilized as an indicator of stress coping. Cortisol reactivity can be determined either pharmacologically, by exposure to real-life stressful events, or experimentally designed stressful events.

The Trier Social Stress Test (TSST) is an example of an experimentally designed tool to stimulate a cortisol stress response [77]. Studies have shown that salivary cortisol levels after the TSST show a two to threefold increase in cortisol levels above baseline within a half hour. Cortisol levels can also be analyzed during hyper-realistic stress inoculation trainings to determine HPA axis reactivity [55]. In addition to cortisol, alpha-amylase has been described as a potential indicator of stress coping through noradrenergic activity and has also been assessed in hyper-realistic stress inoculation trainings [55]. Stress inoculation trainings have shown that stress conditioning is pretty uniform for the sympathetic nervous system, but cortisol reactivity can be stratified into high or low responders, indicating variable stress coping responses [64]. A prospective study conducted with police academy cadets to correlate startle responses to PTSD found that hypersensitivity to contextual threat (indexed by greater fear under low threat), elevated sympathetic nervous system reactivity to explicit threat (indexed by larger responses under high threat), and failure to adapt to repeated aversive stimuli (evidenced by slower habituation) are all unique preexisting vulnerability factors for greater PTSD symptom severity following traumatic stress exposure [66]. Measuring biomarkers indicative of HPA axis or sympathetic activity can provide insight into an individual's stress coping capacity.

Training Is Key

Since stress has been shown to compromise cognitive skills and patient outcomes [63], it is imperative to develop mechanisms for stress conditioning for trauma teams in order to maintain optimal team performance for patients. Trauma team stress inoculation training has been shown to reduce some of these biomarkers associated with low resilience, therefore also lowering probability of development trauma related disorders [51–53]. Multiple medical teams are currently exploring various stress simulations to aid in resilience development [56], including exploring virtual reality immersive simulators [57, 58], emotional excitation simulation [59], and debriefing/communication. Simulation-based training has been found to stimulate cortisol production during stress inoculation training with clinicians [61] and medical students [59, 60] immersed in a hyper-realistic simulation for emergency medical procedures. Interestingly, the hyper-realistic stress training improved self-perception and stress management categories according to results from the EQi-2.0 model of emotional intelligence [62]. Psychological debriefing and positive communication have also shown to reduce stress for individual's teams experiencing trauma. For example, psychiatric morbidity was studied in 106 British soldiers returning from UN peacekeeping duties in the former Republic of Yugoslavia. The group of 106 soldiers received an Operational Stress Training Package prior to their deployment and a randomly selected group also received a post-operational PD. Results show that very low rates of PTSD and other psychopathology were found overall, and the Operational Stress Training Package may have contributed to this. CAGE scores (used to determine substance abuse) diminished significantly in the debriefed group by the end of the follow-up period suggesting that PD may have been of benefit despite the apparent absence of PTSD [50]. Additionally, effect of positive communication during medical handover with anesthesia teams on the subsequent team-based clinical performance in a simulated critical situation has been to decrease the stress response and improve clinical performance [65].

Future of Resilience Building

Newly conducted studies with military medical students at Rocky Vista University and, subsequently, first responders in the fire academy at South Metro Fire Rescue in Colorado to study the stress response and resilience of participating individuals are opening a window to the future of resilience screening. Resilience was assessed by measuring levels of cytokines and steroid hormones from firefighters engaging in fire academy training and comparing those biomarker levels to LEC-5 Life Events Checklist results, resilience scores as determined by the Hardiness Resilience Gauge (HRG) questionnaire, and previous occupational experience in high-stress jobs such as military, EMS, or law enforcement. Results suggested that immune biomarkers and steroid-thyroid hormones correlate with the stress response, resilience scores, and life trauma. More specifically, our preliminary results show that salivary Fgf2 levels may be predictive for cortisol reactivity to stress. Additionally, we were able to show that Fgf2 levels increase following a stressful event. Together, these lead us to conclude that Fgf2 levels exhibited a negative correlation to the cortisol stress response, indicating that Fgf2 is neuroprotective and may represent a novel marker for resilience and stress coping. Finally, analyzing multiple cytokines associated with severity of life trauma experienced by an individual based on a comparison of their LEC-5 results to cytokine levels captured from that same study subject experiencing physical and psychological stress revealed that levels of Fgf2, IL-6, GCSF, and IL-18 correlate with severity of life trauma experienced by the study participants. Ultimately, our preliminary studies have shown that a multitude of immune biomarkers and hormones detected in saliva correlate with the stress response and traumatic life events linked to PTSD and resiliency measures. It is possible from these results to develop a liquid biopsy-screening test to determine risk for poor stress coping and low resilience.

In the future, we will be able to more accurately monitor an individual for stress coping and resilience by combining information from self-reported measures, vital sign and demographic data, psychosocial, stress reactivity, genomics, proteomics, transcriptomics, metabolomics, and epigenetics to apply more of a comprehensive systems approach to diagnosis and treatment of stress-induced disorders. For example, groups are already working on development and validation of an algorithm for prediction of post-traumatic stress disorder with promising results. Results demonstrate externally validated accuracy to discriminate PTSD risk with high precision [74]. In this study, investigators combined measures of vetted mental health screening questionnaires, psychophysiological stress response, threat perception, psychophysiological arousal, immune and inflammatory markers, and psychosocial determinants [74]. More variables to consider here would be brain imaging, both structural and functional MRI, in response to stressful stimuli, with tissue-specific epigenetic data and biomarker levels, in addition to the above-mentioned components. In the future, we will also be able to more accurately determine which stress inoculation or stress simulation tests are the most valuable, by continuing to monitor individuals engaged in these training sessions for stress biomarkers, stress reactivity, and follow-up for mental health related disorders. This will allow development and optimization of the best training curriculum. In the meantime, members of trauma teams must stay committed to staying educated how to best and make sure to build their own individual resilience.

Key Points

- The human response to stress is a homeostatic mechanism allowing adaptation to environmental stressors, involving multiple organ systems and being both adaptive and maladaptive.
- Acute stress involves an immediate, coordinated body response via the SNS and HPA axis, while chronic stress results from prolonged exposure, leading to dysregulation and health issues.
- The SNS, known for the "fight-or-flight" response, releases catecholamines (norepinephrine, epinephrine) to promote survival in stressful situations.
- The HPA axis releases cortisol in response to stress, regulating metabolism, immune responses, and maintaining homeostasis.
- The cardiovascular response to stress includes increased heart rate, blood pressure, and blood glucose levels, with chronic stress contributing to cardiovascular diseases.
- Acute stress enhances humoral immunity while suppressing cellular immunity, whereas chronic stress leads to immunosuppression and increased risk of infection and disease.
- HRV serves as an indicator of autonomic nervous system balance, with low HRV linked to poor health outcomes and increased mortality.
- Psychological stress can mimic physiological stress responses, with the limbic system, especially the amygdala, playing a key role in emotional and stress responses.
- Trauma can lead to long-term psychological and neurobiological changes, with PTSD and burnout being common in high-stress professions like trauma care.
- ACEs are linked to long-term health and psychological issues, with early trauma affecting brain morphology and increasing the risk of substance abuse.
- Resilience training and stress management workshops are effective, with mindfulness, yoga, and other self-care practices improving stress response and resilience.
- Hyper-realistic simulation training improves physiological and psychological responses to stress, helping trauma teams perform better in real-life stressful situations.
- Genetic and epigenetic factors influence individual stress response and resilience, with epigenetic changes being targeted for improving resilience.
- Measuring cortisol, cytokines, and other biomarkers helps assess stress and resilience, guiding personalized interventions for stress management.
- Disruption of circadian rhythms exacerbates the effects of stress, making the maintenance of proper sleep hygiene crucial for health and performance.
- Practical strategies for alleviating stress include individual approaches like mindfulness, emotional regulation, and communication skills training; team approaches such as resiliency training and stress management workshops; and organizational methods like workload and schedule rotations, debriefing sessions, and focus groups.

References

1. Russell G, Stafford L. The human stress response. Nat Rev Endocrinol [Internet]. 2019. Available from: https://www.nature.com/articles/s41574-019-0228-0#citeas.
2. Smith S, Vale W, Clayton Foundation Laboratories for Peptide Biology. The role of the hypothalamic-pituitary-adrenal axis in neuroendocrine responses to stress. Dialogues Clin [Internet]. 2006. Available from: https://doi.org/10.31887/DCNS.2006.8.4/ssmith.
3. Costanzo L. Physiology. Philadelphia: Elsevier – Health Sciences Division; 2018.

4. Pessoa L. Emotion and cognition and the amygdala: from "what is it?" to "what's to be done?". Neuropsychologia [Internet]. 2011;48(12). Available from: https://doi.org/10.1016/j.neuropsychologia.2010.06.038.
5. Das J, Siddiqui W. Kluver Bucy syndrome. In: StatPearls. Treasure Island (FL): StatPearls Publishing; 2020.
6. Gibbison B, Spiga F, Walker J, Russell G, Stevenson K, Kershaw Y, et al. Dynamic pituitary-adrenal interactions in response to cardiac surgery. Crit Care Med [Internet]. 2015. Available from: https://doi.org/10.1097/CCM.0000000000000773.
7. Olff M, van Zuiden M. Neuroendocrine and neuroimmune markers in PTSD: pre-, peri- and post-trauma glucocorticoid and inflammatory dysregulation. Curr Opin Psychol. 2017;14:132–7.
8. Billman G. The LF/HF ratio does not accurately measure cardiac sympatho-vagal balance. Front Physiol. 2013;4:26.
9. Bigger JT, Fleiss JL, Steinman RC, Rolnitzky LM, Kleiger RE, Rottman JN. Frequency domain measures of heart period variability and mortality after myocardial infarction. Circulation. 1992;85(1):164–71.
10. Mølgaard H, Sørensen K, Bjerregaard P. Attenuated 24-h heart rate variability in apparently healthy subjects, subsequently suffering sudden cardiac death. Clin Auton Res. 1991;1(3):233–7.
11. Pulopulos M, Vanderhasselt M-A, De Raedt R. Association between changes in heart rate variability during the anticipation of a stressful situation and the stress-induced cortisol response. Psychoneuroendocrinology. 2018;94:63–71.
12. Stephens MA, Wand G. Stress and the HPA axis: role of glucocorticoids in alcohol dependence. Alcohol Res. 2012;34(4):468–83.
13. Glaser R, Kiecolt-Glaser J. Stress-induced immune dysfunction: implications for health. Nat Rev Immunol. 2005;5:243–51.
14. World Health Organization. (2009). Global health risks : mortality and burden of disease attributable to selected major risks. World Health Organization. https://iris.who.int/handle/10665/44203.
15. Medic G, Wille M, Hemels M. Short- and long-term health consequences of sleep disruption. Nat Sci Sleep [Internet]. 2019;9. Available from: https://doi.org/10.2147/NSS.S134864.
16. Gaba D, Howard S. Fatigue among clinicians and the safety of patients. N Engl J Med [Internet]. 2002. Available from: https://doi.org/10.1056/NEJMsa020846.
17. Chu B, Marwaha K, Sanvictores T, Ayers D. Physiology, stress reaction. In: StatPearls. Treasure Island (FL): StatPearls Publishing; 2020.
18. Lacy BE, Chan JL. Physician burnout: the hidden health care crisis. Clin Gastroenterol Hepatol. 2018;16(3):311–7.
19. Mountfort S, Wilson J. EMS provider health and wellness. In: StatPearls [Internet]. Treasure Island (FL): StatPearls Publishing; 2020.
20. Baier N, Roth K, Felgner S, Henschke C. Burnout and safety outcomes – a cross-sectional nationwide survey of EMS-workers in Germany. BMC Emerg Med. 2018;18(1):24.
21. Crowe RP, Bower JK, Cash RE, Panchal AR, Rodriguez SA, Olivo-Marston SE. Association of burnout with workforce-reducing factors among EMS professionals. Prehosp Emerg Care. 2018;22(2):229–36.
22. Oral R, Ramirez M, Coohey C, Nakada S, Walz A, Kuntz A, Benoit J, Peek-Asa C. Adverse childhood experiences and trauma informed care: the future of health care. Pediatr Res. 2016;79(1–2):227–33.
23. Luftman K, Aydelotte J, Rix K, Ali S, Houck K, Coopwood TB, Teixeira P, Eastman A, Eastridge B, Brown CV, Davis M. PTSD in those who care for the injured. Injury. 2017;48(2):293–6.
24. Sherin JE, Nemeroff CB. Post-traumatic stress disorder: the neurobiological impact of psychological trauma. Dialogues Clin Neurosci. 2011;13(3):263–78.
25. Kirsch DE, Tretyak V, Radpour S, Weber WA, Nemeroff CB, Fromme K, Strakowski SM, Lippard ETC. Childhood maltreatment, prefrontal-paralimbic gray matter volume, and substance use in young adults and interactions with risk for bipolar disorder. Sci Rep. 2021;11(1):123.
26. Boland LL, Mink PJ, Kamrud JW, Jeruzal JN, Stevens AC. Social support outside the workplace, coping styles, and burnout in a cohort of EMS providers from Minnesota. Workplace Health Saf. 2019;67(8):414–22.
27. Yook YS. Firefighters' occupational stress and its correlations with cardiorespiratory fitness, arterial stiffness, heart rate variability, and sleep quality. PLoS One. 2019;14(12):e0226739.
28. Bonanno GA. Loss, trauma, and human resilience: have we underestimated the human capacity to thrive after extremely aversive events? Am Psychol. 2004;59(1):20–8.
29. Lazarus A. Traumatized by practice: PTSD in physicians. J Med Pract Manage. 2014;30(2):131–4.
30. Stuart H. Mental illness stigma expressed by police to police. Isr J Psychiatry Relat Sci. 2017;54(1):18–23.
31. Sandhu HS, Arora A, Brasch J, Streiner DL. Mental health stigma: explicit and implicit attitudes of Canadian undergraduate students, medical school students, and psychiatrists. Can J Psychiatr. 2019;64(3):209–17.
32. Zhang XJ, Song Y, Jiang T, Ding N, Shi TY. Interventions to reduce burnout of physicians and nurses: an overview of systematic reviews and meta-analyses. Medicine (Baltimore). 2020;99(26):e20992.
33. Auxéméry Y. L'état de stress post-traumatique comme conséquence de l'interaction entre une susceptibilité génétique individuelle, un évènement traumatogène et un contexte social [Posttraumatic stress disorder (PTSD) as a consequence of the interaction between an individual genetic susceptibility, a traumatogenic event and a social context]. Encéphale. 2012;38(5):373–80. French.
34. Kim SH, Schneider SM, Kravitz L, Mermier C, Burge MR. Mind-body practices for posttraumatic stress disorder. J Investig Med. 2013;61(5):827–34.
35. Lemay V, Hoolahan J, Buchanan A. Impact of a yoga and meditation intervention on students' stress and anxiety levels. Am J Pharm Educ. 2019;83(5):7001.
36. Pascoe MC, Thompson DR, Ski CF. Yoga, mindfulness-based stress reduction and stress-related physiological measures: a meta-analysis. Psychoneuroendocrinology. 2017;86:152–68.
37. Smith E, Walker T, Burkle FM. Lessons in post-disaster self-care from 9/11 paramedics and emergency medical technicians. Prehosp Disaster Med. 2019;34(3):335–9.
38. Kravits K, McAllister-Black R, Grant M, Kirk C. Self-care strategies for nurses: a psycho-educational intervention for stress reduction and the prevention of burnout. Appl Nurs Res. 2010;23(3):130–8.
39. Ross A, Bevans M, Brooks AT, Gibbons S, Wallen GR. Nurses and health-promoting behaviors: knowledge may not translate into self-care. AORN J. 2017;105(3):267–75.
40. McCue JD, Sachs CL. A stress management workshop improves residents' coping skills. Arch Intern Med. 1991;151(11):2273–7.
41. Schmidt M, Haglund K. Debrief in emergency departments to improve compassion fatigue and promote resiliency. J Trauma Nurs. 2017;24(5):317–22.
42. Schiechtl B, Hunger MS, Schwappach DL, Schmidt CE, Padosch SA. "Second victim": "critical incident stress management" in der klinischen Medizin [Second victim: critical incident stress management in clinical medicine]. Anaesthesist. 2013;62(9):734–41. German.
43. Jacobs J, Horne-Moyer HL, Jones R. The effectiveness of critical incident stress debriefing with primary and secondary trauma victims. Int J Emerg Ment Health. 2004;6(1):5–14.
44. Timms V. BET 1: to debrief or not debrief. Emerg Med J. 2019;36(7):444–5.

45. Dall'Ora C, Ball J, Recio-Saucedo A, Griffiths P. Characteristics of shift work and their impact on employee performance and wellbeing: a literature review. Int J Nurs Stud. 2016;57:12–27.
46. Tahghighi M, Rees CS, Brown JA, Breen LJ, Hegney D. What is the impact of shift work on the psychological functioning and resilience of nurses? An integrative review. J Adv Nurs. 2017;73(9):2065–83.
47. Peterson SA, Wolkow AP, Lockley SW, O'Brien CS, Qadri S, Sullivan JP, Czeisler CA, Rajaratnam SMW, Barger LK. Associations between shift work characteristics, shift work schedules, sleep and burnout in North American police officers: a cross-sectional study. BMJ Open. 2019;9(11):e030302.
48. Wayne DB, Didwania A, Feinglass J, Fudala MJ, Barsuk JH, McGaghie WC. Simulation-based education improves quality of care during cardiac arrest team responses at an academic teaching hospital: a case-control study. Chest. 2008;133(1):56–61.
49. Smith BW, Dalen J, Wiggins K, Tooley E, Christopher P, Bernard J. The brief resilience scale: assessing the ability to bounce back. Int J Behav Med. 2008;15(3):194–200.
50. Schnarrs PW, Stone AL, Salcido R, Georgiou C, Zhou X, Nemeroff CB. The moderating effect of resilience on the relationship between adverse childhood experiences (ACEs) and quality of physical and mental health among adult sexual and gender minorities. Behav Med. 2020;46(3–4):366–74.
51. Costantini L, Pasquarella C, Odone A, Colucci ME, Costanza A, Serafini G, Aguglia A, Belvederi Murri M, Brakoulias V, Amore M, Ghaemi SN, Amerio A. Screening for depression in primary care with Patient Health Questionnaire-9 (PHQ-9): a systematic review. J Affect Disord. 2021;279:473–83.
52. Cooper MA, Clinard CT, Morrison KE. Neurobiological mechanisms supporting experience-dependent resistance to social stress. Neuroscience. 2015;291:1–14. https://doi.org/10.1016/j.neuroscience.2015.01.072.
53. Deahl M, Srinivasan M, Jones N, Thomas J, Neblett C, Jolly A. Preventing psychological trauma in soldiers: the role of operational stress training and psychological debriefing. Br J Med Psychol. 2000;73(Pt 1):77–85.
54. Jackson S, Baity MR, Bobb K, Swick D, Giorgio J. Stress inoculation training outcomes among veterans with PTSD and TBI. Psychol Trauma Theory Res Pract Policy. 2019;11(8):842–50.
55. Zapata I, Farrell J, Morrell S, Ryznar R, Hoang TN, LaPorta AJ. Emotional intelligence, cortisol and α-amylase response to highly stressful hyper-realistic surgical simulation of a mass casualty event scenario. Compr Psychoneuroendocrinol. 2021;5:100031.
56. Stahhl MA. Stress, cognition, and human performance: a literature review and conceptual framework. NASA/TM—2004–212824.
57. Staufenbiel SM, Penninx BWJH, Spijker AT, Elzinga BM, van Rossum EFC. Hair cortisol, stress exposure, and mental health in humans: a systematic review. Psychoneuroendocrinology. 2013;38(8):1220–35.
58. Turner AI, Smyth N, Hall SJ, Torres SJ, Hussein M, Jayasinghe SU, Ball K, Clow AJ. Psychological stress reactivity and future health and disease outcomes: a systematic review of prospective evidence. Psychoneuroendocrinology. 2020;114:104599.
59. Shin R, Nichlany A. The Effects of Stress Inoculation Training in a High Stress Simulated Medical Environment. Western Journal of Emergency Medicine: Integrating Emergency Care with Population Health, 2018; 19(4.1). Retrieved from https://escholarship.org/uc/item/968310s5.
60. Couperus K, Young S, Walsh R, et al. Immersive virtual reality medical simulation: autonomous trauma training simulator. Cureus. 2020;12(5):e8062. Published 2020 May 11.
61. Ignacio J, Dolmans D, Scherpbier A, Rethans JJ, Lopez V, Liaw SY. Development, implementation, and evaluation of a mental rehearsal strategy to improve clinical performance and reduce stress: a mixed methods study. Nurse Educ Today. 2016;37:27–32.
62. Marjanovic NS, Teiten C, Pallamin N, L'Her E. Evaluation of emotional excitation during standardized endotracheal intubation in simulated conditions. Ann Intensive Care. 2018;8(1):117. https://doi.org/10.1186/s13613-018-0460-0. Published 2018 Dec 4.
63. Bong CL, Lightdale JR, Fredette ME, Weinstock P. Effects of simulation versus traditional tutorial-based training on physiologic stress levels among clinicians: a pilot study. Simul Healthc. 2010;5(5):272–8.
64. Zapata, et al. Emotional intelligence, cortisol and α-amylase response to highly stressful hyper-realistic surgical simulation of a mass casualty event scenario. Compr Psychoneuroendocrinol. 2021;5:100031.
65. Laporta A, White A, Lenz A, Ryznar R, Nevins N, Hoang T, Franciose R, Safaoui M, Clegg D, Zapata I. Medical students immersed in a hyper-realistic surgical training environment leads to improved measures of emotional resiliency by both hardiness and emotional intelligence evaluation. Front Psychol. 2020;11:3237.
66. Bertrand B, Evain JN, Piot J, Wolf R, Bertrand PM, Louys V, Terrisse H, Bosson JL, Albaladejo P, Picard J. Positive communication behaviour during handover and team-based clinical performance in critical situations: a simulation randomised controlled trial. Br J Anaesth. 2021;126(4):854–61. S0007-0912(20)30997-1.
67. Paquette AG, Lester BM, Koestler DC, Lesseur C, Armstrong DA, Marsit CJ. Placental FKBP5 genetic and epigenetic variation is associated with infant neurobehavioral outcomes in the RICHS cohort. PLoS One. 2014;9(8):e104913.
68. Pole N, Neylan TC, Otte C, Henn-Hasse C, Metzler TJ, Marmar CR. Prospective prediction of posttraumatic stress disorder symptoms using fear potentiated auditory startle responses. Biol Psychiatry. 2009;65(3):235–40.
69. Pfeiffer JR, Mutesa L, Uddin M. Traumatic stress epigenetics. Curr Behav Neurosci Rep. 2018;5(1):81–93. https://doi.org/10.1007/s40473-018-0143-z.
70. Russo SJ, Murrough JW, Han MH, Charney DS, Nestler EJ. Neurobiology of resilience. Nat Neurosci. 2012;15(11):1475–84. https://doi.org/10.1038/nn.3234. Epub 2012 Oct 14.
71. Schultebraucks K, Shalev AY, Michopoulos V, et al. A validated predictive algorithm of post-traumatic stress course following emergency department admission after a traumatic stressor. Nat Med. 2020;26:1084–8.
72. Yehuda R, Daskalakis NP, Desarnaud F, Makotkine I, Lehrner AL, Koch E, Bierer LM. Epigenetic biomarkers as predictors and correlates of symptom improvement following psychotherapy in combat veterans with PTSD. Front Psych. 2013;4:118.
73. Mehta D, Klengel T, Conneely KN, Smith AK, Altmann A, Pace TW, Rex-Haffner M, Loeschner A, Gonik M, Mercer KB, Bradley B, Müller-Myhsok B, Ressler KJ, Binder EB. Childhood maltreatment is associated with distinct genomic and epigenetic profiles in posttraumatic stress disorder. Proc Natl Acad Sci USA. 2013;110(20):8302–7.
74. Rusiecki JA, Byrne C, Galdzicki Z, Srikantan V, Chen L, Poulin M, Yan L, Baccarelli A. PTSD and DNA methylation in select immune function gene promoter regions: a repeated measures case-control study of U.S. military service members. Front Psych. 2013;4:56.
75. Norrholm SD, Jovanovic T, Smith AK, Binder E, Klengel T, Conneely K, Mercer KB, Davis JS, Kerley K, Winkler J, Gillespie CF, Bradley B, Ressler KJ. Differential genetic and epigenetic regulation of catechol-O-methyltransferase is associated with impaired fear inhibition in posttraumatic stress disorder. Front Behav Neurosci. 2013;7:30.
76. Rebecca Ryznar, Anthony J. La Porta, Ryan Shelton, MarK. Payton, Kelly D. Gubler, Isain Zapata, Amanda Brooks, Identification of the Proteins Involved in Building Resilience Among Surgeons, Medics and First Responders, Journal of the American College of Surgeons, Volume 233, Issue 5, Supplement 2, 2021, Page e125, ISSN 1072-

7515, https://doi.org/10.1016/j.jamcollsurg.2021.08.338. (https://www.sciencedirect.com/science/article/pii/S1072751521015866).
77. Allen AP, Kennedy PJ, Dockray S, Cryan JF, Dinan TG, Clarke G. The trier social stress test: principles and practice. Neurobiol Stress. 2016;6:113–26. https://doi.org/10.1016/j.ynstr.2016.11.001. Published 2016 Nov 12.
78. Bloss EB, et al. Interactive effects of stress and aging on structural plasticity in the prefrontal cortex. J Neurosci. 2010;30:6726–31.
79. McEwen BS. In pursuit of resilience: stress, epigenetics, and brain plasticity. Ann N Y Acad Sci. 2016;1373(1):56–64. https://doi.org/10.1111/nyas.13020. Epub 2016 Feb 25.
80. Ukraintseva S, Arbeev K, Duan M, Akushevich I, Kulminski A, Stallard E, Yashin A. Decline in biological resilience as key manifestation of aging: potential mechanisms and role in health and longevity. Mech Ageing Dev. 2021;194:111418.
81. Wolf EJ, Morrison FG. Traumatic stress and accelerated cellular aging: from epigenetics to cardiometabolic disease. Curr Psychiatry Rep. 2017;19(10):75. https://doi.org/10.1007/s11920-017-0823-5. Published 2017 Aug 29.

Stress Exposure Training

13

Garrett G. R. J. Johnson and Anthony J. LaPorta

Introduction

As illustrated in the previous chapters, quality care of the trauma patient relies not only on the care providers' mastery of technical skills but also on a variety of nontechnical skills [1–3]. Trauma scenarios can be complex, and unexpected situations can arise, which may cause acute psychological stress for healthcare providers [4]. When situational strain causes the perception that demands exceed resources, this will trigger the body's autonomic nervous system to generate a complex hormone cascade leading to the flight-or-flight response. This is responsible at a physiologic level for how a person responds to stress. It has been observed in a variety of fields, including trauma and acute care that high levels of stress are negatively associated with task performance [5–7]. While small increases in stress may actually improve performance, first described by Yerkes-Dodson's law over 100 years ago, higher levels correlate with worse outcomes [8–10]. In trauma, both hospital and prehospital personnel response to high degrees of stress can impair their clinical response by impacting factors such as technical performance, memory, decision-making, communication skills, attention to detail, and error recognition [5–7, 11–13]. Therefore, care providers must train to habituate themselves to stress present in the trauma environment in order to perform effectively.

Stress exposure training (SET) is a type of cognitive-behavioral therapy designed to help individuals cope with stress. It was originally developed by psychologist Donald Meichenbaum and called "stress inoculation training" (SIT) as part of a clinical treatment program to teach patients to cope with pain, anger, and various phobias in response to past psychological traumas [14]. Subsequently, it was adapted by Driskell and Johnson to be applied prophylactically to mitigate the sequelae of stress and augment performance under pressure [15]. For the purposes of this chapter, and for the application in training of trauma team members, we do not differentiate between SIT and SET. SET has been applied in a variety of settings including military training [16], sports [17–19], aviation [20, 21], and medicine [22–25]. In particular, the goal of SET in medicine is to prepare medical personnel to perform tasks effectively under high-demand, stressful conditions, such as in trauma or surgical training, by training under realistic high-pressure environments [23, 25, 26].

Stress Training

SET is distinct from usual training. In usual training programs, the focus is generally on skills acquisition and practice. This is classically done in a quiet environment so that the student may focus on learning without external distractions. However, in reality, many skills must be performed in environments completely different from the classroom. Because of this disparity, training conducted under normal, low-stress conditions may not necessarily improve task performance when performed under stressful conditions [27]. Furthermore, some stress in the learning environment is associated with enhanced memory consolidation [7]. In SET, the focus is to prepare the individual to maintain effective performance in a real-world high-stress environment. As such, effective SET programs are divided into three key components: (1) Knowledge of the real-life stressful environment is provided. (2) Individuals build skills to overcome and manage these stressors. (3) Practice under simulated pressure in order to build confidence and habituate to stress [15].

Information Provision

In this phase, participants receive *preparatory information* designed to convey knowledge of the human stress response, the individual's existing coping skills, and the types of stress-

G. G. R. J. Johnson (✉)
General Surgery and Clinician Investigator Program, University of Manitoba, Winnipeg, MB, Canada
e-mail: umjoh529@myumanitoba.ca

A. J. LaPorta
Rocky Vista University, Parker, CO, USA
e-mail: alaporta@rvu.edu

L. Marshall Gillman, S. Widder (eds.), *Trauma Team Dynamics*, https://doi.org/10.1007/978-3-031-86312-7_13

ors they are likely to encounter during their training. Trainees are taught the rationale for SET so that they may buy in to the concept and understand why it is important to their training. This increases learner attention and motivation in order to acquire the skills required for a particular stressful task environment. Typically anecdotes and empirical data are shared illustrating how stress impacts care, and how the ability to manage stress and act effectively are keys to success. Classically, a Socratic approach is undertaken during this phase in order to build learner engagement [14].

The preparatory information stage enables trainees to form accurate expectations regarding the stress environment and decreases the distraction involved in attending to novel sensations and activities, thus allowing the individual to identify and avoid performance errors that are likely to occur [28].

First, trainees are provided with *sensory information* regarding how the individual is likely to feel when under stress. Participants are provided with accurate information on normal physiological responses to stress, such as increased heart rate, shallow breathing, and emotions like fear, frustration, or confusion, in order to reduce the distraction of having to attend to these unfamiliar reactions in the working environment. These reactions are explained and normalized. Individuals under stress and unfamiliar with their physiologic response tend to assign a heightened importance to physical symptoms, such as a pounding heart, and misinterpret these "normal" stress reactions as catastrophic and expend a disproportionate amount of mental capacity focusing on them, which distracts from task-oriented activity. In contrast, individuals who are able to label or identify physiological reactions are less distressed by those reactions and perform better [15].

Next, *procedural information* is given, in the form of a description of the events that are likely to occur during SET. This may include a description of the environment, the task procedure that participants may be asked to perform, the types of physical stressors that may be encountered, and the effects these may have on participants. Put simply, procedural information warns the participants in advance with what they will be asked to do during simulation [15]. How specific this procedural information needs to be is somewhat controversial, as talking individuals through an entire complex high-fidelity simulation prior to practicing it likely removes much learning associated with decision-making and anticipating the unexpected, which are important tasks to practice under pressure in a trauma environment. However, a general warning to individuals about a stressful environment to come may actually paradoxically serve to increase their levels of "anticipatory" stress. In an ultra-high fidelity trauma simulation, medical students actually had higher levels of stress when their peers warned them of an upcoming stressful scenario, compared to their peers who were not similarly forewarned [23]. A description of the types of events and procedures that a participant might be expected to experience and how this might make them feel, is likely a safe middle ground.

Finally, *instrumental information* is provided, describing strategies for countering the undesirable consequences of stress faced during training. For example, not only are trainees told that the trauma bay can be loud and distracting, but they are given strategies for how to manage this disruption. Specific examples of stress-coping mechanisms are described in the following section.

Skills Acquisition and Rehearsal

The primary focus of the skills acquisition phase is on developing and practicing both technical and non-technical skills that are required to maintain effective performance under pressure. The skills individuals will utilize vary depending on their role and level of experience in the trauma-resuscitation environment. Stress training strategies focus on providing individuals with the skills to become more resistant to the effects of stress and to help them habituate to the effects of stress when they occur. Among stress management strategies, some skills are somewhat generic and are likely to be relevant to most tasks that may be performed under stress conditions, whereas others are task specific and need only be applied in certain situations. Furthermore, individuals' unique strengths and weaknesses may affect how easily they can learn and apply specific stress management strategies. Driskell and Johnston identified several categories of skills training relevant to stress exposure [15]. The following is a description of these skills and how they are applied in trauma resuscitation. Prior to undertaking training under stress, participants should already be facile with the specific medical knowledge and technical skills required in the trauma environment.

Cognitive Control

One of the basic tenets of cognitive behavioral therapy is that a person's thoughts affect how they feel, which in turn affects their behavior. Cognitive control strategies intervene on an individual's thoughts by utilizing a variety of coping strategies with the purpose of providing the participant with control over distracting thoughts and emotions that they may encounter in the stress environment [29]. For SET, the primary goal of these strategies is to replace these negative thoughts with more positive task-focused ones. For example, when faced with a multiple-injured patient, you might feel overwhelmed and experience thoughts of self-doubt, such as "I don't know what to treat first" and "what if I don't succeed." These thoughts are normal but are not helpful to the situation. A cognitive control strategy may be to replace these thoughts with, "I have trained for this. Remember the ABCs. Is he protecting his airway?" and so on. Algorithms or "cheat sheets" with task-oriented information can be used to help with this strategy. In particular, *attentional training* has been shown to be a particularly effective cognitive control strategy, where focus is intentionally narrowed away from task-irrelevant stimuli [30, 31].

One pitfall is to simply replace negative dysfunctional thoughts with more positive thoughts. In the previous example, positive thoughts such as "I can do this" and "I am great" may make the individual feel better but are equally as distracting and unhelpful as the negative thoughts they replaced. In novel environments, individuals expend more cognitive resources on self-attention than usual. They share cognitive resources between the task at hand and worrying about the stress itself. This is thought to be a contributor to how stress negatively affects performance [31–33]. Therefore, in order to be most effective, cognitive control strategies should not only replace negative thoughts with positive ones but also refocus these thoughts onto the task at hand. Participants in training may benefit from a "cheat sheet" or guide to help them with this process.

Physiological Control

The goals of physiological control techniques are to provide the individual with the ability to regulate their own physiologic reactions to stress. The basic premise for this is that if a person's body is relaxed, they are more likely to mentally "feel" relaxed. It has been observed that effective performers, such as high-level athletes under stress tend to display calmness, relaxation, and control—and relaxation techniques attempt to emulate this behavior [15].

One such technique that shows promise for application in trauma and resuscitation scenarios is *controlled breathing*. Breathing is an autonomic function that can be controlled consciously. When using controlled breathing techniques, individuals adjust their breathing rate in order to diminish stress and bring their level of arousal back to a favorable level [34]. This can be applied to trauma personnel in a variety of instances when physiologic arousal is extremely elevated, for example, prior to performing a high-stakes invasive procedure. For an easily learned and applied example, a provider can take a deep breath over the course of four seconds, hold for four seconds, exhale over four seconds, and pause two to four seconds before inhaling again. This may be repeated as required until the desired level of physiologic arousal is attained. While no randomized controlled trials exist demonstrating effectiveness of this technique in trauma and acute medical settings, breathing techniques known as tactical breathing, square breathing, pranayama, or performance enhancing breathing, have been applied in a variety of other high-stakes settings with success [35–38].

Autogenic feedback is another technique, where individuals are taught internal cues in order to modulate reactions to stress. Utilizing principles of operant conditioning, individuals are taught certain cues that are associated with relaxation. Individuals practice controlling their heart rate and blood pressure utilizing these cues, so that when these parameters increase during stress, they can bring these vital signs under control, which can diminish their physiologic stress. This has been shown in nursing students to decrease anxiety and improve performance during medical simulation [39], and has also been used to improve job performance in search and rescue pilots under stressful simulation [40]. A limitation is it takes many hours of training to become proficient at this technique however.

Overlearning

The term overlearning refers to deliberate practice of a skill beyond the level of initial competence. For trauma, examples of skills to which this can be applied will vary depending on the provider's role but could include ensuring equipment is available and functional prior to intubation, or practicing the sequence of steps in central line insertion. However, overlearning strategies should be employed deliberately and thoughtfully in SET programs. While it has been established that overlearning leads to increased knowledge retention, it is also associated with increased rigidity of a response. Individuals experience a loss of flexibility and tend to apply the behavior even when it is not indicated [41]. It is critical that the overlearned task be practiced in a setting that closely approximates the real-life setting—including degrees of stress and distraction. In many aspects, the real-world task environment changes the nature of the task or the types of behavior required for successful performance. Overlearning of a task in a training environment that does not incorporate these factors can lead to the reinforcement of inappropriate or ineffective behavior [15].

Mental Practice

Mental practice refers to the cognitive rehearsal of a task in the absence of overt physical movement. Participants may sit quietly and mentally rehearse their task from beginning to end, allowing them to code components of the task into words or images that can later help with recall. While not as effective as physical practice, as it cannot simulate tactile feedback, mental practice can be particularly useful for tasks that are rare or dangerous [42]. For a trauma setting, there are many examples of procedures that fit into these categories, such as emergency department thoracotomy or cricothyroidotomy. Even for more common scenarios, mental practice can realistically be applied immediately before a patient is wheeled into the resuscitation bay, or before the scene of an accident is approached, as a mental "warm up." In fact, there is some evidence that mental practice has its strongest positive effect when it is performed immediately before the skill must be performed [43]. Care providers could reference a "cheat sheet" to help remind them of the steps of a procedure and guide their mental practice.

Mental practice has been studied most extensively in educational and sports research and shows benefit. It is a component of many cognitive stress reduction techniques [42]. In surgery, it has been employed successfully to improve operative skills [44, 45] and was shown to have some benefit specifically in trauma resuscitation skills training [46].

Decision-Making

High-stress performance environments, such as those that commonly occur in trauma settings, often involve increases in *task load* and *time pressure*. Time pressure is a restriction in time required to perform a task. Time pressure degrades performance primarily due to cognitive demands caused by the requirement to process a seemingly overwhelming amount of information in a limited amount of time [15]. Under time pressure, performance can be further impaired when due to the attentional effects of stress, errors are not recognized and increased time elapses before an error is corrected. Task load refers to the demand of performing multiple tasks simultaneously, or in common vernacular "multi-tasking." It is well established in the education literature that increased task load is associated with worsened performance. Even when performing two simple tasks simultaneously, neither task will be performed as well as if either task were performed in isolation [30]. This holds true for tasks performed in medical settings [47]. Applied to the trauma setting, a possible occurrence is when the trauma team leader attempts to perform a procedure, such as intubation, at the same time as trying to continue to lead the trauma resuscitation, which inevitably causes both responsibilities to suffer.

For specific tasks, two skills can be learned to be performed simultaneously with substantial dedicated practice [48, 49]. However, it is regarded by some authors that a true generalizable timesharing ability does not exist and is not a skill that can be honed [15]. Furthermore, extensive practice of two discrete tasks individually does not appear to enhance performance substantially when these tasks must be performed simultaneously [50, 51]. Following this logic, if tasks are likely to be performed together in a trauma, they must be practiced together extensively in the training environment, so that they can both be performed effectively. It may be more prudent for participants to recognize that they cannot effectively perform two tasks at once and train *prioritization* and *decision-making skills* rather than to focus too much time and energy training dual tasks.

In the stressful environment of trauma resuscitation, usual decision-making strategies that one may employ in other environments may be ineffective. For example, outside of an emergency, the type of clinical reasoning that a physician may typically engage in involves a systematic, organized information search, considers all available alternatives, generates a large differential diagnosis, compares options, and selects an optimal treatment strategy. This is called analytic reasoning. While this process is thorough, it is both mentally exhausting and time consuming [52]. Individuals may have an impaired ability to consider all possibilities when under time pressure and faced with distractions. Utilizing this type of higher level decision-making has its place under stress, although it should be employed selectively, and likely requires practice in this setting [53].

Under stress, a simplified form of decision-making termed hypervigilant decision-making has been observed, in which limited or simplified information is considered, there is a nonsystematic information search, accelerated evaluation of data, and rapid decisions are made [54]. While this type of decision-making can lead to errors, rapid identification of errors and subsequent correction are more critical. In general, this type of decision-making is considered to be inferior to the analytic decision-making process in non-time-sensitive settings; however, it is adaptive in the time-pressured and stressful environment [13]. Furthermore, decision-making under high-stress conditions is an expert skill that can be practiced in order to improve performance [55].

Decision-making can be further adapted through the adoption of various algorithms or heuristics, which can simplify information necessary to perform a given task [13, 56]. This is in essence what Advance Trauma Life Support (ATLS) teaches in the form of the primary survey. Key diagnoses that are rapidly fatal and treatable are examined in a systematic fashion, in the same way every time, in order of priority, to ease cognitive burden and manage time pressure.

Team/Communication Skills

Similar to how individual performance suffers under stress, so does team performance. Etiologic factors include narrowed attention of the individuals, causing their focus to shift from the group to individual goals, which can be inefficient. Furthermore, stress can impair communication, and render individuals less sensitive to social cues [57]. Characteristics of effective teams that perform well under stress conditions include adaptability, effective communication, resource allocation, situational awareness, and clear leadership [13]. Trauma care is delivered in teams, so practice of trauma care delivery, and managing the associated stress should be done in teams as well. Individuals not only must learn to cope with individual stresses that arises, but must be able to manage their teammates' stress. SET has been shown to improve stress adaptation and improve team performance in trauma settings [25].

Some team training strategies to deal with intense stress in trauma settings can be learned from elite military forces. Similar to military operations, medical providers in trauma care must manage the effects of stress in high strakes environments, where the consequences of errors can be devastating, and life threatening. The Israeli special forces employ a technique named for the acronym *iCOVER* (identify, connect, offer, verify, establish, request), where teamwork is applied to administer a physiologic control strategy in order to re-orient team members when they become overwhelmed by acutely stressful events. Soldiers are trained to identify colleagues suffering from the effects of acute stress and employ a structured strategy to reactivate their comrade's frontal cortex, and reorient them to the task at hand. This is a six-step, peer-based intervention that can be completed in under a minute and takes less than an hour of training. Participants are trained to *identify* their colleagues suffering from an acute stress reaction, *connect* with them by speaking their name, or making physical contact, *offer* commitment by reassuring them that they are not alone, *verify* simple facts they are certain to know the answer to (such as their name, or rank), to get their frontal cortex and their thinking re-started, ask them about what is happening around them to "ground" them in the present moment and *establish* an order of events, and then *request* for them to continue productive behavior [58, 59]. While designed for military personnel, such a strategy could be easily applied to medical staff suffering the acute physiologic effects of stress in a trauma-resuscitation setting.

Cross-training, used by elite US military forces in their training programs, is another valuable team lesson that can be applied to trauma teams to manage the effects of stress. Individuals practice to become facile not only with their own roles in the team environment but also in the roles of each of their teammates [60]. This allows each team member to have a shared appreciation of each other's knowledge and expertise and has been shown to diminish stress [61]. Knowing what each of your teammates knows and what exactly they will do in each situation can vastly improve team effectiveness. Other team skills relevant to the care of the trauma patient are discussed elsewhere in this textbook.

Similar to the battlefield, in the high-stakes environment during the care of the multiple-injured trauma patient, stress can be high, and in order to prepare for the deleterious effects, medical staff should be habituated to the stresses of this environment. In the application and practice phase of SET, participants rehearse the skills learned in phase two under stressful conditions. This allows participants to gain familiarity with aspects of the real-life stressful setting under which these skills must be performed. Participants also gain resiliency and confidence as they learn to apply their skills in environments as close to reality as possible [15, 26].

Key to the application and practice phase of SET are not only the provision of realistic stressors to the training environment but also the manner in which trainees approach the scenarios. The classic military mantra "train as you fight" applies. Thus, a core element for maintaining effective performance in a stressful environment is to practice under conditions as similar as possible to those encountered in real-world operational settings. Furthermore, the approach to training must be realistic, especially for tasks that are repetitive, in order to train muscle memory so that the actions are instinctive. Dave Grossman, in his book *On Combat: The Psychology and Physiology of Deadly Conflict in War and in Peace*, illustrates this point with an anecdote. In police training, participants would practice disarming an opponent with a model gun. Once disarmed, they would pick up the weapon from the floor and hand it to their partner to repeat the exercise ad nauseam, in an excellent example of overlearning. When a trainee finally had to apply the exercise in real-life, muscle memory took over, and he knocked the weapon from the aggressor's hand, exactly as practiced. But then, just as he had done in training, he reached down, picked up the weapon, and returned it to the attacker. Grossman argues that police, just as military personnel, should train as though they are in combat. When firing bullets at a range, when a magazine is empty, they should let it drop to the floor and reload as quickly as possible, rather than place it neatly in their pocket. They can worry about the mess once the training is over. Such a mindset could be easily applied to trauma simulation and training, as placing a chest tube for tension pneumothorax in the field should be done as fast as possible, without regard for mess. This may appear very different from how a resident traditionally may have practiced in simulation. Practicing under realistic mindset and training has been done in the US military with great results for decades [62] and has recently been adapted for US military medical training with success [23, 25, 26].

It is integral to the success of SET programs that the information provision and skills acquisition phases are taught prior to practice under simulated stress. Failure to do so carries the risk of causing participants to be confused and frustrated and may damage their confidence. So-called "throwing people in at the deep end" may only benefit those with more instinctive or natural ability to manage stress, or those with previous stress training and experience. The complexity of the stress environment is likely not conducive to the early stages of learning. Expertise in procedural skills of medical knowledge prior to training under stress allows for habituation to the relevant stressors without being overwhelmed. It is possibly for this reason that in medical and surgical education literature, higher fidelity is not necessarily associated with improved learning [63, 64]. The increased complexity of the high-fidelity environment may simply serve as a distraction to the novice learner. They might benefit more from this after they have gained some experience through lower-fidelity alternatives [7].

The benefits of SET for improved performance of specific tasks or specific stressors are quite profound. However, the stressors encountered in trauma are difficult to predict, and the skills that must be performed are myriad. Furthermore, SET is usually performed with a large number of repetitions in order to build expertise and confidence. It would be impractical to practice each and every skill under every possible stressful condition. Fortunately, it has been demonstrated outside of the trauma literature that skills learned in SET are generalizable from one task to another, and between stressors [65].

Limitations of SET

While there are many trials demonstrating the benefits of SET for job performance outside of medical care [66], there are few examining the effect of SET for healthcare providers involved in trauma and acute care. The only randomized control trial of SET in trauma care involved novice application of tourniquets by non-medical practitioners and showed no benefit [24], which may suggest a poor training strategy rather than failure of SET as a technique, as in this study both control and SET groups had abysmal success rates. In non-randomized trials, stress inoculation training does appear to show benefit in training medical personnel for trauma [23, 25, 26].

In a non-trauma medical setting, psychiatric nurses showed some subjective benefit from SET in a randomized control trial [22]; however, this population is quite unlike trauma healthcare providers in that SET employs evidence-based treatment strategies applicable to the management of post-traumatic stress disorder (PTSD) and anxiety disorders [67], so it is conceivable that learning to apply the techniques of this training program in their daily practice may have accounted for some of the improvements in competency that these nurses demonstrated in this study. It is also unclear which components of SET are required for success. Only one study to our knowledge has compared each of the three components and found that skills training (phase 2) had the most profound benefits [68].

Another consideration for SET programs is the negative health effect of repeated and chronic stress exposure. While SET derives from a psychological treatment strategy, SET as a technique in trauma simulation aims only to mitigate the performance issues of stress. There are many non-psychological ill effects of chronic stress, and there is some suggestion that physiologic effects of repeated exposure to stress through simulation can be long-lasting. What effects this has on SET participant long-term health is unknown [69].

Key Points

- Stress is inevitable in the care of severely ill trauma patients.
- Stress is associated with a detriment in both technical and non-technical skills.
- Stress exposure training (SET) is designed to habituate participants to the effects of stress so that they can perform better.
- There are three phases to SET: information provision, skills acquisition, and application and practice. The first two phases are integral prior to practice under stress conditions in the third phase.
- "Train as you fight!" When applying and practicing SET skills, recreate operational conditions as closely as possible.
- Trauma care is delivered in teams, so should practice of trauma care delivery. SET is best practiced in team settings.

References

1. Briggs A, Raja AS, Joyce MF, Yule SJ, Jiang W, Lipsitz SR, et al. The role of nontechnical skills in simulated trauma resuscitation. J Surg Educ. 2015;72(4):732–9.
2. Boet S, Bould MD, Fung L, Qosa H, Perrier L, Tavares W, et al. Transfer of learning and patient outcome in simulated crisis resource management: a systematic review. Can J Anaesth. 2014;61(6):571–82. 3rd ed. Springer US
3. Fung L, Boet S, Bould MD, Qosa H, Perrier L, Tricco A, et al. Impact of crisis resource management simulation-based training for interprofessional and interdisciplinary teams: a systematic review. J Interprof Care. 2015;29(5):433–44.
4. Kent J, Thornton M, Fong A, Hall E, Fitzgibbons S, Sava J. Acute provider stress in high stakes medical care: implications for trauma surgeons. J Trauma Acute Care Surg [Internet]. 2020;88(3):440–5. Available from: https://journals-lww-com.uml.idm.oclc.org/jtrauma/Fulltext/2020/03000/Acute_provider_stress_in_high_stakes_medical_care_.12.aspx
5. Harvey A, Bandiera G, Nathens AB, LeBlanc VR. Impact of stress on resident performance in simulated trauma scenarios. J Trauma Acute Care Surg. 2012;72(2):497–503.
6. Joseph B, Parvaneh S, Swartz T, Haider AA, Hassan A, Kulvatunyou N, et al. Stress among surgical attending physicians and trainees: a quantitative assessment during trauma activation and emergency surgeries. J Trauma Acute Care Surg. 2016;81(4):723–8.
7. Bong CL, Fraser K, Oriot D. Cognitive load and stress in simulation. In: Grant VJ, Cheng A, editors. Comprehensive healthcare simulation pediatric. 1st ed. New York; 2016. p. 3–18.

8. Yerkes RM, Dodson JD. The relation of strength of stimulus to rapidity of habit-formation. J Comp Neurol Psychol [Internet]. 1908;18(5):459–82. Wiley. Available from: https://onlinelibrary.wiley.com/doi/10.1002/cne.920180503
9. LeBlanc V, Woodrow SI, Sidhu R, Dubrowski A. Examination stress leads to improvements on fundamental technical skills for surgery. Am J Surg. 2008;196(1):114–9.
10. Keitel A, Ringleb M, Schwartges I, Weik U, Picker O, Stockhorst U, et al. Endocrine and psychological stress responses in a simulated emergency situation. Psychoneuroendocrinology. 2011;36(1):98–108.
11. LeBlanc VR, MacDonald RD, McArthur B, King K, Lepine T. Paramedic performance in calculating drug dosages following stressful scenarios in a human patient simulator. Prehosp Emerg Care. 2005;9(4):439–44.
12. LeBlanc VR, Regehr C, Tavares W, Scott AK, MacDonald R, King K. The impact of stress on paramedic performance during simulated critical events. Prehosp Disaster Med. 2012;27(4):369–74. Cambridge University Press
13. LeBlanc VR. The effects of acute stress on performance: implications for health professions education. Acad Med. 2009;84(10 Suppl):S25–33.
14. Meichenbaum D, Cameron R. Stress inoculation training. In: Meichenbaum D, Jaremko ME, editors. Stress reduction and prevention. Boston; 1989. p. 115–54.
15. Driskell JE, Johnston JH. Stress exposure training. In: Cannon-Bowers JA, Salas E, editors. Making decisions under stress: implications for individual and team training [Internet]; 1998. p. 191–217. Available from: https://psycnet.apa.org/record/1998-06532-007.
16. Robson S, Manacapilli T. Enhancing performance under stress: stress inoculation training for battlefield airmen [Internet]. Santa Monica: RAND Corporation; 2014. Available from: https://www.rand.org/content/dam/rand/pubs/research_reports/RR700/RR750/RAND_RR750.pdf
17. Mace RD, Carroll D, Eastman C. Effects of stress inoculation training on self-report, behavioural and psychophysiological reactions to abseiling. J Sports Sci. 1986;4(3):229–36.
18. Mace R, Carroll D. Stress inoculation training to control anxiety in sport: two case studies in squash. Br J Sports Med. 1986;20(3):115–7. 33rd ed
19. Mace RD, Carroll D. The effect of stress inoculation training on self-reported stress, observer's rating of stress, heart rate and gymnastics performance. J Sports Sci. 1989;7(3):257–66.
20. McClernon CK, McCauley ME, O'Connor PE, Warm JS. Stress training improves performance during a stressful flight. Hum Factors. 2011;53(3):207–18.
21. Fornette M-P, Bardel M-H, Lefrançois C, Fradin J, El Massioui F, Amalberti R. Cognitive-adaptation training for improving performance and stress management of air force pilots. Int J Aviat Psychol. 2012;22(3):203–23. 3rd ed. Taylor & Francis Group
22. Sargazi O, Foroughameri G, Miri S, Farokhzadian J. Improving the professional competency of psychiatric nurses: results of a stress inoculation training program. Psychiatry Res. 2018;270:682–7. Elsevier
23. LaPorta AJ, McKee J, Hoang T, Horst A, McBeth P, Gillman LM, et al. Stress inoculation: preparing outside the box in surgical resuscitation and education. Curr Trauma Rep [Internet]. 2017;3(2):135–143. Springer. Available from: https://link.springer.com/article/10.1007/s40719-017-0090-2
24. Tsur AM, Binyamin Y, Koren L, Ohayon S, Thompson P, Glassberg E. High tourniquet failure rates among non-medical personnel do not improve with tourniquet training, including combat stress inoculation: a randomized controlled trial. Prehosp Disaster Med. 2019;34(3):282–287. Cambridge University Press
25. Hoang TN, LaPorta AJ, Malone JD, Champagne R, Lavell K, La Rosa De GM, et al. Hyper-realistic and immersive surgical simulation training environment will improve team performance. Trauma Surg Acute Care Open. BMJ Spec J. 2020;5(1):e000393.
26. West E, Singer-Chang G, Ryznar R, Ross D, Czekajlo M, Hoang T, et al. The effect of hyper-realistic trauma training on emotional intelligence in second year military medical students. J Surg Educ. 2020;
27. Zakay D, Wooler S. Time pressure, training and decision effectiveness. Ergonomics. 1984;27(3):273–84.
28. Inzana CM, Driskell JE, Salas E, Johnston JH. Effects of preparatory information on enhancing performance under stress. J Appl Psychol. 1996;81(4):429–35.
29. Regehr C, Glancy D, Pitts A, LeBlanc VR. Interventions to reduce the consequences of stress in physicians: a review and meta-analysis. J Nerv Ment Dis. 2014;202(5):353–9.
30. Ducrocq E, Wilson M, Vine S, Derakshan N. Training attentional control improves cognitive and motor task performance. J Sport Exerc Psychol. 2016;38(5):521–33. Human Kinetics
31. Eysenck MW, Derakshan N, Santos R, Calvo MG. Anxiety and cognitive performance: attentional control theory. Emotion. 2007;7(2):336–53.
32. Wine J. Test anxiety and direction of attention. Psychol Bull [Internet]. 1971;76(2):92–104. Available from: https://psycnet.apa.org/record/1972-02065-001
33. Tryon G. The measurement and treatment of test anxiety. Rev Educ Res. 1980;50(2):343–72.
34. Zaccaro A, Piarulli A, Laurino M, Garbella E, Menicucci D, Neri B, et al. How breath-control can change your life: a systematic review on psycho-physiological correlates of slow breathing. Front Hum Neurosci. 2018;12:353.
35. Deshauer S, McQueen S, Hammond Mobilio M, Mutabdzic D, Moulton C-AE. Mental skills in surgery: lessons learned from Virtuosos, Olympians, and Navy seals. Ann Surg. 2019;
36. Bernier M, Thienot E, Codron R, Fournier JF. Mindfulness and acceptance approaches in sport performance. J Clin Sport Psychol [Internet]. 2009;3(4):320–33. Available from: https://hal-insep.archives-ouvertes.fr/hal-01710619
37. De Couck M, Caers R, Musch L, Fliegauf J, Giangreco A, Gidron Y. How breathing can help you make better decisions: two studies on the effects of breathing patterns on heart rate variability and decision-making in business cases. Int J Psychophysiol. 2019;139:1–9.
38. Ram Bahadur Singh, Agnieszka Wilczyńska-Kwiatek, Jan Fedacko, Daniel Pella, Fabien De Meester. Pranayama: the power of breath. Int J Disabil Hum Dev [Internet]; 2009;8(2):141–154. De Gruyter. Available from: https://www.degruyter.com/view/journals/ijdhd/8/2/article-p141.xml
39. Holland B, Gosselin K, Mulcahy A. The effect of autogenic training on self-efficacy, anxiety, and performance on nursing student simulation. Nurs Educ Perspect. 2017;38(2):87–9.
40. Cowings PS, Kellar MA, Folen RA, Toscano WB, Burge JD. Autogenic feedback training exercise and pilot performance: enhanced functioning under search-and-rescue flying conditions. Int J Aviat Psychol. 2001;11(3):303–15. Taylor & Francis
41. Driskell JE, Willis R, Copper C. Effect of overlearning on retention. J Appl Psychol. 1992;77:615–22.
42. Toth AJ, McNeill E, Hayes K, Moran AP, Campbell M. Does mental practice still enhance performance? A 24 Year follow-up and meta-analytic replication and extension. Psychol Sport Exer [Internet]. 2020;48:101672. Available from: https://www.sciencedirect.com/science/article/pii/S1469029219301530
43. Driskell JE, Copper C, Moran A. Does mental practice enhance performance? J Appl Psychol [Internet]. 1994;79(4):481–92. Available from: https://psycnet-apa-org.uml.idm.oclc.org/doiLanding?doi=10.1037%2F0021-9010.79.4.481
44. Hall JC. Imagery practice and the development of surgical skills. Am J Surg. 2002;184(5):465–70.

45. Arora S, Aggarwal R, Sirimanna P, Moran A, Grantcharov T, Kneebone R, et al. Mental practice enhances surgical technical skills: a randomized controlled study. Ann Surg. 2011;253(2):265–70.
46. Lorello GR, Hicks CM, Ahmed S-A, Unger Z, Chandra D, Hayter MA. Mental practice: a simple tool to enhance team-based trauma resuscitation. CJEM; 2016;18(2):136–142. Cambridge University Press
47. Lee K, Kim MJ, Park J, Park JM, Kim KH, Shin DW, et al. The effect of distraction by dual work on a CPR practitioner's efficiency in chest compression: a randomized controlled simulation study. Medicine. 2017;96(43):e8268.
48. Hirst W, Spelke E, Reaves C, Caharack G, Neisser U. Dividing attention without alternation or automaticity. J Exp Psychol Gen [Internet]. 1980;109(1):98–117. Available from: https://www.semanticscholar.org/paper/Dividing-Attention-Without-Alternation-or-Hirst-Spelke/b5001905e38230c95fc80ff94cd73ff03b8dc2cd
49. Spelke E, Hirst W, Neisser U. Skills of divided attention. Cognition [Internet]. 1976;4(3):215–30. Available from: https://www.sciencedirect.com/science/article/abs/pii/0010027776900184
50. Voelcker-Rehage C, Alberts JL. Effect of motor practice on dual-task performance in older adults. J Gerontol B Psychol Sci Soc Sci. 2007;62(3):P141–8.
51. Damos DL, Bittner AC Jr, Kennedy RS, Harbeson MM. Effects of extended practice on dual-task tracking performance. Hum Factors [Internet]. 1981;23(5):627–31. Available from: https://journals--sagepub-com.uml.idm.oclc.org/doi/10.1177/001872088102300512
52. ten Cate O, Durning SJ. Understanding clinical reasoning from multiple perspectives: a conceptual and theoretical overview. In: Principles and practice of case-based clinical reasoning education [Internet], Innovation and change in professional education, vol. 15. Cham: Springer; 2017. p. 35–46. Available from: https://www.ncbi.nlm.nih.gov/books/NBK543757/.
53. Plessow F, Schade S, Kirschbaum C, Fischer R. Successful voluntary recruitment of cognitive control under acute stress. Cognition. 2017;168:182–90.
54. Johnston JH, Driskell JE, Salas E. Vigilant and hypervigilant decision making. J Appl Psychol. 1997;82(4):614–22.
55. Gamble KR, Vettel JM, Patton DJ, Eddy MD, Caroline Davis F, Garcia JO, et al. Different profiles of decision making and physiology under varying levels of stress in trained military personnel. Int J Psychophysiol. 2018;131:73–80.
56. Hepler TJ, Kovacs AJ. Influence of acute stress on decision outcomes and heuristics. J Sports Med Phys Fitness. 2017;57(3):305–12.
57. Driskell JE, Salas E, Johnston JH. Does stress lead to a loss of team perspective? Group Dyn Theor Res Pract [Internet]. 1999;3(4):291–302. Available from: https://psycnet.apa.org/record/1999-01744-006
58. Adler AB, Start AR, Milham L, Allard YS, Riddle D, Townsend L, et al. Rapid response to acute stress reaction: pilot test of iCOVER training for military units. Psychol Trauma. 2020;12(4):431–5.
59. Svetlitzky V, Farchi M, Ben Yehuda A, Adler AB. YaHaLOM: a rapid intervention for acute stress reactions in high-risk occupations. Military Behav Health. 2019;8(2):232–42. 2nd ed. Routledge
60. Ellis A. System breakdown: the role of mental models and transactive memory in the relationship between acute stress and team performance. Acad Manag J [Internet]. 2006;49(3):576–89. Available from: https://www.jstor.org/stable/20159782?seq=1
61. Ellis APJ, Pearsall MJ. Reducing the negative effects of stress in teams through cross-training: a job demands-resources model. Group Dyn Theor Res Pract. 2011;15(1):16–31.
62. Grossman D, Christensen LW. On combat: the psychology and physiology of deadly conflict in war and in peace [Internet]. PPCT Research Publications; 2007. Available from: https://books.google.ca/books/about/On_Combat.html?id=lJdaAAAAYAAJ
63. Munshi F, Lababidi H, Alyousef S. Low- versus high-fidelity simulations in teaching and assessing clinical skills. J Taibah Univ Med Sci [Internet]. 2015;10(1):12–5. Available from: https://www.researchgate.net/publication/273517582_Low-_versus_high-fidelity_simulations_in_teaching_and_assessing_clinical_skills
64. Steigerwald SN, Park J, Hardy KM, Gillman LM, Vergis AS. Does laparoscopic simulation predict intraoperative performance? A comparison between the Fundamentals of Laparoscopic Surgery and LapVR evaluation metrics. Am J Surg. 2015;209(1):34–9.
65. Driskell JE, Johnston JH, Salas E. Does stress training generalize to novel settings? Hum Factors. 2001;43(1):99–110. 2nd ed
66. Saunders T, Driskell JE, Johnston JH, Salas E. The effect of stress inoculation training on anxiety and performance. J Occup Health Psychol. 1996;1(2):170–86.
67. Bisson JI, Roberts NP, Andrew M, Cooper R, Lewis C. Psychological therapies for chronic post-traumatic stress disorder (PTSD) in adults. In: Cochrane Common Mental Disorders Group, editor. Cochrane database systematic reviews, vol. 12. Wiley; 2013. p. CD003388.
68. West DJ, Horan JJ, Games PA. Component analysis of occupational stress inoculation applied to registered nurses in an acute care hospital setting. J Counsel Psychol [Internet]. 1984;31(2):209–18. Available from: https://asu.pure.elsevier.com/en/publications/component-analysis-of-occupational-stress-inoculation-applied-to-
69. Ghazali DA, Breque C, Sosner P, Lesbordes M, Chavagnat J-J, Ragot S, et al. Stress response in the daily lives of simulation repeaters. In: Puebla I, editor. A randomized controlled trial assessing stress evolution over one year of repetitive immersive simulations, vol. 14(7). PLoS One. Public Library of Science; 2019. p. e0220111.

What Is Mindfulness, and What Role Can It Play in the Mental Health of Health Professionals

14

Rae Paulene Spiwak, Shaan Sareen, Natalie Mota, Justin Gawaziuk, and Sarvesh Logsetty

Introduction

When thinking of mindfulness, an image of a Buddhist monk meditating on a hilltop may come to mind. In fact, this form of mindfulness meditation has existed for nearly 3000 years, yet the popularity of mindfulness to reduce stress and help regulate emotion has only more recently become a popular term or buzzword. Mindfulness, or the state of being present or aware, has been shown to reduce stress, improve attention and memory, reduce anxiety and depression symptoms, and help regulate emotion. This evidence goes back nearly 50 years, beginning with the pioneer of meditation research, Dr. Herbert Benson in 1975. Benson coined this technique as the relaxation response and identified the ability for mindfulness to reduce blood pressure, heart rate, and brain activity, including calming the body's stress or "fight or flight" response. This chapter will help clarify what mindfulness is, as well as identify some of the emerging evidence-based benefits of mindfulness for patients and clinicians. We will review the epidemiology of trauma exposure and other mental health outcomes among health professionals to highlight the important role that mindfulness techniques can play in improving mental health, and we will conclude with concrete tools and tips for health professionals on how to use mindfulness in their daily lives.

R. P. Spiwak · S. Sareen · J. Gawaziuk (✉)
Department of Surgery, Max Rady Faculty of Health Sciences, University of Manitoba, Winnipeg, MB, Canada
e-mail: Rae.Spiwak@umanitoba.ca; justin.gawaziuk@umanitoba.ca

N. Mota
Departments Clinical Health Psychology and Psychiatry, Max Rady Faculty of Health Sciences, University of Manitoba, Winnipeg, MB, Canada
e-mail: natalie.mota@umanitoba.ca

S. Logsetty
Departments of Surgery, Psychiatry, and Pediatrics and Child Health, Max Rady Faculty of Health Sciences, University of Manitoba, Winnipeg, MB, Canada

Firefighters Burn Unit, Health Sciences Centre, Winnipeg, MB, Canada
e-mail: Sarvesh.Logsetty@umanitoba.ca

What Is Mindfulness and How Can It Help Mental Health and Well-Being?

Mindfulness has been referred to as a state of awareness where we aim to pay attention to both internal (e.g., thoughts, feelings, bodily sensations) and external stimuli (e.g., objects, sounds, activities) in a non-judgmental way, from moment to moment, and with total acceptance (Oxford mindfulness center NHS) [1–3]. Mindfulness techniques allow one to be present in the moment and to fully connect with the environment, including enabling the acknowledgment and appreciation of current thoughts and feelings. Such a practice can be helpful in increasing awareness to times of higher stress or anxiety. The practice of mindfulness can also allow the brain to take a break from daily thoughts/stressors by engaging with the world. There are several practices in which an individual can engage to facilitate mindfulness, including yoga, tai chi, and mindfulness meditation. These activities focus on the practice of attending and being aware of the current moment [4].

There are eight pillars or key concepts of mindfulness [5] (Fig. 14.1). The first is attention, in other words, focusing one's attention on the present moment and redirecting the mind away from thoughts about the present or future. Mindfulness training with the inclusion of focusing on the present-moment/experience has been shown to reduce anxiety and depression [5]. The second pillar of mindfulness is automaticity the ability to do tasks and objectives automatically. Mindfulness practice includes recognizing which thoughts and emotions are automatic (the opposite of being mindful) and potentially harmful, then taking steps to reduce automaticity of these thoughts. The third pillar is judgment, which allows the individual to recognize the judgmental nature of their mind and its problematic aspects. Recognizing negative self-talk and transitioning to positive or motiva-

L. Marshall Gillman, S. Widder (eds.), *Trauma Team Dynamics*, https://doi.org/10.1007/978-3-031-86312-7_14

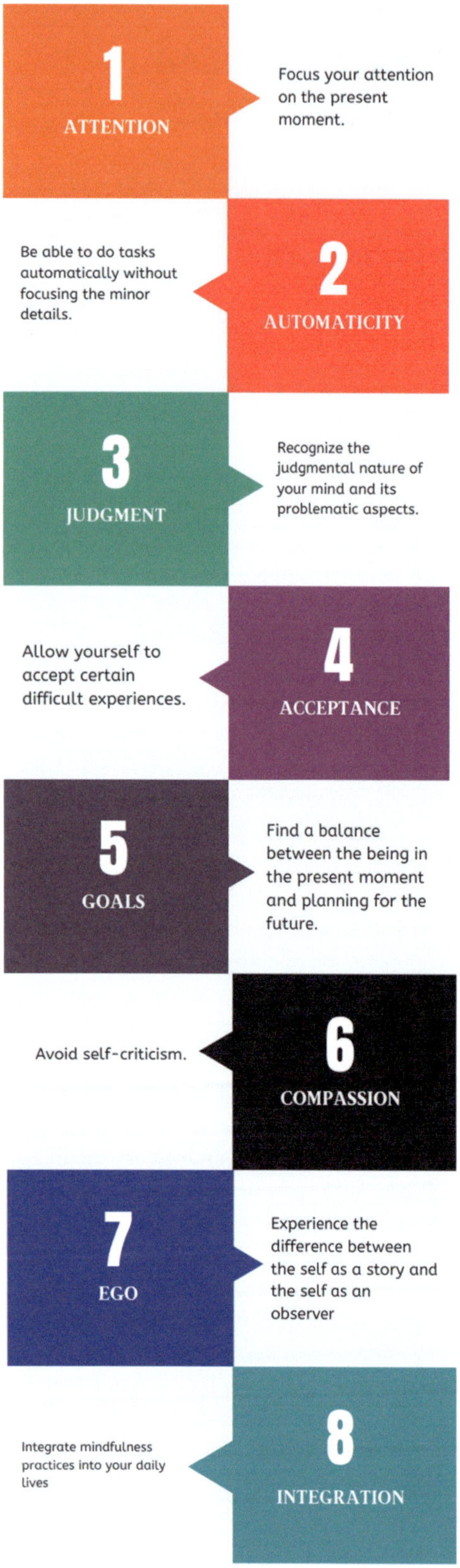
1
ATTENTION
Focus your attention on the present moment.
Be able to do tasks automatically without focusing the minor details.
2
AUTOMATICITY
3
JUDGMENT
Recognize the judgmental nature of your mind and its problematic aspects.
Allow yourself to accept certain difficult experiences.
4
ACCEPTANCE
5
GOALS
Find a balance between the being in the present moment and planning for the future.
Avoid self-criticism.
6
COMPASSION
7
EGO
Experience the difference between the self as a story and the self as an observer
Integrate mindfulness practices into your daily lives
8
INTEGRATION

Fig. 14.1 Eight pillars of mindfulness

tional self-talk has been shown to increase performance in athletes and reduce anxiety [6]. The fourth pillar is acceptance, which enables participants to accept specific difficult and negative experiences as inevitable (not fully within the person's control). Acceptance allows the individual to focus their attention on aspects of life that are within their control. The fifth pillar is goals; participants are encouraged to balance and separate being in the present moment with planning for the future. The sixth pillar is compassion, which discourages self-criticism. Showing oneself compassion can decrease more severe day-to-day negative thoughts and emotions [7]. The seventh pillar is ego, allowing individuals to experience the difference between the self as a story and an observer. This allows the individual to practice an observational relationship with the mind instead of strictly thinking in the first-person. The eighth and final pillar is integration, which emphasizes the integration of mindfulness practice in daily life. While identifying the eight pillars to outline important components of mindfulness is important, developing a mindfulness practice is essential to yield the many evidence-based benefits for both clinicians and non-clinicians.

Some of the empirically supported advantages of mindfulness include reduced rumination, stress, and emotional reactivity, as well as improvements to memory, ability, and focus. For example, a study by Farb et al. (2010) found that individuals who were part of an 8-week mindfulness-based stress reduction group experienced reduced levels of sadness and less neural reactivity (reduced emotional reactivity) as measured by fMRI data when compared to a wait-list control group who did not practice mindfulness [8]. Recent systematic reviews have also supported the global benefits of mindfulness related to depression and anxiety, stress reduction, as well as promising preliminary effects on sleep disturbance, eating disorders, and addiction [9]. While the evidence to support mindfulness in the treatment of post-traumatic stress disorder (PTSD) is developing, overall, it appears that meditation interventions have a positive effect on PTSD; however, due to the vast variability in follow-up time, study quality and overall methodological limitations, more high-quality work is needed to further understand this relationship [9]. Taken together, mindfulness practice may be an important prevention and mental health promotion for both physicians and non-physicians alike.

What Are the Benefits of Mindfulness for Physicians and Health Professionals?

A growing body of literature has demonstrated the effectiveness of mindfulness-based interventions in improving psychological outcomes for health professionals [10]. A recent meta-analysis of 25 studies including both randomized and non-randomized clinical trials found decreases in stress and burnout following completion of mindfulness-based interventions [11]. Other systematic reviews have reached similar conclusions of reduced burnout, improved psychological well-being, and/or decreases in anxiety and depression in physicians participating in interventions with a mindfulness component [12–15]. Reviews have also highlighted the beneficial effects of mindfulness among nurses, suggesting it can be helpful in reducing work-related stress [10]. Emerging evidence in studies of physician samples has also supported a link between mindfulness-based interventions and improvements in other outcomes relevant to well-being, such as loneliness and sleep [16]. One study even identified improvements in heart rate and systolic blood pressure (e.g., biological markers of stress) during participation in a mindfulness-based stress reduction program [17].

Mindfulness-based interventions have additionally led to promising outcomes in some performance indicators among physicians, including improved competencies related to patient safety, more patient-centered communication, and greater empathy, conscientiousness, positive tone, and emotional stability [14, 15, 17–21].

It should be noted, however, that research related to the effectiveness of mindfulness in health professional samples specifically is still limited, the types of mindfulness-based interventions studied in extant research have varied widely, and the methodological rigor of studies has varied equally widely. For example, the overall quality of the evidence in the meta-analysis of physician mindfulness by Fendel and colleagues, for example, was determined to be low (2021). To draw more definitive conclusions in the future for the effectiveness of mindfulness-based interventions among physicians, more randomized clinical trials with greater standardization in length and content of mindfulness practice are needed.

Epidemiology of Trauma Exposure and Mental Health Outcomes

Due to the nature of their employment, healthcare providers including attending and resident physicians are at risk for trauma exposure, including sudden deaths, disaster exposure, and hazard exposures such as COVID-19 [22]. These exposures place health professionals at increased risk for poorer mental health consequences, including PTSD, all of which not only impact well-being but have potential impact on quality of care, healthcare costs, and medical errors [23, 24]. A systematic review of the mental health of doctors in Australia found physician rates of depression ranged from 14% to 60%; anxiety rates ranged between 18% and 55%; and physicians had greater rates of prescription drug use, such as benzodiazepines when compared to other professions [25]. Physicians had greater rates of suicide when compared to the general population, with female physicians having a 146% higher risk of suicide than the general population [25]. Some work suggests that physician trainees may experience even greater mental health consequences of trauma exposures due to being earlier in their training and acquisition of experience, and too often having greater responsibility for providing frontline clinical care with a large patient volume. A recent study of 1134 medical interns found that work-related PTSD occurred three times more often among intern physicians when compared to individuals from the general population. More than half of this group experienced work-related trauma, and of these individuals, almost 20% had possible PTSD [26]. A systematic review of physician and trainee mental health in North America found that most of the existing literature related to physician mental health focused on burnout, with limited work on how physician mental health may impact patients, patient satisfaction, and barriers to help seeking. Future work in these areas is needed [27].

The COVID-19 pandemic has played a large role in the mental health of healthcare providers, with health professionals experiencing higher levels of burnout, insomnia, and mental disorders, including depression [28, 29]. Studies have found that working as a frontline healthcare worker was a risk factor for poor mental outcomes during the pandemic [30, 31]. Certain frontline workers, including those working in emergency, respiratory, infectious disease, and intensive care units, were found to have twice the likelihood of anxiety and depression when compared to non-clinical staff [31]. Whether dealing with traumatic exposures due to death and disease, or due to the pandemic, healthcare providers may benefit from better coping skills to prevent distress and poor mental outcomes. Mindfulness techniques have been shown to reduce distress and improve coping skills [32, 33] and may be a useful way to improve health professional's mental health [34, 35].

Tools for Clinicians: Tips for Mindfulness

Limitations notwithstanding, literature to date supports the benefit of mindfulness-based interventions in improving several outcomes for healthcare providers. As such, several helpful resources have been developed to support greater exposure to mindfulness in this population [36]. The Mindfulness Institute (http://www.mindfulnessinstitute.ca/mindfulness-in-medicine) describes the different institutions with current curricula related to mindfulness in their medical schools, as well as mindfulness-based programs in which physicians can register. The Institute for Physician Wellness also hosts mindfulness-based stress reduction programs specifically for healthcare professionals (https://www.instituteforphysicianwellness.com/mindfulness-in-medicine/). Finally, several books provide excellent starting points for embarking on mindfulness practice, including *Attending: Medicine, Mindfulness, and Humanity* by Dr. Ronald Epstein [37]. In addition, mindfulness applications are readily available on numerous handheld devices [38].

One of the reasons mindfulness is so powerful is because it can be done anytime and anywhere. Practice begins by attending to a chosen stimulus in the present moment, without judgment. It is often recommended that beginners to mindfulness start by focusing on their breath or paying attention to an object or sound in the environment or focusing on the taste and smell of a piece of food (e.g., a mint). The idea is to focus one's attention on the target and really noticing all aspects of it. For example, if it is mindfulness of breath that is being practiced, one might notice whether their breath is deep or shallow, its pace, and whether exhalation occurs through their mouth or nose. It is normal and even expected for the mind to wander during mindfulness practice, for example, to a task that needs completing, to a feeling of stress or anxiety, or to a thought of what is for dinner! Part of mindfulness practice is to gently redirect one's attention to the target, often many times. There is no recommended length of time for a mindfulness practice, but a few minutes in between stressful tasks can be helpful in resetting.

Conclusions, Implications, Next Steps

While much support exists for the practice of mindfulness in improving mental health and well-being, research studies are needed that are of higher quality, with larger sample sizes, appropriate and randomized comparison groups, and with the use of consistent measurement tools and terms [9]. Second, understanding if clinicians and/or individuals who are exposed to trauma regularly through their employment would benefit from mindfulness practice as a form of prevention and mental health promotion is an important future direction. Third, identifying levels of training (e.g., trainees, physicians) and how these individuals respond to traumatic events, including the role of meditation in this response, would be a valuable addition to the evidence base. In conclusion, mindfulness is a powerful and useful tool that is likely to be helpful to health professionals and improve mental health throughout their practice.

Key Points

- Mindfulness may be a useful tool for mental health of health professionals to reducing stress, burnout, anxiety, and depression.
- Mindfulness is maintaining awareness of the present moment in a non-judgmental way.
- Evidence surrounding the effectiveness of mindfulness is still emerging.
- Future research is needed to understand the benefits of mindfulness.

References

1. American Psychological Association. What are the benefits of mindfulness? 2012. https://www.apa.org/monitor/2012/07-08/ce-corner. Accessed 14 Aug 2022.
2. Keng SL, Smoski MJ, Robins CJ. Effects of mindfulness on psychological health: a review of empirical studies. Clin Psychol Rev. 2011;31:1041. https://doi.org/10.1016/J.CPR.2011.04.006.
3. National Health Service. Mindfulness. 2018. https://www.nhs.uk/mental-health/self-help/tips-and-support/mindfulness/. Accessed 14 Aug 2022.
4. Walsh R, Shapiro SL. The meeting of meditative disciplines and Western psychology: a mutually enriching dialogue. Am Psychol. 2006;61:227–39. https://doi.org/10.1037/0003-066X.61.3.227.
5. Parmentier FBR, García-Toro M, García-Campayo J, et al. Mindfulness and symptoms of depression and anxiety in the general population: the mediating roles of worry, rumination, reappraisal and suppression. Front Psychol. 2019:10. https://doi.org/10.3389/FPSYG.2019.00506.
6. Hatzigeorgiadis A, Zourbanos N, Mpoumpaki S, et al. Mechanisms underlying the self-talk–performance relationship: the effects of motivational self-talk on self-confidence and anxiety. Psychol Sport Exerc. 2009;10:186–92. https://doi.org/10.1016/J.PSYCHSPORT.2008.07.009.
7. Jazaieri H, Jinpa GT, McGonigal K, et al. Enhancing compassion: a randomized controlled trial of a compassion cultivation training program. J Happiness Stud. 2013;14:1113–26. https://doi.org/10.1007/s10902-012-9373-z.
8. Farb NAS, Anderson AK, Mayberg H, et al. Minding one's emotions: mindfulness training alters the neural expression of sadness. Emotion. 2010;10:25. https://doi.org/10.1037/A0017151.
9. Zhang D, Lee EKP, Mak ECW, et al. Mindfulness-based interventions: an overall review. Br Med Bull. 2021;138:41–57. https://doi.org/10.1093/BMB/LDAB005.
10. Chmielewski J, Łoś K, Łuczyński W. Mindfulness in healthcare professionals and medical education. Int J Occup Med Environ Health. 2021;34:1–14. https://doi.org/10.13075/ijomeh.1896.01542.
11. Fendel JC, Bürkle JJ, Göritz AS. Mindfulness-based interventions to reduce burnout and stress in physicians: a study protocol for a systematic review and meta-analysis. BMJ Open. 2019;9:e032295. https://doi.org/10.1136/BMJOPEN-2019-032295.
12. Melnyk BM, Kelly SA, Stephens J, et al. Interventions to improve mental health, well-being, physical health, and lifestyle behaviors in physicians and nurses: a systematic review. Am J Health Promot. 2020;34:929–41. https://doi.org/10.1177/0890117120920451.
13. Regehr C, Glancy D, Pitts A, et al. Interventions to reduce the consequences of stress in physicians: a review and meta-analysis. J Nerv Ment Dis. 2014;202:353–9. https://doi.org/10.1097/NMD.0000000000000130.
14. Scheepers RA, Emke H, Epstein RM, et al. The impact of mindfulness-based interventions on doctors' well-being and performance: a systematic review. Med Educ. 2020;54:138–49. https://doi.org/10.1111/MEDU.14020.
15. Tement S, Ketiš ZK, Miroševič Š, et al. The impact of psychological interventions with elements of mindfulness (PIM) on empathy, well-being, and reduction of burnout in physicians: a systematic review. Int J Environ Res Public Health. 2021:18. https://doi.org/10.3390/IJERPH182111181.
16. Thimmapuram J, Pargament R, del Tredici S, et al. Sleep patterns of resident physicians and the effect of heartfulness meditation. Ann Neurosci. 2021;28:47–54. https://doi.org/10.1177/09727531211039070.
17. Amutio A, Martínez-Taboada C, Hermosilla D, et al. Enhancing relaxation states and positive emotions in physicians through a mindfulness training program: a one-year study. Psychol Health Med. 2015;20:720–31. https://doi.org/10.1080/13548506.2014.986143.

18. Beach MC, Roter D, Korthuis PT, et al. A multicenter study of physician mindfulness and health care quality. Ann Fam Med. 2013;11:421–8. https://doi.org/10.1370/AFM.1507.
19. Krasner MS, Epstein RM, Beckman H, et al. Association of an educational program in mindful communication with burnout, empathy, and attitudes among primary care physicians. JAMA. 2009;302:1284–93. https://doi.org/10.1001/JAMA.2009.1384.
20. Liu C, Chen H, Cao X, et al. Effects of mindfulness meditation on doctors' mindfulness, patient safety culture, patient safety competency and adverse event. Int J Environ Res Public Health. 2022:19. https://doi.org/10.3390/IJERPH19063282.
21. Nguyen MC, Gabbe SG, Kemper KJ, et al. Training on mind-body skills: feasibility and effects on physician mindfulness, compassion, and associated effects on stress, burnout, and clinical outcomes. 2019;15:194–207. https://doi.org/10.1080/17439760.2019.1578892.
22. Morganstein JC, West JC, Ursano RJ, et al. Work-associated trauma. Phys Mental Health Well-Being. 2017:33–60. https://doi.org/10.1007/978-3-319-55583-6_2.
23. West CP, Dyrbye LN, Shanafelt TD. Physician burnout: contributors, consequences and solutions. J Intern Med. 2018;283:516–29. https://doi.org/10.1111/JOIM.12752.
24. Fahrenkopf AM, Sectish TC, Barger LK, et al. Rates of medication errors among depressed and burnt out residents: prospective cohort study. BMJ. 2008;336:488–91. https://doi.org/10.1136/BMJ.39469.763218.BE.
25. Elliott L, Tan J, Norris S. The mental health of doctors: a systematic review. 2010. https://www.headsup.org.au/docs/default-source/resources/bl0823-mental-health-of-doctors-report.pdf?sfvrsn=e9fd234d_2. Accessed 16 Jan 2023.
26. Vance MC, Herberman Mash HB, Ursano RJ, et al. Exposure to workplace trauma and posttraumatic stress disorder among intern physicians. JAMA Netw Open. 2021;4:e2112837. https://doi.org/10.1001/JAMANETWORKOPEN.2021.12837.
27. Mihailescu M, Neiterman E. A scoping review of the literature on the current mental health status of physicians and physicians-in-training in North America. BMC Public Health. 2019;19:1363. https://doi.org/10.1186/s12889-019-7661-9.
28. Tiete J, Guatteri M, Lachaux A, et al. Mental health outcomes in healthcare workers in COVID-19 and non-COVID-19 care units: a cross-sectional survey in Belgium. Front Psychol. 2021:11. https://doi.org/10.3389/fpsyg.2020.612241.
29. Varghese A, George G, Kondaguli SV, et al. Decline in the mental health of nurses across the globe during COVID-19: a systematic review and meta-analysis. J Glob Health. 2021;11:05009. https://doi.org/10.7189/jogh.11.05009.
30. Lai J, Ma S, Wang Y, et al. Factors associated with mental health outcomes among health care workers exposed to coronavirus disease 2019. JAMA Netw Open. 2020;3:e203976. https://doi.org/10.1001/jamanetworkopen.2020.3976.
31. Lu W, Wang H, Lin Y, et al. Psychological status of medical workforce during the COVID-19 pandemic: a cross-sectional study. Psychiatry Res. 2020;288:112936. https://doi.org/10.1016/j.psychres.2020.112936.
32. de Vibe M, Solhaug I, Tyssen R, et al. Mindfulness training for stress management: a randomised controlled study of medical and psychology students. BMC Med Educ. 2013;13:107. https://doi.org/10.1186/1472-6920-13-107.
33. de Vibe M, Solhaug I, Rosenvinge JH, et al. Six-year positive effects of a mindfulness-based intervention on mindfulness, coping and well-being in medical and psychology students; Results from a randomized controlled trial. PLoS One. 2018;13:e0196053. https://doi.org/10.1371/journal.pone.0196053.
34. Klatt MD, Bawa R, Gabram O, et al. Embracing change: a mindful medical center meets COVID-19. Glob Adv Health Med. 2020;9:216495612097536. https://doi.org/10.1177/2164956120975369.
35. Marotta M, Gorini F, Parlanti A, et al. Effect of mindfulness-based stress reduction on the well-being, burnout and stress of Italian healthcare professionals during the COVID-19 Pandemic. J Clin Med. 2022;11:3136. https://doi.org/10.3390/jcm11113136.
36. Centre for Mindfulness Studies. CARE EXPANDED – Community & Resiliency for our Healthcare Workers in Ontario. 2022. https://www.mindfulnessstudies.com/care-community-and-resiliency-for-our-healthcare-workers/#:~:text=CARE%20is%20a%20six%2Dweek,being%20during%20these%20turbulent%20times. Accessed 1 Feb 2023.
37. Epstein R. Attending: medicine, mindfulness, and humanity. 1st ed. New York City: Scribner; 2017.
38. Muhiyaddin R, Abd-Alrazaq A, Shah Z, et al. Evaluation of meditation apps available on google play and apple store: an app review. 2022; https://doi.org/10.3233/SHTI210937.

Trauma Video Review

15

Michael A. Vella, Ryan P. Dumas, Zaffer A. Qasim,
Aekta Andrea Miglani, and Daniel N. Holena

Introduction/What Is Trauma Video Review?

Video review technology for use in surgical and emergency medical education was utilized as early as the 1960s [1–3]. Trauma video review (TVR), which specifically describes the process of recording trauma resuscitations for multipurpose review, was first described in 1988 [4]. At that time, researchers used a camera, videocassette recorder, and television mounted on a stand to record over 2500 resuscitations. They showed that implementation of a formal video review conference led to improved patient care delivery.

Modern technology allows for continuous high-definition audiovisual recording of trauma resuscitation bays, encrypted video storage with timed auto-deletion, and the ability to time-stamp, zoom, fast-forward, and rewind recordings [5] (See Fig. 15.1). Integration of video laryngoscopy, ultrasound, and vital sign monitor screens is also possible, while emerging technology allows for video-based activity recognition [6–8].

A central theme of this textbook is the concept that multidisciplinary team simulation and education lead to improved team dynamics, which in turn lead to improved processes of care, which ultimately lead to the common goal of improved patient outcomes. The power of TVR lies in the fact that this technology can be used (and is usually instrumental) in every step of this progression.

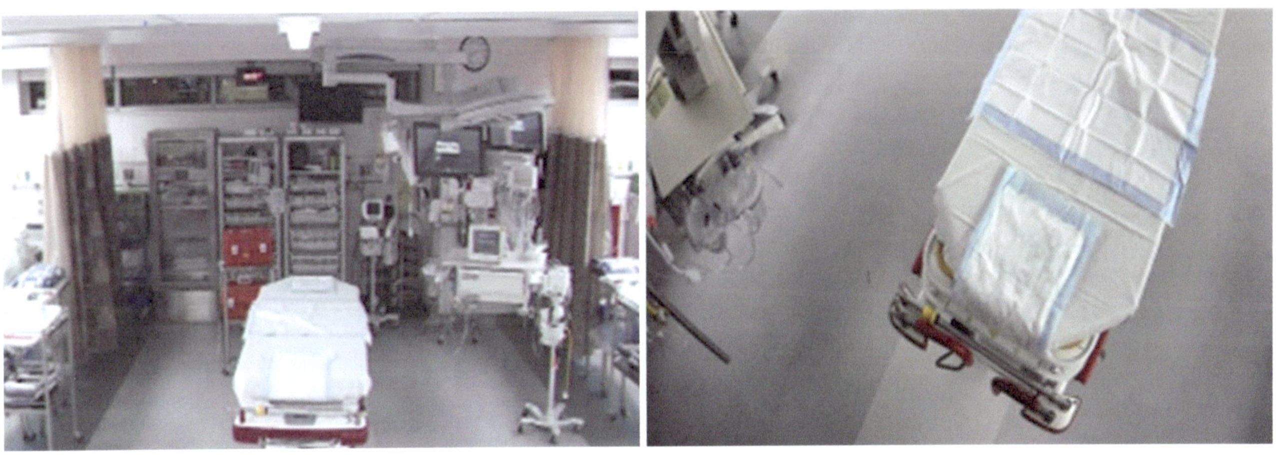

Fig. 15.1 Typical TVR Setup as viewed from cameras (and microphones) located at the foot and head of the bed. This is the view available for those evaluating stored videos

M. A. Vella (✉) · A. A. Miglani
University of Rochester School of Medicine and Dentistry, Rochester, NY, USA
e-mail: michael_vella@urmc.rochester.edu; aekta_miglani@urmc.rochester.edu

R. P. Dumas
Baylor College of Medicine, Houston, TX, USA
e-mail: ryan.dumas@bcm.edu

Z. A. Qasim
University of Pennsylvania Perelman School of Medicine, Philadelphia, PA, USA
e-mail: zaffer.qasim@pennmedicine.upenn.edu

D. N. Holena
University of Pennsylvania Perelman School of Medicine, Philadelphia, PA, USA

Medical College of Wisconsin, Wilwaukee, WI, USA
e-mail: dholena@mcw.edu

L. Marshall Gillman, S. Widder (eds.), *Trauma Team Dynamics*, https://doi.org/10.1007/978-3-031-86312-7_15

This chapter first describes TVR utilization and applications, focusing on the use of TVR for education, performance improvement (PI), and research purposes. Next, the practical considerations of starting or improving an existing TVR program are discussed. Finally, we describe the integration and maintenance of a successful multidisciplinary program as well as emerging opportunities for video-based review in and out of the emergency department.

Historical Trends in TVR Utilization

Despite its potential benefits, utilization of TVR has historically been low. A survey in 1999 of 221 US trauma centers found that only 20% of centers overall and 34% of level one centers were using TVR [9]. Subsequent surveys in 2006 and 2010, albeit with slightly different groups of institutions, found that utilization among level one centers had decreased to and stabilized at 18% [10, 11]. Thirty-five percent of centers in the 2006 study reported that the recently enacted Health Information Portability and Accountability Act (HIPAA) had impacted their TVR programs in some capacity, presumably due to perceived patient privacy and medicolegal concerns [10]. More recently, a 2019 survey of US trauma centers found that overall utilization and use among level one centers had increased to 29% in both groups, and 21% of non-users reported a strong interest in starting TVR program [12].

The most recent survey on TVR practices indicates that the technology is used most commonly for group and individual education and is frequently used to assess trauma team dynamics [12]. Nearly two-thirds of respondents reported that their TVR program has generating PI initiates, with 41% indicating that TVR has led to direct changes in institutional practices. Overall perception of TVR programs among active users was high, with a median score of 8 on a 10-point Likert scale on the domains of overall perception and reliability. These recent findings are consistent with those of older reports, including one study where 100% of respondents indicated that their TVR programs have led to improvement in resuscitation practices [10, 11, 13].

Current Applications and Utilization

Trauma video review has been used to evaluate a multitude of technical and non-technical elements of trauma resuscitation, including but not limited to, airway management, opportunities for improvement in resuscitation, compliance with personal protective equipment, timing of emergent procedures, team dynamics and leadership, and rapid changes in patient condition [8, 12, 14–22]. In these capacities, TVR has been shown to be more reliable than chart review, and video-based feedback has been shown to be more effective than its verbal counterpart [12, 23, 24]. Trauma video review applications can generally be categorized into three broad yet closely related areas, including team simulation/education, performance improvement, and research.

Team Simulation/Education

Evidence suggests that trauma team simulation and leadership training can improve team efficiency, communication, and performance [25–31]. Video equipment can be used to record simulated resuscitations and the associated debriefing sessions, which can be reviewed with the team immediately after the exercise or at a later date. Simulated scenarios can also be used at the outset of new TVR program implementation to improve familiarly with the TVR equipment and video review process. Video-based review of simulated trauma scenarios has also been used to identify latent safety threats that are likely to complicate real trauma resuscitations, such as factors related to communication, physical workspace, and equipment [32].

From an educational perspective, TVR of real trauma resuscitations is ideal for reviewing low frequency, high impact procedures (emergency department thoracotomy, cricothyroidotomy) as well as difficult clinical scenarios like the management of unstable or agitated patients or multicasualty events. The technology allows these "vicarious teachable moments" to be shared with clinicians who were not present during the initial resuscitation and is the arguably the next best thing to standing at the bedside [5]. Trauma video review also allows for evaluation of team dynamics and other "intangibles of resuscitation" that are known to be important but difficult if not impossible to evaluate through traditional means [5]. Various scoring system exist to grade team dynamics during recorded trauma resuscitations, such as the modified Trauma Non-technical Skills (NOTECHS) score [33–35] (See Table 15.1).

Performance Improvement

Trauma resuscitation has been described as a "complex, time critical endeavor requiring the coordinated efforts of a multidisciplinary health care team" [36]. It is imperative that trauma teams function effectively, as 70–80% of healthcare errors in general are related to poor teamwork and communication [37, 38]. Evidence shows that trauma team training improves team performance. In turn, improved team performance has been associated with improved processes of care including faster and more reliable completion of the primary and secondary trauma surveys and patient disposition in both simulated and actual patient scenarios [18, 25, 28, 39–46].

Table 15.1 Description of a Modified Trauma-NOTECHS scoring system

Modified Trauma-NOTECHS			
	1	2	3
Leadership	Team leader clearly recognizable at all times, “birds’ eye” view with delegation, transitions of leadership clear, assignment of roles, excellent time management	Team leader defined but does not fulfill all functions or does procedures meant for others or transitions unclear	Team leader not clear
Cooperation and Resource Management	All team members clearly identified, speak up if help needed, no team members are idle	Role identity of all members not clear, some team members idle some of the time	Role identity of most members not clear, most team members idle most of the time
Communication	Team leader is at the head of the bed, critical communication through the team leader, all orders to team leader, closed loop communication, orders directed to specific people	Communication not always through team leader, orders not always acknowledged	Communication frequently inaudible or incoherent with many simultaneous conversations
Assessment and decision-making	Primary and secondary survey done in order and without omissions, findings summarized, goals and plan communicated to the team	Assessment somewhat out of order, some elements of secondary survey incomplete	Elements of the primary survey incomplete, multiple team members unclear about the next step
Situation awareness	Unforeseen findings, distractions, or change in patient condition did not disrupt orderly evaluation. Team is calm, team plans ahead, awareness of team members emotional condition	Unforeseen findings caused minor delay but did not preclude task completion	Unforeseen events disrupt patient assessment and treatment. Team members stressed, lack of anticipation of next steps

Scoring systems such as this can be used to evaluate trauma team dynamics [33]

TVR allows for the direct evaluation of team performance and was instrumental in many of these studies. For example, one group found that a trauma team leader was not present in 50% of reviewed resuscitations [47]. This finding led to institutional changes in practice as well as implementation of education sessions related to errors in resuscitation. In another study, the implementation of a TVR program was associated with a 17% reduction in resuscitation time as well as improved adherence to resuscitation protocols [4].

Trauma video review is an excellent method to reliably evaluate “known unknowns” like team dynamics and leadership. Interpersonal and qualitative factors such as these are difficult to abstract from medical records and verbal recollections but are believed by expert clinicians to be factors critical to processes of care and patient outcomes [5]. Using a modified T-NOTECHS tool, Dumas et al. evaluated the association between team dynamics and return of spontaneous circulation (ROSC) in patients presenting to a level-one trauma center undergoing emergency department thoracotomy (EDT) [33]. Videos of 61 EDT over a two-year period were reviewed, and the authors found that patients with a “best” score in the domain of “assessment and decision making” were five times more likely to achieve ROSC compared to those with “average” or “worst” scores (See Table 15.1). This was one of the first studies to show an association between team dynamics and a tangible patient outcome. Of note, the median modified T-NOTECHS score for resuscitations in which ROSC was achieved was seven, indicating that even the “best” resuscitations have room for improvement. The presence of a robust TVR program was instrumental in this study.

Resuscitative procedures can also be evaluated with TVR. In one recent study, researchers used TVR to evaluate vascular access strategies in patients arriving in extremis and requiring EDT [19]. Using time-stamped videos, they found that intra-osseous access attempts were as fast as peripheral intravenous access attempts but nearly twice as likely to succeed, and far faster and more successful than central venous access attempts. Efforts such as these may lead to direct changes in institutional resuscitation practices that would be extremely difficult to evaluate without the presence of video review. At another institution, a pre-intubation checklist was evaluated using video review and was found to be associated with fewer errors in trauma airway management [8]. The authors discovered that poor team communication was a major contributor to adverse outcomes, a finding that would not have been evident from medical record review alone. Finally, others have used video review to define standards for procedures such as EDT in an attempt to improve consistency and associate procedural skill with outcomes [16].

Research

The previous sections detail the important role of TVR in research related to simulation/education and performance improvement. The power of TVR for research purposes lies in its ability to reliably and accurately collect data that is not present or incompletely captured in the medical record. Given the fast flow and density of information present in a trauma resuscitation, even traditional gold standards of data capture like prospective real-time in-person collection may fail [5]. For example, in a 2006 study of pediatric trauma resuscitations, only 20% of errors detected on video were found in the medical record [47]. These errors were most commonly related to the physical exam, team dynamics, and delays in therapy, which are ideally suited for video review. In a more recent study utilizing TVR to time EDT, only 57% of patients had any times recorded in the medical record, compared to 97% with TVR [16].

Trauma video review is ideal for research that requires accurate time stamps or the evaluation of rapid changes in patient condition. For example, retrospective studies that evaluate an emerging technology or location of device placement are often confounded by indication related to rapid changes in patient physiology or other logistical factors. While these elements are difficult to capture in a traditional registry, TVR technology may allow for capture of more granular data in order to answer these specific and important research questions.

Practical Considerations When Starting a TVR Program

Although barriers to implementation exist, the success of established and long-standing TVR programs and the increasing utilization of this technology suggest that TVR is safe and feasible. The following sections describe barriers to implementation and other practical considerations.

Potential Barriers

Commonly cited barriers to TVR implementation include medicolegal concerns, staff perceptions, lack of institutional precedent, financial implications, and potential time constraints.

Although medicolegal concerns are often raised in surveys on TVR practices, these reports also highlight the discrepancy between perceived concerns and actual medicolegal cases involving the technology [9, 11, 12]. In the most recent survey of TVR practices, only 2 of 71 (2.8%) centers with active TVR programs reported direct knowledge of *any* case involving TVR [12]. In many states, TVR is protected from discovery as a performance improvement tool, and some have argued that HIPAA does not apply to activities related to provider education and quality improvement. Although HIPAA does not specifically address the video recording of resuscitations, it does allow for data collection and research related to performance and quality improvement [12, 48]. Efforts to start a TVR program should include a detailed review of local and state legal processes along with specific hospital policies from the beginning. Understanding institution-specific medicolegal concerns from the outset helps direct the successful establishment of workflows and protocols. All TVR proposals should be vetted through hospital legal counsel, privacy officers, and hospital and departmental leadership. In some cases, it may be beneficial to provide evidence highlighting the safety and feasibility of successful programs. Contacting and establishing dialogue with similar institutions (or other departments within the same system) that have successfully navigated the process is helpful and prevents the need to "reinvent the wheel." Secure storage of videos, restricting access to recordings, obtaining informed consent, timed auto-deletion of videos, signage in resuscitation areas that indicates active recording is occurring, and separating stored videos from the medical record are some of the strategies that may help to mitigate legal concerns.

Consent Processes

Consent for TVR may not be required in all states, especially because the activity is often related to performance improvement. That said, legal counsel and institutional leadership will need to be involved to help determine both the need for and processes surrounding informed consent. The most recent data on consent practices show that 6% of active users specifically consent for TVR (usually in a retrospective fashion prior to video review but after the recording has occurred), 50% include video recording and review in the general hospital consent, and 30% do not consent at all [12].

Other Considerations

Prior to starting a program, it is important to perform a stakeholder analysis with all involved parties (included but not limited to trauma and emergency department staff, nurses, trainees, pre-hospital providers, and law enforcement) to discuss the benefits of and reasons for starting a program as well as to identify any potential barriers to implementation. It is important to offer opportunities for open discussion in various formats including town halls, emails, small group meetings, and one-on-one conversations when needed. A survey sent to all individuals who will be involved in the TVR process may help to anonymously identify individual staff concerns. While the literature suggests that TVR is well perceived among active users, TVR has been associated with anxiety among providers in at least one study [13]. It is the authors' experience that TVR is overwhelmingly a positive experience for all involved and that initial concerns are often assuaged once the benefits of the process are realized. Those starting a new program may find benefit in initially starting the recording and review process using simulated scenarios.

From a practical standpoint, programs must decide who has video access, how and what videos are chosen for review, what percentage of overall videos are reviewed, and who actually partakes in the review process. The time commitment for video review can be substantial, especially if a program decides to review all trauma resuscitations. Programs must also decide if video recording in the resuscitation bay will be continuous or will start upon manual activation of a button or switch. The most recent survey on TVR practices indicates that most current users continuously record resuscitation areas, store videos less than 30 days, and review <50% of resuscitations [12]. Institutional leadership and staff input should be considered when making these decisions. Finally, programs must decide on when and where to review videos, which is often done in a recurring multidisciplinary conference.

Equipment type and location, storage capacity, and existing building infrastructure should be considered when developing a TVR program. Financial investment for both initial start-up and ongoing maintenance costs is necessary. These factors are extremely important but beyond the scope of this review. Those interested in starting a program should consider reaching out to existing users (including the authors of this chapter) for advice. Potential users should also take advantage of existing infrastructure if similar video equipment and/or vendors are utilized in another area of the institution like the operating room or intensive care unit. Emphasizing the value of a TVR program as a patient safety and educational tool may help to increase support from stakeholders. Those interested in starting a TVR program are also encouraged to pursue available grant funding.

Integrating and Maintaining a Successful TVR Program

Integrating TVR into an existing PI program and maintaining enthusiasm can be challenging but are critically important. The time commitment and resource needs must not be underestimated. In a 2006 survey on TVR practices, 70% of programs that stopped using TVR cited scarce resources and provider time commitment as primary reasons for abandoning a program [10]. More recently, insufficient time was a frequently cited reason for stopping active TVR programs [12]. Resource commitment varies based on the number of individuals who participate in the TVR program as well as the percentage of overall trauma resuscitations chosen for review. These factors can be tailored to institutional needs and constraints.

Setting realistic goals and expectations from the beginning can help prevent the outpacing of resources. The goal of a robust TVR program should not be to review every single case (or even every aspect of a single chosen case), but instead to highlight elements of a trauma resuscitation that hold educational value. We have found that selecting components or certain elements of a resuscitation is most helpful and often choose resuscitations involving critically unstable patients, combative/agitated patients, simultaneous patient arrivals, or challenging airway management. Additionally, we have found that TVR is an ideal avenue to highlight relatively uncommon but high-risk procedures like EDT and cricothyroidotomy and to discuss the intangibles of resuscitation like leadership and team dynamics. Reviewing high-impact but relatively low-frequency procedures allows trainees, nurses, and practicing physicians to discuss procedural steps like positioning and equipment that are often underemphasized but critically important. Re-watching resuscitations on video also allows one to identify potential barriers related to spatial awareness, trauma bay set-up, target fixation, anchor bias, and time mismanagement that can subtly derail an otherwise effective resuscitation and are often not evident from traditional medical record review.

Each individual TVR program must decide the most appropriate venue to review resuscitations. We have found that presenting a small number of resuscitations or components of resuscitations at a recurring multidisciplinary conference with the trauma surgery and emergency medicine services is most educational. Having all members of the trauma team, including trainees, nurses, nurse managers, physicians, advanced practice providers, technologists, and emergency medical services, participate in the conference increases the educational value for all and also helps to achieve and maintain program buy-in and enthusiasm. Involving other specialties like neurosurgery, orthopedic surgery, obstetrics, and radiology may also be beneficial depending on the clinical scenarios presented.

While a TVR conference can be intimidating, especially if you are the one "under the lens," there are several important considerations that can be used to mitigate this anxiety and improve overall buy-in. It is our opinion that team performance rather than individual clinician performance should always be emphasized. As a general rule, all resuscitations contain opportunities for improvement as well as aspects that may have gone exceptionally well. Rather than focusing only on areas where a resuscitation could have been improved, it is important to us TVR as a tool to illustrate outstanding examples of leadership, communication, and teamwork when they occur. Such elements can be brought to light by asking questions such as "was there a clear team leader?", "did the team employ closed-loop communication?", "did physicians and nurses or emergency medicine and trauma surgery communicate effectively?", and "was crowd control managed appropriately throughout the resuscitation?". In general, individual names should not be used, and singling out or targeting individual providers must be avoided. Most providers will be unrecognizable on video when appropriate personal protective equipment is being used. Occasionally, using a proper name to highlight an aspect of a resuscitation that was done well can be used to maintain a positive TVR culture. If there is a particularly challenging case or a case during which a complication or unexpected event occurs, it is advisable to discuss the case with the primary clinician prior to group review; TVR should never surprise those involved on the day of a multidisciplinary conference. Given the high-stakes nature of trauma resuscitations and the interplay between providers that occurs, it is unavoidable that TVR will occasionally capture negative interpersonal interactions. *In such circumstances, we recommend that trauma video review never be used as an arbitration tool, to settle disputes between individuals, or in a punitive manner, as surely conflict resolution can be achieved between professionals without co-opting quality improvement efforts.*

Future Directions

Recent evidence suggests that TVR utilization is likely to increase [12]. Cloud-based storage and online-integrated review platforms (See Fig. 15.2) allow for relatively simple integration of a TVR program into both in-person and virtual conferences. The incorporation of artificial intelligence (AI) with video review is an area of emerging interest, with one recent paper discussing the utilization of these merged technologies to identify the critical view of safety during laparoscopy cholecystectomy [49]. Continued interest in the field of surgical safety and transparency in the operating room has led to the development of platforms that integrate multiple audiovisual feeds with patient data to create a robust timeline of operating room events [50]. This technology is also equipped with multiple AI algorithms to detect intraoperative thermal injuries and bleeding events [51, 52]. As this technology becomes increasingly available, it is likely to reach the trauma resuscitation bay, allowing for important variables like movement in and out of the trauma room, sound, and team dynamics to be studied in ways that were never before possible [6].

Additionally, there is a burgeoning interest in incorporating wearable technology in both the operating and trauma resuscitation rooms for video-based activity recognition and for use in evaluating surgeon ergonomics and technique [7, 53]. Video review technology has also emerged as a valuable tool in the intensive care unit setting, allowing for review of critical ICU events like cardiopulmonary resuscitation, airway management, bedside procedures, and team dynamics [54, 55]. We anticipate that video review technology will have an increasingly important role in the evaluation of non-traumatic yet time-sensitive resuscitations occurring in the emergency department, such as those related to acute coronary syndrome and stroke.

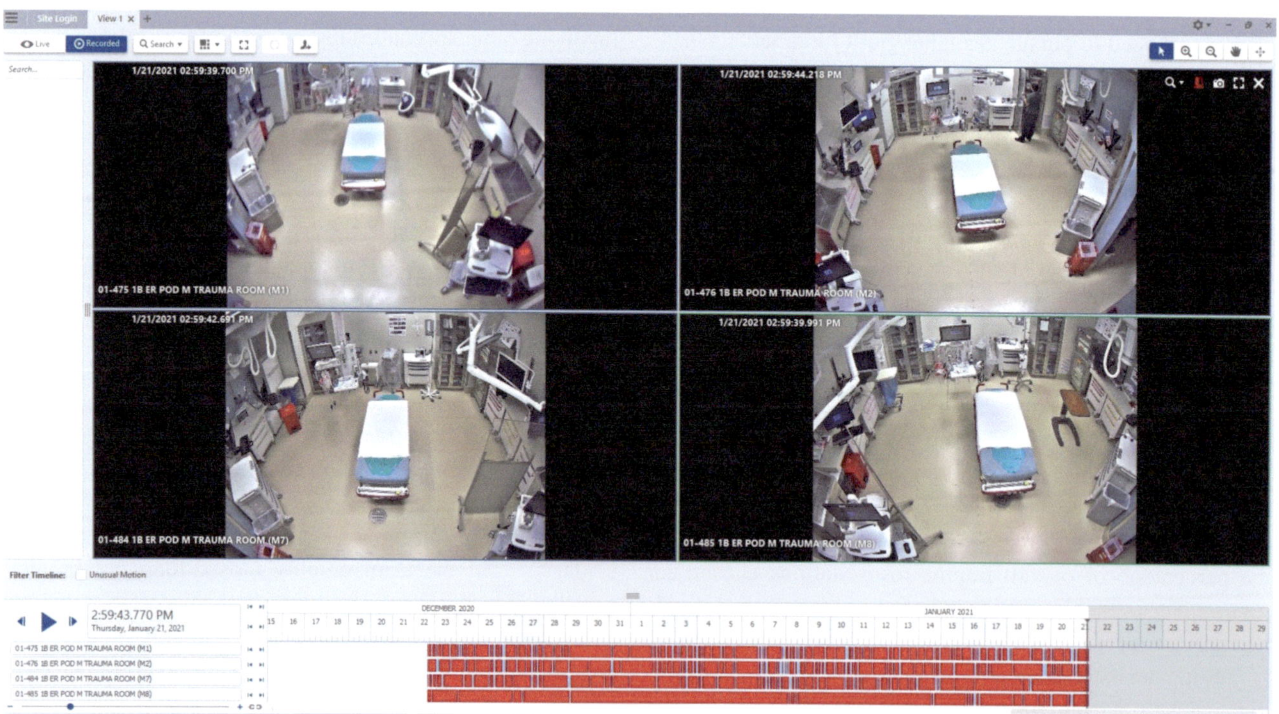

Fig. 15.2 Example of a cloud-based user interface showing camera views for multiple trauma rooms as well as demonstrating the availability of time stamp, fast-forward, and re-wind functions

Conclusion

Video review technology along with video-based trainee education and assessment will only increase over the next decade. This technology and its myriad of applications will undoubtedly improve the quality of care administered to patients in the trauma resuscitation bay, the operating room, and beyond. It is crucial for trauma practitioners to be at the forefront of video review advancement and implementation.

References

1. Williams KS, Pace C, Milia D, Juern J, Rubin J. Development of a video recording and review process for trauma resuscitation quality and education. West J Emerg Med. 2019;20(2):228–31.
2. Goldman LI, Maier WP, Rosemond GP, Saltzman SW, Cramer LM. Teaching surgical technique by the critical review of videotaped performance – the surgical instant replay. Surgery. 1969;66(1):237–41.
3. Goldman LI, McDonough MT, Rosemond GP. Stresses affecting surgical performance and learning. I. Correlation of heart rate, electrocardiogram, and operation simultaneously recorded on videotapes. J Surg Res. 1972;12(2):83–6.
4. Hoyt DB, Shackford SR, Fridland PH, Mackersie RC, Hansbrough JF, Wachtel TL, et al. Video recording trauma resuscitations: an effective teaching technique. J Trauma. 1988;28(4):435–40.
5. Vella MA, Dumas RP, Holena DN. Supporting the educational, research, and clinical care goals of the academic trauma center: video review for trauma resuscitation. JAMA Surg. 2019;154(3):257–8.
6. Nolan B, Hicks CM, Petrosoniak A, Jung J, Grantcharov T. Pushing boundaries of video review in trauma: using comprehensive data to improve the safety of trauma care. Trauma Surg Acute Care Open. 2020;5(1):e000510.
7. Chakraborty I, Elgammal A, Burd RS. Video based activity recognition in truama resuscitation. https://www.computer.org/csdl/proceedings/fg/2013/5545/00/06553758-abs.html. Accessed 1 Nov 2020.
8. Smith KA, High K, Collins SP, Self WH. A preprocedural checklist improves the safety of emergency department intubation of trauma patients. Acad Emerg Med. 2015;22(8):989–92.
9. Ellis DG, Lerner EB, Jehle DV, Romano K, Siffring C. A multistate survey of videotaping practices for major trauma resuscitations. J Emerg Med. 1999;17(4):597–604.
10. Campbell S, Sosa JA, Rabinovici R, Frankel H. Do not roll the videotape: effects of the health insurance portability and accountability act and the law on trauma videotaping practices. Am J Surg. 2006;191(2):183–90.
11. Rogers SC, Dudley NC, McDonnell W, Scaife E, Morris S, Nelson D. Lights, camera, action… spotlight on trauma video review: an underutilized means of quality improvement and education. Pediatr Emerg Care. 2010;26(11):803–7.
12. Dumas RP, Vella MA, Hatchimonji JS, Ma L, Maher Z, Holena DN. Trauma video review utilization: a survey of practice in the United States. Am J Surg. 2020;219(1):49–53.
13. Davis L, Johnson L, Allen SR, Kim PK, Sims CA, Pascual JL, et al. Practitioner perceptions of trauma video review. J Trauma Nurs. 2013;20(3):150–4.
14. Mackenzie CF, Xiao Y, Hu FM, Seagull FJ, Fitzgerald M. Video as a tool for improving tracheal intubation tasks for emergency medical and trauma care. Ann Emerg Med. 2007;50(4):436–42e1.
15. DiGiacomo JC, Hoff WS, Rotondo MF, Martin K, Kauder DR, Anderson HL 3rd, et al. Barrier precautions in trauma resuscitation: real-time analysis utilizing videotape review. Am J Emerg Med. 1997;15(1):34–9.
16. Dumas RP, Chreiman KM, Seamon MJ, Cannon JW, Reilly PM, Christie JD, et al. Benchmarking emergency department thoracotomy: using trauma video review to generate procedural norms. Injury. 2018;49(9):1687–92.
17. Fitzgerald M, Gocentas R, Dziukas L, Cameron P, Mackenzie C, Farrow N. Using video audit to improve trauma resuscitation – time for a new approach. Can J Surg. 2006;49(3):208–11.
18. Sakran JV, Finneman B, Maxwell C, Sonnad SS, Sarani B, Pascual J, et al. Trauma leadership: does perception drive reality? J Surg Educ. 2012;69(2):236–40.
19. Chreiman KM, Dumas RP, Seamon MJ, Kim PK, Reilly PM, Kaplan LJ, et al. The intraosseous have it: a prospective observational study of vascular access success rates in patients in extremis using video review. J Trauma Acute Care Surg. 2018;84(4):558–63.
20. Hoff WS, Reilly PM, Rotondo MF, DiGiacomo JC, Schwab CW. The importance of the command-physician in trauma resuscitation. J Trauma. 1997;43(5):772–7.
21. Hamilton NA, Kieninger AN, Woodhouse J, Freeman BD, Murray D, Klingensmith ME. Video review using a reliable evaluation metric improves team function in high fidelity simulated trauma resuscitation. J Surg Educ. 2012;69(3):428–31.
22. Ritchie PD, Cameron PA. An evaluation of trauma team leader performance by video recording. Aust N Z J Surg. 1999;69(3):183–6.
23. Scherer LA, Chang MC, Meredith JW, Battistella FD. Videotape review leads to rapid and sustained learning. Am J Surg. 2003;185(6):516–20.
24. Prakash S, Bihari S, Laver R, Chandran G, Kerr L, Schuwirth L, et al. Prospective randomized controlled trial of video- versus recall-assisted reflection in simulation-based teaching on acquisition and retention of airway skills among trainees intubating critically ill patients. Crit Care Med. 2020;48(9):1265–70.
25. Capella J, Smith S, Philp A, Putnam T, Gilbert C, Fry W, et al. Teamwork training improves the clinical care of trauma patients. J Surg Educ. 2010;67(6):439–43.
26. Roberts NK, Williams RG, Schwind CJ, Sutyak JA, McDowell C, Griffen D, et al. The impact of brief team communication, leadership and team behavior training on ad hoc team performance in trauma care settings. Am J Surg. 2014;207(2):170–8.
27. Hughes KM, Benenson RS, Krichten AE, Clancy KD, Ryan JP, Hammond C. A crew resource management program tailored to trauma resuscitation improves team behavior and communication. J Am Coll Surgeons. 2014;219(3):545–51.
28. Steinemann S, Berg B, Skinner A, DiTulio A, Anzelon K, Terada K, et al. In situ, multidisciplinary, simulation-based teamwork training improves early trauma care. J Surg Educ. 2011;68(6):472–7.
29. Gjeraa K, Moller TP, Ostergaard D. Efficacy of simulation-based trauma team training of non-technical skills. A systematic review. Acta Anaesth Scand. 2014;58(7):775–87.
30. Knudson MM, Khaw L, Bullard MK, Dicker R, Cohen MJ, Staudenmayer K, et al. Trauma training in simulation: translating skills from SIM time to real time. J Trauma Injury Infect Crit Care. 2008;64(2):255–63.
31. Fernandez R, Rosenman ED, Olenick J, Misisco A, Brolliar SM, Chipman AK, et al. Simulation-based team leadership training improves team leadership during actual trauma resuscitations: a randomized controlled trial. Crit Care Med. 2020;48(1):73–82.
32. Petrosoniak A, Fan M, Hicks CM, White K, McGowan M, Campbell D, et al. Trauma Resuscitation Using in situ Simulation Team Training (TRUST) study: latent safety threat evaluation using framework analysis and video review. BMJ Qual Saf. 2020;
33. Dumas RP, Vella MA, Chreiman KC, Smith BP, Subramanian M, Maher Z, et al. Team assessment and decision making is associated with outcomes: a trauma video review analysis. J Surg Res. 2020;246:544–9.

34. Yule S, Flin R, Paterson-Brown S, Maran N, Rowley D. Development of a rating system for surgeons' non-technical skills. Med Educ. 2006;40(11):1098–104.
35. Sevdalis N, Davis R, Koutantji M, Undre S, Darzi A, Vincent CA. Reliability of a revised NOTECHS scale for use in surgical teams. Am J Surg. 2008;196(2):184–90.
36. Steinemann S, Berg B, DiTullio A, Skinner A, Terada K, Anzelon K, et al. Assessing teamwork in the trauma bay: introduction of a modified "NOTECHS" scale for trauma. Am J Surg. 2012;203(1):69–75.
37. Jeffcott SA, Mackenzie CF. Measuring team performance in healthcare: review of research and implications for patient safety. J Crit Care. 2008;23(2):188–96.
38. Courtenay M, Nancarrow S, Dawson D. Interprofessional teamwork in the trauma setting: a scoping review. Hum Resour Health. 2013:11.
39. Yun S, Faraj S, Sims HP. Contingent leadership and effectiveness of trauma resuscitation teams. J Appl Psychol. 2005;90(6):1288–96.
40. Hjortdahl M, Ringen AH, Naess AC, Wisborg T. Leadership is the essential non-technical skill in the trauma team – results of a qualitative study. Scand J Trauma Resusc Emerg Med. 2009;17:48.
41. Sugrue M, Seger M, Kerridge R, Sloane D, Deane S. A prospective study of the performance of the trauma team leader. J Trauma. 1995;38(1):79–82.
42. Westli HK, Johnsen BH, Eid J, Rasten I, Brattebo G. Teamwork skills, shared mental models, and performance in simulated trauma teams: an independent group design. Scand J Trauma Resus. 2010:18.
43. Rosenbaum L. Divided we fall. N Engl J Med. 2019;380(7):684–8.
44. Pucher PH, Aggarwal R, Batrick N, Jenkins M, Darzi A. Nontechnical skills performance and care processes in the management of the acute trauma patient. Surgery. 2014;155(5):902–9.
45. Briggs A, Raja AS, Joyce MF, Yule SJ, Jiang W, Lipsitz SR, et al. The role of nontechnical skills in simulated trauma resuscitation. J Surg Educ. 2015;72(4):732–9.
46. Park C, Grant J, Dumas RP, Dultz L, Shoultz TH, Scott DJ, et al. Does simulation work? Monthly trauma simulation and procedural training are associated with decreased time to intervention. J Trauma Acute Care Surg. 2020;88(2):242–8.
47. Oakley E, Stocker S, Staubli G, Young S. Using video recording to identify management errors in pediatric trauma resuscitation. Pediatrics. 2006;117(3):658–64.
48. US Department of Health and Human Services. Summary of the HIPAA Privacy Rule. https://www.hhs.gov/hipaa/for-professionals/privacy/laws-regulations/index.html. Accessed 1 Nov 2020.
49. Korndorffer JR, Hawn MT, Spain DA, Knowlton LM, Azagury DE, Nassar AK, et al. Situating artificial intelligence in surgery. Ann Surg. 2020;272(3):523–8.
50. Surgical Safety Technologies. https://www.surgicalsafety.com. Accessed 1 Nov 2020.
51. Goldenberg MG, Jung J, Grantcharov TP. Using data to enhance performance and improve quality and safety in surgery. JAMA Surg. 2017;152(10):972–3.
52. Jung JJ, Juni P, Lebovic G, Grantcharov T. First-year analysis of the operating room black box study. Ann Surg. 2020;271(1):122–7.
53. Kolodzey L, Grantcharov PD, Rivas H. Wearable technology in the operating room: a systematic review. BMJ Innov. 2017;3:55–63.
54. Udeh C, Udeh B, Rahman N, Canfield C, Campbell J, Hata JS. Telemedicine/virtual ICU: where are we and where are we going? Methodist Debakey Cardiovasc J. 2018;14(2):126–33.
55. Barry ME, Hochman BR, Lane-Fall MB, Zappile D, Holena DN, Smith BP, et al. Leveraging telemedicine infrastructure to monitor quality of operating room to intensive care unit handoffs. Acad Med. 2017;92(7):1035–42.

Creating a CRM Toolkit

16

Lawrence Marshall Gillman and Peter G. Brindley

For healthcare professionals who are used to learning facts and "hard" science, Crisis Resource Management (CRM) skills training can sometimes seem vague and theoretical if not presented in a concrete manner. For example, discussing adult learning concepts without offering clear actionable ways, these can be applied in a trauma resuscitation may not be helpful to many learners. For this reason, when teaching the STARTT (Simulated Trauma and Resuscitative Team Training) Course, we like to help learners create their own CRM toolkit with several discrete tools that can be easily retrieved from memory and utilized during stressful trauma resuscitations. In this chapter, we hope to offer some examples of such tools such that the reader may create their own toolkits.

Pre-arrival

While there always will be trauma patients walking in or dropped off at the door, allowing no time for pre-preparation, ideally most trauma patients transported by EMS will allow for a trauma pre-alert based on established trauma team activation criteria, allowing the trauma team members to gather and prepare prior to patient arrival. Pre-arrival checklists allow the team to prepare in a standardized manner to ensure nothing is forgotten in the heat of the moment. These checklists can be easily modified to fit local practices. One such checklist is the zero-point survey discussed in Chap. 11 (Fig. 16.1 and Table 16.1) [1]. Others can help ensure proper equipment and personnel are present (Fig. 16.2).

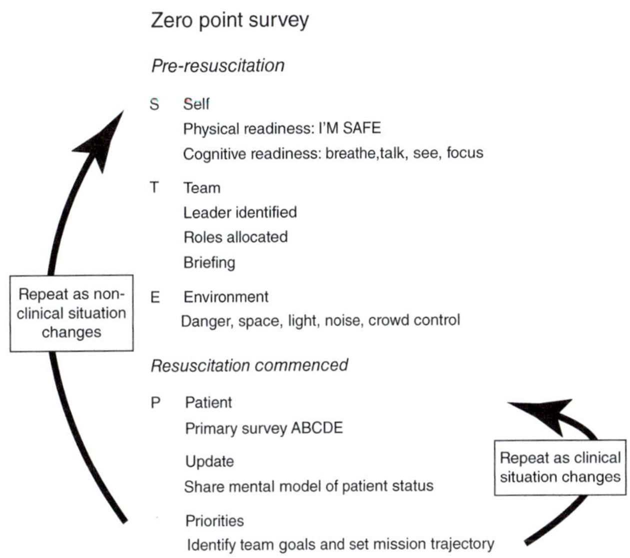

Fig. 16.1 Zero-point survey and the STEP-UP mnemonic

L. Marshall Gillman (✉)
Department of Surgery, Clinical Learning and Simulation Program, University of Manitoba, Winnipeg, MB, Canada
e-mail: Lawrence.Gillman@umanitoba.ca

P. G. Brindley
Department of Critical Care Medicine, University of Alberta Hospital, Edmonton, AB, Canada
e-mail: Peter.Brindley@albertahealthservices.ca

L. Marshall Gillman, S. Widder (eds.), *Trauma Team Dynamics*, https://doi.org/10.1007/978-3-031-86312-7_16

Table 16.1 I'M SAFE checklist

I	Illness
M	Medical
S	Stress
A	Alcohol
F	Fatigue
E	Emotion/Eating

Adapted from Ref. Reid et al. [1]

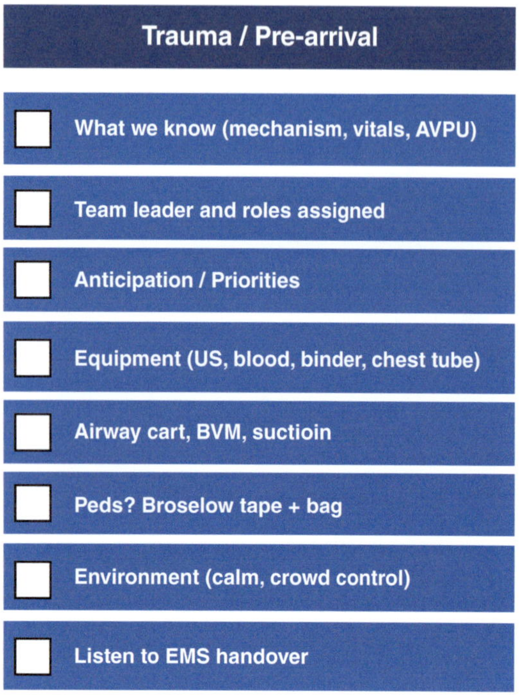

Fig. 16.2 Pre-arrival checklist. (Retrieved from: https://frozendoc.com/2021/03/16/trauma-checklists/, June 14, 2023)

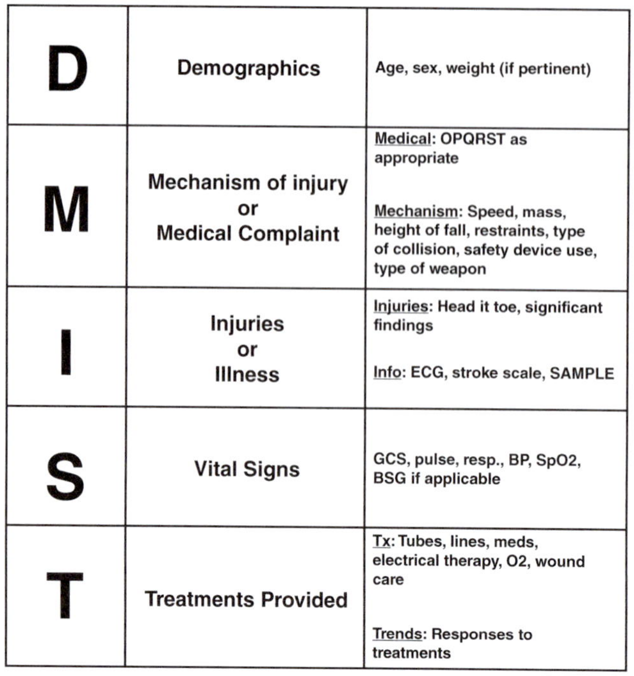

D	Demographics	Age, sex, weight (if pertinent)
M	Mechanism of injury or Medical Complaint	Medical: OPQRST as appropriate Mechanism: Speed, mass, height of fall, restraints, type of collision, safety device use, type of weapon
I	Injuries or Illness	Injuries: Head it toe, significant findings Info: ECG, stroke scale, SAMPLE
S	Vital Signs	GCS, pulse, resp., BP, SpO2, BSG if applicable
T	Treatments Provided	Tx: Tubes, lines, meds, electrical therapy, O2, wound care Trends: Responses to treatments

Fig. 16.3 D-MIST handover. (Retrieved online from: https://www.ptsf.org/wp-content/uploads/2020/10/PA_DMIST_Poster.pdf, June 14, 2023)

Table 16.2 IMIST-AMBO handover protocol

I	Identification
M	Mechanism
I	Injuries
S	Signs
T	Treatment and Trends
A	Allergies
M	Medications
B	Background History
O	Other Information

Adapted from – https://www.slhd.nsw.gov.au/BTF/pdfs/Education/ISBAR/IMIST_AMBO.pdf. June 14, 2023

Patient Arrival

In the absence of an imminent airway emergency or CPR in progress, there is generally time for a pause prior to or following patient transfer from the EMS stretcher to receive EMS handover. A structured handover ensures pertinent data is communicated in a concise and organized fashion. D-MIST is a commonly used tool for this purpose (Fig. 16.3). A variation of this is the IMIST-AMBO handover protocol (Table 16.2).

Resuscitation

During the resuscitation, there are a number of tools that can help prepare the team for procedures and keep the group on track. The most discrete example is an airway timeout. Essential components of an airway time out ensure that medications are prepared, equipment is prepped, and back-up

Fig. 16.4 Example of an airway timeout

PROTECTED INTUBATION CHECKLIST (BRING THIS INTO ROOM)
Airway MD to Read

PATIENT
- □ Position optimized for intubation
- □ O_2 source on the patient
- □ Monitors On and initial Vital Signs documented

MEDICATIONS
- □ Intravenous functional
- □ Consider pretreatments to support hemodynamics: Fluid bolus, Norepinephrine infusion at 0.1 mcg/kg/min prior to RSI
- □ Rapid Sequence Induction (RSI) Drugs ready

EQUIPMENT
- □ Confirm PPE on appropriately
- □ Ventilator ON with initial settings
- □ In-line Suction on circuit
- □ Bag Valve Mask with filter attached
- □ Suction (tested)
- □ Video Laryngoscope
- □ Endotracheal tube (appropriate size, cuff tested, syringe ready)
- □ Bougie
- □ Forceps
- □ PEEP valve
- □ End-Tidal CO_2 Detector
- □ Endotracheal tube holder and bite block
- □ Orogastric tube
- □ Additional rescue airway equipment readily available outside patient room – LMA, cricothyroidotomy kit

PLAN
- □ Reassessment of airway for difficulty
- □ Huddle to review plan for medications and approach to airway and backup approach to airway
- □ 1st attempt using Video Laryngoscopy +/– Bougie
- □ 2nd attempt plan described by Airway MD
- □ Post-intubation management discussed – sedation/analgesia/vasopressors

□ ADDRESS QUESTIONS OR CONCERNS BEFORE PROCEEDING

plans in event of failed airway capture are identified. Figure 16.4 is an example of a comprehensive airway timeout used in our local center during the COVID-19 pandemic.

A simpler example is the SALTED mnemonic (Table 16.3). Again, these can be easily adapted for local use.

A comprehensive ATLS resuscitation checklist may be redundant or unnecessary in a tertiary care center but may be very useful in a smaller center that treats complex trauma patients on a rare or intermittent basis (Fig. 16.5 and Table 16.4). [2]

Table 16.3 SALTED mnemonic

S	Suction
A	Airways (oral airways)
L	Laryngoscope (Video or Direct or Both)
T	Tube (planned size plus size below)
E	End-tidal
D	Drugs and difficult airway needs (if applicable)

Pre-arrival Plan

Check or prepare:
- ☐ Oxygen
- ☐ Suction
- ☐ Bag and mask
- ☐ Intubation tray
- ☐ Intubation medications
- ☐ Defibrillator
- ☐ CPR board

☐ Consider ordering blood

Assign team roles:
- ☐ Airway
- ☐ IV/IO access
- ☐ Primary survey
- ☐ Team leadership

☐ Brief team on incoming patient

☐ Estimate weight:_______ kg

Primary Survey

A	☐ Confirm C-spine is immobilized ☐ Confirm airway is protected
B	☐ Place O_2 mask or connect existing mask to O_2
C	☐ Check pulses ☐ Establish IV/IO access ☐ Consider ordering blood
D	☐ State GCS (eyes, verbal, motor) ☐ State pupil size and response
E	☐ Completely remove patient's clothing ☐ Cover patient with warm blanket
RE-EVALUATE AIRWAY	☐ Evaluate need for intubation ☐ Report FT tube size and depth (if applicable) ☐ Confirm ETCO2 color change (if applicable)
MONITOR	☐ Confirm heart rate is displayed ☐ Confirm pulse ox waveform is displayed
VITALS	State and evaluate whether WNL: ☐ Heart rate ☐ Respiratory rate ☐ Blood pressure ☐ Oxygen saturation ☐ Temperature

Secondary Survey

Evaluate and state findings:
- ☐ Head
- ☐ Ears
- ☐ Eyes
- ☐ Facial bones
- ☐ Nose
- ☐ Mouth
- ☐ Neck//C-spine
- ☐ Chest
- ☐ Abdomen
- ☐ Pelvis
- ☐ Upper extremities
- ☐ Lower extremities
- ☐ Log roll and back exam

Plan of Care

Determine need for:

Laboratory tests	☐ Yes	☐ No
X-rays	☐ Yes	☐ No
CT scans	☐ Yes	☐ No
OR notification	☐ Yes	☐ No
PICU notification	☐ Yes	☐ No

Departure Plan

☐ State patient destination

Prepare patient for travel:
- ☐ Equipment
- ☐ Medications
- ☐ Identify who will travel with patient

Fig. 16.5 ATLS resuscitation checklist. (Retrieved online: https://www.nicepng.com/ourpic/u2w7r5y3i1t4y3u2_trauma-resuscitation-checklist-used-in-the-checklist-atls/, June 14, 2023)

Table 16.4 Trauma transfer checklist

Continue to Care
Establish and maintain spinal motion restriction. Remove scoop stretcher if present and logroll as necessary
Document vital signs and neuro signs q15min
All documentation on trauma notes for CTAS 1 and 2
Airway and breathing
Confirm ability to maintain adequate oxygenation/ventilation
Consider need for endotracheal tube (ETT): Declining GCS, GCS < 8, inhalation injury, maxillofacial injury or other airway concern
Consider need for chest tube: Confirm and document chest tube functioning and placement prior to departure; make necessary adjustments
If intubated
Will require escort for ground transport
Confirm ETT position via: auscultation, end tidal CO_2 and chest x-ray
Secure ETT, monitor O_2 sats and $ETCO_2$
Insert gastric tube
Ensure adequate analgesia and sedation to RASS-4
Circulation
Control all active bleeding sites—apply pressure dressing, sutures, staples; consider tourniquet if indicated
Establish two large bore peripheral IVs (extension tubing required for air transfers)
Pregnancy test for all women of child-bearing years (do not delay transfer for results)
Ensure patient and fluids are warmed
Bleeding or suspected bleeding (adult and pediatric) consider tranexamic acid bolus and infusion if within 3 h from time of injury

(continued)

Table 16.4 (continued)

Consider anticoagulant reversal
Consider blood products
Apply pelvic binder/stabilization, if applicable
Insert Foley catheter with urometer, if applicable
Disability
Review medications proposed for use during transfer with the TCP
Cover open fractures with saline dressing
Reduce and splint extremity fractures (avoid air splints)
Control pain
Prophylaxis
Antibiotics: for all open fractures; consider for all penetrating trauma
Tetanus as required
Check glucose
Expose/Environment
Prevent hypothermia
Document temperature
Assess posterior surfaces; remove from scoop stretcher
Consider Logistics
Team required for transfer: Consider RN, RRT and/or Air Ambulance Crew
RN recommended for analgesia, sedation, blood products, and any transfer when scope of practice exceeds that of transport crew provided
Equipment required for ground transfer:
Airway management/O_2 saturation/$ETCO_2$ monitoring
Blood and blood products properly packaged by lab personnel for transfer, if applicable
Orders required for transfer
Resuscitation: airway control/defibrillation
Medications: including sedation, analgesia, paralytics and anticonvulsant, if applicable
Blood/blood products and I.V. fluid
Confirm targets for O_2 sats, ETCO2, RASS, BP, MAP parameters during transfer
Documentation to accompany patient
Photocopies of all ED physician notes, nurses' notes, and initial ambulance call report
Team leader at sending site to directly contact team leader at receiving site once transfer arrangements are confirmed

Adapted from: TraumaNB Trauma Transfer Checklist https://nbtrauma.ca/wp-content/uploads/2022/02/Trauma-Transfer-Checklist-Nov-2021-bil.pdf

Pre-departure

Prior to leaving the trauma bay, a pre-departure checklist can be helpful to ensure all pertinent exams, and investigations are completed in the trauma bay and that all preparations for transport have been made. This checklist will vary depending on location, for example if transport is within hospital to CT scan, or OR, or interfacility transport (Fig. 16.6).

Fig. 16.6 WHO trauma care checklist. (Reproduced from Trauma Care Checklist, https://www.who.int/publications/i/item/trauma-care-checklist, retrieved online November 13, 2023)

World Health Organization

Trauma Care Checklist

Immediately after primary & secondary surveys:

IS FURTHER AIRWAY INTERVENTION NEEDED? May be needed if: • GCS 8 or below • Hypoxaemia or hypercarbia • Face, neck, chest or any severe trauma	☐ YES, DONE ☐ NO
IS THERE A *TENSION* PNEUMO-HAEMOTHORAX?	☐ YES, CHEST DRAIN PLACED ☐ NO
IS THE PULSE OXIMETER PLACED AND FUNCTIONING?	☐ YES ☐ NOT AVAILABLE
LARGE-BORE IV PLACED AND FLUIDS STARTED?	☐ YES ☐ NOT INDICATED ☐ NOT AVAILABLE
FULL SURVEY FOR (AND CONTROL OF EXTERNAL BLEEDING, INCLUDING:	☐ SCALP ☐ PERINEUM ☐ BACK
ASSESSED FOR PELVIC FRACTURE BY:	☐ EXAM ☐ X-RAY ☐ CT
ASSESSED FOR INTERNAL BLEEDING BY:	☐ EXAM ☐ ULTRASOUND ☐ CT ☐ DIAGNOSTIC PERITONEAL LAVAGE
IS SPINAL IMMOBILIZATION NEEDED?	☐ YES, DONE ☐ NOT INDICATED
NEUROVASCULAR STATUS OF ALL 4 LIMBS CHECKED?	☐ YES
IS THE PATIENT HYPOTHERMIC?	☐ YES, WARMING ☐ NO
DOES THE PATIENT NEED (IF NO CONTRAINDICATION):	☐ URINARY CATHETER ☐ NASOGASTRIC TUBE ☐ CHEST DRAIN ☐ NONE INDICATED

Before team leaves patient:

HAS THE PATIENT BEEN GIVEN:	☐ TETANUS VACCINE ☐ ANALGESICS ☐ ANTIBIOTICS ☐ NONE INDICATED
HAVE ALL TESTS AND IMAGING BEEN REVIEWED?	☐ YES ☐ NO, FOLLOW-UP PLAN IN PLACE
WHICH SERIAL EXAMINATIONS ARE NEEDED?	☐ NEUROLOGICAL ☐ ABDOMINAL ☐ VASCULAR ☐ NONE
PLAN OF CARE DISCUSSED WITH:	☐ PATIENT/FAMILY ☐ RECEIVING UNIT ☐ PRIMARY TEAM ☐ OTHER SPECIALISTS
RELEVANT TRAUMA CHART OR FORM COMPLETED?	☐ YES ☐ NOT AVAILABLE

Communication Skills

During crisis, CRM training can help improve communication and teamwork. There are some discrete tools that can be pulled out in certain circumstances to help facilitate communication and mitigate confusion. The simplest of these is the 3-C's of closed loop communication (Table 16.5).

When team members wish to bring a concern to leader/team's attention, this can sometimes pose a challenge. There are a number of tools that can give members important verbiage that can convey their message in a way that doesn't threaten or undermine the leader's role but still makes their concerns heard by focusing on the patient's safety. These include the PACE levels of graded assertiveness (Table 16.6) and the CUS mnemonic (Table 16.7).

Table 16.5 3 C's of closed loop communication

C—Cite names
C—Clarity of communication
C—Close the loop

Table 16.6 PACE levels of graded assertiveness

P	PROBE—"Did you know that…?"
	"Did you realize the sat probe tracing is poor?"
A	ALERT—"Can we re-assess the situation…?"
	"Can we re-assess the situation as the patient is no longer breathing?"
C	CHALLENGE—"I don't think we should…because"
	"I don't think we should paralyze this burn patient because they may have a difficult airway"
E	EMERGENCY—"Stop what you are doing…"
	"Stop trying to intubate the patient, the patient is hypoxic, we need to proceed with a surgical airway now"

Table 16.7 CUS mnemonic

I am Concerned!
I am Uncomfortable!
This is a Safety Issue!

Structured Handovers

As Chap. 9 discusses, the process of handover is a potentially dangerous time when pertinent information must be communicated in a concise yet comprehensive manner such that important details are both communicated and received. We have already discussed EMS handover, but numerous other handovers exist in hospital during the patient's care journey. In the heat of the moment, the SBAR communicaiton tool represents a tried and proven method of communication (Table 16.8).

Table 16.8 SBAR communication

S	Situation—What is the situation?
	"This is a 29 year old burn patient with a difficult airway"
B	Background—Pertinent background information related to the situation
	"This patient was involved in a house fire in an enclosed space. He has be developing increasing stridor"
A	Assessment—What is your assessment of the situation?
	"I am concerned that his airway is swelling and he requires intubation"
R	Recommendation—What do you want to see happen?
	"I will manage the airway, can you set up for a surgical airway in case it is necessary"

Conclusions

CRM training gives team members a background in non-technical skills and stresses the importance of focussed communication, leadership, and followership skills in times of crisis. However, by offering team members discrete and actionable tools that they can practice in the sim lab and then utilize during real life resuscitations, these CRM theories can then be easily accessed. Thus, all team members can form their very own CRM toolkits.

References

1. Reid C, Brindley P, Hicks C, et al. Zero point survey: a multidisciplinary idea to STEP UP resuscitation effectiveness. Clin Exp Emerg Med. 2018;5(3):139–43.
2. Kulp L, Sarcevic A, Cheng M, Burd RS. Towards dynamic checklists: understanding contexts of use and deriving requirements for context-driven adaptation. ACM Trans Comput Hum Interact. 2021;28(2) https://doi.org/10.1145/3444947.

Part II

Trauma Team Design

Out-of-Hospital Care from Paramedical to Non-medical Personnel

17

Ryan Shelton and Matthew Brock

Origination

Prehospital care has progressed significantly since the first documented ambulance services, organized by Napoleon's chief military physician, Jean Dominique Larrey. Just as EMS began in the military, today's latest lessons learned in trauma remain revolutionized by the military. In recent years, the United States Military has put a significant emphasis on advancing higher levels of care to the point of injury. The goal of all medical treatment is early effective point-of-injury care, transport/extraction, and surgical stabilization at definitive care. For the traumatized patient, this often means a Level 1 Trauma Center. The role of EMS is much more than transport. Appropriate point-of-injury care completed correctly does not lead to a delay in reaching definitive care.

What My Trauma Doctors Need to Appreciate

The *complete trauma team dynamics* concept, or "One Team," as the Colonel Jim Barren of the United States Army team eloquently understood, translates to the medical arena by incorporating key fundamental accomplished objectives to stabilize every trauma patient. The totality of care in a vibrant healthcare system has the entire system of trauma care providing competent care at each level of certification and licensure. This can only be done through a sustained relationship of education and preventative upkeep in the form of continuing education (CE) from the surgeon to the prehospital providers, which includes first responders, emergency medical technicians (EMT), and paramedics.

Paramedics will act quickly in trauma crisis, adapt to less-than-ideal conditions, and operate effectively on critical trauma patients with limited personnel and resources to depend on. Their prehospital environment is heinous at times with challenges of weather, hazardous materials, patient access, extrication complications, and extended patient transport times with hemodynamically unstable patients, and they must consistently operate with comfort in an uncontrolled environment with difficulties of crowds, including violent rapidly erupting scenes. It is important that hospital providers understand prehospital protocols and their limitations with protocols and equipment, while appreciating the environmental constraints they perform their skills in. Many EMS have elevated levels of training in high-performance teams and can manage septic patient in ARDS necessitating 9 IV infusions, vasopressors, chemical sedation, and advanced airway control with two crew in the small quarters of a helicopter or fixed wing, usually staffed by one paramedic and a flight nurse. Cutting-edge prehospital agencies have progressed to utilizing point-of-care-ultrasound (POCUS) to determine termination of resuscitation (TOR), tension pneumothorax confirmation, guided pericardiocentesis, resuscitative endovascular balloon occlusion of aorta (REBOA) zone confirmation, evaluation of inferior vena cava for congestive heart failure, and FAST exams to determine the most appropriate trauma destination. In addition to a widening scope into midlevel knowledge, skills, and abilities (KSA), the prehospital environment continues to evolve. Take the SWAT Paramedic that is staged at a peaceful protest, suddenly turning violent, creating a single gunshot to a patient's mandible necessitating an immediate cricothyrotomy. No hesitation and seconds away security protocols are executed followed by immediate advanced patient care by the SWAT paramedic. What first responders and paramedics

Matt Brock has been a professional firefighter and a paramedic for over 20 years. Over his career, he has been a part of multiple special teams, including USAR, ARFF, HAZMAT, Peer Support, and Pipes and Drums. Matt has been a primary instructor for an EMT-B course for over a decade and remains passionate about not only developing skills but also building resiliency.

R. Shelton (✉)
University of Colorado Hospital, Anschutz, CO, USA
e-mail: ryan.shelton@uchealth.org

M. Brock
South Metro Fire Rescue, Centennial, CO, USA
e-mail: Matt.brock@southmetro.org

L. Marshall Gillman, S. Widder (eds.), *Trauma Team Dynamics*, https://doi.org/10.1007/978-3-031-86312-7_17

do with bleeding control, airway management, or patient temperature management all affect the viability of the patient. Their care can determine whether enough time has been preserved to reach the operating table. The evolution of agencies across the nation is using metrics that capture continuous competency for each paramedic through generated reports and quality assurance programs. Highly functioning Emergency Medical Services (EMS) systems track the first pass success and total intubation rate for each paramedic and system-wide success. In most cases, because our education is not proportionate to our responsibilities and the autonomy related to patient care, a heavy emphasis is placed on capturing procedural statistics and performance metrics for patient protection. The paramedic provider will continue to take on more midlevel scope of practice by necessity of our healthcare system. Cultivating professional relationships of mentoring and education with the prehospital providers of trauma care is imperative. EMS agencies are evolving to becoming evidence-based in their care, like the rest of the field of medicine and appropriately so. A *high-performance trauma team* has no metaphoric walls, and it is inappropriate to operate in silos. It is a choreographed, trained, and performance-driven team responsible for performing within the standard of care maximizing trauma patient survival from the moment the first trained provider is at the patient's side until recovery.

United States Prehospital System Legal Structure

Each state has regulatory power to define a scope of practice for each level of certification that was developed by the National Highway Traffic Safety Administration (NHTSA) standard curriculum. Through the extension of a medical director's licensure, he or she may delegate authority from the state's approved scope of practice list, which includes specified pharmacology, procedures, and protocols within the medical director's local jurisdiction. There are special circumstances where the medical director may petition the state for a "waiver" if a procedure or medication is not on the state's list of acts allowed as a specially approved practice for Paramedics. In that case, the designated state oversight body will allow or reject the waivered request and, if approved, will allow the agency to perform the procedure or medication administration for a specified amount of time. This provides the state with gross oversight and the ability to evaluate trends that may need to be incorporated into the future acts' allowed list, control the complexity and frequency in which a higher skill beyond core curriculum education is performed, and data collection with appropriate reporting to ensure patient safety for skills typically falling outside the acts. Each agency is required to have a medical director who is responsible for the agency-specific protocols. Some medical directors adopt the recommendation from national or state regulatory bodies, while other physicians approve protocols that are either more progressive or more conservative. For these reasons, it is unrealistic to rely on one training curriculum to define the expected standard of care for an EMS system. Instead, the trauma system should look at the evidence-based treatments for trauma patients and determine what can effectively be implemented by the local EMS agencies based on their level of training and equipment carried.

The medical director sets protocols. There are two forms of protocol orders: direct and standing orders. A direct order is obtained directly from the agency affiliation hospital of the medical director by any staffed ED physician. They can approve the requested procedure or medication after receiving a patient report and requested order by an EMT or Paramedic. All procedures and medications that receive approval from the base must be within the scope of practice for that level of provider or have a waiver in good standing. A standing order is an ongoing automatic protocol that allows the paramedic or EMT to provide care within those specific protocol conditions with complete autonomy.

Certification or Licensure

The certification process for First Responders/Emergency Medical Responder, Emergency Medical Technicians (EMT), Advanced EMT, EMT Intermediate, Paramedics, Community Paramedics, and Critical Care Paramedics represent a minimum competency for certification but do not accurately reflect the expectations or capabilities of that same provider once they begin working for an agency. As you can see, there are six levels of prehospital medical providers. These levels of practitioners are complicated and widely variant by state, predominately based on land area make-up (urban, rural) and cost feasibility for the providers. The most functional information is to demonstrate the variance from the lowest level of certification/licensure to the highest level by comparing their scope of practice. The first segment will cover acts allowed for a First Responder or Emergency Medical Responder, which remain mostly in rural volunteer settings and have minimal training, followed immediately by a Critical Care Paramedics scope.

Emergency Medical Responder/First Responder Scope of Practice:

1. Perform initial, focused, and ongoing assessment
2. Provide respiratory assistance utilizing oral and nasal airways, and oxygen delivery system components
3. Apply suctioning techniques to clear airways
4. Apply dressings and bandages for wound care
5. Apply splints and immobilization devices

6. Apply spinal immobilization devices
7. Provide care for obstetrical emergencies including assisting in childbirth
8. Provide ordinary reasonable care for ill and/or injured persons in accordance with established regional protocols
9. Utilize automated defibrillators in accordance with established regional protocols
10. May serve as attendant-in-charge on an EMS Vehicle-Class A
11. May serve as vehicle operator

Critical Care Paramedic Scope of Practice:

1. Video and direct oral laryngoscopy rapid sequence induction (RSI)
2. Supraglottic device insertion (e.g., LMA or KING airway)
3. Needle and surgical cricothyroidotomy
4. Chest/lung compromise needle, simple, and tube thoracostomy with drainage system initiation and management
5. Mechanical ventilation initiation and management of all modes of ventilation; to include but not limited to: high frequency oscillating; volume, pressure, and dual-mode ventilation; non-invasive positive pressure ventilation
6. Cardiovascular management of ventricular assist device (VAD): including but not limited to: percutaneous or central LVAD, RVAD, and BiVAD
7. Management of extracorporeal membrane oxygenation (ECMO) with or without heater/cooler capability
8. Intra-aortic balloon pump (IABP) counter pulsation
9. Perform and interpret 12 Lead ECGs with catheterization lab activation capabilities
10. Intraosseous access (e.g., EZ-IO or FAST1)
11. Indwelling port access (e.g., Hickman, Port-a-Cath, etc.)
12. Transcutaneous, transvenous, and epicardial wire pacemaker capabilities
13. Pericardiocentesis
14. Invasive hemodynamic monitoring (e.g., CVP, pulmonary artery pressures, abdominal pressures, arterial pressures, intracranial pressures)
15. Blood/fluid warming devices and blood product administration (e.g., whole blood, PRBCs, plasma, platelets)
16. Operation of single and multi-channel infusion pump(s), including but not limited to Intravascular, intraosseous, intrathecal, and intra-arterial routes
17. Cardiovascular Doppler/ultrasound monitoring
18. Arterial cannulation, radial and/or femoral
19. Central venous cannulation, femoral, subclavian, and internal jugular
20. Wound closure including but not limited to: suturing, stapling, skinglue
21. Laboratory sampling, point-of-care testing, result interpretation, and treatment
22. Non-invasive tissue oxygenation monitoring
23. Hemorrhage control including but not limited to: tourniquet use, chemical clotting agents
24. Asherman chest seal
25. Tranexamic acid (TXA) and plasma administration
26. Gastric tube placement and management
27. Urinary catheter initiation and management
28. Ability to calculate and independently administer medications applicable to the critical care environment and covered in protocols, guidelines, or standing orders:
    (a) Vasoactive agents, paralytics, anxiolytics, anti-inflammatory, anticonvulsant, narcotics, anesthetics, thrombolytics
    (b) Inhaled gases: Heliox, nitrous oxide, nitric oxide, anesthesia gases
    (c) Nebulized medications
    (d) Antiemetic, antibiotics
    (e) ACLS medications: Epinephrine, lidocaine, atropine, anti-arrhythmic
    (f) Electrolytes: Potassium, magnesium, calcium
    (g) Prostaglandin
    (h) Surfactant blood and blood products
    (i) Tranexamic acid (TXA)
29. Radiographic interpretation
30. Perform and interpret ultrasound imaging including utilization for placement of medical devices, i.e., REBOA
31. Ability to manage and transport any indwelling medical device
32. Invasive and non-invasive temperature monitoring
33. Initiation and management of non-invasive and invasive thermoregulation device
34. Thoracic and extremity escharotomy and fasciotomy
35. Fetal heart/uterine monitoring
36. Umbilical vein/artery cannulation
37. Surfactant administration
38. Esophageal compression tubes
39. Peri-mortem cesarean section
40. Suprapubic cystostomy
41. Esophageal cooling tubes

Association of Critical Care Transport—Critical Care Transport Standards—Version 1.0 ©2016 [1]. The CCT provider may be required to perform skills not otherwise listed in this document via direct or video remote medical oversight. Based on the CCTA's patient population, the need for these skills should be anticipated and included in training and competency assessment.

Paramedic Structure in Canada

Paramedics in Canada are certified as either a primary care paramedic (PCP), a critical care paramedic (CCP), or the advanced care paramedic (ACP). *In order to become a paramedic*, the applicant needs to successfully complete a course of training which can vary in different provinces.

Levels of Paramedics in Canada

- *Primary Care Paramedic*

The PCP is at the entry level of the paramedic profession, with duties that include providing basic medical care, the administration of oxygen, administering IV, cardiac monitoring, semi-automated external defibrillation, administering medications such as aspirin, epinephrine, nitroglycerine, and more for emergency conditions, as well as performing trauma immobilization. If the PCP receives additional training, he or she is authorized to provide medical care on the level of the Advanced Care Paramedic, or ACP.

To become a PCP, the prospective paramedic must take the two-year Primary Care Paramedic Program of training and pass the provincial PCP exam, after which the successful graduate can obtain employment at an ambulance company or a medical institution, first obtaining the approval of the local medical director.

- *Advanced Care Paramedic*

Although jurisdictions and provinces such as New Brunswick and Quebec don't have ACPs, Advance Care Paramedics are greatly in demand in Canada's health professions. ACPs are qualified to carry twenty different medications, although those medications may differ significantly from region to region. ACPs are also trained to perform intubation and intravenous therapy, place external jugular IV lines, perform needle thoracotomy and obstetrical assessment, and administer pain relief. An innovation in Canada that has had a profound effect on patient survival rates allows ACPS discretionary direct 24-h access to cardiac catheterization labs labs, bypassing the hospital emergency departments.

Before becoming an ACP, the paramedic must work as a PCP between 6 and 24 months. The applicant needs to complete the 1200-h ACP training program, passing all required exams and certification programs as required by the Canadian province in which the paramedic is employed.

- *Critical Care Paramedics*

CCPs have prior experience working with ambulances and responding to 911 emergency calls. A CCPs expertise is focused on the critical and intensive unit level care, stabilizing, and transporting patients in hospitals with limited resources to programs that can provide a higher, and in many cases, lifesaving, level of care. A CCP provides care that would otherwise be administered by a physician or nurse. In addition to providing the care levels that are administered by PCPS and ACPs, the CCP is trained to administer medication infusion pumps, mechanical ventilation, and monitor arterial lines.

To be eligible for the CCP program, which takes a year to complete, the applicant must have worked for one year as an ACP, be certified in basic trauma life support and advanced cardiac life support and have aeromedical certification.

As you can see there is a chasm of disparity between the protocols at each level, all grounded by the providers' education, training, knowledge, skills, and abilities. It is up to system administrators to know their local prehospital care limitations.

Science Behind Prehospital Injury Patterns

Largely accepted is the concept of irreversible death in the "immediate" time frame after injury, usually occurring prior to EMS arrival or very shortly thereafter. This is followed by the second peak in the trimodal distribution known as early trauma deaths. This mortality is generally estimated to be around 20-30% [2, 3]. This is where well-choreographed and high-performance prehospital team trauma care can have the greatest impact and is the greatest reversable cause of death post-traumatic injury.

With chest and head injuries leading in patient presentation, providers must be competent with both endotracheal intubation and chest decompression or finger thoracotomy. These are statistically where training will have the most impact on patient outcomes. Unfortunately, many areas struggle with intubation successes, both endotracheal and/or nasal. In business classes, they teach to measure what matters. Here, success in intubation matters so training programs that better identify the airway challenges of every patient encountered and translate that into more successful intubations are preferred. Although volume for skills is down per provider within the 911 system, with evolving technology there is the ability to create life-like task trainers, life-like human-worn simulators for immersion training, 3D-printed anatomy models for skills drills, and both embalmed and flash-frozen cadavers for realistic sequencing and experience training (Fig. 17.1). Each serves a purpose and needs to progress the following route to achieve competency:

We will discuss making an impact reflecting where the data dictates. For trauma patients younger than 65 years, there are nine prehospital deaths for every in-hospital mortality. One estimate suggests that in 2014 alone, 30,000 of 147,000 trauma deaths may have been avoided with timely

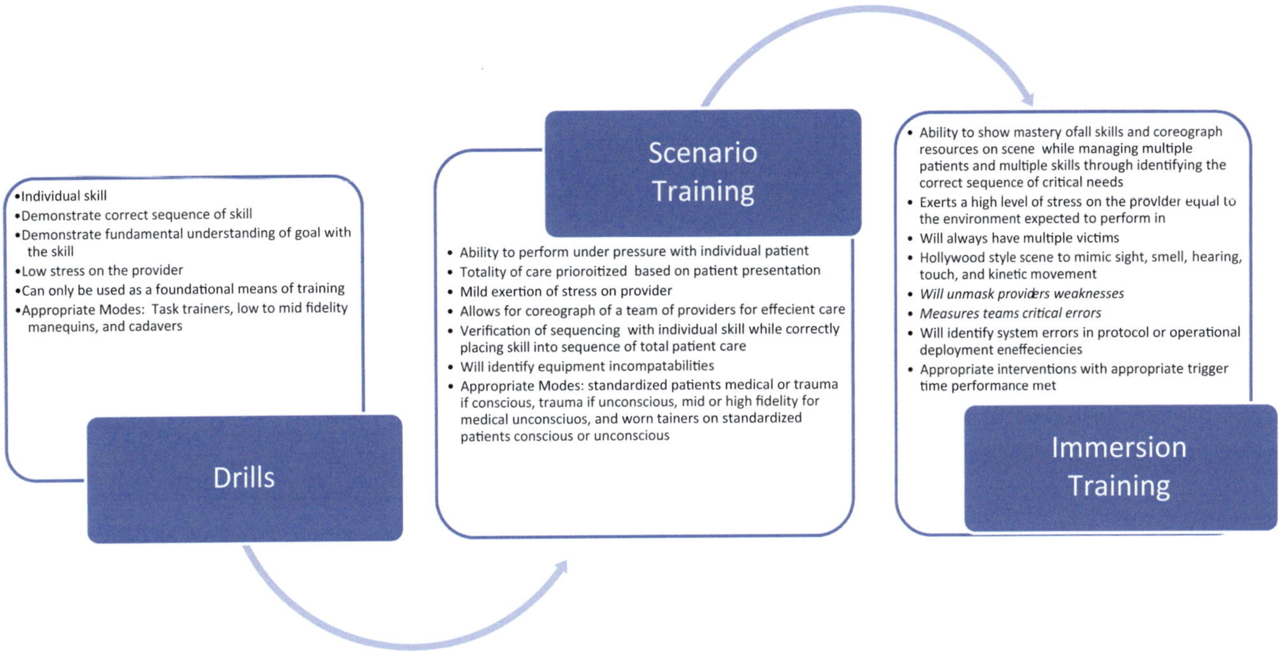

Fig. 17.1 Skills and stress progression corollary. Marks the progressions from static skill mastery under minimal stress to complex deployment of knowledge, skills, and experience for fluent intervention of critical factors that maximizing stabilization increasing survivability in the most challenging environment with multiple patients in a truly dynamic environment. (Source: Shelton 2024)

hemorrhage control [4]. Timely hemorrhage control is a medical intervention that can be performed by both paramedical and non-medical personnel alike. Direct pressure, elevation, and appropriate tourniquet placement are skills taught within basic life support and advanced life support training. These simple interventions can and should be performed long before the patient arrives at the trauma center. In trauma protocols worldwide, control of massive hemorrhage is listed as the first action to be considered and performed if necessary. In the International Trauma Life Support for Emergency Providers, this is laid out using the acronym C-ABC (control bleeding, airway, breathing, circulation). In Tactical Combat Casualty Care Training, this is emphasized using the MARCH acronym (Massive Hemorrhage, Airway, Respirations, Circulation, Hypo/hyperthermia). Paramedical and non-medical personnel play a very large role in external hemorrhage control. External hemorrhage is the easiest to recognize, as the bleeding is both significant and visible.

Concepts in Paramedic Education

Team Synergy vs Rock Star Player

This is an interesting concept for team dynamics and likens to the nature vs nurture debate. In our environment which is most important: a rock star paramedic that can do any skill and catch any abnormal patient presentation or a team with synergy that as individuals intelligence, skill level, and experience is simply average? I have spent thousands of hours teaching thousands of initial certifications for EMT through paramedic and continued education for all prehospital ranks. I can tell you it is impressive to watch a rock star train and do nearly everything by him or herself hitting every benchmark along the way; however, human error increases outside of group dynamics, and the time to critical skills is also much slower for accomplishment. Team synergy is the most important aspect in trauma resuscitation.

Double Checking Is a Sign of Respect

As we talk about this concept, I originally heard it from Steve Markham, 23 years Navy, 19 as Reconnaissance Corpsman with the Marine Corps. It is simple and utilizes the trust and verify concept. The concept comes from a well-intended process to be at the core of any highly functioning team. On all critical tasks, this should be performed. It is preventative in nature, not in the heat of battle. Double check each other with equipment checks, procedural drills, protocol quizzes, and competency scenario performance. The success of the team depends on your preparation.

Medical Errors

In 2016, an article in the *British Medical Journal* written by Martin Makary and Micheal Daniel, titled "Medical Error: The Third Leading Cause of Death in the US," it estimated 251,000 deaths per year were at the hands of medical professionals. This number has been likened to a 737-plane crashing every day, but the math works out to metaphorically crashing over four 737 aircraft with total human life lost every day in the USA. The reason it is frequently compared to the aviation industry is because at one point the aviation industry struggled with increasing examples of human error, climbing crash rates and unacceptable fatality totals. The expert analysts and statisticians for the industry extrapolated that at current growth rate of the aviation industry compared to the amount of human error, there would be one plane crash per month. It was decided within the aviation industry that the projected rates for catastrophic human loss were too great and that aggressive steps needed to be taken to make air travel the safest means to travel. This gave birth to concepts of human error reduction, critical check lists, subservient cultural training, communication training, protocol development, annual competency evaluations, and mentored co-flights. The *Guardian* published that forty commercial passenger planes crashed in 2020 for a .27 fatal accident per million fights. To accomplish such a safety record, the airline industry moved to a risk-based decision-making model with strong regulatory oversight and an incredibly active safety culture within the industry. DeLine Box and Display of Denver has a 2–5% variance with paper material. This allows for human error, humidity, and temperature differences as it reacts with the paper products all to finish with a product within 1/16 of an inch variable. It is important to know your error rates and is a measured standard in nearly every other industry except healthcare, from making packaging to safety in flight. Measuring error is a fundamental principle in high-performance team dynamics and plays a critical role in the reduction of human error. In *Hyper-realistic, Team-Centered Fleet Surgical Team Training Provides Sustained Improvements in Performance,* authored by Tuan Hoang, two critical discoveries were made studying team dynamics: 1. Time for skills performance decreased from 11 min ± 3 min to 3 min ± 1 min and 2. Error rates drastically dropped from 4 errors ± 1 to 1 error ± 1 error. This was directly attributed to a formalized course showing value in improving "teamwork and communication skills of participants" [4]. This course was completely immersive, and every skill had to be performed in realistic conditions. The medical field must follow an example set by the airline industry with a purist safety culture where our performance is measured and trended.

Controversy What Should Our System Implement

"Scoop and Run" Versus "Stay and Play"

The out-of-hospital environment is austere which poses many challenges to initial responders. While principles like "load and go," which minimize scene time and rapid transport to definitive care, are strived for, the reality is the trauma scene is chaotic with multiple competing interests. Limited resources in personnel and equipment can lead to scene departure delays. The identified need for hemostasis or airway/ventilation maintenance should take priority. However, these processes do take time, which is at a premium in the traumatized patient. One of the more time-consuming steps is patient extrication and packaging. Removing an injured patient from a vehicle involved in a collision is inherently time consuming and takes significant personnel and energy. Current rescue dogma is no longer "removing the patient from the vehicle," but rather "removing the vehicle from the patient." This is confounded with an environment of inclement weather, poor lighting, and patient and/or bystander distress. Much of the principles prehospital practitioners follow in managing the trauma scene, and patient is outlined in established curricula in courses like International Trauma Life Support (ITLS) or the American program Prehospital Trauma Life Support (PHTLS). Historically, prehospital care has evolved into paramedical personnel that perform many of life-saving procedures once only employed in hospitals. Procedures like intravenous volume resuscitation or better yet whole blood, needle decompression, and endotracheal intubation can be utilized in the field and delivered to the traumatized patient at the point of injury. Many innovative EMS systems adopted and trained their personnel in these skills and encouraged their use. As evidence-based evaluation of practice migrated to the prehospital world and greater scrutiny was employed, EMS medical directors and practitioners have had to change their standards of practice.

With the evolution and increasing sophistication of EMS systems, medical evidence has weighed in on prehospital care management strategies in trauma. The ongoing debate of "load and go" versus "stay and play" is moot. A strategy of "scoop and treat" is preferred. In the United Kingdom and parts of Europe, physicians can be part of the EMS response. However, even in these systems, where advanced therapeutics and procedures are possible due to the physician present, all practitioners will appreciate that patients need to be transported rapidly from the scene onto a trauma center for definitive care as soon as possible. There will be inherent delays in patient extrication and packaging. Skilled and rapid clinical assessment and patient care should be performed enroute with minimal scene time as the goal. Procedures to optimize the airway, breathing and circulation should be accomplished with minimal delay in transport.

Airway Management Controversy with Paramedics

Conflicting evidence has weighed in on prehospital airway management, which since inception has been the hallmark of the paramedic. There is some evidence showing higher mortality with prehospital intubation of traumatic head injuries

[5]. As a result, there has been a push by some within the medical oversight community to deemphasize airway capture utilizing rapid sequence intubation strategies in the prehospital environment [6]. Furthermore, a recent prospective, randomized, controlled trial showed that prehospital rapid sequence intubation by paramedics increases the rate of favorable neurologic outcome at 6 months compared with intubation in the hospital [7]. It is outside the scope of this text to discuss what a specific agency's protocols should be. This conflicting data allows assessment of not only the paramedic providers but also their role within the entire trauma team. However, these two conflicting studies illustrate a crucial point. The skills, protocols, and effectiveness of EMS systems are variable. As a member of a trauma team, it is crucial to know the protocols and capabilities of the specific EMS systems within that trauma team. With the increase in professionalism and competencies at many prehospital fire departments and EMS agencies, intubation can safely be done in trauma patient care while maintaining proficiency of the skill via tracking of current global agency system success, as well as individual intubation success. This is done through metrics of quality management knowing the systems performance compared to its benchmark for the following criteria: first-time pass, successful intubation acquisition, and second-by-second tracking for capnography during intubation. The system average then gives a direct reflection on your training modality performance. This assures the safest known intubation training, standards, and performance of intubation on our most critical patients of trauma.

It is imperative that the research surrounding a procedure is critically evaluated with the capacity's providers in mind. Common arguments against prehospital advanced airway management include potential delay in transport, studies showing an increase in morbidity or mortality, the belief that EMS providers should wait for the procedure to be done by emergency physicians due to their expertise. Within certain trauma systems, these concerns are valid. However, prehospital advanced airway management can be performed in the prehospital setting without delaying transfer to a trauma center [8, 9]. When performed by skilled emergency medical services (EMS) providers, advanced airway management is associated with a significant decrease in mortality [9, 10]. While it is possible for EMS to wait for the emergency physicians to perform the intubation, in the hospital setting, delayed intubation is associated with increased mortality in non-critically injured trauma patients [11].

The Eastern Association for the Surgery of Trauma (EAST) practice guidelines on Endotracheal Intubation (ETI) immediately following trauma address this contradictory evidence by saying, "No conclusion could be reached regarding prehospital intubation for patients with traumatic brain injury, with or without RSI [rapid sequence intubation]. Diversity of patient population, differing airway algorithms, various experience among emergency medical service personnel in ETI, and differing reporting make consensus difficult" [12].

From the above discussion, we learn that when implemented correctly, advanced airway procedures can be a lifesaving and morbidity-reducing procedure. For this reason, endotracheal intubation *is the standard of care for definitive airway management in hospitals*. When not effectively implemented, advanced airway procedures can end up doing more harm than good by prolonging hypoxia and delaying transport to definitive treatment. There is no indication that the prehospital intubation under the same training and verification procedures is any less impactful. Depending on national, state, and local protocols, a traumatized patient may be received by the trauma team with a wide variety of treatments performed. The Trauma Team should compare the literature with an honest introspective look into the trauma team's capabilities proved by hard numbers of success and failure. The goal of this conversation should be to maximize the efficient treatment, transport, and definitive management of each patient. This involves specific patient-centered protocols based on the capabilities of the EMS system, the local hospitals, and the distance from scene to a trauma center. In one area, a trauma team may receive a patient from the field who has undergone Rapid Sequence Induction followed by being placed on a portable ventilator for a head injury. Another trauma team may receive a traumatized patient directly from the field with only bag valve mask ventilation, the use of supraglottic airway devices, or patients with decreased level of consciousness (GCS < 8) with only supplemental oxygen. Regardless of how the patient arrives, obtaining or confirming definitive airway management, including endotracheal intubation, by receiving trauma teams will need to be a priority.

To Fly or Not to Fly

There are only three circumstances that helicopter transport benefit patients using evidence-based assessment: (1) when time out of physician care is crucial to either patient stabilization efforts or patient survival; (2) if patient access is not available by other means in a timely fashion and the patient is unstable; and (3) if a helicopter has performed a cold landing at a predetermined rendezvous point between the transporting ambulance and trauma center with the load time factored and determined shorter than the ambulance to continue ambulance transport (traffic, time of day, construction). Helicopters are a valuable tool in a trauma system, but it is one of the most misunderstood tools when we look at evidence-based support. Helicopters are most useful for a rural population for the transport of critically ill patients to a larger center [13].

Training Quality

In the book, *Outliers* by Malcom Gladwell, there is a themed concept of the 10,000-h rule as a benchmark for mastery. This was a false conclusion that Gladwell drew from Anders Ericsson's research published in *The Role of Deliberate Practice in the Acquisition of Expert Performance.* Not only was this a misinterpretation of the most important part of the conclusion, but it also took what was a fractionalized concept of hours to aid in expert performance and made it the sole contributor to achieving expert performance. Ericsson's conclusion hinged on a concept of the high quality of instruction and the transferability from the training environment to the expected execution environment with striking similarities as the greatest contributor to mastery. Hours to mastery were discussed at length, but there was no basis for 10,000 h as the actual hour calculations varied from 4000 h to 7000 h without repeated correlation within the research subjects. What matters is simple, as a Paramedic you are expected to do complex tasks in all environments, with varied critical physiological patient presentations, unfavorable weather conditions, and under challenging circumstances. Why do your task trainers exist on a table in a room set at 70 degrees under great lighting? Why do we *ever* have an intubation mannequin on the table? We should not, it does not represent the expected environment we perform in. Your training has set you up for failure if it is not realistic. Human error can be minimized with as realistic as possible training. Each standardized patient must be physiologically modeled after real patients.

Case Study of Effective Trauma System Training: Before the Need

The call came in as a possible shooting in a school in our district. The number of units that were called seemed never-ending. The immediate rush of adrenaline as I heard the tones and information on the radio was nauseating. This was not another training. My mind rushed to make sense of the information and began to create a mental list of what needed to be accomplished. I looked at the MDT to see who was responding, where would I be in the list of units, what might I be assigned to accomplish?

Information that there may be multiple victims and multiple shooters. The first police officers arrived within 2 min and immediately broke into contact teams seeking the shooters. Within 3 min, officers made contact with the shooters and were already providing aid to multiple gunshot victims. Dispatch was getting multiple callers and attempted to make sense of the deluge of information to assist responding units. Students were fleeing the scene, some injured victims, and were desperately seeking safety on this tragic day.

While I drove emergent cars with worried parents followed me as if I was towing them, no doubt trying to make it to help their children. A father myself, with school-age children at a different school not more than a mile away, I understood and felt their pain as I pulled onto the scene. Police were stopping the parents to keep them from going any closer and I could see them screaming at the officer in my rear-view mirror. I parked out of the way to maintain egress for the likely transports to come. As I donned my bulletproof vest and tactical helmet, I could hear screaming parents begging to be allowed to come into the school to find their children. I will never forget the sound of desperation I heard that afternoon.

The sheer number of people and responding vehicles that were at this call was overwhelming. It was difficult to make my way to command to do a face-to-face and get my assignment. Multiple fire engines and trucks were parked well away with the crews already making their way to the scene. Ambulances were staged so that they could take any patients being extracted from the building. Police vehicles were parked near the school, but clear of the road to allow for transporting ambulances to get through. Students were being evacuated in groups, hands in the air, escorted by police in tactical gear. The injured were starting to be extracted from the building to the Casualty Collection Points (CCP).

It was 24 min from the initial 911 call until the last injured patient was transported from the scene, which had fled from the building seeking safety. The 911 call to the first Fire/EMS Rescue Task Force entering the building was 11 min with a transport time from Fire/EMS arrival of 4 min and 32 s for the first two critical patients. Four South Metro Fire Rescue Paramedic Ambulances transported all patients within 13 min of Fire/EMS arrival. Enroute, the victims were treated with skill and precision that helped ensure the best outcome. The hospitals that received these patients were ready and triaged immediately upon activation of the Emergency Management Systems linking prehospital patient needs to hospital resource availability. Each victim, regardless of the hospital, was treated quickly and effectively prevented any further loss of life.

The entire time the radio never stopped buzzing with traffic as command skillfully brought the call first to incident stabilization with no further loss of life, then to an end. With all the victims at the hospitals and the shooters arrested, the first phase of the scene came to a close and all those involved began to process what they experienced. Parents began to be reunited with their children down the street at a nearby church.

Tragically, one student was killed instantly on scene, Kendrick Ray Castillo, after he attempted to stop one of the shooters. His actions allowed other students to disarm the shooter and undoubtably saved multiple lives.

It was no accident or luck that allowed this call to be mitigated with the success that is did. Unfortunately, Colorado has had more than its fair share of school shootings, so experience played a role. We also knew it was only a matter of time before we would have another school shooting, and we needed to prepare for it. We created a large-scale training that included every agency that would be involved, including police, firefighters, EMTs, nurses, and doctors, including surgeons from resident to seasoned. It included a realistic scenario with live victims, from point of injury, extraction, prehospital care, transport, emergency room, and finally ended at the surgical suite in several of our Level I and Level II trauma centers. It was this recent drill that gave us the ability to take command and unify the responders of multiple agencies and disciplines, to work as one unified team to accomplish the one thing that mattered that day in Colorado—saving the kids that were shot.

Active Killer

Realistic Training

At the end of 2018, our fire department decided to break free from the traditional mode of training and bridge to hyper-realistic training. We had created some large-scale trainings that included elaborate scenarios in the past, but we only trained our own people. We realized that we were only one small piece of the puzzle for a patient from injury to discharge from the hospital. We needed to include each element of a patient's success to survive a traumatic injury by truly understanding all the players involved. Dissolve the established silos. We created a training that brought in multiple agencies and disciplines and created "one team" to work synergistically choreographed at accomplishing the missions' objectives to save as many people as possible. It was the ultimate in team dynamics for our community.

It was the multiple mass shootings that were committed in schools, movie theaters, campuses, and on the streets that forced us to look at our response to these events after significant response issues occurred repeatedly across the country. At each event we learned how to do it better and forced us to realize our department's short comings. Despite having this knowledge, it made no difference if all the responders, from law enforcement, Fire/EMS, and hospital staff were trained, a system wide global breakdown occurred with isolation of agencies and hospitals, individualized response plans, and a lack of large scenarios to test the systems process errors. In the end the system errors always outnumbered the individual human errors. Issues with blook bank protocol, like having a nurse check it out for verification who was much more valuable in the ED where the injured were, equipment compatibility, or simply chest tube trays in quantity readily available for the number of patients that these scenes generate. With the help of multiple agencies, we were able to begin piecing together effective training to improve the outcome of these patients using the concepts previously discussed.

This allowed for the creation of Standard Operation Guidelines (SOGs) that were widely accepted over judicial precincts incorporating multiple law enforcement, and Fire/EMS agencies—creating one plan for unified command, defining terminology, declaring tactics that allow for all agencies to work together to complete the mission and assigning responsibilities for every critical factor and objective necessary to stabilize an incident.

Lessons Learned

Again, without breaking from our traditional trainings, we would not have learned so many valuable lessons. Even though we made great strides in working with the police if we had stopped there and had people simply read the new SOGs, we would not have seen such dramatic changes in our operations. A mass scale exercise (not of patients of quality, realism, and follow-through of services) completed with complete emersion and a seamless transition through the entire trauma system from point-of-injury to stabilization in the operation room created a platform for a cultural competency reflecting a shift to a one team philosophy.

Response

We have seen a shift in how we respond to the active shooter incident over the past several years. The Hartford Consensus by the American College of Surgeons implemented the THREAT acronym in 2013 as response to nearly 7000 lessons learned from over a decade of combat studies and the evaluation of over 250 civilian casualties in active shooter events since Columbine in 1999 [14].

- **T**hreat suppression
- **H**emorrhage control
- **R**apid **E**xtrication to safety
- **A**ssessment by medical providers
- **T**ransport to definitive care

Knowing that in an active shooter environment that hemorrhage has always been the single greatest preventable cause of death to our patients. We will flirt with mortality in approximately five minutes post injury and our access to the patients is too slow using our old methodologies of "scene safe," law enforcement brings them to us, or any other outdated practice. If you take 15–23 min trigger time to reach your first patient, you will fail to have any impact on positive patient outcome. You *must* utilize the Hartford recommendations when you train your crews. As Fire/EMS, we will need to operate in the yellow zones which are secure areas from within the building. By secure, I mean vantage points Law Enforcement has given us for the protection of corridors or hallways and/or we have cover if secure ground cannot remain constant. Law Enforcement will have contact teams ahead of us to attain threat contact and then engagement for threat suppression. Other Law Enforcement will be in the function of primary search inadvertently while clearing the building and are mandated to provide hemorrhage control to those in need *as they find them*. Fire/EMS's job is to go in for *known patients* at *known locations* that are relayed to us from Law Enforcement during their clearing and search findings.

The concept of MARCH was developed by the Special Operations Forces in 1996 and has remained unchanged in Tactical Combat Casualty Care and Advanced Trauma Life Support, which outlines the preventable causes of death as follows:

M: Massive hemorrhage
A: Airway
R: Respirations
C: Circulation
H: Head injury and hypothermia

This remains the systemized approach that prioritizes life-threatening interventions.

Nonmedical Personnel

We will explore the role of non-medical personnel within the trauma team, and the roles and responsibilities of the medical personnel within the trauma team that exist in the prehospital environment.

Bleeding control skills are taught in many first aid classes. Non-medical first responders such as police officers, firefighters, schoolteachers, and motorists can all benefit from hemorrhage control training. Members of the trauma team can teach members of the community effective hemorrhage control. According to the CDC unintentional injuries are the leading cause of death for ages 1–44. This information can help the trauma team target training courses to individuals who are within this age group or spend a significant amount of time with individuals in this age group. In some US states, both public and private schools are required by law to train their faculty and staff in hemorrhage control and are required to have bleeding control kits with specific contents outlined within the law. Homeland Security's national awareness campaign, "Stop the Bleed" curriculum, improved the laypersons' self-efficacy and reported willingness to use a tourniquet in an emergency [15]. After a traumatic event, it is likely the first person on scene is not a medical professional. The potential impact of bystander intervention is significant for trauma patients, given the majority of deaths occur before patients reach the hospital.

Conclusion

This is a critical time where effective trauma team dynamics can make a significant impact on the receipt of appropriate, timely care of the traumatized patient. The trauma team dynamics extend beyond individual teams working on a patient to the macro environment of the entire trauma system. Each link in the patient's chain of survival, from point of injury to hospital discharge, should be represented in an evidence-based discussion regarding the expectations of each link within the chain. You must capture preplanning and training on a continual basis as our effectiveness at executing protocols and ability to remain competent as low-frequency, high-risk skills have perishability. This discussion should assess the ability of the providers, equipment, staffing, capabilities of the receiving hospitals and define standards of care that continue to evolve.

Key Terms

- Trauma team dynamics—a multidisciplinary trauma team focused on crisis management strategies to improve teamwork and communication.
- High-performance team—a group of people who work together to achieve exceptional results and outperform other teams. For effective teams, they must have trust, clear goals, well-defined roles, collaboration, and phycological safety and are rooted in a learning culture.
- Waivered medication/procedure—beyond the acts allowed and scope of practice for the provider, which has a state waiver approved to allow acting above their initial training curriculum.
- Medical error—an adverse effect of care that could have been prevented.
- Immersive training—a learning method designed to mimic, as closely as possible, the environment the skills and team is expected to perform in with the intent to reduce human error, eliminate critical errors, improve trigger times, and build high performance teams in stressful environments.
- Rescue task force—a small team with a team leader, law enforcement for a protective element and EMS as the rescue element composing a 4-person team.
- Tactical unit contact team—eliminate threats in the hot zone.

- Active shooter hot zone—direct threat of the shooter and only tactical units are deployed in this area.
- Active shooter yellow zone—indirect threat where risk is mitigated by tactics of a rescue task force for protection or secured ground and corridors establishing tactical advantage to facilitate the treatment and extraction of victims.
- Active shooter green zone—no threat and no need for tactical deployments and will be the location of unified command.

Key Points

- One team concept for trauma care: For the best patient outcomes, trauma surgeons must have ongoing education and training touch points with first responders to deliver best practices and set expectations for regional trauma care.
- Acts allowed by certification/licensure: With each level of certification or licensure, the scope varies widely for procedures and medication administration. It is paramount to ensure protocols align with the providers skill level of competency and the resources available prehospital.
- Critical Care Paramedics: Focus on critical and intensive care that would otherwise be administered by a physician or nurse.
- Primary Causes of Death Prehospital: Hemorrhage, followed by chest and head injuries.
- Progression of Training Concepts: Drills and functions achieved, scenario training and functions achieved, and immersive training with functions achieved and mastery. This progression leads to consciously competent performance by the providers.
- Medical Errors: Medical errors are human errors that are reduced by utilizing effective training modules, and highly effective teams can reduce critical error rates from 4 to 1 per event while cutting the trigger time for a skill in half.
- Scene Philosophy Supporting Survivability: Scoop and run vs. stay and play vs. scoop and treat are the three choices as a philosophy. Utilizing the scoop and treat philosophy maximizes survivability by positively impacting the controllable elements in the prehospital environment.
- Intubation: While presenting both sides of the evidence, pros and cons, for advanced airway management, it is most important to understand the limitations of a studies design, and the correlation and/or causation of the results to the conclusion. Regardless, each agency must have an accurate metric for your providers competency using all facets of airway management tools from basic to advanced tracked not only from the training date but also to patient outcome data. Until science is conclusive and repeatable with a clear indication of increased survivability, it appears the quality of oxygenation and saturation is more important than any specific procedure. Competency is paramount in any airway management and remains a leading cause of traumatic death.
- 10,000 Hours to Mastery: The quality of education and training combined with the transferability from the training environment to the real environment is the most important concept to achieve mastery.
- Rescue Task Forces (RTF): They do not search but will get known victims and start MARCH treatment concepts for extraction to the Casualty Collection Point (CCP). They are shored up with two Law Enforcement personnel for protection in four-person groups.
- Tactical Group and Contact Teams: Stage I is to stop the killers, which will have law Enforcement aggressively contacting the active shooter. Stage II is subsequent officers will shift to a dual objective deployment of stopping the dying, which includes search to coordinate RTF rescue as well as addressing MARCH principles for hemorrhage control while maintaining security of the scene backing up the initial contact teams.
- Metrics: They need to correlate to benchmark trigger times for skills, add objective measures like capnography with intubation or BVM ventilation, and record the success or failure for each critical skill performed prehospital. This data is then run with outcome data to determine competency in the field.

References

1. Kuehl AE. Prehospital systems and medical oversight-national association of EMS physicians. 3rd ed. Dubuque: Kendall Hunt Publishing Co; 2002.
2. Stiell IG, Nesbitt LP, Pickett W, Munkley D, Spaite DW, Banek J, et al. The OPALS Major Trauma Study: impact of advanced life support on survival and morbidity. CMAJ. 2008;178(9):1141–52.
3. Liberman M. Advanced or basic life support for trauma: meta-analysis and critical review of the literature. J Trauma. 2000;49(4):584–99.
4. Hoang TN, Kang J, Siriratsivawong K, LaPorta A, Heck A, Ferraro J, Robinson D, Walsh J. Hyper-realistic, team-centered fleet sur-

gical team training provides sustained improvements in performance. J Surg Educ. 2016;73(4):668–74. https://doi.org/10.1016/j.jsurg.2016.03.004.
5. Murray JA, Demetriades D, Berne TV, Stratton SJ, Cryer HG, Bongard F, et al. Prehospital intubation in patients with severe head injury. J Trauma. 2000;49:1065–70.
6. Bledsoe B. Rethinking ETI: should paramedics continue to intubate. JEMS. 2010;35(7):42–58.
7. Bernard SA, et al. Prehospital rapid sequence intubation improves functional outcome for patients with severe traumatic brain injury: a randomized controlled trial. Ann Surg. 2010;252:959–65.
8. Eckstein M, Chan L, Schneir A, et al. Effect of prehospital advanced life support on outcomes of major trauma patients. J Trauma. 2000;48(4):643–8.
9. Meizoso JP, Valle EJ, Allen CJ, et al. Decreased mortality after prehospital interventions in severely injured trauma patients. J Trauma Acute Care Surg. 2015;79(2):227–31.
10. Lockey DJ, Healey B, Crewdson K, et al. Advanced airway management is necessary in prehospital trauma patients. Br J Anaesth. 2014:1–6. https://doi.org/10.1093/bja/aeu412.
11. Miraflor E, Chuang K, Miranda MA, et al. Timing is everything: delayed intubation is associated with increased mortality in initially stable trauma patients. J Surg Res. 2011;170(2):286–90.
12. Mayglothling J, Duane TM, Gibbs M, et al. Emergency tracheal intubation immediately following traumatic injury: an Eastern Association for the Surgery of Trauma practice management guideline. J Trauma Acute Care Surg. 2012;73(5):S333–40.
13. Cunningham P, Rutledge R, Baker CC, Clancy TV. A comparison of the association of helicopter and ground ambulance transport with the outcome of injury in trauma patients transported from the scene. J Trauma. 1997;43(6):940–6.
14. Jacobs LM, Wade D, McSwain NE, Butler FK, Fabbri W, Eastman A, Conn A, Burns KJ. Hartford consensus: a call to action for THREAT. A medical disaster preparedness concept. J Am Coll Surg. 2014;218(3):467–75. https://doi.org/10.1016/j.jamcollsurg.2013.12.009.
15. Ross EM, Redman TT, Mapp JG, Brown DJ, Tanaka K, Cooley CW, Kharod CU, Wampler DA. Stop the bleed: the effect of hemorrhage control education on laypersons' willingness to respond during a traumatic medical emergency. Prehosp Disaster Med. 2018;33(2):127–32. https://doi.org/10.1017/S1049023X18000055.

18 Trauma Point-of-Care Ultrasound in Prehospital and Austere Environments

Michael Kreiser, Seth Hill, Hunter Barnes, Ryan Shelton, and Amanda Toney

Introduction

The portability and relative affordability of point-of-care ultrasound (POCUS) have made its use in the prehospital environment an increasingly popular area of research. European emergency medical systems (EMS) more commonly have physician responders, who have demonstrated the efficacy of POCUS in prehospital care [1–3]. Despite this utility, surveys of US and Canadian physicians found that only 4.1% of EMS systems are using POCUS [4].

Recent studies have expanded prehospital ultrasound use to non-physician healthcare providers, who demonstrated the ability to obtain adequate scans, interpret images, and adjust medical decision-making accordingly [5–7]. Successful implementation of POCUS into EMS systems, with appropriate training and quality assessment of ultrasound images, affords prehospital providers an additional tool to improve team dynamics and healthcare provision. Critics point to prehospital trials demonstrating delayed patient care with POCUS, while proponents note trials that have implemented the adjunct with minimal obstruction [5–9]. Integrating ultrasound into EMS protocols clearly requires performance metrics to ensure proficiency.

Currently, the American College of Emergency Physicians Ultrasound (ACEP) Guidelines advise a minimum of 25 ultrasound scans per body system prior to field implementation. These scans should be deemed of adequate quality and accurate interpretation per POCUS expert overread [10]. Hands-on and didactic training sessions have been completed over the course of 4–8 h, with some training methods achieving proficiency retention rates of over 1 year [11]. Additional objective measures of ultrasound proficiency have been proposed through hand motion analysis (HMA). Using the Focused Assessment with Sonography in Trauma (FAST), differences in duration of exams, quantity of hand movements, and distances traveled by probes were statistically compared between ultrasound novices and experts. Sonography proficiency was found to have quantifiable metrics from which expertise could be predicted [12].

The HMA technique was successfully trialed in the United States to determine the efficacy of paramedic ultrasound training. Prior to the training, POCUS fellowship-trained physicians had significantly better HMA measurements than 36 paramedics without POCUS experience. Following a 4-h didactic and hands-on ultrasound course, paramedics attained HMA measurements similar to experts, demonstrating the capacity to learn and utilize POCUS. The need for refresher trainings was also illustrated, as paramedics demonstrated degradation in HMA metrics, written examination scores, and objective structured clinical examinations (OSCE) for cardiac POCUS at 2-month and 4-month intervals [13].

Combining traditional simulation sessions with HMA could raise the standard of ultrasound training and better prepare prehospital providers for field implementation. Although training metrics and best practice guidelines are still being standardized, prehospital POCUS trials have already demonstrated improvements in patient care at point-of-injury in well-resourced, under-resourced, austere, and military environments.

M. Kreiser (✉)
Rocky Vista University College of Osteopathic Medicine, Parker, CO, USA

Naval Medical Center Portsmouth, Portsmouth, USA
e-mail: michael.a.kreiser2.mil@health.mil

S. Hill
Rocky Vista University College of Osteopathic Medicine, Parker, CO, USA

The Jewish Hospital, Cincinnati, USA
e-mail: seth.hill@rvu.edu

H. Barnes
Rocky Vista University College of Osteopathic Medicine, Parker, CO, USA

Carl R. Darnall Army Medical Center, Fort Cavazos, USA
e-mail: hunter.barnes@rvu.edu

R. Shelton
South Metro Fire Rescue, Centennial, CO, USA
e-mail: ryan.shelton@southmetro.org

A. Toney
Department of Pediatric Emergency Medicine, University of Colorado and Denver Health Medical Center, Denver, CO, USA
e-mail: Amanda.toney@dhha.org

L. Marshall Gillman, S. Widder (eds.), *Trauma Team Dynamics*, https://doi.org/10.1007/978-3-031-86312-7_18

Prehospital Ultrasound in Well-Resourced Environments

Protocols Streamline Evaluation and Patient Management

Well-resourced EMS systems often take an organized and systematic approach to POCUS. This approach includes the development and implementation of POCUS algorithms for the prehospital setting. These protocols have adapted the FAST exam, combined components of separate exams to differentiate shock and cardiac arrest, and defined methodology for evaluating a mother and fetus.

The Prehospital Focused Assessment with Sonography in Trauma (PFAST) was adapted from the hospital FAST exam. Paramedics in a German multi-center study were able to complete scans on 90% of patients prior to hospital arrival with a 93% sensitivity for intraperitoneal hemorrhage [14]. All paramedics reported that PFAST played a crucial role in team decision-making, with 33% describing changes in on-scene trauma management and 20% noting change in receiving hospital. When a negative exam can be obtained in minutes and a positive exam in only seconds, this protocol requires a small investment for potentially large returns in team dynamics.

Extended Focused Assessment with Sonography in Trauma (eFAST) adds a pneumothorax and hemothorax evaluation to the FAST exam, and the protocol has been successfully deployed in the prehospital environment. One air transport team found that scans obtained by flight paramedics and flight nurses had approximately 100% positive and negative predictive values for torso trauma, which did not statistically differ from the receiving level 1 trauma center teams who repeated the exam [15]. This categorization for blunt trauma patients can help guide prophylactic aggressive treatment while the patient is still hemodynamically stable. In addition to indicating appropriate therapies, POCUS was also useful in avoiding unnecessary interventions and iatrogenic injury when physical exam was misleading. This exam was performed without effect on avionics and without distortion [16, 17]. Prehospital eFAST completion times, performed by aeromedical teams, ranged from 3 to 5 min with a mean completion time of 3 min [16]. The length of these assessments added no meaningful transport time, and the aeromedical teams reported instances in which massive transfusion protocols and surgical team notifications were expedited [15]. Authors suggest that, in some scenarios, POCUS could provide sufficient assessment to forego time-consuming computerized tomography (CT) or surgical team re-evaluation on arrival. This would allow for flight crews and receiving trauma teams to jointly bypass the trauma resuscitation bay and go direct to the operating room.

The Rapid Ultrasound for Shock and Hypotension (RUSH) exam is a three-step algorithm described by Perera and colleagues to evaluate undifferentiated shock [18]. The protocol assesses "the pump," "the tank," and "the pipes," in succession by imaging the cardiac chambers and valves, the lungs and inferior vena cava (IVC), the aorta, the abdomen, and the large blood vessels, respectively. Specific findings for each system are noted and used to categorize shock as hypovolemic, cardiogenic, obstructive, or distributive. Prehospital providers are currently using components of this algorithm through eFAST examinations and aortic evaluations for abdominal aortic aneurysms, and the protocol could be adapted for the prehospital environment. The integration could enhance diagnostic capabilities and improve the delivery rate and fitness of resuscitative interventions, which may require vascular access, volume resuscitation, vasopressors, inotropes, thrombolytics, intubation, needle decompression, pericardiocentesis, thoracentesis, cardioversion, or other life-saving measures [15, 19].

Focused Echocardiographic Evaluation in Life Support (FEEL) is an algorithm for improving resuscitative care currently used by German emergency medicine (EM) physicians that has been deployed in the field with a high degree of diagnostic accuracy [1]. The sequence focuses on reversible causes of cardiac arrest, such as cardiac tamponade, pulmonary embolism, ventricular dysfunction, hypovolemia, ventricular fibrillation, and conditions missed by electrocardiogram. Trauma may precipitate underlying causes of cardiac arrest, making POCUS a valuable tool in discerning these conditions during assessment of the trauma patient. Conversely, an underlying condition may cause a patient to experience trauma, such as lightheadedness or loss of consciousness precipitating a motor vehicle collision (MVC), and the FEEL protocol may discover the more serious illness that might otherwise be missed in the typical evaluation and management of an MVC or other trauma. Prehospital physicians utilizing FEEL reported POCUS-based patient management changes for 78% of patients [1]. The physicians additionally reported detection of pericardial effusions that were previously missed on exam and ECG for 5.4% of patients, the findings of which allowed for rapid pericardiocentesis with improvement in survival to hospital admission [1]. The discerning of treatable conditions allows for the appropriate interventions to be more quickly administered and may better prepare the medical teams at the receiving hospital.

POCUS has also been used in prehospital environments to assess obstetric trauma, a leading precipitant of maternal mortality and still more frequent cause of fetal death [20, 21]. Trauma places the gravid patient at risk for placental abruption, uterine rupture, preterm labor, and other emergencies. The Fetal Evaluation for Transport with Ultrasound (FETUS) protocol has been trialed with an aeromedical team examining fetal position, fetal movements, fetal heart tones, placenta condition, and pelvic fluid [17]. Assessing the sonoanatomy, fetal heart rate, and pelvic region with POCUS can determine viable pregnancies, while levels of free fluid and extent of subchorionic hemorrhage can determine good prognosis versus surgical emergency. Signs and symptoms of shock may not initially be apparent on physical exam, and real-time imaging of the pelvis and abdomen can elucidate fetal distress or maternal complications that indicate more aggressive treatment for hemodynamic instability [22]. This stabilization is integral to the health of the mother and remains the primary means of protecting the pregnancy.

An Adjunct for Adversity

The prehospital environment can be unpredictable and poses challenges to healthcare provision. POCUS has demonstrated utility as an adjunct to the physical exam, supplement to the current diagnostics, and aid to the paramedic's medical decision-making. Physical examination is fallible when compared to the more controlled environment of the hospital. For providers obtaining pulses on patients in cardiac arrest, studies have demonstrated that manual carotid assessment is unreliable even in the more controlled setting of the hospital [23, 24]. Prolonged pulse-checks delay chest compressions and can decrease survival rates [25]. Conversely, false identification of an absent pulse may result in unnecessary CPR and resuscitative medications, which have been associated with poor neurological outcomes [26]. POCUS has helped discern cardiac contractility when the physical exam is equivocal, a scenario not uncommon with the additional challenges of the prehospital environment [1, 5, 6]. Additionally, one random-controlled trial demonstrated that carotid compressibility on ultrasound, a "POCUS pulse-check," had greater first-attempt reliability than manual assessment in obtaining pulses [27].

Because prehospital protocols and diagnostics are also fallible, POCUS offers the provider more versatility for independent investigation. Although the FAST exam is a useful algorithm in discerning the presence of fluid in the chest, pericardium, abdomen, or pelvis, a negative assessment may conceal other serious complications of blunt trauma. A provider with high-suspicion for diaphragmatic rupture may use M-mode to evaluate for liver sliding sign, subphrenic effusion, or absent organ sign [28]. Should internal hemorrhage be suspected, hypovolemia may be assessed by examining IVC diameter and low ventricular end diastolic volume [1, 22]. Studies have projected that up to 86% of cardiac arrest patients initially thought to be in pulseless electrical activity (PEA), based on electrocardiogram and physical exam, demonstrated cardiac motion on ultrasound [29, 30]. Pseudo-pulseless electric activity (PPEA) necessitates treatment that differs from PEA, with improved survival [1, 31].

Paramedics are often faced with difficult decisions in the field, and POCUS has been shown to help guide medical decision-making [1, 14, 15, 31]. During the most critical calls, such as mass casualty incidents (MCI), tactical emergency medical services employ triage algorithms to prioritize, treat, and transport patients. These situations can rapidly evolve and require more than one triage effort. After the definitive patient assignments have been made, POCUS can be employed to evaluate patients with more ambiguous designations, resulting in a more informed triage assessment and plan. The chest, abdomen, IVC, and extremities, in acute triage (CAVEAT) protocol, has been suggested as a triage tool to integrate several current ultrasound algorithms during MCI, but the protocol feasibility requires further investigation [32]. Termination of resuscitation (TOR) is a mentally and emotionally challenging decision for both providers and families. Current research suggests that cardiac standstill on ultrasound has a predictive value as high as 97.5% for patient expiration [33]. Additionally, a multi-center study found that cardiac activity on ultrasound following cardiac arrest was the factor most associated with survival [31]. This predictive value can supplement physical examination to provide a more objective means of TOR. More conclusive decision-making can offer closure to families, while preventing futile emergency transports that would otherwise incur additional costs and risks to healthcare systems and the surrounding community.

Prehospital Ultrasound in Under-Resourced and Austere Environments

Ultrasonography has progressed considerably with technological advancements, especially those in computer science, instrument portability, smartphones, and the Internet. Such advances are opening new opportunities to use POCUS technology outside of well-resourced hospitals and clinics. The benefits that ultrasound brings to rural and remote regions are well documented. Recent discussions with midwives throughout Tanzania highlighted that the technology enabled them to make more informed assessments concerning their patients and even encouraged pregnant women to deliver at a medical center [34]. POCUS use in Rwanda and Liberia influenced medical management for up to 78% of patients, while a study in Cameroon reported ultrasound as the reason for diagnosis in 31% of patients [35–37]. Healthcare providers reported that these diagnoses were not previously on their differential. Implementation of POCUS in the rural Amazon echoes these findings, suggesting that the diagnostic adjunct may significantly improve medical management [38]. A resultant "Magnet Effect" has been documented in communities with ultrasound technology available. Patients had more confidence in the medical team and were more likely to seek care when needed [39]. This ability to screen for internal bleeding, tumors, or other significant findings can ensure a patient with a serious condition makes the necessary but sometimes challenging journey to a medical center. Conversely, POCUS can also help healthy patients in rural regions with minor findings on ultrasound avoid unnecessary travel and expensive procedures with potential complications [38, 40]. Introducing POCUS training and competency programs to rural and remote regions of the globe offers an invaluable tool that improves diagnoses and treatment options for providers and patients alike.

The advantages of ultrasound in rural regions are significant enough that the limitations may not be immediately apparent. However, discussing limitations will help identify how POCUS can improve to accommodate remote and sometimes austere environments. The first limitation of ultrasound in remote areas is that skilled operators are scarce in rural and less economically developed communities. Performing and interpreting ultrasound is a skill that, without training, is useless in practice. Different groups and organizations focus on training local healthcare providers because few of the local providers have prior training or experience [41–44]. Another limitation to accessing ultrasound technology for rural regions is lack of equipment. Even though ultrasound technology is becoming less expensive and more available through mobile computing technology, poorly funded areas still may have only one instrument in an entire hospital or for an entire patient population. The Tanzanian midwives that were interviewed, despite possessing a Doppler ultrasound device, often resorted to a fetoscope because the only hospital Doppler ultrasound was being used for a different patient [34]. Furthermore, austere environments come with their own set of challenges for maintaining and servicing ultrasound equipment. High altitudes, lack of electricity and/or WIFI, extreme temperatures, dirt floors, humidity, sea water, and other environmental hazards may harm the delicate electronics in ultrasound devices. Repairing the device would require delivery or travel to a servicing facility, the receipt of a servicing professional on-site, or additional servicing training for the healthcare provider, each of which are inconvenient and costly options for a remote community [38].

Despite current limitations, ultrasound is still valuable and feasible in remote environments. The dearth of trained personnel may be remedied by teleultrasonography or utilizing existing telecom infrastructure to both train students and review images, as seen in studies in Peru and Ethiopia. The research performed in austere regions of these countries used low-bandwidth internet connections such as 3G, which permitted local ultrasound operators to receive instruction from a physician in another country [44–46]. In locations where even 3G is not available, satellite internet is gradually becoming a more viable option [47]. Geographic limitations of ultrasound devices and access to equipment and repair can be fixed with smaller, more resilient device designs, as seen in those used on Mount Everest [48]. However, there is not yet a clear solution to repairing damaged ultrasound devices. Currently, more durable and portable hand-held models are being investigated as cost-effective options so that any damaged unit can be replaced, rather than sending large equipment for repair or bringing a specialist to the equipment [49].

Ultrasound and the increased use of teleultrasonography will significantly change healthcare team dynamics. Integrating this technology into a community will provide medical teams with additional insight into their patients' health, which may necessitate communication with additional healthcare workers and systems to guarantee optimal care. Another team paradigm shift will involve telemedicine, which links remote providers with a network of colleagues and resources around the globe. Rural practitioners will have new opportunities for medical partnerships and trainings that were previously inaccessible. Consequently, a wider range of specialties and additional expertise will be made available to isolated communities. Preliminary data supports the positive impact of ultrasound on team dynamics, as current surveys report that the technology empowers healthcare providers, improves job satisfaction, and increases retention of skilled teams, all of which are challenges in austere environments [39].

Rural and remote regions traditionally have not had the same level of access to ultrasound technology when compared to regions with more resources. However, the barrier to access is changing with reduction in equipment size and cost. The benefits to patient care and medical team dynamics have been demonstrated, and despite the current challenges of training and equipment repair, ultrasound is rapidly becoming more accessible, utilized, and integral in remote medical care.

Prehospital Ultrasound in the Military

The US military has utilized emergency POCUS since the first Gulf War in 1991. The technology has gradually evolved in its deployment for tactical assessment of combat-related injuries, non-combat-related trauma, guidance for procedures, and aiding resuscitation efforts. Since ACEP released its first guidelines on ultrasound use by Emergency Physicians in 2001, the US military has continued to adapt POCUS for its own use in remote settings [50].

Prehospital ultrasound provides a unique tool to help manage patients in the austere military environment. The practicality, versatility, and portability of ultrasound make this technology ideal for the constantly evolving battlefield. However, it is the accessibility of ultrasound that makes it an ideal tool for dissemination among combat medics. The military has demonstrated that optic nerve sheath diameter (a non-invasive marker of increased intracranial pressure that can present following traumatic brain injury) can be accurately measured by novices after brief didactic and hands-on training [51]. The importance of this technology to the military is evident by its role in Special Operation Medicine, where its effects on team dynamics are even more pronounced. Special Operation Forces (SOF) medics (Role 1 care) are trained in the application of this technology for use in the tactical setting. In addition to diagnosis, the medics also employ POCUS for real-time imaging in procedural guidance such as the removal of shrapnel. In addition, POCUS has allowed for tele-imaging from the field to forward operating bases for expert review. This real-time collaboration allows more flexibility when it comes to the mission at hand and more expedited care when the service member returns to a Role 2 or higher facility (a forward surgical team or beyond) [52].

With the advent of the Space Force and the increasing private sector of space exploration, ultrasound is finding its place among standard medical equipment on space shuttles. The speed and clarity of relayed images in low orbit make the technology practical for telemedicine guidance from flight surgeons at mission control [53]. Ultrasound has allowed for versatile imaging on the International Space Station (ISS), and hand-held models are currently being tested [54]. With limited weight and volume capacities requiring judicious selection of cargo, this transition to POCUS would be ideal. Sonography has been employed clinically on the ISS, largely in evaluation of ophthalmologic, musculoskeletal, and vascular complaints. Ocular changes associated with spaceflight have been well-documented, including globe flattening, cotton wool spots, choroidal folds, retinal thickening, and hyperopic shifts [55]. Ultrasound has been used to evaluate optic nerve sheath diameter and central retinal artery blood flow of crew members to confirm expected microgravity shifts and rule out the need for intervention, which could compromise a mission [54]. Microgravity also affects the musculoskeletal system through gravitational unloading of intervertebral disks, redistribution and alteration of muscle, and demineralization of bone [54]. These effects decrease strength and increase the likelihood of trauma during—and after—a mission. Ultrasound has been used to evaluate the integrity of the multifidus and erector spinae muscles, as well as discern a grade 1 biceps femoris tear. In the latter scenario, an astronaut on the ISS experiencing an injury during physical conditioning was suspected of having a ruptured biceps femoris. However, ultrasound revealed only a minor tear, which decreased the degree of management required [54].

Arguably the most significant clinical use of sonography in space flight medicine occurred when an astronaut with a prominent left external jugular vein was examined. Ultrasound imaging demonstrated an obstructive venous thrombosis in the left internal jugular vein, the scans of which allowed for a multidisciplinary collaboration on optimal therapy. After evaluating the risks of thromboembolism versus anticoagulation without reversal agents aboard the station, an enoxaparin regimen was initiated until apixaban, protamine, and prothrombin complex could be delivered to the station. The plan of care was successful, demonstrating the efficacy of ultrasound in team-driven surveillance, diagnosis, and healthcare during spaceflight [56].

Although clinical sonography has been documented, the scope of space flight ultrasound is limited and largely research oriented. Astronauts receive approximately 40 h of medical training, of which ultrasound comprises 3–4 h [54]. This exposure is shorter in duration—with fewer opportunities to practice—than many proposed EMS training programs for even an isolated system exam. Furthermore, medical equipment, pharmaceuticals, and intervention capabilities are currently limited in spaceflight, and even proficient ultrasound diagnosis does not guarantee healthcare solutions in many scenarios. Perhaps the most limiting factor of clinical use is the minimal data surrounding normal sonoanatomy in microgravity [54]. This incomplete understanding makes research a top priority before expansion of spaceflight clinical applications. Given these limitations, the gold standard of space flight healthcare remains prevention, and intensive physical requirements and screenings are most practical and cost-effective [54]. However, the case reports validate the utility of clinical ultrasound in spaceflight, and improvements in technology, training, and research will only increase its future value as a space flight medicine adjunct.

Using prehospital ultrasound, the military changes the team dynamics of its medical corps by allowing for the transmission of real-time images from the field to medical control. This capability has allowed for immediate management and procedural guidance in austere conditions. During operations that mandate radio silence, the SOF and Space Force teams can make more informed medical decisions that improve triage while deployed. Other missions may find soldiers unable to return to the next level of care and require field procedures, a scenario not uncommon in military medicine. If the next level of care is accessible, the provider can share images and coordinate expedited care with the medical receiving team. In military medicine, the medical corps is often understaffed, requiring providers to assume multiple roles for adequate healthcare provision. Prehospital ultrasound allows the receiving medical team advanced preparation for more organized treatment on patient arrival. Furthermore, when the provider in the field is trusted and competent with ultrasound, the receiving team may agree to bypass the in-house triage system and proceed directly to the operating room. This allows the military medical corps to streamline care, saving valuable time and resources. Thus, POCUS improves the military medical team dynamic through more appropriate and expedited care in transit and more cohesive and resource-conscious care in facility. Prehospital ultrasound use in the military exemplifies the advantages of accurate, low-cost, portable, and versatile technology and how it enhances patient care.

Future Direction

Innovative applications of POCUS are constantly emerging. The versatility of this technology has pioneered and optimized a variety of techniques in emergency and trauma medicine, and this same transformation could extend to the prehospital environment. Uses have been documented for musculoskeletal, genitourinary, cardiovascular, pulmonary, ophthalmologic, and neurological systems, with the potential for numerous applications not yet established.

Trauma can result in a variety of musculoskeletal complaints, and high-frequency linear array ultrasound could be a valuable adjunct in evaluation, stabilization, and pain management [28]. While life-threatening injuries typically indicate resuscitative efforts and rapid transport, lower acuity patients may benefit from additional evaluation and care on-scene. POCUS can discriminate between pulsatile hematoma, pseudoaneurysm, and aneurysm, which may lead to different treatment algorithms. It can also detect hernias, guiding reductions for patient comfort and incarceration prevention. If physical exam is limited by body habitus, swelling, or patient tolerance, findings on ultrasound can safely, reliably, and inexpensively discern the etiology [28]. The hypoechoic foci of tendon and ligament tears differ from arthropathic fluid collections; soft tissue inflammation distortion differs from the cortical disruption in bone fractures. Understanding the source of musculoskeletal pain is crucial to patient care and can help assess whether mild therapy is appropriate or more significant intervention is required, such as long-bone fracture protocol at a trauma facility. Furthermore, POCUS can guide fracture reduction by avoiding neurovascular compromise during bone alignment.

This increased imaging capability may expand therapeutic options in remote or military environments, as the diagnostic adjunct can also guide field musculoskeletal procedures necessitated by scarce medical assistance. Procedures such as arthrocentesis, foreign body localization and removal, steroid injection, nerve block administration, and other interventions have been performed in hospital. Appropriate training could adapt these techniques to remote environments, where patients have significant needs but limited options. Nerve blocks may be especially useful for long transports and manipulative procedures, providing improved localized pain control without the adverse effects of narcotics.

Vascular evaluation and access are an integral part of prehospital emergency care, and POCUS could expand the scope of practice and quality of care provided by paramedics. The use of ultrasound-guided intravenous cannulation is a useful tool for peripheral vascular access in patients with challenging body habitus. When in-hospital ultrasound guidance was compared to palpatory methods of peripheral intravenous cannulation, ultrasound guidance had a greater success rate (97% vs. 33%), shorter completion time (13 min vs. 30 min), fewer percutaneous punctures (1.7 vs. 3.7), and greater patient satisfaction [57]. Prehospital obstructions to peripheral vascular access may exceed those of the hospital environment, yet ultrasound guidance is not a common practice in EMS systems. Using either static or dynamic technique, POCUS can be used to gain access to femoral, jugular, subclavian, or peripheral veins, as well as intraosseous spaces, and studies have demonstrated decreased attempts and increased rates of cannulation with minimal training [57, 58]. In addition to guiding the procedure, the imaging can also serve as placement verification with color Doppler. This additional step is crucial as some researchers note that positioning is not accurately confirmed with presence of blood aspirate or absence of extravasation [59].

Cardiothoracic and vascular procedures with greater risk, such as arterial lines, central vascular access, pericardiocentesis, and thoracentesis including pneumothorax decompression, could also become more feasible and safer in the field with sonography to supplement the traditional use of anatomical landmarks. This utility extends to resuscitative endovascular balloon occlusion of the aorta (REBOA), an intervention used to stabilize patients in hemodynamic shock through temporary interruption of circulation to noncompressible hemorrhages. Animal studies have demonstrated that appropriate application of REBOA results in 74% reduction of mortality during hemorrhagic shock [60]. Ultrasound guidance in cadaver trials has been found to improve incidence of correct zone placement, while decreasing the time to placement [61]. This approach could be adapted to POCUS in the field, potentially improving the care for patients in hemorrhagic shock. Improved vascular visualization and access could improve patient care with more rapid administration of therapies, including necessary fluids, medications, and procedures.

Obtaining an airway in the field may entail working in imperfect environments on patients with challenging body habitus, vomitus, trauma, and other obstructions. Endotracheal tube (ETT) placement may have first-attempt success rates as low as 46%, and esophageal placements necessitate adjustment as quickly as possible [62]. However, physical exam can be equivocal in the best environments, and X-ray confirmation is unavailable. The identification of bilateral lung sliding and diaphragmatic excursion on ultrasound has confirmed ETT position with 100% sensitivity and specificity, making POCUS a useful adjunct in airway confirmation [63]. Furthermore, when ETT placement fails, ultrasound can help obtain an emergency airway via cricothyrotomy. Manual palpation of anatomical landmarks can be unreliable, and studies have found ultrasound guidance to improve success rates and placement times of cricothyrotomy [64, 65].

Early detection and intervention are critical for stroke management. In ischemic stroke, earlier intravenous thrombolysis has been associated with reduced disability and mortality. Hemorrhagic stroke requires prompt surgical intervention, and the time-sensitive nature of these life-threatening events has produced many health system metrics and best practice guidelines regarding rapid patient management. Early studies have suggested that transcranial sonography may have diagnostic value in stroke [66]. Initial scans had a high sensitivity and predictive value for ischemic stroke when color Doppler was applied to the temporal window. Researchers additionally noted high specificity for arterial occlusion, especially with use of contrast agents [67]. Hemorrhagic stroke and vasospasm have also been detected with ultrasound, but determining sensitivity and specificity requires additional investigation [68]. Additional research and training on POCUS could profoundly affect stroke management. Stroke diagnosis can be delayed or missed. The US medical consortium found that fewer than 38% of patients with ischemic stroke reach urban academic medical centers within the window for intravenous thrombolytics. While this analysis considers the urban environment, rural populations may face greater delays. With ultrasound, paramedics could determine the stroke diagnosis and contributing etiologies in the prehospital setting. Transport to the appropriate hospital and mobilization of the appropriate teams would be significantly expedited. With appropriate training and protocols, intravenous thrombolytics could be administered in the prehospital setting to further improve patient outcomes. Some studies have even proposed and trialed the use of sonothrombolysis as a means of managing ischemic strokes [3, 69]. CLOTBUST researchers are trialing a hands-free transducer that may be applied to the temporal window without the need for formal ultrasound training. If sufficiently developed, the technology could revolutionize prehospital stroke management [69].

Ultrasound has been utilized for ophthalmologic complaints of foreign body, globe rupture, lens dislocation, vitreous hemorrhage, and detached retina. While most of the prehospital utility in these evaluations would come from a more rapid notification of ophthalmologists and surgeons, promising trials have used sonography to assess intracranial pressure (ICP) [22]. Optic nerve sheath diameter measurements with ultrasound have a high sensitivity for elevated ICP, and are a quick, non-invasive alternative to waiting for a lumbar puncture or CT scan. Positive findings would guide prehospital care on scene, as well as communications to the appropriate providers during transport, ultimately circumventing time-consuming and expensive diagnostics on arrival.

Although ultrasound often comes to mind for obstetrics, the imaging modality is also useful in evaluating the male reproductive organs. Testicular trauma may involve contusion, obstructive hematocele, fracture, torsion, hernia, or dislocation. Both B-mode and Doppler are useful in discerning the injury location and severity, which can provide surgical teams advance time to prepare for emergency interventions such as decompression, orchiopexy, and repair. Quick activation of the surgical team is important to prevent permanent damage or sterility, and POCUS could facilitate this critical action [70].

Conclusions

Ultrasound is gaining popularity internationally, resulting in frequent innovations. The technology is particularly promising in prehospital and austere environments, where versatility, durability, and mobility are crucial. Prehospital POCUS remains a newly adopted skill, and the education system will need to capture the breadth of POCUS application in future core curriculum. However, paramedic-implemented POCUS is already finding success at its most limited scope, and user proficiency will only improve. With appropriate training, quality review of ultrasound images, and protocol adherence, the adjunct allows for quick, inexpensive, low-maintenance evaluation with decreased risk for iatrogenic injury and ionizing radiation. This enhanced assessment with decreased risk has been shown to improve diagnosis and allow for more rapid administration of appropriate therapies. Real-time determinations improve emergency team organization and surgical team activation, which, in turn, improves patient care. Prehospital studies are currently investigating associations between patient management with POCUS and positive outcomes, including survival following cardiac arrest. Research has already shown high diagnostic sensitivity, specificity, predictive value, and patient management impact, demonstrating great potential for POCUS in the prehospital setting.

With the technology being new to most prehospital providers, proficiency is isolated to specific differentials and the understanding of anatomy in isolated systems. As POCUS becomes more commonly integrated into training programs, paramedics will develop an expertise that allows for the adjunct to be used as intended, a multisystem evaluation that expedites diagnosis and treatment. With a linear progression to POCUS mastery for complex interpretation, beyond the isolated application currently seen with progressive agencies, future uses offer widespread utility. Prehospital application to both medical and trauma patients will mirror practices in major trauma centers, expediting the delivery of more appropriate therapies and optimizing team dynamics from the field to the hospital.

Key Points

- Standardized ultrasound training with performance metrics is crucial to ensuring augmentation—as opposed to impedance—of care.
- Groups who utilize POCUS report positive effects on team dynamics and medical decision-making in the prehospital setting.
- Sonography algorithms are expediting diagnoses and directing management during shock, trauma, and cardiac arrest.
- Expanding diagnostic capabilities of remote providers has improved resource allocation in austere environments.
- POCUS can be a useful adjunct in forward-deployed and aerospace settings, where laypersons can receive telemedicine guidance to make mission-critical decisions.

References

1. Breitkreutz R, Price S, Steiger HV, Seeger FH, Ilper H, Ackermann H, et al. Focused echocardiographic evaluation in life support and peri-resuscitation of emergency patients: A prospective trial. Resuscitation. 2010 Nov;81(11):1527–33.
2. Scharonow M, Weilbach C. Prehospital point-of-care emergency ultrasound: a cohort study. Scand J Trauma Resusc Emerg Med. 2018 Dec;26(1):49.
3. Ketelaars R, Beekers C, Van Geffen G-J, Scheffer GJ, Hoogerwerf N. Prehospital echocardiography during resuscitation impacts treatment in a physician-staffed helicopter emergency medical service: an observational study. Prehosp Emerg Care. 2018 Jul 4;22(4):406–13.
4. Taylor J, McLaughlin K, McRae A, Lang E, Anton A. Use of prehospital ultrasound in North America: a survey of emergency medical services medical directors. BMC Emerg Med. 2014 Dec;14(1):6.
5. Reed MJ, Gibson L, Dewar A, Short S, Black P, Clegg GR. Introduction of paramedic led Echo in Life Support into the pre-hospital environment: the PUCA study. Resuscitation. 2017 Mar;112:65–9.
6. Rooney KP, Lahham S, Lahham S, Anderson CL, Bledsoe B, Sloane B, et al. Pre-hospital assessment with ultrasound in emergencies: implementation in the field. World J Emerg Med. 2016;7(2):117.
7. Kreiser M, Hill B, Karki D, Wood E, Shelton R, Peterson J, et al. Point-of-care ultrasound use by EMS providers in out-of-hospital cardiac arrest. Poster presented at: Association of Military Surgeons of the United States Annual Meeting; 2020; Online.
8. Huis In 't Veld MA, Allison MG, Bostick DS, Fisher KR, Goloubeva OG, Witting MD, et al. Ultrasound use during cardiopulmonary resuscitation is associated with delays in chest compressions. Resuscitation. 2017 Oct;119:95–8.
9. Clattenburg EJ, Wroe P, Brown S, Gardner K, Losonczy L, Singh A, et al. Point-of-care ultrasound use in patients with cardiac arrest is associated prolonged cardiopulmonary resuscitation pauses: a prospective cohort study. Resuscitation. 2018 Jan;122:65–8.
10. Ultrasound Guidelines. Emergency, Point-of-Care and Clinical Ultrasound Guidelines in Medicine. Ann Emerg Med. 2017 May;69(5):e27–54.
11. Heegaard W, Plummer D, Dries D, Frascone R, Pippert G, Steel D, et al. Ultrasound for the air medical clinician. Air Med J. 2004 Mar;23(2):20–3.
12. Ziesmann MT, Park J, Unger B, Kirkpatrick AW, Vergis A, Pham C, et al. Validation of hand motion analysis as an objective assessment tool for the focused assessment with sonography for trauma examination. J Trauma Acute Care Surg. 2015 Oct;79(4):631–7.
13. Ackil DJ, Toney A, Good R, Ross D, Germano R, Sabbadini L, et al. Use of hand-motion analysis to assess competence and skill decay for cardiac and lung point-of-care ultrasound. In: Wagner J, editor. AEM Education and Training; 2020 Dec 15. p. aet2.10560.
14. Walcher F, Weinlich M, Conrad G, Schweigkofler U, Breitkreutz R, Kirschning T, et al. Prehospital ultrasound imaging improves management of abdominal trauma. Br J Surg. 2006 Feb;93(2):238–42.
15. Yates JG, Baylous D. Aeromedical ultrasound: the evaluation of point-of-care ultrasound during helicopter transport. Air Med J. 2017 May;36(3):110–5.
16. Price DD, Wilson SR, Murphy TG. Trauma ultrasound feasibility during helicopter transport. Air Med J. 2000 Oct;19(4):144–6.
17. Polk JD, Merlino JI, Kovach BL, Mancuso C, Fallon WF. Fetal evaluation for transport by ultrasound performed by air medical teams. Air Med J. 2004 Jul;23(4):32–4.
18. Perera P, Mailhot T, Riley D, Mandavia D. The RUSH exam: rapid ultrasound in shock in the evaluation of the critically Ill. Emerg Med Clin North Am. 2010 Feb;28(1):29–56.
19. Heegaard W, Hildebrandt D, Spear D, Chason K, Nelson B, Ho J. Prehospital ultrasound by paramedics: results of field trial: paramedic prehospital ultrasound. Acad Emerg Med. 2010 May 14;17(6):624–30.
20. Varner MW. Maternal mortality in Iowa from 1952 to 1986. Surg Gynecol Obstet. 1989 Jun;168(6):555–62.
21. Lane PL. Traumatic fetal deaths. J Emerg Med. 1989 Sep;7(5):433–5.
22. Cosby KS, Kendall JL. Practical guide to emergency ultrasound. Lippincott, Williams & Wilkins; 2014.
23. Eberle B, Dick WF, Schneider T, Wisser G, Doetsch S, Tzanova I. Checking the carotid pulse check: diagnostic accuracy of first responders in patients with and without a pulse. Resuscitation. 1996 Dec;33(2):107–16.
24. Dick WF, Eberle B, Wisser G, Schneider T. The carotid pulse check revisited: What if there is no pulse? Crit Care Med. 2000 Nov;28(Supplement):N183–5.
25. Larsen MP, Eisenberg MS, Cummins RO, Hallstrom AP. Predicting survival from out-of-hospital cardiac arrest: a graphic model. Ann Emerg Med. 1993 Nov;22(11):1652–8.
26. Fukuda T, Ohashi-Fukuda N, Matsubara T, Gunshin M, Kondo Y, Yahagi N. Effect of prehospital epinephrine on out-of-hospital cardiac arrest: a report from the national out-of-hospital cardiac arrest data registry in Japan, 2011–2012. Eur J Clin Pharmacol. 2016 Oct;72(10):1255–64.
27. Badra K, Coutin A, Simard R, Pinto R, Lee JS, Chenkin J. The POCUS pulse check: A randomized controlled crossover study comparing pulse detection by palpation versus by point-of-care ultrasound. Resuscitation. 2019 Jun;139:17–23.
28. Ma OJ, editor. Ma and Mateer's emergency ultrasound. 3rd ed. New York: McGraw-Hill; 2013.
29. Wu C, Zheng Z, Jiang L, Gao Y, Xu J, Jin X, et al. The predictive value of bedside ultrasound to restore spontaneous circulation in patients with pulseless electrical activity: a systematic review and meta-analysis. Plos One. 2018 Jan 24;13(1):e0191636.
30. Mehta C, Brady W. Pulseless electrical activity in cardiac arrest: electrocardiographic presentations and management considerations based on the electrocardiogram. Am J Emerg Med. 2012 Jan;30(1):236–9.
31. Gaspari R, Weekes A, Adhikari S, Noble V, Nomura JT, Theodoro D, et al. A retrospective study of pulseless electrical activity, bedside ultrasound identifies interventions during resuscitation associated with improved survival to hospital admission. A reason study. Resuscitation. 2017 Nov;120:103–7.
32. Stawicki SP. Portable ultrasonography in mass casualty incidents: The CAVEAT examination. World J Orthop. 2010;1(1):10.
33. Bøtker MT, Jacobsen L, Rudolph SS, Knudsen L. The role of point of care ultrasound in prehospital critical care: a systematic review. Scand J Trauma Resusc Emerg Med. 2018 Dec;26(1):51.
34. Åhman A, Edvardsson K, Lesio Kidanto H, Ngarina M, Small R, Mogren I. 'Without ultrasound you can't reach the best decision' – Midwives' experiences and views of the role of ultrasound in maternity care in Dar Es Salaam, Tanzania. Sex Reprod Healthc. 2018 Mar;15:28–34.
35. Shah SP, Epino H, Bukhman G, Umulisa I, Dushimiyimana J, Reichman A, et al. Impact of the introduction of ultrasound services in a limited resource setting: rural Rwanda 2008. BMC Int Health Hum Rights. 2009 Dec;9(1):4.
36. Kotlyar S, Moore C. Assessing the utility of ultrasound in Liberia. J Emerg Trauma Shock. 2008;1(1):10.
37. Steinmetz JP, Berger JP. Ultrasonography as an aid to diagnosis and treatment in a rural African hospital: a prospective study of 1,119 cases. Am J Trop Med Hyg. 1999 Jan 1;60(1):119–23.
38. Blaivas M, Kuhn W, Reynolds B, Brannam L. Change in differential diagnosis and patient management with the use of portable ultrasound in a remote setting. Wilderness Environ Med. 2005 Mar;16(1):38–41.

39. Eckardt M, Ahn R, Reyes R. The impact of maternal ultrasound in Mali. Poster presented at: American Public Health Association Annual Meeting; 2011; Washington, DC.
40. Kolbe N, Killu K, Coba V, Neri L, Garcia KM, McCulloch M, et al. Point of care ultrasound (POCUS) telemedicine project in rural Nicaragua and its impact on patient management. J Ultrasound. 2015 Jun;18(2):179–85.
41. Sorensen B, Hunskaar S. Point-of-care ultrasound in primary care: a systematic review of generalist performed point-of-care ultrasound in unselected populations. Ultrasound J. 2019 Dec;11(1):31.
42. Ramsingh D, Ma M, Le DQ, Davis W, Ringer M, Austin B, et al. Feasibility evaluation of commercially available video conferencing devices to technically direct untrained nonmedical personnel to perform a rapid trauma ultrasound examination. Diagnostics. 2019 Nov 14;9(4):188.
43. Shokoohi H, Raymond A, Fleming K, Scott J, Kerry V, Haile-Mariam T, et al. Assessment of point-of-care ultrasound training for clinical educators in Malawi, Tanzania and Uganda. Ultrasound Med Biol. 2019 Jun;45(6):1351–7.
44. Marini TJ, Castaneda B, Baran T, O'Connor TP, Garra B, Tamayo L, et al. Lung ultrasound volume sweep imaging for pneumonia detection in rural areas: piloting training in Rural Peru. J Clin Imaging Sci. 2019 Jul;12(9):35.
45. Whitney RE, Riera A, Chen L. Accuracy of remote interpretation of pediatric emergency ultrasound over third generation networks across continents. Pediatr Emerg Care. 2020 Jun;36(6):e340–2.
46. Ferreira AC, O'Mahony E, Oliani AH, Araujo Júnior E, da Silva CF. Teleultrasound: historical perspective and clinical application. Int J Telemed Appl. 2015;2015:1–11.
47. Graydon M, Parks L. 'Connecting the unconnected': a critical assessment of US satellite Internet services. Media Cult Soc. 2020 Mar;42(2):260–76.
48. Otto C, Hamilton DR, Levine BD, Hare C, Sargsyan AE, Altshuler P, et al. Into thin air: extreme ultrasound on Mt Everest. Wilderness Environ Med. 2009 Sep;20(3):283–9.
49. Burleson SL, Swanson JF, Shufflebarger EF, Wallace DW, Heimann MA, Crosby JC, et al. Evaluation of a novel handheld point-of-care ultrasound device in an African emergency department. Ultrasound J. 2020 Dec;12(1):53.
50. Ferre RM, Director EU, Johnson J, Director EUF, Hood F, Hall TB, et al. Military and tactical ultrasound. Am Coll Emerg Physicians [Internet]. Available from: https://www.acep.org/globalassets/uploads/uploaded-files/acep/membership/sections-of-membership/ultra/subcommittees/tactical-us-acep-final.doc
51. Betcher J, Becker TK, Stoyanoff P, Cranford J, Theyyunni N. Military trainees can accurately measure optic nerve sheath diameter after a brief training session. Mil Med Res. 2018 Dec;5(1):42.
52. Hampton KK, Vasios WN, Loos PE. SOLCUS: update on point-of-care ultrasound in special operations medicine. J Spec Oper Med Peer Rev J SOF Med Prof. 2016;16(1):58–61.
53. Feletti F, Mucci V, Aliverti A. Chest ultrasonography in modern day extreme settings: from military setting and natural disasters to space flights and extreme sports. Can Respir J. 2018;2018:1–9.
54. Scheuring R. Personal communication. 2021.
55. Mader TH, Gibson CR, Pass AF, Kramer LA, Lee AG, Fogarty J, et al. Optic disc edema, globe flattening, choroidal folds, and hyperopic shifts observed in astronauts after long-duration space flight. Ophthalmology. 2011 Oct;118(10):2058–69.
56. Auñón-Chancellor SM, Pattarini JM, Moll S, Sargsyan A. Venous thrombosis during spaceflight. N Engl J Med. 2020 Jan 2;382(1):89–90.
57. Costantino TG, Parikh AK, Satz WA, Fojtik JP. Ultrasonography-guided peripheral intravenous access versus traditional approaches in patients with difficult intravenous access. Ann Emerg Med. 2005 Nov;46(5):456–61.
58. Brannam L. Emergency nurses' utilization of ultrasound guidance for placement of peripheral intravenous lines in difficult-access patients. Acad Emerg Med. 2004 Dec 1;11(12):1361–3.
59. Tsung JW, Blaivas M, Stone MB. Feasibility of point-of-care colour Doppler ultrasound confirmation of intraosseous needle placement during resuscitation. Resuscitation. 2009 Jun;80(6):665–8.
60. Chaudery M, Clark J, Wilson MH, Bew D, Yang G-Z, Darzi A. Traumatic intra-abdominal hemorrhage control: Has current technology tipped the balance toward a role for prehospital intervention? J Trauma Acute Care Surg. 2015 Jan;78(1):153–63.
61. Chaudery M, Clark J, Morrison JJ, Wilson MH, Bew D, Darzi A. Can contrast-enhanced ultrasonography improve Zone III REBOA placement for prehospital care? J Trauma Acute Care Surg. 2016 Jan;80(1):89–94.
62. Peters J, van Wageningen B, Hendriks I, Eijk R, Edwards M, Hoogerwerf N, et al. First-pass intubation success rate during rapid sequence induction of prehospital anaesthesia by physicians versus paramedics. Eur J Emerg Med. 2015 Dec;22(6):391–4.
63. Zadel S, Strnad M, Prosen G, Mekiš D. Point of care ultrasound for orotracheal tube placement assessment in out-of hospital setting. Resuscitation. 2015 Feb;87:1–6.
64. Nicholls SE, Sweeney TW, Ferre RM, Strout TD. Bedside sonography by emergency physicians for the rapid identification of landmarks relevant to cricothyrotomy. Am J Emerg Med. 2008 Oct;26(8):852–6.
65. Šustić A, Kovač D, Žgaljardić Z, Župan Ž, Krstulović B. Ultrasound-guided percutaneous dilatational tracheostomy: a safe method to avoid cranial misplacement of the tracheostomy tube. Intensive Care Med. 2000 Sep;26(9):1379–81.
66. Herzberg M, Boy S, Hölscher T, Ertl M, Zimmermann M, Ittner K-P, et al. Prehospital stroke diagnostics based on neurological examination and transcranial ultrasound. Crit Ultrasound J. 2014 Dec;6(1):3.
67. Schlachetzki F, Herzberg M, Hölscher T, Ertl M, Zimmermann M, Ittner KP, et al. Transcranial ultrasound from diagnosis to early stroke treatment – Part 2: prehospital neurosonography in patients with acute stroke – the regensburg stroke mobile project. Cerebrovasc Dis. 2012;33(3):262–71.
68. Lysakowski C, Walder B, Costanza MC, Tramèr MR. Transcranial Doppler versus angiography in patients with vasospasm due to a ruptured cerebral aneurysm: a systematic review. Stroke. 2001 Oct;32(10):2292–8.
69. Barlinn K, Tsivgoulis G, Barreto AD, Alleman J, Molina CA, Mikulik R, et al. Outcomes following sonothrombolysis in severe acute ischemic stroke: subgroup analysis of the CLOTBUST trial. Int J Stroke. 2014 Dec;9(8):1006–10.
70. Jeffrey R, Laing F, Hricak H, McAninch J. Sonography of testicular trauma. Am J Roentgenol. 1983 Nov;141(5):993–5.

19 Prehospital Trauma

Michelangelo Bortolin and Jacopo M. Olagnero

Abbreviations

EMS	Emergency Medical Service
FAST	Focused Assessment with Sonography for Trauma
EMS	Emergency Medical Services
HEMS	Helicopter Emergency Medical Service
HIFU	High-Intensity Focused Ultrasound
IO	Intraosseous (access)
IV	Intravenous
MCVs	Motor Vehicle Crashes
OHCA	Out-of-Hospital Cardiac Arrest
RTA	Road Traffic Accident
TC	Trauma Center
TXA	Tranexamic Acid
US	Ultrasonography

Introduction

The management and treatment of a trauma patient begins immediately at the scene, in the out-of-hospital phase, and determines a significant part of the outcome for the patient and the overall success of the trauma clinical pathway.

When the trauma team enters the scene to take care of the patient, there is a first crucial step to be taken as an immediate priority: the size-up of the scene. This is to guarantee the safety of the team and to understand the scene and the situation of the event. The scene size-up is as essential as the first approach to the scene. When the EMS team first approaches the patient, it is important for a complete assessment to be undertaken as soon as possible: this assessment must establish what and where the problem is, what the impact of the problem is, how to quickly manage the situation, as well as gathering the information needed.

Providers are required to evaluate the patients quickly, address major life threats, and make a full inventory of injuries. Without delay, at the scene healthcare professionals need to be able to handle a broad spectrum of trauma patients and clinical situations. Therefore, it is important for the patient assessment to individuate all of the patients and their critical situations in order to be able to act immediately and in a suitable and timely manner, thus avoiding any further decline. It is essential to understand the basic interventions required in order to minimize the risk of further deterioration and to understand when prioritizing patients and their needs. It is crucial for all healthcare professionals to understand what to look for and how to assess the condition of a patient using a systematic approach. Having a systematic method is essential for a rapid assessment, thus minimizing the chance of failing to spot injuries and avoiding mistakes.

The Trimodal Distribution of Trauma and the Golden Hour

In 1983, Trunkey DD., and several other authors, thereafter, described a trimodal distribution of trauma deaths based upon the time interval from injury to death: immediate, early, and late trauma deaths, respectively, minutes, hours, and weeks after the incident. [1] Referring to this trimodal distribution, it is possible to state that about 50% of deaths related to a traumatic event occur at the scene or in any case up to an hour after the event. Deaths that occur immediately following the accident, and therefore in this first phase, are generally a consequence of severe and non-survivable injuries, and there is no impact of the Emergency Medical Services (EMS) on these situations. These patients are declared dead on the

M. Bortolin (✉)
Disaster Medicine Fellowship at BIDMC (a teaching hospital of Harvard Medical School), Boston, MA, USA

CRIMEDIM – Center for Research and Training in Disaster Medicine, Humanitarian Aid, and Global Health, Università del Piemonte Orientale – UPO, Novara, Italy

J. M. Olagnero
Critical Care Nurse at Humanitas Gradenigo Hospital, Turin, Italy

Temporary Research Fellow in Nursing Science, Università di Torino, Turin, Italy

L. Marshall Gillman, S. Widder (eds.), *Trauma Team Dynamics*, https://doi.org/10.1007/978-3-031-86312-7_19

scene or die shortly after arrival in hospital. In order to reduce the mortality of these traumas, mitigation programs are needed: the international and local development of wide-ranging prevention programs is of absolute priority and validity, that is, both for the population and for the implementation of safety systems [2, 3].

When the mortality of the first phase has not yet affected the outcome of the traumatized patient, the out-of-hospital trauma team must act quickly to ensure the prompt resuscitation of the patient, taking advantage of the short time window to have an impact on the second and third phase of Trunkey's concept. The management must guarantee the swiftest and best definitive treatment while in the field to achieve the best prognosis for the patient. Indeed, in the second phase of the trimodal, mortality from the trauma develops within the first few hours following the accident so the intervention of the trauma team acting directly on the scene is crucial for the immediate and long-term outcome. In this phase, the role of the EMS team is indispensable since the deaths that characterize this phase can be prevented by optimal prehospital care and initial in-hospital care [4]. With reference to the third phase of trauma mortality, it is also undeniable that the action of the prehospital trauma team has repercussions on what the patient's course of recovery will be. In fact, there are studies that underline the possibility of making this last phase of the trimodal distribution minimal, flattening the curve gradient to zero, if the trauma is managed according to the high-quality standards from the first intervention that take place right at the scene of the event [4, 5].

In close relation to this subdivision of trauma mortality into phases is the concept of the "Golden Hour," defined by Cowley. [6]. This assumption is a conceptual reference present in trauma management's way of thinking, which underlines that the vast majority of deaths occur in the first 60 min following injury if prehospital and subsequent emergent trauma care in the hospital are suboptimal [7]. In modern trauma care, this concept of the "Golden Hour" is still acknowledged as valid, though the period of time in question does not really have to be one hour, but rather should be as short as possible, the term "Golden Period" was coined in substitution. In fact, it is known that for many patients 60 min of time between the event and treatment would be too long a period and would be life-threatening, while for others the time that could elapse may be longer. Therefore, the EMS team must act efficiently to reach an ideal balance between the advanced treatment and stabilization of the patient in the field and minimize time spent at the scene in order to achieve the best trauma patient outcomes [8]. The EMS team must always keep in mind these two crucial concepts: trimodal distribution of trauma deaths and the "Golden Period." In order to assure the integrity of these cornerstones, the trauma team must focus on four practical key aspects which must be carried out during the rescue [9]:

- The scene size-up: safety and scene assessment
- Trauma dynamics
- The primary patient assessment and performing lifesaving maneuvers
- The secondary patient assessment before transportation to the hospital

The Scene Size-Up: Safety and Scene Assessment

The first important aspect concerns the scene. Three points are very important in sizing up the scene: the three "S"s—assessment of the scene, the situation, and safety. The consideration of safety is fundamental to avoid going from being the rescuer to being a victim.

Safety

A fundamental element that characterizes the management of out-of-hospital trauma, which is not found in the emergency room, is the need to ensure a safe environment. The safety of the scene is the first aspect to be considered upon arrival at the target of the accident, even before the assessment of the injured [10]. Upon receipt of the emergency call from the Dispatch Center, the rescuer's mind must imagine the types of real dangers they might encounter. The dangers that the scenes of a trauma can show it is good to remember that these are not limited only to road accident situations but are also present in other scenarios, from domestic to rural ones, from industrial ones to disaster situations, up to the possible situations of violence that can also be unleashed on rescuers themselves. The dangers can be represented by different elements, such as people in possession of blades or firearms, dispersed chemical materials, which represent the most frequently encountered category, and the presence of dangerous elements that can fall on the scene. In this context, it is necessary to remember that meteorological situations can also represent a risk. It is necessary to promptly recognize where there may be a potential hazard or risk and adopt valid strategies to mitigate the risk. This must be shared with the team even before reaching the target. Another aspect to improve the safety of operational scenarios is to always entrust the safety of the environment to technical rescue and above all to refrain from maneuvers where sufficient safety conditions are not identified to allow the team to operate.

The last decisive aspect regarding safety is related to the management and positioning of the vehicle, especially in reference to land vehicles such as ambulances. Statistics highlight how EMS personnel have accident rates higher than the general average of workers: it shows that working in out-of-hospital rescue settings is a job with high correlated risks that need to be mitigated [11]. For this reason, it must be a priority to manage the rescue vehicle at the target in a prudent manner, especially when flashing lights and sirens are used [12]. Upon arrival at the scenario, the vehicle must therefore be positioned so that it is visible and that it protects the team from collision with other vehicles [12, 13]. In order to mitigate the risk of road accidents involving EMS personnel, the first incoming emergency vehicles must "draw the line" of the accident, to slow down and direct the oncoming traffic.

Scene Assessment

After putting safety precautions in place, scene assessment means recognizing potential and real hazards, understanding the number of people involved in the event, the number of casualties, and understanding if the team needs more resources and the support of other EMS teams and/or Agencies, such as Fire Brigades or Police. However, the assessment of the scene of the trauma, as well as the preventive recognition of the scenario's potential risks and dangers, must start from the moment of the dispatch.

During approach to the target, the trauma team in the rescue vehicle must begin preparing to ensure adequate performance as well as the necessary equipment. At this juncture it is also possible to devote attention to the division of tasks, especially in cases where the information regarding the mission indicates that a large number of people are involved. To divide the tasks before arrival and on the scene, a team leader should be identified to coordinate the other crew members. The interventions to be implemented should be divided according to a logic that takes into account each team member's technical and non-technical skills.

The first visual assessment of the scenario must begin when the rescue vehicle is about to arrive at the target. From this viewpoint, the rescuers are able to see and begin to think about what may have been the dynamics and kinematics of the trauma, elements which will then be indispensable for conducting a correct and exhaustive general assessment. Looking at the scenario from a distant perspective can allow us to perceive characteristics of the traumatic event that can no longer be seen when the rescuer is immersed in the scene and is dedicated to the patient. An experienced rescuer also gets a general impression in these first moments of rescue, not only for the safety of the scenario but also for the relevance of the trauma. In this context, the rescuer's experience plays an important role since it determines a perception of the contingent situation which is then maintained throughout the mission and which is difficult to abandon. Therefore, the "glance," the experience, and the sharing of information, as well as the collaboration of each team member, are very relevant skills for the overall optimal management of the trauma rescue mission.

The recognition of potential or real hazard is a crucial point because it is important to avoid putting the EMS team in danger and at risk of great vulnerability. To detect the presence or absence of these elements, it is essential that each member of the team uses all their senses and perceives certain details, as well as sounds and smells, maintaining the rationality of not being attracted only by the most obvious.

Trauma Dynamics

A crucial point of a trauma team in the field is to understand the traumatic event, the type of incident, and the trauma dynamics associated.

The traumatic event is described in three different phases: the pre-event, the event itself, and the post-event. The pre-event phase consists of all the factors that can affect the event in varying ways; among these, there may be features that mitigate the effects of the trauma but also those that can worsen the outcome. The pre-event phase can include prevention campaigns regarding road safety, the prevention of domestic accidents, and even new technologies that can help mitigate human errors and their consequences.

The event phase generally begins at the moment of impact between a moving object and a second object. At the moment of impact, various aspects must be considered, such as not only the primary impact of two objects against each other but also the concomitant movement of the organs that occur. There is an exchange of energy between the object and the human body or vice versa in any scenario, from a pedestrian being hit, to falling down stairs, from a stabbing, to a motorcycle collision. The rescuer's assessment takes these aspects into consideration in an important way, including the direction of the energy exchange and, above all, the total sum of the interchanged forces, in order to evaluate the injuries and effects on the victim.

The post-event phase consists of the deductions that the rescuer is able to make from the trauma scenario that has been quickly and carefully assessed. All the features collected are then incorporated into the patient's overall assessment and used for treatment choices; understanding the traumatic event is crucial. For a trauma patient who is walking and is conscious, and appears less severely injured, it is still important to look at the scene and to try to understand what happened. Do not underestimate the patient, as missed injuries and opportunities to treat can occur. A classic example is the patient who is conscious but has head trauma and presents with a "lucid interval." The lucid interval is a period after the trauma in which the patient doesn't show signs of neurological compromise. But after this period, there is neurological deterioration due to delayed secondary neurological damage subsequent to the head injury. "Lucid interval" is observed in 30–40% of severe head-injury patients who finally die. Therefore, do not underestimate trauma patients who are walking and answering questions properly.

Trauma is generally classified as penetrating trauma or blunt trauma. The mechanisms underlying both of these two typologies can be superimposed in terms of the energy exchanged between the two physical systems and the presence of the phenomenon of cavitation. Cavitation is the result of the displacement of the tissues that make up the human body from their physiological position following the exchange of energy between the two bodies following impact. This migration of the tissues can determine a return of the tissues back to the initial position, sustaining however damage (temporary cavity), or it can be characterized by a destruction of the anatomical tissues with the creation of a permanent cavity. A common example of a temporary cavity that causes damage in a road accident is the impact of the driver's abdomen with the steering wheel; a permanent cavity is typically created in the case of a gunshot, in which the bullet penetrates the body, destroying the surrounding tissues. These examples allow us to understand in general how the type of cavitation is determined by the impact area between the object and the human body; on the one hand, in the temporary cavity, the area of the steering wheel that impacts against the abdomen is large and therefore the energy is more widely dispersed and blunt trauma is generated. In the case of the bullet, this has a significantly small impact area, thus releasing a lot of energy in a small space and is able to create more severe injuries.

Trauma dynamics can be different between one trauma and another. The first important step is to understand the mechanism of injury (MOI) and evaluate if it is significant (major trauma supposed) or not (minor). An MOI is significant in the event of: (1) ejection from a vehicle, (2) death in the same passenger compartment, (3) falls >15 feet, (4) rollover mechanism, (5) high-speed vehicle collision, (6) pedestrian versus car, (7) motorcycle crash, (8) bicycle crash, (9) penetrating injury of head, chest, or abdomen.

Moreover, it is possible to categorize trauma dynamics in accordance with the event and, in road traffic accidents (RTAs), by the vehicle involved. This classification into different real situations is somewhat imprecise in completely describing an event: often trauma dynamics are different and intermixed. However, this subdivision can help the rescuer to identify the potential damage that the different impacts can generate [14]. This classification can also be useful in describing potential injuries or damages from types of traumatic events other than RTAs with similar dynamics, such as falls.

Frontal Impact In this type of dynamics, chest damage is frequent with possible fractures to the ribs and, due to the resulting sum of forces, also to internal organs such as the heart and lungs. In frontal impact dynamics, there are also two paths along which the internal occupants of a vehicle move, namely up-and-over and down-and-under. In the up-and-over movement the driver is projected upwards frequently provoking head and neck, as well as abdominal injuries, in which mostly kidneys, liver, spleen are involved but also to large vessels such as aorta and vena cava due to an increase in abdominal pressure. In the down-and-under movement, the occupant of the car is pushed by the impact downward and at the same time forward, inflicting trauma to the coxo-femoral joint and to the knees; fractures of the femurs, tibia, and fibula can be detected in which there is also potentially an injury in the relative blood vessels.

Lateral Impact These typical dynamics are found in road junctions and intersections. In this collision, injuries are mostly found to the two bone girdles with fractures of the collarbone and shoulder but also of the hip and pelvis. The greater the force of the impact more significant the deformation of the affected vehicle, the greater the probability that chest injuries may be encountered, with rib fractures, pulmonary contusions up to aortic shear injuries. Other types of injuries may involve the abdomen (liver and spleen), and the neck and head due to lateral rotational flexions.

Rear Impact A collision occurs between vehicles following the same trajectory at different speeds, identifying a "bullet vehicle" and a "target vehicle." In this dynamic, cervical spine trauma is common and the more serious due to the greater difference in speed between the two cars.

Rotational Impact This occurs when the corner of the vehicle hits an immovable object, resulting in a combined dynamic between the frontal impact and lateral impact injuries. The greatest damage to the occupants of a vehicle that undergoes a rotational impact is borne by the occupant closest to the point of impact with the obstacle.

Rollover In the event of high forces, there may be shearing-type injuries, especially for the occupants of the vehicle who are not restrained to the vehicle by the safety systems. In the event of being unrestrained, ejections from the passenger compartment can occur with consequent serious injuries.

In motorcycle trauma assessment, different and specific dynamics are considered, such as head-on impact, angular impact, and ejection. Commonly to these types of impacts, the different center of gravity of the motorcycle, which is always lower than the occupant, is considered as a feature that distinguishes it from car trauma. Injuries resulting from motorcycle crashes include a wide range such as head, abdominal, thoracic, and vertebral trauma [15]. Injuries to the spine appear to be difficult to mitigate by means of the use of back protectors [16]; therefore, it is advisable, even more so in the case of motorcycle injuries, to invest in preventive road engineering changes in order to reduce resulting mortality and disability [17, 18].

In pedestrian traumas, the dimensions of the vehicle and the victim, together with the intrinsic characteristics of the patient, that is, age and co-morbid states, will determine the injuries and their severity. Often, the first contact between the pedestrian and the vehicle occurs at the knees and the hips, subsequently the pedestrian collides with the hood and the windscreen of the vehicle, and finally the pedestrian falls to the ground, often first hitting the head [14]. Based on the dynamics, traumas are commonly identified in the lower limbs, the spine, and the head. However, the commercialization of SUVs has changed the trauma dynamic and subsequent injuries. Often, the pedestrian is hit at the level of the abdomen and the pelvic area and subsequently falls to the ground.

The Primary Patient Assessment and Performing Lifesaving Maneuvers

In the first approach, in the first seconds, healthcare responders must take a quick look at the trauma patient to have a "first general (field) impression," following the acronym LISA, meaning:

L: Life—Are there any obvious, immediate life threats?
I: I—"I see…" (general impression)
S: Spinal stabilization—consider the need for spinal stabilization
A: AVPU (a quick measure of level of consciousness—Alert, Verbal, Pain, Unresponsive)

The general impression is the starting point in the evaluation of a trauma patient: on the first approach to the patient, it is important to immediately understand whether you are managing a major or a minor case, and so whether the patient needs advanced and quick management and treatment or not.

If the scene size-up and the general impression give you clues as to the mechanism of injury and what is wrong with the patient, then the primary assessment proceeds with the ABCDE (Airway, Breathing, Circulation, Disability, Exposure) standardized trauma approach. All of the steps included in the ABCDE method are performed quickly and efficiently with the goal of minimizing time spent on the scene [14].

A—Airway: The aim is to check, identify, and treat airway obstruction. Always treat airway obstruction as soon as possible: it is an emergency. Untreated airway obstruction leads to hypoxia, and if not treated will cause death.

B—Breathing: Assess the patient's breathing and signs of respiratory distress; both cause hypoxia and so it is important to administer oxygen. In this first assessment, quickly check if the patient has signs of pneumothorax. In this case, the treatment must be immediate and involves performing a needle decompression.

C—Circulation: The most important task in this part is to identify and treat signs of major bleeding or shock. If someone is bleeding, the priority is to stop the blood coming out. Keep in mind: "Stop the bleeding and treat for shock."

D—Disability: The aim is a quick evaluation of the neurological state. If the level of consciousness is reduced, identify and fix the cause. Consider the common causes of a decreased level of consciousness: hypoxemia, hypercapnia, hypotension, hypoglycemia, drugs, and head injury.

E—Exposure: The "E" is particularly important in a trauma case. Examine the patient thoroughly. In a trauma case, full exposure of the body is crucial. However, respect the patient's dignity and minimize heat loss, to avoid hypothermia.

The primary assessment identifies life-threatening conditions, such as pneumothorax or extensive bleeding, which must be detected and treated as a priority.

Later, in order to further reduce the time spent and facilitate rapid evacuation to the most suitable Trauma Center (TC), the secondary survey in many cases is performed during the transport itself.

The Secondary Patient Assessment Before Transportation to the Hospital

One of the aims of the second assessment is to get more information about the patient. The first step is to perform a full "head-to-toe" physical examination. Check every system carefully and then get information about the event and the situation from the patient, if possible. It is crucial to understand the signs and symptoms and the mechanism of the injury, to know whether the patient has any allergies, thus avoiding further side effects and complications during the therapy, whether the patient has some comorbidity, and if any routine medications have been prescribed before the incident.

It is also important, in the second assessment, to evaluate pain. Moreover, the continuous evaluation of pain during monitoring is important in order to understand whether the treatment and/or the pain management is satisfactory. Giving comfort to the patient is fundamental in the practice of every healthcare professional.

At the end of the secondary patient assessment, one must correctly report all the findings, assessment, and therapy concerning the patient in the clinical file. During the first and the second assessment, the healthcare professional must recognize life-threatening situations and treat them accordingly, stabilize the patient, and if possible diagnose potential injuries.

Once the primary and a secondary assessment have been carried out, the patient should be monitored: this means reassessing the patient's condition and vital signs regularly, thus identifying the impact of the treatment and being able to detect any potential deterioration in the patient's condition. The measurement of vital signs and monitoring is mandatory also during transportation. This enables the early detection of the onset and progression of acute situations. Failure to make these measurements could result in both not recognizing patient deterioration and not being able to act correctly to treat it.

New Technology and Treatment Involved in Prehospital Trauma Management

There are several technologies that have been developed in the field of medicine in the last century and in particular in recent years. However, not all of them are always easily applied even in EMS. The equipment available to the trauma teams employed in the out-of-hospital management of trauma is often small and made up of simple and easily transportable equipment. It is this last aspect that is relevant in the choice of aids and technologies, especially where it is necessary to operate in rural scenarios. However, thanks to the introduction of increasingly light, resistant, and small-sized materials, it is increasingly possible to bring technologically advanced tools alongside the traumatized patient at the place of the event, and these can help members of the trauma team improve the outcome of the rescue. However, these technologies must always be combined with an adequate training program capable of developing the appropriate skills in the staff who use the devices. A new technology that is starting to have an important role also in the prehospital setting is the use of ultrasound (US).

Prehospital Ultrasound

Ultrasound is one of the aspects of technological innovation most introduced in EMS. Nowadays, ultrasound scanners are small, comparable to those of a smartphone, thanks to the separation between the probes and the display where the ultrasound images are projected wirelessly. In addition, the ultrasound probes can also communicate with commonly used devices such as smartphones or tablets. This gives the opportunity to send the images to the Dispatch Center or to the TC to receive a second medical opinion or to prepare the in-hospital trauma team that will admit the patient.

The type of modality with which the US is used in the emergency management of trauma patients in the prehospital setting is the "Focused Assessment with Sonography for Trauma" (FAST) and is part of the resuscitation of trauma patients recommended by the international panel consensus. The purpose of FAST is to identify free fluid which in acute trauma patients usually means blood. [19].

Many EMS systems have implemented this equipment on board emergency vehicles, ambulances, and HEMS. Appropriate use of ultrasound can increase patient survival. Several studies showed that prehospital US is feasible, and that the procedure is highly reliable in detection of hemoperitoneum or hemopericardium compared with the low accuracy of physical examination and hemodynamic measurements. An early diagnosis will provide the prehospital physician with the knowledge to prioritize the relevant initial treatment and to choose the closest appropriate hospital and transportation form [20]. Prehospital emergency ultrasound can be introduced into an EMS as a diagnostic modality that can benefit patients, especially in rural areas with longer transport routes and journey times [20, 21]. Overall, the prehospital US appears to have a high diagnostic accuracy. In particular, US is also characterized in EMS by high sensitivity and high specificity on different endpoints [22]:

- Pneumothorax
- Free abdominal fluid
- Hemoperitoneum (both on site and during transport)

An aspect that must always be considered a priority in the use of technology must be the training of EMS providers. Those using the US must be specifically trained and must participate in continuous education activities [19].

In addition to a bleeding diagnosis, the US also potentially finds other fields of use in the prehospital emergency. Although these practical applications are rarely mentioned in the literature, it is also possible to apply the US in the retrieval of an IV access. Another potential application of US concerns the diagnosis of pneumothorax, for which US has proved to be an effective tool even in the case of traumatized patients [23]. Still further applications of the US are also possible in the prehospital field among which the confirmation of endotracheal tube placement, the diagnosis of intracranial bleeding, the diagnosis of fractures in austere environment [22], everything as long as it is always closely related to the patient's condition, to priority clinical needs, avoiding time wasting, and the organization of the EMS, also in terms of distances to the TC.

Trauma Management: Tranexamic Acid (TXA) Administration

It is well known that a considerable number of preventable deaths caused by trauma are due to the onset of states of shock [24]. For many years in the past, the focus of the advanced intervention of health care has been placed on volume replacement, but in recent years it has been noted that the priority should be to control bleeding. This practice is also accompanied by the administration of tranexamic acid (TXA), a clot-stabilizing medication, which has also been introduced in the context of prehospital trauma management. TXA is able to interfere with the remodeling process of the clot being formed which is simultaneous with the coagulation cascade, necessary for stopping the bleeding, stabilizing the new clot.

The first significant study regarding the use of TXA in prehospital trauma management was the CRASH-2 study [25] which demonstrated that this drug is able to significantly reduce bleeding and therefore reduce mortality. In the CRASH-2 study, a loading dose of 1 g over 10 min and then infusion of 1 g over 8 hours was administered; currently, the EMS are introducing this treatment worldwide as an integral part of the management of polytrauma.

Conclusion

The management and treatment of a trauma patient is always a challenge. And it starts at the scene, in the prehospital setting. The out-of-hospital phase determines a significant part of the final outcome for the patient and the overall success of the trauma clinical pathway. And it is fundamental in guaranteeing the best prognosis for the patient. Therefore, prehospital management and treatment is a key aspect in the management of trauma.

To achieve the best results, the EMS team must follow a systematic approach to evaluating the scene and the patient. A systematic method is very useful in the evaluation of a patient in every situation, a method that helps the healthcare professional to recognize situations and priorities in order of importance.

***

Key Points

- The management and treatment of a trauma patient begins at the scene, in the out-of-hospital phase, and determines a significant part of the final outcome for the patient and the overall success of the trauma clinical pathway.
- When the trauma team enters the scene, it must size up the scene to guarantee the safety of the team itself and to understand the scene and the situation of the event.
- When approaching the patient, it is crucial that all healthcare professionals have a systematic method for a rapid assessment, thus minimizing the chance of failing to spot injuries and avoiding mistakes and wasting time.
- The primary and secondary assessment must establish what and where the problem is, what the impact of the problem is, how to quickly manage the situation, as well as gathering the information needed.
- Healthcare providers are required to evaluate trauma patients quickly, address major life threats, and make a full inventory of injuries.

References

1. Trunkey DD. Trauma. Sci Am. 1983;249(2):28–35.
2. World Health Organization. Road safety is no accident. https://www.who.int/world-health-day/previous/2004/en/. Published February 9, 2004. Accessed 23 Aug 2020.
3. Schermer CR. Alcohol and injury prevention. J Trauma. 2006;60:447–51.
4. Regel G, Stalp M, Lehmann U, Seekamp A. Prehospital care, importance of early intervention on outcome. Acta Anaestesiol Scand Suppl. 1997;110:71–6.
5. Cuschieri J, Johnson JL, Sperry J, et al. Benchmarking outcomes in the critically injured trauma patient and the effect of implementing standard operating procedures. Ann Surg. 2012;255(5):993–9.
6. History of the Shock Trauma Center: Tribute to R Adams Cowley, MD. Available at web address: https://www.umms.org/ummc/health-services/shock-trauma/about/history (last view: 2020/12/26).
7. Forrester JD, August A, Cai LZ, Kushner AL, Wren SM. The golden hour after injury among civilians caught in conflict zones. Disaster Med Public Health Prep. 2019 Dec;13(5-6):1074–82.

8. Cornwell EE 3rd, Belzberg H, Hennigan K, Maxson C, Montoya G, Rosenbluth A, Velmahos GC, Berne TC, Demetriades D. Emergency medical services (EMS) vs non-EMS transport of critically injured patients: a prospective evaluation. Arch Surg. 2000 Mar;135(3):315–9.
9. American College of Surgeons Committee on Trauma. Resources for optimal care of the injured patient. Chicago: American College of Surgeons Committee on Trauma; 2006.
10. Williams J, Ndum O, Goldstein S. EMS, tactical, personal, patient, and team safety. 2020 Sep 20. In: StatPearls [Internet]. Treasure Island: StatPearls Publishing; 2020.
11. Maguire B, Smith S. Injuries and fatalities among emergency medical technicians and paramedics in the United States. Prehosp Disaster Med. 2013;28(4):376–82.
12. Murray B, Kue R. The use of emergency lights and sirens by ambulances and their effect on patient outcomes and public safety: a comprehensive review of the literature. Prehosp Disaster Med. 2017 Apr;32(2):209–216. De Anda HH, Moy HP. EMS Ground Transport Safety. 2020 Jul 2. In: StatPearls [Internet]. Treasure Island (FL): StatPearls Publishing; 2020 Jan–.
13. Biggers WA Jr, Zachariah BS, Pepe PE. Emergency medical vehicle collisions in an urban system. Prehosp Disaster Med. 1996 Jul-Sep;11(3):195–201. https://doi.org/10.1017/s1049023x00042941.
14. Pollak et al. PHTLS PreHospital trauma life support, 9th ed.
15. Markogiannakis H, Sanidas E, Messaris E, Koutentakis D, Alpantaki K, Kafetzakis A, Tsiftsis D. Motor vehicle trauma: analysis of injury profiles by road-user category. Emerg Med J. 2006 Jan;23(1):27–31.
16. Ekmejian R, Sarrami P, Naylor JM, Harris IA. A systematic review on the effectiveness of back protectors for motorcyclists. Scand J Trauma Resusc Emerg Med. 2016 Oct 4;24(1):115.
17. Gonzales MM, Dickinson LM, Di Guiseppi C, Lowenstein SR. Student drivers: a study of fatal motor vehicle crashes involving 16-year-old drivers. Ann Emerg Med. 2005 Feb;45(2):140–6.
18. Demetriades D, Murray J, Martin M, Velmahos G, Salim A, Alo K, Rhee P. Pedestrians injured by automobiles: relationship of age to injury type and severity. J Am Coll Surg. 2004 Sep;199(3):382–7.
19. Savatmongkorngul S, Wongwaisayawan S, Kaewlai R. Focused assessment with sonography for trauma: current perspectives. Open Access Emerg Med. 2017 Jul 26;9:57-62. doi: https://doi.org/10.2147/OAEM.S120145. PMID: 28794661; PMCID: PMC5536884.
20. Jørgensen H, Jensen CH, Dirks J. Does prehospital ultrasound improve treatment of the trauma patient? A systematic review. Eur J Emerg Med. 2010 Oct;17(5):249–53.
21. Weilbach C, Kobiella A, Rahe-Meyer N, Johanning K. Einführung der präklinischen Notfallsonographie in einem ländlichen Notarztdienst-Bereich [Introduction of prehospital emergency ultrasound into an emergency medical service area]. Anaesthesist. 2017 Jan;66(1):21–27. https://doi.org/10.1007/s00101-016-0248-2. Epub 2016 Dec 9.
22. van der Weide L, Popal Z, Terra M, Schwarte LA, Ket JCF, Kooij FO, Exadaktylos AK, Zuidema WP, Giannakopoulos GF. Prehospital ultrasound in the management of trauma patients: systematic review of the literature. Injury. 2019 Dec;50(12):2167–2175. https://doi.org/10.1016/j.injury.2019.09.034. Epub 2019 Sep 28.
23. Staub LJ, Biscaro RRM, Kaszubowski E, Maurici R. Chest ultrasonography for the emergency diagnosis of traumatic pneumothorax and haemothorax: a systematic review and meta-analysis. Injury. 2018 Mar;49(3):457–466. doi: https://doi.org/10.1016/j.injury.2018.01.033. Epub 2018 Feb 8.
24. Napolitano LM, Kurek S, Luchette FA, Anderson GL, Bard MR, Bromberg W, Chiu WC, Cipolle MD, Clancy KD, Diebel L, Hoff WS, Hughes KM, Munshi I, Nayduch D, Sandhu R, Yelon JA, Corwin HL, Barie PS, Tisherman SA, Hebert PC, Practice Management Workgroup EAST, American College of Critical Care Medicine (ACCM). Taskforce of the Society of Critical Care Medicine (SCCM). Clinical practice guideline: red blood cell transfusion in adult trauma and critical care. J Trauma. 2009 Dec;67(6):1439–42.
25. Roberts I, Shakur H, Coats T, Hunt B, Balogun E, Barnetson L, Cook L, Kawahara T, Perel P, Prieto-Merino D, Ramos M, Cairns J, Guerriero C. The CRASH-2 trial: a randomised controlled trial and economic evaluation of the effects of tranexamic acid on death, vascular occlusive events and transfusion requirement in bleeding trauma patients. Health Technol Assess. 2013 Mar;17(10):1–79.

Transport Medicine

20

Michelangelo Bortolin and Jacopo M. Olagnero

Introduction

The right patient in the right place at the right time—this is a fundamental principle to guarantee the swiftest and best definitive treatment, as well as the best outcome for the patient. This will ensure that a healthcare system is able to manage patients with a high level of efficiency and efficacy. Often, in the case of a trauma, much attention is paid to the aspects of the treatments that can be practiced in the field, in the emergency room, or in the operating theater; however, this principle indirectly demonstrates and highlights the key role of the patient's transportation from the field or from another healthcare facility to the right hospital and in a specific time. And so, transportation becomes a key aspect in the management of trauma and indispensable in maintaining the continuity of care.

The transportation and the management of a trauma patient in the correct diagnostic and clinical pathway involve different aspects:

- The establishment and the importance of a Trauma Clinical Network (TCN) between the Emergency Medical Services (EMS), trauma hospitals of different levels, and also rehabilitation trauma centers
- Classification of the transport: definition and difference between direct and inter-hospital transportation, and transportation in emergency or non-emergency situations
- Transportation of critically ill patients
- Means of transportation
- The trauma team in transportation

M. Bortolin (✉)
Disaster Medicine Fellowship at BIDMC (a teaching hospital of Harvard Medical School), Boston, MA, USA

CRIMEDIM - Center for Research and Training in Disaster Medicine, Humanitarian Aid, and Global Health, UPO - University of Eastern Piedmont, Novara, Italy

J. M. Olagnero
Critical Care Nurse at Humanitas Gradenigo Hospital, Turin, Italy

Temporary Research Fellow in Nursing Science, Università di Torino, Turin, Italy

The Trauma Clinical Network (TCN)

A Clinical Network is defined as an organizational model that ensures patient care by interconnecting via formalized and coordinated methods, healthcare professionals, healthcare facilities, and services providing health and social health interventions of different types and levels. This interconnection will be in compliance with continuity of care and clinical and organizational appropriateness. The Clinical Network identifies the nodes and the related connections of the network, defining the rules of operations, the monitoring system, the quality and safety requirements of the processes and care pathways, and the roles and responsibilities of the healthcare professionals. [1]

In the establishment of a Trauma Clinical Network (TCN), it is crucial that overall quality is improved and that there is a successful outcome in the supply of trauma patient care [2, 3]. The network will involve EMS, hospitals of different levels, from rural or local hospitals to highly specialized hospitals (Trauma Centers, TC), and then from the hospital discharge to the rehabilitation trauma center. Usually, the TCN is established regionally.

The mission, stakeholders, rules, roles, responsibilities, and Key Performance Indicator (KPI) of the TCN must be revised systematically and improved according to evidence-based guidelines.

Classification of the Transport

The transport can be classified as direct or inter-hospital transport and emergency or non-emergency transport.

L. Marshall Gillman, S. Widder (eds.), *Trauma Team Dynamics*, https://doi.org/10.1007/978-3-031-86312-7_20

Direct Transport

Direct transport, or primary transport, is patient transportation managed by the EMS, from the field to the hospital, in agreement with the TCN. Direct transport is, by definition, always carried out in an emergency situation. Direct transport involves a field triage and a first assessment and stabilization of the patient on the scene in order to proceed with the patient's evacuation to the most suitable hospital. Assuming an accurate field triage and first assessment by the EMS team on the scene, which recognizes and initiates the initial treatment of a trauma, the transportation of a major trauma patient directly to a TC can consensually be considered optimal, bypassing the nearest rural or local hospital. But this is not always possible. For example, in rural areas, the TC is often some distance away and an Advanced Life Support (ALS) team is not always available. Therefore, to be compliant with the golden hour, a Basic Life Support (BLS) team is dispatched to the scene and the patient is then transported by the BLS team to the nearest hospital, even if rural. This is to allow the initial ATLS stabilization of the patient and then, at a later stage, proceed with the transfer to a specialized center with an ALS team [4]. This is an example of a so-called inter-hospital transport: it is the movement of patients from one healthcare facility to another.

Inter-hospital Transport

Any transfer of a patient from a hospital with a low or insufficient level of care to the nearest facility providing the highest level of specialized care and/or between two hospitals due to the unavailability of diagnosis and treatment facilities is called inter-hospital transport, also known as inter-facility or secondary transfer.

Generally, the following indications are recognized for the activation of inter-hospital transport:

- Specialized expertise unavailable
- Resources not available
- Specialized investigations not available
- Unavailability of beds

Inter-hospital patient transfer should aim at maintaining optimal health, and the transport between hospitals must take place when the benefits for the patient outweigh the risks of the transfer. It should be considered that the transfer of a sick patient may induce various physiological alterations and that this is a moment of potential serious criticality which may adversely affect the prognosis of the patient [5, 6].

Emergency or Non-emergency Transportation

Direct transport is always carried out in an emergency situation, but secondary transportation can be both in an emergency or also in a non-emergency situation.

Secondary transfer becomes an emergency when the already hospitalized patient has health and trauma-related problems that are time-dependent, and in order to provide a definitive treatment, the patient requires a higher level of specialized care in a different hospital, such as TC, that for a number of reasons could not be provided at the first stage. For example, it is very different managing a major trauma in the Australian desert where distances are enormous, or on a small island, such as Capri (Italy), or in the Alps during a winter storm when a helicopter is not fit-to-fly and only BLS teams on the ambulance are available, compared to the same event in other places such as cities like New York, Tokyo, or Paris. So, in some situations, the patient is first transported to a local hospital for ATLS stabilization and later, in a second phase, to the TC. Management always aims to provide the best care for the patient, but the ways of achieving this can differ substantially, depending on a number of different circumstances.

In all the other cases, when the patient's situation is not time-dependent but will at some point require a transfer to other healthcare facilities, this is defined as non-emergency transportation.

Transportation and Effects of Transportation on a Critically Ill Patient

Transportation is a very important procedure for every patient and particularly so for critical patients. Critically ill patients have an increased risk of morbidity and mortality during inter- and/or intra-hospital transportation. Beforehand, the physician must evaluate the benefits and risks involved in transportation. But when transportation is deemed to be necessary, the healthcare professional must take every precaution against possible complications. Here, new technologies, new devices, and new processes have an important role in being able to minimize the risks inherent in transportation.

Pre-transport: Preparation and Planning

The preparation and planning of inter-hospital transport are essential and crucial for ensuring the best and safest care for the traumatized patient, by avoiding adverse events. The first step is the evaluation of the patient's clinical situation, to understand which hospital is able to take definitive care of the patient, which risks exist in inter-hospital transportation, which healthcare professionals can perform the transporta-

Table 20.1 Eherenwerth classification

Class	Clinical features
I	Patient ambulates autonomously Does not require monitoring of vital signs Clinical stability does not depend on oxygen therapy Must not be transferred to an Intensive Care Unit
II	Patient does not ambulate Rarely requires monitoring of vital signs Clinical stability does not depend on oxygen therapy Must not be transferred to an Intensive Care Unit
III	A (Airways) Presents no risk of airway obstruction, Patient who does not need Guedel cannula or orotracheal intubation B (Breathing) May have mild or moderate respiratory distress May have a respiratory rate of <36 acts / min and> 8 acts min It may require continuous administration of O2 to obtain a SpO2 of at least> 92% (in the absence of chronic pathologies such as COPD), but it is not in assisted ventilation C (Circle) May have peripheral vascular access It is hemodynamically stable, does not present arrhythmias, does not require pharmacological support May require continuous electrocardiographic monitoring It doesn't need any invasive monitoring Does not have a temporary pacemaker D (Disability) May present a compromised state of consciousness (GCS>9) May present an anatomically stable or unstable lesion of the spinal cord below T9 E (Exposure) Any uncontrolled bleeding
IV	The patient must be included in class IV if it is characterized by the need for frequent monitoring of vital signs such as class III and if the following criteria are added: Requires tracheal intubation Requires ventilatory support It needs two venous lines or CVC to keep the cardiovascular parameters stable May present with severe respiratory distress Impairment of the state of consciousness may be present, with GCS </= 8 May require continuous administration of artificial or supportive drugs or substitute treatments without which the patient's hemodynamic or respiratory failure occurs It is transferred to the general ICU. In this case, the cases of transfers between two ICUs of stabilized patients that do not require life support treatments or continuous infusion of life-saving drugs are excluded Presents an anatomically unstable spinal cord injury above T9
V	Assigned for a patient for whom there is a high risk of mortality during transport

tion, and the equipment required. To do so, it is important to pay attention to important elements such as:

- The primary traumatological condition
- Any comorbidities
- Transportation risk classification (usually with an appropriate evaluation tool)

In order to plan transport in an accurate way, there are different methods and systems to assess and classify transportation risk. An example is the Eherenwerth Classification (see Table 20.1). The Eherenwerth Classification [7] analyzes the patient condition and potential evolutions of the clinical situation. This classification is not specific for trauma, but it is comprehensive and broad to include any medical and surgical condition.

Table 20.2 Risk score for transport patients (RSTP)

Measurement	Indicators	Score
Hemodynamics	Stable Moderately stable (requires volume <15 ml/min in adults) Unstable (requires volume >15 ml/min or inotropics or blood)	0 1 2
Arrhythmias (existing or probable)	No Yes, not serious (and AMI after 48 h) Serious (and AMI in the first 48 h)	0 1 2
ECG monitoring	No Yes (desirable) Yes (essential)	0 1 2
Intravenous line	No Yes (desirable) Pulmonary artery catheter	0 1 2
Provisional pacemaker	No Yes (not invasive). Always AMI in the first 48 h Yes (endocavitary pacemaker)	0 1 2
Respiration	Respiratory rate between 10 and 14 breaths/min in adults Respiratory rate between 15 and 35 breaths/min in adults Apnea <10 or >36 or irregular breathing	0 1 2
Airway	No Yes (Guedel tube) Yes (intubation or tracheostomy)	0 1 2
Respiratory support	No Yes (oxygen therapy) Yes (mechanical ventilation)	0 1 2
Assessment	GCS=15 GCS 8–14 GCS <8 and/or neurological disorder	0 1 2
Prematurity	Newborn >2000 g Newborn between 1200 and 2000 g Newborn <1200 g	0 1 2
Pharmacological and/or medical device support (current or en route) (see Appendix A)	None Group I* Group II**	0 1 2

Another transportation risk classification is the Risk Score for Transport Patients (RSTP) [8] that suggests which type of ambulance and team is required for transportation in agreement with the patient's clinical condition. To RSTP, the cut-off that best identifies the critically ill patient and seems to be able to better predict which patients may be susceptible to complications during transport is RSTP ≥ 7 (see Table 20.2 with appendices).

Appendix A: Medication for Risk Groups

Group I*		Group II**	
	Inotropics Vasodilators Antiarrhythmics Bicarbonate Analgesics Antiepileptics Steroids Mannitol 20% Thrombolytics Thoracic tube Suction		Inotropics + vasodilators MAST Infant incubator General anesthetics Uterine relaxants

Appendix B: Management of At-Risk Patients

Points	Group	Vehicle	Staff
3–6	0	Conventional ambulance	Technicians (EMT)
3–6	I	Conventional ambulance	Nurse
Over 6	II	ICU ambulance	Physician and nurse

The TCN is very useful in quickly identifying the receiving hospital or facility appropriate for the patient as well as the transportation risk classification. The referring physician will identify and contact the admitting physician at the receiving hospital to confirm their acceptance of the patient in transfer and to confirm, before the transfer takes place, that the appropriate higher-level resources are available [9]. If not already established by the TCN, both physicians will determine the accompanying personnel and the mode of transportation appropriate for the case.

During the preparation and planning phase, the team must check the equipment and ensure adequate supplies of the required drugs. Often, many instruments and materials are required during the transport of a critically ill patient to the accepting hospital. In order to make sure that everything necessary is available and ready to use, protocols and checklists are useful tools to mitigate any safety events. It is essential to prepare ALS drugs for the transport, according to the most up-to-date international guidelines, drugs to ensure correct analgesia and sedation and infusions for volume resuscitation. To ensure the safety of the patient and the operators' effectiveness and to avoid the necessity for dilutions during transport, drugs in a ready-to-use formulation may be preferred. These are thermostable and therefore less subject to environmental conditions, their effects can easily be controlled by parenteral route, and they are in single doses and concentrations to avoid confusion for the operators who administer them.

It is also a good idea to avoid bringing material that is not useful for the specific transport, as this could incur unnecessary confusion. Many unforeseen events, accidents, and adverse events that occur during both primary and secondary medical transport are due precisely to the organization of the aids and equipment for transport. Therefore, it is essential that a checklist of all drugs and electromedical devices is made before transport or at the beginning of the service shift, both to verify the appropriate quantities and correct functionality. Several studies report that the majority of adverse events can be prevented simply by following existing checklists; for example, deterioration in a patient's clinical conditions, equipment failures, incomplete supplies, shortage of oxygen or batteries, and drug administration errors or delay [6, 10].

At the end of this phase, the team leader takes charge of the patient. The team leader must have thorough knowledge of the trauma case, the patient's clinical condition, and the documentation.

In the case of secondary transport, the "scoop and run" approach is unacceptable: the team has the time to plan in advance and to be prepared. The team must, however, avoid unnecessary delays.

The patient's medical record documentation and the investigation reports of procedures that the patient has undergone in the healthcare facility are crucial. The trauma team leader of the transport must guarantee that the documentation follows the patient until arrival at the receiving hospital, where the medical records of the transfer process must also be handed over. This is important for the overall diagnostic and clinical pathway of the patient, for audit and medical-legal purposes.

Monitoring During Transport

Accurate monitoring throughout the entire duration of the transport is mandatory for the transfer of all critically ill patients. The minimum standard of monitoring recommended for critical patient transfer includes respiratory rate, heart rate, blood pressure, oxygen saturation, temperature, continuous evaluation of the Glasgow Coma Scale (GCS), and electrocardiogram monitoring. Additional monitoring may be required, such as end-tidal carbon dioxide (in ventilated patients), invasive (intra-arterial) blood pressure, central venous, or intracranial pressure.

The patient must be monitored and re-evaluated for the complete time of the transport while en route. Monitoring is essential to verify that the patient is stable and is not deteriorating or, should this be the case, changes in clinical stability must be promptly corrected. Furthermore, continuous monitoring is also important to reveal conditions that may have been overlooked during the first assessment and that may be manifested during transport.

The End of Transportation

Upon arrival at the receiving hospital, the healthcare team must provide patient monitoring, assistance, and support until the receiving physician and his team are ready to take care of the patient. This moment will be the handover. The transportation team that had performed the transportation must deliver all of the medical documentation: all the medical records, the investigation reports, and the transportation medical report. These are important for maintaining the continuity of the patient's medical care and for medico-legal purposes.

Effects of Transportation on a Critically Ill Patient

Within an accurate transport plan, the influences of the transport itself on the traumatized patient cannot be neglected: these are the changes that a critically ill patient could experience during transportation. Indeed, the different features of the kinematics of the means of transport can cause changes to the patient's stability, to his vital parameters and even cause damage.

Transportation could involve all the systems and all the organs of the body. Indeed, for example, the heart rate could be influenced, and also arrhythmias, or changes in intracranial pressure, blood pressure, or oxygen saturation.

The team must take into account all these characteristics in order to limit them and mitigate their consequences where possible. Knowledge of this transport pathophysiology is essential in helping the operator both anticipate and recognize the presence of new pathological conditions, or their worsening, as soon as possible and to hasten their treatment.

The characteristics of transport that can cause changes to the clinical stability of the patient transported by any means are essentially five:

1. Changes in patient's position
2. The presence of inertial forces
3. The mechanical vibrations of the vehicle
4. The noises, lights, and sirens
5. The microclimate

All these elements are found in and are common to all means of transport, both in motor vehicles such as ambulances, and on aircraft such as helicopters and airplanes or other rescue vehicles, such as boats. Inevitably, the proportion of these elements will vary according to the means of transport in question. In general, since it is known that transport can cause a variation in a patient's stability, it is advisable for the traumatized patient to be satisfactorily stabilized before the start of transport.

1. Changes in the patient's position: During transportation by road, such as by ambulance, the patient usually assumes a supine position with the head facing, in most cases, in the opposite direction of travel. This can lead to greater sensitivity to road surface irregularities and sudden movements as well as a greater risk of motion sickness.

   Two other undesirable events that can occur in supine transport are alterations in the microcirculation with a reduction in tissue perfusion due to the disappearance of flow fluctuations in the capillary circulation and the alteration of the relationship between ventilation and perfusion in the most declining lung portions.

   Especially in the case of steep inclines and descents, the possibility of dislocation of the abdominal viscera must be considered and the change in position of the vehicle positions the patient in the Trendelenburg and anti-Trendelenburg position. An ambulance that travels a prolonged downhill stretch with a medium-high slope involves the patient in an imposed Trendelenburg position, in which consequently the chest is located lower than the abdomen; this consequently leads to an increase in preload, ICP and PVC, as well as a reduction in the expansion of the lung bases.

   On the other hand, the road travel of a prolonged uphill stretch with a medium-high slope means that the patient is in an imposed anti-Trendelenburg position in which the head is higher than the chest, and this can involve the displacement and accumulation of blood in the more caudal areas, relative hypovolemia, reduction of cardiac output, and therefore reduced peripheral and cerebral perfusion.
2. The presence of inertial forces occurs when the body's state of motion varies with the decrease or increase in speed or change in direction of the means of transport. These forces are exerted when the means of transport makes sudden movements when changing gear, or in acceleration and deceleration, braking, and steering. These influencing elements on transport concern not purely transport in land vehicles such as ambulances, but also in aircraft or boats or any other means of transportation. Inertial forces can cause the abdominal masses to compress between themselves and against the bones and muscles. The same forces are capable of producing displacements of the blood mass, given its liquid nature, which characterizes an easy translocation. For example, in a helicopter take-off, the force is applied upward and the blood mass, accordingly, moves downward. In the case of an ambulance, road jolts determine an inertial force upward, while the blood mass remains in the sloping spaces; in both cases, the result is a reduction in cardiac preload. Similarly, when a vehicle brakes, the blood mass is projected forward, in the braking direction, with the effects depending on the duration and application of the force; in particular, a sudden stop is capable of causing a cerebral blood overflow, or, in contrast, a sudden acceleration can induce a blood overflow in the peripheral areas of the body. Likewise, the sudden changes in direction of an aircraft vehicle such as a helicopter can induce a centrifugal movement of the blood mass that tends to maintain the initial direction of motion.

   Inertial forces also have an effect on patients in the case of irregularities of the road (jolts on a bumpy road) or during the phases of loading and unloading the patient. Other adverse effects on the body in these situations are, for example, an increase in pain (in particular for patients with fractures: it is particularly painful for patients with a fracture of the pelvis), or there is the risk of aggravating spine injuries.
3. Vibrations that can affect the transport of a victim of trauma patient mostly originate from a disconnected road network in the case of ambulances, while in the case of helicopters, from the rotor, turbines, and turbulence typical of low altitude. The range of vibrations within which biological damage typically occurs is between 4 and 12 Hz: vibrational frequencies are capable of causing resonance to internal organs. The vibrations of any means of transport are transmitted to the patient mostly from the support surface; therefore, in order to limit the potential damage of these phenomena, it is necessary to stabilize at best, also using a vacuum mattress where available. The main adverse effects due to vibration frequencies on the patient can be the appearance of general disturbances to the autonomic nervous system with headache, reflex vasoconstriction induced by alterations of the hypothalamic function, worsening of aneurysm or hemorrhagic foci in previously stabilized bleeding, mobilization of the stumps of displaced fractures, and abdominal pain by torsion of the abdominal viscera. More in detail, some organs and systems resonate at certain frequencies generated by vibrations: the respiratory system resonates

between 1 and 4 Hz potentially causing dyspnea and chest tightness, the heart resonates between 4 and 8 Hz with the appearance of precordial pains, cardiac arrhythmias, pressure changes, and the digestive tract, depending on the filling, resonates between 4 and 8 Hz stimulating abdominal pain and vomiting. Another phenomenon that vibrations may generate is alterations in the signals detected by the monitors that can record artifacts, and, in general, can influence all electro-medical devices and equipment.

4. Noise is another influencing element related to transport, common to almost all rescue vehicles of any type, both by land, and even more so with aircraft. Among the main negative effects, noise favors the development of motion sickness on the transported patient but, potentially, also on the other team members, reducing their performance; among the team members, noise can also make communication difficult, as well as the performance of some medical maneuvers such as auscultation and hearing the audible alarms of electromedical devices. Finally, sirens' lights may cause seizures in patients with neurological diseases: sirens and alarm lights are particularly irritating not only for the team but also for the patient. Furthermore, an alarm light can cause significant stress and could be a trigger for seizures. Flickering or flashing lights can be responsible for the onset of a tonic-clonic, absence, or myoclonic seizure.
5. The microclimate is a final aspect to consider in the context of the elements that influence transport. First of all, ambient temperature finds its optimal value around 22°C, while brightness around 1000 lm. The first fundamental problem with regard to temperature is to find a temperature which permits a better enzymatic activation, which is not inhibited by too low temperatures, that inhibit blood coagulation. It is crucial to consider how the microclimate can have an impact on the transportation of the patient: several studies describe and explain how hypothermia is the first indirect cause of complications during the transport of a patient. Hypothermia could promote bleeding, it has effects on the pH, increasing the excretion of acid into the blood, and it has an influence on the respiratory and coagulative pattern. Therefore, in order to avoid detrimental effects, it is necessary to appropriately increase or decrease the temperature inside the vehicle, cover the patient with an isothermal blanket, and evaluate the advisability of administering heated infusions. Moreover, even if the administration of oxygen is necessary, especially in the case of prolonged journeys, it ideally should be humidified and warmed.

Another important factor regarding the microclimate, typical of air transportation, is altitude: the effect of an increase in altitude on the human body is mainly related to a decrease in inspired oxygen levels. Indeed, according to Dalton's Law or the Law of Partial Pressures, stating that the total pressure exerted by a mixture of gases is equal to the sum of the partial pressures of the gases in the mixture, it follows that as the altitude increases, the partial pressure of the gases, including oxygen, is reduced.

$$\mathbf{P}_{\text{total}} = \mathbf{P}_{\mathrm{A}} + \mathbf{P}_{\mathrm{B}} + \mathbf{P}_{\mathrm{N}}$$

Law of Partial Pressures

The aircraft affected by this physical law are non-pressurized ones, including helicopters, which are widely used in the EMS systems. However, this effect does not apply to fixed-wing aircraft having a pressurized cabin in which the gas mixture is controlled, although, during the flight, aircraft pressurized maintains a pressure level equivalent to that of 5000 to 8000 ft above sea level.

Another physical law that is related to air transport management is Boyle's law which affirms that as barometric pressure increases decreases, gas volume increases.

$$\mathbf{P}_1\mathbf{V}_1 = \mathbf{P}_2\mathbf{V}_2$$

Boyle's Law

The clinical implications of these altitude-related changes in pressures are: the expansion of intracranial air can lead to brain herniation, pneumothorax, dehiscence of surgical wounds, expansion of intestinal and gastric air causing a decreased capacity of the lungs, and hypoxia until respiratory failure. Trauma team can predict these changes: a better understanding of altitude-related volume changes will help decision-making before transportation. Therefore, it is highlighted that it is appropriate to plan a flight at lower altitudes if one of these causes can evolve, be suspected, or confirmed [11]. The trauma team has to consider clinical characteristics and inflight physiological stressors, prescribing specific interventions such as a cabin altitude restriction (CAR) to ensure patient safety and clinical stability [12].

Another implication of flight altitude for non-pressurized aircraft to be observed concerns medical devices, especially mechanical ventilators. In fact, not all pulmonary ventilators are able to keep the tidal volume output constant as the altitude and barometric pressure vary. The trauma team has to be aware of these potential problems related to ventilator performance in order to compensate for physical variation and ready to modify the parameters set in order to maintain the patient's clinical stability [13]. Regarding instead changes in endotracheal tube (ETT) cuff pressure during HEMS transport, there is insufficient evidence to support the hypothesis that the effects of transient increase in ETT intracuff pressure are clinically significant [14]. Therefore, the effects of the microclimate, and in particular of temperature and altitude, are substantial during helicopter transportation, while jet aircraft have pressurized air cabins, also permitting a precise regulation of the temperature, not to mention also less noise and vibration.

All members of the trauma team must have an overall knowledge of all these influencing elements on transport that can actively contribute to a change in the clinical stability of the patient in order to permit rapid recognition and consequently an equally rapid response to preserve the clinical conditions of the patient transported.

Means of Transportation

The two modes of transfer used most for medical transportation are on ground or by air. On ground is by ambulance. By air, the transportation can be performed by rotary-wing aircraft, such as helicopters, or by fixed-wing aircraft, which include propeller-driven or jet engine powered and include commercial flights as well as private jets set up as an Intensive Care Unit (ICU). Helicopters are used for shorter travel distances, local or regional distances. Jet aircraft are used for long distances, including intercontinental flights. This mode of transportation requires more infrastructures (airports) and a stronger logistic support. In some particular places, such as Venice (Italy), transportation is often carried out by boat.

The choice of the means of transport must also be meticulously assessed on the basis of the following main elements:

- The nature of the trauma, the patient's condition, and potential evolution of the clinical situation
- The urgency of transfer
- The distances to be covered and the relative times
- Contingent availability of resources
- Environment and geomorphology
- Traffic conditions
- Weather conditions
- Transportation costs

Transport by means of an ambulance allows it to be activated even in adverse weather conditions, has lower costs and often faster activation times, is more familiar to operators, and allows easier patient monitoring. However, when the travel times for an ambulance are too long or the geomorphological conditions are unfavorable, transfer is preferable by air, which has reduced transport times and does not have the sudden linear and angular accelerations and decelerations of ground vehicles. Air travel, however, has considerable disadvantages, such as being subjected to weather conditions and higher costs. In addition, it is important to consider for air vehicles, in particular for helicopters, elements such as noise, lack of space and visibility, potential various physiological phenomena related to flight, and the difficulty to perform many medical procedures, as additional elements that can affect the transportation of the patient.

The Trauma Team in Transportation

The patient's transfer outcomes depend on the expertise of the healthcare personnel performing the transportation and, in the case of direct transportation, of the EMS team performing the field triage, first assessment, stabilization of the patient on the scene, and evacuation to the hospital. It is generally recommended to have at least two healthcare professionals accompanying the patient being transferred, in addition to the vehicle operators.

An optimal trauma team recognizes and organizes itself both in the in-hospital and out-of-hospital settings, recognizing a trauma team leader. Competence and leadership skills are crucial: the leader's competence must be such as coordinating and managing the team in situations where speed, organization, and rapid response to prevent, prepare for, or fix problems are a priority. In direct transport, the leader of the EMS team can be an emergency physician in a Franco-German EMS model system, or a paramedic in an Anglo-American EMS model system.

Differently, in inter-hospital transportation: the leader of the trauma team can be a physician, usually an anesthesiologist, an emergency physician or surgeon, or even a critical-care nurse, a paramedic, or EMT, in accordance with the TCN and the transportation risk classification.

It has been identified that the quality of the transport and reduced adverse effect of any type, medical or technical, depend on the trained and skilled healthcare professional. The trauma transport team should be trained to anticipate or solve complications and provide care to the needs of the patient.

Communication is fundamental for the team and in all the phases of transportation. There must, therefore, be good communication between the members of the trauma team themselves but also between the team leader and the other healthcare professionals who are involved in the management of the transportation such as, for example, EMS Dispatch Center personnel, the referring hospital and physician, and the accepting hospital and physician.

Conclusion

The transportation of the patient to the right hospital, from the field or from another healthcare facility, is fundamental in guaranteeing the best definitive treatment and prognosis for the patient. Therefore, transportation becomes a key aspect in the management of trauma and is indispensable in maintaining the continuity of care.

Key Points

- "The right patient, in the right place, at the right time."
- Transportation becomes a key aspect in the management of trauma, indispensable in maintaining the continuity of care, to guarantee the best prognosis for the patient, and to assure a high level of efficiency and efficacy of a healthcare system.
- The transportation and the management of a trauma patient in the correct diagnostic and clinical pathway involve different aspects: the establishment of a Trauma Clinical Network (TCN), the effects of transportation on a critically ill patient, the means of transportation, the place and the weather, and the trauma team during the transportation.

The type and clinical condition of the patient, the TCN, the team, the variety of characteristics typical of the operational territory, from a geographical and environmental point of view, the weather, and the type of vehicle used (ambulance, helicopter, boat, plane) are crucial elements to consider for a patient's transportation.

***

References

1. AGENAS. Linee Guida per la Revisione delle Reti Cliniche D.M. n.70/2015 – Le Reti tempo dipendenti. 2016, pg.5
2. Regional Office for Europe of the World Health Organization (WHO). Emergency medical services systems in the European Union – Report of an assessment project co-ordinated by the World Health Organization – Data Book, 2008
3. MacKenzie EJ, Rivara FP, Jurkovich GJ, Nathens AB, Frey KP, Egleston BL, et al. A national evaluation of the effect of trauma-center care on mortality. N Engl J Med. 2006;354:366–78.
4. Hamada SR, Delhaye N, Degoul S, et al. Direct transport vs secondary transfer to level I trauma centers in a French exclusive trauma system: impact on mortality and determinants of triage on road-traffic victims. PLoS One. 2019;14(11):e0223809. Published 2019 Nov 21. https://doi.org/10.1371/journal.pone.0223809.
5. Kulshrestha A, Singh J. Inter-hospital and intra-hospital patient transfer: recent concepts. Indian J Anaesth. 2016;60(7):451–7. https://doi.org/10.4103/0019-5049.186012.
6. Droogh J. Interhospital transport of the critically ill patient: focus on the journey. Doctor of Philosophy. University of Groningen, [S.l.]; 2014.
7. Ehrenwerth J, Sorbo S, Hackel A. Transport of critically ill adults. Crit Care Med. 1986 Jun;14(6):543–7. https://doi.org/10.1097/00003246-198606000-00005.
8. Markakis C, et al. Evaluation of a risk score for interhospital transport of critically ill patients. Emerg Med J. 2006;23:313–7. https://doi.org/10.1136/emj.2005.026435.
9. Warren J, Fromm RE Jr, Orr RA, Rotello LC, Horst HM, American College of Critical Care Medicine. Guidelines for the inter- and intrahospital transport of critically ill patients. Crit Care Med. 2004;32(1):256–62. https://doi.org/10.1097/01.CCM.0000104917.39204.0A.
10. Sethi D, Subramanian S. When place and time matter: How to conduct safe inter-hospital transfer of patients. Saudi J Anaesth. 2014;8(1):104–13. https://doi.org/10.4103/1658-354X.125964.
11. Knotts D, Arthur AO, Holder P, Herrington T, Thomas SH. Pneumothorax volume expansion in helicopter emergency medical services transport. Air Med J. 2013 May-Jun;32(3):138–43. https://doi.org/10.1016/j.amj.2012.10.014.
12. Butler WP, Steinkraus LW, Burlingame EE, Smith DE, Fouts BL, Serres JL, Burch DS. Clinical impact of cabin altitude restriction following aeromedical evacuation. Mil Med. 2018 Mar 1;183(suppl_1):193–202. https://doi.org/10.1093/milmed/usx171.
13. Rodriquez D Jr, Branson RD, Dorlac W, Dorlac G, Barnes SA, Johannigman JA. Effects of simulated altitude on ventilator performance. J Trauma. 2009 Apr;66(4 Suppl):S172–7. https://doi.org/10.1097/TA.0b013e31819cdbd1.
14. Weisberg SN, McCall JC Jr, Tennyson J. Altitude-related change in endotracheal tube cuff pressures in helicopter EMS. West J Emerg Med. 2017 Jun;18(4):624-629. https://doi.org/10.5811/westjem.2017.3.32078. Epub 2017 May 15. PMID: 28611883; PMCID: PMC5468068.

Trauma Team Structure and Organization

21

Eric Walser, Paul T. Engels, J. Damian Paton-Gay, Homer C. Tien, and Patrick B. Murphy

Introduction

The American College of Surgeons (ACS) and its Committee on Trauma (COT) have developed the Advanced Trauma Life Support (ATLS) program to guide healthcare professionals in the care of the injured patient [1]. The ATLS program provides a safe, reliable method for immediate management of the severely injured patient. Tasks are performed in sequence, in a programmatically defined order of priority. While the ATLS program provides the backbone of trauma resuscitation, it is important to remember it was conceived and has been developed for individuals working in a setting with limited resources, including limited healthcare personnel.

Ideally trauma care should be a team sport [2]. It is well established that care of the severely injured trauma patient is best accomplished by an organized team [3, 4] that may consist of physicians, nurses, and allied health personnel [5]. A team approach can greatly improve the efficiency and efficacy of resuscitation, as tasks can be performed in parallel, as opposed to in sequence.

In 1976, the American College of Surgeons Committee on Trauma published the first resource guide for care of the injured patient that described the concept of trauma care in a team setting [6]. The document has evolved significantly, as has the "Trauma Team." A modern definition of a Trauma Team is a group of doctors, nurses, and support staff whose primary responsibility is to receive and care for severely injured trauma patients in a comprehensive and multidisciplinary manner. This includes personnel removed from the initial patient encounter, including registry staff, quality improvement nurses, and intensive care unit staff. The Trauma Team is an integral part of any Trauma System. Resuscitation by a specific group of healthcare professionals, with clearly defined roles, led by an experienced Trauma Team Leader (TTL), has been demonstrated to improve patient care and outcomes [7–12] and forms the backbone of care in major trauma centers [5, 13].

Teamwork is recognized as an essential component in ensuring the best outcomes in patient safety and is encouraged to achieve optimal performance [14]. Despite the protocol-driven nature of ATLS, [1] human factors may affect team structure [15], leadership, communication, [16] and effectiveness [17]. As outlined in Section 1, non-technical skills, or Crisis Resource Management (CRM) skills, are increasingly recognized as being invaluable components for optimal team function [18], and the deliberate teaching of CRM skills has been shown to improve team performance. [19] Trauma team training programs have been shown to improve team knowledge and performance in a multitude of settings ranging from US civilian trauma centers [20], to developing countries [21–23], and the military. [24] The most recent edition of ATLS clearly recognizes the importance of the Trauma Team and its function—and the

E. Walser
Department of Surgery & Division of Critical Care Medicine, Western University, London, ON, Canada
e-mail: eric.walser@lhsc.on.ca

P. T. Engels
Department of Surgery, Faculty of Health Sciences, McMaster University, Hamilton, ON, Canada
e-mail: engelsp@mcmaster.ca

J. D. Paton-Gay
Department of Surgery, Faculty of Medicine and Dentistry, University of Alberta, Edmonton, AB, Canada
e-mail: patongay@ualberta.ca

H. C. Tien
Division of General Surgery, University of Toronto, Toronto, ON, Canada
e-mail: homer.tien@sunnybrook.ca

P. B. Murphy (✉)
Department of Surgery, Division of Trauma and Acute Care Surgery, Medical College of Wisconsin, Wisconsin, WI, USA
e-mail: pmurphy@mcw.edu

L. Marshall Gillman, S. Widder (eds.), *Trauma Team Dynamics*, https://doi.org/10.1007/978-3-031-86312-7_21

necessity of training to optimize performance—in order to best care for the injured trauma patient [1].

Ideally, the Trauma Team should be present before arrival of the trauma patient, but this requires both advance warning of arrival and available personnel. In the absence of a Trauma Team, the Emergency Department (ED) response to an injured patient typically begins with an assessment by an Emergency Medicine (EM) physician, who may have several other patients to follow and can accomplish tasks in succession only. In this setting, ATLS dictates the sequence of care and should be followed until the patient stabilizes. Consultation of additional surgical specialties might only occur if deemed necessary after the assessment, thereby delaying any response. Trauma patients frequently present in physiologic extremis and require urgent diagnostic and therapeutic interventions immediately upon arrival. The implementation of dedicated Trauma Teams has been shown to improve patient outcomes [11, 12, 25] and is the standard of care in North American trauma centers [5, 13].

A Trauma Team Activation (TTA) is the logistical sequence of notification of members of the team, as well as other key members of an institution that may not attend the trauma but are frequently involved in the care of the severely injured patient. Criteria for a TTA should be tailored to a particular institution's resources and setting, and selection of these criteria dictates which patients will be cared for by the Trauma Team as opposed to EM physicians [5]. As even delayed TTA has been associated with prolonged hospital stay [26], the balance between over- and under-triage must be continuously monitored [5, 27]. How a medical facility meets the needs of the trauma patients will vary among countries; however, the ATLS [1] and WHO guidelines [28] form the backbone of the standards of care for any trauma facility (Table 21.1).

The goal of early Trauma Team Activation (TTA) is to mobilize the team members and hospital resources before the patient arrives, so that life- and limb-saving interventions can be provided immediately upon arrival. As well, it is also

Table 21.1 Composition of trauma team in a high-income country [43]

Role	Responsibility	Position	Personnel
Activation			
Team Leader	Coordinate team activities, review all data, formulate definitive plans. In lower resource setting, may also perform primary survey	Foot of the bed	EM Physician or Surgeon
Airway	Establish a clear airway, intubate as required	Head of the bed	EM Physician or Anesthesia or Surgeon
Respiratory Therapist	Assist in intubation and ventilator setup	Head of the bed	Respiratory Therapist
First Assistant	Primary and Secondary Survey, assist in procedures if not additional physicians	Patient right	EM Physician or Surgeon
Second Assistant	Procedures (chest tubes, lines, FAST. Assist with log roll	Patient left	EM Physician or Surgeon
Primary Nurse	First set of vitals, intravenous access, drawing of bloodwork	Patient left	Nurse
Secondary Nurse	Medication draw-up and administration, assisting primary	Patient left or right	Nurse
Recorder	Documentation of resuscitation	Computer	Nurse
X-Ray Technician	Performs X-rays as dictated by team leader	Away from patient until needed	Technician
Additional members			
Service		**Responsibility**	
Orthopedic Surgery		Consult as needed for the management of traumatic fractures	
Neurosurgery		Consult as needed for the management of traumatic brain injury	
Social Worker		Coordinate family care and support	
Chaplain		Coordinate family care and support	
Trauma Floor Nursing		Provide care on the trauma floor (lab draws, vitals, medication administration)	
Intensive Care Unit Nursing		Provide care in the intensive care unit (lab draws, vitals, medication administration)	
Trauma Registrars		Data-drive feedback to the Trauma Team	
Blood Bank/Lab Technicians		Participate in development and implementation of transfusion protocols	

Adapted from Hoff et al. and the WHO "Guidelines for essential trauma"
EM Emergency Medicine, *FAST* Focused Assessment with Sonography for Trauma

important to share pre-hospital information with the team in preparation for the patient arrival, and allow members of the multidisciplinary team to garner personal protective equipment, including lead shielding.

The size and composition of the Trauma Team may vary with hospital size and resources; additionally, institutions may define different levels of activation based on the severity of injury. Most high-level TTAs within a resource-rich environment include core team members from anesthesia, emergency medicine, general surgery, neurosurgery, orthopedic surgery, respiratory therapy, and nursing. The personnel attending TTA varies by level of activation, institution, country, and accreditation [5]. Airway obstruction is a rare but exceedingly rapid cause of trauma-related death. Severe brain injury and torso exsanguination cause the vast majority of all trauma-related deaths [25]. Extremity injuries are among the leading causes of disability after injury [29, 30]. Other individuals not directly involved in resuscitation are activated such as social work and security. Given the frequent need for rapid access to resources, notification of radiology (technicians and physicians), blood bank, operating room, and critical care leadership is prudent. Smaller hospitals may only be able to mobilize smaller team, and less-severely injured patients may only lower-tier activations.

All team members, including surgical specialists, perform their investigations and interventions in accordance with established principles and guidelines. The TTL's purpose is to coordinate the activities of all Trauma Team members and to ensure that each phase of care is performed thoroughly and rapidly, from the resuscitative phase, to the imaging or operative/intervention phase, and finally to the transfer of care to the ward, operating room, or intensive care unit. This role requires medical knowledge, technical skill, and ability to lead a team in a high-stress environment.

Team Members and Roles

As discussed previously, the composition of the Trauma Team is variable. Table 21.1 lists typical members of the Trauma Team. Depending on the level of TTA, members may be added or subtracted according to institutional guidelines and accreditation of centers. There really is no right or wrong formula; the Trauma Team composition should be based on specialties and personnel available as well as resources.

Trauma Team Leader (TTL)

The Trauma Team Leader is an experienced physician or surgeon that is the "captain" of the Trauma Team [5]. The leader provides expert management of the trauma patient during the resuscitative phase of their care. This includes preparing the team prior to the patient's arrival (pre-hospital background such as number of individuals involved, mechanism of trauma, severity of trauma, and/or injuries), managing the patient in the trauma bay, caring for the patient during transport and during diagnostic imaging, and providing care until a satisfactory handover has occurred to appropriately skilled personnel, who will continue managing ongoing care requirements. The TTL must have the experience and medical expertise to guide the trauma patient through these phases of care, as well as exhibit the ability to work within a team framework and be able to assume its leadership. [31]

The training background of the TTL varies by center, but the TTL is often a surgeon, emergency physician, or another acute care physician with an interest/additional training in trauma. Several studies have compared the outcomes of patients treated by surgeon- and non-surgeon TTLs. There were no differences in survival or length of stay, but one study identified a higher rate of missed injury in patients treated by non-surgeon TTLs [32, 33]. In the United States, trauma surgeons serve as the predominant TTLs at Level I/II centers, although the use of emergency medicine TTLs in this setting is still supported [34]. This likely reflects the much higher rate of penetrating injuries in the United States, which are more likely to require immediate surgical intervention. [35] In settings where the TTL is not a surgeon, there must be a robust protocol in place to rapidly activate a surgical team.

The TTL must have exceptional skills as a communicator, manager, and collaborator to effectively lead the Trauma Team. The TTL is generally positioned at the foot of the patient's bed and away from direct patient contact, with a direct view of the vital signs monitor. This allows the individual to maintain situational awareness and direct all the activity of the other team members. As highlighted in Chap. 8, this global focus minimizes the likelihood of committing a fixation error (persistent failure to revise a diagnosis or plan in the face of readily available evidence that suggests that a revision is necessary) [36]. The TTL is responsible for generating a shared mental model for Trauma Team members, as well as directing communication with the operating room, radiology department members, and critical care unit staff. The individual will decide which diagnostic and therapeutic interventions need to be performed and in what order. The TTL is also responsible for ensuring that the major findings, summary of injuries, and treatment plan are documented in the medical record. In the event that a patient is accompanied by Police or presents with a stab or gunshot wound, the TTL is responsible for interacting with any officer and ensuring compliance with any jurisdictional requirements to notify Police in the setting of such wounds, as well as protecting the safety of Trauma Team members [37, 38].

Airway

Assessment of the airway is the first step of ATLS in single-provider environments, and in well-resourced settings, a single provider should focus on this critical system. While this role is generally filled by an Emergency Medicine Physician or Anesthetist, any provider highly skilled in airway management can take on the role; often Trauma Surgeon or Critical Care attending or senior residents. This person should be positioned at the head of the bed and will be delegated with managing most "Airway" issues often with the help of a respiratory therapist. Part of this position includes communicating airway concerns with the TTL and identifying the need for securing an airway. One exception to the responsibilities for the Airway provider may be in the "difficult airway" that requires cricothyrotomy. In many trauma centers, a trauma or general surgery senior team member is responsible for performing surgical airways. In conjunction with other members of the team, the Airway provider may also be asked to help with managing "circulatory issues." Particularly, they may be asked to place central venous catheters, transfuse blood products (along with nursing team members), and place arterial lines. Also, as part of the adjuncts to the primary survey of ATLS, the Airway provider may be asked to place orogastric or nasogastric tubes. In the event that the airway provider is not from Anesthesia, this service should be involved immediately for patients requiring operative intervention.

Respiratory Therapy

The Respiratory Therapist works with the Airway provider to assist in assessment and management of the airway. They are specifically responsible for setting up equipment including airway devices and adjuncts, ventilators, arterial lines, end-tidal CO2 monitoring, and drawing and running arterial blood gases. This role will be discussed further in Chap. 22.

Emergency Medicine Physician

The role of the Emergency Medicine varies greatly depending on the hospital and even country, but in almost all instances the Emergency Medicine physician will be the first responder to trauma activations without advance warning, and in some circumstances remains the lynchpin of the Trauma Team in the TTL role. This is often the case in non-trauma center hospitals. Once other members of the team arrive, their broad skillset allows them to effectively substitute for many other team members. Airway management, fluid resuscitation, performing FAST (Focused Assessment with Sonography for Trauma), and even some emergency surgical procedures such as cricothyroidotomy and thoracotomy fall within the scope of a skilled emergency medicine physician. The role they fill as part of the Trauma Team is therefore variable and often dependent on local medical culture. Some countries involve Critical Care physicians to fulfill this role.

General Surgery

The General Surgery representation on the Trauma Team typically consists of a junior and/or senior resident. In some countries General Surgery presence has been completely replaced by Trauma Surgery. They should be positioned at the patient's sides. Using the ATLS paradigm, the general surgery team members function as first assistant and are usually asked to perform the primary survey of trauma patients. A second member of the general surgery team (often replaced by an Emergency Medicine Physician or resident) is usually responsible for placing chest tubes to relieve hemo/pneumothoraces. For "Circulation," the general surgery team usually participates in the resuscitation of patients in hemorrhagic shock, along with the Airway provider and nursing. As part of the resuscitative efforts, the general surgery team is often responsible for placing central venous catheters (subclavian/femoral). More importantly, the TTL usually delegates the responsibility of localizing and definitively stopping major sources of hemorrhage to the general surgery team; performing the FAST exam is an important part of the general surgery exam for major sources of hemorrhage. When FAST is unavailable or non-diagnostic, Diagnostic Peritoneal Lavage or Aspiration may be performed by general surgery in the unstable patient. Major sources of hemorrhage include the thorax, abdomen, retroperitoneum (including pelvis), extremity, and external sites of bleeding. General surgery, therefore—in collaboration with the TTL—determines whether the patient requires a trip to the operating room for laparotomy, thoracotomy, or neck exploration, to angiography for embolization, should remain in the trauma bay for additional interventions, or can proceed with cross-sectional imaging. In addition, general surgery is responsible for reviewing any CT imaging of the torso, abdomen, and soft tissues of the limbs (including blood vessels) and neck with radiology.

Orthopedic Surgery

The Orthopedic Surgery representation on the Trauma Team may consist of a junior resident, but often a senior resident may be required especially for the placement of advanced skeletal traction. They are often not part of the initial resuscitation but are consulted for the management of traumatic fractures. If part of the initial resuscitation, they should be positioned at the patient's pelvis and will be delegated specific roles in the assessment and management of "Circulatory" issues in addition to maintaining primary responsibility for "Disability" issues in the injured patient. Regarding "Circulation," orthopedics usually will be asked to identify and bind unstable pelvic fractures, and identify and splint grossly angulated extremity fractures. For "Disability and Exposure," the orthopedic team will specifically examine all extremities, the pelvis and spine. The orthopedic team will be responsible for performing a detailed secondary survey of the musculoskeletal system and will review all extremity imaging and spine imaging. In the event of an injury to the spine, either orthopedics or neurosurgery is generally responsible for managing this injury based on local agreements. While not all trauma systems include orthopedics in the core Trauma Team, it is essential that they are readily available to participate if required based on identified or suspected injuries.

Neurosurgery

The Neurosurgery representation on the Trauma Team typically consists of a resident and, similar to orthopedics, is often absent from the initial trauma resuscitation until a relevant injury is identified. If part of the resuscitation, the individual is responsible for the "Disability" component of ATLS, including assessment of the spine on log roll when appropriate. They may make recommendations to the TTL regarding the management of any increased intracranial pressure. They are responsible for immediate interpretation of the CT/CT Angiogram and discussion with their attending surgeon regarding any operative management or ventricular drainage. Traumatic brain injury is a major cause of death in multiply injured patients, and early neurosurgical evaluation is essential [25]. Similar to Orthopedics, if Neurosurgery is not a part of the core team, they must be able to respond quickly if required.

Primary and Secondary Nurses

Trauma nurses are generally drawn from the Emergency Department nursing staff, and a high-tempo trauma will often require two or more skilled nurses as an absolutely essential component of the team. Their roles are exceptionally broad but generally include placing appropriate patient monitoring, obtaining the first set of vitals, inserting peripheral intravenous catheters, obtaining blood samples for the laboratory, assistance in patient manipulation including log-rolling, and acting as non-sterile assistant to a member of the team who is performing an invasive procedure such as chest tube or central line insertion. They are generally responsible for administrating any medications or vaccinations. Nursing roles will be further outlined in Chap. 22. Their importance to the functioning of the team is difficult to understate.

Recording Nurse

The role of the recording/documenting nurse is just that: to document, on an appropriate trauma medical record, the important findings of the Trauma Team in their assessment of the patient. This includes recording vital signs, assessments, and nature and type of procedures performed. This nurse is typically situated near the foot of the bed, in proximity to the TTL, so as to gain a view of the monitors and be able to hear the Trauma Team's assessment as it is relayed to the TTL. Often acting as a nursing team lead, they are often the most senior nurse on the team and work in conjunction with the TTL to facilitate team communication and task delegation, especially with services/resources not directly present in the trauma bay. As mentioned previously, nursing roles will be further discussed in Chap. 22. The electronic medical record has greatly changed the role of the recording nurse, and this individual is paramount to quality improvement initiatives for the injured patient. Accurate data is paramount in root-cause analysis.

Trauma Team Activation

The Trauma Team is called into action with a Trauma Team Activation (TTA). The TTA may be in response to pre-hospital information or information obtained when the patient first arrives to the ED. The value of having a Trauma Team ready and awaiting the arrival of a severely injured patient cannot be understated, as it allows for appropriate preparation of the room and equipment, introduction and organization of the Team, and preparation based on the anticipated injuries of the patient from any pre-hospital information.

A TTA may occur in a tiered fashion, or have graded "levels" of response [39, 40]. Tiers should be organized based on the requirement for immediate or subsequent intervention and the resources required in your care. Triage should be based on injury mechanism and clinical status, either from pre-hospital reports or once the patient arrives in the trauma bay. Triage systems will vary based on systems, but general criteria for the highest-level response include but are not limited to traumatic arrest, hypotension (systolic blood pressure < 90 mmHg), GCS < 9, penetrating neck, abdomen or torso trauma, transfusion of blood to maintain vitals, intubated patients, or physician discretion. For these patients, in addition to the standard Trauma Team, the Trauma Surgeon,

Table 21.2 American college of surgeons committee on trauma minimally acceptable criteria for highest level of Trauma Team activation [5]

1. Confirmed blood pressure <90 mm Hg at any time in adults and age-specific hypotension in children
2. Gunshot wounds to the neck, chest, or abdomen
3. GCS<8 with mechanism attributed to trauma
4. Transfer patients from other hospitals receiving blood to maintain vital signs
5. A) Intubated patients transferred from the scene
OR
B) Patients with respiratory compromise or obstruction (includes intubated patients who are transferred from another facility, with ongoing respiratory compromise but does not include patients intubated at another facility and are now stable from a respiratory standpoint)
6. Emergency Physician's discretion

Operating Theatre, Blood Bank, and Intensive Care Unit may also be notified. For other patients that have evidence of multisystem trauma but are hemodynamically normal, a lesser activation comprising the TTL and the core Trauma Team members may occur at the discretion of the TTL, charge nurse, or emergency physician.

Each institution will have its own method for TTA, which may include dedicated pagers, overhead pages, or even "walkie-talkies" for immediate notification. Notification may either alert the Trauma Team member to proceed immediately to the Trauma Bay or provide an update on an anticipated trauma with an estimated time of arrival. The developing field of pre-hospital telemedicine and teleradiology may, in the future, facilitate the transmission of important diagnostic information to the awaiting hospital Trauma Team so that they may better prepare for the patient's specific injuries [41].

The criteria for a graded activation must be clearly defined by the trauma center and continuously evaluated by the performance improvement and patient safety program [5]. Inevitably, over-triage (triage decision that classifies a patient as requiring TTA when, in fact, they do not) and under-triage (triage decision that classifies a patient as not requiring TTA when, in fact, they do) will occur, but a trauma system should establish and monitor acceptable rates for these. Obviously, under-triage carries a greater threat to patient care than over-triage. Suggested rates for TTA are >95% of patients with an ISS> = 16, and in <30% of patients with an ISS = < 9. The ACS/COT suggested TTA criteria are listed in Table 21.2 [5]. Newer methods of determining TTA include the need for emergent invention within 6 h [27].

The Trauma Bay

The Trauma Bay, or resuscitation area of the Emergency Department, is where major trauma patients should be received and is the primary location where trauma patients are initially treated. The ideal Trauma Bay has the following characteristics: easily accessible to EMS personnel, well lit (with OR-quality overhead lights), spacious enough to accommodate the Trauma Team and necessary equipment, have the ability to perform plain film radiography, be close to a CT Scanner, and be in reasonable proximity with direct access to the Operating Rooms and Intensive Care Unit. Many trauma centers have a dedicated area in, or adjacent to, their emergency department with the ability to care for two or more severely injured patients simultaneously. A typical arrangement of a Trauma Bay is depicted in Fig. 21.1, with a picture of a typical Trauma Bay in Fig. 21.2. It is important that all potentially required equipment be located *within* the Trauma Bay to avoid unnecessary delays. Equipment should also be grouped together by the requirements for performing each procedure. For example, a "chest tube package" may include a sterile cut-down tray containing appropriate instruments, with a suture, scalpel, chest tube, sterile gown, and gloves taped on top of it, already sitting on its own moveable table with a chest tube drain and antiseptic solution on the lower shelf. Similar packages should exist for central venous catheters, thoracotomy sets, surgical airways, and arterial catheters. The contents and accessibility of these packages must be reviewed on a regular basis by physicians participating in the care of trauma patients. These packages should also be ergonomically placed in the Trauma Bay, i.e., the chest tube packages should be placed on either side of the patient's stretcher. A complement of airway management devices must be immediately accessible at the head of the bed; many centers have a standardized "difficult airway cart" placed within the trauma bay. An adequate supply of individual lead-lined protective garments must also be available to facilitate care while plain radiographs are obtained. Ideally, these garments are donned underneath personal protective equipment (gown, gloves, full-face mask) by all members of the Trauma Team as they arrive into the trauma bay, so that trauma patient care is not interrupted when X-rays are performed. An in-depth discussion of the trauma bay environment and its design can be found in Chapters 23 and 24.

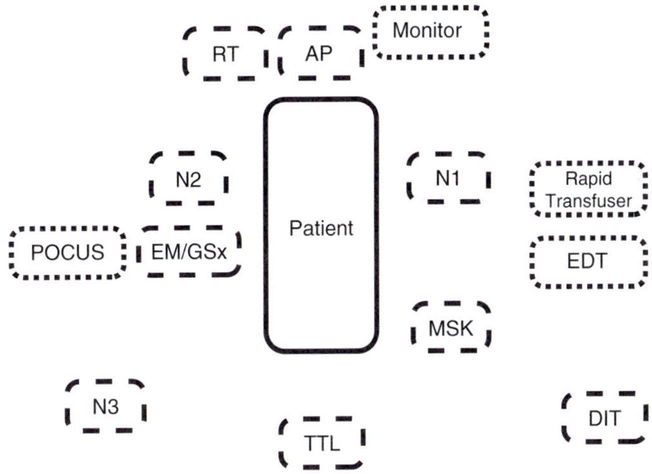

Fig. 21.1 Trauma Team positioning in the trauma bay. *TTL* Trauma Team Leader, *EM/GSx* Emergency Medicine or General Surgery Provider, *MSK* Musculoskeletal Provider, *AP* Airway Provider, *RT* Respiratory Therapist, *N1* and *N2* Circulating Nurses, *N3* Recording Nurse, *DIT* Diagnostic Imaging Technician, *EDT* Emergency Thoracotomy Tray, *POCUS* Point of Care Ultrasound Unit

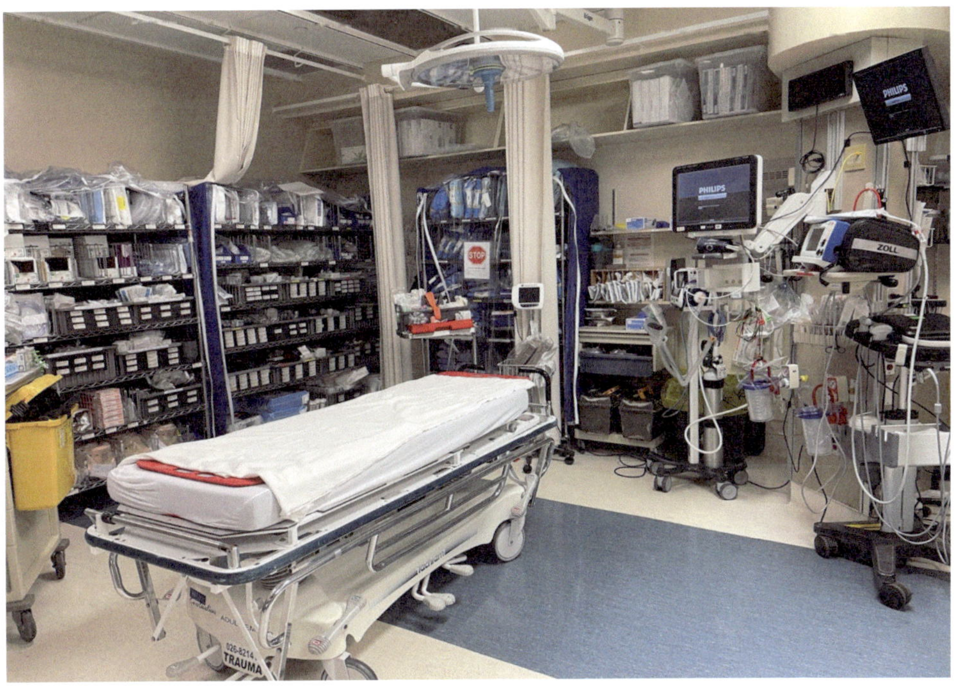

Fig. 21.2 Representative trauma bay. (London Health Sciences Center/Western University)

Trauma Team Function

Above all else, the Trauma Team must function as a *team*. During the resuscitation of a severely injured trauma patient, a large amount of information is rapidly gathered about the patient's injuries and physiologic condition, and management decisions are similarly rapidly made based on this information, often in a near-simultaneous fashion. The presence of a team allows multiple actions to be accomplished at once compared with a serial or vertical approach required when only one physician is available to treat such a patient. This departure from primary-care emergency care provision in a small hospital is important to note.

To function properly as a team, the team needs clear leadership. All information must be passed to the TTL and all high-level decisions must be made by the TTL; otherwise, the Team function becomes chaotic. For example, if only one nurse is available, and both the anesthesia resident and the orthopedic residents are demanding nursing assistance for procedures (arterial catheters versus splints), the requests should go through the TTL, and the TTL must prioritize the order of work and decisively delegate the nurse to one or the other resident's aid.

Ideal destinations after leaving the Trauma Bay are: the OR, the angiography suite, the ICU, or the Trauma Ward. However, if their condition allows, many patients may be required to return to the ED while awaiting bed availability. Many trauma centers have time-driven goals to measure delays in care and time to definitive investigations/treatment. Commonly cited time goals include: handover (< 60 s), primary survey (< 5 min), CT scan (< 15 min), admission/operating room (< 1 h) [42]. Reviewing these metrics on a regular basis can identify opportunities for improvement.

Summary

The optimal care of the severely injured trauma patient is predicated on the seamless function of a multidisciplinary Trauma Team under the effective leadership of an expert trauma clinician. Team and venue preparation are key components for success, and attention to the appropriate training—including education, simulation, and quality improvement processes—will allow a Trauma Team to excel in its care for these patients.

Key Points

- Treatment of a severely injured trauma patient is a complex process.
- Optimal resuscitation is best accomplished with a multidisciplinary team.
- Team function is dependent on technical as well as non-technical skills.
- To optimize team function, it must be practiced.

References

1. American College of Surgeons Committee on Trauma. In: Merrick C, Stewart RM, Rotondo MF, Henry SM, Drago M, editors. Advanced trauma life support. 10th ed. Chicago: American College of Surgeons; 2018.
2. Civil IDS. Trauma care—a team sport in the 21st century. Injury. 2007;38(1):5–6. https://doi.org/10.1016/J.INJURY.2006.11.013.
3. Adedeji OA, Driscoll PA. The Trauma Team–a system of initial trauma care. Postgrad Med J. 1996;72(852):587–93. https://doi.org/10.1136/PGMJ.72.852.587.
4. Driscoll PA, Vincent CA. Organizing an efficient Trauma Team. Injury. 1992;23(2):107–10. https://doi.org/10.1016/0020-1383(92)90043-R.
5. American College of Surgeons Committee on Trauma. Resources for optimal care of the injured patient. Chicago; 2022.
6. Optimal hospital resources for care of the seriously injured. Bull Am Coll Surg. 1976;61(9):15–22. Accessed 9 Sept 2022.
7. Cole EM, West A, Davenport R, Naganathar S, Kanzara T, Carey M, Brohi K. Can residents be effective Trauma Team leaders in a major trauma centre? Injury. 2013;44(1):18–22. https://doi.org/10.1016/J.INJURY.2011.09.020.
8. Rainer TH, Cheung NK, Yeung JHH, Graham CA. Do Trauma Teams make a difference? A single centre registry study. Resuscitation. 2007;73(3):374–81. https://doi.org/10.1016/J.RESUSCITATION.2006.10.011.
9. Nathens AB, Jurkovich GJ, Gummings P, Rivara FP, Maier R, v. The effect of organized systems of trauma care on motor vehicle crash mortality. JAMA. 2000;283(15):1990–4. https://doi.org/10.1001/JAMA.283.15.1990.
10. MacKenzie EJ, Rivara FP, Jurkovich GJ, Nathens AB, Frey KP, Egleston BL, Salkever DS, Scharfstein DO. A national evaluation of the effect of trauma-center care on mortality. N Engl J Med. 2006;354(4):366–78. https://doi.org/10.1056/NEJMSA052049.
11. Leung GKK, Ng GKB, Ho W, Hung KN, Yuen WK. Impact of a multidisciplinary Trauma Team on the outcome of acute subdural haematoma. Injury. 2012;43(9):1419–22. https://doi.org/10.1016/J.INJURY.2011.03.017.
12. Gerardo CJ, Glickman SW, Vaslef SN, Chandra A, Pietrobon R, Cairns CB. The rapid impact on mortality rates of a dedicated care team including trauma and emergency physicians at an academic medical center. J Emerg Med. 2011;40(5):586–91. https://doi.org/10.1016/J.JEMERMED.2009.08.056.
13. TRAUMA SYSTEM ACCREDITATION GUIDELINES. Trauma Association of Canada Association Canadienne de Traumatologie Fourth Revision. 2011. www.traumacanada.org. Accessed 9 Sept 2022.
14. Clancy CM, Tornberg DN. TeamSTEPPS: assuring optimal teamwork in clinical settings. Am J Med Qual. 2019;34(5):436–8. https://doi.org/10.1177/1062860619873181.
15. Xiao Y, Seagull FJ, Mackenzie CF, Klein K, Ziegert J. Adaptation of Team Structure of Trauma Resuscitation Teams. Proc Hum Factors Ergon Soc Annu Meet. 2016;46(3):569–73. https://doi.org/10.1177/154193120204600374.
16. Xiao Y, Mackenzie CF, Patey R. Team coordination and breakdowns in a real-life stressful environment. Proc Hum Factors Ergon Soc Annu Meet. 2016;1:186–90. https://doi.org/10.1177/154193129804200301.
17. Marshall S, Miller A, Xiao Y. Development of team coordination and performance measures in a trauma setting. Proc Hum Factors Ergon Soc Annu Meet. 2016;2:717–21. https://doi.org/10.1177/154193120705101124.
18. Brindley PG, Reynolds SF. Improving verbal communication in critical care medicine. J Crit Care. 2011;26(2):155–9. https://doi.org/10.1016/J.JCRC.2011.03.004.
19. Hicks CM, Kiss A, Bandiera GW, Denny CJ. Crisis Resources for Emergency Workers (CREW II): results of a pilot study and simulation-based crisis resource management course for emergency medicine residents. CJEM. 2012;14(6):354–62. https://doi.org/10.2310/8000.2012.120580.
20. Holcomb JB, Dumire RD, Crommett JW, Stamateris CE, Fagert MA, Cleveland JA, Dorlac GR, Dorlac WC, Bonar JP, Hira K, et al. Evaluation of Trauma Team performance using an advanced human patient simulator for resuscitation training. J Trauma. 2002;52(6):1078–86. https://doi.org/10.1097/00005373-200206000-00009.
21. O'Reilly GM, Fitzgerald M, Dewan Y, Chou K, Mathew J, Peters N. The alfred Trauma Team training program in India and Sri Lanka. Emerg Med Australas. 2011;23(5):632–9. https://doi.org/10.1111/J.1742-6723.2011.01459.X.
22. Pemberton J, Rambaran M, Cameron BH. Evaluating the long-term impact of the Trauma Team training course in Guyana: an explanatory mixed-methods approach. Am J Surg. 2013;205(2):119–24. https://doi.org/10.1016/J.AMJSURG.2012.08.004.
23. Bergman S, Deckelbaum D, Lett R, Haas B, Demyttenaere S, Munthali V, Mbembati N, Museru L, Razek T. Assessing the impact of the Trauma Team training program in Tanzania. J Trauma. 2008;65(4):879–83. https://doi.org/10.1097/TA.0B013E318184A9FE.

24. McLaughlin T, Hennecke P, Garraway NR, Evans DC, Hameed M, Simons RK, Doucet J, Hansen D, Annand S, Bell N, et al. A predeployment Trauma Team training course creates confidence in teamwork and clinical skills: a post-Afghanistan deployment validation study of Canadian Forces healthcare personnel. J Trauma. 2011;71(5 Suppl 1):S487–93. https://doi.org/10.1097/TA.0B013E318232E9E7.
25. Solagberu BA, Adekanye AO, Ofoegbu CPK, Udoffa US, Abdur-Rahman LO, Taiwo JO. Epidemiology of trauma deaths: a reassessment. J Trauma. 1995;38(2):177–81. https://doi.org/10.1097/00005373-199502000-00006.
26. Ryb GE, Cooper C, Waak SM. Delayed Trauma Team activation: patient characteristics and outcomes. J Trauma Acute Care Surg. 2012;73(3):695–8. https://doi.org/10.1097/TA.0B013E31825ABF6F.
27. Morris RS, Karam BS, Murphy PB, Jenkins P, Milia DJ, Hemmila MR, Haines KL, Puzio TJ, de Moya MA, Tignanelli CJ. Field-triage, hospital-triage and triage-assessment: a literature review of the current phases of adult trauma triage. J Trauma Acute Care Surg. 2021;90(6):E138–45. https://doi.org/10.1097/TA.0000000000003125.
28. World Health Organization. Guidelines for essential trauma care / World Health Organization, International Society of Surgery/Société Internationale de Chirurgie and the International Association for the Surgery of Trauma and Surgical Intensive Care (IATSIC). 2004. http://apps.who.int//iris/handle/10665/42565. Accessed 9 Sept 2022.
29. Soberg HL, Finset A, Bautz-Holter E, Sandvik L, Roise O. Return to work after severe multiple injuries: a multidimensional approach on status 1 and 2 years postinjury. J Trauma. 2007;62(2):471–81. https://doi.org/10.1097/TA.0B013E31802E95F4.
30. Holtslag HR, Post MW, van der Werken C, Lindeman E. Return to work after major trauma. Clin Rehabil. 2007;21(4):373–83. https://doi.org/10.1177/0269215507072084.
31. Hjortdahl M, Ringen AH, Naess AC, Wisborg T. Leadership is the essential non-technical skill in the Trauma Team–results of a qualitative study. Scand J Trauma Resusc Emerg Med. 2009;17(1):48. https://doi.org/10.1186/1757-7241-17-48.
32. Hajibandeh S, Hajibandeh S. Who should lead a trauma team: surgeon or non-surgeon? A systematic review and meta-analysis. J Inj Violence Res. 2017;9(2):107–16. https://doi.org/10.5249/JIVR.V9I2.874.
33. Leeper WR, Leeper TJ, Vogt KN, Charyk-Stewart T, Gray DK, Parry NG. The role of Trauma Team leaders in missed injuries: does specialty matter? J Trauma Acute Care Surg. 2013;75(3):387–90. https://doi.org/10.1097/TA.0B013E31829CFA32.
34. Grossman MD, Portner M, Hoey BA, Stehly CD, Schwab CW, Stoltzfus J. Emergency traumatologists as partners in trauma care: the future is now. J Am Coll Surg. 2009;208(4):503–9. https://doi.org/10.1016/J.JAMCOLLSURG.2009.01.013.
35. Richardson EG, Hemenway D. Homicide, suicide, and unintentional firearm fatality: comparing the United States with other high-income countries, 2003. J Trauma. 2011;70(1):238–43. https://doi.org/10.1097/TA.0B013E3181DBADDF.
36. Rall M, Gaba D, Howard S, Dieckmann P. Chapter 6: human performance and patient safety. In: Miller's Anesthesia. Churchill Livingstone; 2009.
37. Mandatory Gunshot Wounds Reporting Act, 2005, S.O. 2005, c. 9. https://www.ontario.ca/laws/statute/05m09. Accessed 9 Sept 2022.
38. GUNSHOT AND STAB WOUND MANDATORY DISCLOSURE ACT. 2010. www.qp.alberta.ca. Accessed 9 Sept 2022.
39. Claridge J, Golob J Jr, Leukhardt W, Kan J, Como J, Malangoni M, Yowler C. Trauma Team activation can be tailored by prehospital criteria. Am Surg. 2010;76(10):1401–7.
40. Kohn MA, Hammel JM, Bretz SW, Stangby A. Trauma Team Activation Criteria as Predictors of Patient Disposition from the Emergency Department. Acad Emerg Med. 2004;11(1):1–9. https://doi.org/10.1111/J.1553-2712.2004.TB01364.X.
41. McBeth P, Crawford I, Tiruta C, Xiao Z, Zhu GQ, Shuster M, Sewell L, Panebianco N, Lautner D, Nicolaou S, et al. Help is in your pocket: The potential accuracy of smartphone- and laptop-based remotely guided resuscitative telesonography. Telemed J e-Health. 2013;19(12):924–30. https://doi.org/10.1089/TMJ.2013.0034/ASSET/IMAGES/LARGE/FIGURE3.JPEG.
42. Mark A, Taylor I, Hewes HA, Bolinger CD, Fenton SJ, Russell KW. Established time goals can increase the efficiency of trauma resuscitation. Cureus. 2020;12(8):e9524. https://doi.org/10.7759/CUREUS.9524.
43. Hoff WS, Reilly PM, Rotondo MF, DiGiacomo JC, Schwab CW. The importance of the command-physician in trauma resuscitation. J Trauma. 1997;43(5):772–7. https://doi.org/10.1097/00005373-199711000-00007.

Interprofessional Team Roles

22

Elaine Sigalet and Mirette Dubé

Trauma patients are complex. Rapid assessment and surgical intervention of seriously injured trauma patients can influence the patient's outcome: morbidity and mortality [1]. To optimize outcomes in this cohort of patients, it is important to have a highly trained team of experts who can be rapidly assembled to ensure these patients get "effective" and "time-critical" care [2]. This team of professionals is called a trauma team (TT).

Membership of a TT can vary nationally and internationally [3]. Membership can depend on the level of trauma center, an institution's resources, professional practice roles, and the practice model. According to the Advanced Trauma Life Support Course (ATLS), membership should include a team leader, usually an Emergency (EM) physician or trauma surgeon, an airway specialist, a circulating nurse and physician, a scribe or documenter (nurse), and a social worker. In our experience, it is helpful to have an extra nurse assigned to medications, a dedicated porter, and unit clerk to facilitate the transfer of information and resources as needed. In North America, the respiratory therapist is the airway specialist. The addition of a nurse practitioner is becoming more common especially in smaller trauma centers. With Pediatric Trauma, depending on the level of consciousness, it may be helpful to have a child life specialist. Today, regardless of the profession, TT members are expected to complete advanced certification in courses such as the Advanced Cardiac Life Support Course (ACLS) and Pediatric Advance Life Support Course (PALS). Furthermore, nurses are often required to complete additional courses like the Trauma Nursing Core Course (TNCC), the Advance Trauma Care Nursing Course (ATCN), the Certified Emergency Nurse (CEN), and the Emergency Nursing Pediatric Course (ENPC). Specific requirement for trauma team nurses varies by institution, organization, and level of trauma center. Respiratory therapists are often regulated and licensed and can hold a variety of professional designations or titles such as a respiratory therapist (RT), registered respiratory therapist (RRT), respiratory care practitioner (RCP), and or anesthesia or advanced practice respiratory therapist (APRT) [4]. Where there is no integration of the profession in critical care settings, this role may be carried out by other experienced team members. Regardless of professional designation, nurses and respiratory therapists are expected to recertify in the advanced courses as dictated by the course, licensing body, and/or organization. The concept of effective teamwork is a core element in all these courses, yet practice is still frequently restricted to intraprofessional practice often because of course logistics and the clinical demands. This underpins the need for incorporating simulation as a platform for streamlining the interprofessional task interdependence needed to optimize "time-critical" assessment and intervention with seriously injured trauma patients [5]

Effective and time-critical care is optimized when team members can complete the taskwork in their role competently and confidently to reduce the time to definitive care [1, 3]. Honing task interdependence, the completion of several tasks simultaneously or in a horizontal fashion is optimized when team members have opportunities to practice together. The interdependence of taskwork is also referred to as teamwork. The outcome of teamwork is often referred to as team performance [6]. Simulation creates a platform for deliberate practice. Providing team members with this opportunity is critical. Team members should be given opportunities to practice task interdependence without any risk to the real trauma patient. Research suggests teams who work together frequently, without changes in membership, are more effective [7]. Simulation as a training platform for postgraduates has been shown to decrease the time to critical operations for trauma patients [8]. Teams who practice together learn with each other, about each other, and from

E. Sigalet (✉)
Founding Partner Healthcare Systems Simulation International Inc, Adjunct Assistant Professor, Department of Community Health Sciences, University of Calgary, Calgary, AB, Canada

M. Dubé
Healthcare Systems Simulation International Inc., Cochrane, AB, Canada
e-mail: Mirette@HealthcareSSI.com

L. Marshall Gillman, S. Widder (eds.), *Trauma Team Dynamics*, https://doi.org/10.1007/978-3-031-86312-7_22

each other to optimize efficiency and quality in the care [6, 9, 10]. In care processes where emotion plays a role, deliberate practice becomes even more important. With the serious nature of injuries in the trauma patient and the risk of exsanguinating, time pressure to perform competently in roles becomes a source of emotion for many team members. Emotion can interfere with how we store, process, and retrieve information. Illeris refers to this as the tension triangle [11]. Our knowledge and skills, and our emotion is dynamic and differs for each team member. When a team member is functioning with a high emotional load, it may be difficult for them to retrieve and apply information in the moment. Most professionals will recognize a time when this happened to them. This can lead to feelings of shame, perceived incompetence, and perceptions of feeling judged, which can impede the success of the team. This has been the impetus behind the development and use of cognitive aids in addition to engaging in simulated deliberate practice. This is real and a vulnerability associated with being human. Preventing these circumstances is fueled by establishing strong team skills and a sense of psychological safety among team membership. Psychological safety is the internal feeling team members have, but rarely express in front of colleagues, especially if they perceive judgment, or there is an explicit power gradient [12].

Teamwork skills are underpinned by communication, coordination, and collaboration to ensure role clarity, effective leadership, closed-loop communication, situational awareness, mutual support, and effective resource utilization [2, 6]. Communication errors inclusive of missing information play a key role in hospital deaths [13]. According to the joint commission, 66% of in-hospital deaths are attributed to communication errors, and this can amount to up to 10% of seriously injured trauma patients who may have presented with survivable injuries [13]. These skills, in addition to a sense of psychological safety, are improved through opportunities for deliberate practice. It provides opportunities for team members to engage in care process discussions using teamwork skills and ask for help when in doubt without feeling judged with effective facilitation of the simulation. Teamwork skills create a common language and expectation for membership task interdependence. Today, in most undergraduate education and training programs, students are introduced to these concepts, and in many programs, they have had opportunities for application in simulation. They are developed in further postgraduate opportunities in the real clinical practice contexts and in simulation.

To appreciate the dynamics within the TT membership, it is helpful to reinforce the concept of inclusive leadership. Inclusive leadership is a style developed to impart psychological safety amongst team members. With this style, leaders encourage team members to ask questions and support decision-making, making it explicit that they will not be judged [14]. An inclusive leader recognizes the vulnerability associated with our human nature and calls on team members to work together using established teamwork skills to ensure the care process is appropriate and timely. As already stated, the respiratory therapy role and nursing roles are vital to effective team performance. Each role has specific taskwork, which we will detail below.

Respiratory therapists are often required to cover large emergency departments including all incoming trauma admissions autonomously within their role. In smaller hospitals, there may only be one or two therapists working at a time for the entire hospital. This requires the RRT to maintain situational awareness and coordination with other team members to ensure resources are balanced for patients requiring acute respiratory care. During trauma admission, the respiratory therapist often assumes a position at the head of the bed near the airway and can be called upon to manage many different tasks in trauma. During a trauma admission, the RRT will rapidly assess and manage the immediate respiratory and airway needs alongside the trauma or emergency designated physician. The RRT specializes in advanced airway management, including intubation and mechanical ventilation strategies. Their expertise includes the initiation, maintenance, and discontinuation of mechanical ventilation, as well as the administration of oxygen (dry and heated humidification systems) and other aerosol therapies. They are often responsible for the administration of medical gases such as Heliox, inhaled Nitric Oxide, and Epoprostenol, a pulmonary vasodilator [15]. They specialize in difficult airway manipulation and capture techniques. In some situations, and centers, RRTS may be the assistant to the person intubating, and in others, they may be designated to perform the intubation [15]. Regardless of who performs the intubation, the RRT's expertise is critical to locating, preparing, and inserting all airway devices such as video laryngoscopy and alternative airways. During intubation, an RRT prompts and facilitates plans for the intubation; whether this is through following a specified airway management/intubation team brief or checklist that exists in a center, or through ensuring a clear intubation plan A, B, and C is established in advance with the team. These airway management team briefings ensure strategies, equipment, and human resources are discussed should an airway attempt become difficult. This enables anticipation and planning and allows opportunity for team suggestions. Another responsibility in this role is to align optimal ventilation strategies to the patient condition (e.g., blood gas analysis, work of breathing, pulmonary mechanics) and monitor physiologic response to the changes made while clearly communicating these to the interprofessional team. It is critical that the RRT and RN communicate any changes occurring, as one change to mechanical ventilation parameters or medication administration, for example, can have a profound impact on the overall patient condition, including hemodynamic stability and respiratory status. Understanding the measurement and analysis of pulmonary mechanics is key to effective ventilation strategies. These measurements often performed by the RRT include plateau pressures, total and optimal positive end-expiratory pressure (peep) studies, driving pressure (defined as plateau pressure minus total PEEP), and lung recruitment maneuvers. In consultation with the physician, they monitor the status of ventilation alerting team members to the level of sedation and other observations required. RRT's autonomy includes the implementation of RRT-driven protocols in the trauma setting such as lung protective strategies (i.e., ensuring safe plateau pressures), ventilation for traumatic brain injury, chest trauma, and other trauma epidemiology to optimize outcomes. The RRT cross-monitors and shares roles and responsibilities related to preparation, insertion, and monitoring of arterial lines. They assist with cardiopulmonary resuscitation, chest tube setup and monitoring, and patient transport and provide mutual support to other team members to ensure a high-performing team. How these tasks are shared can depend on available personnel, the workload, the situation, and the local practice model. The RRT is required to relay urgency and gain the attention of other team members to ensure timely action for the most critical patients. This skill is especially helpful in the complex trauma care environment.

The nursing roles on the TT are often identified by the associated taskwork. Roles include a documenter, a procedure/circulating nurse, and a medications nurse. In line with the ATLS recommendations, nursing membership on a TT ranges from 2 to 4 nurses depending on the practice model, department workload, and available personnel [2]. This number is not influenced by the NP role, as that role often acts as a physician assist supporting all aspects of trauma management. The documenter usually assumes a position at the foot of the bed close to the TTL, to keep a 40,000-foot view of the care process. Responsibilities in this role include documentation of history, assessments, all interventions, and timekeeping. As a timekeeper, the documenter alerts team members to time lapses associated with interventions and medication. Some TTLs prefer to write down necessary interventions and empower the documenter to assign taskwork to the relevant team member based on priority. This strategy can decrease the leader's cognitive load. This primarily relates to frequent interruptions that are a reality as team members seek input about patient status to inform taskwork. Lastly, the documenter participates in all handovers. Handovers will always be vulnerable points in the care process for communication errors [16]. With seriously injured patients, the management is complex, there can be tremendous distractions as patients are moved along the care pathway, and the list of findings and interventions can be long [16]. Loss of information can negatively influence ongoing management [17]. In a study by Zakrison and colleagues [13], chart audits exposed missed injuries in 24% of trauma patients admitted to ICU and clinical information was inconsistent between the Emergency and ICU department in 48% of patients. Management was changed for almost 33% of patients when information was reconciled. The authors note that standardizing handover in trauma patients remains a shortcoming that must be addressed to reduce communication errors that impact clinical outcomes.

The medication nurse works from the side of the bed closest to the medication cart. Administration of rapid sequence intubation medications, vasopressors to hemodynamic support, volume expanders, antibiotics, tetanus, administration of anticoagulation reversal protocols (ACRP), tranexamic acid (TXA), and sometimes resuscitation drugs are common in trauma. Vulnerabilities in this role are associated with the necessary actions the nurse takes to focus and ensure the medication dose, route, and timing are accurate. Research suggests this role can experience a high cognitive load which can create vulnerability to error [18]. For this reason, some trauma teams assign two nurses to this role or have this role supported by the documenter. This role is vulnerable to the loss of situation awareness. Preparation of the medication requires focus. The nurse often does this with their back to the patient. Unfortunately, this can lead to the loss of situation awareness as the patient's condition may have changed in the time lapse of preparing a medication. To ensure the medication is still needed, the nurse should verbalize intention to administer the drug and wait for affirmation before giving it. Fortunately, today many of the medications are standardized for adults and can be prepared in advance; this can often be done upon receiving the pre-arrival notification call from emergency services. A recent simulation study showed that having medication and oral tracheal intubation equipment prepared and organized prior to the task, compared to on scene, resulted in improved time to intubation, a decrease in associated errors, and decreased cognitive load especially for the person assisting with the intubation [18].

The third nursing role is a procedure nurse. This nurse usually works on the opposite side of the bed to the medication nurse to reduce congestion around the patient. Responsibilities in this role include attaching the patient to the cardiac monitor, vital signs inclusive of temperature, vascular access, trauma labs inclusive of glucose, initiation of two large bore intravenous catheters and infusion of crystalloid blood products, and, when required, initiation and administration of the massive transfusion protocol (MTP). When fluid resuscitation requires the use of the rapid pressure infuser, a fourth nurse is often utilized. Other responsibilities include the insertion of an oral gastric tube post intubation, a urinary catheter to monitor output, wound care, and splinting. In centers where there is no respiratory therapist, responsibilities would extend to supporting endotracheal intubation.

In different parts of North America, the role of nursing on the TT continues to evolve. At the University of California, San Diego, trauma NPs typically work in Emergency or ICU departments and are educated to work independently and collaboratively with other team members. This is similar in Canada, with the exception that they are either Adult or Pediatric NPs. The scope of practice for the NP includes ordering medical tests, initiating emergency care, evaluating treatment, caring for wounds, monitoring trauma patient progress, completing discharges, and communicating with the families of trauma patients. Additionally, they can insert or remove chest tubes, take out foreign objects, manage ventilators, address complex injuries, and act as first assist to other physicians on the team [3, 19]. The level of engagement in scope is dependent on the institution's trauma management practice model. In North Carolina, trauma centers are using a new role, identified as a trauma nursing lead (TNL) [20]. In this State, the TT has two TNLs instead of the more familiar 2–4 nurse model. This designation of nurses has completed specialty training (certification in some of the courses detailed above), have extensive experience in trauma nursing, and some hold paramedic licenses. Nursing taskwork is shared between the two TNL roles: assistance with primary or secondary surveys, vital signs, vascular access, fluid resuscitation including the massive transfusion protocol (MTP), administration of ACRP, TXA, medications, wound care, splinting, documentation, and handovers. In this center, the 11 employed TNLs, all pursing advanced education, are an integral part of the multidisciplinary trauma team. As such, they participate in trauma rounds, oversee the care for admitted trauma patients, accompany trauma patient to CT scan, and support all MTP and ACRP infusions in the hospital. Lastly and as important, they ensure patients receive family-centered care and families become an integral part of the patient journey [21]. Research at this center suggests many advantages of using this role. Patients cared for in these centers after this role was started had better outcomes. Time to the operating theater decreased by 20 min. The length of stay (LOS) decreased by 1 day and up to 2.5 days for patients in ICU. The LOS for patients in hospital who had received MTP decreased from 36 days to just under 22 days [21].

Nursing and respiratory therapy play pivotal roles on the TT. As such they must be afforded opportunities to engage in simulation to optimize the teamwork skills and task interdependence required in management of a seriously injured trauma patient. In both professions, team members are expected to use the teamwork skills to support team communication, coordination, and collaboration in preparing for an incoming trauma patient, during the care process, and all handovers. Family-centered care, as with other medical emergencies, is important to embrace in these care processes. All team members have a role to play. Trauma patients present with a broad range of pathologies. Communication, coordination, and collaboration will always be the cornerstones of effective management of both the patient and family.

Key Points

- Trauma team (TT) membership includes nurses, nurse practitioners, and respiratory therapists in North America.
- Nursing specialists and respiratory therapists play a key role in a high-functioning trauma team.
- In North America, the registered respiratory therapist (RRT) is the airway specialist.
- The RRTs are responsible for initiation, maintenance, and discontinuation of mechanical ventilation, administration of oxygen, other aerosol therapies, and medical gases such as Heliox, inhaled Nitric Oxide, and Epoprostenol.
- Nursing roles include documentation, procedures, medication administration, and general support of all procedures as requested by the team leader.
- It is important to create opportunities for the interprofessional trauma teams to engage in simulation-based practice to hone communication, coordination, and collaboration among the team members to ensure the team can provide timely, effective trauma care.

Acknowledgments The author team would like to acknowledge Peter Dhillon and Tona Laerz who provided their expertise and experience as Respiratory Therapists.

References

1. Gerardo CJ, Glickman SW, Vaslef SN, Chandra A, Pietrobon R, Cairns CB. The rapid impact on mortality rates of a dedicated care team including trauma and emergency physicians at an academic medical center. J Emerg Med. 2011;40:586–91.
2. Trauma, American College of Surgeons. Committee on. (2018) Subcommittee on Advanced Trauma Life Support (ATLS) of the American College of Surgeons (ACS), Committee on Trauma, 1987–1988. Advanced Trauma Life Support Course for Physicians. Chicago, Ill. Committee on Trauma, American College of Surgeons, 1989. (vol. 10th edn). Chicago: American College of Surgeons.
3. Tiel Groenestege-Kreb D, van Maarseveen O, Leenen L, Howell SJ, Trauma team, Br J Anaesth 2014 Aug;113(2):258–265. Available from: https://doi.org/10.1093/bja/aeu236
4. Alismail A, Lopez D. Clinical competencies in advanced practice respiratory therapy education: is it time to entrust the learner? Adv Med Educ Pract. 2020;11:83–9. Available from: https://www.ncbi.nlm.nih.gov/pmc/articles/PMC6986539/ARC

5. Brown CW, Howard M, Morse J. The use of trauma interprofessional simulated education (TIPSE) to enhance role awareness in the emergency department setting. J Interprof Care. 2016 May;30(3):388–90.
6. Salas E, Cooke NJ, Rosen MA. On teams, teamwork and team performance: discoveries and developments. Human Factors. 2008;50(3):540–7.
7. AbdelFattah K, Gardner AK. Should they stay or should they go now? Exploring the impact of team familiarity on interprofessional team training outcomes. Am J Surg. 2018 Feb;215(2):243–9. https://doi.org/10.1016/j.amjsurg.2017.08.048.
8. Murphy M, Curtis K, Lam MK, Palmer CS, Hsu J, McCloughen A. Simulation-based multidisciplinary team training decreases time to critical operations for trauma patients. Injury. 2018 May;49(5):953–958. https://doi.org/10.1016/j.injury.2018.01.009. Epub 2018 Jan 8.
9. Ericcson K, Krampe R, Tesch-Romer C. The role of deliberate practice in the acquisition of expert performance. Psychol Rev. 1993;100(3):363–406.
10. Barr H. An interprofessional journey: a valedictory editorial. J Interprof Care. 2020;34(6):719–25. https://doi.org/10.1080/13561820.2020.1853015.
11. Illeris K. Towards a contemporary and comprehensive theory of learning. Int. J. Lifelong Educ. 2003 July-Aug;22(4):396–406.
12. Edmondson AC. Psychological safety, trust, and learning in organizations: a group-level lens. In: Kramer RM, Cook KS, editors. Trust and distrust in organizations: dilemmas and approaches. Russell Sage Foundation; 2004. p. 239–72.
13. Zakrison TL, Rosenbloom B, McFarlan A, Jovicic A, Soklaridis S, Allen C, et al. Lost information during the handover of critically injured trauma patients: a mixed-methods study. BMJ Qual Saf. 2016;25(12):929–36.
14. Ahmed F, Zhao F, Faraz NA, Qin YJ. How inclusive leadership paves way for psychological well-being of employees during trauma and crisis: a three-wave longitudinal mediation study. J Adv Nurs. 2020;00:1–13.
15. Health Profession Act Respiratory Therapy Alberta. 2021. Available from: https://www.qp.alberta.ca/documents/Acts/H07.pdf
16. Young JQ, Wachter RM, Ten Cate O, O'Sullivan PS, Irby DM. Evidence for validity for the cognitive load inventory for handoffs. Med Educ. 2020;55(2):222–32.
17. Weigl M, Heinrich M, Keil J, Wermelt JZ, Bergman F, Hubertus J et al. Team performance during postsurgical patient handovers in paediatric care. Eur J Pediatr. 2020 Apr;179(4):587–596. https://doi.org/10.1007/s00431-019-03547-w. Epub 2019 Dec 19.
18. Swinton P, Corfield AR, Moultrie C et al. Impact of drug and equipment preparation on pre-hospital emergency Anaesthesia (PHEA) procedural time, error rate and cognitive load. Scand J Trauma Resusc Emerg Med. 2018;28(82). Available from: https://doi.org/10.1186/s13049-018-0549-3
19. Wright A. Day in the life of a trauma nurse practitioner. 2020, Oct. Available from https://www.nursepractitionerschools.com/blog/day-in-the-life-of-trauma-np/
20. Clements A, Curtis K, Horvat L, Shaban RZ. The effect of a nurse team leader on communication and leadership in major trauma resuscitations. Int Emerg Nurs. 2015 Jan;23(1):3–7 https://doi.org/10.1016/j.ienj.2014.04.004. Epub 2014 May 9.
21. Polovitch S, Muertos K, Burns A, Czerwinski A, Flemmer K, Rabon S. Trauma nurse leads in a level 1 trauma center: roles, responsibilities, and trauma performance improvement outcomes. J Trauma Nurs. 2019;26(2):99–103. https://doi.org/10.1097/JTN.0000000000000431. Available from: https://pubmed.ncbi.nlm.nih.gov/30845009/

The Trauma Bay Environment

23

Rondi Gelbard and Kenji Inaba

Introduction

The purpose of the Trauma Resuscitation area is to receive and triage patients that present to the Trauma Center with injuries of varying severity. The area is used to initiate resuscitation and facilitate the correct disposition of these patients. The Trauma Resuscitation area should be designed to accommodate high patient turnover and allow a single team to concurrently manage multiple patients. Its design must take into consideration such factors as accessibility, imaging needs, and procedural capability, as well as employee and patient safety. This chapter will discuss the physical design of the ideal Trauma Resuscitation area and Trauma bay, and the necessary equipment for successful trauma resuscitation. This chapter will also review the importance of direct patient triage from EMS to OR, as well as the benefits of a hybrid trauma/OR suite for the optimal care of the critically injured patient.

General Design of a Trauma Resuscitation Area

Trauma accounts for over 42 million emergency department visits and two million hospital admissions annually across the United States [1]. It is essential that all Trauma centers have an efficient system in place in order to adequately receive and manage critically injured patients [2, 3]. In order to accomplish this, trauma centers should have a designated Trauma Resuscitation area, often housed within or in close proximity to the Emergency Department (ED). The design of the Trauma Resuscitation area should take into consideration the hospital's annual and average daily census and should be of sufficient size to accommodate all admissions and inter-hospital transfers requiring a higher level of care. In many centers, especially those with lower trauma volumes, these rooms are utilized for the resuscitation of all patients, both trauma and non-trauma, surgical and medical, and this must also be taken into consideration. The overall number of individual Trauma bays within the Resuscitation area will also be influenced by factors such as inpatient bed accessibility and available staffing, and should be capable of temporary expansion as part of the hospital's surge capacity plan in case of a disaster.

The Los Angeles County + University of Southern California (LAC+USC) Medical Center is among the busiest Level I trauma centers in the United States. Located east of downtown Los Angeles, LAC+USC is a 650-bed hospital that admits over 6000 trauma patients annually. At LAC+USC, the multi-use Resuscitation area is situated within the Emergency department and consists of individual rooms each capable of physiologic monitoring and a wide range of invasive procedures, including thoracotomies and laparotomies. Other functional areas include a decontamination area, the Triage/Waiting area, and staff workstations. In addition, a pharmacy, clean and dirty utility rooms, and an adjoining Radiology suite are all considered part of the Resuscitation area. Each of these components and their spatial arrangement within the Resuscitation area are discussed separately within this chapter.

Access to the Resuscitation Area

The Resuscitation area should be located on the ground floor for easy access. The layout of the Resuscitation area should allow easy access for ground EMS crews and direct access from the helicopter-landing pad for efficient patient inflow. An elevator for direct transportation to and from a

R. Gelbard
Division of Acute Care Surgery, University of Alabama at Birmingham, Birmingham, AL, USA
e-mail: rgelbard@uabmc.edu

K. Inaba (✉)
Division of Trauma Surgery and Surgical Critical Care, University of Southern California, Los Angeles, CA, USA
e-mail: kinaba@surgery.usc.edu

L. Marshall Gillman, S. Widder (eds.), *Trauma Team Dynamics*, https://doi.org/10.1007/978-3-031-86312-7_23

helicopter pad is critical for patients arriving via rotary wing transport. For patient outflow, there should be access to the radiology suite, operating room, and the Intensive Care Unit. The routes should minimize distance and travel through non-patient care areas where there is public access protecting patient privacy and promoting public safety. All elevators in the pathway should be large enough to accommodate the team, patient, and ventilator, and be card-access controlled to minimize any delay. The access area must be well lit, and protected parking areas for consultants as well as EMS and law enforcement should be available. Appropriate physical barriers should designate "drop off" zones for ambulances and other transport vehicles. The entire access area should be secured and large enough to be used as an external decontamination and triage area in case of a disaster.

Immediate access to CT scanning improves efficiency, and a system for the electronic display of images (i.e. Picture Archiving Communications System or PACS) should be accessible from the Trauma bays and the administrative areas [4]. The CT scanner should be located adjacent to or within the Resuscitation area. A radiology technician must be notified of the patient's imminent arrival and be readily available during the initial evaluation and management of the patient. Rapid access to the Intensive Care Unit and a designated Trauma Operating Room is important for minimizing transfer times of critically ill patients.

Entry to the Pharmacy/medication room should be clearly marked and secure. The area should be accessible to all clinical areas and have sufficient space to accommodate a pharmacy preparation area. Warmed fluids should be housed centrally. For higher volume centers, a satellite blood refrigerator containing O^- or O^+ blood and thawed group AB or low titer group A plasma should be considered. This refrigerator should be located in close proximity to the Resuscitation area. In an emergent situation, when the patient's blood type is not known or compatibility testing has not been completed, these emergency release products can be used.

There should be a room for the storage of equipment and disposable medical supplies that are not currently being used. There should also be a clean utility room of sufficient size for the storage of clean and sterile supplies, and this should have adequate workspace for the preparation of procedure trays and equipment. Access to a dirty utility or disposal room should be available from all clinical areas. The physical design of the Resuscitation area should allow for rapid access to additional equipment if needed. There must be an emergency power supply for the entire Resuscitation area, and a backup system for lighting should be immediately available in the event of a total power failure.

Patient Flow and Disposition

All patient flow upon entry should be directed toward the Reception/Triage area from which the ambulance entrance should be clearly visible [5]. From here, critically ill patients can then be directed to the Resuscitation area. At LAC+USC once the initial assessment and all necessary imaging is completed, the patient is transported via elevator to one of several different locations depending on their injury: the patient ward, ICU, Observation Unit, or the Operating Room. The initial resuscitation should be performed as rapidly as possible. Once the primary survey has been completed and all immediately life-threatening injuries have been addressed, patients requiring surgery should be transferred immediately to the Operating Room or to definitive care without further delay.

It is important to have a designated transport protocol in place for moving the patient rapidly and safely to these areas [2]. The protocol must ensure that the benefits of the transport outweigh the potential risks, and that the same standards of care employed in the trauma bay are also in place during transport. Prior to intra-hospital transport, all life-threatening injuries must be addressed and the patient must be deemed stable enough to withstand transport. A checklist for ensuring that all safety and monitoring issues have been addressed should be considered. There must be an adequate oxygen supply for the duration of the transport as well as a self-inflating bag with PEEP valve, facemask, and oral airway. It is essential that the patient be connected to a portable monitor at all times, with pulse oximetry, blood pressure, and electrocardiography capabilities. Transport equipment should also include basic intubation equipment, resuscitation medications, and IV fluids. A fully equipped Trauma team, including a physician, trauma nurse, and respiratory therapist, must accompany the patient to their next destination and be prepared to administer further resuscitation or transport the patient back to the Trauma bay or to the OR immediately if necessary.

Surge Capacity

The physical plan of the Trauma Resuscitation area should allow for temporary expansion in the setting of mass casualty events [2]. In the setting of a major disaster, other patient assessment areas within the Emergency Department should have the capacity to be converted into functional Trauma bays and the potential to serve as post-anesthesia care units if necessary. In the event that patient assessment areas within the ED cannot be used, waiting rooms, parking areas, and other access areas can be set up outside to receive and triage these patients. A hospital-wide disaster plan should be in place to streamline this process in the event of an emergency

[6]. This requires communication and cooperation among other services within the hospital. Medical and surgical teams must be prepared to decompress the ED and create space for casualties as quickly as possible.

Decontamination

Although covered in greater detail in Sect. 6, a decontamination area is an essential component of the Trauma Resuscitation environment. In the event of chemical/biological disasters or radiation incidents, a plan should be in place for wet and dry decontamination to occur outside of the main Resuscitation area. An internal decontamination room that is directly accessible from the Ambulance bay without entering other parts of the Resuscitation area must also be available. This room must be equipped with running water, a floor drain, and a trap for contaminated water, as well as adequate storage space for personal protective equipment.

Communication

Maintaining clear lines of communication in the Trauma Resuscitation area is essential for maximizing efficiency and minimizing stress in this busy environment. Telephones should be available within each Trauma bay and at each clerical area in order to facilitate this. Direct radio communication should be available to the local EMS services, and an intercom or public address system that can reach all areas of the Resuscitation area (including Reception/Triage and the Radiology suite) [6]. Not only is communication between members of the Trauma team essential, but key personnel including CT scan technicians, Radiologists, and the OR teams, for example, must be notified of the patient's arrival. All key personnel involved in the care of the critically injured patient should be kept apprised of changes in the patient's condition as well as other important events as they occur. In designing the optimal resuscitation area, clear sight lines between Trauma Bays can be extremely beneficial when overseeing the concurrent resuscitation of multiple patients.

Communications systems that involve mobile phones, radios, and pagers are likely to be overwhelmed during a mass casualty or active shooter incident. Therefore, a backup system for ensuring internal and external communication is essential. This may include overhead speaker alert, mass text message, or hospital-wide email alert to disseminate critical information. In the event that all communication systems fail or are overwhelmed, alternative options include a courier service or "runners" to deliver important information. A third-party, off-site source of information, such as the Red Cross, should also be included in the mass casualty preparedness plan to prevent overloading the hospital's telephone system. In the setting of an active shooter incident, dedicated lines of communication with law enforcement agencies are a critical part of the planning process. All emergency departments should work closely with the closest law enforcement agencies prior to an incident to ensure the responding units know the response plan as well as the location of and access points to the critical patient care areas.

Control Center

A central Medical Alert Center (MAC) should be in place for coordinating the distribution of critically injured patients to the closest regional Trauma Center. This will be dictated by the local trauma center availability. In LA County, for example, the MAC serves 13 Trauma Centers with over 20,000 trauma activations annually [7]. Communication begins when the MAC center receives a call from the emergency medical service regarding a critically injured patient. The MAC will then alert the Trauma center that a patient is en route to the hospital. The Trauma center should then have a system in place for announcing the arrival of the injured patient to the Trauma team at any time of day or night, in order to ensure their timely arrival to the Trauma bay. The MAC center is also responsible for coordinating the distribution of patients in a mass casualty incident. Coordinated and timely communication between the MAC and Trauma center is essential for notifying the Trauma team of patient injuries and giving all personnel adequate time to prepare.

Security Considerations

Every Trauma center should ensure the safety and security of the employees, as well as the patients and their visitors. The entrances to the Trauma Resuscitation area must be monitored at all times and access from waiting areas to the treatment areas should be restricted. Security personnel should be immediately available to the Resuscitation area in case a safety or security issue arises, and have the ability to remotely monitor the remainder of the patient care areas and waiting room [8]. Access to the Trauma Center should be secure with an enclosed area that can be used for external triage, mass decontamination, or for high-profile patient management.

Having a secured entrance area is also critical as hospitals and healthcare facilities are high-risk targets for active shooter incidents [9]. In addition, the possession of weapons, even among trauma victims who come through the Emergency Department, is not uncommon [10]. Having a security plan in place to screen all patients entering the trauma bay, using metal detectors or physical examination, will allow for weapons to be detected and secured prior to them entering patient care areas [10].

In the event of an active shooter event, it is essential to have a response plan in place. In non-healthcare settings, the "run, hide, fight" strategy has been shown to be effective. However, many of the patients in the emergency department and trauma bay will not be able to comply with this. Instead, a "secure, preserve, fight" strategy has been proposed as an alternative approach in the healthcare setting [9]. Patient care areas where life-sustaining treatments can be provided during the incident must be identified and secured with locking devices or barricades. The optimal design of the emergency department and trauma bay areas will allow for compartmentalization, with access points that can be rapidly sealed, allowing this life-sustaining patient care to continue.

The Trauma Bay

Resuscitation areas will vary in the number of individual "Trauma bays" that they contain. These are often separated by movable partitions in order to maintain patient privacy but allow communication and direct sight lines in cases of multiple casualty incidents. The physical layout of a typical civilian trauma bay is shown in Fig. 23.1.

Each Trauma bay should have a bed in the center that allows for complete access to the patient from all directions. The Trauma bay must have adequate lighting and sufficient space to allow for movement of staff and equipment around the work area. A portable ventilator is usually located at the head of the bed, along with a large monitor that is clearly visible to all Trauma team members. The monitor should be capable of displaying hemodynamic parameters including electrocardiogram (ECG) tracings, non-invasive blood pressure (NIBP), pulse oximetry, respiratory rate, and body temperature [11]. Lab values including thromboelastography (TEG) tracings can also be projected for the team to see. Each bed space should be equipped with a wall-mounted ophthalmoscope and otoscope, and might contain infusion pumps, fluid warming devices, rapid infusion systems, and a portable monitor/defibrillator. At LAC+USC, a boom-mounted ultrasound machine is located at the head of the bed in each Trauma bay, allowing for immediate Focused Assessment with Sonography for Trauma (FAST) and eFAST during the initial assessment of the patient.

Each Trauma Bay must be equipped for the active resuscitation of at least one patient. If the surge capacity plan involves housing multiple patients in a single room, redundancy in the resuscitation equipment must be considered. Equipment and supplies should be organized on clearly labeled shelves or mobile carts. Mobile carts allow for convenient one-stop shopping and minimize wastage of actions and time of the trauma team. These might include an airway cart, surgical procedure cart, and an IV access cart [2]. The airway cart contains equipment such as laryngoscopes with various blades, masks, bag-valve-mask devices, suction devices, carbon dioxide detectors, stylets, and endotracheal tubes of different sizes. Equipment for difficult airway situations, including cricothyrotomy, should also be readily available.

The procedure cart must contain sterile gloves, masks, gowns, and eye protection, as well as equipment for the insertion of central venous catheters, thoracostomy tubes, nasogastric tubes, and bladder catheters. The cart should also contain pre-labeled sterilized trays with supplies for diagnostic peritoneal lavage, thoracostomy tubes, and resuscitative thoracotomies. These procedure carts must be checked for

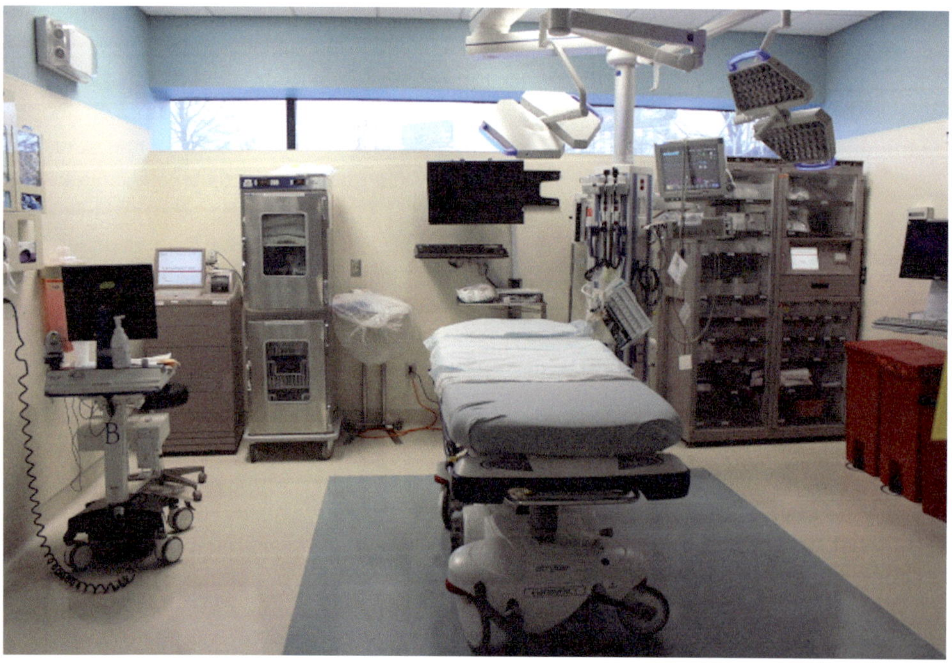

Fig. 23.1 Photograph of the physical layout of a typical trauma bay. A bed is shown in the center of the room. A monitoring display, IV poles, and a wall-mounted ophthalmoscope and otoscope are located at the head of the bed. Equipment and supplies are located on clearly labeled shelves at the back of the room. Off to the right, there is a workstation containing a computer and forms for documentation, and to the left, disposal containers for used needles and other sharp objects

inventory and replenished immediately after use. The IV access cart contains the necessary supplies for the insertion of peripheral venous catheters, arterial catheters, central venous catheters, and intra-osseous catheters, as well as blood sampling tubes and IV fluids. Disposal containers for used needles and other sharp objects should be accessible within each room, and a cart containing suture materials, splinting materials, and immobilization devices such as cervical collars and pelvic binders should be located nearby. Each Trauma bay should contain a sink for hand washing as well as dispensers with non-sterile latex gloves, gowns, masks, face shields, and shoe covers to assist with personal protection. At LAC+USC, there is also a pneumatic tube system within the Resuscitation area for the rapid transport of blood samples to the central laboratory. The use of pneumatic tubes has been found to significantly decrease turnaround times for laboratory results and to improve the overall efficiency of patient care [4].

Trauma Observation Unit Setup

A Short Stay or Observation Unit is an effective way of managing patients with an expected length of stay less than 24 h. At LAC+USC, the Surgical Observation Unit (SOU) contains 10 beds and is staffed by nurses in a 2:1 ratio, as well as mid-level providers. It is easily accessed from the Resuscitation area and is adjacent to the OR. Patients who require close serial clinical examinations as part of non-operative management of a penetrating injury, or who require resuscitation prior to operation, can be moved here, decompressing the resuscitation areas.

Special Situations

Noise Discipline in Trauma Resuscitation

According to Chhangani et al., the level of ambient noise is inversely related to the coordinated activity of the trauma team [2]. A professional environment without excessive noise should be maintained at all times within the Trauma Resuscitation area. Keeping ambient noise to a minimum will minimize patient anxiety, improve team efficiency, and allow the Trauma team leader to be heard by all those participating in the resuscitation. This is particularly important in Mass Casualty Incidents.

Resuscitation in the Operating Room

The unstable patient with a clear mechanism of injury requiring operative intervention may bypass the Trauma bay and proceed directly to the Trauma Operating Room. The Trauma OR is ideally located near or adjacent to the Resuscitation area to minimize transportation times, and should be appropriately staffed by a dedicated team that includes an Anesthesiologist, circulating nurse, scrub nurse, and additional OR personnel depending on the nature of the injury. The Trauma OR should be immediately available 24 h per day and be prepared to accommodate an unstable patient with little advanced notice [12]. In addition to the equipment found in the Trauma bay, the Trauma OR also contains an anesthesia machine, multiple infusion pumps, auto-transfusion devices, and access to sterilized surgical supplies.

Hybrid Operating Rooms

Over the past several years, hybrid operating rooms have emerged that combine interventional and surgical procedures for the care of the critically injured patient. The hybrid OR, equipped with a fixed C-arm and angiography table, allows for specialized interventions to be carried out simultaneously and therefore maximizes efficiency [13–15]. Unstable patients with significant hemorrhage from pelvic fractures, for example, can be transported to the hybrid OR for pelvic packing and internal iliac artery control followed by angioembolization without ever leaving the Operating Room. The layout of a typical hybrid Trauma OR is depicted in Fig. 23.2. Hybrid ORs will be covered furtherin Chap. 25.

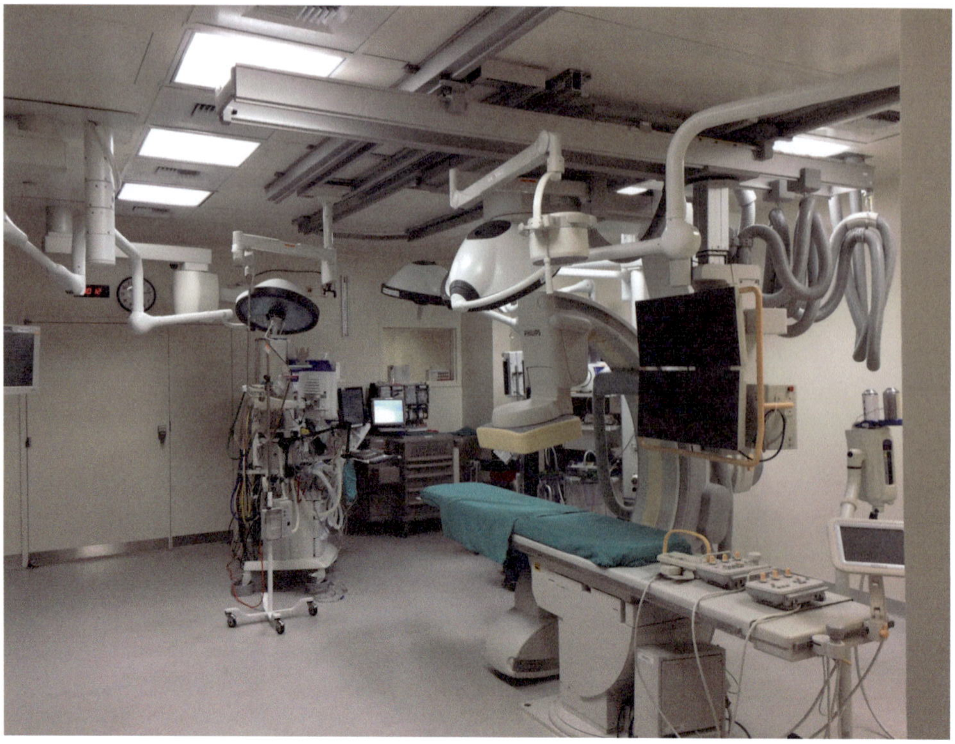

Fig. 23.2 Photograph of a typical hybrid operating room at a Level I trauma center. The OR contains the same equipment and materials as the Trauma bay, all arranged around a centrally placed operating room table. The hybrid OR is also equipped with a fixed C-arm and angiography table that allows for specialized interventions to be carried out simultaneously

Conclusion

A well-designed Trauma Resuscitation area facilitates the rapid mobilization of personnel and resources, and streamlines the evaluation, resuscitation, and treatment of critically injured patients. The physical design of the space not only impacts staff workflow and communication but also directly affects all steps of the patient triage and resuscitation. In this era of cost containment, building flexibility into the design will ensure maximal efficiency in usage of the space while allowing for rapid ramp-up in case of mass casualties. As future technological advances occur, flexibility in design will also allow the resuscitation area to adapt and continue providing optimal care.

Key Points

- The design of the Resuscitation area should allow for efficient patient inflow and outflow.
- The entrance to the Resuscitation area should be well lit with designated "drop off" zones; it must be secure and large enough to be used as an external decontamination and triage area in case of a disaster.
- The physical plan of the Trauma Resuscitation areas should allow for temporary expansion as part of a surge capacity plan.
- An Observation Unit is an effective way of managing patients who require close serial examinations or resuscitation prior to surgery and can decompress the Resuscitation area.
- Preparation is critical and the Resuscitation area should include all necessary equipment and supplies for the physiologic monitoring and active resuscitation of the trauma patient.
- Communication is key, and the design of the Resuscitation area must ensure clear lines of communication at all stages of patient triage and resuscitation.
- A strategic response plan and specific security measures should be in place to reduce potential harm in the event of an active shooter incident.

References

1. National Trauma Institute. "Trauma Statistics." http://www.nationaltraumainstitute.org/home/trauma_statistics.html [online]. Accessed 26 Oct 2013.
2. Chhangani SV, et al. Resuscitation suite and operating room readiness. In: William CW, Grande CM, Hoyt DB, editors. Trauma: emergency resuscitation, perioperative anesthesia, surgical management. New York: Informa Healthcare USA, Inc; 2007.
3. Markovchick VJ, Moore EE. Optimal trauma outcome: trauma system design and the trauma team. Emerg Med Clin N Am. 2007;25:643–54.
4. McKay JI. Building the emergency Department of the Future: philosophical, operational and physical dimensions. Nurs Clin North Am. 2002;37(1):111–22.

5. Huddy J, McKay. The top 25 problems to avoid when planning your new emergency department. J Emerg Nurs. 1996;22(4):296–301.
6. Hoyt DB, Coimbra R. Trauma systems. Surg Clin N Am. 2007;87:21–35.
7. Cryer HG, Hiatt JR. Trauma system: the backbone of disaster preparedness. J Trauma. 2009;67(2):S111–3.
8. Kennedy MP. Violence in emergency departments: under-reported, unconstrained, and unconscionable. Med J Aust. 2005;183:362–5.
9. Inaba K, Eastman AL, Jacobs LM, Mattox KL. Active-shooter response at a health care facility. NEJM. 2018;379:583–6.
10. Smalley C, O'Neil M, Engineer R, Simon E, Snow G, Podalsky S. Dangerous weapons confiscated after implementation of routine screening across a healthcare system. Am J Emerg Med. 2017;36:1497–520.
11. Parlak S, Sarcevic A, Marsic I, Burd RS. Introducing RFID technology in dynamic and time-critical medical settings: requirements and challenges. J Biomed Inform. 2012;45(5):958–74.
12. Brasel KJ, Adason J, Weigelt JA. Dedicated operating room for trauma: a costly recommendation. J Trauma. 1998;44(5):832–8.
13. Pryor JP, Braslow B, Reilly PM, Gullamondegi O, Hedrick JH, Schwab CW. The evolving role of interventional radiology in trauma care. J Trauma. 2005;59:102–4.
14. Cate G, Fosse E, Hol PK, Samset E, Bock RW, McKinsey JF, et al. Integrating surgery and radiology in one suite: a multicenter study. J Vasc Surg. 2004;40(3):494–9.
15. Calligaro KD, Dougherty MJ, Patterson DE, Raviola CA, DeLaurentis DA. Value of an endovascular suite in the operating room. Ann Vasc Surg. 1998;12(3):296–8.

24 Trauma Bay Development and Design Designed to Perform: How Simulation Can Inform the Design of Elite Trauma Resuscitation Environments

Andrew Petrosoniak, Frank Panici, and Christopher Hicks

Introduction

Poor design in healthcare is common [1, 2]. Design flaws are more than simple nuisances but rather require constant improvised or ad hoc work-around solutions that expose patients and providers to risks and safety hazard [3]. During a trauma resuscitation when the chest tube equipment is laid out over the patient instead of a purposely design procedure cart, situated in a room designed to facilitate trauma care, the reflex should be to recognize how the system fails to promote the safe performance of the procedure.

In contrast, most healthcare workers, including those who care for the critically injured, are not conditioned to respond by asking how the system design failed the patient and the team. We have been socialized to *take pride* in our ability to overcome poor designs and *just make things work*. In most modern healthcare systems, the onus for avoiding hazards and safety threats falls almost exclusively on the provider [4, 5]—a model that is both unethical and unsustainable. Ask any trauma systems provider: barriers to safe and effective care consistently arise from systemic encumbrances that impact their energy and impair their determination [6]. It is not unusual for trauma clinicians to be searching for the patient's source of bleeding while searching even harder for the life-saving equipment they need to stop it.

Trauma resuscitation exemplifies the complexity that exists within healthcare [7]. Clinicians are faced with competing priorities, diagnostic uncertainty, and dynamic clinical situations accentuated by critical illness. This culminates in challenges linked to logistics, processes, and systems as much as the inherently difficult diagnostic and management decisions. A rational and sustainable way forward for the engineering of resilient trauma systems requires up-front investments in understanding system complexity and potential vulnerabilities. This approach places the end-user, both patients and clinicians, at the center of the design process [8]. At every point in the design process, the question should be asked: "Is the choice we're making increasing safety or increasing risk?" [9].

In this chapter, we describe a framework for the design of trauma resuscitation environments that emphasizes the needs of the end-users (patients and providers) linked to a systems-thinking perspective. This process builds on our own experience in the design of a new trauma bay combined with evidence-based design principles. In summary, this four-phased approach (design-build-train-excel) systematically supports the conceptualization (*design*), prototyping (*build*), orientation and utilization of high-performance teams (*train*), and constant evaluation (*excel*) necessary to create a highly functional space.

Design

Formalizing Clinician-Designer-Builder Partnerships

The typical process for the design and construction of trauma resuscitation environments can be described as "fragmented" at best [2]. It is not uncommon for an entire clinical space to be constructed by teams working in silos with little communication between them. Siloed processes may result in clinical environments that lack usability especially when seconds are the difference between life and death.

The success of any project is tightly linked with the quality of the team responsible for its completion. In trauma care, the design of a trauma resuscitation space requires expertise in clinical care, logistics, and architecture. Clinicians are not

A. Petrosoniak (✉) · C. Hicks
Department of Medicine, University of Toronto, Toronto, ON, Canada

Department of Emergency Medicine, St. Michael's Hospital, Toronto, ON, Canada
e-mail: Christopher.Hicks@unityhealth.to

F. Panici
Health Sciences, NORR Architects & Engineers Ltd., Toronto, ON, Canada
e-mail: Frank.Panici@norr.com

L. Marshall Gillman, S. Widder (eds.), *Trauma Team Dynamics*, https://doi.org/10.1007/978-3-031-86312-7_24

architects, contractors, or project managers, nor should they pretend to be. Formalizing partnerships between builders and end-users is absolutely critical. To be effective, trauma bay design can't happen in a bubble, but rather it should bring all relevant parties to the table to co-create, prototype, and test solutions prior to implementation. A nurse with a design idea for a resuscitation room layout needs to be able to interface with an architect to create a rendering, simulationists to test and generate feedback, and project managers to cost, plan, and implement solutions.

In our experience, engagement with the architectural design team is critical upon project conception. This provides ample opportunity for architects, project managers, and other non-clinical personnel to deeply understand the needs, workflows, and challenges of the end-users. These early conversations, facilitated through multiple techniques that will be discussed below, will ensure even the earliest plans and designs will be informed by end-user feedback.

A Human-Centered Approach

A purposefully designed trauma bay may be the difference between life and death when a team is required to respond in a rapid and coordinated fashion to a hemodynamically unstable patient requiring a sequence of time-sensitive interventions. The inherent challenges of trauma care are amplified when they occur within poorly designed clinical spaces. Providers have become accustomed to overcoming such safety threats and inefficiencies, relying on their individual and team resilience. The link between the physical space and care delivery cannot be overstated. As eloquently stated by author James Clear:

> The environment is the invisible hand that shapes human behavior

Increasingly, healthcare has followed the way of other domains by adopting a human-centered design processes [10, 11]. This approach involves applying the human perspective throughout all steps of the problem-solving process. This links closely with *participatory ergonomics* whereby people are involved in the planning of their own work, resulting in improved productivity [12]. This deeper understanding of *work as done* has been achieved recently using simulation in several case studies of assembly line and healthcare systems design [13–16].

Participatory ergonomics and human-centered design, well studied in several domains, have yet to be robustly applied within the design of the trauma care environment. We advocate for an easily implementable framework to support these principles by way of simulation-informed clinical design. This puts the patient, clinician, and other involved care providers front and center in the design process [17]. Within this process, we utilized design thinking methodology, a toolkit familiar to those in technology and business, to create end-user optimized designs [18–20]. Simulation-informed clinical design places a significant emphasis on understanding the needs of the end-user. This upfront investment pays dividends later through design solutions that are iteratively prototyped, achieving proven benefits for patient, provider, and system [21].

The Missing Link

Business and technology sectors have long understood the importance of the customer experience [22]. The patient experience during healthcare delivery is the subject of increasing interest among healthcare organizations as they integrate patient-centered metrics in their evaluation processes [23]. Much of this focus relates to patient-provider interactions and processes to improve pain control or wait times. There is a lack of well-formulated mechanisms, however, to integrate the patient perspective during the design of new healthcare infrastructure, including those for trauma care. The importance of creating positive patient experiences cannot be discounted as it serves to enhance trust among clinicians, reduce posttraumatic stress disorder, and improve patient outcomes [24].

An illustrative example of the positive impact of integrating the patient experience into the design process comes from Doug Dietz, an executive at General Electric [25, 26]. He was tasked with designing a new MRI machine for pediatric patients. When he observed the machine in use, he saw children so scared and anxious that many required sedation. While satisfied with the technical outputs of the machine, he realized it did not meet the needs of the "end-user," in this case the children. Using principles of human-centered design and design thinking methodology, he re-designed the experience to feature "adventure" environments that resonated with children, like an MRI room to mimic a pirate ship. Multiple iterations of child-friendly designs were created and the experience was completely re-imagined and re-designed. These designs may sound great, but is there a clinically relevant outcome? Interestingly, this project resulted in a substantial reduction in the need for sedation, both a safety and patient-centered outcome [27]. An amazing result from a seemingly simple yet elegant design.

How can we translate the patient perspective into the trauma bay design process? Following the design thinking methodology, the first step is *empathize*, whereby the designers seek to better understand the needs of the user. There is growing research about the emotions experienced by trauma patients [24]. Semi-structured interviews can offer designers a unique lens through the eyes of the patient and how the care process can be improved without compromising efficacy. Additionally, standardized patients can provide their insights during the debriefing phase of a simulation session. Ensuring the architects and design team are present only further enhances the value of the session.

We believe that each trauma program should seek to understand the unique aspects of the patient experience at their institution to inform future designs, and we summarize some common themes from both the literature and our personal experiences: [24, 28, 29].

1. Trauma patients experience a range of emotions that may impact their understanding of the steps taken during a resuscitation.
2. Pain is nearly ubiquitous in trauma and will substantially impact the patient experiences.
3. Exposure to strangers while necessary to provide care creates a vulnerable environment.
4. Uncertainty and concern about the patient's clinical condition are common among family members.

It is our contention that these themes, while not all-encompassing, represent a starting point to inform unique design features to enhance the patient experience. For example, it may be possible to mitigate some of the negative emotions inherent with serious injuries with adjustments in noise and wall color or perhaps calming images on the ceiling that serve to reassure the patient that they will be cared for with dignity and respect. Additional design features might serve to support patient-oriented outcomes such as timely analgesia delivery.

The Case for Less

In a healthcare system hungry for additional capacity, the desire for more can drive decision-making, without considering if more translates to better. At St Michael's Hospital in Toronto, the design for a new trauma bay included expanding from two to three stretchers, ostensibly to care for 50% more critically injured patients at any given time.

Added capacity has advantages but presents challenges as well, many of which are difficult to see. These latent hazards are threats to patient and provider safety that aren't easily identified until they create a problem, which carries the potential for adverse events and harm [30–32].

We used simulation-informed clinical design to put both our old and new trauma bays through their paces [17, 32–35]. To do so, we brought a number of simulation modalities to bear, selected based on the task at hand:

- Current state analysis: In situ simulation exercises based on known difficult trauma cases, run with the full team in the "old" trauma room
- Hazard matrix, framework analysis, and video review with the help of human factors engineers
- Table-top talk simulations of the new space, using scale models and design schematics
- Full-scale simulations in mock-ups of the proposed new space, pre-construction
- In situ simulation in the constructed new space, prior to opening for clinical care

At every step, our findings were shared with the design and project management teams. It turns out that the crowding of three stretchers created a series of negative trade-offs and limited the ability to deliver safe and timely care. What followed was a reworking of the space and design to feature a two-stretcher steady state with the ability to flex up to three if necessary; clear floor markings to preserve the circle of care around the patient's head, neck, and torso; and clinical logistics to support bedside critical care procedures.

Evidence-Based Design

With growing research in healthcare design, evidence-based healthcare design (EBD) has emerged as an important influence as new facilities are built. The Center for Health Design, an organization that supports this approach, defines EBD as "the process of basing decision about the built environment on credible research to achieve the best possible outcomes" [36].

Although it seems obvious that resuscitation spaces for critically injured patients should be designed using research and end-user input, the use of EBD in this area is still relatively new. The Agency for Healthcare Research and Quality (AHRQ) partnered with the Centre for Health Design and proposed 10 evidence-based design considerations. While these represent generic principles, each is backed by evidence that it positively impacts healthcare outcomes [37]. We describe how these 10 principles are relevant to the built environment of the trauma bay (Table 24.1). Notably, institutions may prioritize each principle differently based on their current environment, culture, and user perspectives. We advocate that these principles be included in the design process which may occur in several ways including:

1. Conversation guide between designers-builders-clinicians
2. Checkpoints for clinicians to ensure appropriate elements considered
3. Content to inform and support the design evaluation process

Table 24.1 Evidence-based design principles applied to the trauma resuscitation environment

Evidence-based design principles	Examples relevant to trauma bay design
Standardization	Implementation of pre-arrival/pre-departure checklists to ensure key aspects of care completed
Staff fatigue	Optimize layout of the space to ensure high-use items are near the bedside and easily accessible while less frequently used items placed further to minimize encumbrances to movement around the patient
Enhance visibility to patients	Vital sign monitors in multiple locations (e.g., head of bed, foot of bed) to enhance visibility
Reduce noise	Ventilation systems that function quietly to minimize additional noise Floor markings and crowd control designs that ensure efficient workflows resulting reductions in unnecessary noise and chatter
Reduce communication breakdown	Ergonomically optimized labeling of equipment to help retrieval of necessary equipment Personnel stickers for each team member denoting name/role/specialty to improve intra-team communication
Control/eliminate sources infection	Designs that promote the easy application of PPE Keep space around the patient clear, promoting both free movement of team members and minimizing splatter onto equipment
Minimize environmental hazards	Optimize moveable procedure carts that can be brought to the bedside when needed Floor markings that designate a "circle of care" or lines indicating care team and support team Flat workspaces for equipment during procedures
Automate where possible	Integration of vital signs and laboratory results into clinical design support tools (e.g., triggers for massive hemorrhage protocol activation) Motion sensors to trigger device activation (e.g., clinical timers, video recordings) High-risk tasks (e.g., blood product checks and administration)
Support patient and family involvement in care	Space for family to wait with dedicated trauma team members to liaise with family/friends Physical designs that serve to calm and reassure patients (e.g., calming images on ceilings)
Consider adjacencies	Construction trauma bay near EMS entry; planning for CT scanner adjacent to trauma bay

Design Priorities Specific to Trauma

Based on our research studying trauma teams within their authentic workplace, we have established more specific design priorities that align with the broad evidence-based design principles from AHRQ [32]. Building on the work of other groups and based on our own observations, we identified several recurrent latent safety threat (LSTs) themes that manifest during trauma care [5, 30, 32, 33, 38, 39]. LSTs can be defined as "previously unrecognized system-based conditions that under certain circumstances manifest and threaten patient safety" [30]. These LSTs include the physical workspace and interpersonal and team communication, establishing shared mental models, infection prevention/safety, equipment, and procedural/process-based issues. By understanding the frequency of such safety threats, design teams can look to proactively "design out" these hazards from occurring. More simply, design features can be included that serve to eliminate or mitigate LSTs.

Importantly, these themes, while likely generalizable may not apply to every institution or organization. An in-depth analysis by the design team using a multi-modal approach including simulation within the existing space, stakeholder and end-user interviews, morbidity and mortality reports, and adverse event reviews will help form a comprehensive understanding of the design priorities needed. At our institution, we applied a detailed workplace analysis using these methods before we began construction of our new trauma bay (Fig. 24.1). Through this process, we identified several unique design features relevant to trauma care:

1. *Ensure 360° access to the patient*: Critically injured patients require a range of time-sensitive interventions, including intubation, intravenous access, chest tubes, and extremity splints, and optimizing access to the entire body is essential.
2. *Optimize sightlines to vital sign monitors*: Conventional resuscitation designs use a single monitor at the head of the bed. The addition of vital sign monitors at the side and foot of the bed increases visibility among team members of key physiologic parameters that will dictate management interventions.
3. *Use modular and moveable task-based carts*: To ensure easy access around the patient, the space should not be cluttered with equipment. To facilitate this, modular and moveable task-based carts can be stationed outside of the immediate care space and brought to the bedside on an as-needed basis.
4. *Design room layout and equipment placement according to frequency of use*: There is predictable equipment that will be needed frequently while other equipment rarely. A prioritization strategy should balance frequency of use with urgency (e.g., thoracotomy kit while rarely used should be positioned relatively near the bedside, while orthopedic supplies, which are less urgent items, can be placed further away).

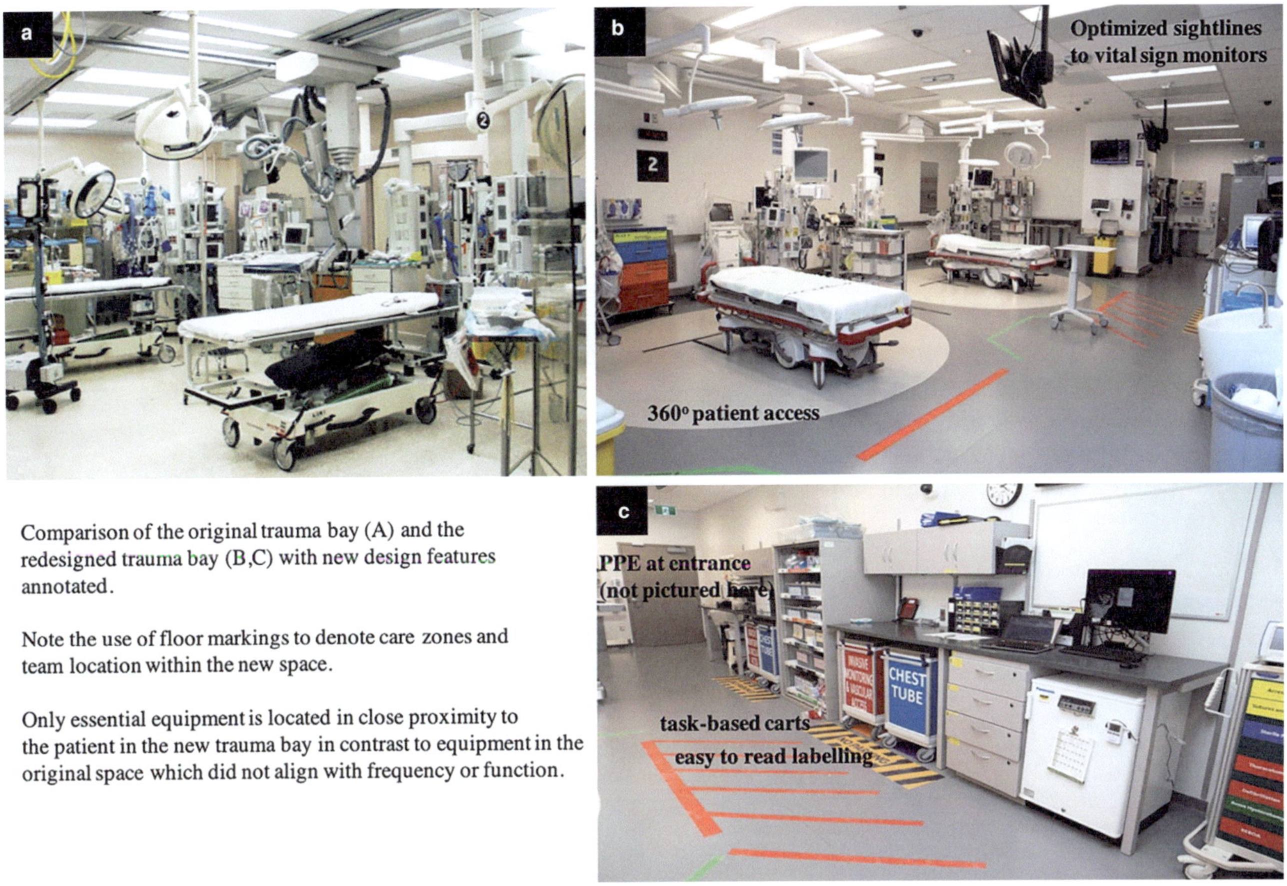

Fig. 24.1 A comparison of the original trauma bay with the newly redesigned trauma bay using a comprehensive design strategy including simulation-informed design. (Location: St. Michael's Hospital, Toronto, Canada; photo credit: Katie Cooper)

5. *Apply an equipment labeling approach that is clinician focused*: Easily readable, color-coded, and appropriately positioned to facilitate rapid location and acquisition of necessary equipment while under stress.
6. *Promote PPE application and personnel identification*: Position PPE at the entrance in easily accessible locations to improve compliance and safety for team members. The use of identification stickers can further improve team communication and promote a shared understanding of management plans.

Build

The transition from the design phase to the build phase is described as discrete for the purposes of this chapter; however, it may overlap substantially as the design team will toggle between each phase. The initial principles and features that emerged from the design phase, during the build phase, are prototyped and more closely evaluated in a manner that establishes their utility within the local institution. For example, the design team will apply the principle of creating a physical layout that aligns with frequency and urgency of use of equipment. During the build phase, prototyping of this layout may determine that assumptions and design decisions do not function optimally once simulated and minor design changes are required.

To accomplish much of the work during the build phase, we apply simulation-informed clinical design in a more detailed manner using a range of simulation techniques, following the functional requirements or objectives of the project [40]. This approach is growing in its application; however, it remains novel within the trauma community. Several groups have described their experience with various forms of simulation-informed clinical design. This spans its application to guide the early design throughout the design process and ultimately testing the clinical space prior to opening for patient care [37, 41–46]. A common thread among each group is the continued involvement of the design team who are invited and participate in the simulation-informed clinical design process.

In our experience, the presence of architects and the construction team during simulations of design prototypes promotes a shared mental model of features that are and are not functional. More specifically, the design team comes to understand how "work as imagined" may differ with "work as done." The net result is an increased probability that the final product will function optimally for the end-users, both clinicians and patients alike.

Simulation involves the re-creation of real-world events, using a variety of techniques and tools like high-tech patient simulators, partial task trainers, and patient actors. This suite of options allows the simulation to immerse the trauma team in a realistic environment to elicit reflection and promote learning. When simulation is used to support design of new clinical infrastructure, the unit of analysis is the physical space and the systems within it. This "allows for reliable and repeatable analysis of hazards and the design and testing of controls to mitigate those hazards at a system level" [9].

There are multiple simulation techniques, each serving a specific purpose, that can be applied throughout the project. Below, we describe four common techniques used during simulation-informed clinical design projects (Table 24.2).

Each technique described in Table 24.2, alone, will not provide sufficient information to inform the entire design of a new trauma environment, but rather we advocate that a combination of techniques be used to provide a comprehensive understanding and evaluation of the design. Which technique is used depends on several factors, including:

1. Session objectives
2. Time, personnel, and equipment resources available to the team
3. Expertise to conduct the session(s)
4. Project timeline (Fig. 24.2)

Table 24.2 Descriptions of simulation modalities and application within the design of trauma infrastructure

Simulation modality	Application in trauma care design
Tabletop simulation *Small-scale replica of the clinical space to evaluate workflows, systems, and spaces, contributing to a macro-understanding of the physical space*	A resource-efficient simulation modality that enables the design team to observe high-level trauma workflows and processes using blueprints or plans of the new space Adjacency considerations, including patient transport to the OR and/or CT scan, are easily evaluated
Mock-up simulation *Replica of the clinical environment to evaluate personnel movement, equipment location, and clinical care within a space similar or identical in size to the final product*	A technique that allows trauma clinicians to immersively experience a replica of the new design A trauma team can practice diagnostic and management strategies with real or replica equipment to evaluate the adequacy of the physical space, the location of equipment, and their abilities to provide time-sensitive care The environmental fidelity may vary from tape on the floors denoting equipment and walls to an identical recreation of the soon-to-be-constructed trauma environment
In situ simulation *Simulation within the authentic clinical environment*	This modality can be used to understand the existing trauma space, including current workflows, deficiencies, and areas for opportunity Additionally, this technique can be used to "crash" test equipment and workflows (e.g., thoracotomy, intubation) within the newly constructed trauma bay to ensure all elements required for trauma care are fully functional before opening day
Computer-based simulation *Clinical environments recreated using computer-based technology*	An effective technique to design and iteratively refine a new trauma bay before investing in the actual construction of the space Trauma clinicians can be provided tasks (e.g., chest tube insertion) within the virtual environment and provide feedback on feasibility, space optimization, and placement of equipment

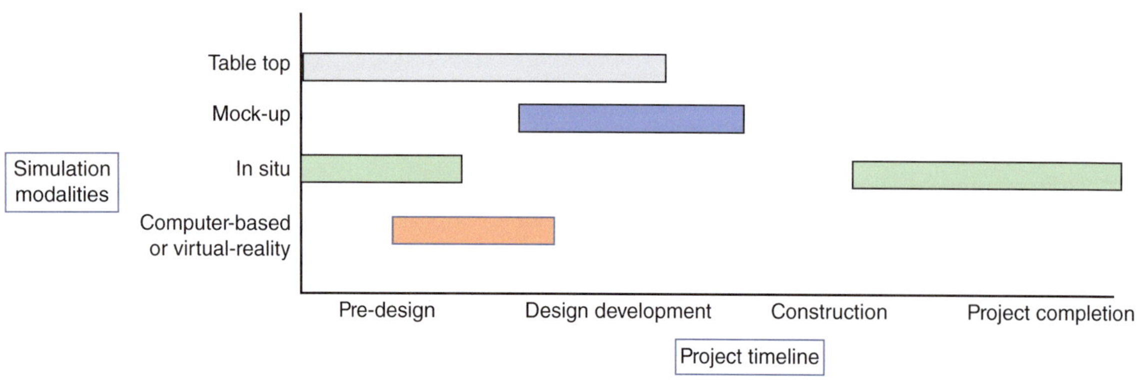

Fig. 24.2 Proposed sequence of simulation techniques applied during the design of a new trauma resuscitation environment

How Can Simulation-Based Movement Tracking Be Integrated into Healthcare Design?

As our modes of healthcare delivery become increasingly complex, more advanced techniques to understand, study, and optimize care are needed. Efficiency is even more important when patients are in the throes of a life-threatening condition. The last thing that any team needs is to be searching for equipment scattered around the room while a patient is lying on the stretcher waiting for a life-threatening intervention. One tool to combat these inefficiencies and improve the design of clinical spaces is movement tracking. That is, technology that allows for removing extraneous information to highlight locations where clinicians move and concentrate their time.

Non-healthcare industries have long understood the value of movement tracking. Look no further than UPS, which studied the movement of their delivery vans [47]. At first glance, it would seem to make sense that vans take the most direct route. Faster is better right? Think again. The company extensively studied delivery routes and realized they could make substantial gas savings by routing their vehicles to avoid left turns. It may add extra miles on individual routes, but overall speed increased and both total mileage and gas consumption decreased. Why? Because left turns result in increased accidents and longer waits at lights. The result: 1110 fewer trucks and ten million fewer gallons of fuel. This counterintuitive initiative only resulted from focused movement tracking data.

We used in situ simulation coupled with movement tracking to study how a high-performance trauma team interacted with the clinical environment (Fig. 24.3) [34]. We conducted the exact same simulation several times over the course of a year within our trauma bay. What did we find?

1. There are substantial differences in the distance traveled between clinicians even when they're performing the same task. Why?
2. Small design changes can drastically alter how far people move. Not surprisingly, packaging essential equipment to perform a life-threatening procedure resulted in more efficient movement than if the equipment was scattered around the room.
3. Just studying the movement of people proved to be eye-opening, as clinicians suddenly realized how often they found themselves walking aimlessly around the room searching for equipment. The opportunity to observe movement tracking maps was the light bulb that many needed to prompt important design changes.

In addition to our work, other researchers and design groups now use similar movement tracking techniques (also described as link analyses) [44, 46, 48, 49]. Given the effort and resources required for these investigations, the design team should rightly ask whether it is worth it? Specifically, do participants move and behave in the same way during mock-up simulations as within the actual space? If the answer is yes, then important information can be gained to guide the design of a new clinical space without investment in construction costs. Researchers from Alberta, Canada, investigated this question by evaluating newly constructed medication rooms in a hospital space [46]. They built a high (detailed) and low (simple) fidelity mock-up along with a virtual reality version of the space and compared movement from various tasks with video recordings within the actual clinical after it opened to patient care (Fig. 24.4). They concluded the "workflow within each of the three mock-up types accurately represents realistic workflow in a medication room." Our own observations and research in the trauma

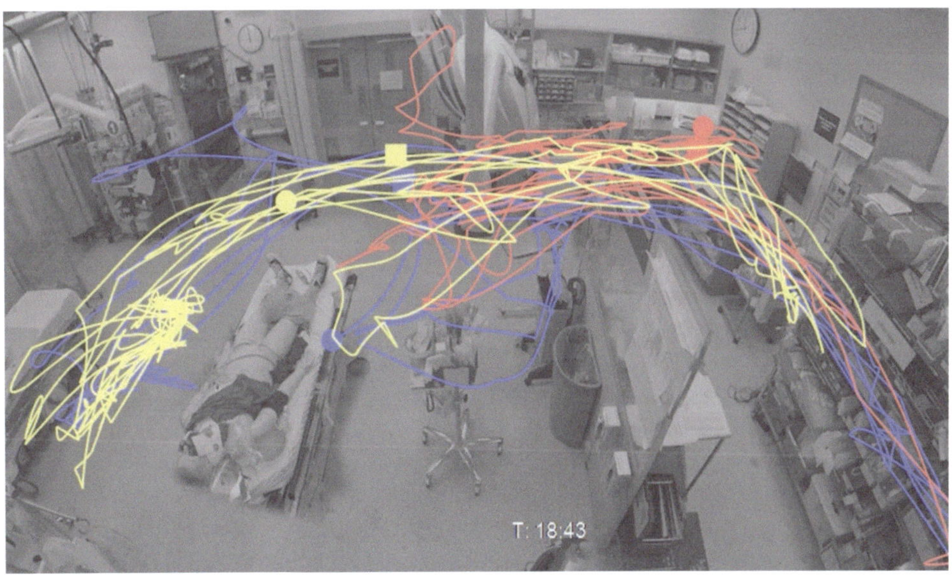

Fig. 24.3 Movement tracking diagram during a simulated trauma resuscitation. Each line represents the movement of a clinical team member over the course of the 18-min simulation

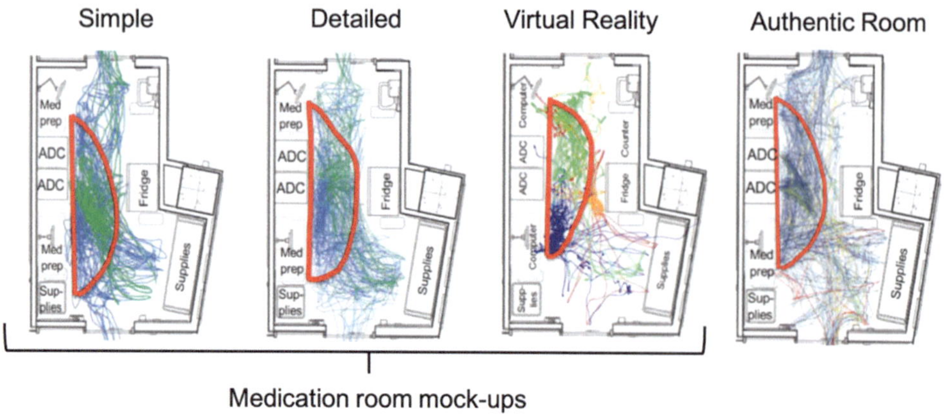

Fig. 24.4 Movement tracking data within three mock-ups (simple, detailed, virtual reality) of a medication room compared to the actual clinical space (authentic room). (Modified from Alberta HQCo [46])

resuscitation environment support these findings. It is very likely that well-developed simulations within trauma mock-ups will provide accurate and representative data of actual trauma resuscitation workflows.

A key aspect to any design project is understanding the end-user. Movement tracking provides a unique look at how the end-user interacts with their space, a perspective that simply is not possible when the individual is questioned directly. When we asked clinicians about how long it took to find equipment or how far they traveled, their estimates were not even close. It is clear that people find it conceptually difficult to accurately recall movement, especially under times of stress. Tracing maps clearly illustrate points of congestion and opportunities for design improvements.

The future of clinical space design includes a deeper appreciation of "how" work is done. What better way to understand the "how" than directly observing the path required to make it happen? Objective and focused efforts to track movement are essential design tools to optimize spatial utilization, reduce time, and save money.

Train

A simulation-informed clinical design approach to the construction of a new trauma resuscitation environment is closely linked to the team training plans once the space is operational. While a detailed overview of trauma team training is published elsewhere and beyond the scope of this chapter [50], there is no doubt that the built environment is closely linked to team performance.

Look no further than the Formula 1 racing industry [51, 52]. The sport's pit crews have become the archetype of team performance. In pairs, the team can remove and replace four tires, a remarkable feat and one that is only achieved with intense training. While training is critical, the teams could not perform tasks with such speed without perfectly designed equipment and team members perfectly positioned around the car. This link between design and function is a key to success that many industries have long appreciated. In acute care medicine, we are only now beginning to realize the importance of form-fitting function, and once optimized, team performance and ultimately patient outcomes improve [53].

In trauma training, we focus extensively on teaching crisis resource management (CRM) strategies to support teams during high-stress, time-sensitive situations [50, 54]. The principles of CRM include an emphasis on team communication and effective teamwork strategies [55–59]. For example, two team members using closed-loop communication might sound like the following:

Please get the chest tube cart
Where is the chest tube cart?
Behind the door on the other side of the room
OK, I see it, I'll grab it. Here it is
Thank you, chest tube cart received

In this situation, the team members are using closed-loop communication, and this is effective in obtaining the necessary equipment. This type of communication is effective, but it requires practice. What is apparent, however, in this example and typical of many trauma resuscitations is that communication becomes the backstop for poorly designed spaces. Teams rely on highly effective communication skills to overcome the deficiencies of the clinical environment [32, 33]. If the trauma resuscitation environment was designed more intuitively, team training could focus on more patient-centered elements rather than ensuring they can effectively request and describe the location of poorly located equipment.

Imagine how the communication between team members may take place in a space where the chest tube cart was located in a more appropriate location. It may eliminate the need to ask a fellow team member for the cart, and the clinician may be immediately ready to perform the procedure:

Team lead, I have the chest tube cart and I'm ready to proceed on your call
Thank you, go ahead with the chest tube insertion now

At our institution, we have observed that when the layout and usability of the space are intuitive, less time is required to teach people about how to use the space, and greater effort is directed toward optimizing patient care. The downstream impact of highly functional clinical design should be considered as a significant return on investment (ROI) for future training plans. The built environment cannot be separated from the training process. By optimizing the physical space and equipment within it, through intuitive designs, the emphasis of team training can be shifted toward the nuanced aspects of clinical decision-making and team performance.

Excel

The transition from construction to beginning clinical care is exciting and ultimately represents the culmination of an extensive project. Once the construction of the trauma resuscitation environment is, however, it is not sufficient to stop the design process [42, 43]. While there is a higher probability that design flaws have been identified and mitigated using simulation-informed clinical design, latent safety threats may still pose risks to patients. Additionally, changes in processes and systems may not have been considered during the design process, thus requiring updates.

The construction of a new trauma resuscitation environment should be paired with ongoing evaluation strategies to monitor for issues and recognize successes. The latter represents the traditional approach to safety (Safety I), whereby the unit of analysis is the "accident" or the harm [8]. In Safety I, safety is defined by the absence of harm, we seek to learn from our errors, and the system is designed to avoid errors. In contrast, Safety II, an approach popularized by Braithwaite and colleagues, emphasizes the protective factors and decisions that support successes [8]. In Safety II, safety is defined as the presence of "what goes right" and we reorient our perspective to design our systems to support these successful behaviors.

A well-designed trauma program and trauma environment will include both Safety I and Safety II perspectives. The physical structure of the environment can do so using built-in technology like video and audio recording devices that allow for periodic case review. We believe that both successful cases and those involving adverse events be subject to review as learnings will be found in both instances. During case review, specific attention should be paid toward the design features that supported specific behaviors. Video review of trauma resuscitations is discussed further in Chap. 15.

Emerging technology, such as artificial intelligence, may enhance our ability to improve by providing unique insights into behaviors, systems, and infrastructure that are otherwise difficult to appreciate. For example, the Black Box, technology that is now in place in operating rooms, has the ability to capture multiple environmental factors (conversations, decibel levels, team movement) and link them to the patient's clinical status, team decisions, life-saving procedures, and ultimately patient outcomes [60, 61]. This in-depth understanding has the potential to completely alter our ability to reflect, refine, and improve our systems and clinical designs. The learnings from these outputs can then be integrated into the trauma system and, when possible, used to redesign the clinical environment.

Return on Investment

The costs associated with building elite trauma resuscitation environments are not insignificant, and it behooves the design team to complete at or under the budget available. At first glance, the methods we describe in this chapter may seem overwhelming in terms of human, equipment, and financial resources. The evidence suggests these upfront costs, however, are quickly mitigated given the benefits of simulation-informed and design thinking processes. This is supported by the concepts described in the MacLeamy Curve (Fig. 24.5) which speaks to a very simple but important principle in architectural and project management: design changes become more costly and less effective the farther along they occur, underscoring the importance of *getting it right* from the beginning [62].

While the MacLeamy Curve and its associated concepts seem intuitive, it may not be obvious to clinicians, funders, and the design team when developing and evaluating the initial project plan. We propose that an early meeting explicitly addresses in part the following:

- Introduce this concept to clinicians, the design team, and the funders
- Acknowledge that upfront costs will have downstream savings (both time and economic)
- Heavy investment in understanding the needs of end-users (patients and clinicians), the potential future of trauma care, the potential to adapt for rare events (pandemic, mass casualties)

Upon acknowledging the value of front-loaded work to yield dividends long term, the plan for simulation-informed design can begin. In our experience, findings from a simulation-informed design process can be broken down into two general categories:

The known unknowns: Data is a more powerful driver for change than anecdote. Codifying and quantifying known issues by way of a current state analysis can inform process improvement to a greater extent than incident reports and hallway conversations. Even if everyone already knows there's an issue: "It takes way too long to get blood to the bedside in trauma." The data from targeted in situ

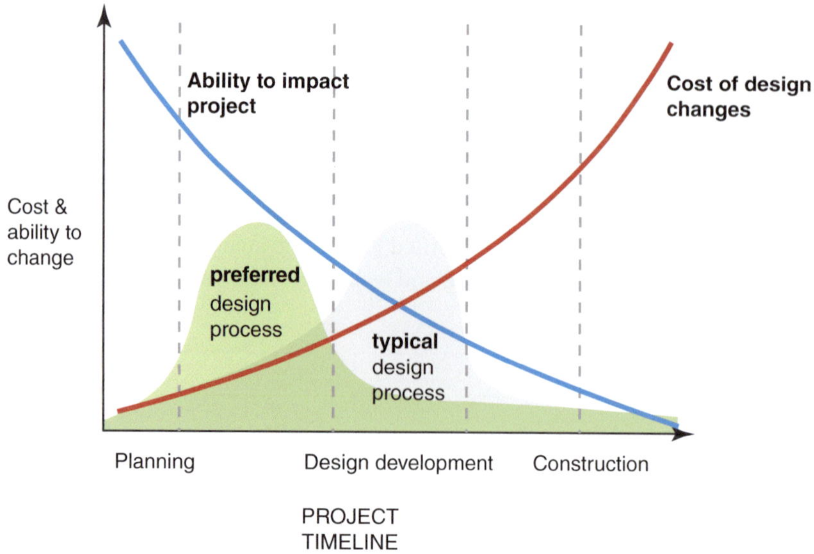

Fig. 24.5 MacLeamy curve. The preferred design process emphasizes upfront investment during project planning and design development. This maximizes the ability to make project changes while minimizing the cost of such changes. (Modified from Overbey [63])

simulations can substantiate those observations in ways that are hard to ignore: "Our simulations demonstrated an average delay to blood product delivery of X minutes, which is associated with an increase in patient mortality of Y."

The unknown unknowns: Sometimes, you don't know something is a problem until it's a problem. Once you know there's an issue, simulation can help you get to the root of the problem. Turns out, delays in blood product delivery were due in part to the circuitous path our blood runners had to take to get to the blood bank, and not knowing how or when to announce themselves when they got back.

Data and observation inform better decisions for process improvement. At our institution, the case of improving blood product delivery times and revising the massive hemorrhage protocol would have done nothing to make the process better or faster. Instead, a human-focused solution to shorten the distance traveled and facilitate awareness upon arrival decreased blood product delivery times from 11.5 min to 9 min, an improvement that is associated with a 12.5% decrease in mortality for trauma patients [35, 64].

There is growing evidence that these forward-thinking and innovative approaches to clinical design yield substantial dividends later on in the project. Several groups have described their findings using both simulation-informed clinical design and the design thinking process.

A Canadian group of researchers conducted a detailed ROI analysis of using simulation-based mock-ups to mitigate the need for future renovations of medication rooms (Fig. 24.4) [46]. They concluded a return on investment (in percentage) between 506% and 2685%, depending on the simulation technique used. Translated into dollar savings, for every dollar invested in mock-up simulations, between $5.06 and $26.85 can be saved after the investment is recovered. The authors described additional intangible benefits that included design interventions that were applied following the mock-up evaluation process, resulting in fewer interruptions, potential for fewer errors, and faster preparation time for medications.

An independent ROI analysis of IBM's design thinking strategy concluded that its application reduced design time of new products by 75%, doubled the speed to move products to market, decreased product testing times, and ultimately increased profits by >$100,000 for small projects and >$1,000,000 for large projects [21].

In our experience and upon review of broader literature using these methods, the return on investment (ROI) is substantial and favors the use of simulation-informed and design thinking-based processes.

Putting It Together

This chapter describes a detailed and practical approach to the design of trauma resuscitation environments using simulation-informed clinical design. Based on our experience, our research, and the work of others, this represents a robust and highly usable framework. Linked closely to our approach is design thinking methodology which we have used to test, evaluate, and modify new clinical infrastructure [17].

This human-centered process is used in numerous non-healthcare domains to support the design and testing of new products [65]. A key difference to this methodology compared to others is the focus on the "end-user." In trauma care, the "end-user" is not a single individual but rather comprises groups of people from patients/families to clinicians to non-clinical staff. The design thinking process consists of five steps that promote a human-centered focus, and simulation is integrated throughout (Fig. 24.6).

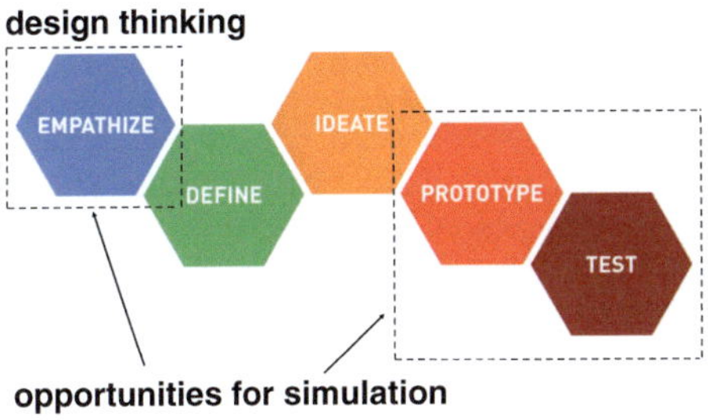

Fig. 24.6 A framework for design thinking, central to the simulation-informed clinical design concept. (Modified from Standford d. school [66])

A detailed review of design thinking is beyond the scope of this chapter [20]; however, we offer a brief summary of the steps:

1. *Empathize*: Develop an understanding of the end-user(s) through a comprehensive process that may include direct observation of trauma teams within the existing space, simulation, interviews, and case reviews.
2. *Define*: Building on the findings from the empathy step, the design team identifies and defines the issues related to the delivery of trauma care within the clinical environment.
3. *Ideate*: This step is typically undertaken by a multidisciplinary team (including clinicians, support staff, and patient advocates), and solutions are brainstormed using alternative and creative ways to solve problems.
4. *Prototype*: Ideas are piloted using multiple methods and scaled up over time. During this phase, we advocate for simulation methods that include tabletop simulation, mock-ups, and in situ simulation.
5. *Test*: Finally prototypes are tested prior to patient care beginning. In the context of opening a new trauma resuscitation environment, in situ simulation of the space is undertaken with authentic teams and actual equipment.

The principle that no patient will be the first test of a new clinical space is applied.

While these are listed in a sequence, they can be applied in a non-linear and iterative manner. Design teams may toggle between steps (back and forth between define and ideate) before moving on, based on the outputs of their process. Design teams may find this process helpful to include within their own structure of design, build, train, and excel.

Summary

The dynamic and complex interactions inherent to trauma resuscitation require a purposefully built environment that supports the delivery of time-sensitive and life-saving interventions. The historic and siloed approach frequently applied to the design of clinical infrastructure rarely considered the nuanced and specific needs of the end-user. In this chapter, we advocate for a deeper understanding of the end-user (both patients and providers) in the design process, ultimately resulting in the construction of a space that efficiently and effectively supports high-performing teams in delivering high-quality care. We describe a framework of design-build-train-excel that can be applied under various circumstances within the design and/or re-design of a trauma resuscitation environment. Key techniques in this framework include simulation-informed clinical design and design thinking methodologies. The process begins by formalizing partnerships between the clinical and architectural design teams. This is followed by simulation-based prototyping, iteratively refining and testing the clinical space. The end result is a built environment that is highly functional, fully tested, and patient/provider-focused—key ingredients for exceptional trauma care.

Key Points

- Trauma care is a complex process, and its inherent challenges are amplified when they occur within poorly designed clinical spaces.
- The design of physical spaces for trauma care should employ a human-centered design focus with an emphasis on patient experience.
- Evidence-based design is critical to ensure the design of a functional clinical space, and this should be guided by the 10 principles of EBD proposed by the Centre for Health Design.
- A four-phased approach (design-build-train-excel) systematically supports the conceptualization (*design*), prototyping (*build*), orientation and utilization of high-performance teams (*train*), and constant evaluation (*excel*) necessary to create a highly functional space.
- The return on investment of a systematic and structured approach to building a trauma bay is high, resulting in cost savings, improved patient outcomes, and an accelerated design/build process.

References

1. Anaker A, Heylighen A, Nordin S, Elf M. Design quality in the context of healthcare environments: a scoping review. HERD. 2017;10(4):136–50.
2. Ibrahim AM, Dimick JB, Joseph A. Building a better operating room: views from surgery and architecture. Ann Surg. 2017;265(1):34–6.

3. Ulrich RS, Zimring C, Zhu X, DuBose J, Seo HB, Choi YS, et al. A review of the research literature on evidence-based healthcare design. HERD. 2008;1(3):61–125.
4. Hayden EM, Wong AH, Ackerman J, Sande MK, Lei C, Kobayashi L, et al. Human factors and simulation in emergency medicine. Acad Emerg Med. 2018;25(2):221–9.
5. Kobayashi L, Parchuri R, Gardiner FG, Paolucci GA, Tomaselli NM, Al-Rasheed RS, et al. Use of in situ simulation and human factors engineering to assess and improve emergency department clinical systems for timely telemetry-based detection of life-threatening arrhythmias. BMJ Qual Saf. 2013;22(1):72–83.
6. Reith TP. Burnout in United States healthcare professionals: a narrative review. Cureus. 2018;10(12):e3681.
7. Wooldridge A, Carayon P, Hoonakker P, Hose BZ, Ross J, Kohler JE, et al. Complexity of the pediatric trauma care process: implications for multi-level awareness. Cogn Technol Work. 2019;21(3):397–416.
8. Braithwaite J, Wears RL, Hollnagel E. Resilient health care: turning patient safety on its head. Int J Qual Health Care. 2015;27(5):418–20.
9. Petrosoniak A, Hicks C. Design, build, train, excel: simulation and the creation of elite trauma systems. Int Anesthesiol Clin. 2021;59:58.
10. Barbé J, Wolff M, Mollard R, editors. Human centered design approach to integrate touch screen in future aircraft Cockpits. Berlin, Heidelberg: Springer Berlin Heidelberg; 2013.
11. Zachry M, Spyridakis JH. Human-centered design and the field of technical communication. J Tech Writ Commun. 2016;46(4):392–401.
12. Imada AS. Participatory ergonomics: past, present and future. J Hum Ergol (Tokyo). 2011;40(1–2):85–9.
13. Andersen SN, Broberg O. Participatory ergonomics simulation of hospital work systems: the influence of simulation media on simulation outcome. Appl Ergon. 2015;51:331–42.
14. Broberg O, Andersen V, Seim R. Participatory ergonomics in design processes: the role of boundary objects. Appl Ergon. 2011;42(3):464–72.
15. Sundin A, Christmansson M, Larsson M. A different perspective in participatory ergonomics in product development improves assembly work in the automative industry. Int J Ind Ergon. 2004;33(1):1–14.
16. Wilson J. Ergonomics and participation. In: Wilson JR, Corlett EN, editors. Evaluation of human work: a practical ergonomics methodology. London: Taylor & Francis Ltd; 1995. p. 1071–96.
17. Petrosoniak A, Hicks C, Barratt L, Gascon D, Kokoski C, Campbell D, et al. Design thinking-informed simulation: an innovative framework to test, evaluate, and modify new clinical infrastructure. Simul Healthc. 2020;15(3):205–13.
18. Altman M, Huang TTK, Breland JY. Design thinking in health care. Prev Chronic Dis. 2018;15:E117.
19. Luna DR, Rizzato Lede DA, Otero CM, Risk MR, Bernaldo G, de Quiros F. User-centered design improves the usability of drug-drug interaction alerts: experimental comparison of interfaces. J Biomed Inform. 2017;66:204–13.
20. Roberts JP, Fisher TR, Trowbridge MJ, Bent C. A design thinking framework for healthcare management and innovation. Healthcare. 2016;4(1):11–4.
21. The Total Economic Impact™ Of IBM's Design Thinking Practice 2018 Oct 24, 2020. Available from: https://www.ibm.com/design/thinking/static/Enterprise-Design-Thinking-Report-8ab1e9e1622899654844a5fe1d760ed5.pdf.
22. Becker L, Jaakkola E. Customer experience: fundamental premises and implications for research. J Acad Mark Sci. 2020;48(4):630–48.
23. Bastemeijer CM, Boosman H, van Ewijk H, Verweij LM, Voogt L, Hazelzet JA. Patient experiences: a systematic review of quality improvement interventions in a hospital setting. Patient Relat Outcome Meas. 2019;10:157–69.
24. Kaufman EJ, Richmond TS, Wiebe DJ, Jacoby SF, Holena DN. Patient experiences of trauma resuscitation. JAMA Surg. 2017;152(9):843–50.
25. Talks T. Transforming healthcare for children and their families; 2012. https://www.youtube.com/watch?v=jajduxPD6H4.
26. Kelley T, Kelley D. Chapter 1. Creative confidence: unleashing the creative potential within us all. New York: Crown; 2013.
27. Matheson GO, Pacione C, Shultz RK, Klugl M. Leveraging human-centered design in chronic disease prevention. Am J Prev Med. 2015;48(4):472–9.
28. Beaton A, O'Leary K, Thorburn J, Campbell A, Christey G. Improving patient experience and outcomes following serious injury. N Z Med J. 2019;132(1494):15–25.
29. Sanders SB, Santry HP. The myth of patient centeredness in the Trauma Bay. JAMA Surg. 2017;152(9):851.
30. Patterson MD, Geis GL, Falcone RA, LeMaster T, Wears RL. In situ simulation: detection of safety threats and teamwork training in a high risk emergency department. BMJ Qual Saf. 2013;22(6):468–77.
31. Wheeler DS, Geis G, Mack EH, LeMaster T, Patterson MD. High-reliability emergency response teams in the hospital: improving quality and safety using in situ simulation training. BMJ Qual Saf. 2013;22(6):507–14.
32. Petrosoniak A, Fan M, Hicks CM, White K, McGowan M, Campbell D, et al. Trauma resuscitation using in situ simulation team training (TRUST) study: latent safety threat evaluation using framework analysis and video review. BMJ Qual Saf. 2020;30:739.
33. Shah S, McGowan M, Petrosoniak A. Latent safety threat identification during in situ simulation debriefing: a qualitative analysis. BMJ Simul Technol Enhanc Learn. 2020;7:194.
34. Petrosoniak A, Almeida R, Pozzobon LD, Hicks C, Fan M, White K, et al. Tracking workflow during high-stakes resuscitation: the application of a novel clinician movement tracing tool during in situ trauma simulation. BMJ Simul Technol Enhanc Learn. 2019;5(2):78.
35. Petrosoniak A, Gray A, Pavenski K, McGowan M, Chartier L. The clock is ticking: using in situ simulation to improve time to blood delivery in bleeding trauma patients. CJEM. 2019;21(supplement S1(May)):S40–S1.
36. Design TCfH. What is Evidence-Based Design (EBD)? Available from: https://www.healthdesign.org/certification-outreach/edac/about-ebd.
37. Colman N, Doughty C, Arnold J, Stone K, Reid J, Dalpiaz A, et al. Simulation-based clinical systems testing for healthcare spaces: from intake through implementation. Adv Simul (Lond). 2019;4:19.
38. Couto TB, Barreto JKS, Marcon FC, Mafra A, Accorsi TAD. Detecting latent safety threats in an interprofessional training that combines in situ simulation with task training in an emergency department. Adv Simul (Lond). 2018;3:23.
39. Minor S, Green R, Jessula S. Crash testing the dummy: a review of in situ trauma simulation at a Canadian tertiary Centre. Can J Surg. 2019;62(4):243–8.
40. Hamstra SJ, Brydges R, Hatala R, Zendejas B, Cook DA. Reconsidering fidelity in simulation-based training. Acad Med. 2014;89(3):387–92.
41. Bender GJ. In situ simulation for systems testing in newly constructed perinatal facilities. Semin Perinatol. 2011;35(2):80–3.
42. Colman N, Stone K, Arnold J, Doughty C, Reid J, Younker S, et al. Prevent safety threats in new construction through integration of simulation and FMEA. Pediatr Qual Saf. 2019;4(4):e189.

43. Kaba A, Barnes S. Commissioning simulations to test new healthcare facilities: a proactive and innovative approach to healthcare system safety. Adv Simul (Lond). 2019;4:17.
44. Shultz J, Borkenhagen D, Rose E, Gribbons B, Rusak-Gillrie H, Fleck S, et al. Simulation-based mock-up evaluation of a universal operating room. HERD. 2020;13(1):68–80.
45. Ventre KM, Barry JS, Davis D, Baiamonte VL, Wentworth AC, Pietras M, et al. Using in situ simulation to evaluate operational readiness of a children's hospital-based obstetrics unit. Simul Healthc. 2014;9(2):102–11.
46. Alberta HQCo. Healthcare facility mock-up evaluation guidelines: using simulation to optimize return on investment for quality and patient safety; 2020.
47. Writer US. ORION: the algorithm proving that left isn't right: UPS; 2016. Available from: https://www.ups.com/us/en/services/knowledge-center/article.page?kid=aa3710c2.
48. Bayramzadeh S, Joseph A, Allison D, Shultz J, Abernathy J, Group ROS. Using an integrative mock-up simulation approach for evidence-based evaluation of operating room design prototypes. Appl Ergon. 2018;70:288–99.
49. Peavey EK, Zoss J, Watkins N. Simulation and mock-up research methods to enhance design decision making. HERD. 2012;5(3):133–44.
50. Hicks C, Petrosoniak A. The human factor: optimizing trauma team performance in dynamic clinical environments. Emerg Med Clin North Am. 2018;36(1):1–17.
51. Stavropoulos V. A thorough analysis of the pit stop strategy in formula 1 Statathlon; 2018. Available from: https://statathlon.com/analysis-of-the-pit-stop-strategy-in-f1/.
52. Medeiros J. How McLaren learned to treat its pit crew like athletes: wired.com; 2018.
53. Buljac-Samardzic M, Doekhie KD, van Wijngaarden JDH. Interventions to improve team effectiveness within health care: a systematic review of the past decade. Hum Resour Health. 2020;18(1):2.
54. Petrosoniak A, Hicks CM. Beyond crisis resource management: new frontiers in human factors training for acute care medicine. Curr Opin Anaesthesiol. 2013;26(6):699–706.
55. Howard SK, Gaba DM, Fish KJ, Yang G, Sarnquist FH. Anesthesia crisis resource management training: teaching anesthesiologists to handle critical incidents. Aviat Space Environ Med. 1992;63(9):763–70.
56. Entin EE, Serfaty D. Adaptive team coordination. Hum Factors. 1999;41(2):312–25.
57. Mathieu JE, Heffner TS, Goodwin GF, Salas E, Cannon-Bowers JA. The influence of shared mental models on team process and performance. J Appl Psychol. 2000;85(2):273–83.
58. Hollenbeck JR, Moon H, Ellis AP, West BJ, Ilgen DR, Sheppard L, et al. Structural contingency theory and individual differences: examination of external and internal person-team fit. J Appl Psychol. 2002;87(3):599–606.
59. Burke CS, Salas E, Wilson-Donnelly K, Priest H. How to turn a team of experts into an expert medical team: guidance from the aviation and military communities. Qual Saf Health Care. 2004;13(Suppl 1):i96–104.
60. Jung JJ, Juni P, Lebovic G, Grantcharov T. First-year analysis of the operating room black box study. Ann Surg. 2020;271(1):122–7.
61. Nolan B, Hicks CM, Petrosoniak A, Jung J, Grantcharov T. Pushing boundaries of video review in trauma: using comprehensive data to improve the safety of trauma care. Trauma Surg Acute Care Open. 2020;5(1):e000510.
62. Davis D. The MacLeamy curve; 2011. Available from: https://www.danieldavis.com/macleamy/.
63. Overbey D. Five diagrams every design team should know building enclosure online; 2018. Available from: https://www.buildingenclosureonline.com/blogs/14-the-be-blog/post/87371-five-diagrams-every-design-team-should-know.
64. Meyer DE, Vincent LE, Fox EE, O'Keeffe T, Inaba K, Bulger E, et al. Every minute counts: time to delivery of initial massive transfusion cooler and its impact on mortality. J Trauma Acute Care Surg. 2017;83(1):19–24.
65. Cross N. Design thinking: understanding how designers think and work. Oxford: Berg Publishers; 2011.
66. Design thinking process: Stanford d school. Available from: https://dschool.stanford.edu/.

Operating Room Setup and Design

25

Chad G. Ball and Andrew W. Kirkpatrick

Introduction

The construction of a modern operating theatre (OR) requires experienced input from a number of collaborators. The specific background and composition of this expert team varies depending on if the operating environment is being constructed de novo (new building or operating rooms) or involves a renovation of an already existing OR structure. It must be cautioned, however, that retrofitting an existing OR structure in the context of developing a hybrid environment (open and percutaneous capabilities) in particular can often be financially and/or engineering prohibitive. Team planning members may include, but are not limited to, experts in construction/renovation (electrical, plumbing, heating, ventilation and air conditioning (HVAC), flooring, carpentry), architecture, administrating, funding, clinical care (trauma surgery, anesthesia, nursing, interventional radiology, emergency medicine, and respiratory therapists), information technology, custodial care, and human factor analysis (i.e., trained in environment efficiency, work flow, physical spacing, and factor improvements). Despite the variability and unique skill sets of each member, the primary goal of the team must be regularly re-emphasized: to develop the best possible *clinical* workspace with the broadest range of potential therapies possible.

In the development of a hybrid operating environment (i.e., aimed at arresting ongoing hemorrhage), many of these decisions become increasingly complex due to the number of stakeholders and varied opinions on technology selection and positioning. The team must remember to ensure a collaborative and safe environment in order to achieve maximum group intelligence. Additional technology decisions for a hybrid OR include selection of a preferred angiography unit (typically ceiling mounted), hybrid surgical operating table, surgical lights/booms, potential computed tomography accessory, and control room hardware and software.

C. G. Ball (✉) · A. W. Kirkpatrick
University of Calgary, Foothills Medical Centre, Calgary, AB, Canada
e-mail: Andrew.kirkpatrick@ahs.ca

Human Factor Analysis

The role of human factor analysis experts deserves particular attention. More specifically, these highly trained professionals have expertise in quality and patient safety, and contribute heavily to the design of any OR (especially hybrid environments) by addressing the integration of clinical teams who are highly dedicated to clinical care but unfamiliar with working as a team within the same time and physical space. In most advanced human factor analyses, simulation remains an incredibly helpful tool. The primary goals of simulation are identifying latent threats to both patient safety and efficient group function. Human factor analysis further focuses on subsequent clinician training and teamwork skills to both evaluate and refine the practicalities of a physical OR environment. This role must not be understated, as the more complex the interaction, the greater the likelihood of miscommunication, conflict, and flawed decision-making. It has been reported that more than half of errors leading to preventable trauma deaths even in mature trauma systems occur during the initial evaluation, resuscitation, and transport to, or during, the initial interventions and activities, which are particularly error prone.

This reality seems especially topical for a hybrid OR, which is even more complex, as trauma resuscitations are typically performed by teams assembled on an ad hoc basis without opportunities for regular structured team training. User input during the design phase is always essential, and human factors evaluation methodologies allow for a systematic approach to: [1] better understand how proposed workspaces will be utilized and [2] incorporate user feedback during the design stage. Using patient simulation to evaluate "mock-up" rooms (i.e., physical models within the actual proposed space) has thus been previously employed in the design of intensive care unit patient rooms, emergency department examination rooms, inpatient hospital rooms, designated assisted living resident rooms, and now complex operating theatres. In an optimal scenario, the initial evaluation involves designing realistic clinical scenarios which are

L. Marshall Gillman, S. Widder (eds.), *Trauma Team Dynamics*, https://doi.org/10.1007/978-3-031-86312-7_25

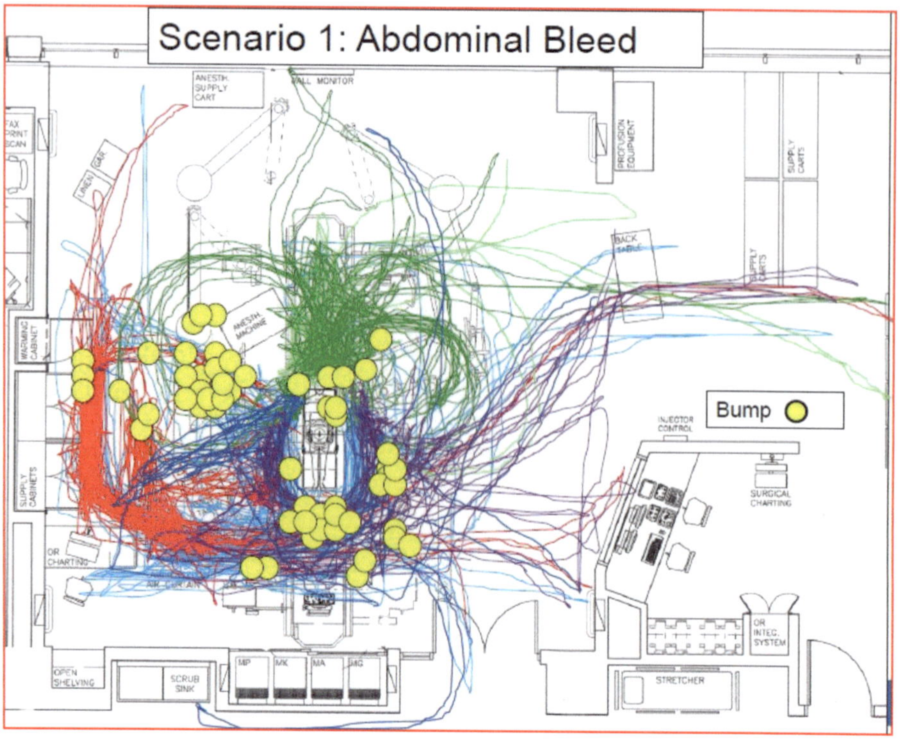

Fig. 25.1 Workflow patterns during a simulated trauma laparotomy followed by DI procedure. Bumps, pinch-points, and general inefficiencies in the progenitor RAPTOR candidate during the HF simulation of a trauma laparotomy followed by an interventional angiographic procedure. Bumps are denoted by circles. (Reprinted with permission from: Kirkpatrick et al. [16])

then enacted by a team of healthcare professionals using patient simulation. This event is then followed by extensive debriefing sessions within a full-scale mock-up environment in the planned hybrid footprint. Evaluations should include workflow, team integration, and identified barriers to optimal inter-professional care during resuscitations/procedures. The simulations also allow various clinical teams to "test drive" the space early in the room design process so that changes are still possible prior to the final build, recognizing that once constructed, the lifespan of healthcare spaces is typically decades. Concepts of high importance include evaluating the physical space, equipment access, staff workflow efficiencies, patient monitoring, and team interactions. Attention to the realities of physical congestion and "bumping" between clinicians is also mandatory. For example, in the design of our own hybrid theater, these congestion points were physically located in the nursing areas at the bottom and side of the OR table (Fig. 25.1). The planned location of the supply cabinets forced nurses to walk back and forth repeatedly around the sterile surgical supplies. Furthermore, the charting table at the foot of the bed created a pinch point. These challenges were corrected and modified in the final design and construction. It must also be stated that repeated simulation in potentially new environments, which may be inherently stressful and acute, provides opportunities for evaluation of targeted communications issues, default room configuration prior to patient arrival, role clarity, environmental factors, adopting the use of new and expanded roles, and further evaluation of patient and clinician safety risks.

Unique Realities for the Hybrid Operating Environment

Although many of the previously mentioned planning concepts remain universal to the design of all operating theatres, their importance is even more critical in the context of building a hybrid operating environment. More specifically, realities such as hemorrhage control, gastrointestinal containment, hostile patient physiology therapy (i.e., resuscitation and critical care), and critical patient imaging can all coincide on a truly emergent and synchronous basis. Without question, however, ongoing massive hemorrhage remains the dominant etiology of patient death following severe injury in those who survive to hospital admission [1–8]. Fortunately, we have an increasing variety of instruments aimed at technical hemorrhage control and concurrent resuscitation [6, 9]. As discussed above, one of these paradigm-shifting concepts is the hybrid operating environment (RAPTOR: *R*esuscitation with *A*ngiography, *P*ercutaneous *T*echniques, and *O*perative *R*epair) [7, 9–12]. This tool allows a transition in care from a location-based approach to a truly disease- and urgency-based algorithm [11]. Despite the tremendous financial and human resource costs of developing a hybrid suite, the utility of this technology is becoming more clear. Publications have now confirmed improved morbidity and mortality within a hybrid suite in patients with continued bleeding [7, 11]. In addition to patient outcomes, the specific terminology and technical details that surround truly hybrid operating environments remain heterogeneous and unclear in the literature.

Table 25.1 RAPTOR (hybrid OR) terminology/lexicon

Simultaneous	Two separate teams (surgical and percutaneous) are both scrubbed and operating at precisely the same time
Concurrent	Synonymous with "simultaneous"
Synchronous	One team performs its procedural component first, followed rapidly by a second team.
Serial	Synonymous with "synchronous."

Hybrid Operating Environment Lexicon

In numerous publications, the term "simultaneous" is employed to describe the ability of clinicians to arrest ongoing hemorrhage and resuscitate patients in a single interventional location (i.e., RAPTOR) [12]. Similar to our oncologic colleagues, other authors have also utilized the term "synchronous." [7, 11] The reality is that very few of these potentially life-saving trauma procedures are truly "simultaneous." They are better described as rapid serial interventions (open surgical procedures immediately followed by percutaneous endovascular techniques; or vice versa) that are performed within the same location and visit (Table 25.1). A similar scenario occurs during "synchronous" hepatic and intestinal resections for colorectal liver metastases [13]. These "combined" interventions do not occur at precisely the same time within the context of the overall procedure. Truly simultaneous/concurrent open and percutaneous procedures are therefore distinct from those that occur in a rapid sequential/synchronous manner. As a result, the specific technical nuances required for making these combined interventions effective and efficient are also different.

Technical Optimization Within the RAPTOR

The optimal RAPTOR working environment should include: [1] standard hybrid operating theater components (carbon fiber table, fixed angiographic capabilities) [2], preparation of two full instrument setups (open and percutaneous) at the beginning of the case [3], dual "scrub" nurses [4], two circulating nurses and one radiology technician [5], surgical team positioned on the left of the patient with angiography monitors near the feet end of the bed (this allows subsequent rapid access to the left thorax if needed); percutaneous team positioned on the right of the patient (this allows direct visualization of the monitors) [6], cautery machine, suction device(s), ventilator, ultrasound each positioned on the right of the patient above the arm board [7], power contrast injector on the left of the patient [8], early patient arterial access (i.e., for both monitoring and therapeutic interventions) [9], standard patient trauma skin preparation (rapidly from the angle of mandible to ankles), and [10] strategizing groin (or alternative) arterial access in patients who require pelvic binders. All team members (anesthesia, nursing, percutaneous, and surgical teams) should wear lead aprons/garments/eye protection. Closed-loop communication in a quiet and efficient working environment is critical.

If truly simultaneous/concurrent surgical and endovascular procedures are engaged, radiation protection for the entire healthcare team, with a focus on the surgeon, is essential. All percutaneous endovascular interventions require fluoroscopy. For example, if a significant liver injury requires rapid and sustained manual packing, as well as arterial embolization, the surgeons' hands are at risk of being irradiated if left in place within the abdomen. The simultaneous treatment of an unstable patient, therefore, works best when separate body areas are being treated at the same time (e.g., high-grade splenic injury requiring splenectomy, as well as active hemorrhage within the pelvis; the surgical team can remove the spleen while the IR team embolizes the arterial pelvis). Another optimized simultaneous example is embolization of a bleeding thoracic artery or aortic stent-grafting while the surgical team works within the abdomen or pelvis). Safe radiation practices require the surgeon to remove his/her hands out of the fluoroscopic field. Another factor to consider in ensuring optimal surgical intervention is the physical positioning of the image intensifier ("C-arm") itself.

Percutaneous access warrants a distinct comment. Left radial access is the preferred site for percutaneous body procedures, as it precludes crossing the aortic arch (i.e., as in right radial access) and lessens the chance of a stroke (especially in a trauma patient where anticoagulation may be an issue). Left-sided radial access involves some arm/wrist placement issues to facilitate good ergonomics and proper visualization of the abdomen and pelvis. More specifically, once the left arm is completely prepped in a sterile manner, it can then be bent 90 degrees at the elbow (i.e., the left wrist is positioned close to the right hip). Radial access can then be performed in a conventional manner, or with distal left radial access. This position will then allow excellent visualization of the upper solid organs (spleen, liver, kidneys). For visualization of the pelvis, the left wrist is moved superiorly to the upper abdomen. Both positions allow the operator to work on the "normal" right side of the patient (and therefore surgical team on the left side if necessary). This can also be achieved with the abdomen exposed and the arm/wrist moved as needed. It should be noted that although it is possible for the percutaneous team to work from the left side of the patient, this alignment becomes much more ergonomically challenging (i.e., due to equipment issues such as C-arm and screen positioning).

Patient Outcomes and Flow

Preceding publications have confirmed that a subset of critically injured patients *clearly* benefit from access to a RAPTOR hybrid trauma suite [7, 11]. It is also evident that despite the significant financial costs associated with RAPTOR technology [7, 9–12], patients who require nearly concurrent emergent percutaneous and open procedures to arrest ongoing hemorrhage may be "saved" by this resource [7, 11]. More specifically, improving efficiencies for patients with continuous bleeding who would have traditionally required transportation between venues (angiography suite and operating theater) [7, 9–12] has been transformational.

Despite the clear advantage of a RAPTOR, the lexicon describing its technical use remains heterogeneous. As mentioned, multiple terms such as synchronous, simultaneous, serial, and concurrent have each been used to define both similar and differing events within the RAPTOR suite. Simultaneous (synonymous with "concurrent") RAPTOR procedures refer to scenarios where two separate teams (surgical and percutaneous) are both scrubbed and operating at precisely the same time (including associated nursing teams). Rapid serial (synonymous with "synchronous") RAPTOR interventions refer to scenarios where one team performs its procedural component first. This initial procedure is then followed by a second team (i.e., once the first team has stopped). This scenario may repeat itself again depending on the complexity and demands of the given patient's injuries.

In a prospective comparison of patients who required truly simultaneous versus rapid serial/synchronous procedures to arrest ongoing hemorrhage, it is evident that patients requiring care from both teams at the same time were more severely ill. More specifically, they are more often hemodynamically unstable (92%), require damage control (83%), undergo more frequent massive transfusions (67%), less frequently receive the benefit of preoperative CT (25%), and are transferred from the ambulance to the RAPTOR suite in a much more rapid interval (31 min). Despite this difference, the mortality rate among this patient cohort remains similar to patients who underwent a serial procedure (17% vs. 13%). This observation suggests that trauma surgeons were able to identify more critically ill patients with ongoing hemorrhage and expedite their care *to* the RAPTOR suite. In the context of previous publications confirming both improved survival and more efficient care *within* the RAPTOR suite for patients with ongoing hemorrhage (49% mortality in pre-RAPTOR vs. 42% in pre-RAPTOR following quality improvements vs. 22% in RAPTOR patients (excluding stable EVAR patients) vs. 16% in all RAPTOR patients) [7, 11], it should be reinforced that it is of the utmost importance to eliminate any obstacles in the pre-hospital setting, trauma bay/emergency department, and/or patient transfer process that slow the ability of the trauma surgeon to make an initial disposition decision for every bleeding patient [14].

It is also evident that 92% of the patients treated in a truly simultaneous manner *clearly* benefit from a *concurrent* hybrid procedure. The definition of *clear* remains the very high likelihood that the patient would have died in the absence of the simultaneous nature of both procedures [7, 11].

A specific commentary regarding the importance of moving patients as rapidly as possible from the moment of injury through to the arrest of ongoing hemorrhage is also warranted. Upon review of the data from a well-known institution, the time interval from arrival at the trauma bay to procedural intervention decreased from 212 (angiography suite) to 148 (angiography suite with quality improvements) to 101 (operating theater) to 90 (operating theater with quality improvements) to 82 (RAPTOR available) to 31 min (RAPTOR for the most critically ill patients requiring truly simultaneous procedures) [7, 11, 15]. As previously mentioned [7, 11], this decrease in time is a direct result of the ability of the operating theater staff and surgeon to mobilize effective resources and destination access at a much greater speed than was available within an isolated angiography suite. Unfortunately, it must also be stated that maintaining rapid patient-focused care for critically injured victims of ongoing hemorrhage requires the frequent and perpetual revisitation of specific clinician roles within the team, "direct to RAPTOR" and patient transfer indications, patient outcomes, and obstacles to efficient patient care.

Summary

Despite the descriptions above, the specific technical setup for both operative and percutaneous interventions will vary across institutions and clinicians in both traditional and hybrid operating rooms [11, 12]. It must be noted, however, that trauma surgeons have now become central to the design and construction of many of these operating environments (i.e., both hybrid and non-hybrid) throughout the world (e.g., Australia, Finland, Germany, and the United States).

In summary, the development of hybrid operating environments will require the best of collaborative teamwork, thoughtful planning, and patience. Critical concepts must be considered in an environment where two separate teams with unique equipment and operating requirements will be working in a simultaneous manner. In addition to the specific recommendations listed above, these principles include: [1] adequate nuanced communication between the trauma surgeon (open team) and the percutaneous team (typically interventional radiologist) [2], a rapid pre-procedural briefing for all team members of the planned interventional and care sequence [3], the ability to rapidly obtain/set up both open and percutaneous equipment with adequate patient access points for both teams [4], a quiet working environment that facilitates communication between the anesthesiologist, surgical, and percutaneous teams [5], a clear division of space around the patient to facilitate simultaneous procedures (which must be flexible when required), and [6] specific protections to avoid unnecessary ionizing radiation exposure to the team (especially the surgeon).

It can be surmised that up to 18% of patients requiring an emergent procedural intervention benefit from utilizing a hybrid environment such as the RAPTOR. Patients who require truly simultaneous hybrid procedures (i.e., even more critically ill) will benefit from access to the RAPTOR hybrid suite to an even greater extent. Outcomes associated with these patients can achieve equivalence to their less injured counterparts with rapid trauma surgeon efficiency and the employment of specific techniques among both the open surgical and percutaneous interventional teams. Use of the RAPTOR suite considerably shortens the time interval to both percutaneous and open procedures, as well as reduces the required rate of blood transfusion. Data also suggests that a RAPTOR environment may result in a substantially decreased mortality rate among our most critically injured patients who display ongoing hemorrhage. It must be acknowledged, however, that this patient cohort is only a small proportion of all injured patients admitted to a busy trauma service (1–3%), and therefore, the frequency of these events may not justify institutional investment in RAPTOR suites.

Key Points

A. RAPTOR: *R*esuscitation with *A*ngiography, *P*ercutaneous *T*echniques, and *O*perative *R*epair.
B. The optimal construction of a new operating environment requires a multidisciplinary team with expertise in clinical care, physical construction, human factor analysis, and resource allocation.
C. "Simultaneous" (synonymous with "concurrent") RAPTOR procedures refer to scenarios where two separate teams (surgical and percutaneous) are both scrubbed and operating at precisely the same time.
D. Rapid serial (synonymous with "synchronous") RAPTOR interventions refer to scenarios where one team performs its procedural component first.
E. Up to 18% of patients requiring an emergent procedural intervention benefit from utilizing a hybrid environment such as the RAPTOR.

References

1. Kahl JE, Calvo RY, Sise MJ, Sise CB, Thorndike JF, Shackford SR. The changing nature of death on the trauma service. J Trauma Acute Care Surg. 2013;75:195–201.
2. Holcomb JB, Fox EE, Scalea TM, Napolitano LM, Albarado R, Gill B, Dunkin BJ, Kirkpatrick AW, Cotton BA, Inaba K, et al. Current opinion on catheter-based hemorrhage control in trauma patients. J Trauma Acute Care Surg. 2014;76:888–93.
3. Holcomb JB, del Junco DJ, Fox EE, Wade CE, Cohen MJ, Schreiber MA, Alarcon LH, Bai Y, Brasel KL, Bulger EM, et al. The prospective, observational, multicenter, major trauma transfusion (PROMMTT) study: comparative effectiveness of a time-varying treatment with competing risks. JAMA Surg. 2013;148:127–36.
4. Ball CG. Damage control resuscitation: history, theory and technique. Can J Surg. 2014;57:55–60.
5. Ball CG, Das D, Roberts DJ, Vis C, Kirkpatrick AW, Kortbeek JB. The evolution of trauma surgery at a high-volume Canadian centre: implications for public health, prevention, clinical care, education and recruitment. Can J Surg. 2015;58:19–23.
6. Darrabie MD, Croft CA, Brakenridge SC, Mohr AM, Rosenthal MA, Mercier NR, Moore FA, Smith RS. Resuscitative endovascular balloon occlusion of the aorta: implementation and preliminary results at an Academic Level I Trauma Center. J Am Coll Surg. 2018;227:127–33.
7. Fehr A, Beveridge J, D'Amours S, Kirkpatrick AW, Ball CG. The potential benefit of a hybrid environment among severely injured patients with persistent haemorrhage: how often could we get it right? J Trauma Acute Care Surg. 2016;80:457–60.
8. Roberts DJ, Harzan C, Kirkpatrick AW, Dixon E, Grondin SC, McBeth PB, Kaplan GG, Ball CG. One thousand consecutive in-hospital deaths following severe injury: has etiology of traumatic inpatient death changed in Canada? Can J Surg. 2018;61:150–2.
9. Ball CG. The R.A.P.T.O.R. suite: resuscitation with angiography, percutaneous techniques, and operative repair. J Trauma. 2011;70:1579–80.
10. Kirkpatrick AW, Vis C, Dube M, Biesbrek S, Ball CG, Laberge J, Shultz J, Rea K, Sadler D, Holcomb JB, et al. The evolution of a purpose designed hybrid trauma operating room from the trauma service perspective: The RAPTOR (resuscitation with angiography percutaneous treatments and operative resuscitations). Injury. 2014;45:1413–21.
11. Carver D, Kirkpatrick AW, D'Amours S, Hameed SM, Beveridge J, Ball CG. A prospective evaluation of the utility of a hybrid operating suite for severely injured patients. Overstated or underutilized? Ann Surg. 2020;271(5):958–61.
12. Ito K, Nagano T, Nakazawa K, Numasawa Y, Watanabe M, Akoi S, Mizusawa H, Ishiai S, Yokota T. Simultaneous damage control surgery and endovascular procedures for patients with blunt trauma in the hybrid emergency room system: new multidisciplinary trauma team building. J Trauma Acute Care Surg. 2019;86:160–2.
13. Howard C, Clements TW, Edwards JP, MacLean AR, Buie WD, Dixon E, Grondin SC, Gomes A, McColl M, Cleary S, et al. Synchronous colorectal liver metastases: a national survey of surgeon opinions on simultaneous resection and multidisciplinary cooperation. Hepatobiliary Surg Nutr. 2018;7:242–50.
14. Clements TW, Vogt K, Hameed SM, Parry N, Kirkpatrick AW, Grondin SC, Dixon E, McKee J, Ball CG. Does increased prehospital time lead to a "trial of life" effect for patients with blunt trauma? J Surg Res. 2017;216:103–8.
15. Smith A, Ouellet JF, Niven D, Kirkpatrick AW, Dixon E, D'Amours S, Ball CG. Timeliness in obtaining emergent percutaneous procedures in severely injured patients: how long is too long and should we create quality assurance guidelines? Can J Surg. 2013;56:154–7.
16. Kirkpatrick AW, Vis C, Dube M, Biesbrek S, Ball CG, Laberge J, Shultz J, Rea K, Sadler D, Holcomb JB, et al. The evolution of a purpose-designed hybrid trauma operating room from the trauma service perspective: The RAPTOR (resuscitation with angiography percutaneous treatments and operative resuscitations). Injury. 2014;45:1413–21.

26 Systems-Focused Simulation and Debriefing to Improve Patient Safety, Quality Care, Environments, and Processes

Mirette Dubé, Shaunna Milloy, Jennifer Jordan, Tona Laerz, Sara Nosworthy, James Huffman, Jonathan Gaudet, Bryan Weber, and Barbara Blackie

Introduction

The use of simulation is well suited for training healthcare teams and individuals to improve knowledge and skills and to practice effective teamwork behaviors. The necessary evolution of simulation to expand beyond its use to close individual knowledge and skill gaps is well aligned with patient safety science. Patient safety science research suggests that despite healthcare improvement efforts over the past decade, inadvertent harm in healthcare continues to be the third leading cause of death behind heart disease and cancer [1, 2]. Organizations that primarily take a "person-centered" approach to problem-solving around such harms may unduly focus on individual factors and rely heavily on interventions such as education and training to address them. Conversely, including the "system-approach" to exploring patient safety liabilities allows consideration of complex influences on the overall environment and system surrounding the individual.

> Your system is perfectly designed to give you the results you are getting. [3]

Systems engineering, the science of designing and managing complex systems throughout their life cycle, also considers that errors and adverse events are often not due to individual deficits. Instead, gaps in elements of the complex healthcare system that surround individuals while they work are considered. Systems integration is an engineering term to describe many sub-systems coming together into one better functioning whole [4]. Therefore, simulation for systems integration, also known as **system-focused simulation** or *translational simulation*, moves away from solely focusing on individual knowledge and skills and takes a systems approach to understanding complex healthcare systems [5–7].

Using this approach, high priority objectives are identified in consultation with all stakeholders (i.e., expert representatives of their professional role) who may be impacted by a simulation evaluation [8–11]. This approach works on the premise that spaces or processes (e.g., protocol, pathway) should not be tested on real patients for the first time [12–14]. Furthermore, simulation is ideally enacted in the in situ or actual clinical care environments, with real teams and without the potential for harm to patients [15].

M. Dubé (✉)
Alberta Simulation Program, Foothills Medical Center, Alberta Health Services, Calgary, AB, Canada
e-mail: Mirette.Dube@albertahealthservices.ca

S. Milloy
Provincial Patient Safety, Alberta Health Services, Calgary, AB, Canada
e-mail: Shaunna.Milloy@ahs.ca

J. Jordan
Emergency Department, Foothills Medical Centre, Calgary, AB, Canada
e-mail: Jennifer.jordan@ahs.ca

T. Laerz
Respiratory Services, Foothills Medical Centre, Alberta Health Services, Calgary, AB, Canada
e-mail: Tona.Laerz@ahs.ca

S. Nosworthy
Cardiac Sciences, Foothills Medical Centre, Calgary, AB, Canada
e-mail: Sara.nosworthy@ahs.ca

J. Huffman · B. Weber
University of Calgary, Calgary, AB, Canada
e-mail: jlhuffma@ucalgary.ca; Bryan.weber@ucalgary.ca

J. Gaudet
Department of Critical Care Medicine, University of Calgary, Calgary, AB, Canada
e-mail: jgaudet@ucalgary.ca

B. Blackie
Division of Emergency Medicine, Institution Sidra Medicine, Doha, Qatar
e-mail: bblackie@sidra.org

L. Marshall Gillman, S. Widder (eds.), *Trauma Team Dynamics*, https://doi.org/10.1007/978-3-031-86312-7_26

Stakeholders may include expert representatives from clinical and non-clinical care areas such as managers, educators, physicians, nurses, respiratory therapists, unit clerks, porters, and hospital administrators. Inclusivity is important to ensure all perspectives are heard and considered for a realistic and integrated approach to systems testing. Following stakeholder consultation and determination of evaluation objectives, relevant workflows are identified and translated into a simulation scenario(s), striving to recreate a realistic context with actual teams, equipment, and spaces.

Simulation allows for the recreation of these complex systems and represents as closely as possible how work is actually happening versus how we may perceive it is happening to better assess risk, mitigate harm, and proactively improve systems and processes of care delivery [16]. System-focused debriefing (SFD) differs in purpose and approach to debriefing focused on individual learner knowledge and skills [17]. It is a purposeful exploration of the highest priority objectives identified. These elements may include the physical workspace/environment, tasks, tools, technology, people, and organizations that interact to enable safe and effective care processes and optimize outcomes [18].

Using observations from the simulation exercise and pre-identified objectives from stakeholder consultation helps guide the debrief and elicit feedback from the end users of the system. Positive system function is highlighted and reinforced as well as a collection of gaps and threats are identified to subsequently inform future improvement work. Hearing from all relevant stakeholders is a key part of systems integration, where different groups have opportunity to understand how any one workflow or process impacts the whole team and other sub-systems.

Growing evidence continues to accrue for the use of system-focused simulation to reduce organizational costs, proactively improve safety and efficiency, inform and reduce risk, and solve clinical challenges [12, 18]. This chapter will highlight several examples of these principles to test and revise trauma and difficult airway protocols. Examples include the arrival of a single trauma patient contrasted to activation of mass casualty incident protocols; how to incorporate human factors methods and system simulation to test the usability of difficult airway carts and airway management pause checklists; and the commissioning of new spaces such as emergency rooms and trauma room bays.

Case Study 1: Standardizing the Level 1: Acute Trauma Admission Process Using Systems Simulations

In a complex healthcare system, a change to one element of the system may have large effects on others. This is especially relevant in time-pressured situations where teams comprised of multiple healthcare professionals are required to form rapidly and come together quickly to manage the sickest trauma patients with time-sensitive conditions. Trauma protocols or pathways are intended to help organize team roles, establish workflow to align with evidence-based standards, and rapidly enable safe diagnosis and delivery of treatment.

Testing these processes is essential in order to prepare the team within their roles, test the many interactions between the people and their care environment, and proactively identify and mitigate systems issues.

Our first case study focuses on a protocol designed to guide the admission, initial assessment, rapid diagnosis, and treatment for a trauma patient arriving to an Emergency Department.

In our tertiary care trauma center, both evidence from Trauma Quality data indicators and information received from staff debriefing sessions indicated multiple factors that may have led to less-than-optimal trauma care. Working groups were created with frontline staff to provide input for a major renovation in the trauma rooms at the Foothills Medical Centre in Calgary, Alberta. Information gathering during the working groups identified several areas of process improvement. This required the Emergency Department to further examine their trauma protocols and test targeted improvements using simulation. An improved process was needed to help with crowd control and to implement clearer communication strategies, including a consistent pre-arrival briefing that better enabled role clarity, identified clear leadership, and ultimately reduced chaos frequently encountered in these situations. The overall goal for the project was to improve trauma patient mortality, and to build safer and more efficient trauma team practice(s).

The interprofessional trauma team prioritized five targeted process steps to lead to potential improvement in trauma resuscitation. The five process steps that were deemed key to evaluation were (1) the trauma pre-brief, (2) imminent life-threat survey, (3) primary survey, (4) a clear leader is identified, and (5) an EXIT or pre-transport checklist. Each of these steps needed to be embedded in the trauma guideline and tested in simulation.

Project Implementation

A working group was formed in early 2019 which included interdisciplinary team members from the Emergency Department (ED), Respiratory Therapy, Emergency Medical Services (EMS), and Trauma Services with the goal of improving trauma care in the ED.

The working group collaborated to develop a Level 1 Trauma Guideline. Once the guideline was developed, it was tested through iterative cycles of refinement using simulation to assess for systems issues including latent safety threats. The simulations included over 40 individuals in each simulation from all teams involved in trauma including the ED, operating room, site leadership, transfusion medicine, bed placement, surgery, and more. The objectives of the simulations and debriefs were focused on the five process steps and included testing checklists and aids such as the pre-brief checklist, a standardized EMS handover tool, and EXIT checklist. All tools and the overall guideline were revised and refined based on user feedback from the debriefings. The findings from these simulations were used to finalize the Level 1 Trauma Guideline. Implementation included bi-weekly simulations for all staff with the opportunity to apply the Guideline and share information with content leaders.

Simulation and debriefing are powerful mediators of quality improvement, change, and implementation science. This project included strategies to ensure a lens of continuous quality improvement using clinical event debriefing after trauma admissions to elicit further feedback from team members, bi-weekly trauma-focused simulations with debriefing targeting the five process steps, and ongoing data analysis post implementation.

Results

Success of this approach was underpinned by the collaboration of interprofessional teams and individuals committed to improving patient care. This was achieved by comprehensive planning, open communication, proper risk management, integration of system simulations, and preparation for implementation for frontline staff.

Successes enabled by standardization included the following: the reduction in the number of staff in the trauma room with effective crowd control, improved communication techniques with the use of the pre-brief and EXIT checklists, and an observable improvement in role definition most important with respect to having a clear trauma team leader. Feedback from team debriefs and ongoing reports at Trauma Quality Council Meetings reported a decrease in ambient environmental noise during resuscitations leading to easier team communication.

Case Study 2: Foothills Emergency Response Activation for Multi-Trauma (FERA-Trauma) Testing and Implementation

Our next case study builds on complexity of situations where there are multiple incoming trauma patients simultaneously or disaster events. System integration is often challenging in these situations due to the many roles, teams, tasks, and vital communications happening at the same time. These situations are often described as high-stress and time-pressured.

Level 1 Trauma activation at our large tertiary care center (i.e., Foothills Medical Centre: FMC) is modelled around the care of a single trauma patient. Although, there are instances when multiple trauma patients requiring resuscitation and operative intervention will simultaneously arrive or present in rapid succession to the FMC ED. The Foothills Emergency Response Activation for Trauma (FERA Trauma) protocol was developed to help guide the FMC team in the care and resource management for these patients. This process was designed as a first step in a scalable response in what may become a Code Orange, or disaster event activation.

The criteria for activation of FERA Trauma is three or more patients meeting Level 1 criteria within 1 h. The criteria for activation were simplified to ensure the decision to activate could be made in a timely fashion. Like Level 1 Trauma activations, it was anticipated that a certain percentage of the FERA Trauma activations would be "stood down".

Implementation and Evaluation

An interdisciplinary project team collaborated with representation from: Trauma Services, ED, Intensive Care Unit (ICU), Operating Room (OR), Anesthesia, General Surgery, Site Administration, Respiratory Therapy, Bed Placement, and Transfusion Medicine to develop a process for times when multiple trauma patients present concurrently to the FMC ED but fall short of activation of a code orange (disaster).

After the process was drafted, simulations were used to test the FERA Trauma processes and communication to identify any latent threats to patient and staff safety and to make system improvements before implementation in July 2020. Iterative Plan, Do, Study, Act (PDSA) testing cycles through simulation helped to ensure a safe and quality-driven approach and to identify the most important issues.

The simulations identified several opportunities for improvement. The initial pager script and membership of the page-out were refined to ensure the right teams appeared for the huddle as soon as possible. Checklists were developed for each team and refined through simulation to prepare for an incoming FERA Trauma. Clear communication and handover were key to improve patient care and a clear leader was required. As a result of simulation and debriefing of actual cases, it was identified that this leader should be a physician that was not involved in direct patient care, was a clear communicator, and must be able to work closely as a dyad with the ED charge nurse. Through this, process gaps were identified in the Transfusion Medicine process, and as a result, the teams refined the process to improve timely communication to Transfusion Medicine.

Further implementation and education of the process was completed using the following communication strategies: emails, grand rounds, and presentations at leadership and staff meetings. Each of the services involved in FERA Trauma protocol was responsible for their own internal staff education and rollout plan.

Clinical event debriefing is another tool to ensure continuous quality improvement to review clinical events and enable team members to share reflections and ideas on improvement. These debriefs were built into the FERA Trauma process to allow for post-event evaluation. The FERA Trauma committee decided that debriefs must occur after the FERA Trauma had also been "stood down" to identify continuing opportunities for improvement. It was felt that all findings needed to be brought to the FERA Trauma Committee to ensure a process existed for review and further improvement. In the first year following implementation, several improvements were implemented including the revision of pager scripts, an additional focus on the dyad leadership model, improved huddle effectiveness, the use and design of cognitive aids, and standardized communication. Staff reported improved communication with the OR, a consistent membership for the FERA Trauma activation, and identified the importance of including the hospital administrator on call and ED managers for both initial activation and employing the stand-down process for FERA trauma protocol.

The extra resources mobilized by the FERA Trauma activation help to expedite patient care and transfers out of the ED in preparation for potential increased need in capacity. These improvements have helped to make the FERA Trauma activation more effective and acceptable to all stakeholders involved. This example serves to highlight the use of simulation-based methods to design protocols, test them with the clinical teams, take end-user feedback to make iterative refinements prior to implementation, and then use multiple communication strategies and an ongoing clinical event debriefing program to establish a culture and means of continuous quality improvement.

Case Study 3: The Use of System Simulation with Usability Testing (Difficult Airway Management (DAM) Algorithm, Airway Management Pause (AMP) Checklist, and DAM Cart)

The use of system simulation in tandem with human factors methods such as usability testing is an effective way to enable user-centered design.

Usability testing is best described as a "systematic way of observing actual users trying out a product and collecting information about the specific ways in which the product is easy or difficult for them" [19]. Central to usability testing is end users using the product as they normally would in clinical practice to gain an understanding of how effective, efficient, safe, and how satisfied they are with a specific piece of equipment. Facilitating usability testing helps to inform purchase and design decisions, and support implementation. Usability depends on defining the appropriate user, having a specified goal and objectives surrounding the tasks of the user, and ensuring alignment within the environment and context where use of the equipment or tools will occur.

When looking at usability testing for a complex healthcare trauma team, one application may be the testing of new carts used within the trauma bay. This serves as one example of many other potential healthcare environments and applications [20, 21]. Simulation to create a real-to-life clinical situation allows evaluation of where a cart would need to be accessed, and what supplies are chosen and used in the context of caring for a traumatic or neonatal patient. Observable behaviors and self-reported user feedback can be collected through debriefing, and additional data around timed metrics, number and type of errors, and other measures may be chosen to evaluate usability.

We share a case study of a wholesale revision to the approach and management of difficult endotracheal intubation outside the OR through the development of a suite of new difficult airway management tools and a Difficult Airway Management (DAM) Cart. After iterative refinement and testing, the algorithm and suite of airway tools were implemented in four adult acute care hospital sites including an acute trauma center in the Calgary Zone of Alberta Health Services.

Through a needs assessment, it was identified that existing DAM cart contents and layout needed to be revised to reflect evolving DAM equipment and practices and to better marry with the development and adoption of a new algorithm for difficult endotracheal intubation. A DAM algorithm (Fig. 26.1) was adapted from an existing DAM algorithm in the existing literature to focus airway management teams on a clear progression through airway management techniques when difficult intubation is identified in order to improve endotracheal intubation success and mitigate patient harm [22]. This included various oxygenation methods with prompts to progress to the next step of the algorithm (i.e., Plan A, Plan B, Exit) and to proceed to an Emergency strategy requiring front of neck access or surgical airway for failed oxygenation. The Airway Management Pause (AMP), a pre-intubation communication checklist, was also integrated in the revision as a strategy to standardize terminology and facilitate development and communication of an airway management plan that would help to move the team from one strategy to the next in the event of difficult or failed endotracheal intubation.

Organization and layout of the DAM cart were configured to mirror the DAM algorithm so that the two tools can be

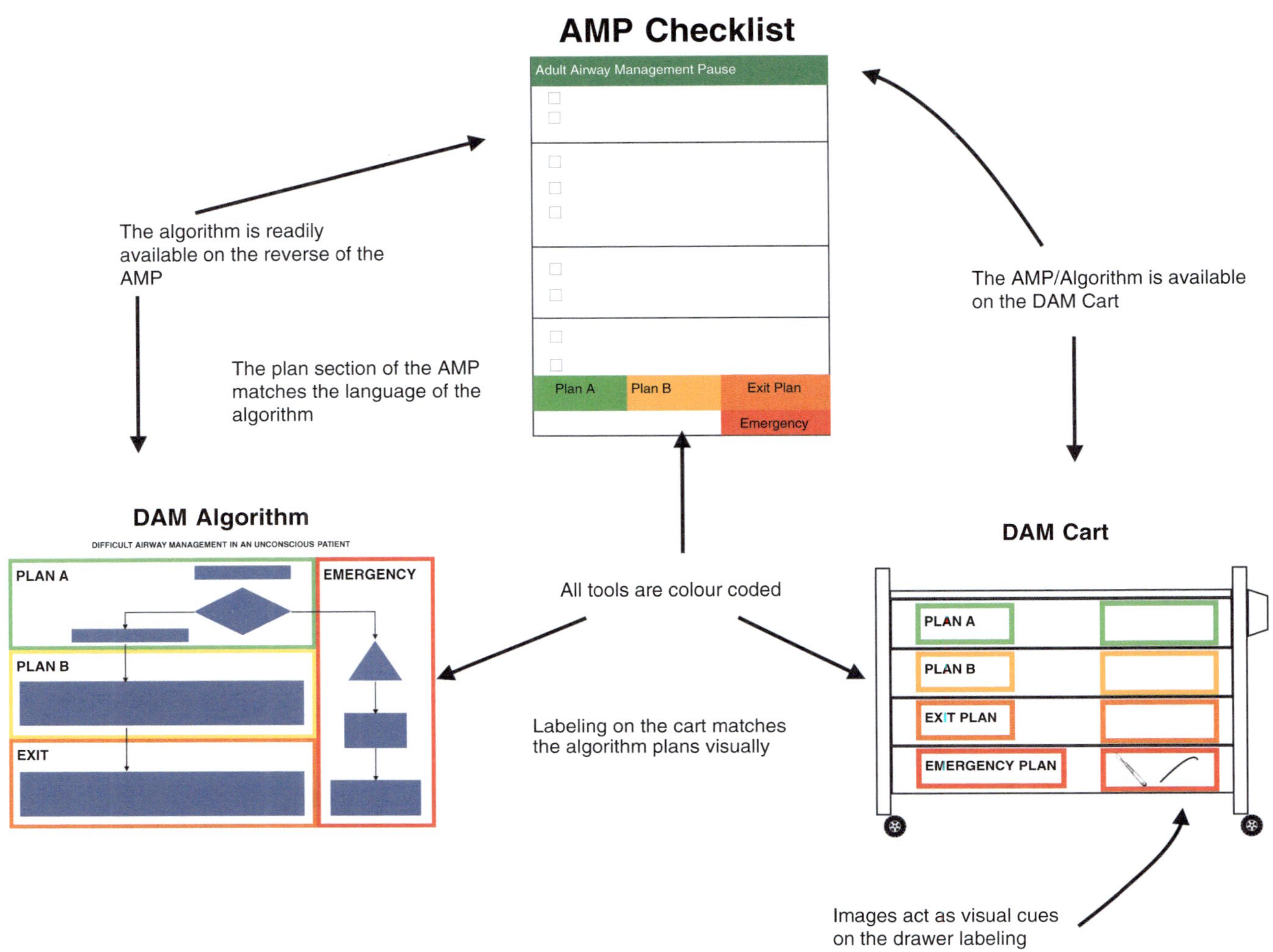

Fig. 26.1 Difficult Airway Management (DAM) Algorithm, Airway Management Pause (AMP) Checklist, and Difficult Airway Management (DAM) Cart we designed to support each other functionally

used together seamlessly when managing a difficult airway. Specifically, the cart was organized by airway plan and the color coding and wording on the DAM algorithm and AMP was mirrored on the cart (e.g., Plan A in text and green color swatch on the outside drawer of the DAM cart to align with Plan A on the DAM algorithm and AMP (Fig. 26.1). In addition, images of select equipment housed within the drawers were displayed on the outside of the cart to aid fast recognition (e.g., laryngoscope blade to indicate initial intubation strategy equipment). Equipment needed for that step in the algorithm was placed inside the corresponding drawer. Cart contents were also streamlined by standardizing equipment necessary for where it would be used (i.e., Emergency Departments (ED) and Intensive Care Units (ICU)), and incorporating human factors principles such as the functional grouping principle, sequence of use principle, and clutter-avoidance principle [23].

Simulation was used in usability testing where seven physicians and six respiratory therapists from multiple sites and care areas (i.e., ED, ICU, OR) used the AMP, the DAM algorithm, and DAM cart in a simulated difficult airway management scenario in a hospital simulation lab with a patient mannequin. This was the first step of usability testing prior to using it in the in situ clinical environment. A trauma scenario of a gunshot wound to the face was used as an anticipated difficult airway scenario where the patient's condition worsened progressively through the scenario to increase the urgency for decision-making and airway management actions. Participants were told that intubation attempts were unsuccessful to encourage movement through the DAM algorithm and the use of specific plans and tools in the DAM cart that mirrored the patient's condition (e.g., Plan B, Exit, Emergency). Following the simulation, participants were debriefed and completed a questionnaire about the DAM algorithm, DAM cart, and AMP which included a mix of Likert and open-ended questions (Appendix A).

Usability testing provided the opportunity for clinicians to try the new DAM equipment and tools in a realistic fashion and provide feedback. Through a combination of observational data and end-user feedback, small changes were made to the DAM cart, DAM algorithm, and AMP to ensure they would meet clinical user needs. Some examples include more closely aligning the colors assigned to each plan between the algorithm, the cart, and the AMP, increasing contrast on the algorithm by using the colors as a border around each plan. Additional changes included adding items such as anti-fog gel for the disposable bronchoscope (Ambu aScope), pediatric stylets, and a "call for help" sign to the outside of the cart to mirror the algorithm.

Implementation of the revised DAM carts was supported by the simulation team and multiple simulation labs, and funding was obtained to upgrade existing DAM carts throughout the Zone. This upgrading included replacement of drawers, the addition of labelling, and the purchase of additional equipment. Funds were also used to facilitate the training of end users and to support ongoing interprofessional team training.

Respiratory Therapists (RT) are the primary hands-on users of the DAM carts, with the need to locate and prepare equipment rapidly in emergency situations. The simulation lab carts were revamped prior to clinical implementation to allow for RTs and clinicians from all professions to familiarize themselves with and use the tools in a safe environment with no risk to actual patients.

Case Study 4: New Clinical Environments and Programs

System simulation is paramount to the safe testing and opening of new clinical environments and programs prior to use with actual patients [24]. Guidelines suggest that for every dollar invested in simulation-based mock-up evaluations, somewhere between $5.06 and $26.85 can be saved through the avoidance of future renovations [24]. In addition to cost savings, these methods improve patient and staff safety, afford greater efficiency in operations, improve utilization of space, and promote better overall function.

In newly developed centers and programs, the following case study highlights the use of simulation to standardize, test, and implement a new pediatric trauma program. In this context, a combined focus and scaffolded approach to individual and team training, in combination with systems and workflow testing, was required to meet the needs of many new team members coming together in a new program and space.

Our acute level 1 and subacute level 2 team consisted of trauma team leads (i.e., a mix of experienced emergency physicians and pediatric trauma surgeons), clinical pharmacists, respiratory therapists, nurses, social workers, radiology technicians, and child life specialists. Additionally, Orthopedics and Neurosurgery consultants would be directly called when indicated, and Transfusion Medicine and the OR would be notified for all acute traumas.

As part of pre-opening, several trauma clinical practice guidelines were developed, using Advanced Trauma Life Support (ATLS) principles, key landmark studies, and other published guidelines. These clinical practice guidelines were approved by all stakeholders involved in the trauma program at Sidra Medicine, and are the foundations for most of the level 1 and 2 care for pediatric trauma patients cared for in the ED and beyond.

This program consisted of several implementation phases to scaffold learning and complexity during clinical commissioning. First, it was important to ensure that nursing and physician staff were similarly qualified in baseline skills and courses (i.e., ATLS). The second phase included site-specific equipment training for key pieces of trauma equipment such as intravenous hotlines/fluid warmers, the Level 1 rapid infuser, application of site-specific pelvic binders, cervical collars, femoral splints, and backboards and scoops. It was also important to train providers on the equipment and consumables used for a variety of trauma-related procedures including chest tube insertion, femoral nerve blocks, intraosseous insertion, and airway management. The third phase included a simulation curriculum than was facilitated over 12 weeks designed to incorporate increasing complexity (i.e., individual, team, and systems complexity) and emotional intensity to align with realistic trauma scenarios.

Simulation scenarios were designed to focus on trauma and injury profiles including road collisions, ATV injuries, falls resulting in isolated head injuries, head injuries with pneumothorax, abdominal trauma, poly trauma, spinal trauma, and traumatic cardiac arrest. Where appropriate, clinical practice guidelines were used in the development of cases with the expectation that the teams providing care would incorporate these guidelines as part of their management. Initially, cases focused heavily on non-technical skills, such as Crisis Resource Management (CRM), in addition to the initial medical stabilization and management of pediatric trauma patients. CRM skills were key as none of the teams had worked together prior to the hospital opening. CRM topics included elements of teamwork, problem-solving, closed-loop communication, and the use of other TeamSTEPPS strategies and tools [25]. The goal was to enhance communication, leadership, and resource management. Most cases were 15–30 min long, depending on complexity and workflow, and the debrief post event ran for 45 min.

The curriculum then transitioned to a greater focus on workflow and systems testing. For example, one of the polytrauma cases included activation of the massive transfusion protocol as well as testing the workflow from the ED resuscitation area to the OR. For other cases, the focus was on the workflow and transfer of patients to diagnostic imaging for computed tomography (CT) or the Pediatric Intensive Care Unit (PICU). Scenarios that tested workflows of ED trauma bay to diagnostic imaging or to OR ran as much as 45 min or more. On average, 8–12 scenarios were facilitated per week.

Debriefing was aligned to the objectives of each scenario using a mixed method of debriefing to elicit feedback from the participants. Questions centered on what happened, what was learned from the event, and what should be changed or done differently for the next event. Feedback was collected, and task assignments were made after each debrief to ensure that potential changes would be prioritized and completed.

Several measures were collected to assess outcomes of the program. Key indicators included a shortened time to complete the primary and secondary survey; time to the OR, CT, and PICU; and time to lab results and time to transfusion. The number of missed injuries in complex cases was recorded and reduced over time, and a noted decrease in the number of deviations from the trauma clinical practice guidelines was observed. Team communication also improved dramatically.

Conclusion

The use of simulation for systems integration, including the design and testing of new and used spaces and processes, has been shown to reduce organizational costs, improve safety and efficiency, and lead to better implementation. This takes a shift in mindset that moves us away from a primary focus on the individual healthcare provider to thinking about the healthcare system and the factors that impact our ability to function within our role(s). These can include factors such as the environment (e.g., noise, lighting, distractions, physical layout and design), the physical tasks (e.g., difficulty, complexity, sequence, variety), the tools and technology (e.g., usability, functionality, accessibility, level of automation), or broader organization features (e.g., staffing, workloads, day versus night differences, work culture).

This "approach" to simulation can be referred to variably in existing literature, and can be referenced as system-focused simulation, design thinking approach to simulation, translational simulation, and simulation-based clinical systems testing, to name a few. As this science evolves, principles can be applied from various other disciplines such as patient safety science and quality improvement, human factors, project and change management, design thinking, process improvement, and implementation science.

It is advantageous to think of focused systems events as *ongoing tests of change* and improvement, which can help both facilitators and participants establish a system thinking mindset. One such idea is to consider plan-do-study-act cycles in the context of simulation projects. This helps to prepare teams for the work and change that most often follows the simulation and debrief. Having a project manager role, or someone to take on related project tasks, is very helpful to manage the planning of communications, scenario co-development process, logistics, event planning, and follow-up work. Some simulation programs may be armed with dedicated simulation personnel who can manage both the project and simulation work, while others may be a collaboration between educators, simulationists, and project managers. Lastly, it is important to have the "sponsorship" from healthcare leadership required to enable the work to happen, implement the changes that may be required, and to support staff to engage in the process.

Taking a "systems thinking" approach is key from the planning stages through to the simulation, debriefing, and improvement stages. This supports effective scenario design, ensures debriefing focused on systems rather than individuals, and captures the feedback used to inform change.

Consider starting with a small project, perhaps a process change on one unit with just a few stakeholders, and then increase complexity to larger system-based projects over time. These more complex projects may include multiple user groups, complex spaces (i.e., building a new unit or hospital), and processes (i.e., complex multi-user disaster events, protocols).

What is evident is that taking any small step to get your system-focused simulation program operational will be a step in the right direction to enable user-centered design and improved safety and efficiency of your healthcare system.

Key Points

- The objectives, design, and debriefing of systems-focused simulation differs in primary purpose and approach from traditional simulation in that it is focused on the system elements surrounding the healthcare team, such as the physical environment, tasks, tools, technology, people, processes, and organization, to enable safe and effective care.
- Simulation allows for the recreation of complex systems and represents as close as possible how work is actually happening versus how we may perceive it is happening to better assess risk, mitigate harm, and proactively improve systems and processes of care delivery.
- System-focused simulation can reduce organizational costs, improve safety and efficiency, inform and reduce risk, as well as solve clinical challenges.
- This chapter highlights several examples of the real-world utilization and outcomes of systems simulation and human factors including protocols to improve the initial arrival of a single trauma patient contrasted to activation of mass casualty incident protocols; how to incorporate human factors and system simulation to test the usability of difficult airway management carts and airway management pause checklists; and the commissioning of new spaces such as emergency rooms and trauma room bays.

Acknowledgments The authors would like to recognize Dr. Andrea Boone, Elaine Sigalet, Jason Laberge, Chris Cuthbert, and all project sponsors for their support for this work.

Appendix A: Dam Tools Usability Testing Questionaire

Role:	❑ RT ❑ Physician ❑ Resident
Primary Care Area:	❑ Emergency Department ❑ ICU ❑ Other:________
Primary Site:	❑ FMC ❑ PLC ❑ RGH ❑ SHC
Name (optional):	

This is a feedback form to provide your assessment of the standardized Difficult Airway Management (DAM) tools that are being developed (i.e. DAM cart configuration, DAM algorithm, Airway Management Pause). Your participation in completing this form is valued to help assist in determining how these tools might work in practice and if any further changes are required before rollout and implementation.

Thank you in advance for your feedback.

Please indicate your responses with a ✓ in the appropriate field using the following scale:

1= Strongly Disagree; 2= Disagree; 3= Neutral; 4= Agree; 5= Strongly Agree

Criteria – DAM Cart Configuration	1	2	3	4	5	N/A
1. The configuration (layout) of contents in the DAM cart is intuitive						
2. It is difficult to find items in the DAM cart						
3. Items that are used together are stored together in the DAM cart						
4. The labelling and pictures on the outside of the DAM cart drawers is helpful to locate specific supplies						
5. I prefer the new configuration of the DAM to the current layout at my site						
Criteria – DAM Algorithm	**1**	**2**	**3**	**4**	**5**	**N/A**
6. The DAM algorithm is intuitive and easy to use						
7. The DAM algorithm matched the DAM cart set up						
8. It is unclear when to move to the next step in the algorithm						
9. I feel the DAM algorithm would help guide my practice for difficult airway management						

Please continue on back of the page

Have you responded to any difficult airway management situations in the past year? YES NO

If yes, how many? ____________________

General comments on the DAM cart configuration (likes, dislikes, anything you would change)

____

____

____

____

____

General comments on the DAM algorithm (likes, dislikes, anything you would change)

____

____

____

____

____

Please indicate your responses with a ✓ in the appropriate field using the following scale:

1= Strongly Disagree; 2= Disagree; 3= Neutral; 4= Agree; 5= Strongly Agree

Criteria – Airway Management Pause	1	2	3	4	5	N/A
The layout of the AMP checklist is easy to follow						
The process of talking through the intubation plan with the whole team using a communication pause is a waste of time						
The AMP checklist fits well with the DAM Cart set up						
The AMP checklist fits well with the DAM algorithm						
There are_______________ items on the AMP checklist (*please explain your answer in the comments below*)	❑ Too many		❑ The right amount		❑ Not enough	

General comments on the AMP (likes, dislikes, anything you would change)

____

____

____

____

____

References

1. Baker GR, Norton PG, Flintoft V, Blais R, Brown A, Cox J, Etchells E, Ghali WA, Hébert P, Majumdar SR, O'Beirne M, Palacios-Derflingher L, Reid RJ, Sheps S, Tamblyn R. The Canadian Adverse Events Study: the incidence of adverse events among hospital patients in Canada. Can Med Assoc J. 2004;170(11):1678–86.
2. Committee on Quality of Health Care in America. In: LT CJK, Donaldson MS, editors. To err is human: building a safer health system. Washington: Institute of Medicine (US), National Academies Press (US); 2000. PMID: 25077248.
3. Deming. Available from: https://deming.org/quotes/10141/.
4. Lopreiato JO. Healthcare simulation dictionary. Rockville: Agency for Healthcare Research and Quality. AHRQ Publication No. 16(17)-0043; 2016.
5. Dube M, et al. COVID-19 pandemic preparation: using simulation for systems-based learning to prepare the largest healthcare workforce and system in Canada. Adv Simul (Lond). 2020;5:22.
6. Mirette Dubé BJ, Kaba A, Cunnington W, France K, Lomas K, Novick RJ, Robertson K, Coltman C, Ferland A. Preventing harm: testing and implementing health care protocols using systems integration and learner-focused simulations: a case study of a new postcardiac surgery, Cardiac Arrest Protocol. Clinical Simulation in Nursing. X:1–9. Available at https://doi.org/10.1016/j.ecns.2019.10.00 May 2020 Special Patient Safety Issue.
7. Brazil V. Translational simulation: not 'where?' but 'why?' A functional view of in situ simulation. Adv Simul (Lond). 2017;2:20.
8. Dubé M, et al. Building impactful systems-focused simulations: integrating change and project management frameworks into the pre-work phase. Adv Simul (Lond). 2021;6(1):16.
9. Colman N, et al. Simulation-based clinical systems testing for healthcare spaces: from intake through implementation. Adv Simul (Lond). 2019;4:19.
10. Dubé M, et al. Goals, recommendations, and the how-to strategies for developing and facilitating patient safety and system integration simulations. HERD. 2020;13(1):94–105.
11. Stone KP, et al. Systems integration, human factors, and simulation. In: Comprehensive healthcare simulation: pediatrics. Springer; 2016. p. 67–75.
12. Dubé M, et al. Evaluations for new healthcare environment commissioning and operational decision making using simulation and human factors: a case study of an interventional trauma operating room. HERD. 2021;14(4):442–56.
13. Colman N, et al. Prevent safety threats in new construction through integration of simulation and FMEA. Pediatr Qual Saf. 2019;4(4):e189.
14. Kaba A, Barnes S. Commissioning simulations to test new healthcare facilities: a proactive and innovative approach to healthcare system safety. Adv Simul (Lond). 2019;4:17.
15. Auerbach M, Kessler DO, Patterson M. The use of in situ simulation to detect latent safety threats in paediatrics: a cross-sectional survey. BMJ Simul Technol Enhanc Learn. 2015;1(3):77–82.
16. Brazil V, Purdy EI, Bajaj K. Connecting simulation and quality improvement: how can healthcare simulation really improve patient care? BMJ Qual Saf. 2019;28(11):862–5.
17. Dubé MM, et al. PEARLS for systems integration: a modified PEARLS framework for debriefing systems-focused simulations. Simul Healthc. 2019;14(5):333–42.
18. Holden RJ, et al. SEIPS 2.0: a human factors framework for studying and improving the work of healthcare professionals and patients. Ergonomics. 2013;56(11):1669–86.
19. Dumas JF, Redish J. A practical guide to usability testing. Greenwood Publishing Group Inc; 1993.
20. Lefebvre MS, Milloy S, Joynt C. Optimal crash cart configuration for a surgical NICU: utilizing human factors principles. Adv Neonatal Care. 2021;21(4):289–396.

21. Milloy S, Bubric K. A four-stage method for optimizing and standardizing a crash cart configuration. IISE Trans Occup Ergon Hum Factors. 2018;6(3–4):157–64.
22. Law JA, et al. The difficult airway with recommendations for management–part 1–difficult tracheal intubation encountered in an unconscious/induced patient. Can J Anaesth. 2013;60(11):1089–118.
23. Lee J, et al. Introduction to Human Factors Engineering. 2nd ed; 2003.
24. Healthcare facility mock-up evaluation guidelines: using simulation to optimize return on investment for quality patient safety; 2016.
25. Quality, A.F.H.R.A. Team strategies and tools to enhance team performance and safety. [cited 23 Jan 2023]. Available from: https://www.ahrq.gov/teamstepps/index.html.

Quality Improvement and Trauma Quality Indicators

27

Nori L. Bradley and Sandy Widder

> Measurement is the first step that leads to control and eventually to improvement. If you can't measure something, you can't understand it. If you can't understand it, you can't control it. If you can't control it, you can't improve it.—H. James Harrington

Introduction

Quality in the healthcare system is being increasingly questioned [1]. The oft-cited report "To Err Is Human" by the Institute of Medicine indicates up to 98,000 people die annually in US hospitals because of injuries during their care [2]. This has been a strong impetus for the public to demand better quality from their healthcare system and their providers at an affordable cost [3]. Trauma is the leading cause of death in the first four decades of life, the fourth leading cause of death overall in North America, and a significant contributor to potential years of life lost. Overall, major trauma patients have a 20% mortality rate, while survivors often sustain permanent disability [4]. Acute trauma care providers share the same attitude as the public: that systems and healthcare teams can be further improved to benefit patients and population health.

It is standard for healthcare organizations to measure quality data regularly and rigorously, but it takes more than just measurement to determine whether targeted changes are truly leading to improvements and prolonged success. Many interventions are reactive to critical incidents or high-profile issues, and sustainability may not have been factored in during the change design. This chapter will discuss healthcare quality as it relates to trauma, current measurement systems and indicators, and the potential benefits that can be derived from contributing to a trauma data registry.

N. L. Bradley (✉)
Department of Surgery, University of Alberta, 2D Walter Mackenzie Centre, University of Hospital, Edmonton, AB, Canada

S. Widder
Department of Surgery, University of Alberta, Edmonton, AB, Canada
e-mail: sandy.widder2@albertahealthservices.ca

Healthcare Quality and Relevance to Trauma

A widely accepted definition states *quality of care* is "care that results in desired health outcomes and is consistent with best professional practice" [5]. In order to delineate an abstract concept like quality into a measurable framework, six dimensions of quality have been proposed under the Institute of Medicine (IOM)'s "Aims for Improvement" [2]:

1. *Safe*: Care in healthcare facilities should be free from harm.
2. *Effective*: Evidence-based practice should be the standard of care.
3. *Efficient*: Care should be cost-effective with minimal waste in the system.
4. *Timely*: Waits and delays to care/treatment should be minimized.
5. *Patient-centered:* Care should focus on the patient, respecting personal preferences and supporting patient control during treatment.
6. *Equitable*: Disparities in care should be eradicated.

Ideally, specific performance measures that align with these six dimensions of quality healthcare will drive improvement in patient care within each healthcare discipline. However, a recent report highlighted a gap within trauma care for quantifiable metrics in the areas of patient-centeredness and equity. Performance measures may be categorized as those reflecting *structure*, *process*, and *outcomes*, relying on the Donabedian model. Briefly, structure refers to the physical environment of a healthcare facility, process refers to clinical interventions for a given patient, and outcome refers to the patient status after completing an episode of care. See Table 27.1 for definitions and trauma-specific examples. With respect to the IOM aims, a process measure

L. Marshall Gillman, S. Widder (eds.), *Trauma Team Dynamics*, https://doi.org/10.1007/978-3-031-86312-7_27

Table 27.1 Performance measures: descriptions and examples

Measure	Description	Trauma examples
Structure	Measures of the static characteristics of the individuals providing care (e.g., education, certification) and the settings where care is provided (e.g., equipment, staffing levels)	Proportion of ATLS-trained healthcare providers Level of the trauma center
Process	Measures of what takes place during the delivery of care. It can reflect both appropriateness of an action (e.g., ordering the right test) and skill for properly performing the action in a timely fashion	Obtaining a CT head for GCS ≤8 within 30 min of arrival to a healthcare facility Proportions of patients who received DVT prophylaxis
Outcome	Measures of whether healthcare goals were achieved, which can include cost, patient satisfaction, or disease control	30-day mortality or Return to work within 3 months of injury

reflecting "timely" and "effective" care would be getting trauma patients to the operating theatre within 60 min. A process measure reflecting "safe" care would be the proportion of trauma patients receiving appropriate deep vein thrombosis prophylaxis. Defined and meaningful trauma quality indicators allow for identification of appropriate interventions and subsequent change management.

Trauma patients are inherently at risk for harm in healthcare. While they are generally young with minimal co-morbidities, trauma patients can present to healthcare in physiological extremis, have above-average rates of untreated mental health and addiction issues, and are often socially disadvantaged. Great variability in clinical outcomes has been observed across hospitals that treat trauma patients, including Level I centers [7]. Even in countries with mature trauma systems, up to 50% of major trauma patients do not receive recommended care, and preventable trauma deaths still occur in hospital [8]. In Canada, adherence to ATLS guidelines appears low in rural settings [9]. Furthermore, medical errors are common in critically ill trauma patients [8]. Review of in-hospital trauma deaths has found 2.5–14% of medical errors were preventable [10]. Quality improvement can support positive and sustainable change for trauma systems.

The Evolution of Quality Indicators in Trauma

The use of quality indicators in trauma care is an evolving process. Ideal quality indicators should have high reliability, sensitivity, and specificity, while process measures should have empirical links with patient outcomes [11]. With respect to trauma, ideal quality indicators should apply to a significant number of cases, rely on current and best practice, consider a specific/appropriate population, include a risk adjustment strategy, and reflect outcomes other than mortality [12]. Most of us have experienced cases where good patient outcomes have occurred despite poor care (i.e., faulty process or inadequate structure) and cases when poor outcomes have occurred despite optimal care in well-equipped facilities. Thus, any measure that assesses quality must be designed such that it truly captures the aspect of the healthcare system/patient care that it is thought to capture.

Table 27.2 Ten most common quality indicators identified from 247 trauma centers (Santana and Stelfox [13])

Quality indicator	Percentage of centers
Appropriate admission service/physician	53
Hospital mortality	43
Secure airway in comatose patient	40
Time to laparotomy	39
Scene time	38
Time to craniotomy in severe traumatic brain injury	36
Length of stay	35
Reintubation within 48 h of extubation	34
Nonsurgical management of gunshot wound	32
Unplanned return to operating room	30

The American College of Surgeons Committee on Trauma (ACS-COT) used expert consensus to create a set of quality indicators (audit filters) in 1987 to facilitate quality improvement from the peer review process [6]. Since then, a plethora of indicators have been implemented in a variety of jurisdictions, which allows for standards to be set, and for other organizations to strive for to improve trauma patient care. In a recent survey of Trauma Centers in Canada, the USA, and Australasia, 10,587 quality indicators were identified from 242 institutions, including 1102 unique indicators. The 10 most common quality indicators identified are listed in Table 27.2 [13].

Several limitations in these reported quality indicators were noted. Most quality indicators were not well specified, meaning a descriptive statement was included but little detail regarding data elements or construction of the measure, which impacts reliability and validity of the indicator. Furthermore, not all aspects of trauma care were captured with these measures. While many indicators reflected hospital process and outcomes for trauma care, few measured pre-hospital care and even fewer measured post-hospital care or secondary prevention. In all phases of trauma care, structure-based quality indicators were rarely used. With respect to the Institute of Medicine's six aims for improvement (described earlier in this chapter), patient-centered care and equitable care were measured by less than 1% of the 10,587 quality indicators reported [13]. Process measures put forth by ACS-COT were also questioned in their ability to reflect patient outcomes [14]. A review of current ASC-COT quality indicators found that those that are strongly associated with clinical outcomes lacked face validity to identify poor-quality care for complex multi-trauma patients [7]. Thus, gaps existed in assessments of trauma quality.

Considering these gaps, several initiatives in North America have advanced the measure of quality in trauma. In 2006, the American College of Surgeons created the Trauma Quality Improvement Program (TQIP) to move forward from ASC-COT audit filters and provide reliable, high-quality, and risk-adjusted data for mortality rates, common in-patient complications (e.g., deep venous thrombosis), and trauma processes of care across participating trauma centers [15]. Rigorous standardization of the National Trauma Data Standard (how hospital data is collected) has allowed TQIP to provide benchmarking measures such that individual trauma hospitals can compare themselves to other centers and identify areas of strength and weakness in pre-specified areas [15, 16]. As well, there is the ability for institutions to network to facilitate and offer mentorship around QI initiatives. This allows institutions to focus QI efforts in addressing areas of sub-standard performance. It also highlights best practices of care, which can be shared among institutions, and can influence funding in pay-for-performance models. Currently, over 900 institutions in North America are using TQIP [17].

Currently, TQIP relies on ordinary logistic regression to compare institutions. Ongoing work in Quebec, Canada, to assess inter-hospital mortality suggests that hierarchical logistic regression may be a better method to assess hospitals given the relationship among patients treated at the same institution [18]. Related work suggests that risk-adjusted models for length of stay [19] and unplanned readmissions [20] are valid quality indicators to reflect acute trauma care. These models are based on routinely collected registry and administrative data and can be used to drive performance improvement. However, this method is more complex than ordinary logistic regression, and the implications of widespread implementation are still being evaluated. Another method to increase the reliability of trauma quality indicators has been the development of composite measures for predicting mortality. Computation of composite scores, based on multiple indicators, takes interactions between processes into account and may better reflect the complexity of trauma care [21]. Composite measures have been used to identify top hospital performers in management of medical issues such as: congestive heart failure, pneumonia, and acute myocardial infarction [22]. In the setting of trauma care, performance on nine process measures, i.e., CT head within 2 h of injury, combined as a composite measure successfully predicted mortality rates at the individual hospital level (Table 27.3) [12]. However, composite measures are sensitive to the methodology used in their construction, and different approaches can yield different results. This limitation was highlighted in a recent review of the Michigan Trauma Quality Improvement Program. Applying different weights to metrics included in the composite score revealed variability in scores, which could be viewed more favorably by providers in one calculation, or by patients or institutions in other calculations.

Table 27.3 Quality indicators included in composite score (Willis et al. [7])

Quality indicator
Team activated for major trauma patients
Fixation of femoral diaphyseal fracture in adult trauma patients
Head CT received within 2 h
GCS score <13 and head CT received within 2 h
Sub/epidural hematoma receiving craniotomy within 4 h
Cranial surgery <24 h
Abdominal surgery <24 h
Interval <8 h between arrival and treatment of blunt, compound tibial fracture
Laparotomy performed less than 2 h after arrival at ED

The TQIP program, hierarchical logistic regression, and development of composite measures are important steps to improve the validity of quality indicators in trauma. Unfortunately, many of these initiatives have focused on identifying factors associated with in-hospital mortality. Development of trauma systems over the past four decades has contributed to significant reductions in mortality. However, decreases in mortality rates do not necessarily reflect lower morbidity rates, and may overlook deficiencies in caring for those who survive and miss opportunities for quality improvement [23]. Several groups [10, 18, 24] have shown that other important aspects of trauma care are worthy of—and deserve—rigorous assessment. These groups advocate for additional outcome measures to evaluate the quality of trauma care, such as health-related quality of life [10], length of stay [19], and unplanned readmissions [20]. A recent review and consensus manuscript suggested internationally accepted quality indicators for trauma management. However, definitions and thresholds were not included, and alignment with the IOM's six aims for improvement was not described. As the science of QI continues to evolve and lessons are learned from the refinement of mortality-based quality indicators, a standardized and complete approach to QI in trauma care can be established. As leaders and advocates for the provision of trauma care, it is our responsibility to participate in this process.

Quality indicators help us establish that there is a problem, but these measures do not tell us how to fix the problem or whether the changes we implement are actually leading to an improvement. Here is where knowledge of quality improvement science can be of tremendous value. QI fundamentals, which include defining the problem, identifying the root cause, and using the Plan–Do–Study–Act Cycle to operationalize change, underlie how we can move forward to standardize and improve trauma care.

Quality Improvement and Change Management

Quality improvement (QI) is an approach that originated in industry during the 1920s and has been more recently applied to the healthcare system. It is both a method and cultural movement for all stakeholders including healthcare providers, management, patients, and families to evaluate and improve processes of patient care to achieve better patient outcomes, system performance, and professional development [25].

Five key steps to a successful QI initiative are as follows: (1) Stakeholder engagement. (2) Aligning with organizational needs and priorities. (3) Aim statement a priori. (4) Implementing the QI tool appropriate for your identified problem. (5) Incorporating change management principles. QI failure is often due to not following these key steps, and although some success might be attained, true sustainability and change are often not.

Before beginning any improvement initiative, *stakeholder engagement* is vital to understand where the problems are, why they might be occurring, and what changes might lead to successful improvements. Most individuals are "status quo" when it comes to the introduction of QI initiatives; if one can inspire these individuals, the QI sphere of influence and chances of successful implementation and sustainability greatly increase. To do this, it is important to understand human nature and some basic change management principles. Firstly, change is specific and different with everyone. Change might threaten those who favor the current state, or it may encourage those who see a need for change. Improving success with implementing QI initiatives, it is important to create awareness for the need to change. Building and creating awareness cannot be accomplished through one single medium such as a memo or newsletter but needs a multifaceted approach such as face-to-face communications, newsletters, huddles, social events, and video conferencing, for example [27]. When introducing QI initiatives, change often happens too quickly and at a high frequency which can lead to anger, frustration, and disengagement, which in turn can lead to barriers and resistance. To mitigate change resistance, it is important to give people time to contemplate and reflect on the problem at hand. Early conversations and dissemination of information in a timely manner give a sense of control, and stakeholders are not taken by surprise. Face-to-face conversations and visibility by change leaders are essential to make stakeholders feel supported and valued. As always, there will be resistors within the group, and it is critical to find out what their values are to find common ground with a shared interest. Encouraging participation, including sharing of thoughts and ideas so that individuals feel valued and empowered, is also key. The biggest resistors can occasionally become the QI initiative's biggest ally as these individuals will often bring innovative solutions that others have not thought of. It is important to not just hear what people are saying but truly listen as key change ideas will come from the grassroots of the organization.

Alignment with organizational needs is critical to obtain leadership support for the QI initiative but also for ongoing success and sustainability [27]. Executive sponsorship can help remove barriers, provide linkages to key stakeholders, and accessibility to resources. To be strategic, understand what is important for the leaders within your organization, select a QI initiative that is in line with priorities and vision, and ensure it is of clinical significance and will make a difference to the lives of patient and families. What is a priority for an individual may not be a priority for everyone else, and ultimately will not be successful [27].

Once a QI initiative has been decided on, it is important to communicate what the goals are in a clear manner a priori. An aim statement describes the project's desired outcomes in a measurable and time-specific way such that there is a shared mental model, and everyone understands what they are working toward [28]. Without this clear and concise statement, it will be difficult to work collaboratively and effectively toward a goal. The aim statement should be clear and unambiguous with end goals, specify a time period, and be ambitious. The aim statement should answer the questions: "How much? By when? For whom? For goals, consider standards that may already be established, or if there are no examples of leading practices, aim to decrease suboptimal care or adverse events by no less than 50% as an initial step. A small incremental change will not represent a sustainable change in quality or performance, and may not justify the resources or people required [29].

A variety of *QI tools* exist to evaluate a system for improvement, including cause and effect diagram (Fishbone) and failure mode effects analysis (FMEA). For this chapter, we will be focusing on a commonly used tool for improvement: the Shewhart Cycle/Plan–Do–Study–Act (PDSA) cycle (Fig. 27.1) [26]. Before performing a PDSA cycle, we must define the project aim, components to measure, and intervention for change by answering three key questions: [1] What are we trying to accomplish? (Aim), [2] How will we know that a change is leading to an improvement? (Measure), and [3] What change can we make that will result in improvement? (Change). Once a change and its measure are defined (Plan), it is tested on a small scale in a real setting (Do). Successes and failures of the intervention are analyzed with frequent modifications made in response to observations (Study). The inter-

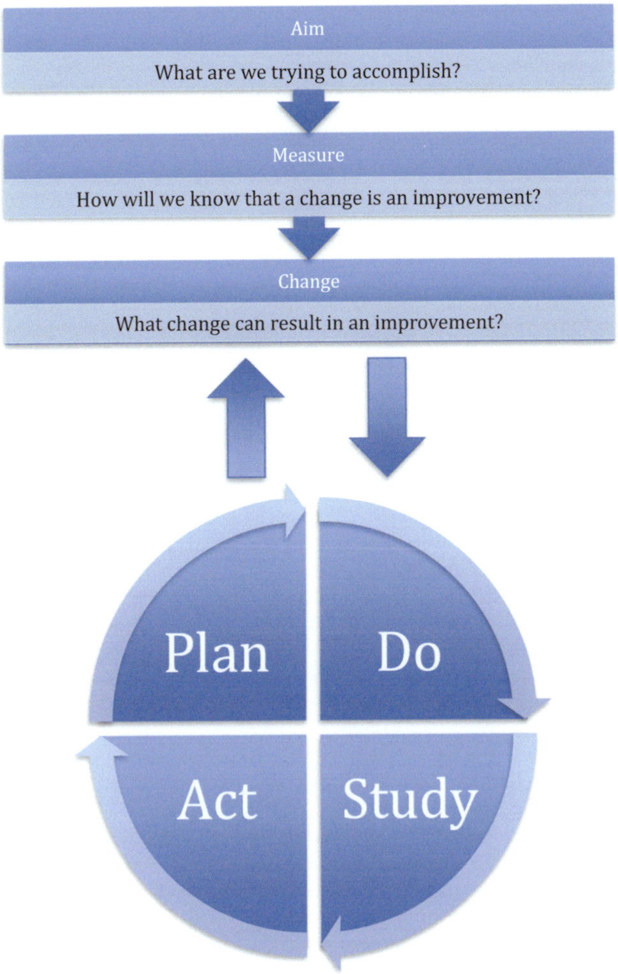

Fig. 27.1 Shewhart/Plan-Do-Study-Act Cycle

vention is tested repeatedly with these improved variations (Act) before being implemented on a broader scale. While scientifically grounded, such an approach is inherently different from that used in conventional randomized controlled studies because modifications to the intervention are continuous, and we begin to make improvements in the system before the intervention itself is perfected. In this way, a PDSA cycle allows us to exact change quickly while adapting interventions to suit the needs of the users and system.

The PDSA model for improvement can be seen in the following example. Plan—To improve compliance with administration of deep venous thrombosis (DVT) prophylaxis in trauma patients. Do—A monthly educational seminar to new residents orienting on the trauma service. Study—Audit charts on a weekly basis and determine compliance rates after 3 months. Act—Compliance rates have not improved to targeted goal, prompting another change intervention, i.e., a standardized order set including DVT prophylaxis. The cycle is then repeated until the target goal is achieved. Failure of quality improvement projects is most often due to lack of rigorous testing and introduction of change too early in the process.

When initiating a PDSA cycle, it is important to develop a family of performance measures. In addition to choosing an outcome and process measure, i.e., percent of trauma patients with pulmonary embolism complications and percent of patients getting DVT prophylaxis, respectively, one must also consider a balancing measure. A balancing measure is an outcome that is measured to ensure that the impact of changes to one part of the system does not cause changes (positive or negative) to another aspect of the system (e.g., increased bleeding with higher rates of DVT prophylaxis).

After choosing appropriate measures, an improvement plan requires that data is collected on a regular basis and audited. Results should be analyzed in meaningful intervals so that data is displayed over time. Quality tools such as run charts or control charts, which are beyond the scope of this review, are powerful methods to visualize the impact of a change. Sharing results in a transparent manner will also inspire new change ideas and also improvements.

To ensure small wins, and early successes to drive larger organizational projects, several principles should drive any QI initiative:

1. Select an issue that is feasible and within your area of influence.
2. Choose targets that are easy to measure at baseline and over time.
3. Ensure that data is being collected and reviewed on a regular basis.
4. Find commonalities and relate microsystem quality data and projects to organizational initiatives to help build support for future projects.

Opportunities for Improvement

We will leave you with several clinical questions to reflect how the Institute of Medicine's Six Aims for Improvement can be applied to trauma care at your institution:

1. *Safe*: What is the mortality rate and the adverse events rate for trauma patients treated at your facility?
2. *Effective*: Do all trauma patients with a GCS ≤ 8 get a head CT within 2 h of injury? What is the rate of compliance with DVT prophylaxis in trauma patients at your institution?
3. *Efficient*: Is there significant duplication of imaging and tests for patients transferred from other facilities?
4. *Timely*: How long does it take for trauma patients within your catchment area to obtain definitive care?

5. *Patient-centered:* What proportion of patients and families are provided with clear information during transitions between facilities or hospital departments?
6. *Equitable*: Are certain trauma patient populations that you treat (e.g., rural patients, First Nations) having worse outcomes that may be attributable to disparities in care?

Approaching these questions requires targeted audits of your trauma registry and appropriate application of QI tools to identify root causes that can be targeted for intervention. Ongoing critical evaluation of your current level of care will allow you to identify opportunities to improve quality of trauma care for your patients, and ultimately change outcomes for your population.

Key Notes

- When building a quality improvement initiative, think about the six aims for improvement (safe, effective, efficient, timely, patient-centered, equitable).
- Use of trauma quality indicators allows one to regularly measure and gauge quality improvement initiatives, including whether standards of care are being achieved.
- Process quality indicators are easier to measure short term than outcomes and can be early markers of improvement.
- Apply change management principles when translating improvement projects into practice.

References

1. Berwick DM, Nolan TW, Whittington J. The triple aim: care, health, and cost. Health Aff. 2008;27(3):759–69.
2. Institute of Medicine. Crossing the quality chasm: a new health system for the 21st century. Washington: Institute of Medicine, National Academies Press; 2001.
3. National strategy for quality improvement in health care: agency-specific quality strategic plans; 2011. http://www.ahrq.gov/workingforquality/nqs/nsqplans.pdf. Accessed 14 Oct 2013.
4. Evans C, Howes D, Pickett W, Dagnone L. Audit filers for improving processes of care and clinical outcomes in trauma systems. Cochrane Database Syst Rev. 2009;4
5. National Research Council. America's health in transition: protecting and improving quality. Washington: Institute of Medicine, National Academies Press; 1994.
6. Nayduch D, Moylan J, Snyder BL, et al. American College of Surgeons trauma quality indications: an analysis of outcome in a statewide trauma registry. J Trauma. 1994;37:565–73.
7. Glance LG, Dick AW, Mukamel DB, Turner MO. Association between trauma quality indicators and outcomes for injured patients. Arch Surg. 2012;147(4):308–15.
8. Gruen RL, Jurkovich GJ, McIntyre LK, et al. Patterns of error contributing to trauma mortality: lessons learned from 2,594 deaths. Ann Surg. 2006;244:371–80.
9. McCrum ML, McKee J, Lai M, Staples J, Switzer N, Widder SL. ATLS adherence in the transfer of rural trauma patients to a level I facility. Injury. 2013;44(9):1241–5.
10. Stelfox HT, Bobranska-Artiuch B, Nathens A, et al. Quality indicators for evaluating trauma care: a coping review. Arch Surg. 2010;145:286–95.
11. Freeman T. Using performance indicators to improve health care quality in the public sector: a review of the literature. Health Serv Manag Res. 2002;15:126–37.
12. Willis CD, Gabbe BJ, Cameron PA. Measuring quality in trauma care. Injury. 2007;38:527–37.
13. Santana MJ, Stelfox HT. Quality indicators used by trauma centers for performance measurement. J Trauma. 2012;72(5):1298–303.
14. Willis CD, Stoelwinder JU, Cameron PA. Interpreting process indicators in trauma care: contstruct validity versus confounding by indication. Int J Qual Health Care. 2008;20:331–8.
15. Hemmila MR, Nathens AB, Shafi S, et al. The Trauma Quality Improvement Program: pilot study and initial demonstration of feasibility. J Trauma. 2010;68:253–62.
16. Nathens AB, Cryer HG, Fildes J. The American College of Surgeons trauma quality improvement program. Surg Clin N Am. 2012;92:441–54.
17. ACS Trauma Quality Improvement Program. https://www.facs.org/quality-programs/trauma/quality/trauma-quality-improvement-program/. Accessed 30 June 2022.
18. Moore L, Hanley JA, Turgeon AF, Lavoie A. Evaluating the performance of trauma centers: hierarchical modeling should be used. J Trauma. 2010;69(5):1132–7.
19. Moore L, Stelfox HT, Turgeon AF, Nathens AB, Lavoie A, Emond M, et al. Derivation and validation of a quality indicator of acute care length of stay to evaluate trauma care. Ann Surg. 2014;00:1–7.
20. Moore L, Stelfox HT, Turgeon AF, Nathens AB, Lavoie A, Bourgeois G, Lapointe J. Derivation and validation of a quality indicator for 30-day unplanned hospital readmission to evaluate trauma care. J Trauma Acute Care Surg. 2014;76:1310–6.
21. Willis CD, Stoelwinder JU, Lecky FE, Woodford M, Jenks T, Bouamra O, Cameron PA. Applying composite performance measures to trauma care. J Trauma. 2010;60:256–62.
22. Ashish KJ, Orav EJ, Zhonghe L, Epstein AM. The relationship between mortality rates and performance in the hospital quality alliance measures. Health Aff. 2007;26(4):1104–10.
23. Hashmi ZG, Schenider EB, Castillo G, Jaut ER, Zafar SN, Cornwell EE 3rd, Mackenzie EG, Latif A, Haider AH. Benchmarking trauma centers on mortality alone does not reflect quality of care: implications for pay-for-performance. J Trauma Acute Care Surg. 2014;76(5):1184–91.
24. Moore L, Lavoie A, Sirois M-J, Swaine B, Murat V, Le Sage N, Emond M. Evaluating trauma centre structural performance: the experience of a Canadian provincial trauma system. J Emerg Trauma Shock. 2013;6:3–10.
25. Batalden PB, Davidoff F. What is "quality improvement" and how can it transform healthcare? Qual Saf Health Care. 2007;16:2–3.
26. Langley GL, Moen R, Nolan KM, Nolan TW, Norman CL, Provost LP. The improvement guide: a practical approach to enhancing organizational performance. 2nd ed. San Francisco: Jossey-Bass Publishers; 2009.
27. Hiatt J. ADKAR: a model for change in business, government, and our community. Colorado: Prosci Research; 2006.
28. Kotter JP. Leading change. Harvard Business Press; 2012.
29. Health Quality Ontario. http://www.hqontario.ca.

Putting It All Together: Quality Control in Trauma Team Training

28

Corry J. Kucik, Polly A. Haskins, and William P. Mulvoy III

Introduction

Quality control (QC) is a term originating in business and manufacturing. QC is increasingly being applied to "production lines" in medicine and is a process by which companies review the quality of all the factors contributing to "their" performance. The following factors are important to achieve and maintain quality: standards (recognized best practices), review of individual cases, individual qualifications and competence, healthy team interactions and relationships ("esprit de corps"), and organizational culture or climate. A supportive system will catch and correct [most] mistakes in patient care; however, a deficiency in any single aspect of these criteria can contribute to conditions leading to potential avoidable adverse outcomes [1].

Just as in business, medicine's "product" [patient care and outcome] is increasingly being evaluated by "inspectors," such as the Joint Commission, representatives of the insurance industry, and state and federal health regulators. Careful attention to detail and willingness to engage in the betterment of teamwork and communication are absolutely required to achieve optimum performance of a trauma team, which may mean the difference between life and death for our patients, and continued employment for teammates and ourselves.

The Institute of Medicine's (IOM) "Six Domains of Health Care Quality" (Table 28.1) serve as a useful educational tool to consumers (patients) on the quality of care they will receive, as well as an excellent guide to providers (physicians, nurses, techs, and the teams they comprise) as to the criteria upon which their performance will be "graded" by the healthcare system.

As one can see, the IOM asserts that safe and effective care is the sine qua non [the thing that is absolutely necessary] of all patient care, including trauma medicine. However, such other quality metrics as efficiency, patient satisfaction, and culturally appropriate care, will drive healthcare decisions, providing optimal care to trauma patient [2, 3].

C. J. Kucik (✉)
Department of Anesthesiology and Pain Medicine, University of Washington School of Medicine, Seattle, WA, USA

P. A. Haskins
US Naval Reserve, Norfolk, VA, USA

W. P. Mulvoy III
Department of Anesthesiology, Division of Cardiac Anesthesiology, Division of Critical Care Medicine, University of Florida College of Medicine, Gainesville, FL, USA
e-mail: wmulvoy@anest.ufl.edu

L. Marshall Gillman, S. Widder (eds.), *Trauma Team Dynamics*, https://doi.org/10.1007/978-3-031-86312-7_28

Table 28.1 Institute of Medicine's Six Domains of Health Care Quality

Safe: Avoiding harm to patients from the care that is intended to help them
Effective: Providing services based on scientific knowledge to all who could benefit and refraining from providing services to those not likely to benefit (avoiding underuse and misuse, respectively)
Patient-centered: Providing care that is respectful of and responsive to individual patient preferences, needs, and values and ensuring that patient values guide all clinical decisions
Timely: Reducing waits and sometimes harmful delays for both those who receive and those who give care
Efficient: Avoiding waste, including waste of equipment, supplies, ideas, and energy
Equitable: Providing care that does not vary in quality because of personal characteristics such as gender, ethnicity, geographic location, and socioeconomic status

Defining Quality in the Team Context

Trauma and critical care teams have required "interdisciplinary" medical teams much longer than this term has been used in the medical context. Interdisciplinary or multidisciplinary (transdisciplinary) teams are defined as multiple specialized professionals working together under a shared model with a common language [4]. Team-based workflow is essential in trauma and critical care for several factors:

1. Increasing complexity of skills and knowledge required to provide complex care to patients
2. Increasing specialization in health professions and a corresponding fragmentation of disciplinary knowledge, resulting in no single healthcare professional being able to meet all the complex needs of the patient
3. Policy emphasis on multi-professional teamwork and development of shared knowledge
4. Pursuit of continuity of care moving toward continuous quality improvement

Cross-disciplinary collaboration in the realm of patient safety has been emphasized in the IOM's "To Err is Human: Building a Safer Health System [5]." One of this report's landmark recommendations advocated that "Patient safety programs should establish interdisciplinary team training programs for providers that incorporate proven methods of team training, such as simulation." The report further asserted that considering how people interact with each other in teams, as well as counting technology as a member of the work team, should be integral in designing safer healthcare systems. To that end, Nancarrow et al. proposed ten "Interdisciplinary Team Competencies" to guide the formulation, operation, and quality control of such teams [14]:

1. An identified leader who provides clear direction and vision for the team as well as listening, support, and supervision
2. Incorporation of a set of values that provide direction for team's service, which should be visible
3. Demonstration of team culture and an interdisciplinary atmosphere of trust, wherein contributions are valued and consensus fostered
4. Appropriate processes and infrastructure to uphold the vision of service (communication, equipment, referral, transfer to next echelon of care)
5. Provision of quality patient-focused services with documented outcomes, utilizing feedback to improve quality
6. Use of strategies that improve intra-team communication, collaborative decision making, and effective team processes
7. Sufficient team staffing to integrate appropriate mix of competencies, skills, and personalities to meet needs of all patients
8. Recruitment of staff who demonstrate interdisciplinary competencies including team functioning, collaborative leadership, communication, professional knowledge, and experience
9. Promotion of role interdependence while maintaining respect for individual roles and autonomy
10. Facilitation of personal development through appropriate training, rewards, recognition, and career opportunities

The Military-Medical Overlap: Some Quality Control Principles in Trauma Teams

Successful teams display five characteristics: *commitment*, *common goals*, *competence*, *performance consistency*, and *communication* [6]. Commitment by all members, both to a common goal and to each other, can be cultivated by clear expectations, unequivocal leadership, a history of shared experiences, and basic trust and respect for each other's diverse skills. Experienced, effective teams adapt to changing patient requirements, can anticipate clinical activities, monitor interventions, are familiar with each other's roles, and offer corrective action when necessary. In such teams, suggestions and corrections are welcome from all, regardless of rank or station, and are made without fear of reprisal.

Table 28.2 Crew Resource Management principles and Analogous TeamSTEPPS principles

Decision-Making	Leadership, Mutual Support
Assertiveness	Leadership, Attitudes
Mission Analysis	Situation Monitoring, Attitudes
Communication	Communication
Leadership	Leadership
Adaptability/Flexibility	Attitudes
Situational Awareness	Situation Monitoring

Teaching the multitudes of comprehensive leadership training and team management models is beyond the scope of this work, and there are important principles that are easily elucidated for incorporation into the trauma team concept. Many of these principles have been developed not only in industry but also in "high-reliability organizations [7]" such as commercial aviation, aircraft carrier flight decks, and nuclear power reactors. The ability to process large amounts of information quickly and then act effectively on it (faster than one's enemy, in military parlance) has been codified in the "Boyd Cycle" or "OODA Loop" (Observe, Orient, Decide, Act) advocated by air combat pioneer Col. John Boyd [8]. Models such as aviation's Crew Resource Management (CRM) sprang from such innovations, and have been effectively adapted into medical practice, including the Team Strategies and Tools to Enhance Performance and Patient Safety (TeamSTEPPS) (Table 28.2).

A variation on CRM, Trauma Crew Resource Management (TCRM) evolved from the UK Ministry of Defense aviation training CRM programs of the 1980s and emphasized communication and teamwork to increase safety of military air operations. TCRM was initially adopted by anesthesia teams in immersion-type simulation training, utilizing fast-moving scenarios, debriefing, and analysis of team performance. CRM courses have now been adapted to trauma and critical care teams and teach essential skills such as adaptability; task prioritization; shared situational awareness; workload distribution; team communication before and after patient arrival; mobilization of resources in trauma bay, operating room (OR), intensive care unit (ICU) and diagnostics; performance monitoring and cross-checking of data; command, communication, and feedback coordination; leadership and management of team member followership; willingness to challenge each other; and conflict resolution skills [9]. With training, processes become planned and standardized, and each member knows not only his or her own responsibilities but also those of his teammates, and can anticipate actions due to repetition and practice.

TeamSTEPPS evolved from the Joint Commission's 2008 National Patient Safety Goal 16: Improve recognition and response to changes in a patient's condition. It was developed by the Agency for Healthcare Research and Quality (AHRQ) for training teamwork tools and strategies to healthcare professionals (available at http://teamstepps.ahrq.gov/). Several important innovations of the program have already reached prominence in medical practice and are increasingly being incorporated into trauma care. Rapid Response Systems (RRS) were the inaugural medium used to incorporate inter-team knowledge, "boundary spanning" transition support, and communication utilizing a specific framework. Inter-team knowledge supports continuity of care between different levels or types of care within the hospital (e.g., from the OR to the Post Anesthesia Care Unit), and expects that team members will have an understanding of roles and responsibilities within the team. The "SBAR" framework provides a standardized communication format for passing patient information, and consists of the components Situation (What is going on with the patient?), Background (What is the clinical background or context?), Assessment (What do I think the problem is?), and Recommendations/Request (What would I do or ask that my teammate do?). Evidence supports the positive impact of implementation of RRS and TeamSTEPPS [10], and various "how-to" guides are available to assist [11, 12].

MedTeams, a training medium developed by The Society of Trauma Nurses, similarly converts these concepts to apply to healthcare. The curriculum teaches teams to clarify the medical situation, use a callback system to enhance communication, support a culture of challenge (validate decisions by team members), delegate tasks to a specific people, and communicate the plan to the entire team [13].

Individual Qualifications and Team Training

Appropriate individual education, training, and baseline qualifications are a requisite starting point for building the successful trauma team. However, individual qualifications alone are not enough; indeed, poorly coordinated or even conflicting experts in their field may produce inferior patient outcomes when compared to a well-rehearsed team whose individuals, while competent, may be mediocre by comparison. Emergency physicians, trauma surgeons, anesthesia providers, additional consultants, nursing staff, respiratory therapists, and medical technicians (like the Navy Hospital Corpsman) must converge upon the patient in a well-choreographed effort to save a life. No single specialty can do it all, and trauma is indeed a team sport [13]. A team is essentially defined as a small group of people with corresponding, complementary skills, all working together to achieve a common goal. Effective teams are scalable and dynamic, performing both independent behaviors as well as interdependent and coordinated series of tasks [14].

Team-Based Principles

Again, a full discussion of principles such as *leadership*, *adaptability*, and *assertiveness* are included in earlier chapters. Many of these characteristics are not easily taught but must be developed through experience, introspection, and careful study. Thus, there is need for simulations, drills, reviews, and feedback. Indeed, some principles, most notably leadership and decision-making, are the focus of advanced study in many fields. While some have argued that traits such as leadership and adaptability are innate, growing evidence [15] suggests that even among those not so inclined, these skills can at least to some degree be learned. In many ways, leadership will "declare" itself in a trauma team, and team members will adapt to its presence (or absence) over time. Anyone who wishes to exert leadership within a trauma team should expect not only to know his or her field well but should also commit to continuously revisiting the study of leadership in adversity, human behavior, and communication.

Maintaining good *situational awareness* as well as a healthy appreciation for how quickly the clinical (or operational) situation can change (*adaptability*) are critical, especially in a combat or mass casualty environment. The trauma team must not only anticipate the likely course of a specific injury but also respond seamlessly when the information changes—especially for the worse—and must do so in a non-accusatory manner if trust and communication are to be reinforced. Situational awareness generally involves three (or four) levels: perception, comprehension, and projection. *Perception* encompasses monitoring, cue detection, and simple recognition, and leads to an individual awareness of current objects, events, people, systems, and environmental influences. *Comprehension* involves integration of the many varied perceived components, as well as an appreciation for how these factors may influence individual or team goals, objectives, and outcomes. *Projection* is achieved through taking the knowledge gained from perception and comprehension and then extrapolating their likely impact on the patient or operational environment in a timely manner [16]. Personnel and supply status, the likelihood of additional incoming casualties, Operating Room availability, blood supply, En-route-care capability, evacuation assets, weather conditions, and the current tactical or security situation must all be within the "scan" of the modern trauma team's situational awareness, particularly when making patient care decisions in a deployed environment [17]. The trauma environment, much like the combat setting, implies dynamic conditions that routinely change in a split-second, and therefore, situational awareness becomes a product of the team, whereby "distributed cognition" becomes the team's expected norm, significantly augmenting their previous performance.

Good *communication* naturally lends itself to distributed situational awareness, augmented trust, and teamwork. Familiarity as a team can also lead to the ability to "read" unspoken communication factors; body language, task distribution, command structure, team history, and individual personality considerations all play a role. It is broadly documented that errors in communication are responsible for approximately 60–80% of all healthcare errors. Communication between team members must be clear and unambiguous, and is most effective when members feel respected and empowered to participate [18].

Communication must be in a language all team members can understand and not be "profession-specific" (sometimes interpreted as condescending). Ideally, the communicator will make eye contact, will stop distractions or other tasks if possible, and will check understanding on the part of the intended receiver (e.g., by having them repeat back the information or request that was passed), all while minimizing any emotional factors. Unequivocal ("autocratic") communication from a defined trauma team leader has been shown to contribute to improved team coordination, ATLS adherence, and secondary survey [9] performance, and is often called for during stressful phases of initial evaluation and resuscitation. Conversely, once the patient has been stabilized and admitted, the multidisciplinary trauma/critical care team (intensivists, nurses, respiratory and physical therapists, pastoral care, interpreters, and many others) can ideally operate under a more collaborative governance [18].

Most successful team leaders promote "psychological safety," encouraging all team members to express their observations and opinions without fear. This, however, must be balanced with the responsibility of each member to be accountable for, and competent in, their actions, and to perform them well in a stressful, fast-paced environment. Team-wide familiarity with each member's skillsets, norms, and role expectations increases cohesiveness, communication, and ultimately, performance. Additionally, leaders who utilized cross-disciplinary leadership, collaborative decision making, and clear communication tended to benefit more from team feedback and inspire motivation, leading to overall improvement in team performance [14]. *Flexibility* of all members between the autocratic (trauma team leader) and the empowering (intensivist leader) styles reflects trust and suggests a "flat hierarchy," one in which the leader is part of the interdisciplinary team, information is disseminated without restraint, and all members regardless of rank or position can express concerns or make suggestions [19]. Taking full advantage of the abilities of team members to communicate, both within and external to the team, will improve team performance. For instance, nurses are a valuable asset as they not only bring a highly developed clinical skill set but also serve as key communicators both within the team as well as to ancillary staff and family. Nurses demonstrate collaboration, credibility, compassion, and coordination when communicating with the healthcare team [20].

As mentioned earlier, communication in the trauma bay must be clear, direct, and often autocratic in order to avoid confusion and ensure tasks are accomplished expeditiously. *Communication errors* are often divided into "sender" and "receiver" errors. Sender errors include those pertaining to delivery (too quiet, too fast), clarity (Who's the intended receiver?), context confusion (Which arm?), detail and timing questions (dosages and order of ACLS drugs), lack of non-verbal communication (sense of urgency), and failure to check to see if directions were understood. Receiver errors include a lack of preparation to receive message, preconception as to what the message is (bias), distractions, task saturation, and failure to confirm for accuracy. Noise, lighting, ancillary equipment, communication devices, additional people, the need to protect certain patient information, interruptions, and other occurrences (both clinical and security-related) can all degrade communication flow. Emotional factors such as staff anxiety about the situation/role/rank, disagreements with other team members, personal concerns at home or even hunger, feeling tired, or even being late for duty can also influence the receiver's ability to process information. Increased training, experience, and team familiarity can mitigate these factors over time [21].

Other Factors Affecting Team Performance

There are many other factors that may adversely affect trauma team dynamics and the work they produce [9]. Individual (or human) factors such as clinical knowledge, fatigue, external workload demands, sleep deprivation [5], stress, personal concerns, and patient deaths may cloud judgment or contribute to task saturation. Noise, lighting, temperature, motion (e.g., on a ship or aircraft), noxious fumes (e.g., field generators, vehicle exhausts), administrative distractions, tactical situation, and physical/space constraints may all impinge on the care environment. Equipment factors such as maintenance, familiarity, usability, and the need for personal protective equipment (e.g., infectious disease or Weapons of Mass Destruction (WMD) concerns) can degrade performance markedly. Policy and procedures, documentation, staffing demands, safety, pressure to produce, and training comprise the organizational climate, which can influence morale and work ethic. A high staff turnover, over-reliance on short-term staff, and poor organizational management can lead to a lack of collective focus and have negative influences on teamwork [14] and effectiveness.

The "problem physician" (or other team member) is a dreaded contingency that may cause interpersonal problems, avoidance, suboptimal team performance, and even legal issues. Such issues may stem from personal or marital problems, feelings of insecurity or superiority, substance abuse, or even psychiatric diagnoses. Dealing with difficult personalities is never easy, but again, the team's preparation can make dealing with such problems much more effective. Getting the team member the help he or she needs quickly and in a non-accusatorial fashion should be the team's collective goal. Knowing both internal (e.g., chaplain, psychiatry, risk management) and external (financial or marriage counseling, substance abuse treatment) resources before a problem presents offers the best chance for good outcomes for all involved.

Continuous Improvement Processes

Finally, effective trauma teams will pursue some form of feedback incorporation in order to iteratively improve their performance. Several methods exist to accomplish this goal, including simulation, videotaped review, performance metrics measurements, and iterative incorporation of best practices into a set of guidelines.

Several studies demonstrate that patient *simulation* teaches and reinforces clinical skills, decision-making, cooperation, leadership, and communication in a safe and increasingly realistic environment [5, 13, 22] and calls for feedback at the end of training sessions to encourage continuing improvement. Clinical training and education are essential to cultivate a culture of safety in healthcare. Moving forward, computerized simulators plus CRM principles may be incorporated into all aspects of transdisciplinary team training courses. Simulation training can help trauma teams overcome these challenges, and should concentrate on meeting these specific competencies and practicing team decision-making [9]. Advanced Trauma Life Support (ATLS), Tactical Combat Casualty Care (TCCC), and Trauma Nursing Core Course (TNCC) are all examples of clinical skill-based training that utilizes patient simulation scenarios to teach decision-making and basic initial resuscitation skills. "Train in teams those who are expected to work in teams [5]."

Video analysis of trauma team performance provides real-time feedback and allows reviewers to analyze individual performance, teamwork/communication, and leadership, as well as adverse events that may affect team performance. Video review can be utilized as a tool for quality assessment and to determine whether teams are following "best practice" guidelines (ATLS, JTS CPGs). In the future, process (activities) and patient outcomes can be identified and measured using videotaping resuscitations and can be translated into trauma team performance metrics [9]. Patient confidentiality/medicolegal and logistical/resource issues are some of the barriers to videotape review of trauma resuscitations.

Performance tools and metrics, such as the Trauma Team Performance Observation Tool (TPOT), can be used to assess leadership, situation monitoring, mutual support and teamwork, communication quality, and overall team performance [23]. The evolution and incorporation of best practices into *standards and checklists* have become proven, well accepted [24] (and even expected as their use has entered popular literature [25], and will likely continue to grow as a benchmarking measure in trauma care. Many organizations are compiling, publishing, and iteratively revisiting/revising checklists and guidelines, fine-tuning their recommendations as evidence accumulates. One such system that has grown from recent conflict is the US military's Joint Trauma System (JTS) Clinical Practice Guidelines (CPGs), available to the public online at http://www.usaisr.amedd.army.mil/clinical_practice_guidelines.html. Based on a significant body of evidence from trauma cases in both Iraq and Afghanistan, the CPGs undergo periodic review and continuous process improvement, and where applicable, their tenets have even begun to influence civilian practice, for instance, with the concept of damage control resuscitation.

Conclusion

The importance of monitoring quality, from all aspects and vantage points, cannot be understated in trauma team dynamics. The standardization of best practices, timeliness of interventions, effectiveness of communication, and continuous improvement through avenues such as simulation will all coalesce into the early recognition of clinical outliers and the mitigation of unnecessary variance and avoidable adverse outcomes. Improved team performance and outcome-based metrics will become increasingly mandatory in a resource-constrained practice environment.

Key Points

- Quality control is the process by which an organization reviews all the factors contributing to performing and production outcomes.
- Healthcare quality defined by safe, effective, patient-centered, timely, efficient, and equitable criteria for healthcare and provider evaluation.
- Crew resource management is a methodology to effectively adapt team strategies, tools, and patient safety measures to ensure engagement of the trauma team and improve quality patient outcomes.
- Leadership is earned and adapted from historical shared experiences within the organization and team allowing for constructive open communications and corrections without reprisal.
- Team performance should be constantly evaluated and discussed to improve communication, effectiveness, and motivation of all members of the trauma team.

References

1. Reason J. Human error: models and management. BMJ. 2000;320(7237):768–770.
2. Institute of Medicine (IOM). Crossing the quality Chasm: a new health system for the 21st century. Washington, D.C: National Academy Press; 2001.
3. Institute of Medicine (IOM). Performance measurement: accelerating improvement. Washington, D.C: National Academy Press; 2005.
4. Institute of Medicine (IOM). Establishing Transdisciplinary Professionalism for Health Workshop. May 14–15, 2013. Available at http://books.nap.edu/openbook.php?record_id=18398&page=121.
5. Institute of Medicine (IOM). To Err is human: building a safer health system. Washington, D.C: National Academy Press; 2000.
6. Weingar MB. Enhancing you power and influence on the OR team. Refresh Courses Anesthesiol. 1999;27:199–210.
7. Baker D, Day R, Salas E. Teamwork as an essential component of high-reliability organizations. Health Serv Res. 2006;41(4 Pt 2):1576–98.
8. Coram R. Boyd: the fighter pilot who changed the art of war. New York: Little, Brown; 2002.
9. Barach P, Weinger M. Trauma team performance. In: Wilson W, Grande C, Hoyt D, editors. Trauma: emergency resuscitation, perioperative anesthesia, surgical management, vol. 1. New York: Informa Healthcare; 2007.
10. Massoud MR, et al. A framework for spread: from local improvements to system-wide change. IHI Innovation Series white paper. Cambridge, MA: Institute for Healthcare Improvement; 2006.
11. Running a successful campaign in your hospital, how-to guide, institute for healthcare improvement 100,000 Lives Campaign; 2006.
12. Getting started kit: sustainability and spread, how-to guide, institute for healthcare improvement 100,000 lives campaign; 2006.
13. Harkins D. Trauma is a team sport. J Traum Nurs. 2009;16:2.
14. Courtenay M, Nancarrow S, Dawson D. Interprofessional teamwork in the trauma setting: a scoping review. Hum Resour Health. 2013;11:57.
15. Snook S, Khurana R, Nohria N. The handbook for teaching leadership: knowing, doing, and being. Thousand Oaks: SAGE Publications; 2012.
16. Pew R, Mavor A. Modeling human and organizational behavior: application to military simulations. Washington DC: National Academy Press; 1998.
17. Beekley A, Bohman H, Schindler D. Modern Warfare. In: Savitsky E, Eastridge B, editors. Combat casualty care: lessons learned from OEF and OIF. Washington, DC: Office of the Surgeon General, Department of the Army; 2012.
18. Manthous C, Hollingshead A. Team science and critical care. Am J Respir Crit Care Med. 2011;184:17–25.
19. Hunt E, Mininni N, DeVita M. Simulation training programs for rapid response or medical emergency teams. In: Riley R, editor. Manual of simulation in healthcare. New York: Oxford UP; 2008.
20. Apker J, Propp K, Zabava Ford W, Hofmeister N. Collaboration, credibility, compassion, and coordination: professional nurse communication skill sets in health care team interactions. J Prof Nurs. 2006;3:180–9.
21. Horne S, Hicks A, Moor P, McConnell D. Trauma team training workbook. Plymouth: Department of Emergency Medicine, Derriford Hospital. Available at http://media.wix.com/ugd/c16455_7ffb9f4f029ac8cf19a51be9b87b0d47.pdf.
22. Georgiou A, Lockey D. The performance and assessment of hospital trauma teams. Scand J Trauma Resusc Emerg Med. 2010;18(66):2010.

23. Capella J, Smith S, Philp A, et al. Teamwork training improves the clinical care of trauma patients. J Surg Educ. 2010;67:439–43.
24. Pronovost P, et al. An intervention to decrease catheter-related bloodstream infections in the ICU. N Engl J Med. 2006;355:2725–32.
25. Gawande A. The checklist manifesto. New York: Metropolitan Books; 2009.

Part III

Trauma Resuscitation

Trauma Resuscitation

29

Paul M. Cantle and John B. Kortbeek

Epidemiology of Trauma

Throughout history, injury, both intentional and unintentional, has been among the leading causes of premature death and disability. Today trauma continues to be the primary cause of death and disability in the first four decades of life. The impact of injury continues to rise with the increasing motorization in developing countries. The World Health Organization (WHO) estimates that injury is responsible for 10% of annual deaths worldwide, with youth and young adults being the predominant victims (WHO) [1]. Road traffic crashes, suicide, and homicide are each expected to increase in rank among the global causes of death. The number of victims suffering disability following trauma increases the injury burden. The global macroeconomic costs of road injuries alone from both direct healthcare costs and indirect loss of productivity are estimated to be over 100 billion dollars annually [2].

Recognition of the impact of trauma has resulted in significant strides in injury control. Over time, the combined work of both the public and private sectors, including the efforts of healthcare workers, public health professionals, police forces, the automotive industry, traffic and road engineers, insurance companies, and government ministries, have, and continue to, significantly reduced the burden of injury. The introduction of formal trauma systems has been dramatic, with successful examples in developed nations demonstrating significant reductions of years of life lost due to injury nearing 50% [3]. The four Es of injury control: engineering, enforcement, education, and economics are a powerful combination [4]. Healthcare practitioners providing daily care for the injured can increase their impact by partnering with and advocating for injury control organizations.

P. M. Cantle
Clinical Lecturer Department of Surgery, University of Calgary, Peter Lougheed Centre, Calgary, AB, Canada
e-mail: paul.cantle@albertahealthservices.ca

J. B. Kortbeek (✉)
Department's of Surgery and Critical Care, University of Calgary, Calgary, AB, Canada
e-mail: John.Kortbeek@AlbertaHealthServices.Ca

Death Due to Injury

Historically, death following injury follows a tri-modal distribution. Catastrophic injury including aortic disruption, cardiac rupture, massive hemorrhage, brain injury with herniation, atlanto-occipital dislocation, brainstem injury, and complete airway disruption/obstruction are major causes of non-preventable death at the scene [5]. These fatalities can only be avoided through primary prevention measures such as eliminating impaired and distracted driving, seatbelt laws, and motor vehicle safety. Patients who survive the initial trauma can be salvaged through prompt attention to maintaining or establishing the airway, restoration of inadequate ventilation and oxygenation, and early hemorrhage control. Patients who survive beyond the first day may still succumb to severe traumatic brain injury and sepsis/multi-organ failure. However, effective initial resuscitation and management including minimizing delayed diagnosis and treatment of injuries enhances survival. Current literature suggests that mature trauma systems have minimized the third peak of "late" trauma deaths leading to a bimodal distribution of injury deaths as a more common current trend [6, 7]. Coordinated multidisciplinary trauma teams, proficient critical care, and established trauma systems are the foundations for maximizing survival in these patients. Modern trauma systems have reduced late deaths and disability due to early recognition and management of injury and hemorrhage control.

L. Marshall Gillman, S. Widder (eds.), *Trauma Team Dynamics*, https://doi.org/10.1007/978-3-031-86312-7_29

Mechanisms

Injury may be intentional or unintentional, and due to blunt, penetrating, and/or blast mechanisms. Knowledge of the circumstances leading to the injury can serve as important clues to occult trauma at presentation. Secondary factors, such as alcohol, drug, and toxin ingestion, are also essential considerations in the initial management of the trauma patient. Environmental exposure is an important concern and determinant of risk at presentation. Hypothermia should be suspected with prolonged pre-hospital times, particularly in cold climates. Burns, smoke inhalation, and carbon monoxide poisoning are often present when patients present following extraction from enclosed settings during fires.

Blunt mechanisms have characteristic injury patterns. Falls from a height of 5 m or more are often associated with extremity, spine, and solid organ injury. Falls down greater than several stairs are associated with upper extremity, face, head, and neck trauma. Auto-pedestrian collisions have a high risk of head and neck injuries. Young children frequently present with isolated head injury following pedestrian motor vehicle crashes [8]. Elderly patients frequently present with intracranial hemorrhage, torso, and extremity injury and have a significant increase in morbidity and mortality [9]. Side impact collisions are usually associated with solid organ injury as well as extremity and rib fractures, and chest trauma on the affected side [10–12].

Injuries sustained from penetrating trauma vary considerably with the speed of the projectile. Knives and low-velocity handguns tend to cause injury along the missile's trajectory. Higher-velocity weapons such as hunting and assault rifles additionally cause significant cavitation due to the associated pressure wave. This can disrupt tissue many centimeters away from the missile's trajectory and significantly increase the severity of injury [13].

Blast injuries can cause overpressure injuries affecting the middle ear, lungs, and hollow viscous, penetrating injuries due to shrapnel, and blunt force trauma as the victim is struck by large objects or thrown due to the force of the blast [14].

Host factors are equally important when considering potential injuries. Children and toddlers have a wide range of normal age-specific physiology. They often harbor significant internal injury with less apparent external trauma. Based on size alone, they are more susceptible to multisystem injury [15]. Their physiologic reserve tends to be greater but can dramatically and rapidly deteriorate once exhausted.

The elderly often present with significant occult injury despite experiencing relatively low energy. A frequent example is the ground-level fall. Furthermore, injury response may be masked, due to both a lack of extreme physiologic reaction and underlying co-morbidity, such as atrial fibrillation or the presence of a pacemaker. Cirrhosis, congenital coagulopathy, chronic obstructive pulmonary disease, ischemic heart disease, and diabetes mellitus in particular increase the mortality of the geriatric trauma patient. Medication effects may also be significant (e.g., beta blockers, anticoagulants) and must be considered. Non-reversible anticoagulants, now popular in the management of atrial fibrillation, pose significant challenges in managing trauma related hemorrhage in the elderly [16]. Further elaboration on this topic can be found in Chap. 42.

Trauma Teams and Preparation

Physicians, nurses, and other health care providers may encounter injured patients in a variety of settings ranging from the pre-hospital environment, rural hospitals with teams consisting of a doctor, nurse, and X-ray technician, to tertiary care facilities with dedicated trauma teams and all specialties immediately available. Regardless of the setting, preparation is critical to success. Poor planning and execution can delay effective assessment, resuscitation, and definitive care of the injured.

Because of local and regional variations, it is imperative that trauma practitioners understand the workings and agreements of their own trauma systems. Practitioners should be able to easily answer the following questions: Which patients can be definitively managed in your institution? What are the pre-hospital triage and bypass criteria? What happens when a case is mistriaged? What happens when a multi- or mass casualty event occurs? What are the criteria for activating the trauma team in your hospital? What is the composition of the team ?[17, 18].

In jurisdictions with formalized trauma systems, a tremendous amount of work has occurred to effectively coordinate a response that maximizes the survival of the injured. While many of these systems seem intuitive, they require continued support, organization, and advocacy. Within a facility, trauma team individual practitioners should be clear on their role. They should inform themselves of the resuscitation setup and the location of all essential equipment in the area prior to patient arrival. Where is the difficult airway cart? What is in it?—including special intravenous (IV) equipment, central line trays, and intra-osseous equipment. Pediatric resuscitation kits, the Breslow tape? Chest tubes, insertion trays, and pleural drains? Where is the ultrasound unit for performing focused assessment with sonography in trauma (FAST) or eFAST? Does it work and where is the on switch? How are stat radiographs, operating room (OR) access, and patient transport arranged? These are simple questions that a brief walk through of the resuscitation bay can answer. Being prepared lays the stage for a smooth coordinated resuscitation with effective team leadership and a minimum of chaos and conflict [19–22].

Assessment and Priorities: xABCDE

The ATLS® course fundamentally changed the initial assessment and management of trauma [23]. The course was introduced in North America in 1980 by the American College of Surgeons following development of the prototype in Nebraska. It standardized a single safe approach to trauma care and introduced a common language. The course along with ACLS® (Advanced Cardiac Life Support) also introduced large-scale simulation to medical training. A parallel curriculum and certification program for course instructors promoted quality and consistency. By 2006 the program trained over a million physicians and currently has expanded to over 80 countries. Programs such as PHTLS® (Prehospital Trauma Life Support) and ATCN® (Advanced Trauma Care for Nurses) also expanded the audience for the ABCDE approach to trauma care. The principles of ATLS® are relevant to both practitioners who infrequently manage the severely injured and trauma teams in large urban trauma centers where the initial priorities are applied simultaneously. The goal is to manage the greatest threat to life first and to do no further harm to the patient.

The priorities, making up the primary survey, are as follows: (and have recently change to xABCDE in the 11th edition of ATLS)

- Control of eXanguinating external hemorrhage (recently added to the 11th Edition of ATLS)
- Airway assessment and management with attention to cervical immobilization (when relevant)
- Breathing (Assessment and management of oxygenation and ventilation)
- Circulation (Assessment and management of shock states)
- Disability (Assessment and management of neurologic injury)
- Exposure (Assessment and management of the back and extremities)

The patient should be approached from the head of the bed by whoever is responsible for performing the initial assessment. The findings should be clearly communicated to the team. This assessment and the initiation of resuscitation should take one to two minutes to complete [24–26].

A typical sequence in approaching a suspected major trauma patient would be as follows:

1. Ask the patient his or her name, apply oxygen, and if no response proceed to more definitive airway maneuvers while simultaneously ensuring that the cervical spine is immobilized where appropriate.
2. Inspect and auscultate the chest, palpate and percuss where findings warrant.
3. Palpate a pulse to establish rate and caliber. Ask for a set of vital signs including heart rate, blood pressure, temperature, and respiratory rate. Ask for initiation of two large bore IVs (18 gauge minimum) and initiate warmed intravenous fluids or, if a patient is hypotensive and in shock, early blood products where appropriate.
4. Check the patient's pupils. Estimate the Glasgow coma scale (GCS).
5. Expose the patient. This is a great time to log roll, remove the backboard, and perform a rectal examination when indicated.

The key findings requiring intervention during the initial assessment are as follows:

1. Identifying airway obstruction, either anatomic, mechanical, or due to coma, that requires an airway maintenance technique.
2. Identification of large or tension pneumothoraces requiring needle decompression or finger thoracostomy, and chest tube insertion.
3. Identification of shock and consideration of the etiology.
4. Identification of coma and especially impending herniation evidenced by a dilated pupil requiring urgent neurosurgical assessment and temporizing medical decompression.
5. Identification of life- or limb-threatening extremity injuries.

The most useful investigations that should be performed immediately are the chest X-ray, which identifies hemo-pneumothoraces, an EFAST (Extended Focused Assessment with Sonography for Trauma) (as discussed later in Chaps. 44 and 45) for identifying potential sources of hemorrhage and cardiac tamponade for patients in shock, as well as screening for pneumothoraces and hemothoraces, and a blood gas, which provides an immediate estimate of adequacy of oxygenation and ventilation, the level of base deficit and serum lactate, and an early hemoglobin (Hgb). In the case of major blunt force mechanisms, the inclusion of a pelvic X-ray is also very useful to screen for open book and vertical sheer pelvic fractures (important sources of hemorrhage) [27]. A trauma lab panel including a type and screen and/or cross match should also be drawn during this process. Serum alcohol (ETOH) levels are often routinely performed to assist in assessment of depressed level of consciousness and to aid with future trauma prevention initiatives. Drug and toxin screening may also be very useful at this stage.

The primary survey and resuscitation including all of these investigations should be completed within 15 minutes or less. Clear communication of actions and findings will speed the process and allow earlier intervention when required. Agreeing on the sequence of these steps by team members before the resuscitation is very advantageous. Remember that the *greatest threat to life should be treated first*. A patient who presents with obvious major hemorrhage from a scalp or extremity wound should have direct pressure applied to arrest the bleeding while approaching the airway assessment. Immediate application of a tourniquet in the field for blast or high-velocity extremity wounds in the combat arena has proven life-saving. As in all aspects of medicine, clinical judgment and experience are important.

Once the initial assessment is complete and initial resuscitation has commenced, a quick repeat of the ABCs is very useful. At this point, unless immediate surgical intervention is required, the team can proceed to a complete head-to-toe examination (the secondary survey) and more definitive investigations. Early transfer should be considered at this point if this initial patient management is occurring at a site that is not resource intensive (blood products, surgical specialties, necessary imaging, personnel). CT imaging should not delay transport to tertiary care unless it will impact the transfer decision.

Airway: Assessment and Management

Following control of exanguinating hemorrhage, the airway is the priority in assessment and management. Patients with airway obstruction have moments to live. The obstruction may be mechanical due to soft tissue injury or swelling or may be functional, associated with depressed levels of consciousness including coma. Airway obstruction may be obvious or subtle, especially in the case of impending obstruction, which can occur following an inhalation injury in a closed space during fires [28].

In all cases where cervical spine injury is suspected or possible, the cervical spine must be immobilized during airway assessment and management. Theis includes virtually all blunt force trauma patients with a significant mechanism of injury. It also includes penetrating trauma with a trajectory that may involve the cervical spine, penetrating trauma that may be associated with unwitnessed blunt trauma, blast injuries where multiple mechanisms are evident, and patients presenting with coma where trauma is within the differential.

The best initial approach to the airway is simply to introduce yourself to the patient and ask the patient their name. The ability to respond indicates a patent airway, reasonable ventilation, circulation adequate to perfuse the brain, and the absence of major traumatic brain injury. For patients able to speak, the most useful follow-up questions are asking them their Allergies, Medications, Past medical history, Last meal, and what happened (Events) (AMPLE history). Oxygen should be applied in all suspected cases of major trauma until a thorough assessment of the magnitude of injury is complete.

In patients where airway obstruction may be impending, consider the following rules. GCS < 8 = intubate. If patients have a potential impending airway obstruction with intermediate levels of GCS 9–12, inhalation injury, or neck hematoma, then ask yourself the following. What is my experience? What assistance and backup are available? Where will the patient be monitored? In cases of transport, who is travelling with the patient? What equipment do they have and how long will it take? All of these factors should be considered when planning a definitive or temporizing airway.

Once a decision has been made that the patient requires an airway, then assess for difficulty. If the patient is dying from airway obstruction and you are the only help available, then attempt intubation and/or proceed directly to a surgical airway. In other cases, airway maintenance techniques including jaw thrust, chin lift, insertion of an oral or nasal airway, and bag mask ventilation should be performed next.

In all other cases, assess the difficulty of intubation. Remember that cervical spine immobilization will shift the spectrum of airway control towards more difficult. This may increase the need for airway adjuncts such as intubating video laryngoscopes. Forming an opinion of the difficulty of airway capture is important. An easy airway typically would be recognized by a wide mouth, normal-sized and placed dentition, a large chin and jaw, and a lack of facial and neck soft tissue trauma or swelling. Clues to a difficult airway include small mouth, chin, jaw, significant overbite, and facial/neck trauma. The LEMON pneumonic is a useful reminder.

- Look
- Evaluate
- Mallampatti Score
- Observe
- Neck

In cases of an easy airway with fairly straightforward anatomy, proceeding to drug-assisted intubation, after preoxygenation with an appropriately sized cuffed tube is recommended for all practitioners who have had adequate training [29]. Appropriate equipment including suction, oxygen, oropharyngeal airways, nasopharyngeal airways, bag-mask, laryngoscope, bougie, supra-glottic devices, endotracheal tubes, pulse oximetry, CO2 detections devices, and a surgical airway kit should all be close at hand.

Where a difficult airway is suspected, temporizing with bag mask ventilation and oxygen is the next step. In regional or urban institutions, asking for experienced help should be next. In rural and remote locations, bag mask ventilation until the arrival of an experienced aero medical transport crew may be appropriate [30].

In difficult airway cases, the application of a variety of airway tools and devices to assist intubation is critical to success. A variety of approaches and devices have been described by various specialty organizations. The best approach is the one which your center and team are most familiar and comfortable with. A simple and inexpensive device, which often allows capture of a more difficult airway, is the gum elastic bougie. It is a long slender rod with a hook or hockey stick at the end. Simply visualize the epiglottis, hook it underneath, and advance. Correct tracheal positioning is confirmed by feeling the bougie bounce along the tracheal rings. When advanced, gentle resistance will be encountered when it reaches the secondary and tertiary bronchi. The absence of resistance and tracheal ring sensation suggests esophageal intubation.

The laryngeal mask airway (LMA) can provide reasonable ventilation and oxygenation when this is difficult to achieve using bag mask ventilation. In experienced hands, the intubating LMA can be very useful. However, the LMA does not protect the airway in cases of aspiration and may be easy to dislodge.

Recently, the introduction of the video laryngoscope has revolutionized the management of the difficult airway and greatly facilitated capture on these patients. Intubation over a fiberoptic bronchoscope remains an option in the right hands.

Regardless of approach, if the airway is not captured and the patient is desaturating, proceed immediately to a surgical airway. Surgical airways will be discussed further in Chap. 33.

Once an airway is placed, always confirm correct position using these five techniques:

1. Look for symmetrical chest wall expansion.
2. Listen and auscultate for breath sounds.
3. Feel—palpate the chest wall for symmetrical expansion.
4. Oxymetry—confirm adequacy of oxygenation.
5. Capnometry—confirm adequacy of ventilation.

Remember that an AP chest X-ray (CXR) cannot confirm the correct positioning in the trachea vis-a-vis the esophagus. Look for evidence of right mainstem bronchus intubation, due to the lesser angulation and more direct descent compared to the left. Typical endotracheal tube sizes would be 7 mm for females and 8 for males. Average distance from the teeth would be 22 cm for females and 24 cm for males for correct tracheal positioning 3–4 cm above the carina. Confirm this position on the chest X-ray.

Breathing: Oxygenation and Ventilation

Assessment of the chest initially by inspection and auscultation is performed early in the primary survey. The goal is to confirm the presence of bilateral breath sounds. Simultaneous oxymetry and, in the case of airway capture, capnometry are very useful. If breath sounds are absent, check the vitals and pulse oxymeter—if both are adequate take the time to complete the remainder of the primary survey and obtain a CXR. EFAST (see Chap. 22) in experienced hands can be a useful aid in detecting large hemo–pneumothoraces. If the patient is desaturating or hypotensive, then immediate decompression is required. While large pneumothoraces can develop in spontaneously breathing patients leading to air hunger and desaturation, pneumothoraces with mediastinal displacement and tension physiology leading to hypotension are most likely in patients who have had positive pressure ventilation of any means.

If the patient has already been intubated and breath sounds are absent on the left, always confirm that this is not due to right main stem intubation. Simply check the endotracheal-tube (ETT) position, and if it seems well-advanced, try pulling it back 1–3 cm and repeat the auscultation. When absent breath sounds are confirmed and persistent and the patient is desaturating or hypotensive, perform needle decompression with a large over-the-needle catheter in the 5th intercostal space just anterior mid axillary line. In an overweight or obese patient, perform needle decompression in the 2nd intercostal space in the midclavicular line [31]. If the needle fails due to chest wall thickness or kinking, consider performing a finger thoracostomy followed with a chest tube (28–32 French). The chest tube should be placed in the mid-anterior axillary line, above the rib to avoid the neurovascular bundle. Useful landmarks are to remain above the nipple in males and above the inframammary fold in females. This should avoid inadvertent injury to the diaphragm and intra-abdominal organs. A sharp trochar should not be used for chest tube placement. Good sterile technique with complete barrier precautions should be used whenever possible to mitigate the risk of empyema and its associated morbidity. The chest tube should be connected to 20 cm underwater suction, and outputs closely measured.

Hemorrhage of >1500 cc, or >200 cc/hour for four consecutive hours or more are indications for thoracotomy. If the chest tube drainage stops, beware, it may simply be clotted. Persistent evidence of shock with a large hemothorax on EFAST/CXR are also indications for surgery.

At the completion of the primary survey, a CXR should be obtained and a more thorough exam performed. Simple pneumothoraces, particularly those that occupy 2 cm or less from the chest wall or apex, or occult pneumothoraces (pneumothoraces seen only on computerized tomography (CT) occupying less than 1/3rd of the pleural cavity) may be observed in stable patients. Repeat CXR should be performed within approximately 6 hours. In patients requiring transport, placement of a chest tube is advised.

Additional injuries should be identified on the CXR including rib, clavicle, scapular, and vertebral fractures, wide mediastinum, pneumo-mediastinum, pulmonary contusion or aspiration, elevated or obvious ruptured hemidiaphragms, and subcutaneous emphysema. The presence of these abnormalities provides important clues to the severity of injury, necessary additional investigations, and treatment plans.

CT of the cervical spine is increasingly being performed for cervical spine clearance in major mechanisms of injury. CT of the abdomen and pelvis is likewise routinely performed to identify occult intra-abdominal injury. Together these tests will also identify all cases of occult pneumothorax. CT of the chest should be added to these investigations where the mechanism is high impact/rapid deceleration and could be associated with blunt traumatic aortic injury. CT of the chest combined with CT of the C Spine and CT of the abdomen and pelvis allows complete reformatting and inspection of the cervical, thoracic, and lumbar spine improving both the accuracy and timeliness of spinal clearance. This is important for early mobilization, initiation of physiotherapy, and prevention of respiratory failure in patients with blunt chest trauma. In patients with multiple rib fractures and significant chest pain, mobilization and pain control should be a priority.

At the completion of the secondary survey, an electrocardiogram (ECG) should be performed. Significant cardiac contusion leading to pathologic arrhythmias and heart failure or hypotension typically occurs in patients with severe polytrauma and abnormal vital signs on presentation. Patients may present following an acute myocardial infarction or arrhythmia as the initiating event that led to syncope that in turn resulted in a traumatic event causing injury. This should be screened for by obtaining the ECG. Wide QT and QRS may be seen in patients with co-existent toxic ingestion. Troponins are of little value in acute chest trauma. In the absence of a suspected acute coronary syndrome, they are not predictive of outcomes in trauma [32].

Circulation: Recognition of Shock and Control of Hemorrhage

Once airway and breathing have been attended to and obvious sources of external hemorrhage are compressed, the vital signs should be reviewed. Quick palpation of a pulse for caliber and rate and assessment of skin temperature provide valuable information. The most common cause of patients in shock following trauma is hemorrhage. Other potential causes of shock to consider include obstructive shock due to tension pneumothorax or cardiac tamponade, distributive shock due to spinal injury (or sepsis when presentation is delayed), and cardiogenic shock due to an underlying acute coronary event/myocardial infarction. The history of the event, combined with pulse, blood pressure, skin temperature, and examination of the neck veins, will usually help identify the cause of shock (Table 29.1).

Two large bore IVs, 18 gauge or larger, should be initiated. If they cannot be inserted and the patient is in profound hypovolemic shock, then one should move onto a different form of access and consider an intraosseous line, central venous access, or a venous cutdown based on the expertise of the clinician. Options for venous access and considerations for choice will be elaborated on in Chap. 33. Warm intravenous fluid, such as crystalloid or blood products, should be initiated, but the primary goal is to find and stop the bleeding or correct the underlying cause of shock. An initial crystalloid bolus of up to 1 liter may be necessary, but aggressive fluid resuscitation has been shown to increase mortality and therefore should be used judiciously. In patients with traumatic brain injuries, hypotension should be avoided as it worsens outcomes. In penetrating trauma with ongoing hemorrhage, aggressive resuscitation prior to surgical control of bleeding may in fact further exacerbate hemorrhage, increase coagulopathy, and worsen outcomes. Damage Control Resuscitation will be considered in Chap. 30.

If a patient is hypotensive and in suspected hemorrhagic shock, a massive transfusion protocol should be activated. These protocols have streamlined resuscitation and help avoid coagulaopathy and thrombocytopenia through the early administration of packed red blood cells, plasma, and platelets in predefined low ratios [33]. This will be discussed further in Chap. 30. Tranexamic acid is also now an accepted adjunct. It is an antifibrinolytic which is cheap, safe, and potentially effective if used within the first 3 hours of injury.

Always remember that hypotension is a late sign of shock and, in the case of hemorrhage, typically does not occur until the loss of one third or more of the blood volume. Early signs are anxiety, confusion, tachycardia, and narrowed pulse pressure. Repeat the vital signs to follow trends and monitor resuscitation. Useful ways to evaluate the adequacy of resuscitation include the cardiac rhythm, GCS, and urine output.

Ultimately, the goal is to find and correct the cause of shock. In the case of hemorrhage, identifying the source and rapidly stopping the bleeding is the key. ATLS® teaches "blood on the floor and four more." In addition to external hemorrhage from lacerations, principal sites of blood loss are the chest, pelvis, abdomen, and long bones. A CXR,

Table 29.1 Shock, physical findings

Etiology of shock	Pulse	BP	Skin	Jugular venous pressure
Hemorrhagic	Rapid, thready	Low with reduced pulse pressure	Cool	Low
Tension pneumothorax	Rapid, thready	Low with reduced pulse pressure	Cool	Elevated
Tamponade	Rapid, thready	Low with reduced pulse pressure	Cool	Elevated
Spinal	Normal, slow, full	Low with wide pulse pressure	Warm	Low
Cardiogenic	Rapid, thready	Low with reduced pulse pressure	Cool	Elevated

Pelvic X-ray, EFAST exam, and palpation of the extremities will review the potential sources of blood loss. EFAST can also demonstrate cardiac tamponade and identify pneumothoraces, both potential sources of obstructive shock.

A patient in shock due to hemorrhage or tamponade requires immediate definitive management. With external hemorrhage, direct pressure, compressive dressings, hemostatic agents, extremity tourniquets, and junctional tourniquets are among the tools to be considered [34]. In the case of pleural hemorrhage or cardiac tamponade, a thoracotomy should be performed. In cases of positive abdominal FAST exam, the treatment is immediate laparotomy. With long bone fractures, splinting and resuscitation should be definitive [35].

Pelvic fractures represent a special challenge. The three patterns of pelvic trauma are lateral compression with pubic rami fractures, open book fractures, and vertical sheer injury. Lateral compression fractures are associated with pubic rami and acetabular fractures but usually do not present with massive hemorrhage. These patients often can have urethral or extraperitoneal bladder injury. Open book fractures frequently have major bleeding. Compression with a binder or sheet to temporize is useful. Vertical shear fractures usually present in hemorrhagic shock. Pelvic binders are less practical and often have to be combined with axial traction. Early orthopedic consultation is very helpful. In cases where shock is present, a decision is required on whether the next step is surgery with packing and pelvic stabilization followed by angio-emolization, immediate embolization, or CT first to plan therapy followed by either surgery and or angio-embolization. This can be difficult as angiography, while particularly useful for retroperitoneal or solid organ arterial hemorrhage, does not stop venous bleeding and can miss low flow bleeding. In profound shock, patients should go directly to the operating room. Patients who respond to initial resuscitation may be reasonable candidates to be taken by the team to CT. Patients with partial or transient response can be divided into FAST positive or negative groups. FAST positive should have laparotomy first, FAST negative can be managed initially with angio-embolization. Pelvic fractures may be associated with intra-abdominal hemorrhage in which case initial management should be in the OR [36–38]. These challenging scenarios will be further highlighted in Chaps. 32 and 33.

Patients in neurogenic shock should receive initial 1–2 L boluses of crystalloid but then frequently require pressor therapy and ICU monitoring. Patients with co-existent cardiac pathology due to an MI or severe contusion will need to be supported in an ICU with close cardiac monitoring and physiological adjuncts such as inotropes.

It is important to not get fixated on a single body cavity or single cause of shock. Trauma patients can have multiple causes of shock and multiple sources of hemorrhage. Traumatic brain injury does not cause shock. In addition, a wide mediastinum with a suspected blunt aortic injury is also almost never the source of hemorrhagic shock as frank aortic rupture usually leads to immediate death. In these situations, look elsewhere for a source of hemorrhage. Patients who are relatively stable during resuscitation are candidates for truncal CT to help with definitive diagnosis and to exclude occult injury. Abdominal examination is unreliable in patients following major trauma especially when associated with multiple extremity or spine injuries. FAST is not sensitive for solid or hollow viscous injury. It simply identifies free fluid, which may indicate bleeding.

Neurologic Injury

The goal during the disability portion of the primary survey is to recognize life-threatening neurologic injury, particularly severe traumatic brain injury. Pupils and GCS should be inspected and estimated during the initial assessment. Severe traumatic brain injury is characterized by GCS less than or equal to 8. Asymmetric pupils may indicate mass effect with impending transtentorial herniation. The presence of either mandates prompt neurosurgical consultation. The most effective initial management is to ensure that viable brain is preserved by maintaining oxygenation and perfusion. In these patients, vigorous resuscitation to avoid or correct hypotension is a priority. Systolic blood pressure target should be greater than 110 mmHg as this may decrease mortality and improve outcomes. Resuscitation for patients with hemorrhagic shock should employ a massive transfusion protocol. Mannitol 0.–1 g/kg may be an effective temporizing maneuver in order to control ICP and avoid arterial hypotension and, as a result, transiently minimize brain swelling and herniation. The same is true of temporary hyperventilation when used in moderation for as short a period as possible. Prolonged hyperventilation, with a PCO2 < 25mmHG, should be avoided. In most cases, normal PaCO2 levels are desirable to avoid cerebral vasoconstriction, but in the case of impending herniation, this can be life-saving.

CT of the head should be performed as soon as possible. However, treatment of hemorrhage in order to maintain cerebral perfusion still takes precedence. Patients presenting with hemorrhagic shock still need to have the bleeding stopped first, before brain imaging, in most cases. Patients who respond to resuscitation and who in the judgment of the trauma team leader will maintain perfusion while undergoing CT may have an expedited CT performed first [39].

Traumatic brain injury (TBI) may be characterized as severe (GCS </= 8), moderate (GCS 9–12), and mild (GCS 13–15) including concussion. Patients with moderate traumatic brain injury should undergo CT. Patients with mild TBI should be assessed in accordance with the Canadian CT

head rule to determine whether CT vs. simple observation and follow-up is required. See Chaps. 46 and 47 for an evidence-based discussion of imaging in stable patients. CT is required for patients with evidence of open, depressed, or basal skull fracture, persistent GCS < 15 beyond 2 hours, age >65 with loss of consciousness, amnesia, or disorientation, and/or vomiting two or more times. Consideration should be given to imaging those with dangerous mechanisms or amnesia for events >30 minutes [40, 41].

Musculoskeletal Trauma Including Spine

The priority during the exposure portion of the primary survey is to identify long bone fractures. Patients are initially exposed, log rolled, and extremities are inspected and rapidly palpated. Management of fractures is by immobilization and splinting. During the secondary survey, all extremities and joints should be examined, in detail, including sensory, motor, and neurovascular examination.

The entire spine, cervical, thoracic, and lumbar should be immobilized until spinal column injury has been ruled out. In most cases of major blunt mechanisms or penetrating injury with trajectory near the spine, X-rays are required. CT is not required for all injured patients but has proven invaluable for major blunt trauma patients, particularly those that also require truncal CT. If CT of the chest and abdomen/pelvis are not being performed, then plain radiographs should be obtained. For patients who did not have major mechanism, the Canadian C Spine rule [42] provides guidelines on when to request C spine x rays and when clinical exam is sufficient. If clinical exam is being relied upon, patients must have a GCS of 15, be stable, be younger than 65, must not have been exposed to a dangerous mechanism, and must not have any extremity paresthesias. They should be alert, and cooperative, have no midline pain, and be able to actively rotate to 45 degrees in both directions, extend, and flex the neck comfortably [43].

Patients who present with spinal cord or peripheral nerve injury should have initial findings carefully documented, and the injured part should be protected through immobilization. The primary management of these injuries in early trauma care is preservation of oxygenation, ventilation, and perfusion while taking care to do no further harm [44].

Management of extremity fracture is by splinting and immobilization. As already noted, direct compression of bleeding and/or application of a pelvic binder should already have been performed as part of the circulation portion of the primary survey. Open fractures should receive antibiotic and tetanus prophylaxis as well as prompt orthopedic consultation. Dislocated joints should be recognized and reduced emergently, ideally in the trauma resuscitation room. If operative reduction is required, this should be performed emergently [45, 46].

Musculoskeletal injuries in major trauma patients are frequently not recognized during initial trauma assessment. A thorough secondary assessment when appropriate, as well as routine performance and documentation of a tertiary survey within 24–36 hours, is important to identify these injuries. Reassessment, particularly when level of consciousness improves if initially compromised, will enhance detection rates and prevent morbidity due to delayed recognition.

Conclusions

An organized, consistent approach by trauma practitioners and trauma teams will allow effective and safe management of the severely injured. Early identification and management of shock is critical. In cases of hemorrhage, the priority is to stop the bleeding. Rapid performance of an xABCDE assessment accompanied by a CXR, Pelvic XR, and EFAST exam simplifies decision-making in blunt trauma. Operative control, angio-embolization, and musculoskeletal stabilization, when required, should occur immediately in tertiary care trauma centers. In referring centers, well-organized trauma systems will focus on early injury identification, efficient but thorough communication, and prompt arrangement of transport.

Repeating the ABCs serially, as well as point-of-care testing with ABGs initially and as required, will allow all patients with evolving shock to be readily identified and appropriately resuscitated. Massive transfusion protocols and attention to avoidance of hypothermia, acidosis, and coagulopathy are keys to success [47, 48].

Patients who suffer trauma through a significant mechanism and in whom major injury is obvious or suspected require a thorough head to toe assessment, full head, neck, thoracic, abdominal, and pelvic CT, when hemodynamically stable, to rule out truncal and spine injury and the liberal use of plain radiographs for all extremities and joints with pain or abnormal physical findings [49].

Trauma systems and teams are designed to ensure that resources and infrastructure are available to support safe care. Trauma is not a solo sport; early engagement of the system and team saves lives [49–51]. Trauma care continues to evolve and adapt to changing technology, medical advances, and systems and team dynamics [52].

Key Points

- Organized trauma systems and trauma care significantly reduce injury death and morbidity.
- The ATLS® system provides a common global approach to trauma resuscitation. It allows teams and centers to speak a common language.
- The ABCDE principles of trauma resuscitation are equally valid when practiced sequentially or simultaneously by a trauma team.
- Trauma teams function optimally when members are prepared, leadership is clear, and communication is encouraged.
- Trauma resuscitation continues to improve with the adoption of balanced resuscitation, massive transfusion protocols, and adjuncts for rapid and definitive control of hemorrhage.

References

1. WHO. WHO library cataloguing-in-publication data injuries and violence: the facts. WHO Press, © World Health Organization; 2010.
2. Chen S, Kuhn M, Prettner K, Bloom DE. The global macroeconomic burden of road injuries: estimates and projections for 166 countries. Lancet Planet Health. 2019;3(9):e390–8.
3. Gabbe BJ, Lyons RA, Fitzgerald MC, Judson R, Richardson J, Cameron PA. Reduced population burden of road transport-related major trauma after introduction of an inclusive trauma system. Ann Surg. 2015;261(3):565–72.
4. Mace SE, Gerardi MJ, Dietrich AM, Knazik SR, Mulligan-Smith D, Sweeney RL, et al. Injury prevention and control in children. Ann Emerg Med (United States). 2001;38(4):405–14.
5. Evans JA, van Wessem KJ, McDougall D, Lee KA, Lyons T, Balogh ZJ. Epidemiology of traumatic deaths: comprehensive population-based assessment. World J Surg (United States). 2010;34(1):158–63.
6. Demetriades D, Kimbrell B, Salim A, Velmahos G, Rhee P, Preston C, et al. Trauma deaths in a mature urban trauma system: is "trimodal" distribution a valid concept? J Am Coll Surg (United States). 2005;201(3):343–8.
7. Gunst M, Ghaemmaghami V, Gruszecki A, Urban J, Frankel H, Shafi S. Changing epidemiology of trauma deaths leads to a bimodal distribution. Proc (Bayl Univ Med Cent). 2010;23(4):349–54.
8. Jones S, Tyson S, Young M, Gittins M, Davis N. Patterns of moderate and severe injury in children after the introduction of major trauma networks. Arch Dis Child. 2019;104(4):366–71.
9. Bauzá G, Lamorte WW, Burke PA, Hirsch EF. High mortality in elderly drivers is associated with distinct injury patterns: analysis of 187,869 injured drivers. J Trauma (United States). 2008;64(2):304–10.
10. Demetriades D, Gkiokas G, Velmahos GC, Brown C, Murray J, Noguchi T. Alcohol and illicit drugs in traumatic deaths: prevalence and association with type and severity of injuries. J Am Coll Surg (United States). 2004;199(5):687–92.
11. Kent A, Pearce A. Review of morbidity and mortality associated with falls from heights among patients presenting to a major trauma centre. Emerg Med Australas (Australia). 2006;18(1):23–30.
12. Yoganandan N, Pintar FA, Maltese MR. Biomechanics of abdominal injuries. Crit Rev Biomed Eng (United States). 2001;29(2):173–246.
13. Volgas DA, Stannard JP, Alonso JE. Ballistics: a primer for the surgeon. Injury (England). 2005;36(3):373–9.
14. Plurad DS. Blast injury. Mil Med (United States). 2011;176(3):276–82.
15. Bayreuther J, Wagener S, Woodford M, Edwards A, Lecky F, Bouamra O, et al. Paediatric trauma: injury pattern and mortality in the UK. Arch Dis Child Educ Pract Ed (England). 2009;94(2):37–41.
16. Siram SM, Sonaike V, Bolorunduro OB, Greene WR, Gerald SZ, Chang DC, et al. Does the pattern of injury in elderly pedestrian trauma mirror that of the younger pedestrian? J Surg Res (United States). 2011;167(1):14–8.
17. Kortbeek J, Buckley R. Trauma Care Systems in Canada. Injury. 2003;34(9):658–63.
18. Kortbeek J. From Anthony Henday to Big Box superstores: trends in Canadian trauma care. J Trauma. 2003;55(3):395–8.
19. Knudson MM, McGrath J. Improving outcomes in pediatric trauma care: essential characteristics of the trauma center. J Trauma (United States). 2007;63(6 Suppl):S140-2.
20. Turner L, Kenward G, Hodgetts T. Preparing to receive patients with trauma. Nurs Times (England). 2002;98(37):34–6.
21. Horne S, Smith JE. Preparation of the resuscitation room and patient reception. J R Army Med Corps (England). 2011;157(3 Suppl 1):S267–72.
22. Schmidt J, Moore GP. Management of multiple trauma. Emerg Med Clin North Am (United States). 1993;11(1):29–51.
23. Committee on Trauma. ATLS: Advanced Trauma Life Support for doctors (Student Course Manual). 10th ed. Chicago: American College of Surgeons, Committee on Trauma; 2018.
24. Kortbeek JB, Al Turki SA, Ali J, Antoine JA, Bouillon B, Brasel K, et al. Advanced trauma life support, 8th edition, the evidence for change. J Trauma (United States). 2008;64(6):1638–50.
25. Dollery W, Driscoll P. Resuscitation after high energy polytrauma. Br Med Bull (England). 1999;55(4):785–805.
26. Carmont MR. The Advanced Trauma Life Support course: a history of its development and review of related literature. Postgrad Med J (England). 2005;81(952):87–91.
27. Kool DR, Blickman JG. Advanced trauma life support. ABCDE from a radiological point of view. Emerg Radiol (United States). 2007;14(3):135–41.
28. McGill J. Airway management in trauma: an update. Emerg Med Clin North Am (United States). 2007;25(3):603–22, vii.
29. Reed MJ, Dunn MJ, McKeown DW. Can an airway assessment score predict difficulty at intubation in the emergency department? Emerg Med J (England). 2005;22(2):99–102.
30. Boet S, Bould MD, Diemunsch P. Evolving challenges and opportunities for difficult airway management guidelines. Can J Anaesth (United States). 2011;58(8):703–8.
31. Azizi N, ter Avest E, Hoek AK, et al. Optimal anatomical location for needle chest decompression for tension pneumothorax: a multicenter prospective cohort study. Injury (United States). 2020:2–7. In-Press
32. Hameed M, Kortbeek J. Chest injuries. Orthopaedics and Trauma (England). 2003;17(4):260–73.
33. Holcomb JB, Tilley BC, Baraniuk S, et al. Transfusion of plasma, platelets, and red blood cells in a 1:1:1 vs a 1:1:2 ratio and mortality in patients with severe trauma: the PROPPR randomized clinical trial. JAMA (United States). 2015;313:471–82.
34. Cantle PM, Roberts DJ, Holcomb JB. Damage control resuscitation across the phases of major injury care. Curr Trauma Rep (United States). 2017;3:238–48.
35. Garcia A. Critical care issues in the early management of severe trauma. Surg Clin North Am (United States). 2006;86(6):1359–87.

36. Grotz MR, Allami MK, Harwood P, et al. Open pelvic fractures: epidemiology, current concepts of management and outcome. Injury (England). 2005;36(1):1–13.
37. Lopez PP. Unstable pelvic fractures: the use of angiography in controlling arterial hemorrhage. J Trauma (United States). 2007;62(6 Suppl):S30–1.
38. Kregor PJ, Routt ML. Unstable pelvic ring disruptions in unstable patients. Injury (England). 1999;30 Suppl 2:B19–28.
39. Bratton SL, Chestnut RM, Ghajar J, et al. Guidelines for the management of severe traumatic brain injury. J Neurotrauma (United States). 2007;24 Suppl 1:S1–95.
40. Papa L, Stiell IG, Clement CM, Pawlowicz A, Wolfram A, Braga C, et al. Performance of the Canadian CT Head Rule and the New Orleans Criteria for predicting any traumatic intracranial injury on computed tomography in a United States Level I trauma center. Acad Emerg Med (United States). 2012;19(1):2–10.
41. Bouida W, Marghli S, Souissi S, Ksibi H, Methammem M, Haguiga H, et al. Prediction value of the Canadian CT head rule and the New Orleans criteria for positive head CT scan and acute neurosurgical procedures in minor head trauma: a multicenter external validation study. Ann Emerg Med (United States). 2013;61(5):521–7.
42. Stiell IG, Wells GA, Vandemheen KL, Clement CM, Lesiuk H, De Maio VJ, et al. The Canadian cervical spine radiography rule for alert and stable trauma patients. J Am Med Assoc (United States). 2001;286:1841–8.
43. Chittiboina P, Cuellar-Saenz H, Notarianni C, et al. Head and spinal cord injury: diagnosis and management. Neurol Clin (United States). 2012;30(1):241–76, ix.
44. O'Dowd JK. Basic principles of management for cervical spine trauma. Eur Spine J (Germany). 2010;19 Suppl 1:S18-22.
45. Abdelgawad AA, Kanlic EM. Orthopedic management of children with multiple injuries. J Trauma (United States). 2011;70(6):1568–74.
46. Pape HC, Giannoudis P, Krettek C. The timing of fracture treatment in polytrauma patients: relevance of damage control orthopedic surgery. Am J Surg (United States). 2002;183(6):622–9.
47. Cantle PM, Cotton BA. Balanced resuscitation in trauma management. Surg Clin North Am (United States). 2017;97(5):999–1014.
48. Hardy JF, De Moerloose P, Samama M. Massive transfusion and coagulopathy: pathophysiology and implications for clinical management. Can J Anaesth (Canada). 2004;51(4):293–310.
49. Eurin M, Haddad N, Zappa M, Lenoir T, Dauzac C, Vilgrain V, et al. Incidence and predictors of missed injuries in trauma patients in the initial hot report of whole-body CT scan. Injury (Netherlands). 2012;43(1):73–7.
50. Sakran JV, Finneman B, Maxwell C, Sonnad SS, Sarani B, Pascual J, et al. Trauma leadership: does perception drive reality? J Surg Educ (United States). 2012;69(2):236–40.
51. Georgiou A, Lockey DJ. The performance and assessment of hospital trauma teams. Scand J Trauma Resusc Emerg Med (England). 2010;18:66.
52. Brasel K, et al. (ATLS subcommittee and ATLS international working group) Advanced trauma life support (ATLS): the ninth edition. J Trauma Acute Care Surg (United States). 2013;74(5):1363–6.

30 Damage Control Resuscitation

Chad G. Ball

Introduction

Damage control is a Navy term defined as "the capacity of a ship to absorb damage and maintain mission integrity" [1]. Although the adaption of this term to the field of traumatology can be credited to Dr. Schwab and colleagues in 1993 [2], its dominant principles are more accurately rooted in Dr. Lucas and Ledgerwood's 1976 address to the American Association for the Surgery of Trauma [3]. More specifically, they described a small series of patients who underwent sponge-based packing of major liver injuries [3]. This concept was reiterated shortly thereafter by Calne [4], as well as Feliciano and Mattox [5] in 1979 and 1981, respectively. Despite these small series outlining the success of perihepatic packing, the visionary extrapolation of this principle to patients with multiple concurrent life-threatening injuries and major coagulopathy was not published until 1983 [6]. Harlan Stone retrospectively described 31 patients who developed major bleeding diatheses [6]. Of these, 17 patients underwent the modern damage control principles of arresting surgical hemorrhage and abbreviating the subsequent operative intervention. This led to the survival of 11 patients who were predicted to have a lethal coagulopathy.

The natural extension and further development of DCS have been damage control *resuscitation* (DCR). This concept includes not only DCS but also the early initiation of blood product transfusions and massive transfusion protocols, reduced crystalloid fluid administration, permissive hypotension in selected populations, and immediate hemorrhage control (whether operative or angiographic). In other words, DCR is a structured intervention that is mobile and can be delivered to a critically ill patient in any location (Emergency Department, interventional radiology suite, operating theater, and/or intensive care unit). Regardless of their destination, arresting hemorrhage, restoring blood volume, and correcting coagulopathy are ongoing.

C. G. Ball (✉)
Foothills Medical Centre, Calgary, AB, Canada

Massive Transfusion

Although the traditional definition of a massive transfusion is ≥10 units of red blood cells (RBC) in a 24-hour period, this term has been modified with regard to both the amount of blood product and the time interval to better reflect true coagulation biochemistry [16, 19]. The 3% and 8% of civilian and military injuries, respectively, who require a massive transfusion are predictably associated with high mortality rates (27% to 51%) [19]. Furthermore, the early coagulopathy of trauma is a well-recognized entity that is present upon admission of over 25% of injured patients with a base deficit greater than 6 [20]. Although coagulopathy was historically viewed as a byproduct of resuscitation, hemodilution, and hypothermia, the bloody vicious cycle is now understood to be significantly more complex [21]. Tissue trauma, shock, hemodilution, hypothermia, acidemia, and inflammation all play key trigger roles in the acute coagulopathy of trauma-shock [21]. The improved understanding of inter-relationships and recognition of these six key initiators of coagulopathy support the modern use of massive transfusion protocols (MTPs) (Table 30.1).

A modern MTP aims to approximate delivery of 1:1:1 ratio of RBC:fresh frozen plasma:platelets [21]. By addressing the early coagulopathy of trauma, MTPs have been shown to improve mortality in multiply injured populations [20, 22]. While the specific structure of MTPs varies slightly from center to center [23], they are all approximations of Sheldon's fresh whole blood resuscitation principles from 1975 [24]. Additional benefits of a formal MTP include earlier administration of blood products during resuscitations, improved blood banking efficiency, decreased total blood product utilization during a hospital stay, and significant economic savings [25]. It must also be noted, however, that reasonable scientific concern remains with regard to the apparent improvement in survival via MTPs [26]. The possibility of a strong survival bias based on survivorship (i.e., surviving long enough to receive the most RBC units) remains [26]. It should also be noted that although the potential benefits of

L. Marshall Gillman, S. Widder (eds.), *Trauma Team Dynamics*, https://doi.org/10.1007/978-3-031-86312-7_30

Table 30.1 Massive transfusion protocol: package contents[a]

Package	PRBCs	Plasma	Platelets	Cryoprecipitate
Initiation	6 units (UD/TS)	6 units (UD)		
1 (0.5 hr)	6 units (UD/TS)	6 units (UD)	1 apheresis[b]	
2 (1 hr)	6 units (UD/TS)	6 units (TS)		20 units
3 (1. 5 hr)[c]	6 units (UD/TS)	6 units (TS)	1 apheresis[b]	
4 (2 hr)	6 units (UD/TS)	6 units (TS)		10 units
5 (2.5 hr)	6 units (UD/TS)	6 units (TS)	1 apheresis[b]	
6 (3 hr)[d]	6 units (UD/TS)	6 units (TS)		10 units

PRBCs Packed red blood cells, *UD* Universal donor, *TS* Type-specific
[a]PRBCs and plasma can be doubled to 12 units each per cycle by request
[b]1 apheresis unit of platelets considered to equal 8–10 standard units
[c]Recombinant Factor VIIa may be used at attending physician discretion (Dose: 3.6 mg, one repeat dose as needed in 30 minutes)
[d]If protocol still active, alternate packages identical to packages 5 and 6 until protocol terminated

MTPs have been widely publicized, numerous theoretical and observational complications have been linked to MTPs using retrospective registry data. These include, but are not limited to, potentially increased risks of acute lung injury (ALI), acute respiratory distress syndrome (ARDS), and hypothermia, and other risks associated with the transfusion of any blood product [27–29]. Further study is clearly warranted and ongoing.

Another major benefit of an MTP is the avoidance of excess crystalloid fluid administration [30]. This reduction in crystalloid volume during the resuscitation period minimizes multiple associated side effects including reperfusion injury, increased leukocyte adhesion and inflammation, associated acidosis, and resultant acute respiratory distress syndrome, systemic inflammatory response syndrome, and multi-organ failure [31–33]. On an anecdotal platform, excess crystalloid administration also remains an obstacle to obtaining early definitive fascial closure of the abdominal wall secondary to both visceral and abdominal wall edema.

Permissive Hypotension

Further mention of the concept of permissive hypotension is also prudent and must reference the original randomized controlled trial by Mattox and colleagues in 1994 [17]. More specifically, this trial successfully challenged the dogma of restoring a patient's blood pressure to physiologic levels in scenarios defined by ongoing hemorrhage. While this study was also heavily criticized due to the dominance of penetrating injuries and the proximity of patients to the trauma center, an updated prospective randomized trial has recently supported this initial observation in a multitude of injured patients [18]. This recent study noted that hypotensive resuscitation (MAP goal of 50 mmHg) is a safe strategy for injured patients that results in less overall blood product and intravenous fluid administration, decreased postoperative coagulopathy, and reduced early postoperative death [18]. It should be emphasized that this applies only to patients who are imminently going for definitive surgical repair and should not be applied to patients with potential delays to management and/or anticipated long transport times. Other patient populations where this may be contraindicated include elderly patients, patients with pre-existing hypertension, and head-injured patients.

Damage Control Surgery and Its Indications

Once damage control surgery (DCS) was born, it was quickly marketed into other disciplines that included, but were not limited to, neck [7], vascular [8], orthopedic [9], thoracic [10], and military injuries [11]. The conceptual maturation of DCS has led to fundamental tenants that include: (1) arresting surgical hemorrhage, (2) containment of gastrointestinal spillage, (3) surgical sponge insertion, and (4) temporary abdominal closure. This sequence is followed by immediate transfer to the intensive care unit with subsequent re-warming, correction of coagulopathy, and hemodynamic stabilization. Return to the operating theater is then pursued 6 to 48 hours later for a planned re-exploration that includes definitive repair and primary fascial closure if possible. It is clear that the DCS approach leads to improved survival for both blunt and penetrating injuries in patients who are approaching physiologic exhaustion [12].

Despite the clear utility of DCS, its widespread propagation throughout the trauma community has led to a clear over-utilization of this technique. More specifically, multiply injured patients who are *not* approaching physiologic exhaustion are often exposed to the potential risks associated with an open abdomen. As a result, the pertinent question remains: Who needs DCS? The succinct response is "patients who are more likely to die from uncorrected shock states than from failure to complete organ repairs." Depending on the center, these "metabolic cripples" encompass 3–8% of all *severely* injured patients (penetrating vs. blunt; military vs. civilian). In essence, they continue to suffer the sequelae of tissue shock that is manifest as *persistent* hypothermia, *persistent* metabolic acidosis, and non-mechanical (i.e., non-surgical) bleeding. More specifically, DCS triggers include core temperature <35 °C, pH < 7.2, base deficit > −15, and/or significant coagulopathies. [13–16] It must be emphasized, however, that not all patients with initial physiologic deficits as significant as these values mandate DCS. With rapid arrest of hemorrhage, as well as ongoing resuscitation, some patients will improve dramatically in all parameters on repeated intra-operative blood gases. These patients stabilize and begin to recover. It should also be stated that patients with multiple intra-abdominal injuries are not always in metabolic failure.

Vascular Damage Control Techniques

Although it is clear that arresting ongoing hemorrhage is the most crucial of damage control tenants, *vascular* damage control has been traditionally limited to vessel ligation. More recently, however, balloon catheter tamponade and temporary intravascular shunts (TIVS) have increased in popularity. The impressive utility of balloon catheters for tamponade of exsanguinating hemorrhage has a long history dating back more than 50 years [34]. Although this technique was originally described for esophageal varices [35], it was quickly extended to patients with traumatic vascular and solid organ injuries [36]. Since the initial treatment of an iliac arteriovenous lesion in 1960 [3], balloon catheters have also been used for cardiac [37], aortic [38], pelvic [39], neck (carotid, vertebral, and jugular) [40, 41], abdominal vascular [42], hepatic [43], subclavian [44], vertebral [34], and facial trauma [45]. While this technique was originally intended as an intraoperative endovascular tool [34], it has since been employed as an emergency room maneuver with the balloon being placed outside of the lumen of the injured vessel [46, 47].

Modern indications for this damage control technique are limited. This is primarily because routine methods for controlling hemorrhage, such as direct pressure, are typically successful. As a result, indications for catheter tamponade include: (1) inaccessible (or difficult to access) major vascular injuries, (2) large cardiac injuries, and (3) deep solid organ parenchymal hemorrhage (liver and lung) [34, 37]. Of interest, the type of balloon catheter (Foley, Fogarty, Blakemore, or Penrose with red rubber Robinson), as well as the duration of indwelling, can vary significantly. In conclusion, balloon catheter tamponade is a valuable tool for damage control of exsanguinating hemorrhage when direct pressure fails, or tourniquets are not applicable. It can be employed in multiple anatomic regions and for variable patterns of injury. Prolonged catheter placement for maintenance of hemostasis is particularly useful for central hepatic gunshot injuries [47].

Temporary intravascular shunts (TIVS) are intraluminal synthetic conduits that offer non-permanent maintenance of arterial inflow and/or venous outflow [48]. As a result, they are frequently life- and limb-saving when patient physiology is hostile. By bridging a damaged vessel and maintaining blood flow, they address both acute hemorrhage and critical warm ischemia of distal organs and limbs. Although Eger and colleagues are commonly credited for pioneering the use of TIVS in modern vascular trauma [49], this technique was initially employed by Carrel in animal experiments [50]. The first documented use in humans occurred in 1915 when Tuffier employed paraffin-coated silver tubes to bridge injured arteries [51]. This technique evolved from glass to plastic conduits in World War II [52], and continues to vary both in structure and material amongst today's surgeons [53].

Modern indications for TIVS include the following: (1) replantation, (2) open extremity fractures with concurrent extensive soft tissue loss and arterial injury (Gustilo IIIC), (3) peripheral vascular damage control, (4) truncal vascular damage control, and (5) temporary stabilization prior to transport [48, 54]. While the understanding of TIVS use for military and civilian settings is increasing [53], the optimal shunt material, dwell time, and anticoagulation requirements remain poorly studied. It can be noted, however, that TIVS are remarkably durable and rarely clot unless they: (1) are too small (diameter), (2) kink because of inappropriate length, and/or (3) are placed in an extremity without appropriate (or shunted) venous outflow (venous hypertension leads to arterial thrombosis) [54].

Despite the penetrating mechanism dogma associated with TIVS over the past 40 years, the majority (64%) of TIVS in a large National database (National Trauma Data Bank—NTDB) were used in patients injured via a blunt mechanism [55]. Although the kinetic force of an MVC or MVC-pedestrian collision can be tremendous, TIVS is often discussed in the context of extremity damage control for gunshot wounds in patients with hostile physiology [55]. This NTDB analysis, however, indicated that most extremity TIVS are actually placed for blunt vascular trauma associated with extensive orthopedic and/or soft tissue injuries (74%). They are also most often used as a temporizing maneuver to provide distal flow to a limb while orthopedic injuries are assessed and fixated. The use of TIVS for this scenario is well recognized and documented to significantly reduce the rate of amputation. In the patients who did not undergo TIVS for fractures and soft tissue defects, it appears that shunting was employed as an extremity damage control technique in those who presented with hemodynamic instability and severe base deficits (26%) [55]. These patients displayed a much lower level of subsequent amputation when compared to cases of blunt trauma with concurrent fractures and soft tissue trauma. In addition to using TIVS in blunt injured patients, the NTDB also indicates this technique is being performed relatively uncommonly across a wide range of hospitals [55]. Of 111 trauma centers employing TIVS, only 6 used 5 or more shunts throughout the study period. Additionally, only 3 centers employed more than 10 shunts. TIVS appear to be useful in any scenario with a major vascular injury and hostile patient physiology. This includes cases of blunt MVC trauma with concurrent severe extremity fractures and/or soft tissue injuries. In spite of their simplicity, however, they are underutilized.

Non-vascular Damage Control Techniques

Two additional components to damage control surgery must also be addressed: (1) non-vascular ongoing hemorrhage and (2) hollow viscous contamination. Non-vascular persistent abdominal bleeding is most commonly related to the liver, spleen, pancreas, and/or kidney. Unlike the spleen and kidney, the liver and pancreas cannot generally be resected in a rapid, on-demand basis. It should be noted, however, that prior to the removal of any kidney, palpation for a normal-sized contralateral kidney must be completed.

Technical details surrounding hepatic hemorrhage include leaving the falciform ligament intact to provide a medial wall against which to improve packing pressure (especially in blunt trauma). If hemorrhage continues, an early Pringle maneuver (clamping of the porta hepatis with a vascular clamp) is mandated as both a diagnostic and potentially therapeutic technique. If bleeding continues despite application of a Pringle clamp, a retrohepatic IVC or hepatic venous injury is likely. It should be noted that critically injured patients in physiologic extremis do not tolerate extended Pringle maneuvers to the same extent as patients with hepatic tumors undergoing elective hepatic resection (40 minute upper limit). If the liver hemorrhage responds to packing, but continues to hemorrhage when unpacking is completed, the patient should be repacked and transferred to the ICU with an open abdomen once damage control of concurrent injuries is complete. Covering the liver with a plastic layer of sterile X-ray cassette material avoids capsular trauma/oozing upon eventual unpacking. If control of the liver hemorrhage is dependent upon maintenance of a Pringle maneuver despite packing, call for senior assistance, mobilize the right lobe, and suture the IVC or hepatic veins with 4-0 prolene on SH needles. These patients also typically require total vascular exclusion (TVE) of the liver (complete occlusion of the infrahepatic IVC, suprahepatic IVC, porta hepatis (Pringle maneuver), as well as an aortic cross-clamp within the abdomen). If TVE is pursued without concurrent clamping of the aorta, the patient will arrest due to a lack of coronary perfusion. Technically savvy surgeons prefer to obtain suprahepatic IVC control within the abdomen in patients with a normal length of IVC inferior to the diaphragm. A good alternative option includes accessing the IVC as it enters the heart within the pericardium. This 2 cm length of IVC is easily accessible by opening the pericardial sac after dividing the diaphragm (it can also be accessed from the thorax if a thoracotomy has already been performed). Veno-veno bypass is also a theoretical damage control option, but rarely used due to a lack of transplant training in most trauma/general surgeons. In the case of central hepatic gunshot wounds or deep central lacerations where access and exposure are difficult, ongoing hemorrhage should be stopped with balloon occlusion as previously described. Return to the operating suite in patients with packed livers should occur in 72 hours (assuming hypothermia, coagulopathy, and acidosis are corrected). If an atrial-caval shunt is contemplated, two experienced surgical teams (one for the thorax and one for the abdomen) are essential. The decision to pursue this damage control shunt must be made early in the exploration process as they rarely result in patient salvage.

It should be noted that although the published history of hepatic trauma is littered with descriptions of various technical maneuvers ordered in a hierarchical scheme, very few are relevant in context of modern trauma care. More specifically, damage control packing of hepatic hemorrhage controls the vast majority of ongoing bleeding in critically ill patients.

Damage control pancreatic maneuvers are extremely limited and revolve around drainage of nearly all pancreatic injuries (either with a closed suction drain and an open abdomen, or simply open abdomen alone). The dominant associated life-threatening scenario for peripancreatic injuries involves hemorrhage from the portal and superior mesenteric veins. Although these veins can be ligated, repairs are generally performed with 5-0 or 6-0 prolene once control is obtained. Clamps above and below the injury are essential for visualization. Alternate damage control options include TIVS with a small chest tube conduit or ligation (assuming the hepatic artery is intact) [56]. Damage control maneuvers for the splenic vein are generally limited to bulk ligation.

Damage control technique for hollow viscous organs requires ligation and subsequent exclusion of injured and/or leaking segments. This is typically performed using gastrointestinal staplers. The supplying mesenteries can be ligated in a rapid fashion using clamps or vascular staplers. In the case of gastric division, the proximal stomach should be decompressed by a nasogastric tube. Small bowel and colon can be left in discontinuity for up to 48 hours with minimal sequelae.

Abdominal Compartment Syndrome

Abdominal compartment syndrome (ACS) is defined as sustained intra-abdominal pressure greater than 20 mmHg that is associated with new organ dysfunction/failure [57–62]. ACS differs from intra-abdominal hypertension (IAH) which is a graded (I-IV) and sustained pathological elevation greater than 12 mmHg. Symptoms of ACS are extensive and impact every major system within the human body. These include, but are not limited to, cardiovascular (hypotension), renal (acute kidney injury), and respiratory (failure) elements. It is interesting to note that many of the dominant risk factors for developing ACS mirror the physiologic triggers for engaging in DCS/DCR [57, 58]. This observation supports these physiologic variables (pH, base deficit, core temperature) as clear markers for the absolute "sickest of the sick." Closing the abdomen in patients manifesting physiologic extremis often leads to ACS, as first demonstrated by Morris Jr and colleagues in 1993 [59]. With closure, these authors described severe abdominal distension in concert with raised peak airway pressures, CO2 retention, and oliguria [59]. Their observed 63% mortality rate associated with reperfusion injury after unpacking was also dramatic, and currently emphasizes the importance of "recurrent" or "tertiary" ACS [60]. While the incidence of primary ACS has decreased dramatically over the past decade [57], continued vigilance is crucial to guard against secondary and recurrent ACS. Despite the increased understanding surrounding this anatomic and physiologic complication, it is clear that the actual practice of clinicians requires more education with regard to both monitoring and treating ACS [61]. This reality has led to a recent evidence-based update of both definitions of primary, secondary, and recurrent ACS, as well as of an expert society's therapeutic recommendations [62]. More specifically, in addition to multiple "suggestions," the World Congress of the Abdominal Compartment Syndrome (WCACS) strongly recommends: (1) measuring IAP when any known risk factor for IAH/ACS is present in a critically ill or injured patient using a trans-bladder technique (GRADE 1C), (2) utilizing protocolized monitoring and management of IAP (GRADE 1C), (3) engaging in a decompressive laparotomy for cases of overt ACS (GRADE 1D), (4) attempting to ensure same-hospital-stay abdominal fascial closure (GRADE 1D), and (5) utilizing negative suction therapy in patients with open abdominal cavities (GRADE 1D) [62]. It should also be noted that some patients may adequately respond to decompression (nasogastric, colonic, intraperitoneal (i.e., ascites), increased sedation, and/or paralysis as primary therapeutic maneuvers). Failure to resolve ACS with these medical therapies, however, should lead to rapid surgical decompression. Measuring intra-abdominal pressures can be easily performed at the bedside with a three-way Foley catheter, pressure transducer, and intravenous tubing. The probe should be zeroed at the phlebostatic angle in the supine position.

Open Abdominal Management

The concept of delaying abdominal wall closure is credited to Dr. Stone at Grady Memorial Hospital in 1981 [63]. Among 167 patients, mortality approximated 85% in those whose abdomens were closed under tension, compared to only 22% who underwent delayed fascial closure. This truly remarkable report altered the DCS landscape dramatically. Unfortunately, the open abdomen is also responsible for significant short-term (fluid and protein loss, sepsis, intestinal fistulae, nursing care challenges, economic costs) and long-term (chronic physical discomfort, physique embarrassment, delayed return to work, poor quality of life) morbidity [64–67]. Although multiple techniques are described for managing the open abdomen (Table 30.2), it is clear that intestinal coverage (via endogenous abdominal wall or skin or split-thickness skin graft) must be achieved as soon as possible to limit subsequent fistulae. It is also evident that regardless of technique, severely injured patients more commonly achieve fascial closure during their initial hospital stay than their non-trauma, acute care surgery counterparts. If closed too early, however, ACS, fascial dehiscence, necrotizing fasciitis, and ventilation challenges are notable complications.

Despite the poor methodology inherent in the open abdomen literature (i.e., mixed patient cohorts, lack of complete inclusion, ignorance of non-survivors, variable individual surgeon effort and interest), it is evident that negative suction dressings have improved closure rates, and reduced complications such as intestinal fistulae. Whether home-grown [68] or commercially derived [69], these technologies have advanced to the point where they have now become commonplace. The two dominant principles when utilizing negative suction therapy remain: (1) maintenance of the peritoneal/abdominal domain and (2) continuous and progressive tension on the midline abdominal wall. These goals are achieved by insertion of a plastic barrier deep into the paracolic gutters (maximally lateral to prevent adhesions

Table 30.2 Open abdomen coverage techniques

Skin only	Polypropylene mesh
Towel clip	Polyglycolic/Polyglactic acid mesh
Silastic sheet	Polytetrafluoro-thylene mesh
Bogota bag	Parachute Silk
3-liter genitourinary bag	Hydrogel/Aquacel
Steri-drape / X-ray cassette	Ioban
Zippers	Vacuum pack
Slide fasteners	Abdominal wound VAC
Velcro analogue/Wittmann	Bioprosthetics

between the colon and abdominal wall) and generation of midline abdominal wall tension using non-fascial retention sutures or commercial systems. It should also be noted that intra-abdominal pressures often exceed "normal" (>20 mmHg) immediately after progressive increases in tension at the midline during repeat laparotomy and attempted closure. This typically abates over the subsequent few hours, and is considered acceptable in the absence of end organ ischemia (decreased urine output, increased airway pressures). As a result, it is considered fundamentally different from the acute phase of ACS. If the intra-abdominal pressure does not normalize however, the abdomen must be reopened to prevent recurrent ACS.

An individual patient with an open abdomen will either continue to improve, mobilize fluid, and allow gradual abdominal closure via repeat laparotomies, or they will continue to be challenged with sepsis and multi-organ failure, will not mobilize fluid, and will eventually require skin graft coverage. Entero-atmospheric fistulae must also be prevented at all costs. This morbidity complicates not only short-term management but also eventual abdominal wall reconstruction (component separation, modified component separation). If present, these fistulae are best intubated by soft rubber catheters placed within the sponge material of negative pressure suction dressing [70]. Over time, this will allow the clinician to develop a granulation plate around the fistulae appropriate for a skin graft (i.e., conversion into a stoma).

A detailed discussion of the tiered algorithm for abdominal wall reconstruction, as well as the indications for occasional use of biologic materials, is beyond the goals of this review. Clearly, the appropriate timing of reconstruction (8–12 months) is crucial to the success of the repair (adhesions vs. rectus muscle lateral retraction). Extensive experience in reconstructive techniques is crucial to ensure acceptable outcomes. These principles include, but are not limited to, timing, sequencing (stoma reversal, fistula closure), ensuring adequate skin coverage, sparing of periumbilical perforators, minimally invasive lateral releases, and management of wound complications.

In conclusion, DCR includes early blood product transfusion, arrest of ongoing hemorrhage, and restoration of patient blood volume and physiologic/hematologic status. As a result, it recognizes and addresses the early coagulopathy of trauma, avoids massive crystalloid resuscitation, and leaves the peritoneal cavity open when a patient approaches physiologic exhaustion without improvement. DCS vascular techniques include balloon tamponade, as well as temporary intravascular shunts.

Damage Control Environments

Although damage control is a process that should be specific to a given patient (i.e., the need to arrest ongoing hemorrhage, contain gastrointestinal contamination, and restore patient physiology and biochemistry as individually needed), the trauma surgeon must also consider the environment within which they are providing care. More specifically, the concepts of operational and occupational workflow includes considerations that are unique to standard operating rooms, hybrid (Resuscitation with Angiography, Percutaneous Techniques and Operative Repair (RAPTOR)) theaters, and extreme environments (e.g., care under fire, zero gravity, remote terrestrial) [71, 72]. Access to hybrid operating theatres, for example, now shows clear associated peer-reviewed evidence that the time from patient arrival to intervention (and arrest of hemorrhage), morbidity, and mortality are each improved in patients who require both open and percutaneous approaches for hemorrhage control [73]. Whether truly simultaneous (operating surgical and percutaneous teams performing procedures at precisely the same time) or synchronous (one team completes their damage control procedure, followed immediately by the second team), the hybrid (RAPTOR) environment benefits the damage control process via increased capacity, capability, and optimization of patient care within a single location (resuscitation, imaging, open and percutaneous therapies, critical care) [74]. Operating room design, including hybrid OR suites, are discussed further in Chap. 25.

Unique challenges and obstacles specific to more exotic environments must also be considered for any clinician engaging in damage control procedures [75]. These include damage control resuscitation during spaceflight (i.e., zero gravity) and within military conflicts [76–78]. These scenarios are highlighted by the trauma team's need to "think innovatively" in addressing issues that include, but are not limited to, patient (body fluid and physical body) restraint, limited resources, clinician/team safety, timeliness of extraction to better equipped staging medical facilities, mission critical goals, and potential time/transfer challenges. In these austere damage control scenarios, leadership and teamwork will be tested and require thoughtful, directive, and close communication among all team members [79, 80].

Key Notes

1. Damage control resuscitation incorporates principles of early blood product transfusion, minimization of crystalloid administration, permissive hypotension, abbreviated operative interventions, and sustained critical care with early re-operation.
2. Vascular damage control techniques include the placement of balloon tamponade and temporary intravascular shunts.
3. Successful closure of the fascia in open abdomens during the same hospital stay requires perseverance by the surgeon to apply progressive midline tension and maintain abdominal domain.

References

1. Manual for Naval warfare. United States of America Navy; 1996.
2. Rotondo MF, Schwab CW, McGonigal MD, Phillips GR 3rd, Fruchterman TM, Kauder DR, et al. Damage control: an approach for improved survival in exsanguinating penetrating abdominal injury. J Trauma. 1993;35:375–83.
3. Lucas CE, Ledgerwood AM. Prospective evaluation of hemostatic techniques for liver injuries. J Trauma. 1976;16:442–51.
4. Calne RY, McMaster P, Pentlow BD. The treatment of major liver trauma by primary packing with transfer of the patient for definitive treatment. Br J Surg. 1979;66:338–9.
5. Feliciano DV, Mattox KL, Jordan GL Jr. Intra-abdominal packing for control of hepatic hemorrhage: a reappraisal. J Trauma. 1981;21:285–90.
6. Stone HH, Strom PR, Mullins RJ. Management of the major coagulopathy with onset during laparotomy. Ann Surg. 1983;197:532–5.
7. Firoozmand E, Velmahos GC. Extending damage control principles to the neck. J Trauma. 2000;48:541.
8. Granchi T, Schmittling Z, Vasquez J, Schreiber M, Wall M. Prolonged use of intraluminal arterial shunts without systemic antigoagulation. Am J Surg. 2000;180:493–6.
9. Scalea TM, Boswell SA, Scott JD, Mitchell KA, Kramer ME, Pollak AN, et al. External fixation as a bridge to nailing for patients with multiple injuries and with femur fractures: damage control orthopedics. J Trauma. 2000;48:613–23.
10. Vargo DJ, Battistella FD. Abbreviated thoracotomy and temporary chest closure: an application of damage control after thoracic trauma. Arch Surg. 2001;136:21–4.
11. Holcomb JB, Helling TS, Hirshber A. Military, civilian and rural application of the damage control philosophy. Mil Med. 2001;166:490–3.
12. Nicholas JM, Rix EP, Easley KA, Feliciano DV, Cava RA, Ingram WL, et al. Changing patterns in the management of penetrating abdominal trauma: the more things change, the more they stay the same. J Trauma. 2003;55:1095–108.
13. Lier H, Krep H, Schroeder S, Stuber F. The influence of acidosis, hypocalcemia, anemia, and hypothermia on functional hemostasis in trauma. J Trauma. 2008;65:951–60.
14. Wyrzykowski AD, Feliciano DV. Trauma damage control. In: Feliciano DV, Mattox KL, Moore EE, editors. Trauma. 6th ed. New York: McGraw-Hill Medical; 2008. p. 851–70.
15. Cushman JG, Feliciano DV, Renz BM, Ingram WL, Ansley JD, Clark WS, et al. Iliac vessel injury: operative physiology related to outcome. J Trauma. 1997;42:1033–40.
16. Holcomb JB, Jenkins D, Rhee P, Johannigman J, Mahoney P, Mehta S, et al. Damage control resuscitation: directly addressing the early coagulopathy of trauma. J Trauma. 2007;62:307–10.
17. Bickell WH, Wall MJ Jr, Pepe PE, Martin RR, Ginger VF, Allen MK, et al. Immediate versus delayed fluid resuscitation for hypotensive patients with penetrating torso injuries. N Engl J Med. 1994;27:1105–9.
18. Morrison CA, Carrick MM, Norman MA, et al. Hypotensive resuscitation strategy reduces transfusion requirements and severe postoperative coagulopathy in trauma patients with hemorrhagic shock: preliminary results of a randomized controlled trial. J Trauma. 2011;70:652–63.
19. Como JJ, Dutton RP, Scalea TM, Edelman BB, Hess JR. Blood transfusion rates in the care of acute trauma. Transfusion. 2004;44:809–13.
20. Brohi K, Singh J, Hern M, Coats T. Acute traumatic coagulopathy. J Trauma. 2003;54:1127–30.
21. Hess JR, Brohi K, Dutton RP, Hauser CJ, Holcomb JB, Kluger Y, et al. The coagulopathy of trauma: a review of mechanisms. J Trauma. 2008;65:748–54.
22. Borgman MA, Spinella PC, Perkins JG, Grathwohl KW, Repine T, Beekley AC, et al. The ratio of blood products transfuse affects mortality in patients receiving massive transfusions at a combat support hospital. J Trauma. 2007;64:805–13.
23. Dente CJ, Shaz BH, Nicholas JM, Harris RS, Wyrzykowski AD, Patel S, et al. Improvements in early mortality and coagulopathy are sustained better in patients with blunt trauma after institution of a massive transfusion protocol in a civilian level I trauma center. J Trauma. 2009;66:1616–24.
24. Sheldon GF, Lim RC, Blaisdell FW. The use of fresh blood in the treatment of critically injured patients. J Trauma. 1975;15:670–7.
25. O'Keeffe T, Refaai M, Tchorz K, Forestner JE, Sarode R. A massive transfusion protocol to decrease blood component use and cost. Arch Surg. 2008;143:686–90.
26. Snyder CW, Weinberg JA, McGwin G Jr, Melton SM, George RL, Reiff DA, et al. The relationship of blood product ratio to mortality: survival benefit or survival bias? J Trauma. 2009;66:358–62.
27. Park PK, Cannon JW, Ye W, Blackbourne LH, Holcomb JB, Beninati W, et al. Transfusion strategies and development of acute respiratory distress syndrome in combat casualty care. J Trauma Acute Care Surg. 2013;75(S):S238–46.
28. Inaba K, Branco BC, Rhee P, et al. Impact of plasma transfusion in trauma patients who do not require massive transfusion. J Am Coll Surg. 2010;210:957–65.
29. Sharpe JP, Weinberg JA, Magnotti LJ, Fabian TC, Croce MA. Does plasma transfusion portend pulmonary dysfunction? A tale of two ratios. J Trauma Acute Care Surg. 2013;75:32–6.
30. Cotton BA, Guy JS, Morris JA, Abumrad NN. Cellular, metabolic, and systemic consequences of aggressive fluid resuscitation strategies. Shock. 2006;26:115–21.
31. Rhee P, Koustova E, Alam HB. Searching for the optimal resuscitation method: recommendations for the initial fluid resuscitation of combat casualties. J Trauma. 2003;54:S52.
32. Pruitt BA Jr. Protection for excessive resuscitation: "pushing the pendulum back". J Trauma. 2000;49:567–8.
33. Ball CG, Kirkpatrick AW. Intra-abdominal hypertension and the abdominal compartment syndrome. Scand J Surg. 2007;96:197–204.
34. Feliciano DV, Burch JM, Mattox KL, Bitondo CG, Fields G. Balloon catheter tamponade in cardiovascular wounds. Am J Surg. 1990;160:583–7.

35. Myhre JR. Balloon tamponade of hemorrhagic esophageal varices. Tidsskr Nor Laegeforen. 1958;78:511–3.
36. Taylor H, Williams E. Arteriovenous fistula following disk surgery. Br J Surg. 1962;50:47–50.
37. Pearce CW, McCool E, Schmidt FE. Control of bleeding from cardiovascular wounds: balloon catheter tamponade. Ann Surg. 1966;166:257–9.
38. Foster JH, Morgan CV, Threlkel JB. Proximal control of aorta with a balloon catheter. Surg Gynecol Obstet. 1971;132:693–4.
39. Sheldon GF, Winestock DP. Hemorrhage from open pelvic fracture controlled intraoperatively with balloon catheter. J Trauma. 1978;18:68–70.
40. Belkin M, Dunton R, Crombie HD, Lowe R. Preoperative percutaneous intraluminal balloon catheter control of major arterial hemorrhage. J Trauma. 1988;28:548–50.
41. Brendahan J, Swanepoel E, Muller R. Tamponade of vertebral artery bleeding by Foley's catheter balloon. Injury. 1994;25:473–4.
42. Smiley K, Perry MO. Balloon catheter tamponade of major vascular wounds. Am J Surg. 1971;121:326–7.
43. Morimoto RY, Birolini D, Junqueira AR Jr, Poggetti R, Horita LT. Balloon tamponade for transfixing lesions of the liver. Surg Gynecol Obstet. 1987;164:87–8.
44. DiGiacomo JC, Rotondo MF, Schwab CW. Transcutaneous balloon catheter tamponade for definitive control of subclavian venous injuries: case reports. J Trauma. 1994;37:111–3.
45. Sing RF, Sue SR, Reilly PM. Balloon catheter tamponade of exsanguinating facial hemorrhage: a case report. J Emerg Med. 1998;16:601–2.
46. Navsaria P, Thoma M, Nicol A. Foley catheter balloon tamponade for life-threatening hemorrhage in penetrating neck trauma. World J Surg. 2006;30:1265–8.
47. Ball CG, Wyrzykowski AD, Nicholas JM, Rozycki GS, Feliciano DV. A decade's experience with balloon catheter tamponade for the emergency control of hemorrhage. J Trauma. 2011;70:330–3.
48. Frykberg ER, Schinco MA. Peripheral vascular injury. In: Feliciano DV, Mattox KL, Moore EE, editors. Trauma. 6th ed. New York: McGraw-Hill Medical; 2008. p. 956–7.
49. Eger M, Golcman L, Goldstein A, Hirsch M. The use of a temporary shunt in the management of arterial vascular injuries. Surg Gynecol Obstet. 1971;132:67–70.
50. Makins GH. Gunshot injuries to the blood vessels. London: Simpkin, Marshall, Hamilton, Kent & Co; 1919. p. 109–11.
51. Tuffier. French surgery in 1915. Br J Surg. 1916;4:420–32.
52. Matheson NM, Murray G. Recent advances and experimental work in conservative vascular surgery. In: Bailey H, editor. Surgery of modern warfare, vol. 1. Baltimore: Williams and Wilkins; 1941. p. 324–7.
53. Ding W, Wu X, Li J. Temporary intravascular shunts used as a damage control surgery adjunct in complex vascular injury: collective review. Injury. 2008;39:970–7.
54. Ball CG, Feliciano DV. Damage control techniques for common and external iliac artery injuries: have temporary intravascular shunts replaced the need for ligation? J Trauma. 2010;68:1117–20.
55. Ball CG, Kirkpatrick AW, Rajani RR, Wyrzykowski AD, Dente CJ, Vercruysse GA, et al. Temporary intravascular shunts: when are we really using them according to the NTDB? Am Surg. 2009;75:605–7.
56. Ball CG, Kirkpatrick AW, Smith M, Mulloy RH, Tse L, Anderson IB. Traumatic injury of the superior mesenteric vein: ligate, repair or shunt? Euro J Trauma Emerg Surg. 2007;43:1–3.
57. Balogh ZJ, van Wessem K, Yoshino O, Moore FA. Postinjury abdominal compartment syndrome: are we winning the battle? World J Surg. 2009;33:1134–41.
58. Balogh Z, McKinley BA, Holcomb JB, Miller CC, Cocanour CS, Kozar RA, et al. Both primary and secondary abdominal compartment syndrome (ACS) can be predicted early and are harbingers of multiple organ failure. J Trauma. 2003;54:848–59.
59. Morris JA Jr, Eddy VA, Blinman TA, Rutherford EJ, Sharp KW. The staged celiotomy for trauma: issues in unpacking and reconstruction. Ann Surg. 1993;217:576–86.
60. Ball CG, Kirkpatrick AW, Karmali S, Malbrain ML, Gmora S, Mahabir RC, et al. Tertiary abdominal compartment syndrome in the burn injured patient. J Trauma. 2006;81:1271–3.
61. Kirkpatrick AW, Laupland KB, Karmali S, Bergeron E, Stewart TC, Findlay C, et al. Spill your guts! Perceptions of Trauma Association of Canada member surgeons regarding the open abdomen and the ACS. J Trauma. 2006;60:279–86.
62. Kirkpatrick AW, Roberts DJ, De Waele J, et al. Intra-abdominal hypertension and the abdominal compartment syndrome: updated consensus definitions and clinical practice guidelines from the World Society of the Abdominal Compartment Syndrome. Intensive Care Med. 2013;39:2290–06.
63. Stone HH, Fabian TC, Turkleson ML, Jurkiewics MJ. Management of acute full-thickness losses of the abdominal wall. Ann Surg. 1981;193:612–8.
64. Balogh ZA, Moore FA, Goettler CE. Surgical management of the abdominal compartment syndrome. In: Ivatury RR, Cheatham ML, Malbrain MLNG, et al., editors. Abdominal compartment Syndrom. Georgetown: Landes Biomed; 2006. p. 266–9.
65. Ball CG, Kirkpatrick AW, McBeth PB. The secondary abdominal compartment syndrome: not just another post-traumatic complication. Can J Surg. 2008;51:399–405.
66. Cheatham ML, Safcsak K, Llerena LE, Morrow CE Jr, Block EF. Long-term physical, mental and functional consequences of abdominal decompression. J Trauma. 2004;56:237–41.
67. Cheatham ML, Safcsak K. Long-term impact of abdominal decompression: a prospective comparative analysis. J Am Coll Surg. 2008;207:573–9.
68. Brock WB, Barker DE, Burns RP. Temporary closure of open abdominal wounds: the vacuum pack. Am Surg. 1995;61:30–5.
69. Garner GB, Ware DN, Cocanour CS, Duke JH, McKinley BA, Kozar RA, et al. Vacuum-assisted wound closure provides early fascial reapproximation in trauma patients with open abdomens. Am J Surg. 2001;182:630–8.
70. Al-Koury G, Kaufman D, Hirshberg A. Improved control of exposed fistula in the open abdomen. J Am Coll Surg. 2007;206:397–8.
71. Ball CG. The R.A.P.T.O.R. suite: resuscitation with angiography, percutaneous techniques, and operative repair. J Trauma. 2011;70:1579–80.
72. Kirkpatrick AW, Vis C, Dube M, Biesbroek S, Ball CG, Laberge J, et al. The evolution of a purpose designed hybrid trauma operating room ffrom the trauma services perspective: the RAPTOR (resuscitation with angiography, percutaneous treatments and operative resuscitations). Injury. 2014;45:1413–21.
73. Carver D, Kirkpatrick AW, D'Amours S, Hameed SM, Bevereidge J, Ball CG. A prospective evaluation of the utility of a hybrid operating suite for severely injured patients: overstated or underutilized? Ann Surg. 2020;271:958–61.
74. Ball CG, Kirkpatrick AW, Wong J, Clements T. Simultaneous versus serial/synchronous interventions in a hybrid operating suite for severely injured patients: a prospective evaluation of differences in R.A.P.T.O.R. outcomes and techniques. J Trauma Acute Care Surg. 2021; In Press.
75. Roberts DJ, Ball CG, Feliciano DV, Moore EE, Ivatury RR, Lucas CE, et al. History of the innovation of damage control for management of trauma patients: 1902-2016. Ann Surg. 2017;265:1034–44.
76. Kirkpatrick AW, McKee JL, Tien CH, LaPorta AJ, Lavell K, Leslie T, et al. Abbreviated closure for remote damage control laparotomy in extreme environments: a randomized trial of sutures versus wound clamps comparing terrestrial and weightless conditions. Am J Surg. 2017;213:862–9.
77. Kirkpatrick AW, McKee JL, Tien H, LaPorta AJ, Lavell K, Leslie, et al. Damage control surgery in weightlessness: a comparative

study of simulated torso hemorrhage control comparing terrestrial and weightlessness conditions. J Trauma Acute Care Surg. 2017;82:392–9.

78. Kirkpatrick AW, McKee JL, McBeth PB, Ball CG, LaPorta A, Broderick T, et al. The damage control surgery in Austere Environments Research Group (DCSAERG): a dynamic program to facilitate real-time telementoring/telediagnosis to address exsanguination in extreme and austere environments. J Trauma Acute Care Surg. 2017;83(Suppl 1):S156–63.
79. Ball CG. Leadership during the COVID-19 crisis and beyond. Can J Surg. 2020;63:272–3.
80. Ball CG. Do we need to reassess the meaning of "team" in our health care environments? Can J Surg. 2020;63:94–5.

Special Trauma Cases and Damage Control Surgery

31

Caitlyn McCall and Lisa L. Schlitzkus

Trauma patients present with unique physiology anatomy and circumstances that challenge the trauma team. Injuries can be highly destructive and distort the anatomy and minor or sensational injuries can distract the team from the life-threatening ones. Multiple cavities can be involved and prioritizing operative interventions must be undertaken with little patient or clinical data. Further complicating the clinical picture is the delayed presentation of the trauma patient whether due to environmental transport or patient factors. Delay can lead to physiologic derangements from uncontrolled bleeding and/or contamination. Historically the surgeon would complete the operation including all bowel and vascular anastomoses and close the abdomen. Complications such as abdominal compartment syndrome the classic triad of death—hypothermia coagulopathy and acidosis—and later multisystem organ failure would ensue [1, 2]. This led surgeons to challenge the traditional approach by aborting the operation early and creating a staged approach in a concept termed "damage control". First described in 1983 [3] damage control demonstrated improved outcomes in 1993 [4]. Improvements in certain stages have been described and recognition that many physiologic challenges begin the moment injury occurs has led to implementing changes in the prehospital setting [5, 6]. Initially damage control surgery was applied to intra-abdominal injuries but now has been expanded to include thoracic vascular and extremity injuries [7, 8]. The military uses damage control across theaters—temporizing on the front lines at a forward operating base resuscitating the patient then transporting to a higher level of care at a well-established military base in another country or even continent [9–11].

C. McCall
Department of Surgery, Denver Health Medical Center, Denver, CO, USA

Division of Gastrointestinal, Trauma, and Endocrine Surgery, Department of Surgery, University of Colorado Anschutz Medical Center, Aurora, CO, USA
e-mail: Caitlyn.mccall@cuanschutz.edu

L. L. Schlitzkus (✉)
UCHealth Memorial Hospital Central, Colorado Springs, CO, USA
e-mail: Lisa.schlitzkus@uchealth.org

Indications for Damage Control Surgery

The goal of damage control surgery is to recognize patients who are physiologically deranged, need second explorations, or are at risk for poor outcomes if the traditional approach with closure is undertaken. Classically, the lethal triad of hypothermia, coagulopathy, and acidosis appears as the patient reaches physiologic exhaustion. Waiting for physiologic exhaustion to develop and then undertaking damage control defeats the purpose of damage control. Bleeding and contamination are controlled in the first operation. The patient is then taken to the intensive care unit (ICU) for resuscitation, allowing time to recapture the patient's physiology.

Identification of patients who benefit from damage control surgery is an art that requires experience and depends on communication of vital information. Prior to arrival, emergency medical services (EMS) communicating prehospital hypotension, hypothermia, blood loss at the scene or ongoing, and transfusions can trigger the trauma team to entertain damage control. Patient selection also plays a role. Older age is an independent predictor of mortality due to lack of physiological reserve [2, 12]. pH and temperature also are independent predictors of survivability; both affect enzyme, clotting, and myocardial function [12]. In fact, age, temperature, and pH have been tested in predictive equations to preoperatively provide a survivability percentage [12]. The ethical ramifications of treating patients with extremely low chances of survival are debatable—false hope for patients and family, resource utilization, etc.; however, it does demonstrate that there is a group of patients who are unsalvageable and that damage control surgery is futile [12].

While more than 115 indications for damage control have been published, there are only 59 unique indications [13]. Of

L. Marshall Gillman, S. Widder (eds.), *Trauma Team Dynamics*, https://doi.org/10.1007/978-3-031-86312-7_31

those, only six have strong evidence that damage control may improve survival: hypothermia, acidosis, coagulopathy that develops during an operation, an abdominal vascular injury with a pancreatic injury, ≥ 1 major abdominal vascular injury, and two or more abdominal visceral injuries in patients who have received >10 units pRBCs [13]. For the last three indications, injury patterns that require a prolonged definitive repair should undergo damage control. When surveyed, most trauma surgeons utilized temporary abdominal closure when fascia could not be closed (subjectively tight), subjective massive visceral edema, for a planned reoperation (pack removal, second look), or when abdominal compartment syndrome developed during attempted fascia closure [13]. Constant and effective communication with anesthesia is necessary to ensure frequent monitoring, guide resuscitation, and communicate the decision to abort the operation and rapidly proceed to the ICU [14].

Patients with multiple cavity injuries are ideal candidates for damage control. Ongoing bleeding can hasten physiologic exhaustion, so hemorrhage control must be expeditiously undertaken, leaving no opportunity for definitive repair. For example, a patient with a thoracoabdominal or multiple stab wounds may need both the abdomen and mediastinum or thorax explored, and the surgeon must make a judgment about which cavity is the primary source of bleeding or life-threatening injury. Once bleeding is controlled in one cavity, the surgeon must rapidly examine the next. Other situations that lend themselves to damage control are those where endovascular techniques may achieve hemorrhage control more effectively, such as severe liver or pelvic bleeding. While waiting for the endovascular team to arrive, the surgeon may explore the abdomen and pack the liver or pelvis and even isolate and temporarily occlude the porta hepatis or internal iliac arteries. Once the endovascular team is available, the surgeon and radiologists can work together to combine operative and endovascular interventions to stop bleeding. Operations that require extensive reconstruction or anastomoses such as a "trauma Whipple" are ideal for damage control. Given that tissues and anatomy are generally destroyed, prompting these operations, a damage control sequence allows the surgeon to return and examine the tissue for further necrosis and ensure that the final anastomosis is with the healthiest tissue. Ultimately, the earlier the decision is made to undertake damage control, the less physiologically deranged the patient becomes with hope for a better chance of salvaging the patient.

Ground Zero: Scene to Emergency Department

Prehospital Trauma Life Support (PHTLS) is the backbone of prehospital treatment. Transport to a definitive trauma center without delay is the primary goal of PHTLS and prehospital care, with a goal of less than 30 min from call initiation to arrival at the trauma center. An airway must be established if a patient cannot protect his own. Needle decompression or tube thoracostomy may be performed for hypoxia and loss of breath sounds. Large bore IVs should be placed, and resuscitation should begin with isotonic crystalloid. If IV access cannot be obtained, intraosseous (IO) access is an effective alternative that provides rapid access for fluids and medications. Hemorrhage can be controlled with tourniquets or digital pressure. Data suggest that tourniquets are underutilized, and when applied in the prehospital setting can result in a sixfold mortality reduction in patients with peripheral vascular injuries [15].

Fractures can be splinted to provide stability and decrease ongoing bleeding. Previously, two liters of isotonic crystalloid were given, and then more crystalloid or blood products, if available, to achieve the desired response in vital signs. As discussed in Chap. 30, data now suggest that a systolic blood pressure of 80–90 mmHg may be more ideal in a severely injured patient until hemorrhage is controlled under certain circumstances [16]. Administration of prehospital plasma for traumatically injured patients with hemorrhagic shock does have a survival benefit, and benefits outweigh the risk if the transport time is >20 min [17]. Certainly, early administration of blood and blood products should be undertaken if available in the prehospital setting in a trauma patient with hemorrhage, and prehospital resuscitation is an area that continues to be highly researched.

Frequent, effective communication is imperative between the prehospital and emergency department teams. Utilizing prehospital care protocols and live online medical direction can improve the prehospital care. Updating the receiving facility on vital signs and physical findings allow emergency department personnel to mobilize resources. Necessary equipment can be gathered and procedure trays opened. Radiology technicians can be at the bedside waiting with portable X-rays and expedite any other radiological interventions such as computed tomography (CT). The blood bank can be notified if a massive transfusion is planned in order to begin thawing products. Most importantly, roles during the hospital triage are assigned and performed in an organized manner. Mobilization of the team prior to patient arrival decreases evaluation time and eliminates delay to imaging or the operating room.

Failure to relay important clinical information can result in undertriage. The American College of Surgeons Committee on Trauma (ACS-COT) has six minimum criteria to activate a full trauma team (confirmed blood pressure <90 mmHg at any time in adults; gunshot wound to neck, chest, abdomen, or extremities proximal to elbow/knee; Glasgow Coma Scale (GCS) <9 with mechanism attributed to trauma; patients transferred from other hospitals receiving blood to maintain vitals; intubated patients who have respiratory compromise or in need of emergent airway; and emergency physician discretion) [18]. Compliance is highly variable for numerous reasons, but if one triage criteria is met, the patient is significantly more likely to undergo an intervention (79%) with 35% being an emergent operation. Undertriaged patients are more likely to die than appropriately triaged patients [18].

The patient should spend as little time as possible—certainly no more than 20 min—in the emergency department resuscitation/trauma area, including procedures and adjuncts (see Fig. 31.1). The trauma surgeon working with the emergency department team must decipher what the life-threatening injuries are in order to determine the next stage of damage control. In trauma patients with blunt mechanisms, multiple cavities may be involved, and the sources of hemorrhage are difficult to identify as they may not be visible. Penetrating traumas are much easier to triage, given the external wound. It is important to determine trajectory; the external wound may appear to lie within a single cavity but may involve multiple cavities. It is important to place a marker such as a paperclip or an electrocardiogram (EKG) lead on the external wound prior to imaging to help determine trajectory.

The majority of hypotensive trauma patients are in hemorrhagic shock. A patient may exsanguinate externally or internally (thorax, abdomen, pelvis, retroperitoneum, soft tissues). If life-threatening bleeding is ongoing in one of the abovementioned cavities and/or the patient unstable, the surgeon should proceed rapidly to the operating room. Should a patient arrest just prior to arrival or in the resuscitation bay, an emergent resuscitative thoracotomy may be performed to release a cardiac tamponade and/or occlude the aorta in order to maintain perfusion to the heart and brain. Since endovascular technology has further evolved, the use of resuscitative endovascular balloon occlusion of the aorta (REBOA) in trauma is being revisited [19]. While it cannot relieve a cardiac tamponade, REBOA can be used in blunt or penetrating trauma prior to arrest to manage non-compressible hemorrhage at multiple levels of the aorta without the morbidity of a large chest wound [19]. The femoral artery may be accessed percutaneously, or by cut down, and balloon placement does not require fluoroscopy. This is much easier to do prior to an arrest and, in some institutions, is performed in every trauma patient or those with an SBP <90 mmHg [9, 20]. REBOA is discussed further in Chap. 34.

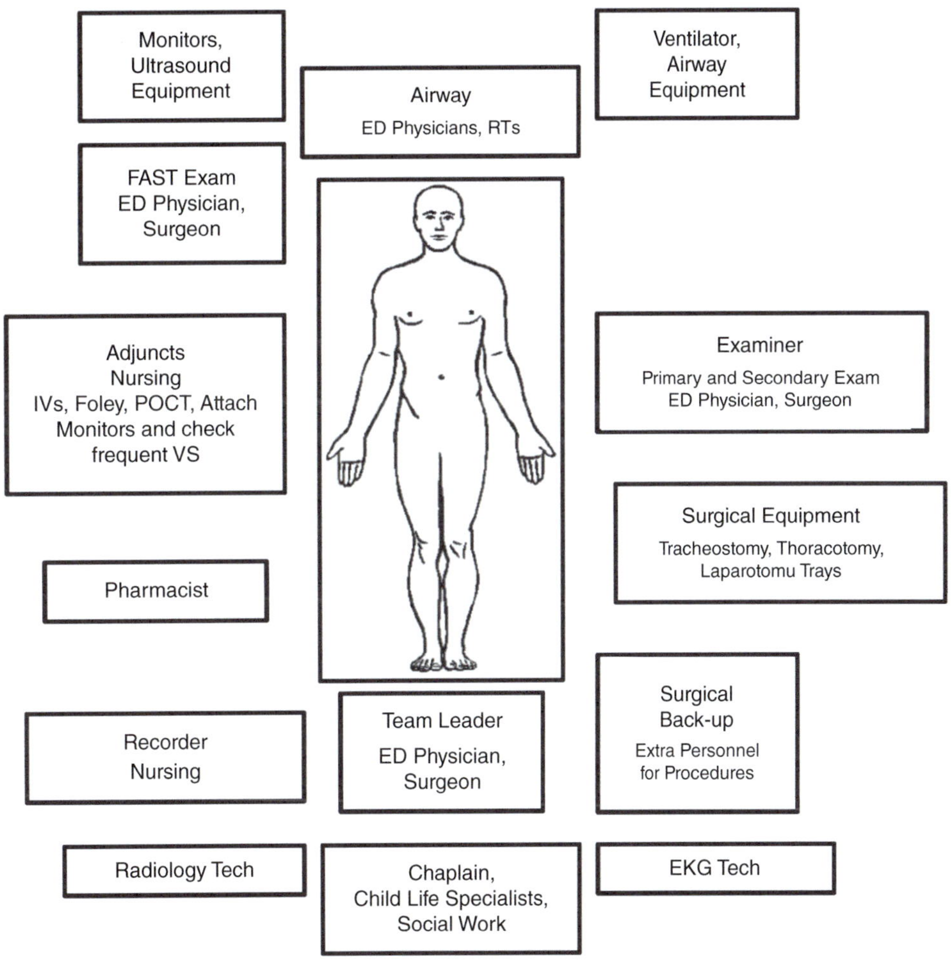

Fig. 31.1 Arrangement of Emergency Department resuscitation area conducive to effective communication. Note that the recorder is adjacent to the Team Leader to read back information. Examiner should be on patient's left side to facilitate Emergency Department (ED) Thoracotomy and other surgical procedures if necessary. Supply carts and medication dispensers/storage should be in close proximity if not in the same room along the walls. RT Respiratory Therapist, POCT Point-of-Care Testing, VS Vital Signs, EKG Electrocardiogram

Massive transfusion protocol (MTP) should be implemented as soon as deemed necessary to ensure products are available as soon as possible. MTPs are low risk and associated with a significant survival benefit (15.5). Smaller, rural, or critical access hospitals may need time to thaw product, so triggering the initiation of an MTP may be based on prehospital report. Larger institutions with high volumes usually have immediate access to the initial round of blood products in a fridge near or in the resuscitation area. Whole blood is now being utilized prior to component therapy. MTPs ensure a 1:1:1 (Plasma:Platelets:pRBC) resuscitation [21].

Depending on patient stability and resource availability, the team may elect to obtain a CT to gain further information. If a liver injury or pelvic fracture with bleeding is found, the team may proceed to a hybrid operating and endovascular room (when available) to control hemorrhage operatively while mobilizing the endovascular team.

Again, effective communication is of utmost importance in efficient patient flow. The CT technologist should be notified that the patient will be arriving momentarily. Radiology technicians (CT and X-ray) are paged/notified along with the trauma team at some institutions and respond to the resuscitation area to ensure a seamless flow. The ordered scans should be discussed and clarified. It helps the technologist and radiologist reading the images to know the history and physical exam findings as well as injuries the treating team is concerned about because the radiologists/technicians may recommend arterial and venous phased scans, thinner slices through worrisome areas, or additional scans while the patient is still on the table. If there is a possibility the patient may be proceeding to the operating room, notifying the operating room team at the earliest opportunity is ideal. Some centers place the OR staff on standby when the trauma team is activated in the emergency department or OR staff respond to the resuscitation area like radiology. While a trauma-ready operating room is always available at an ACS-verified Level 1 trauma center, the lights can be turned on, the room and bed warmed, and the nurse, scrub technician, and anesthesia team mobilized to prepare for a case. A trauma cart with basic supplies (shunts, staplers, tubes, drains, vacuum dressings), various trays (vascular, thoracotomy, laparotomy), and a trauma suture tree should already be available in the room or just outside. In large institutions, these supplies are kept in a specific room, but also on a portable cart that can be transported.

Damage Control Part 1: Operative Intervention

There are two goals in damage control Part 1: control of bleeding and contamination. The patient should spend no longer than 90 min in the operating room, so the team must act and communicate efficiently. Upon arrival to the room, the surgeon should give the team a brief history, interventions undertaken thus far, lines and tubes in place or still needed, and the overall plan for the operation. It can be extremely helpful if anticipated problems are vocalized so that anesthesia staff can prepare for resuscitation and allow time for the nurses to have rapid transfusers and an abundant supply of sponges, basins, and large volume suction available. In extreme situations, intubation may be occurring while prepping and draping the patient if the patient is not already intubated. In some instances, time will only permit splash prep. Assigning roles ensures that perceived, insignificant jobs are not overlooked, resulting in patient decompensation and a confusing clinical picture. For example, failure to hook up chest tubes to suction could result in re-accumulation of a tension pneumothorax and a hypotensive patient.

The positioning of the patient is dependent on which cavities or extremities need to be explored, as previously determined in the emergency department. Generally, the trauma patient is supine with both arms abducted at 90 degrees and prepped from chin to knees and laterally to the bed. If a combined thoracotomy and laparotomy is entertained and the hemithorax previously determined, a modified taxi cab hailing position is ideal. The patient is primarily supine, but on the ipsilateral side of the thorax to be entered, the chest wall is rotated medially about 30 degrees to the coronal plane and supported with a roll. The ipsilateral arm is abducted at 90 degrees, and the elbow flexed at 30 degrees. Any extremity may be prepped, draped, and included in the operative field. If a vascular injury is suspected, both legs and the lower abdomen from the umbilicus to knees should be prepped in the event that vein graft is needed. The general rule of thumb is always prep more than what is anticipated to be accessed.

Once a cavity is opened, hematoma and blood should be evacuated (usually manually due to clot), and the cavity packed with lap sponges. Compression of the aorta may be necessary to halt blood loss. If exsanguination is temporized, the surgeons should pause and allow anesthesia to aggressively resuscitate the patient. Unfortunately, we do not know an optimal systolic blood pressure (SBP) or mean arterial pressure (MAP) in early resuscitation [14]. All injuries must be fully exposed to localize hemorrhage and contamination. Bleeding organs on a pedicle (spleen, kidney) should be sacrificed in less than 10 min per organ. Liver and lung resections are non-anatomical and usually performed with staplers. Finger occlusion of a pedicle, the Pringle maneuver for the liver, or twisting the lung at its hilum are fast techniques to control significant bleeding. Various maneuvers (Kocher, Mattox, Cattell-Braasch) expose the retroperitoneum. Most vessels may be ligated. If a vessel supplies an end organ or extremity, the vessel should be shunted [22–25]. However, in life-threatening situations, even the inferior vena cava may be ligated at its bifurcation.

Visceral contamination can initially be controlled with a clamp and then later during the operation, by stapling and removing the injured segment of bowel or simply whip stitching the injury closed. If a segment is removed, the patient is left in discontinuity due to time and the need for a second look, given the possibility of further necrosis. If an ostomy is planned, maturing the ostomy should not be undertaken during the initial operation. A temporary abdominal, chest, or extremity dressing is placed, allowing for rapid re-entry or examination while preserving the fascia and skin for definitive closure. These may be manufactured or homemade with negative pressure applied. Incorrect counts are common due to the emergent nature of the operation. While attempts are made to count the number of sponges and instruments left in a packed, open cavity, the count should never delay placement of a temporary dressing and transport to the ICU.

Again, communication with bed control to ensure an ICU bed is available as well as with the ICU nursing and physicians facilitates the transition to the next stage of damage control. It may take time to move another patient out of an ICU room, clean the room, and bring the hospital bed to the operating room. Report can be called about 20–30 min prior to leaving the operating room, which allows the ICU staff time to set up suctioning, warming, and massive transfusion equipment, gather pumps, tubing, and supplies, and prepare for the patient as well as notify respiratory therapy to bring a ventilator to the ICU room.

Damage Control Part 2: Resuscitation

The goal of Part 2 is aggressive, rapid resuscitation in order to correct physiologic derangements. Upon arrival to the ICU, the surgical team should communicate the brief history, interventions, what needs to happen immediately, and what the team should be assessing for. A full laboratory panel should be sent upon arrival to the ICU, including a complete blood count (CBC) with differential, complete metabolic panel (CMP) with all electrolytes, creatinine kinase (CK), lactic acid (LA), arterial blood gas (ABG), and coagulation panel including fibrinogen and repeated every 4–6 h to guide resuscitation and organ perfusion endpoints. Viscoelastic assays—rotational thromboelastometry (ROTEM) and rapid thromboelastography (TEG)—are becoming gold standard testing since results are real-time and provide more information about clot stability and lysis, leading to a more tailored resuscitation [14]. Serial troponins and electrocardiograms may also be included. Core temperature should be monitored, and rewarming measures such as blankets and warmed fluids used because hypothermia can inactivate the clotting cascade and impede the body's ability to coagulate blood.

While the resuscitation ratio is debated, a 1:1:1 ratio of fresh frozen plasma (FFP) to platelets to packed red blood cells (pRBCs) is the current recommendation [21]. The goal of resuscitation is to achieve a hemoglobin ≥7 mg/dL, INR <1.5, maintain platelets >100,000, and cryoprecipitate or fibrinogen concentrate may need to be given if the fibrinogen is <200 mg/dL (<2 g/L). If these goals are met, isotonic crystalloid may be used, but be mindful that normal saline may lead to a non-anion gap metabolic acidosis, worsening coagulopathy. Lactated Ringer's is more physiologic, but animal evidence suggests it may activate the immune system, causing damage at the cellular level.

An adjunct to massive transfusion that should be considered in severely injured trauma patients is tranexamic acid (TXA). One gram is given over 10 min, followed by 1 g given over the next 8 h with initiation of administration within 3 h of injury [26]. TXA has been associated with lower mortality [26, 27]—most pronounced in the patients undergoing massive transfusion and those demonstrating hyperfibrinolysis [27]. While the CRASH-2 trial found no adverse events related to TXA administration [26], the MATTERs study found a low but significantly increased risk of PE (2.7%) and DVT (2.4%) [27]. Military data have demonstrated that TXA was independently associated with survival and improved coagulopathy in massively transfused patients [27]. TXA inhibits fibrinolysis, is inexpensive, and has been deemed relatively safe; thus, its use has been growing [27, 28]. Based on a systematic review, the Eastern Association for the Surgery of Trauma practice management guideline could not identify a universal mortality benefit to TXA, but "the safety profile...seems to be favorable when used early after injury (within 3 hours)"; thus, they conditionally recommend TXA in a hospital setting [21]. After publication of the practice management guideline, a multicenter, retrospective study was performed, powered sufficiently, and demonstrated no increased risk of VTE, MI, or CVA and is associated with lower mortality and transfusion need [29]. Prehospital TXA trials are pending, but a meta-analysis seconds that prehospital TXA administration also significantly reduces mortality without an increased risk of VTE [21, 30].

Initially, the use of recombinant factor VIIa, a procoagulant used in hemophilia, appeared promising for coagulopathic blunt trauma patients, reducing the number of transfusions and the need for massive transfusion [31]. Unfortunately, it did not affect mortality or reach statistical significance for penetrating trauma [31]. Subsequently, its safety was questioned when data demonstrated an increased risk of thromboembolic events [32]. The CONTROL trial, a prospective, randomized, double-blinded, multicenter study attempting to determine the efficacy and safety of Factor VIIa, was terminated early when it did not demonstrate mortality benefit with questionable enrollment [33]. Ultimately, future studies should be directed at answering these questions [21]. In the interim, factor VIIa is reserved for patients in extremis, usually undergoing massive transfusion, with 200 micrograms/kg given at hour 0 and 100 micrograms/kg at post-injury hours 1 and 3. Again, it has not demonstrated a mortality benefit, and, if given early, may decrease the need for massive transfusion, but the safety particularly with regard to VTE rates is unknown [21].

There is no single resuscitative endpoint. Clinically, urine output may be measured, stabilization in vital signs with titration of pressors off, and improvement in laboratory values are indicative end organ perfusion is being achieved. The characteristic of the output from the temporary vacuum dressing and the amounts from the drains and tubes should be monitored. Ultrasound can help guide resuscitation, as the intravascular volume can be based on inferior vena cava (IVC) collapsibility and cardiac contraction. Correction of the coagulopathy, hypothermia, and acidosis are guidance parameters.

Another important role of the ICU provider is to perform a thorough tertiary survey, including physical examination and review of the data to ensure that no injuries or wounds have been missed. Once resuscitation endpoints are met, ideally within 24–36 h, the patient is returned to the operating room for a second look, or Part 3—definitive repair. If at any point during Part 2 the acidosis or coagulopathy is not correcting or was trending in the correct direction, but then regresses, or if there is clinical evidence of ongoing, rapid hemorrhage, the patient should be immediately returned to the operating room as this is indicative of a missed injury or ongoing, uncontrolled bleeding.

Finally, complications of resuscitation can arise. Acute respiratory distress syndrome (ARDS) and transfusion-related acute lung injury (TRALI) can result from aggressive resuscitation and blood product administration. One should, however, consider other differential causes for persistent hypoxemia, i.e., abdominal compartment syndrome. In the event of persistent hypoxemia, lung protective strategies such as ARDS Net ventilation should be implemented.

Compartment syndrome may develop in the abdomen even with a temporary dressing in place. It should be suspected if the cardiac return is low, the IVC is collapsed on ultrasound, the urine output decreases when previously appropriate, or in the event of persistent hypoxia or hypercarbia. Bladder pressures should be measured frequently. If pressures remain high, the dressing may need to be modified, loosened, or reapplied.

For extremities, a Stryker needle can be used to objectively quantify the pressure; rapid, significant increases in compartment pressures, a measured compartment pressure >30 mmHg, or <30 mmHg difference in the diastolic blood pressure and measured compartment pressure should prompt fasciotomies. Ultimately, compartment syndrome both in the abdomen and extremities is a clinical diagnosis.

Damage Control Part 3: Definitive Repair

Once the patient is resuscitated as defined by meeting end organ and hemodynamic endpoints, the patient is returned to the operating room for definitive repair. The temporary dressing and all packs are removed. The cavity should be thoroughly explored. If at any point the patient becomes hemodynamically unstable or physiologically deranged as in Part 1, begins re-bleeding, or demonstrates they are unable to undergo a lengthy operation, the temporary dressing may be reapplied, and the patient returned to the ICU for further resuscitation. Definitive repair entails restoring bowel continuity, tissue debridement, and vascular grafts and anastomoses. Prior to closing the abdomen, an X-ray should be obtained and confirmed with radiology that no foreign bodies remain in the cavity. If multiple cavities are left open in Part 1, all cavities may be closed in Part 3 or only one, and Part 3 is repeated for each cavity.

Damage Control Strategy Under Special Circumstances

The following represents specific treatment strategies for unique conditions. The ultimate goal of each strategy is to implement the damage control concept early in care, combat the lethal triad, and transport victims safely to the hospital setting where definitive management can be provided.

Blast Injuries

Blast injuries are challenging as patients can suffer from both penetrating and blunt mechanisms. Treatment goals remain the same, and ABCs initially assessed. The provider should not become distracted by the often unsightly injury but rather focus on treatment according to protocol and standard practice. The airway is managed in the same manner, with oxygen supplementation and intubation if needed. Cricothyroidotomy may be necessary with a blast to the face. Breathing, circulation, and IV or IO access are addressed per ATLS recommendations. Damage control with the blast-injured patients is done in large part by controlling hemorrhage. Hemorrhage sites are either anatomically compressible (e.g., extremity or axillary/groin vascular injuries) or completely non-compressible (e.g., truncal injuries). Patients with non-compressible hemorrhage sources receive the highest priority for immediate transport to a hospital, as there are few tools available to prehospital care providers to manage such bleeding. Compressible hemorrhage sites are amenable to direct digital pressure or tourniquet control, which can be instituted by first responders. Control of bleeding with proximal arterial compression is not advised as it does not address venous hemorrhage. Using large stacks of gauze or additional dressings in lieu of manual compression should be avoided, as this technique dissipates the pressure applied directly to the bleeding site and may delay identification of ongoing bleeding [34].

While the use of tourniquets has been controversial in the damage control situation, multiple reports in the literature on tourniquet use have defined their advantages [37–42]. These include improved hemorrhage control upon patient arrival, decreased incidence of shock in those casualties treated with tourniquets, improved survival, and acceptably low tourniquet-related complications. Tourniquets should be applied to exsanguinating extremities as soon as possible in damage control situations. It is generally recommended that restoration of arterial blood supply must be completed within 6 h from placement of the tourniquet [34]. Prior to patient arrival, it is helpful for the emergency department personnel to know if a tourniquet was placed and when, the characteristic of bleeding (dark non-pulsatile versus bright red, pulsatile), and a description of the injuries. When giving report at patient arrival, the transport team should include the time of injury and the approximate amount of blood loss at the scene. If the patient's bleeding is controlled upon arrival, the primary and secondary surveys should be rapidly conducted in the usual fashion, and the four remaining cavities assessed for hemorrhage with the adjuncts as described above. Given the potential injuries to extremities, these patients may benefit from central venous access placed in the resuscitation bay or immediately upon arrival to the operating room.

Blast injuries can create penetrating wounds from shrapnel but can strike a patient with great force, causing blunt injuries such as intraabdominal hemorrhage and contamination concurrently. Military personnel frequently encounter dismounted complex blast injury (DCBI), an explosion to a foot patrol troop with a specific pattern of injury—traumatic amputation of at least one leg, severe injury to another extremity, and pelvic, abdominal, or urogenital injuries due to an improvised explosive device (IED) and land mines [35]. This is the ideal situation for damage control. Prior to proceeding to the operating room, the staff should be told to obtain a sterile pneumatic tourniquet and prepare for abdominal and extremity exploration and temporary dressings. If extremity hemorrhage is controlled with a tourniquet and the patient's FAST is positive, and if two teams are available, both the extremity and abdomen may be explored concurrently. If only one operative team is available, they should begin with abdominal exploration if the extremity hemorrhage is controlled with a tourniquet. All exsanguination must be expeditiously stopped [36].

Traumatic amputations should be completed or revised as distal as possible with vessels ligated. External fixation should be placed on the pelvis and long bones to prevent ongoing hemorrhage as well as pain control. Soft tissue damage is associated with many blast injuries; frank necrosis should be debrided, and contamination burden decreased through irrigation and debridement at the initial operation. Soft tissue damage evolves and the goal should be to preserve as much healthy tissue for reconstruction so if tissue is questionable and not contaminated, do not debride it [36]. Should blood supply to an extremity be compromised for greater than 4–6 h, or if there is already concern for compartment syndrome, fasciotomies should be undertaken in Part 1. If fasciotomies are not performed, it should be relayed to the ICU team to clinically assess the compartments hourly.

Burns

Many providers hesitate to treat burn patients as they are not comfortable and confident. The same ATLS principles apply. Burn patients, too, can suffer from multiple mechanisms as an explosion may cause a burn, produce shrapnel and penetrating injuries, and throw the patient back, causing a blunt mechanism. As with any other trauma patient, the standard primary and secondary survey should be followed to identify life-threatening injuries.

Burn care commences at the scene. As in all circumstances, personal protection is paramount. The provider must ensure that the scene is safe and the care team is not in harm's way. Personal protection equipment should be applied. After self, the first priority is to stop the burning process and remove the patient from the source [43]. Patients should be immediately placed on 100% O_2 as the adequacy of the airway is evaluated. The provider should pay particular attention to signs of impending airway edema or collapse, such as hoarseness. Patients will often have singed nasal and facial hair or eyebrows. While these findings are important to note and represent a significant injury to the face, they are not specific for airway compromise. Hoarseness, on the other hand, is representative of vocal cord injury or edema and should prompt rapid intubation in the setting of a significant mechanism.

After an airway is established, it is important to check the adequacy of ventilation by watching the chest rise and fall. Patients may have circumferential third-degree burns, which ultimately limit the expansion of the chest. In some circumstances and under the direction of a physician, sharp release of the constricting skin may be necessary to allow for adequate chest expansion [43].

The American Burn Association (ABA) recommends that if prehospital personnel are unable to establish IV access, hospital transport should not be delayed. IV access ideally should be through unburned skin. IO access should be considered to expedite the timeliness of resuscitation and transport. In the adult, heart rates can range from 100 to 120 due to catecholamines; higher than 120 may indicate hypovolemia. Lactated Ringer's is preferred (or an isotonic crystalloid equivalent) and should be run at 500 cc/h. in patients over the age of 14, at 250 cc/h. for patients between the ages of 6 and 14, and at 125/h. if the patient is 5 years or younger [43, 44]. IVs must be frequently assessed because aggressive resuscitation can lead to rapid edema, IV dislodgement, and subsequent subcutaneous infiltration.

The patient should be completely exposed and all jewelry, watches, rings, belts, and diapers removed. Remove contact lenses. A clean, dry dressing, such as a sterile sheet, should be applied. The patient should be wrapped in warm blankets to prevent heat loss. The trauma resuscitation area should be warmed above 80 degrees Fahrenheit. No attempt should be made to cool the patient to counter the burning process; this may be a potentially lethal intervention. Patients have lost the barrier needed for thermoregulation, and despite the appearance of burned skin, patients are often hypothermic [43, 44].

Burn patients at the extremes of age, with significant, multiple co-morbidities, with obvious >10% second and third-degree burns or inhalational injury or burns to sensitive areas such as the face, hands, feet, or genitalia should be directly transported to a burn center if possible. All others may be taken to the closest trauma center. Again, communication between the care components and damage control parts is imperative. A good report from the transport crew includes if the burn occurred in a closed space (potential inhalation injury), if an explosion occurred (multiple mechanisms), if the patient experienced a loss of consciousness (carbon monoxide poisoning or anoxic brain injury), and most importantly, the time of the injury to calculate resuscitation recommendations. The airway and face should be described as intubation may need to be undertaken rapidly and may be extremely difficult due to edema. Knowledge prior to the patient's arrival allows for extra supplies to be gathered, including a tracheostomy tray and a wide range of endotracheal tube sizes, extra clean sheets, and warming of the room. A Rule of Nines figure (used to calculate burned body surface area) should be posted in the emergency department and reviewed prior to patient arrival. Documentation in the patient's chart should be completed as precisely as possible.

Resuscitation in burn patients is based primarily on urine output (0.5 cc/kg/h. in adults, 1 cc/kg/h. in children <30 kg), so an indwelling bladder catheter is needed early. The Parkland formula—2 cc/kg/percentage of second and third-degree burns of Lactated Ringer's with half given in the first 8 h from the time of injury and the remaining in the following 16 h—is a guideline of how to initiate resuscitation and may be adjusted to achieve urine output goals. It should be noted this is only a guide and often overestimates fluid requirements. Early communication with the burn center is imperative as they may adjust resuscitation and recommend tetanus administration. It is imperative that all team members monitor end organ perfusion, recognize resuscitation goals, and communicate about changes needed to achieve those goals.

If a burn patient is found to have a concomitant life-threatening injury such as intra-abdominal hemorrhage, the patient should be taken to the operating room and explored and undergo the damage control sequence as any other trauma patient would prior to transportation to the burn center. The patient can be transferred with an open abdomen, a temporary abdominal dressing in place, and still needing a definitive operation. Resuscitation goals must be clarified with anesthesia because these patients require a significant amount of fluid and often leave the operating room under-resuscitated.

Burn injuries are discussed further in Chap. 55.

Head Injury

Traumatic brain injury (TBI) continues to lead trauma statistics with high mortality rates and long-term disabling outcomes [45, 46]. Primary injury occurs at the time of the traumatic event; however, secondary injury, whether progression of the disease process or iatrogenic, can be minimized. By preventing or recognizing the sequelae of the primary injury and avoiding clinical situations that worsen the secondary injury, providers have a unique opportunity to impact outcomes. As always, no interventions should delay transfer to a neurotrauma center. While the Brain Trauma Foundation (BTF) guidelines [47]. support advanced life support as opposed to basic life support transport, no data support this statement. Ultimately, transport should be efficient and uphold the two main principles of the BTF guidelines: preventing hypoxia (SpO2 < 90%) and hypotension (SBP < 90 mmHg). Both oxygenation and blood pressure should be managed continuously or as frequently as possible with the most accurate equipment available. A large prospective database has demonstrated that a single episode of hypotension or hypoxemia, the strongest independent predictors of outcome, can double mortality and increase morbidity [48–51].

Management of the prehospital airway in a TBI patient is controversial and is dependent on the initial assessment of the patient. If the patient is being transported by ground in an urban environment and able to maintain SpO2 > 90% with only supplemental oxygen, data suggest that intubation with paralytics demonstrates equivocal or even worse outcomes [52–54]. Unfortunately, much of the remaining data on intubation and paralytics are observational, retrospective, and controversial leading to no best practice guidelines [55]. Risks of intubation include esophageal intubation with failure of recognition, aspiration, delay in transport, and may place personnel who do not frequently intubate in a high-stress situation, potentially worsening patient outcome. Hypotension with induction medications and respiratory arrest should intubation fail are the downfalls of prehospital rapid sequence intubation (RSI).

These risks should not deter intubation in a severely injured TBI patient (GCS <9) as on-scene intubation may improve outcomes in the sicker patient [56, 57]. Should the patient require intubation, the responder with the most experience should intubate and use RSI if needed [58]. Historically, ketamine has not been used in TBI patients as it was thought to elevate ICPs. However, recent data suggest it may be a viable option to etomidate, which causes vasodilatory effects leading to hypotension [59]. Successful intubation should be confirmed with both clinical exam and end-tidal carbon dioxide (CO_2) detection.

Traditionally, TBI patients would be hyperventilated to a partial pressure of carbon dioxide ($PaCO_2$) <30 mmHg, inducing vasoconstriction. We now know that maintaining a normal $PaCO_2$ of 35–40 mmHg improves outcomes. Only in the setting of acute neurological change or impending herniation with signs such as unequal or fixed and dilated pupils, extensor posturing, or a decrease in Glasgow Coma Scale (GCS) >2 points should hyperventilation briefly be undertaken with a goal of $PaCO_2$ of 30–35 mmHg. Continuous end-tidal CO_2 monitoring is recommended in the prehospital setting, although still not widely available. If not available, generally 20 breaths per minute for an adult or 25 breaths for a child will achieve these goals.

Ideally, a Glasgow Coma Score (GCS) should be determined prior to administering sedatives or paralytics to the patient. While airway, breathing, and circulation should be addressed prior to determining GCS, an experienced provider can assign a GCS rapidly while multi-tasking. Pupil exam should also quickly be performed, noting orbital trauma, asymmetry (>1 mm difference in diameter), or fixed pupils (<1 mm change with bright light). Resuscitation should be undertaken utilizing isotonic fluids. In a patient with a GCS <8 or with signs of impending herniation, hypertonic saline may be given. Other maneuvers that can be beneficial in the treatment of TBI patients include minimizing noise and light stimulation, elevating the head of the bed/stretcher using reverse Trendelenburg, and loosening a constricting cervical collar (C-collar) to encourage venous drainage.

The CRASH-3 trial evaluated mortality of patients with TBI who were given TXA. In patients presenting with GCS 3 or bilateral unreactive pupils, no mortality difference was found; however, in patients with mild to moderate TBI (GCS 9–15), mortality was significantly less in the group that received TXA. CRASH-3 further demonstrated that early treatment (first 3 h after injury) is superior to later treatment in the mild to moderate TBI group. Again, there was no increased risk of vascular occlusive events or increased rate of seizures in the TXA group [60]. Ultimately, outcomes following TBI are dependent on rapid transport to a neurotrauma facility with CT scanning capability, intracranial pressure (ICP) monitoring and treatment, and available neurosurgical care.

Risk versus benefit must be weighed in patients with concomitant injuries such as multiple penetrating injuries or a combined blunt mechanism with traumatic brain injury. The same primary and secondary survey with adjuncts to determine cavity involvement should proceed rapidly. Any indication, such as a single episode of hypotension, a bleeding wound, or a positive FAST, should prompt rapid transport to the operating room for exploration and damage control initiation prior to imaging. The neurosurgical team should be notified as soon as possible as this is an indication for intracranial pressure monitoring at a minimum. The monitor may be placed intra-operatively at the same time the abdomen is being explored. The goals of avoiding hypoxia and hypotension must be communicated to all involved in the care across the realms of the damage control sequence. If the patient is hemodynamically unstable following exploration with control of hemorrhage, other causes of shock should be explored while in the operating room. Instability due to TBI should be a diagnosis of exclusion. If no other interventions are to be undertaken in the OR, Part 2 of damage control with rapid transport to the ICU and aggressive resuscitation should begin given the instability; an unstable patient should never be taken to imaging. If stable following exploration, CT scans may be performed next, which may prompt return to the operating room if further neurosurgical intervention is warranted or to the ICU depending on patient stability and radiologic findings. Ultimately, hemorrhage control trumps imaging, but not intracranial pressure monitoring, which can be placed concurrently and requires communication with neurosurgical consultants.

Further discussion on the treatment of traumatic brain injury can be found in Chap. 43.

Crush Injury

Crush syndrome is greatly underappreciated in trauma care. Specific compartments or the entire body may be crushed. It is the second most common cause of death after an earthquake, following asphyxia [61]. Much of the literature is a result of worldwide learning experiences following mass casualties such as earthquakes. However, many prehospital and hospital personnel are not aware of specific interventions that can affect outcomes.

When approaching a victim of a crush injury, medical personnel should ensure their own safety first. If multiple victims are involved, medical attention should be directed to patients already freed, allowing rescue providers to extricate additional victims. First-line providers should be familiar with basic life support measures and ATLS principles. If the patient can be reached without endangering the medical provider or hindering rescue efforts, ideally, they should be assessed prior to extrication coupled with frequent re-assessment. Rescue deaths are patients that appear stable prior to extrication, but rapidly deteriorate following extrication thought to be due to reperfusion and systemic dissemination. Attention should first be directed at establishing large-bore intravenous access. Any limb may be utilized, IO access if no IV can be established, and even subcutaneous infusion at 1 cc/min if absolutely no other options exist is an option. Isotonic crystalloids should be used; Lactated Ringer's is preferable in an acidemic patient but even the minimal potassium in Lactated

Ringer's can contribute to life-threatening hyperkalemia; usually normal saline is more readily available [62]. Dextrose 5% may be added to either normal saline or Lactated Ringer's as it supplies calories and can mitigate hyperkalemia [63]. While trapped, adults should be given 1 L/h; children 15–20 cc/kg/h. If extrication takes longer than 2 h, fluids should be reduced to 0.5 L/h. The elderly, children, and patients with congestive heart failure and chronic kidney disease require less fluid. Other patient factors that may need more fluid include higher body mass indices, severely injured patients, delayed extrication, and higher fluid losses due to bleeding or hot weather. The goals of fluid resuscitation are intravascular resuscitation and to dilute nephrotoxic myoglobin and enhance its clearance [62].

On-scene amputation should not be performed to prevent crush injury—only to free a patient in a threatening situation such as impending structural collapse. A tourniquet may be placed just proximal to the amputation site to control bleeding. The most distal guillotine amputation should be performed, and intravenous ketamine may be used.

Communication with rescue personnel must be precise, and extrication must be deliberate, as life-threatening situations (bleeding, airway compromise) can arise. Patients who are trapped in Trendelenburg positions are especially at risk for rapid pulmonary edema and airway compromise. Once extricated, tourniquets may be applied for lethal bleeding, not to prevent the release of metabolites from the crushed tissue, and the usual precautions (spinal, airway, etc.) with rapid transport may commence. Hyperkalemia precipitating dysrhythmias often develop <1 h after extrication [63].

Upon arrival to the trauma facility, assessment should follow the standard approach of primary and secondary exams with imaging and laboratory adjuncts. Any life-threatening situations should be addressed immediately. All wounds should be considered dirty with antibiotics and tetanus administered appropriately. Hypothermia should be avoided or corrected.

Consequences of crush syndrome include rhabdomyolysis, acute kidney injury (AKI), hyperkalemia, and compartment syndrome. Routine labs, specifically including basic metabolic function (BMP), lactic acid (LA), creatinine kinase (CK), and urine pH, should be checked frequently, usually every 4–6 h. A CK >5000 is an independent risk factor for acute kidney injury in traumatically injured patients, but unfortunately, CK levels in isolation are a poor prognostic indicator [62, 64]. Hence, an indwelling bladder catheter should be placed to accurately measure urine output (UOP). Urine output for adults should be a minimum of 50 cc/h, ideally 100 cc/h. Isotonic crystalloids are the preferred resuscitative fluid, and there are no data to support alkalinization of the urine with a bicarbonate drip or administration of Mannitol to prevent AKI, need for renal replacement therapy, or improvement in mortality [62]. Mannitol should not be used in anuric or hypotensive patients, but may have a role as a free radical scavenger and in decreasing compartment pressures. If given, assess the response to a small (25–50 grams) dose; maximum benefit is achieved in about 40 min. Blood products should only be used to correct a coagulopathy or treat a symptomatic hemoglobin <7 g/dL. Hyperkalemia is treated in the usual fashion, administering calcium to stabilize cardiac cell membranes. EKGs should be frequently utilized. Emergent dialysis may be necessary. Improved mortality has been demonstrated in trauma patients when dialysis has been started prior to a BUN >60 mg/dL [65]. Absolute indications for dialysis in the setting of crush injury include: serum potassium ≥6.5 mmol/L or rapidly rising not responsive to other measures; refractory acidosis (serum pH ≤7.1); serum blood urea nitrogen (BUN) ≥100 mg/dL (30 mmol/L); serum creatinine ≥8 mg/dL (700 μmol/L); uremia with volume overload, pericarditis, bleeding diastasis, or unexplained altered mental status; oliguria or anuria despite adequate fluid resuscitation [63]. Loop diuretics [63] and low-dose renal dopamine have demonstrated no benefit. Nephrotoxic agents, hypotension, bleeding, and anemia should all be avoided in the oliguric phase.

Surgical treatment of crush injury includes fasciotomies and amputations. Fasciotomies can result in infection, increasing the risk of amputation, serous drainage and bleeding, and sensory and motor loss. Measurement of compartment pressures (>30 mmHg or <30 mmHg difference between the compartment and diastolic pressure) is the only objective indication for a fasciotomy. Subjectively fasciotomies may be performed if pain is out of proportion on exam or with passive flexion, loss of pulses, paresthesias, or if debridement of necrotic tissue is needed. If there is an underlying fracture, performing a fasciotomy converts this to an open fracture, and orthopedic consultation may be indicated prior to performing the fasciotomy as it may alter the incision and definitive repair of the fracture. Delaying fasciotomies can lead to muscle loss and permanent sensory and motor deficits. If the indication for fasciotomies is soft and Mannitol is given to reduce compartment pressures, surgical planning should begin and commence if no response within 1 h of administration of Mannitol.

Amputations are performed in extremis situations—overwhelming rhabdomyolysis, myoglobin release, hyperkalemia, sepsis, or impending death. They should not be performed to prevent crush syndrome and the sequelae. If guillotine amputation is to be undertaken, it should be performed as soon as the above is recognized and often at the bedside due to patient instability. If the patient is too unstable, a tourniquet can be placed and the extremity iced for a physiological amputation. Elective amputations, also guillotine, may be performed if a combination of major nerve, vascular, bone, or soft tissue trauma is present, usually rendering the extremity non-functional.

Conclusions

Damage control was first described as a surgical concept in an attempt to intercede prior to a patient reaching physiological exhaustion. This concept has since evolved into a resuscitative strategy from the time of injury until definitive surgical repair. Of utmost importance to employing damage control as a concept is team collaboration that ensures efficient flow and care of the severely injured patient. It is essential to adhere to the damage control concept, especially during special situations such as blast, burn, and crush injuries where the soft tissue destruction may distract from the life-threatening injuries.

Key Notes

- Damage control surgery is the concept of staging interventions with early implementation to provide the best opportunity of salvaging a critically ill trauma patient.
- Effective communication is the cornerstone of providing a seamless transition from the scene to the emergency department, control of bleeding and contamination in Part 1, resuscitation in Part 2, to achieving definitive repair in Part 3.
- Special circumstances such as burns, blast injuries, and traumatic brain injuries are evaluated in the same methodical manner, recognizing multiple cavities and life-threatening injuries can be present concurrently.
- Burns require aggressive resuscitation. The goal in traumatic brain injury treatment is to avoid secondary injury by preventing hypoxia and hypotension.

References

1. Cinat ME, Wallace WC, Nastanski F, West J, Sloan S, Ocariz J, et al. Improved survival following massive transfusion in patients who have undergone trauma. Arch Surg. 1999;134:964–70.
2. Krishna G, Sleigh JW, Rahman H. Physiological predictors of death in exsanguinating trauma patients undergoing conventional trauma surgery. Aust N Z J Surg. 1998;68:826–29.
3. Stone HH, Strom PR, Mullins RJ. Management of the major coagulopathy with onset during laparotomy. Ann Surg. 1983;197: 532–35.
4. Rotondo MF, Schwab CW, McGonigal MD, Phillips GR 3rd, Fruchterman TM, Kauder DR, et al. "Damage Control": an approach for improved survival in exsanguinating penetrating abdominal injury. J Trauma. 1993;35:375–82.
5. Johnson JW, Gracias VH, Schwab CW, Reilly PM, Kauder DR, Shapiro MB, et al. Evolution in damage control for exsanguinations penetrating abdominal trauma. J Trauma. 2001;51:261–69.
6. Hoey BA, Schwab CW. Damage control surgery. Scand J Surg. 2002;91:92–103.
7. Porter JM, Ivatury RR, Nassoura ZE. Extending the horizons of "Damage Control" in unstable trauma patients beyond the abdomen and gastrointestinal tract. J Trauma. 1997;42:559–61.
8. Pape HC, Giannoudis P, Krettek C. The timing of fracture treatment in polytrauma patients: relevance of damage control orthopedic surgery. Am J Surg. 2002;183:622–29.
9. Sebesta J. Special Lessons Learned from Iraq. Surg Clin N Am. 2006;86:711–26.
10. Holcomb JB, Helling TS, Hirschberg A. Military, Civilian, and rural application of the damage control philosophy. Military Medicine. 2001;166:490–93.
11. Eiseman B, Moore EE, Meldrum DR, Raeburn C. Feasibility of damage control surgery in the management of military combat casualties. Arch Surg. 2000;135:1323–27.
12. Kairinos N, Hayes PM, Nicol AJ, Kahn D. Avoiding futile damage control laparotomy. Injury, Int. J. Care Injured. 2010;31:64–8.
13. Roberts DJ, Bobrovitz N, Zygun DA, Kirkpatrick AW, Ball CG, Fair, PD, et al. Evidence for use of damage control surgery and damage control interventions in civilian trauma patients: a systematic review. World J of Emergency Surgery. 2021;16:10.
14. Fort AC, Zack-Guasp. Anesthesia for Patients with Extensive Trauma. Aneshtesiology Clin. 2020;38:135–48.
15. Teixeria PGR, Brown CVR, Emigh B, Long M, Foreman M, Eastridge B, et al. Civilian Prehospital Tourniquet Use Is Associated with Improved Survival in Patients with Peripheral Vascular Injury. J Am Coll Surg. May 2018;226(5):769–761.e1.
16. Holcomb JB. Damage Control Resuscitation. J Trauma. 2007; 62:S36–S37.
17. Pusateri AE, Moore EE, Moore HB, Le TD, Guyetter FX, Chapman MP, et al. Association of Prehospital Plasma Transfusion With Survival in Trauma Patients With Hemorrhagic Shock When Transport Times Are Longer Than 20 Minutes: A Post Hoc Analysis of the PAMPer and COMBAT Clinical Trials. JAMA Surg. Feb 1 2020;155(2):3195085.
18. Tignanelli CJ, Vander Kolk WE, Mikhail JN, Delano MJ, Hemmila MR. Noncompliance with American College of Surgeons Committee on Trauma recommended criteria for full trauma team activation is associated with undertriage deaths. J Trauma. 2018; 84(2):287–94.
19. Stannard A, Eliason JL, Rasmussen TE. Resuscitative endovascular balloon occlusion of the aorta (REBOA) as an adjunct for hemorrhagic shock. J Trauma. 2011;71:1869–72.
20. Brenner ML, Teeter W, Hoehn M, Pasley J, Hu P, Yang S, et al. Use of Resuscitative Endovascular Balloon Occlusion of the Aorta for Proximal Aortic Control in Patients With Severe Hemorrhage and Arrest. JAMA Surg. 2018;153(2):130–35.
21. Cannon JW, Khan MA, Raja AS, Cohen MJ, Como JJ, Cotton BA, et al. Damage control resuscitation in patients with severe traumatic hemorrhage: A practice management guideline from the Eastern Association for the Surgery of Trauma. J Trauma. March 2017; 82(3):605–17.
22. Reilly PM, Rotondo MF, Carpenter JP, Sherr SA, Schwab CW. Temporary vascular continuity during damage control: intraluminal shunting of proximal superior mesenteric artery injury. J Trauma. 1995;39:757–60.
23. Rasmussen TE, Clouse WD, Jenkins DH, Peck MA, Eliason JL, Smith DL. The Use of Temporary Vascular Shunts as a Damage Control Adjunct in the Management of Wartime Vascular Injury. J Trauma. 2006;61:8–15.
24. Chambers LW, Green DJ, Sample K, Gillingham BL, Rhee P, Brown C, et al. Tactical Surgical Intervention with Temporary Shunting of Peripheral Vascular Trauma Sustained during Operation Iraqi Freedom: One Unit's Experience. J Trauma. 2006;61:824–30.
25. Starnes BW, Beekley AC, Sebesta JA, Anderson CA, Rush Jr RM. Extremity Vascular Injuries on the Battlefield: Tips for Surgeons Deploying to War. J Trauma. 2006;60:432–42.
26. CRASH-2 trial collaborators, Shakur H, Roberts I, Bautista R, Caballero J, Coats T, et al. Effects of tranexamic acid on death, vascular occlusive events, and blood transfusion in trauma patients with significant haemorrhage (CRASH-2): a randomized, placebo-controlled trial. Lancet. 2010;376:23–32.

27. Morrison JJ, Dubose JJ, Rasmussen TE, Midwinter MJ. Military application of tranexamic acid in trauma emergency resuscitation (MATTERs) study. Arch Surg. 2012;147:113–19.
28. Nishida T, Kinoshita T, Yamakawa K. Tranexamic acid and trauma-induced coagulopathy. J Intensive Care. 2017;5:5.
29. Rivas L, Estroff J, Sparks A, Nahmias J, Allen R, Smith SR, et al. The incidence of venous thromboembolic events in trauma patients after tranexamic acid administration: an EAST multicenter study. Blood Coagul Fibrinolysis. 2021;32:37–43.
30. Almuwallad A, Cole E, Ross J, Perkins Z, Davenport R. The Impact of Pre-Hospital TXA on Mortality among Bleeding Trauma Patients: A Systematic Review and Meta-Analysis. J Trauma. 2021. Publish Ahead of Print. https://doi.org/10.1097/TA.0000000000003120.
31. Boffard KD, Riou B, Warren B, Choong PIT, Rizoli S, Rossaint R, et al. Recombinant Factor VIIa as Adjunctive Therapy for Bleeding Control in Severely Injured Trauma Patients: Two Parallel Randomized, Placebo-Controlled, Double-Blind Clinical Trials. J Trauma. 2005;59:8–18.
32. Levi M, Levy JH, Andersen HF, Truloff D. Safety of Recombinant Activated Factor VII in Randomized Clinical Trials. NEJM. 2010;363:1791–800.
33. Hauser CJ, Boffard K, Dutton R, Bernard GR, Croce MA, Holcomb JB, et al. Results of the CONTROL trial: efficacy and safety of recombinant activated Factor VII in the management of refractory traumatic hemorrhage. J Trauma. 2010;69;489–500.
34. Perkins, J. Beekley A. "Damage Control Resuscitation." 22 Jan 2013. http://www.cs.amedd.army.mil/borden/book/ccc/UCLAchp4.pdf.
35. Dismounted Complex Blast Injury: Report of the Army Dismounted Complex Blast Injury Task Force. 18 June 2011. https://armymedicine.health.mil/-/media/Files/ArmyMedicine/Reports/DCBITaskForceReportRedactedFinal.ashx?la=en&hash=8E5DFE19DF70E9FAC7E046D6E468FFABD713F4A2A9115FCEA102A99CBC103233.
36. Gordon W, Talbot M, Fleming M, Shero J, Potter B, Stockinger Z. High Bilateral Amputations and Dismounted Complex Blast Injury (DCBI). Military Medicine. Sept-Oct 2018;183(2):118–22.
37. Kragh JF Jr, Walters TJ, Baer DG, Fox CJ, Wade CE, Salinas J, et al. Practical use of emergency tourniquets to stop bleeding in major limb trauma. J Trauma. 2008;64:S38–49.
38. Beekley AC, Sebesta JA, Blackbourne LH, Herbert GS, Kauvar DS, Baer DG, et al. Prehospital tourniquet use in Operation Iraqi Freedom: effect on hemorrhage control and outcomes. J Trauma. 2008;64:S28–37.
39. Brodie S, Hodgetts TJ, Ollerton J, McLeod J, Lambert P, Mahoney P, et al. Tourniquet use in combat trauma: UK military experience. J R Army Med Corps. 2007;153:310–13.
40. Kragh JF Jr, Baer DG, Walters TJ. Extended (16-hour) tourniquet application after combat wounds: a case report and review of the current literature. J Orthop Trauma. 2007;21:274–78.
41. Lakstein D, Blumenfeld A, Sokolov T, Lin G, Bssorai R, Lynn M, et al. Tourniquets for hemorrhage control on the battlefield: a 4-year accumulated experience. J Trauma. 2003;54:S221–S225.
42. Mabry RL. Tourniquet use on the battlefield. Mil Med. 2006; 171: 352–56.
43. Herndon, David N. Total Burn Care. Fifth Edition. China: Elservier, Inc. 2017.
44. American Burn Association. Advanced Burn Life Support Course, Provider Manual. Chicago, Il: American Burn Association, 2018.
45. Stein SC, Georgoff P, Meghan S, Mizra K, Sonnad SS. 150 years of treating severe traumatic brain injury: a systematic review of progress in mortality. J Neurotrauma. 2010;27:1343–53.
46. Andriessen TM, Horn J, Franschman G, van der Naalt J, Haitsma I, Jacobs B, et al. Epidemiology, severity classification, and outcome of moderate and severe traumatic brain injury: a prospective multicenter study. J Neurotrauma. 2011;28:2019–31.
47. Brain Trauma Foundation. Guidelines for Prehospital Management of Traumatic Brain Injury, 2nd ed. Prehosp Emerg Care. 2007:12;S1–S52.
48. Chesnut RM, Marshall LF, Klauber MR, Blunt BA, Baldwin N, Eisenberg HM, et al. The role of secondary brain injury in determining outcome from severe head trauma. J Trauma. 1993;34: 216–22.
49. Marmarou A, Anderson RL, Ward JD, et al. Impact of ICP instability and hypotension on outcome in patients with severe head trauma. J Neurosurg. 1991;75:S159–66.
50. Fearnside MR, Cook RJ, McDougall P, McNeil RJ. The Westmead Head Injury Project outcome in severe head injury. A comparative analysis of pre-hospital, clinical, and CT variables. Br J Neurosurg. 1993;7:267–79.
51. Stocchetti N, Furlan A, Volta F. Hypoxemia and arterial hypotension at the accident scene in head injury. J Trauma. 1996;40:764–67.
52. Davis DP, Dunford JV, Ochs M, Park K, Hoyt DB. The use of quantitative end-tidal capnometry to avoid inadvertent severe hyperventilation in patients with head injury after paramedic rapid sequence intubation. J Trauma 2004;56:808–14.
53. Davis DP, Dunford JV, Poste JC, Ochs M, Holbrook T, Fortlage D, et al. The impact of hypoxia and hyperventilation on oucome after paramedic rapid sequence intubation of severely head-injured patients. J Trauma. 2004;57:1–10.
54. Davis DP, Hoyt DB, Ochs M, Fortlage D, Holbrook T, Marshall LK, et al. The effect of paramedic rapid sequence intubation on outcome in patients with severe traumatic brain injury. J Trauma. 2003;54:444–53.
55. Bochicchio GV, Ilahi O, Joshi M, Bochicchio K, Scalea TM. Endotracheal intubation in the field does not improve outcome in trauma patients who present without an acutely lethal traumatic brain injury. J Trauma. 2003;54:307–11.
56. Davis DP, Koprowicz KM, Newgard CD, Daya M, Bulger EM, Stiell I, et al. The relationship between out-of-hospital airway management and outcome among trauma patients with Glasgow Coma Scale Scores of 8 or less. Prehosp Emerg Care. 2011;15:184–92.
57. Bernard SA, Nguyen V, Cameron P, Masci K, Fitzgerald M, Cooper DJ, et al. Prehospital rapid sequence intubation improves functional outcome for patients with severe traumatic brain injury: a randomized controlled trial. Ann Surg 2010;252:959–65.
58. Davis DP, Peay J, Sise MJ, Kennedy F, Simon F, Tominaga G, et al. Prehospital airway and ventilation management : a trauma score and injury severity score-based analysis. J Trauma 2010;69: 294–301.
59. Jabre P, Combes X, Lapostolle F, Dhaouadi M, Ricard-Hibon A, Vivien B, et al. Etomidate versus ketamine for rapid sequence intubation in acutely ill patients: a multicenter randomized controlled trial. Lancet. 2009;374:293–300.
60. The CRASH-3 trial collaborators. Effects of tranexamic acid on death, disability, vascular occlusive events and other morbidities in patients with acute traumatic brain injury (CRASH-3): a randomized, placebo-controlled trial. Lancet. 2019;394(10210):1713–23.
61. Ukai T. The great Hanshin-Awaji earthquake and the problems with emergency medical care. Ren Fail. 1997;19:633–45.
62. Cote DR, Fuentes E, Elsayes AH, Ross JJ, Quraishi SA. A "crush" course on rhabdomyolysis: risk stratification and clinical management update for the perioperative clinician. J Anesthesia. 2020; 34:585–98.
63. Lameire N, Sever MS, Van Biesen W, Vanholder R. Role of the International and National Renal Organizations in Natural Disasters: Strategies for Renal Rescue. Semin Nephrol. 2020; 40:393–407.
64. Brown CV, Rhee P, Chan L, Evans K, Demetriades D, Velmahos GC. Preventing renal failure in patients with rhabdomyolysis: do bicarbonate and mannitol make a difference? J Trauma. 2004;56;1191–96.
65. Gettings LG, Reynolds HN, Scalea T. Outcome in post-traumatic acute renal failure when continuous renal replacement therapy is applied early vs. late. Int Care Med. 1999;25:805–13.

32 Trauma Team Decision-Making

Nada Gawad, Nori L. Bradley, Larissa Roux, and S. Morad Hameed

We choose to go to the moon in this decade ... not because it is easy but because it is hard and because that goal will serve to organize and measure the best of our energies and skills because that challenge is one that we are willing to accept one we are unwilling to postpone and one which we intend to win [1]. (John F. Kennedy, Rice University, 1962)

Introduction: A Well-Planned Journey into the Unknown

Trauma team activations exemplify the potential of health-care systems to synthesize and move beyond individual excellence, to become high reliability organizations. Trauma teams must assemble rapidly and harness multidisciplinary and multimodal resources in acute and extraordinarily complex clinical situations, and under conditions of extreme uncertainty. Successful resuscitation depends on the efficient acquisition and analysis of clinical data, and the rapid formulation of safe and actionable plans. Trauma teams must seamlessly transition from assessment and thoughtful planning to decisive action, which requires tight integration of multidisciplinary efforts, and clear forward communication. Although the flow of trauma resuscitation is based on algorithms and standards, the best trauma teams are adaptive—responding to new information and correcting errors in real time, before those errors reach clinical significance. This chapter starts by introducing the thought processes underlying decisions and the unique challenges posed in trauma. Then, we focus on the critical transitions in acute trauma care and how adherence to the principles of trauma resuscitation can form the foundation of effective decision-making under conditions of uncertainty and inform the coordination of complex teams in the pursuit of critical and time-dependent priorities.

The Anatomy of a Decision

A 32-year-old male who is involved in a high-speed motorcycle crash on a highway outside a major city. He is initially assessed by a local emergency medical services (EMS) crew, and is found to be obtunded and hypotensive, with a deep laceration over his anterior abdominal wall. Resuscitative measures are initiated, and a helicopter team is activated for rapid transport. The patient is transferred by air to a waiting trauma center, where he is initially found to be hemodynamically unstable, with a small amount of fluid on the FAST ultrasound examination and a pelvic fracture. The trauma team must decide what to do next.

A decision is defined as a commitment to a course of action that is intended to yield results that are satisfying for specified individuals [2]. In trauma, the specified individual is first and foremost the patient, and the intended results are to minimize the duration and consequences of shock. Modern decision-making theory is known as the dual process theory, and consists of using a combination of non-analytic (System 1) and analytic (System 2) reasoning to solve complex problems. System 1 thinking is quick and automatic, relying on pattern recognition and stored memories [3]. System 2 thinking is slow and deliberate [3, 4]. Although the two decision-making systems are interdependent, one system may predominate, depending on factors such as time pressures or the experience of the decision-maker [3–5]. For example, an expert trauma team leader (TTL) may skillfully and subconsciously use experiential knowledge stored in long-

N. Gawad
Department of Surgery, University of Ottawa, Ottawa, ON, Canada
e-mail: nada.gawad@mail.utoronto.ca

N. L. Bradley
Department of Surgery, University of Alberta, Edmonton, AB, Canada

L. Roux
T6 Health Systems, Brookline, MA, USA

S. M. Hameed (✉)
Department of Surgery, University of British Columbia, Vancouver, BC, Canada
e-mail: morad.hameed@vch.ca

L. Marshall Gillman, S. Widder (eds.), *Trauma Team Dynamics*, https://doi.org/10.1007/978-3-031-86312-7_32

term memory and rapidly retrieved through System 1 thinking to recognize that the above patient may need to go straight to the operating room without a CT scan [3, 6]. An important pitfall to recognize for novice TTLs and trainees observing apparently spontaneous decisions, however, is that trauma represents one of the most challenging decision-making environments for physicians.

In the absence of experience, novices rely on conceptual knowledge to analytically reason through decisions [4]. Inexperienced, intuitive (System 1) decisions have low accuracy [6]. To improve accuracy, non-experts must slow down their decision-making and allow System 2 thinking to predominate. But time is a luxury that we lack in trauma, thus affecting the quality of decision-making [4, 7]. In addition, most trauma patients present in what is known as *indeterminate zones of practice*, as trauma is laden with uncertainty, may have conflicting values, and is often ill-defined [8]. For example, the etiology of shock may be unclear, there may be multiple forms of shock present, or potential substance use could be clouding the clinical picture of shock. These muddy, indeterminate zones of practice further increase the TTL's cognitive load, decrease situational awareness, and make decision-making more challenging.

While an expert TTL may make seemingly effortless decisions based on instinct, they are actually relying on years of formed experiences to allow them to quickly and accurately recognize patterns (System 1) [3, 4]. The expert TTL has also developed the wisdom to recognize when a patient's unique presentation does not quite fit with known patterns, thus signaling the need to slow down and allow System 2 thinking to predominate [3]. On the other hand, non-experts have limited experience to draw on and thus require more time and use a greater cognitive load to make the same decisions [7]. The time pressures and indeterminate zones of practice of the trauma bay result in decreased accuracy and situational awareness as decisions are made [3, 4]. Trauma is therefore the perfect storm of decision-making. The TTL is at the eye of this storm, analyzing and reanalyzing information, determining a course of action, uniting the team around a common purpose, and lighting the way forward.

Early Data Acquisition: The Primary Survey as a Decision-Making Tool

The handover from EMS is the first key transition point in the trauma resuscitation and can provide critical data on a trauma patient's ultimate disposition. A clear and concise handover is also the launch point for the primary survey and may direct the trauma team to issues requiring special focus and attention to detail.

The primary survey and its adjuncts are designed to provide high-priority and immediately actionable clinical data, particularly regarding the presence or absence of shock and its likely causes [9, 10]. Focused patient assessment and clear reporting of findings by a single designated clinician are at the core of the trauma team response. This communication is a key source of raw data that will guide the team in the major decisions that lie ahead. In some cases, as few as two data points are sufficient to prompt decisive action; for example, the presence of penetrating chest trauma and profound hypotension may trigger a decision to initiate a resuscitative thoracotomy. The primary survey should be concurrently completed and reported within minutes and should be repeated until a clear injury pattern has emerged, key assessments have been completed, critical interventions have been performed, a measure of stability has been attained, and onward disposition has been determined. The adjuncts to the primary survey (Table 32.1), once completed, are important sources of information in the resuscitation effort. Their results should be announced and documented as each becomes available and, where possible, should be prominently displayed.

Table 32.1 Adjuncts to the primary survey as shock resuscitation tools

Adjunct	Application in shock resuscitation
ECG	Blunt cardiac injury, acute versus cardiac disease (e.g., acute coronary syndrome)
Sa02	Peripheral perfusion
BP	Presence of shock
ABG	Base deficit—Presence of shock Lactate—Presence of shock
EtCO2	Tube placement, adequacy of circulation
Gastric	–
Foley	Urine output for severity of shock
CXR	Evaluate sources of hemorrhagic shock
PXR	Evaluate source of hemorrhagic shock
EFAST	Evaluate source of hemorrhagic shock
T	Adjunct treatment in hemorrhagic shock

Abbreviations: *SaO2* arterial saturation, *BP* blood pressure, *ABG* arterial blood gas, *EtCO2* end tidal carbon dioxide, *CXR* chest X-ray, *PXR* pelvic X-ray, *EFAST* extended focused assessment with sonography for trauma

The primary survey and its adjuncts should begin to create a clear picture of a trauma patient's clinical status and should begin to outline and prioritize available courses of action. Each new data point will further support or refute a TTL's hypothesis regarding the nature and severity of shock and will refine the decision-making process.

Weighing the Options

While the emergency department (ED) is an appropriate place for the initial assessment and early resuscitation of trauma patients, it is not a place for definitive diagnosis or treatment, and no strong gains in either area will be made as long as patients are left there. In general, time in the ED should be minimized. However, as soon as a patient is moved from the resuscitation area, he or she will encounter new risks that must be weighed against the benefits of this movement.

For hemodynamically unstable patients, the choice of transfer destination is relatively straightforward. Shock patients who are non-responders or are transient responders to early resuscitative measures should be taken immediately to the operating room (OR). A single hypotensive episode, which reflects over 1500 mL of blood loss, may be enough to determine the presence of hemodynamic instability, although some clinicians will add an assessment of metabolic acidosis (base deficit, lactate) to more definitively confirm the presence of shock before making a commitment to go to the OR [11]. The decision to go to the OR with an unstable patient can occur early on in the course of the resuscitation, often on the basis of only a few data points, and in this case, the remainder of the resuscitative effort is dedicated to getting the patient ready to move, ensuring that key details of the resuscitation are completed (e.g., adjuncts to primary survey, cross match), and preparing the accepting team in the operating room for the next phase of patient care. The transition to the operating room is described in more detail below.

For patients with relative hemodynamic stability, the decision to pursue an operative intervention is not as urgent, and there are more diagnostic and therapeutic options available. It should be remembered, however, that many of these patients, particularly those who have been injured recently, may be in compensated shock and have undetected ongoing bleeding. Any evidence of hemodynamic deterioration should redirect patients to an operative algorithm. Until such deterioration occurs, trauma teams will be faced with the following six options:

1. *Sit tight and wait for a signal*: When a patient's hemodynamic status is unclear, a period of intense watchful waiting in the secure surroundings of the trauma resuscitation area may be warranted. It should be emphasized that this is a period of active observation, with serial determination of vital signs, repetition of the physical examination, and serial determination of the presence of occult shock through the measurement of base deficit and lactate, with special focus on how these parameters respond to initial resuscitation. The primary survey should be iterative, and the results of the adjuncts should be carefully reviewed to determine potential etiologies for shock. During a brief period of watchful waiting, the appropriate transfer destination may become clear—a patient considered to be a transient responder may need to go to the operating room, while a stable patient may be safely transferred to CT for definitive imaging.
2. *Computed tomography*: Taking a trauma patient to CT is a well-known pitfall in trauma care. Trauma teams should always recognize the potential for a patient in (undetected) compensated shock to decompensate in the scanner, where access to the patient can be limited, and resuscitative equipment and personnel less available. However, the speed of modern CT scanners and their geographic location—often steps away from the resuscitation area—have reduced the risk of a trip to CT. There can be multiple advantages of CT, both for blunt trauma as a definitive imaging tool, and penetrating trauma to map trajectory and establish follow-up diagnostic and therapeutic approaches. Still, trauma teams must confirm hemodynamic stability before traveling to CT.

Since CT is a default path for the majority of stable multitrauma patients, and since it is a time-dependent priority in patients with traumatic brain injuries, resuscitative efforts in the primary survey are often directed toward moving the patient efficiently from the trauma bay to CT. The TTL should remain vigilant and immediately address lulls in the progress of this transfer. If there is any concern about the need for operative intervention after CT scan, the OR and relevant surgical services (e.g., neurosurgery) should be informed and on standby so that a time-consuming transfer back to the ED can be avoided.

3. *Angiography*: The role of angiography in unstable patients is limited to very few clinical scenarios. Some groups of investigators have advocated for the use of angiography for the control of hemorrhage in patients with solid organ and pelvic injuries whose hemodynamics can be maintained with active resuscitation (transient responders) [12, 13]. However, extreme caution must be exercised when contemplating such a move, and the full spectrum of resuscitative capabilities and personnel should be transferred to the angiography suite along with the patient. Resuscitation can be difficult under these circumstances, with a sterile field and radiography limiting access to the patient, and without the usual equipment available for resuscitative procedures. Furthermore, since most hemorrhagic injuries of the liver and pelvis are venous, angiography may be of limited utility in many of these injuries. That said, if no surgically accessible injuries are identified in the primary survey, and a patient's hemodynamic stability can be maintained with a carefully controlled resuscitation, the risks of angiography may be justifiable. In general, angiography usually follows CT, where contrast extravasation in the arterial phase pinpoints specific areas of active arterial hemorrhage, and CT rules out the immediate need for operative intervention [14]. For patients with suspected pelvic fractures and bladder injuries, pelvic angiography should be completed before retrograde urethrograms or cystograms to ensure vascular contrast extravasation in the pelvis can be detected.

4. *Operating room*: The operating room is an ideal destination for patients in shock. With dedicated surgeons, anesthesiologists, and nurses present, and a full spectrum of resuscitative options and equipment available, resuscitation can be intensified and titrated against continuous hemodynamic monitoring. With better lighting, sterile technique, and equipment, procedures such as chest tube and line placement, exploration of wounds, and completion of resuscitative thoracotomy can be done more safely and more precisely. However, for unstable patients, a partially unmonitored move to an incompletely prepared operating theater can be hazardous. Transfer to the operating theater is a critical transition (Fig. 32.1), whose benefits can be maximized by careful mitigation of risks. Some trauma centers have full operating theater capabilities in the resuscitation area, allowing the resuscitation to blend seamlessly with definitive surgery for damage control. Locating surgical capabilities in the resuscitation area has been associated with better outcomes for some of the most unstable patients [15]. When such capabilities are not available, it may still be possible to create a smooth transition between the trauma bay and the operating room. The OR should be part of the trauma activation call out and OR personnel, including anesthesia and nursing, should begin to arrange operative capacity for a potential imminent transfer. The TTL and the OR should be in close communication throughout the resuscitation, and the decision to transfer to the OR and the anticipated resource and equipment needs should be specified as early as possible (Fig. 32.2). Some operating theaters have pre-specified trauma laparotomy trays, complete with vascular and thoracic instruments, along with appropriate retractors, and even sternal saws that can be rapidly opened as needed. It is important that the OR setup for trauma is pre-defined, but even if it is, it is useful for the surgeon to conduct a briefing to ensure that the assembled team has a shared mental model of the risks, expected operative strategies, and anticipated equipment needs. Ideally, the trauma patient will arrive from the trauma bay to a fully staffed, warm operating room, with monitoring interfaces and operative instruments set up and ready to go. Even, or perhaps especially, in this operative crisis situation, a preoperative briefing and a time out, as defined by the WHO Safe Surgery Saves Lives Campaign, is essential to set the direction for the case [16]. We have found that a clear and deliberate briefing, summarizing clinical findings and anticipated operative strategies and tactics, should occur just as the trauma team and patient roll into the operating room. The receiving anesthesia and nursing teams, deeply engaged with preparation until that moment, are often very receptive to this moment of situation awareness and opportunity to create a shared mental model of the operative intervention ahead.

   In some cases, a thorough primary survey, including chest and pelvic X-rays and an extended Focused Assessment with Sonography in Trauma (eFAST) ultrasound exam of the chest and abdomen, may not reveal a clear, single cause of hemodynamic instability, and an unstable patient may arrive in the operating room without a clear operative plan. Some operating rooms are equipped with diagnostic modalities and expertise, including transesophageal echocardiography, X-ray, ultrasound,

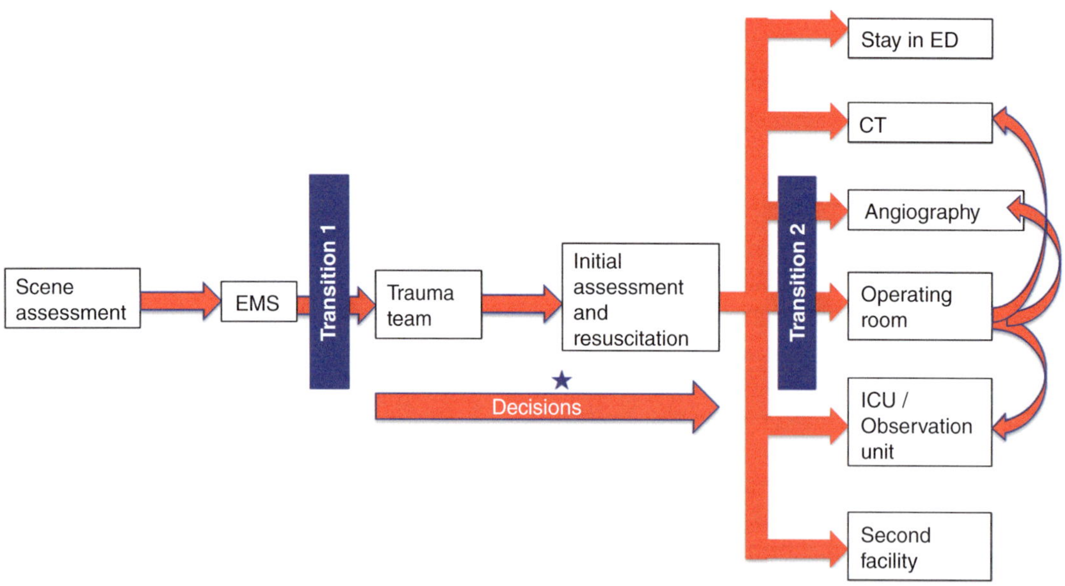

Fig. 32.1 The process of trauma care—key transitions and decision points. Early decisions regarding the need for damage control resuscitation, massive transfusion, and disposition from the trauma bay and (onward) can be made very early in the course of resuscitation

Fig. 32.2 An example of a checklist describing key priorities before transfer from the trauma bay to the operating room

CHECKLIST
preparation for damage control surgery

- Pre operative briefing: case discussed with OR and anesthesia
- Advise blood bank of move to OR
- Thoracic, cardiac and vascular instruments
- Cell saver
- Warm room
- Perfusion technician notified if needed?

interventional radiology, and upper and lower gastrointestinal endoscopy to quickly repeat or intensify the workup of undifferentiated trauma patients. When the source of hemorrhage is difficult to identify (when diagnostic imaging is not directive or not performed), the abdomen is the usual suspect. Investigators at the University of Southern California (USC) observed that exploratory laparotomy was required much more frequently than exploratory thoracotomy (89% versus 1.9%) for unstable patients with thoracoabdominal trauma. They suggested abdominal exploration should be prioritized over thoracic exploration in this instance [17]. The team should, however, be prepared to do both, although this was rarely required in the USC series (2.1%).

Operative interventions in hemodynamically unstable patients should have defined objectives, and clear onward disposition options. Hemodynamic instability is often associated with acidosis, coagulopathy, and hypothermia, which justify a damage control surgical approach that prioritizes early control of hemorrhage and contamination, and abbreviation of operative efforts [18]. Trauma surgeons can decide on this course of action even before a patient's arrival in the operating room, and should know the onward disposition from the operating theater even before a patient arrives there. For example, if a traumatic brain injury was suspected, but a CT head could not be obtained in advance of an urgent exploratory laparotomy, arrangements can be made for immediate postoperative transfer to CT. Alternatively, if a patient with a complex pelvic fracture is taken to the operating room for thoracic or abdominal injuries, the interventional radiologists and angiography suite can be readied in advance for possible direct transfer from the operating room to the angiography suite. Finally, if operative intervention has been successful in controlling hemorrhage, aggressive restoration of homeostasis is best accomplished by rapid, seamless transfer to a briefed and prepared intensive care unit (ICU).

5. *Intensive care unit:* The ICU is almost inevitably the ultimate target for trauma patients with hemodynamic instability. It is here that oxygen delivery, especially within the first few hours after injury, can be promptly and judiciously restored, where hypothermia, acidosis, and coagulopathy can be readily corrected, and where organ injury and organ failure can be supported. The ICU team should be aware of the arrival of critical trauma patients in the ED and should track their progress through the first phases of assessment and treatment. Failure to engage the ICU team early will result in poor appreciation of the pattern and severity of injury, which may lead to delays in achievement of resuscitation targets. In a damage control surgery/resuscitation situation, onward disposition from the ICU is a critical matter as well. Surgical teams may require staged operative approaches to ensure hemostasis, complete repairs, and accomplish abdominal or thoracic closure. In recent years, close collaboration between ICU and trauma teams with respect to fluid balance, and increased dedication to abdominal wall closure have, in some series, led to near universal abdominal closure rates [19]. Surgical teams should be prepared to return their patients to the operating room for definitive repairs the moment physiologic derangements have been normalized, and should return at high frequency until reconstructions are complete. For evidence of persistent hemorrhage, as evidenced by ongoing high transfusion requirements, surgical teams should have a low threshold to return to the operating room, in particular if bleeding continues after the correction of coagulopathy and hypothermia.
6. *Transfer out:* One of the key priorities in the initial assessment of trauma patients is to determine whether definitive care of all of the injuries will be possible at the admitting facility. TTLs should make themselves familiar with local and regional trauma expertise and resources ahead of time and, as soon as the injury pattern is established, determine the need for and the mechanics of transfer to a

Fig. 32.3 An example of a checklist describing key priorities before inter-facility transfer of a critically injured trauma patient

CHECKLIST
preparation for trauma patient transfer

EMS report included

Primary and secondary survey documents completed

Radiology findings documented and images uploaded

Spine precautions for transportation documented

Verbal handover completed. Name of accepting physician:__________

referral facility. Transfers should be initiated early and should occur along pre-established referral pathways in an integrated trauma system, where the capabilities and roles of each hospital are already known and designated. The arrangement of transfers has two logistical challenges: arranging the transport and communicating initial findings to the receiving hospital. Both of these challenges must be addressed early, concurrently with resuscitation, so that once the initial phases of resuscitation have been completed, patients are ready to move in a controlled fashion and without significant delay. A safe and seamless transfer depends on accurate and complete communication between referring and receiving facilities. Often, in the heat of resuscitation, and the push to move patients out, the completion or communication of certain details can be missed [20]. In a survey of trauma personnel in our trauma system, 67% of respondents felt that incomplete communication at the time of trauma patient transfer was a potential source of critical delays in appropriate care and serious adverse events. We also found that inter-facility trauma patient transfer was often characterized by loss of information from the scene and/or the referring hospital. In an already high acuity and indeterminate zone of practice, transfer protocols and checklists may help to ensure completeness of care, documentation, and forward communication, and may therefore make trauma care safer and more seamless (Fig. 32.3).

The Physiology of a Decision

A thorough understanding of physiological principles and the available options for definitive care are the basic prerequisites for effective decision-making in trauma resuscitation. All of the transfer destinations outlined above are legitimate options under the right circumstances, and very often, a combination of destinations must be selected. TTLs and trauma teams must carefully weigh incoming physiologic and anatomic data in order to define the best possible course (and specific sequence) of action. In general, clinical decision-making must merge available patient data with the best available scientific evidence, plotting a course based on unique patient circumstances, efficacy and safety of competing therapies, as well as local care pathways. In trauma, this decision-making process has heightened importance and is greatly accelerated.

TTLs and trauma teams making critical transfer decisions under conditions of extreme uncertainty have several decision support tools at their disposal. While no two trauma patients are identical, these tools apply the best available evidence and thought processes to standardized situations that may help to inform real-world decision-making. We will briefly consider three types of tools: predictive scores, clinical practice guidelines, and decision analysis methods.

Predictive Scores

Predictive scores help to process raw clinical data in order to inform complex decisions. One of the most familiar of these, the Glasgow Coma Scale, merges neurologic findings to give healthcare teams an indication if a trauma patient is alert enough to protect his/her airway and if a definitive airway might be urgently needed. Similarly, the ABC score (penetrating mechanism, blood pressure, heart rate, FAST ultrasound [21]) and the TASH score (sex, blood pressure, heart rate, FAST ultrasound, hemoglobin, base deficit, fractures) [22] combine physiologic and anatomic data to bring evidence and clear rationale to the activation of trauma exsanguination (massive transfusion) protocols.

These scores may focus resuscitation teams on key, predictive variables, thereby facilitating more evidence-based decisions. For example, a male patient with a hemoglobin <9 g/dL (90 g/L), base excess < -6, SBP <100 mmHg, HR <120, and a positive FAST exam has a TASH Score of 17/28, and would be expected to have a 43% chance of requiring a massive transfusion [23]. While this probability on its own may not be compelling enough to prompt activation of a trauma exsanguination protocol, it does bring a constellation of data into an evidence-based decision process.

Clinical Practice Guidelines (CPGs)

CPGs are algorithms [24] for the major possible trauma scenarios and attempt to synthesize the best available evidence and the best available judgment into safe and efficient strategies to advance patient care (Fig. 32.4).

But the decision to transfer a patient out of the trauma bay toward more definitive care is not easily informed by simple or even multivariate scores, and the specific decision points within CPGs still depend on the analysis of data and individual judgment (Fig. 32.4). Data points used to inform the decision arrive in real time, can rapidly change over time, and can be unreliable. The decisions themselves, even if based on perfect data, are complex. While all clinical decisions are made under conditions of uncertainty, decision-making in trauma often occurs under conditions of extreme uncertainty, making judgment and experience big factors in the determination of strategy.

The science of *decision analysis* applies explicit and quantitative methods to analyze decisions made under conditions of uncertainty. Figure 32.5 explores the decision to move a patient from the trauma bay to the CT scanner or to the operating room, a frequent challenge encountered by TTLs. While all the inputs into this decision and the consequences of this decision are difficult to map out in an embedded figure, the exercise of doing so can help decision-makers gain some depth of understanding about the decision-making process. The raw data to calculate the probabilities for the chance nodes of this decision tree already exist in the literature. Decision-making tools in the future may be able to harness the data collection, computing, and analytic power of new information technology tools not only to populate the probabilities but also to modify these probabilities and inform clinical decisions based on accumulating data in real time.

Regardless of what decision-making strategy is used, TTLs must take an active role in the decision-making process to progress the trauma patient through resuscitation and toward definitive management. Even incorrect decisions will provide information that will shape subsequent decisions. Decision-making is a dynamic and iterative process that requires close observation and continuous refinement. For example, if a patient's blood pressure drops as they are being readied for CT and outcome probabilities change, the decision-making process and the team should be agile enough to rapidly re-direct them to a waiting operating room. The team would have been observing the patient intently during the transfer process, watching for new information,

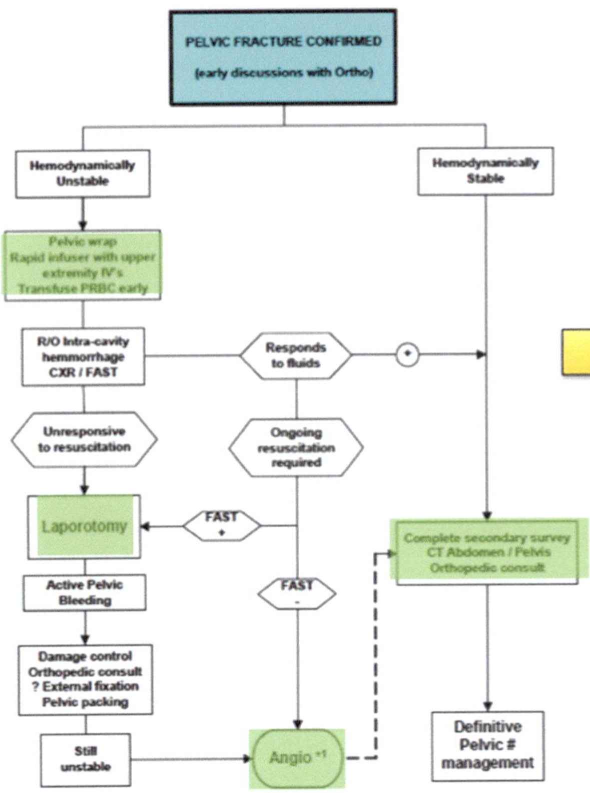

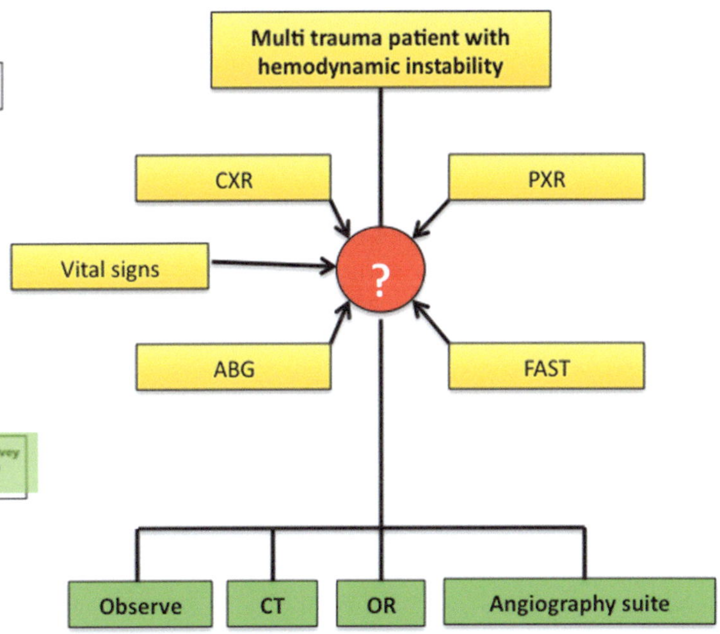

Fig. 32.4 Clinical decision-making under conditions of uncertainty—integration of anatomic data (chest X-ray (CXR), pelvic X-ray (PXR), FAST), and physiologic data on response to resuscitation (arterial blood gas (ABG), vital signs) guides movement down the clinical pathways and to the ultimate destinations (shown in light green)

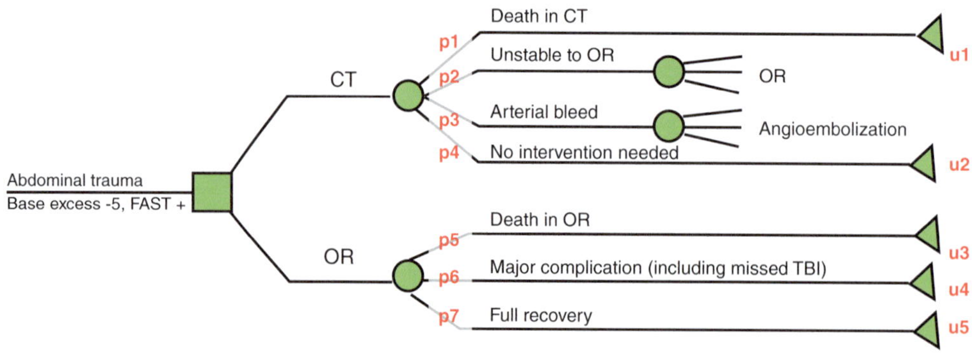

Fig. 32.5 The anatomy of a decision—lessons from decision analysis. This is the age-old decision about whether to take a transiently responsive trauma patient to CT or to the OR. While critical decisions in the trauma bay are often made based on judgment and pattern recognition, every major decision can be broken down into its component elements, and analyzed based on the best available probability and outcomes data. The probabilities "p" will be modified based on emerging physiologic data and will in turn influence the proportion of patients reaching each health utility "u" state. In this example, indicators of shock (base deficit) or active bleeding (FAST exam) may make p1 and p2, and their outcomes prohibitively higher than p5 and p6, supporting a decision to go to the OR. Currently, TTLs weigh these probabilities subconsciously, but information technologies may eventually be able to provide and adjust probabilities in real time, to increase the objectivity of decision-making. Square = decision node, circle = probability node, triangle = outcome node

keeping options open, and modifying the plan accordingly. As long as TTLs and trauma teams are keenly aware of emerging data and the effect of decisions, a wrong decision is better than no decision.

Trauma Team Leadership: Translating Decisions into Action

There are three essential aspects of trauma team leadership: continuously gathering and processing information from an array of sources to create a clear vision about the priorities of care, making decisions based on this information, and inspiring and coordinating the trauma team to enact these decisions. The process of transforming raw data to clear vision and finally to concerted action is examined in Endsley's exploration of the concept of *situation awareness*, which he defines as "the perception of elements in the environment within a volume of time and space, the *comprehension* of their meaning, and the projection of their status in the near future." This process, which involves taking disjointed data elements regarding the status and dynamics of a situation, integrating them into a comprehensive picture, and then predicting and addressing future developments, is a fundamental responsibility of the TTL. To do this well, the TTL must promote an environment of open and clear communication, and must be able to step back from the resuscitation enough to achieve and act on situation awareness [25].

It is helpful for both inexperienced and experienced trauma teams to be aware of all relevant data as these data are collected, and periodic summaries of clinical status can reduce uncertainty and anxiety, and inspire confidence in team leadership considerably. It is also extremely helpful for the team (and the TTL) to communicate the anticipated threats and the rationale for decision-making, even if the decision may subsequently be revised. A decision-making rationale statement may be something like this:

> This is a 32-year-old man involved in a motorcycle crash with transiently responsive hemodynamic instability, possibly due to intra-abdominal hemorrhage or pelvic fracture based on our FAST exam and pelvic X-ray. We have secured his airway and have good IV access, with O negative blood infusing. CT is ready for us. Our priorities are to log roll him, place an orogastric tube and a foley catheter, and prepare him for transfer to CT within the next 5 min. I am still worried about ongoing bleeding, and we should keep an OR on standby.

This statement clarifies the TTL's thinking and priorities and brings the team in on the decision-making process creating a shared mental model (Chaps. 4, 5, 6, 8), thus allowing the team to simultaneously prepare for multiple possible scenarios. Synthesizing gathered information into a plan of action, rather than simply summarizing, is an essential way to prepare a complex resuscitation and multidisciplinary team to transition seamlessly between therapeutic alternatives.

The style of leadership that engages the vision and talents of team members and unifies them behind a singular purpose has been described by Collins in a study of highly successful companies. Collins' research team noted that companies that were able to negotiate adversity to achieve dramatic growth consistently had leaders with a "paradoxical" combination of great personal humility and strong professional will to achieve sustained results. The researchers considered this combination to be at the pinnacle of the hierarchy of leadership attributes, and called it Level 5 leadership. The ability of a trauma team to acquire and share knowledge and to seamlessly deliver complex, integrated, life-saving care may depend on a similar style of open and humble leadership and an unwavering focus on process and goals [26].

Forward Communication and Handover

One of a TTL's essential roles is to pave the way forward for the patient and the team. Forward communication should commence even before a patient's arrival, or very early during a patient's assessment. Vital time is lost, and the duration of shock prolonged, if this role is neglected. Forward communication starts with the automatic alerts of all essential services, including emergency medicine and surgical teams, radiology, lab, blood bank, OR, and ICU. However, as therapeutic priorities become clearer, the TTL must move beyond the automatic alerts to customize the response. This may mean ensuring that the CT scanner is clear and that the radiologists are aware of the studies needed and the suspected injuries. It may include ensuring that an operating room is being prepared and that the anesthesiologist is aware of the status of the resuscitation. It may include letting the interventional radiologist know that the patient may be coming to the angiography suite directly from CT. Besides being the architect of a dynamic plan, the TTL must coordinate seamless transitions in resuscitation and definitive care. As noted, this forward facilitation may save hours of shock and its many downstream complications.

Special Considerations in Mass-Casualty Situations

Mass-casualty situations are discussed in detail elsewhere in this text (Chap. 49). By definition, these events overwhelm the usual processes of emergency trauma and surgical care [27]. However, the essential considerations for transfer to definitive care remain the same. Individual trauma teams designated for each arriving patient must assess their patients and develop specific strategies. The overall TTL, who must remain above the fray of individual trauma resuscitations, will pave the way forward for each team by activating all potential downstream pathways simultaneously, then directing patients forward based on level of acuity and other considerations. A considerable part of the TTL's time will be spent activating pathways and providing forward communication, thereby ensuring that an institution-wide response flows as seamlessly and efficiently as possible. The same principles of identifying the presence of shock and minimizing its duration and making the best decisions possible under dynamic and uncertain considerations still apply, only on a larger scale and with the added layer of decision-making regarding prioritization and resource allocation in the presence of multiple patients.

The Role of Information Technology

The formulation of trauma resuscitation and transfer strategies represents the pinnacle of multimodal patient assessment, decision-making under conditions of uncertainty, and team leadership. A wealth of experience has accumulated in each of these areas, and trauma centers around the world have applied this experience, increasingly combining it with predictive tools and decision-making algorithms, to address shock from complex, multisystem trauma with a prompt, aggressive, high-quality response (Table 32.2). New information technology tools, including artificial intelligence and machine learning algorithms, may have the capacity to optimize the use of data in clinical decision-making, bring tailored trauma response algorithms to the bedside, and enhance communication at the critical periods of transition between the emergency department and definitive care [28, 29].

Table 32.2 Early resuscitation process measures from the American College of Surgeons Trauma Quality Improvement Program

Trauma quality improvement process measures
Measurement of best Glasgow coma scale (GCS)
Time to operating room for hemorrhage control
Time to angiography for hemorrhage control
Transfusion in the first 4 hours (packed red blood cells (pRBCs) and fresh frozen plasma (FFP))

Table 32.3 Features of high-reliability organizations

Sensitivity to operations
Reluctance to simplify
Preoccupation with failure
Deference to expertise
Commitment to resilience

Future Directions: Toward High Reliability Organizing

High reliability organizations (HROs), such as aircraft carriers and nuclear power plants, are those with complex operations that function under extraordinarily high-risk conditions, where errors have potentially catastrophic consequences, and yet almost never experience catastrophic failures [30]. They expect and are preoccupied by failure, but they strive to contain and minimize the consequences of those failures. Studies of HROs reveal some common features (Table 32.3) that together create mindfulness, collective intelligence, and, ultimately, resilience. In healthcare, trauma teams exemplify many defining features of HROs and have evolved with many HRO features. At the core of this evolution has been the recognition that trauma care is complex with high stakes and that successful teams require the engagement of all members to minimize or avoid pitfalls. Similar considerations (shared understanding of expected progress, early recognition of worrisome trends, vigilance against cognitive biases, clear communication in flattened hierarchies, and strong organizational culture) define the emerging concept of rescue. Failure to rescue, defined as the ratio between mortality and total number of complications, is increasingly seen as an important indicator of healthcare performance. As complex adaptive systems and HROs, trauma systems should embrace complexity and risk, but have a strong ability to minimize failure to rescue [31]. As the complexity of trauma resuscitation and the capability of trauma teams increase, trauma systems would benefit from measuring and optimizing their collective intelligence, reliability, and resilience.

Conclusions

Each trauma resuscitation is a coordinated, multidisciplinary effort and a powerful application of healthcare resources in a complex and time-dependent situation. Trauma resuscitation serves "to organize and measure the best of our energies and skills" in healthcare. Decision-making in trauma, incorporating anatomic and physiologic data, integrating technology, and creating culture that is greater than the sum of its parts, represents a rapidly evolving and exciting frontier in healthcare.

Key Points

- Trauma team leadership, decision-making, and organization are based on fundamental physiological principles including prompt reversal of shock and minimization of secondary injuries.
- A picture of trauma patient disposition often develops early as primary survey data accumulate. Early diagnostic imaging adjuncts to the primary survey may also be directive. The trauma team should gear itself toward one of six disposition strategies very early on in order to avoid potentially life-threatening situations and logistical delays: watchful waiting, CT, interventional radiology, operating room, ICU/trauma unit, or transfer to another facility for definitive care.
- Unstable patients are best managed in the operating room.
- Forward planning and forward communication should begin very early in the course of assessment and resuscitation.
- Decision-making under conditions of uncertainty can be guided by careful consideration of risks, benefits, and probabilities of the various possibilities based on emerging information. These decisions are often based on judgment and experience, but may increasingly be informed by predictive analytic tools.
- Trauma team leaders should maintain situation awareness and pursue an open model of leadership that encourages communication, engages team members to maximize their potential, and establishes and pursues a clear and shared purpose. These are key aspects of mindful, high reliability organizations that recognize deviations from expected trajectories and failures and that continuously adapt to mitigate risks.

References

1. Kennedy J. Rice stadium moon speech. Presented at: Houston, Texas: https://er.jsc.nasa.gov/seh/ricetalk.htm.
2. Yates JF, Tschirnhart MD. Decision-making. In: Ericsson K, Charners N, Feltovich P, Hoffman R, editors. The Cambridge handbook of expertise and expert performance. Cambridge University Press; 2006. p. 421–37.
3. Moulton CAE, Regehr G, Mylopoulos M, MacRae HM. Slowing down when you should: a new model of expert judgment. Acad Med. 2007;82(10):109–16. https://doi.org/10.1097/ACM.0b013e3181405a76.
4. Brush JE, Sherbino J, Norman GR. How expert clinicians intuitively recognize a medical diagnosis. Am J Med. 2017;130(6):629–34. https://doi.org/10.1016/j.amjmed.2017.01.045.

5. Pelaccia T, Tardif J, Triby E, Charlin B. An analysis of clinical reasoning through a recent and comprehensive approach: the dual-process theory. Med Educ Online. 2011;16(1):1–9. https://doi.org/10.3402/meo.v16i0.5890.
6. Way LW, Stewart L, Gantert W, et al. Causes and prevention of laparoscopic bile duct injuries. Ann Surg. 2003;237(4):460–9. https://doi.org/10.1097/01.SLA.0000060680.92690.E9.
7. Stiegler MP, Gaba DM. Decision-making and cognitive strategies. Simul Healthc. 2015;10(3):133–8. https://doi.org/10.1097/SIH.0000000000000093.
8. Schön DA. Educating the reflective practitioner: toward a new design for teaching and learning in the professions. Jossey-Bass; 1987.
9. Ali J, Adam R, Stedman M, Howard M, Williams J. Advanced trauma life support program increases emergency room application of trauma resuscitative procedures in a developing country. J Trauma Inj Infect Crit Care. 1994;36(3):391–4.
10. Kortbeek JB, Al Turki SA, Ali J, et al. Advanced trauma life support, 8th edition, the evidence for change. J Trauma Inj Infect Crit Care. 2008;64(6):1638–50. https://doi.org/10.1097/TA.0b013e3181744b03.
11. Tisherman SA, Barie P, Bokhari F, et al. Clinical practice guideline: endpoints of resuscitation. J Trauma Inj Infect Crit Care. 2004;57(4):898–912. https://doi.org/10.1097/01.TA.0000133577.25793.E5.
12. Stassen NA, Bhullar I, Cheng JD, et al. Nonoperative management of blunt hepatic injury: an Eastern Association for the Surgery of Trauma practice management guideline. J Trauma Acute Care Surg. 2012;73(5):S288–93. https://doi.org/10.1097/TA.0b013e318270160d.
13. Cullinane DC, Schiller HJ, Zielinski MD, et al. Eastern association for the surgery of trauma practice management guidelines for hemorrhage in pelvic fracture—update and systematic review. J Trauma Inj Infect Crit Care. 2011;71(6):1850–68. https://doi.org/10.1097/TA.0b013e31823dca9a.
14. Mohseni S, Talving P, Kobayashi L, et al. The diagnostic accuracy of 64-slice computed tomography in detecting clinically significant arterial bleeding after pelvic fractures. Am Surg. 2011;77(9):1176–82. https://doi.org/10.1177/000313481107700930.
15. Karmy-Jones R, Nathens A, Jurkovich GJ, et al. Urgent and emergent thoracotomy for penetrating chest trauma. J Trauma Inj Infect Crit Care. 2004;56(3):664–9. https://doi.org/10.1097/01.TA.0000068238.74552.4B.
16. Haynes AB, Weiser TG, Berry WR, et al. A surgical safety checklist to reduce morbidity and mortality in a global population. N Engl J Med. 2009;360(5):491–9. https://doi.org/10.1056/NEJMsa0810119.
17. Berg RJ, Okoye O, Teixeira PG, Inaba K, Demetriades D. The double jeopardy of blunt thoracoabdominal trauma. Arch Surg. 2012;147(6):498. https://doi.org/10.1001/archsurg.2011.2289.
18. Rotondo M, Schwab W, McGonigal M, et al. "Damage control" an approach for improved surviv in exsanguinating pentrating abdominal injury. J Trauma Inj Infect Crit Care. 1992;33(1):161.
19. Cothren CC, Moore EE, Johnson JL, Moore JB, Burch JM. One hundred percent fascial approximation with sequential abdominal closure of the open abdomen. Am J Surg. 2006;192(2):238–42. https://doi.org/10.1016/j.amjsurg.2006.04.010.
20. McCrum ML, McKee J, Lai M, Staples J, Switzer N, Widder SL. ATLS adherence in the transfer of rural trauma patients to a level I facility. Injury. 2013;44(9):1241–5. https://doi.org/10.1016/j.injury.2012.05.009.
21. Nunez TC, Voskresensky IV, Dossett LA, Shinall R, Dutton WD, Cotton BA. Early prediction of massive transfusion in trauma: simple as ABC (assessment of blood consumption)? J Trauma Inj Infect Crit Care. 2009;66(2):346–52. https://doi.org/10.1097/TA.0b013e3181961c35.
22. Yücel N, Lefering R, Maegele M, et al. Trauma associated severe hemorrhage (TASH)-score: probability of mass transfusion as surrogate for life threatening hemorrhage after multiple trauma. J Trauma Inj Infect Crit Care. 2006;60(6):1228–37. https://doi.org/10.1097/01.ta.0000220386.84012.bf.
23. Maegele M, Lefering R, Wafaisade A, et al. Revalidation and update of the TASH-score: a scoring system to predict the probability for massive transfusion as a surrogate for life-threatening haemorrhage after severe injury: score to predict massive transfusion after severe injury. Vox Sang. 2011;100(2):231–8. https://doi.org/10.1111/j.1423-0410.2010.01387.x.
24. Civil I. Guidelines, protocols and checklists: do we need them to provide good trauma care? Injury. 2010;41(1):8–9. https://doi.org/10.1016/j.injury.2009.11.003.
25. Endsley MR. Toward a theory of situation awareness in dynamic systems. Hum Factors. 1995;37
26. Collins J. Good to great. HarperCollins; 2001.
27. Ball CG, Kirkpatrick AW, Mulloy RH, Gmora S, Findlay C, Hameed SM. The impact of multiple casualty incidents on clinical outcomes. J Trauma Inj Infect Crit Care. 2006;61(5):1036–9. https://doi.org/10.1097/01.ta.0000231764.00067.54.
28. Sucher JF, Moore FA, Todd SR, Sailors RM, McKinley BA. Computerized clinical decision support: a technology to implement and validate evidence based guidelines. J Trauma Inj Infect Crit Care. 2008;64(2):520–37. https://doi.org/10.1097/TA.0b013e3181601812.
29. Zargaran E, Schuurman N, Nicol AJ, et al. The electronic trauma health record: design and usability of a novel tablet-based tool for trauma care and injury surveillance in low resource settings. J Am Coll Surg. 2014;218(1):41–50. https://doi.org/10.1016/j.jamcollsurg.2013.10.001.
30. Sutcliffe KM, Paine L, Pronovost PJ. Re-examining high reliability: actively organising for safety. BMJ Qual Saf. 2017;26(3):248–51. https://doi.org/10.1136/bmjqs-2015-004698.
31. Ghaferi AA, Wells EE. Improving postoperative rescue through a multifaceted approach. Surg Clin North Am. 2021;101(1):71–80. https://doi.org/10.1016/j.suc.2020.09.004.

Emergency Critical Care Procedures

33

Paul B. McBeth and S. Morad Hameed

Introduction

The purpose of this chapter is to provide a review of selected emergency critical care procedures. A generalized approach and description of indications, contraindications, controversies, and common pitfalls are provided. Topics covered include: surgical airway management, vascular access, tube thoracostomy, resuscitative thoracotomy, and diagnostic peritoneal lavage. Detailed descriptions of individual procedures are referenced and detailed elsewhere.

Emergency Procedures and Team Dynamics

The team architecture and dynamic is centered around a trauma team leader (TTL) whose responsibility is to provide oversight in the management of critically ill patients. The TTL directs the flow of resuscitative efforts, including the selection and prioritization of life saving procedures, based on the patient's presentation and information gathered by other care providers—making closed-loop communication practices essential. When possible, the TTL should avoid engagement in specific procedures in order to facilitate a cohesive flow of the resuscitation, but should remain aware of the capabilities of team members and stay up to date on procedural progress and success. Since emergency procedures conducted on critically ill or injured patients require speed and efficiency, the most skilled team member is usually selected to carry out these procedures in order to provide the greatest chance of successful patient outcome. Specific roles of each team member should be determined and rehearsed beforehand. Regular simulation-based training is helpful to establish these roles as well as to determine group dynamics, closed-loop communication with specific emphasis on procedure delegation and reporting, familiarization with equipment, and awareness of institutional protocols. Clear communication is essential when resuscitating a critically ill patient and performing emergency procedures. All reasonable efforts should be made to ensure emergency procedures remain controlled and organized, incorporate sterile techniques, and consider patient safety and comfort. The health and safety of each team member are also paramount. Personal protective equipment should be worn in all emergency procedures including gowns, gloves, eye wear, and when appropriate lead aprons. In the era of the COVID-19 pandemic, N-95 respirators in addition to appropriate PPE should be worn for any aerosol-generating medical procedures (AGMP). Post-procedure debriefings are helpful to support learning and ensure quality assurance for improved patient outcomes.

Airway Management

Emergency surgical airway management is an essential skill required by providers of critically ill patients. A surgical airway is generally considered a procedure of last resort when alternative attempts to capture a patient's airway have failed. The criteria prompting the need for surgical airway management is best summarized by the "can't intubate, can't ventilate" dictum where the care provider is unable to intubate or provide effective bag mask ventilation. In particular, sustained hypoxemia during intubation efforts provides justification for initiation of surgical airway procedures. Other indications for surgical airway management include: severe facial or nasal injuries, massive facial trauma, possible cervical spine trauma preventing adequate ventilation, anaphylaxis, and chemical inhalation injuries. There are no absolute contraindications to surgical airway management; however, caution should be considered in patients with known underlying anatomical abnormality, tracheal transection, and acute

P. B. McBeth (✉)
Alberta Health Services | South Health Campus, Calgary, AB, Canada

S. M. Hameed
Trauma Services VGH, Vancouver, BC, Canada
e-mail: morad.hameed@vch.ca

L. Marshall Gillman, S. Widder (eds.), *Trauma Team Dynamics*, https://doi.org/10.1007/978-3-031-86312-7_33

laryngeal disease due to infection or in small children under the age of 10 years [1, 2].

Emergency surgical airway management is often performed in critically ill patients, necessitating time-sensitive management of the airway in an often austere environment [3]. Given the urgent need for the procedure, availability of resources is often limited. If time permits, the ideal location for surgical airway management is in the operating room (OR) where appropriate access to surgical instruments, anesthetic supplies, support teams, and lighting is available.

A cricothyrotomy is the procedure of choice in an emergent situation when unable to intubate. This is done by securing an airway passage through the cricothyroid membrane, which in most patients is straightforward to identify on direct palpation of the neck. This technique allows avoidance of the vocal cords, thyroid isthmus, and associated vessels. There are three main approaches to cricothyroidotomy: needle cricothyroidotomy, percutaneous cricothyroidotomy using the Seldinger technique, and surgical cricothyroidotomy. Descriptions of these procedures can be found elsewhere [4]. The decision of which approach to use is guided by both the patient's condition and the familiarity of the care provider with the procedure. The needle cricothyroidotomy technique is limited by the volume of gas exchange through the catheter and the need for a high-pressure gas source for jet ventilation; therefore, its effectiveness at ventilation is limited while its capability to provide oxygen delivery is favorable. This technique serves as a useful time bridge toward establishing a definitive endotracheal intubation and is the preferred method of securing a crash airway in infants and young children where surgical cricothyrotomy is contraindicated. Percutaneous cricothyroidotomy using the Seldinger technique and surgical cricothyroidotomy are both equally effective at securing an airway. It should be noted that some commercially available percutaneous cricothyroidotomy sets do not have cuffed tubes, which may limit airway protection and ventilation until conversion to a more definitive airway is possible. In the authors' experience, percutaneous cricothyroidotomy, which requires some force for tube placement over the wire, without direct visualization of the airway, is a less controlled procedure than open cricothyroidotomy. A more simple surgical cricothyroidotomy can be successfully completed using only a scalpel, bougie, and an endotracheal tube. For both procedures, we recommend a vertical incision, which can be extended based on palpation of anatomic landmarks and which may help avoid inadvertent injury to the anterior jugular veins. Once a vertical incision is made, palpation for the cricothyroid membrane is completed. A scalpel is used to make an incision into the cricothyroid membrane being mindful not to plunge the scalpel into the posterior airway. Using the blunt end of the scalpel handle, open the cricothyroid membrane and advance the bougie along the side of the scalpel handle. The bougie should advance easily if it is within the airway; then advance an endotracheal tube over the bougie. The selection of percutaneous or open methods is dependent on the availability of equipment and skill of the operator. Once the procedure is complete, confirmation of location is essential prior to commencement of ventilation to avoid insufflation of false passages. This can be done using a bronchoscope for direct visualization, in-line capnography for confirmation of end-tidal CO_2, or small volume ventilation with an ambu-bag with bilateral lung auscultation [2].

Once the surgical airway has been captured, the cricothyroidotomy should be evaluated by a surgeon to assess for injury to the airway and neighboring anatomical structures. This assessment is conducted in the OR followed by conversion to a tracheostomy. This helps to avoid the long-term complications of glottis or subglottic stenosis, laryngeal stenosis, tracheomalacia, and dysphonia [4]. Early post-procedure complications include: bleeding, subcutaneous emphysema, obstruction, esophageal or mediastinal perforation, aspiration, vocal cord injury, pneumothorax, and posterior tracheal wall perforation [4, 5].

Surgical airway management is a potentially life-saving skill and should be part of the training repertoire of any surgeon, emergency medicine, or critical care physician. Given the low incidence of surgical airway management, alternative training and credentialing modalities are needed, including phantom model, human cadaver, and animal simulation [6].

Tube Thoracostomy

Tube thoracostomy is the insertion of a tube into the pleural cavity to facilitate the drainage of air and fluid. This procedure serves as both a diagnostic and therapeutic intervention. In critically ill patients with undifferentiated shock, rapid bilateral finger thoracostomy followed by chest tube insertion, even before chest X-ray evaluation, is a useful procedure for guiding diagnostic evaluation. Other indications for tube thoracostomy include: pneumothorax, hemothorax, hemopneumothorax, hydrothorax, chylothorax, empyema, pleural effusion, and prophylactic decompression for patients undergoing air transport [7–9]. There are no absolute contraindications, but relative contraindications include: coagulopathy, pulmonary bullae, loculated pleural effusion, empyema, or pulmonary, pleural, or thoracic adhesions. The size of the tube placement dictates the surgical technique used. Small pigtail drains are placed using CT or ultrasound guidance using the Seldinger technique [10]. Larger surgical drains are placed under direct visualization with a surgical approach involving tissue dissection. Detailed descriptions of procedural steps for tube thoracostomies are provided elsewhere [11].

Controversies

Despite numerous studies, the use of prophylactic antibiotics, appropriate tube size selection, and management of occult pneumothorax remain controversial topics.

Antibiotics

The need for prophylactic antibiotics prior to thoracostomy tube placement is controversial and is dependent on the clinical situation. Several studies have been conducted to evaluate the need for prophylactic antibiotic use prior to chest tube placement. The majority of these studies have been limited by heterogenous population mix and lack power to demonstrate a clinically significant difference. The Eastern Association for the Surgery of Trauma guidelines does not support the use of prophylactic antibiotics [12]. Patients with non-traumatic spontaneous pneumothorax do not require prophylactic antibiotics prior to chest tube insertion. A recent systematic review and meta-analysis of patients with penetrating thoracic trauma demonstrated significant reductions in the risk of empyema (OR 0.28, 0.14–0.57) [13]. This is supported by a meta-analysis by Sanabria, which demonstrated that the use of prophylactic antibiotics in patients with chest trauma decreased the incidence of post-traumatic empyema (RR 0.19, 0.07–0.50) and pneumonia (RR 0.44, 0.27–0.73) [14]. Despite these studies, the question of prophylactic antibiotics remains controversial. Infectious complications of tube thoracostomies can be minimized by ensuring adequate drainage of hemopneumothorax, using appropriate sterile techniques for tube placement, and appropriate securing of the chest tube to ensure unintentional dislodgement.

Tube Selection

Adequate drainage of traumatic hemothoracies is essential in order to prevent retained hemothoraces, complications of additional tube thoracostomy, infection, and trapped lung. The optimal tube size for drainage of pneumo- or hemothoraces is unknown. A recent study by Inaba demonstrated no clinically significant difference between 28–32 and 36–40 French chest tube size [15]. A smaller study by Kulvatunyou demonstrated 14 Fr pigtail catheters could be effectively used to drain hemothoracies in stable trauma patients [16]. However, pigtail catheters should be reserved for stable patients only and avoided in urgent/emergent situations where time is of the essence. In addition, these require adequate training and experience in both image guidance and appropriate patient selection. Patients at risk of a large air leak due to a bronchial-pleural fistulae should have a larger bore tube (20-28Fr).

Occult Pneumothorax

Occult pneumothorax is defined as a pneumothorax detected with thoracic or abdominal CT, and not diagnosed on preceding supine anteroposterior chest X-ray. Patients with small occult pneumothoraces in the absence of positive pressure ventilation can be managed safely without tube thoracostomy. The optimal treatment of patients with occult pneumothoraces requiring positive pressure ventilation is unknown. Recent retrospective data suggest tube thoracostomy may not be required. However, data from two small randomized control trials suggest otherwise [17–20]. The authors of this document support close monitoring of occult pneumothoraces in the setting of positive pressure ventilated patients.

Complications and Post-tube Thoracostomy Management

Close observation of patients following chest tube placement is needed to ensure resolution of the initiating reason for tube placement and for monitoring of immediate or delayed complications. Complications of tube thoracostomy include: unresolved or re-accumulation of pneumothorax or hemothorax, improper placement (pleural positioning, lung fissure or parenchyma, intra-abdominal), bleeding, organ penetration, tube dislodgement, and empyema. Many of these complications can be avoided by appropriate training and rigorous attention to surgical techniques, including consideration of using prophylactic antibiotics, careful chest X-ray review and landmarking, sterile technique, and a mindful finger sweep of the pleural space before tube introduction. Hemothoraces should be monitored with daily chest X-rays to ensure appropriate resolution of the chest drainage. Retained blood in the chest after chest tube placement increases the risk of empyema and fibrothorax by as much as 20%, prompting additional drain placement or surgical decortication [21]. Retrospective and randomized control trial data support the use of early (less than 5 days post injury) video-assisted thoracoscopic surgery (VATS) for evacuation of retained hemothoraces [21–23].

Timing of chest tube removal is dependent on the resolution of the original clinical presentation. Chest tube drainage less than 100 cc/day with complete radiographic improvement of hemo/pneumothorax may prompt tube removal in the absence of positive pressure ventilation. Caution should be used in patients under positive pressure ventilation as chest tube removal may increase the risk of recurrent pneumothorax, leading to possible tension pneumothorax.

Vascular Access

Early establishment of vascular access in patients who are critically ill is essential for both volume expansion and medication delivery. Selection of vascular access sites is dependent on the goals of resuscitation. Large volume resuscitation is best achieved using large bore peripheral access. Central access is usually reserved for medication delivery; however, large volume resuscitation can also be achieved.

Large volume resuscitation is restricted by the size of the intravenous access. The flow is determined by the Hagen-Poiseuille equation, which states:

$$Q = \Delta P \times \left(\pi r4 / 8\mu\text{L}\right)$$

where:

Q = Flow in Liters/second.
μ = Viscosity in Pa.s,
P = Pressure in Pascals.
r = Radius of the tube in meters,
L = Length of the tube in question in meters.

Essentially, large bore size and short length are needed to maximize flow. Tables 33.1 and 33.2 outline typical flows seen with catheters.

Peripheral Intravenous Access

Peripheral intravenous access is the mainstay of early fluid resuscitation of critically ill patients. Indications for peripheral intravenous access include: venous blood sampling, intravenous fluid and medication infusion, blood transfusion, and intravenous contrast administration. Access points include both upper and lower limbs, including the long saphenous, cephalic, basilic, and median cubital veins. Contraindications to intravenous access include: extremity with significant edema, burns, sclerosis, phlebitis, or thrombosis, and ipsilateral radical mastectomy. Early complications include bruising infiltration, interstitial fluid/medication delivery, and air embolism. Late complications include thrombophlebitis, infection, nerve damage, and thrombosis [24].

Central Intravenous Access

Central venous catheterization is used to access central veins for medication and fluid delivery and patient monitoring of central venous pressures and right heart catheterization. A variety of sites can be used, including femoral, subclavian, and internal/external jugular veins. Each site has its own set of advantages, disadvantages, and risk of complications outlined in Table 33.3.

Table 33.1 Flow characteristics in peripheral vascular catheters

Gauge size	Inside diameter (mm)	Length (mm)	Flow rate (mL/min)
16 (gray)	1.3	30	220
18 (green)	1.0	30	105
		50	60
20 (pink)	0.8	30	60

Abbreviations: *mm* millimeters, *mL/min* milliliters per minute

Table 33.2 Selected characteristics of triple-lumen central venous catheters and intraosseous access

Size (Fr)	Length (cm)	Lumens	Lumen size (Ga)	Flow rate (mL/min)
7	16	Distal	16	57
		Medial	18	30
		Proximal	18	32
7	20	Distal	16	52
		Medial	18	25
		Proximal	18	27
7	30	Distal	16	38
		Medial	18	17
		Proximal	18	18
8.5 (Cordis)	10	Single	8.5 Fr	333
Intraosseous [24]	5	Single	15	165

Abbreviations: *Fr* French, *Ga* Gauge, *cm* centimeters, mL/min milliliters per minute

Table 33.3 Central line placement

Site	Advantages	Disadvantages	Complications
Internal jugular	Anatomic landmarks are easy to identify with ultrasound Head-of-table access Can recognize and control bleeding with direct pressure Minimal risk of pneumothorax Malposition of catheter placement is rare	Difficult to access during emergency airway management Risk of carotid artery puncture Patient discomfort Vein prone to collapse with hypovolemia Avoid if concern about cerebral perfusion Avoid in cervical trauma patients	Pneumothorax Hemothorax Chylothorax Neck hematoma and tracheal obstruction Endotracheal cuff perforation Tracheal perforation Brachial plexus injury Air embolism Cardiac dysrhythmia Thrombosis
Subclavian	Good external landmarks Improved patient comfort Easier to maintain dressings Accessible during airway management or patients with C-spine collars	Unable to compress bleeding vessels Blind procedure Experience related success rate Longer path from skin to vessel Catheter malposition	Pneumothorax Hemothorax Brachial plexus injury Hematoma Air embolism Cardiac dysrhythmia Thrombosis
Femoral	Good external landmarks allowing for rapid access Technically easy Does not interfere with CPR Useful alternative with coagulopathy Trendelenburg position not required	Limits patient mobilization Delayed circulation of drugs during CPR Difficult to keep site sterile Increased risk of iliofemoral thrombosis Not reliable for CVP of central venous gas measurements	Arterial puncture Bowel injury Retroperitoneal hematoma Psoas abscess Bladder injury Air embolism

Abbreviations: *CPR* cardiopulmonary resuscitation, *CVP* central venous pressure, *PA* pulmonary artery

Indications for central venous access include: emergency venous access; high-volume/flow resuscitation; central venous pressure monitoring; inability to obtain peripheral venous access; repetitive blood sampling; administration of hyperalimentation, caustic agents, or concentrated fluids; hemodialysis or plasmapheresis; and placement of transvenous cardiac pacemakers or pulmonary artery catheters. Contraindications for central venous access include: infection over the placement site; distortion of landmarks by trauma or congenital anomalies; coagulopathies, including anticoagulation and thrombolytic therapy; pathologic conditions, including superior vena cava syndrome; current venous thrombosis in the target vessel; prior vessel injury or procedures; morbid obesity; and uncooperative patients. Complications for central venous access are outlined in Table 33.3. Infection rates for internal jugular, subclavian, and femoral central lines are reported as 8.6, 4.0, and 15.3 per 1000 catheter-days, respectively [24]. Thrombosis rates of internal jugular, subclavian, and femoral central lines are reported as 1.2–3, 0–13, and 8–34 per 1000 catheter-days, respectively [24].

Intraosseous Access

Intraosseous (IO) access is a technique where a needle is advanced into the bone marrow to achieve an entry point into the systemic venous system. IO route provides a rapid and effective means of administering drugs, fluid, and blood. Blood can also be drawn from an IO device and used for blood gases, electrolyte and hematologic evaluation, and blood cultures [25–27]. This technique is indicated for adult patients in whom attempts at peripheral or central venous access have been unsuccessful. This may include adult patients with burns, trauma, shock, dehydration, or status epilepticus [28]. Multiple sites, including the iliac crest, femur, proximal and distal ends of the tibia, radius, clavicle, and calcaneus may be used [29–32]. A wide variety of commercial IO devices are currently available. It is important that the provider is familiar with local hospital practice and equipment. Detailed description of IO placement is provided elsewhere [33]. IO devices should be avoided in patients with orthopedic or vascular trauma because of the risk of extravasation. Other contraindications include cellulitis or burns over the insertion site, patients with known underlying bone disease such as osteogenesis imperfect, and previous IO attempts on the ipsilateral side. Technical difficulties are the most common complications and are associated with equipment unfamiliarity. Complications of IO devices include malposition resulting in skin and bone trauma, compartment syndrome from unrecognized extravasation, epiphyseal injuries, and fat embolism. Prior to using an IO site, 10 cc of normal saline should be flushed through the line. Infusion of fluids through the needle at high rates is sometimes associated with patient discomfort. IO access is meant only for temporary access and should be removed when definitive intravenous access is established.

Ultrasound

The use of ultrasound-guided central line placement has become a standard of care. Ultrasound provides a real-time window of vascular anatomy with the ability to directly visualize placement of central lines into a vessel. Traditional use of anatomical-based land marking for central venous access has resulted in failure, and complication rates are as high as 19% and 30%, respectively [32]. Ultrasound-guided CV line placement has been demonstrated to significantly decrease the failure rate, complication rate, and number of attempts required for successful access [34–36].

A recent randomized, multicenter trial using ultrasound-guided CV cannulation reported ultrasonographic guidance had an odds improvement of 53.5 (6.6–440) times higher than landmark-based technique for success of cannulation [37]. The average number of cannulation attempts was also significantly lower in the ultrasound-guided group. The frequency of complications related to line placement is reduced with the use of ultrasound. For internal jugular line placement, arterial punctures are reduced from 9.4% to 1.8%, hematomas 2.2% to 0.4%, and pneumothorax 0.2% to 0% [38–40].

Resuscitative Thoracotomy

A resuscitative thoracotomy (RT) is an emergency procedure used to gain access to the chest in severely injured patients. The decision to perform an RT should be guided by consideration of mechanism of injury and signs of life. The rationale for performing an RT is: (1) release of cardiac tamponade, (2) control intrathoracic hemorrhage, (3) evacuation of air embolism, (4) performance of open cardiac massage, and (5) cross-clamping the descending thoracic aorta [41, 42]. Given the potential risk involved to healthcare workers, the decision to undertake an RT must be made in the context of an anticipated successful clinical outcome. Trauma patients arriving to the emergency department (ED) pulseless should be assessed for clinical history, cardiac rhythm, and a brief neurologic examination prior to commencement of an RT. Patient management is guided initially by mechanism of injury, downtime, and ECG recording. Victims of blunt trauma with no signs of life upon arrival to the ED universally have poor survival rates (<1%) [42, 43]. The authors suggest RT should not be performed in this population when the duration of downtime is greater than 5 min. Patients with penetrating thoracic injury with previously witnessed cardiac activity within 15 min of presenting to a trauma center or unresponsive with hypotension (SBP <70 mmHg) despite ongoing resuscitation with a narrow complex ECG rhythm should be considered for an RT. Relative indications for RT include: penetrating thoracic injury with traumatic arrest with previously witnessed cardiac activity, and penetrating non-thoracic injury with traumatic arrest with previously witnessed cardiac activity (pre-hospital or in-hospital). Other indications for urgent thoracotomy include (1) chest tube output >1000 mL, (2) evidence of ongoing bleeding following placement of a tube thoracostomy at a rate of 200 to 300 mL/h for 4 h, (3) massive chest tube air leak, (4) cardiac tamponade, and (5) air embolism [41–43]. Despite these indications, providers must also consider the patient disposition for definitive surgical repair following a successful RT. Limitations in hospital infrastructure and personnel may prevent successful outcomes. An RT is conducted through anterolateral thoracotomy along the fifth intercostal space on the side of the injury. Detailed surgical steps of an RT are provided in Table 33.4 [44].

Table 33.4 Operative technique for resuscitative thoracotomy

Surgical step	Description	Equipment
Sterilization of skin	Application of Chlorhexidine to the skin surface Draping as appropriate	Chlorhexidine Surgical draps
Surgical incision	Anterolateral incision at the fourth or fifth intercostal space Division of the intercostal muscles Placement of the rib spreader with ratchet mechanism facing downward	#10 Scalpel blade Mayo scissors Rib spreader
Mobilization of the lung	Divide the inferior pulmonary ligament	Metzenbaum scissors
Bleeding control	Apply digital control or pack the chest with surgical sponges	Surgical sponges
Pericardiotomy	Lift the pericardial sac with forceps and cut pericardium with scissors Extend incision caudal-to-cephalad to avoid injury to the phrenic nerve	Metzenbaum scissors
Aortic cross-clamping	Bluntly dissect surrounding tissue. Identify esophagus Apply temporary vascular clamp to aorta	Vascular clamp
Hilar cross-clamping	Identify the pulmonary hilum Apply temporary vascular clamp	Vascular clamp Surgical sponges
Cam-shell exposure	Anterolateral incision across the sternum to the right fourth or fifth intercostal space Divide the sternum with a Lebsche sternal knife Reposition rib spreader as appropriate	#10 Scalpel blade Lebsche sternal knife Rib spreader

Outcomes

A clinically successful RT in the setting of blunt trauma is rare (<1%); therefore, the authors advocate its use in only selected situations. Improved outcomes are seen in patients with penetrating (8–10%) injuries. The greatest survival advantage is an RT performed for stab wounds (18–24%). Survival following a gunshot wound with an RT is 4–5% [45].

Contraindications

Contraindications for an RT include: blunt injury without witnessed cardiac activity, penetrating trauma without cardiac activity (CPR > 15 min) with no signs of life (pupillary response (in the absence of epinephrine administration), respiratory effort, or motor activity), asystole or wide complex rhythm, non-traumatic cardiac arrest, severe head injury, severe multisystem injury, improperly trained team, and insufficient equipment [42, 43].

Volume Expansion

Patients presenting with the need for an RT are often volume-depleted and require fluid resuscitation. As such, appropriate IV access is required to achieve administration of crystalloid or blood products. Fluid administration is titrated to achieve end organ perfusion. The use of vasopressor support should be limited and used only as a temporary measure to support blood pressure in a crashing patient, especially in the setting of pure hemorrhagic shock [46]. The use of vasopressors has been shown to be deleterious [47].

Management

The decision to perform an RT should be guided by the algorithm outline above. Once the decision for an RT is made, OR staff should be put on hold in anticipation of definitive management in the OR. Team dynamics and organization is orchestrated by the TTL in order to maximize patient and healthcare provider safety. As described above, each team member should have pre-defined roles within the resuscitation team. Protective equipment should be worn by all team members. The patient-directed goal of RT in the ED should be to temporize thoracic injury and re-establish systemic oxygen delivery. Temporizing measures in the ED should be limited to digital compression of cardiac or vascular injuries, aortic or pulmonary hilar cross clamping, or packing of chest wall injuries with definitive repair and continued resuscitation done in the controlled confines of the OR. There is no role for a trauma laparotomy in the ED. In pre-arrest patients, the decision for transfer to a standby OR for definitive management should be considered. This decision is based on the injury patterns of the patient, anticipated clinical course, and availability of an OR and support staff. A recent study by the Western Trauma Association demonstrated improved outcomes when patients were managed in the OR or in the ED with equipment setup similar to the OR [48]. Successful RT requires definitive surgical repair in the OR. Management of cardiac injuries, injuries of the great vessels, lung, tracheobronchial tree, esophagus, and thoracic aortic rupture should be definitively managed in the OR [44, 49]. This should be done by a trained trauma surgeon or cardiothoracic surgeon.

Diagnostic Peritoneal Lavage

Diagnostic peritoneal lavage (DPL) is a diagnostic procedure used to provide information in the evaluation of patients with blunt or penetrating trauma. With the widespread integration of FAST ultrasound and improved resolution of computed tomography (CT), some believe DPL has become a lost procedure [50–53]. This has led to a poor understanding of current indications for DPL [54]. Despite the low frequency of use, DPL remains the most sensitive test to identify mesenteric and hollow viscus injury [55].

In the era of modern trauma care, DPL may be indicated in the following clinical circumstances [54–57]:

- Hemodynamically unstable patients with suspected multicavitary bleeding but with negative or indeterminate FAST.
- Stable patients with anterior abdominal stab wounds with proven peritoneal violation in the absence of peritonitis.

A variety of surgical techniques have been described for performing a DPL. The most commonly used are the open and Seldinger techniques. These methods are described elsewhere [58]. A supraumbilical approach should be considered in patients with pelvic fractures, pre-existing lower midline surgical incisions, or early pregnancy. Decompression of the stomach and bladder is important to prevent iatrogenic injury.

Interpretation of Results

If the initial aspiration of peritoneal fluid yields 5–10 cc of gross blood, the test is positive. In the absence of gross blood on the initial aspiration, 1 L of normal saline is infused into the peritoneal cavity. The mixed fluid is then sampled. The following is suggestive of a positive test: in the setting of blunt abdominal trauma a red blood cell count (RBC) more than 100,000/cc is considered a positive test; for penetrating trauma, there is no consensus; however, for anterior abdominal injuries more than 100,000/cc, RBC is considered positive; other positive results include more than 500/cc white blood cell count or the presence of gross or microscopic enteric contents [55–57].

Complications of DPL include: catheter misplacement, vascular injury, intrabdominal or retroperitoneal organ injury, and wound infection.

In summary, DPL is a useful adjunctive diagnostic test despite the widespread use of FAST ultrasound and CT scans. Knowledge of the different diagnostic criteria based on the mechanism of injury is required [54].

Summary

In summary, this chapter provides an integrated approach to emergency critical care procedures including surgical airway management, vascular access, tube thoracostomy, resuscitative thoracotomy, and diagnostic peritoneal lavage. The combination of teamwork, organization, closed-loop communication, and uncompromising attention to technical detail are essential for successful management of critically ill patients.

Key Notes

Key notes of this chapter are as follows:

- The team architecture and dynamic is centered around a trauma team leader (TTL) whose responsibility is to provide oversight in the management of critically ill patients.
- A generalized approach and description of indications, contraindications, controversies and common pitfalls of surgical airway management, vascular access, tube thoracostomy, resuscitative thoracotomy, and diagnostic peritoneal lavage are outlined.
- Clear communication is essential when resuscitating a critically ill patient and performing emergency procedures.
- The health and safety of each team member are critical. Personal protective equipment should be worn in all emergency procedures. In the era of the COVID-19 pandemic, N-95 respirators should also be worn for any aerosol-generating medical procedures.
- Post-procedure debriefings provide opportunities for learning and evaluation of quality healthcare delivery.

References

1. Nolan JP, Kelly FE. Airway challenges in critical care. Anaesthesia. 2011;66(Suppl. 2):81–92.
2. Reid LA, Dunn M, Mckeown DW, Oglesby AJ. Surgical airway in emergency department intubation. Eur J Emerg Med. 2011;18(3):168–71.
3. Macdonald JC, Tien HCN. Emergency battlefield cricothyrotomy. Can Med Assoc J. 2008;178(9):1133–5.
4. Hebert RB, Bose S, Mace SE. Chapter 6: Cricothyrotomy and percutaneous translaryngeal ventilation. In: Roberts JR, Hedges JR, editors. Clinical procedures in emergency medicine. 5th ed; 2009. p. 120–33.
5. Cook TM, MacDougall-Davis SR. Complications and failure of airway management. Br J Anaesth. 2012;109(S1):i68–85.
6. Shetty K, Nayyar V, Stachowski E, Byth K. Training for cricothyroidotomy. Anaesth Intensive Care. 2013;41(5):623–30.
7. Bailey RC. Complications of tube thoracostomy in trauma. J Accid Emerg Med. 2000;17(2):111–4.
8. Leigh-Smith S, Harris T. Tension pneumothorax—time for a re-think? Emerg Med J. 2005;22(1):8–16.
9. Tsukahara K, Kawabata K, Mitani H, Yoshimoto S, Sugitani I, Yonekawa H, et al. Three cases of bilateral chylothorax developing after neck dissection. Auris Nasus Larynx. 2007;34(4):573–6.
10. Seldinger SI. Catheter replacement of the needle in percutaneous arteriography; a new technique. Acta Radiol. 1953;39(5):368–76.
11. Kirsch TD, Sax J. Chapter 10: Tube thoracostomy. In: Roberts JR, Hedges JR, editors. Clinical procedures in emergency medicine. 5th ed; 2009. p. 189–211.
12. Luchette F, Barie P, Oswanski M. Practice management guidelines for prophylactic antibiotic use in tube thoracostomy for traumatic hemopneumothorax: EAST Practice Management Guidelines Work Group. J Trauma. 2000;48(4):753–7.
13. Bosman A, de Jong MB, Debeij J, van den Broek PJ, Schipper IB. Systematic review and meta-analysis of antibiotic prophylaxis to prevent infections from chest drains in blunt and penetrating thoracic injuries. Br J Surg. 2012;99(4):506–13.
14. Sanabria A, Valdivieso E, Gomez G, Echeverry G. Prophylactic antibiotics in chest trauma: a meta-analysis of high-quality studies. World J Surg. 2006;30(10):1843–7.
15. Inaba K, Lustenberger T, Recinos G, Georgiou C, Velmahos GC, Brown C, Salim A, Demetriades D, Rhee P. Does size matter? A prospective analysis of 28–32 versus 36–40 French chest tube size in trauma. J Trauma Acute Care Surg. 2012;72(2):422–7.
16. Kulvatunyou N, Joseph B, Friese RS, Green D, Gries L, O'Keeffe T, Tang AL, Wynne JL, Rhee P. French pigtail catheters placed by surgeons to drain blood on trauma patients: is 14-Fr to small? J Trauma Acute Care Surg. 2012;73(6):1423–7.
17. Ball CG, Hameed SM, Evans D. Occult pneumothorax in the mechanically ventilated trauma patient. Can J Surg. 2003;46:373–9.
18. Ball CG, Kirkpatrick AW, Laupland KB. Incidence, risk factors and outcomes for occult pneumothoraces in victims of major trauma. J Trauma. 2005;59:917–25.
19. Enderson BL, Abdalla R, Frame SB, Casey MT, Gould H, Maull. Tube thoracostomy for occult pneumothorax: a prospective randomized study of its use. J Trauma. 1993;35:726–30.
20. Brasel KJ, Stafford RE, Weigelt JA, et al. Treatment of occult pneuothoraces from blunt trauma. J Trauma. 1999;46:987–91.
21. Drummond DS. Traumatic hemothorax: complications and management. Am Surg. 1967;33:403–8.
22. Meyer DM, Jessen ME, Wait MA, Estrera AS. Early evacuation of traumatic retained hemothoraces using thoracoscopy: a prospective, randomized trial. Ann Thorac Surg. 1997;64(5):1396–400.

23. Smith JW, Franklin GA, Harbrecht BG, Richardson JD. Early VATS for blunt chest trauma: a management technique underutilized by acute care surgeons. J Trauma. 2011;71(1):102–5.
24. McNeil CR, Rezaie SR, Adams BD. Chapter 22: Central venous catheterization and central venous pressure monitoring. In: Roberts JR, Hedges JR, editors. Clinical procedures in emergency medicine. 5th ed; 2009. p. 397–431.
25. Brickman KR, Krupp K, Rega P, Alexander J, Guinness M. Typing and screening of blood from intraosseous access. Ann Emerg Med. 1992;21:414.
26. Johnson L, Kissoon N, Fiallos M, Abdelmoneim T, Murphy S. Use of intraosseous blood to assess blood chemistries and hemoglobin during cardiopulmonary resuscitation with drug infusions. Crit Care Med. 1999;27:1147.
27. Fiorito BA, Mirza F, Doran TM, Oberle AN, Cruz EC, Wendtland CL. Intraosseous access in the setting of pediatric critical care transport. Pediatr Crit Care Med. 2005;6:50.
28. Frascone R, Kaye K, Dries D, Solem L. Successful placement of an adult sternal intraosseous line through burned skin. J Burn Care. 2003;24:306.
29. Ong ME, Chan YH, Oh JJ, Ngo AS. An observational, prospective study comparing tibial and humeral intraosseous access using the EZ-IO. Am J Emerg Med. 2009;27(1):8–15.
30. Valdes M. Intraosseous fluid administration in emergencies. Lancet. 1977;235:1235.
31. Calkins MD, Fitzgerald G, Bentley TB, Burris D. Intraosseous infusion devices: a comparison for potential use in special operations. J Trauma. 2000;48:1068.
32. Clem M, Tierney P. Intraosseous infusions via the calcaneus. Resuscitation. 2004;62:107.
33. Deitch K. Chapter 25: Intraosseous infusion. In: Roberts JR, Hedges JR, editors. Clinical procedures in emergency medicine. 5th ed; 2009. p. 455–68.
34. Sznajder JI, Zveibil FR, Bitterman H, Weiner P, Bursztein S. Central vein catheterization. Failure and complication rates by three percutaneous approaches. Arch Intern Med. 1986;146(2):259–61.
35. Abboud PA, Kendall JL. Ultrasound guidance for vascular access. Emerg Med Clin North Am. 2004;22(3):749–73.
36. Denys BG, Uretsky BF, Reddy PS. Ultrasound-assisted cannulation of the internal jugular vein. A prospective comparison to the external landmark-guided technique. Circulation. 1993;87(5):1557–62.
37. Verghese ST, McGill WA, Patel RI, Sell JE, Midgley FM, Ruttimann UE. Ultrasound-guided internal jugular venous cannulation in infants: a prospective comparison with the traditional palpation method. Anesthesiology. 1999;91(1):71–7.
38. Milling TJ Jr, Rose J, Briggs WM, Birkhahn R, Gaeta TJ, Bove JJ. Randomized, controlled clinical trial of point-of-care limited ultrasonography assistance of central venous cannulation: the Third Sonography Outcomes Assessment Program (SOAP-3) Trial. Crit Care Med. 2005;33(8):1764–9.
39. Oguzkurt L, Tercan F, Kara G, Torun D, Kizilkilic O, Yildirim T. US-guided placement of temporary internal jugular vein catheters: immediate technical success and complications in normal and high-risk patients. Eur J Radiol. 2005;55:125.
40. Merrer J, De Jonghe B, Golliot F, Lefrant JY, Raffy B, Barre E. Complications of femoral and subclavian venous catheterization in critically ill patients: a randomized controlled trial. JAMA. 2001;286:700.
41. Burlew CC, Moore EE, Moore FA, Coimbra R, McIntyre RC Jr, Davis JW, Sperry J, Biffl WL. Western Trauma Association critical decisions in trauma: resuscitative thoracotomy. J Trauma Acute Care Surg. 2012;73(6):1359–63.
42. Søreide K, Petrone P, Asensio JA. Emergency thoracotomy in trauma: rationale, risks, and realities. Scand J Surg. 2007;96(1):4–10.
43. Buchman TG. Emergency department resuscitative thoracotomy. J Am Coll Surg. 2005;200(1):148.
44. Jones RF, Rivers EP. Chapter 18: Resuscitative thoracotomy. In: Roberts JR, Hedges JR, editors. Clinical procedures in emergency medicine. 5th ed; 2009. p. 325–39.
45. Cothren CC, Moore EE. Emergency department thoracotomy for the critically injured patient: objectives, indications, and outcomes. World J Emerg Surg. 2006;1:4.
46. Beloncle F, Meziani F, Lerolle N, Radermacher P, Asfar P. Does vasopressor therapy have an indication in hemorrhagic shock? Ann Intensive Care. 2013;3(1):13.
47. Sperry JL, Minei JP, Frankel HL, West MA, Harbrecht BG, Moore EE, Maier RV, Nirula R. Early use of vasopressors after injury: caution before constriction. J Trauma. 2008;64(1):9–14.
48. Karmy-Jones R, Nathens A, Jurkovich GJ, Shatz DV, Brundage S, Wall MJ Jr, Engelhardt S, Hoyt DB, Holcroft J, Knudson MM, Michaels A, Long W. Urgent and emergent thoracotomy for penetrating chest trauma. J Trauma. 2004;56(3):664–8.
49. Moore EE, Knudson MM, Burlew CC, Inaba K, Dicker RA, Biffl WL, Malhotra AK, Schreiber MA, Browder TD, Coimbra R, Gonzalez EA, Meredith JW, Livingston DH, Kaups KL, WTA Study Group. Defining the limits of resuscitative emergency department thoracotomy: a contemporary Western Trauma Association perspective. J Trauma. 2011;70(2):334–9.
50. McKenney M, Lentz K, Nunez D, Sosa JL, Sleeman D, Axelrad A, Martin L, Kirton O, Oldham C. Can ultrasound replace diagnostic peritoneal lavage in the assessment of blunt trauma? J Trauma. 1994;37(3):439–41.
51. Soto JA, Anderson SW. Multidetector CT of blunt abdominal trauma. Radiology. 2012;265(3):678–93.
52. Fang JF, Wong YC, Lin BC, Hsu YP, Chen MF. Usefulness of multidetector computed tomography for the initial assessment of blunt abdominal trauma patients. World J Surg. 2006;30(2):176–82.
53. Cha JY, Kashuk JL, Sarin EL, Cothren CC, Johnson JL, Biffl WL, Moore EE. Diagnostic peritoneal lavage remains a valuable adjunct to modern imaging techniques. J Trauma. 2009;67(2):330–4.
54. Rhodes CM, Smith HL, Sidwell RA. Utility and relevance of diagnostic peritoneal lavage in trauma education. J Surg Educ. 2011;68(4):313–7.
55. Whitehouse JS, Weigelt JA, Scand J. Diagnostic peritoneal lavage: a review of indications, technique, and interpretation. Trauma Resusc Emerg Med. 2009;17:13.
56. Wang YC, Hsieh CH, Fu CY, Yeh CC, Wu SC, Chen RJ. Hollow organ perforation in blunt abdominal trauma: the role of diagnostic peritoneal lavage. Am J Emerg Med. 2012;30(4):570–3.
57. Biffl WL, Kaups KL, Cothren CC, Brasel KJ, Dicker RA, Bullard MK, Haan JM, Jurkovich GJ, Harrison P, Moore FO, Schreiber M, Knudson MM, Moore EE. Management of patients with anterior abdominal stab wounds: a Western Trauma Association multicenter trial. J Trauma. 2009;66(5):1294–301.
58. Runyon MS, Marx JA. Chapter 43: Peritoneal procedures. In: Roberts JR, Hedges JR, editors. Clinical procedures in emergency medicine. 5th ed; 2009. p. 852–72.

REBOA and Novel Hemorrhage Control Methods

34

Nori L. Bradley, Shaun Cowan, and Megan Brenner

Introduction

Hemorrhage is a leading cause of mortality in trauma [1, 2]. New and emerging technologies and devices are broadening the trauma resuscitationists' toolbox with options to control a variety of challenging bleeding injuries [3, 4]. The basic principles of managing massive bleeding include hemorrhage control and hemostatic resuscitation. The latter refers to the maintenance of thermoregulation and protection from heat loss, balanced blood product resuscitation (including whole blood) with point of care-directed factor resuscitation, where available, and correction of coagulopathy. This chapter will focus on hemorrhage control; hemostatic resuscitation is detailed in the Damage Control Resuscitation chapter.

When considering the options for hemorrhage control, it is useful to consider compressible versus incompressible sites of hemorrhage to select appropriate and effective interventions [5, 6]. In general, compressible hemorrhage occurs in extremities, while non-compressible hemorrhage is truncal. The junctions between the neck, axilla, and groins are referred to as junctional hemorrhage, and can be compressible or not, depending on the anatomical location and severity of the injury. Non-compressible hemorrhage is difficult to control quickly but can be managed with the implementation of effective teams and appropriate tools. In this chapter, we discuss a variety of hemorrhage control adjuncts for both massive compressible and non-compressible hemorrhage (Table 34.1).

N. L. Bradley (✉)
Department of Surgery, University of Alberta, Edmonton, AB, Canada

Department of Medicine, University of British Columbia, Vancouver, BC, Canada
e-mail: Nori.Bradley@albertahealthservices.ca

S. Cowan
Department of Surgery, University of Alberta, Edmonton, AB, Canada

Department of Critical Care Medicine, University of Alberta, Edmonton, AB, Canada
e-mail: cowan@ualberta.ca

M. Brenner
School of Medicine – Surgery, University of California Riverside School of Medicine, Riverside, CA, USA
e-mail: MBrenner@mednet.ucla.edu

L. Marshall Gillman, S. Widder (eds.), *Trauma Team Dynamics*, https://doi.org/10.1007/978-3-031-86312-7_34

Table 34.1 Non-operative/procedural hemorrhage control tools for trauma resuscitation

Compressible hemorrhage sites		
Extremity hemorrhage	Junctional hemorrhage	Non-compressible hemorrhage sites
Digital/manual pressure	Packing gauze[a]	Pelvic binder
Packing gauze	Hemostatic gauze[a]	External aortic manual compression
Hemostatic gauze	Hemostatic powders[a]	Abdominal aortic tourniquet
Hemostatic powders	Foley catheter	Intra-abdominal foam[b]
Tourniquets	Pelvic binder	REBOA
Pneumatic	Abdominal aortic tourniquet	
Strap and windlass style	Junctional tourniquet	
	REBOA	

[a]If wound accessible for compression
[b]In development

Resuscitative Endovascular Balloon Occlusion of the Aorta

Resuscitative Endovascular Balloon Occlusion of the Aorta (REBOA) is a well-described percutaneous approach to non-compressible torso hemorrhage, as an alternative to traditional open aortic cross-clamping [7]. The original report from Lieutenant Colonel Carl Hughes in 1954 described internal aortic balloon occlusion as an approach for managing abdominal trauma during the Korean War [8]. Fifty years later, endovascular aortic balloon occlusion was described for emergent management of ruptured abdominal aortic aneurysms [9]. Subsequent military interest in endovascular hemorrhage control and military-civilian partnerships led to trauma surgeons utilizing the available technology in civilian trauma centers [10, 11]. While early reports supported REBOA as an alternative to resuscitative thoracotomy in shock from hemorrhage below the diaphragm, the development of smaller 7 French sheath introducers and wireless technology has led to international uptake of REBOA as part of hemorrhage control protocols in high and low-to-middle income countries [12–15]. Use of REBOA has been described in austere, pre-hospital, rural, and transfer environments [16–21]. The recent report of a new, smaller COBRA-OS device—a 4 French Control of Bleeding, Resuscitation, Arterial Occlusion System—may also extend the role of aortic occlusion in a variety of clinical settings [22].

Clinical algorithms for REBOA have been well described (Fig. 34.1) [23, 24]. Trauma patients in hemorrhagic shock without suspected major thoracic vascular injury (e.g., aortic, cardiac, major thoracic vascular) may be candidates for REBOA. Chest X-ray should be performed urgently to identify or rule out a treatable cause of shock (e.g., tension pneumothorax, hemothorax). If there are no indications for tube or finger thoracostomy, Focused Abdominal Sonography for Trauma (FAST) should be performed to assess for intra-abdominal hemorrhage and rule out pericardial tamponade. Patients with persistent hypotension (sBP <90 mmHg) despite blood product resuscitation with positive FAST or compressible source of hemorrhage (e.g., pelvic fracture) are potential candidates for REBOA. Balloon deployment within the aorta is either within Zone 1 or Zone 3. Zone 1 of the aorta extends from the left subclavian to the celiac artery. Zone 3 extends from the lowest renal artery to the aortic bifurcation [24] (Fig. 34.1). Patients in cardiac arrest or with non-compressible hemorrhage below the diaphragm warrant Zone 1 deployment, while those with hemorrhage due to pelvic fracture warrant Zone 3 deployment.

Specific details regarding the technical aspects of REBOA deployment are described elsewhere [25]. The basic steps include: insertion of arterial sheath (size dependent on device being used), insertion of REBOA catheter to appropriate location, confirmation of position, balloon inflation, balloon deflation, catheter removal, and sheath removal.

Arterial access to deploy REBOA should be via the common femoral artery (CFA) [22]. Obtaining CFA access is the rate-limiting step in deployment, and introducing the device through non-CFA sites increases complications [26]. Early reports from the AORTA registry noted 50% open surgical cut-down for CFA access [27], which decreased to 17–24% in more recent reports [15, 28]. However, surgical cut-down is more likely to be required for patients in cardiac arrest [29]. Percutaneous approaches relied on landmarks more often than ultrasound, 51% versus 21%, respectively [28]. Small studies in laboratory or animal settings have suggested longer time to access but potentially higher CFA access success rates using ultrasound for percutaneous access. Thus, a pre-assembled kit for REBOA deployment containing all supplies required to gain access (open or percutaneous), deploy the balloon, and secure the device must be available in areas where REBOA will be deployed [30].

Insertion depth of the REBOA catheter should be based on pre-assessed external landmarks. Newer generation catheters have standard distance markings for Zone 1 and Zone 3, but data for validation in clinical use is not yet available [31]. At this time, X-ray or fluoroscopy should be used to confirm position prior to balloon inflation. Ultrasound may identify wire position within the aorta but has limitations in identifying balloon position [32]. Deferring radiographic confirmation should be limited to exceptional circumstances

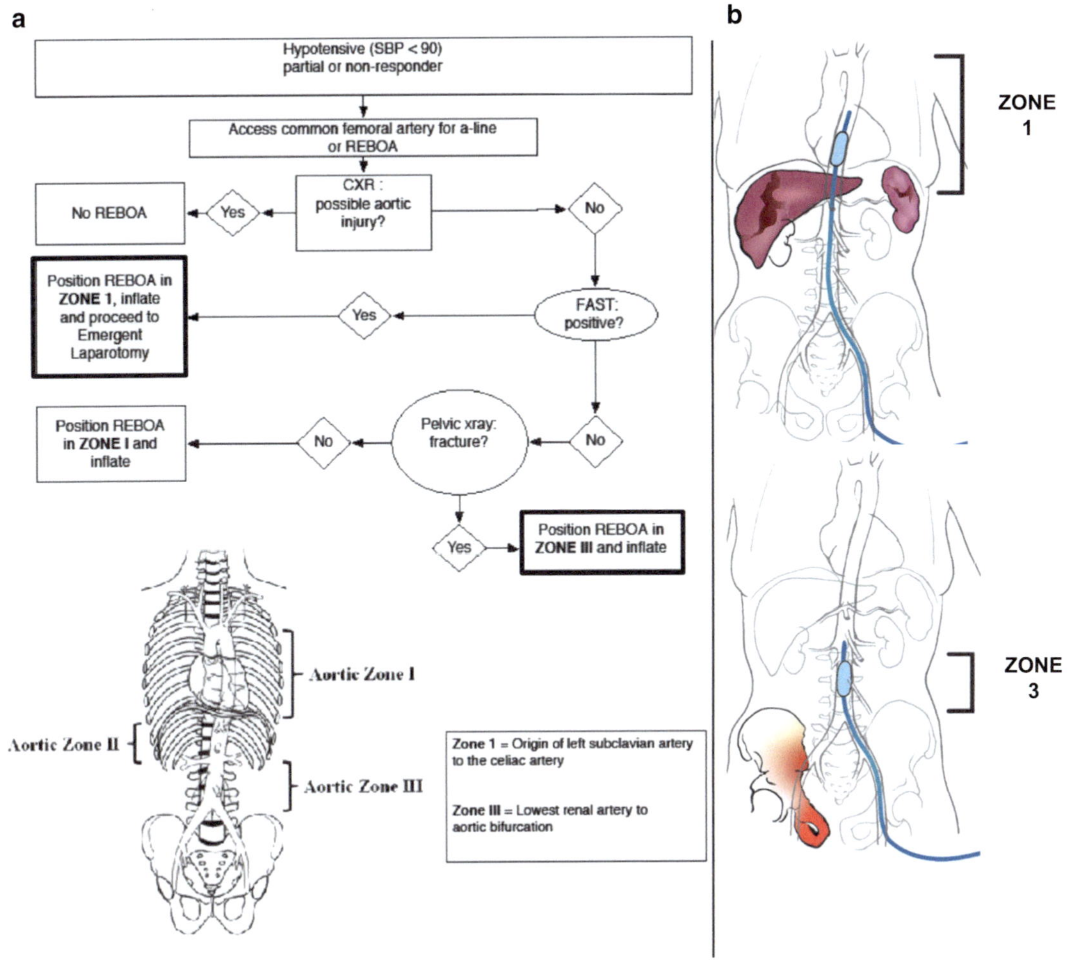

Fig. 34.1 Algorithm for Zone 1 and Zone 3 REBOA , insertion with relevant trauma anatomy highlighted. Panel a STC REBOA Algorithm from Trauma Acute Care Surg. 2014 Aug;77 (2):286–91, with permission. Panel b demonstrates placement zone 1 versus zone 3 ballon placement from BEST© course content, with permission.

(such as active cardiopulmonary resuscitation); confirmation should then be obtained as soon as possible [33].

Balloon inflation should follow manufacturer's instructions for use and avoid over-inflation. Balloon rupture, arterial rupture, and death have been associated with over-inflation [34]. Real-time feedback with increase in blood pressure via arterial line tracing from above the balloon should be observed. Loss of the contralateral femoral pulse should also be confirmed in the absence of cardiac arrest. Documentation of balloon inflation time is required, and updates to commercially available catheters have made this process more user-friendly.

Once the balloon has been inflated, definitive hemorrhage control must be obtained as soon as possible. Guidelines based on physiologic end-points in animal research and clinical use recommend Zone 1 inflation no more than 30 minutes and Zone 3 inflation no more than 60 minutes [33, 35–38]. Institutional pathways to facilitate these timelines should be in place and reviewed regularly for optimization. Balloon deflation should occur as soon as hemorrhage control is obtained. The time of deflation should be documented. If partial REBOA is utilized, this should also be part of the documentation [31].

Removal of the catheter from the sheath should occur as soon as possible. Distal blood flow should be confirmed and documented, ideally with angiography prior to leaving the OR, IR, or hybrid suite. The sheath should also be removed as soon as possible. This may not be feasible at the time of hemorrhage control due to coagulopathy, need to transfer to intensive care, or other logistical constraints. However, increased duration of sheath dwell time increases the risk of limb complications. The limb and access site should be monitored regularly for 24 hours, and a CFA US should be performed within 72 hours in order to assess for hematoma, CFA pseudoaneurysms, or arteriovenous fistulas [33].

Complications associated with REBOA use have been well described [34, 39]. In general, these can be classified as balloon deployment related or access site related. As mentioned, balloon deployment complications can lead to arterial injury (e.g., dissection) or rupture (aorta, iliac artery) and devastating hemorrhage. Inappropriate locations for deployment can also result in mesenteric ischemia or acute kidney injury due to visceral or renal artery occlusion. Access site-related complications can include bleeding/hematoma (including retroperitoneal), or arterial injury such as pseudoaneurysm or dissection both at the arteriotomy site or more proximally into the iliac vessels. Thrombus from the access site or along the balloon catheter can embolize, leading to limb ischemia or even limb loss. Awareness of the complications and rigorous protocols for assessment and treatment are critical to prevent and mitigate complications.

REBOA Programs

Implementation of REBOA within a healthcare and/or hospital system requires a thoughtful, multidisciplinary approach. Credentialing, equipment resources for balloon insertion and deployment, human resources for balloon deployment, monitoring, and post-removal care, patient pathways, and quality assurance and quality improvement need to be considered [40]. Multidisciplinary training, both via formalized courses and ongoing system learning, is key for successful program implementation and maintenance [23, 40]. A local REBOA coordinator, such as a surgeon champion, can bridge the gaps between the stakeholder departments and is recommended. A multidisciplinary approach with surgical presence during deployment is critical to a successful program [30].

Partial REBOA

Partial REBOA is defined as partially deflating the REBOA balloon to allow for some distal flow [41]. Some centers and providers have reported experience with partial REBOA [42]. However, partial inflation of a REBOA balloon can result in balloon migration and intimal injuries [43]. It also requires continuous blood pressure monitoring above and below the balloon [42]. Despite some successful reports in military contexts [44], data to guide partial REBOA in civilian settings are limited [42]. A recent report using partial REBOA in a high volume trauma center supported feasibility but failed to show a survival benefit [45]. At this time, partial REBOA is not recommended in multiple national civilian REBOA consensus guidelines and should be considered with caution [33, 38]. New products with balloons specific for partial REBOA and subsequent dedicated research may modify these recommendations.

Intermittent REBOA

Intermittent REBOA is periodic deflation of the REBOA balloon and is hypothesized to extend the therapeutic time frame of REBOA by allowing transient distal flow with cyclic balloon inflation and deflation [41]. Reports from swine models have shown mixed results. Small studies have reported improved survival [46] and distal ischemia [47] or no improvement when compared with partial REBOA [48]. Further translational research will be required to determine the role of intermittent REBOA in human trauma resuscitation.

Pre-hospital and Transfer REBOA

The use of REBOA in a pre-hospital setting may have a role where expedited transport (i.e., achieve Zone 1 and 3 target timelines) to an appropriate facility with immediate surgical capabilities exists and can be rapidly mobilized. US Special Forces medical providers have reported success with field implementation of this technique as a bridge for transport [17, 19]. European civilian EMS systems have also successfully deployed the technology, with physician presence [19, 20]. Use of REBOA has also been described in a US rural civilian setting where transfer to higher level of care was achieved [19]. Limitations of pre-hospital and transfer REBOA use include exceeding recommended balloon inflation times, and the logistics plus human resources required to successfully transport a patient to definitive surgical intervention and reperfusion. Bringing REBOA closer to the point of injury means taking it farther away from hemorrhage control. The significant coordination and resources required for pre-hospital and/or transfer REBOA exceeds local capabilities in most non-military jurisdictions. Overall, we support Lamhaut and colleagues (2018) who caution that it is "imperative REBOA is developed within a system that can rapidly transport to definitive repair."

Vena Cava Occlusion

Major trauma that results in inferior vena cava (IVC) injuries has not shown the same reduction in mortality as severe hepatic injuries over time, especially for retrohepatic caval injuries [49]. Given the challenging exposure for more cranial IVC injuries, endovascular approaches have been described in a small number of animal studies. Resuscitative

Endovascular Balloon Occlusion of the Vena Cava (REBOVC) prolonged time to death and decreased blood loss in a swine model [50]. More recently, a swine model using a combined approach with REBOVC plus REBOA to achieve total hepatic isolation provided superior hemodynamic stability than REBOVC alone or with a Pringle maneuver [49]. While significant physiologic derangements were observed, both studies concluded that REBOVC could potentially "buy time" while obtaining definitive surgical bleeding control. More research is needed in this area. The advantages to balloon occlusion in this setting include a potential reduction in trauma to the IVC during clamping, as well as the ability to allow partial flow remotely. Disadvantages can be life-threatening, as the reduction in preload can have dire consequences, some of which can be avoided with central resuscitation.

Aortic Occlusion in Non-trauma Settings

REBOA use has been reported in non-traumatic hemorrhage, such as massive gynecological bleeding (active or anticipated) during morbidly adherent placenta [15], massive gastrointestinal bleeds [51, 52], visceral artery and aneurysm rupture, and hemorrhagic necrotizing pancreatitis [52]. Similar to trauma, use of REBOA in these settings serves as a temporizing bridge to definitive control via interventional radiology or surgical bleeding control and repair. Also similar to trauma, the institutional considerations mentioned above still apply to REBOA use in non-trauma settings in order to optimize patient safety and clinical performance.

Tourniquets

While conceptually not new, the resurgence of tourniquets has occurred over the last several decades due to the military experiences caring for casualties in Afghanistan and Iraq [53]. In both the military and civilian prehospital setting, tourniquet use temporarily controls extremity hemorrhage, allowing for evacuation to definitive care. In civilian settings, pre-hospital tourniquet placement significantly decreases mortality and volume of blood transfusions compared to waiting until arrival to hospital for tourniquet application [54, 55]. Within the hospital, tourniquet use can temporarily control extremity hemorrhage, allowing the resuscitation team to focus on identifying and addressing other threats to life associated with multi-system trauma. This is especially relevant during multi- or mass-casualty situations so that limited provider resources can temporize extremity hemorrhage and continue to support disaster management [56].

The trauma resuscitationist should understand considerations for tourniquet use and removal. In orthopedic surgery, tourniquets are routinely used to create a blood-free surgical field and are often in place for up to two hours [57]. Data from combat injuries note good outcomes with tourniquet times up to four hours of duration, and in select patients and circumstances [55], limb recovery is documented for tourniquet times up to 16 hours, although outcomes beyond four hours are variable [58]. The goal should be to obtain hemorrhage control while minimizing tourniquet time.

Considerations in Tourniquet Use

Placement of an arterial tourniquet should be 3–5 cm above the injury on the affected extremity, and as distal as possible, while avoiding positioning over a joint. Extremity bony anatomy consists of two-bone (distal) and one-bone (proximal) compartments. Tourniquet effectiveness is relative to tissue volume and is most effective more distal than proximal as a function of the lesser compressed tissue volume in two-bone compartments. Upper thigh tourniquet placement can often require the placement of two or more windlass-style tourniquets for effective hemorrhage control [56, 59].

There are two hard endpoints of tourniquet tightening: (1) cessation of bleeding and (2) obliteration of distal arterial circulation. The latter can be confirmed by assessing for the absence of a distal pulse by palpation (e.g., in field settings), Doppler ultrasound, or using cuff pressures of 20% above systolic pressure (e.g., using a pressure-controlled pneumatic tourniquet). Blood pressure cuffs and improvised tourniquets offer suboptimal performance and should be avoided in tourniquet management of traumatic injuries. Improvised devices as tourniquets are shown to be less effective than commercial devices and should not be relied upon [56].

An injured extremity with a tourniquet in situ can draw significant attention upon arrival to the Emergency Department. The temptation for early release of a tourniquet should be resisted and focus shifted to the usual ATLS© approach to trauma care. Release of an extremity tourniquet should only be attempted once a primary survey is complete and adequate resuscitation, including reliable vascular access, access to surgical support, and blood products, is available. Clean dressings, hemostatic gauze, and suturing supplies should be present. Hasty release of tourniquets can exacerbate blood loss, and removal should follow a controlled and planned approach. Of note, the tourniquet should remain on the limb—not be cut or removed—in preparation for tightening if hemorrhage recurs. The time of tourniquet release should be documented. Further, removal after prolonged occlusion can be accompanied by washout of cellular metabolites such as potassium and lactate, which can contribute to hemodynamic instability or even arrest. Appropriate team communication and preparation can mitigate these physiologic complications.

Many EMS and police departments across North America carry commercial tourniquets, and the use of these devices is becoming more widespread. International programs, such as Stop the Bleed™, are teaching and advocating layperson use of these devices as well [60].

Junctional Tourniquets

The concept of junctional tourniquets is best thought of as a pressure device more so than a true circumferential tourniquet. Junctional tourniquets are a collection of mechanical devices that replace manual pressure for either direct or indirect hemorrhage control in junctional anatomical locations—groin, buttock, axillary, and clavicular regions—in which bleeding is often difficult to control [20]. Several commercial devices available are designed and promoted to free up manual pressure in junctional areas where pressure for temporizing control is needed for field or inter- or intra-hospital transportation to definitive hemorrhage control [19, 28, 29]. These devices, like many novel hemorrhage control devices, are limited by distribution and availability at the point of use, as well as cost. Additionally, there is a paucity of effectiveness data during live patient transport or in the field [61].

Abdominal Aortic Compression.

External compression of the abdominal aorta for control of distal pelvic or junctional groin bleeds has been described using manual techniques and purpose-built devices [61, 62] (Fig. 34.2).

The objective of this technique is to compress the aorta (anterior) against the body of the spine (posterior) to occlude distal flow and hemorrhage. Successful manual occlusion of the aorta through trans-abdominal pressure has been demonstrated [63]. An attendant can apply fists or a knee to the mid-abdomen in order to compress the aorta between the fists/knee and the vertebral bodies to achieve aortic occlusion [62]. This technique has been successfully simulated in a mannequin model, sustaining pressure up to 20 minutes, but it could not consistently be sustained during patient transport [64].

Several commercial devices are in use in military and prehospital settings and have been successfully deployed in prehospital settings. Duration of occlusion data suggests that a "balloon-time" of external compression target maximum of 60 minutes is supported, and occlusion times beyond 1 hour are associated with intra-abdominal organ injury [65, 66]. These abdominal aortic tourniquets are currently in use in military medical systems and may be encountered in arriving trauma patients as availability and data supporting use expand [67].

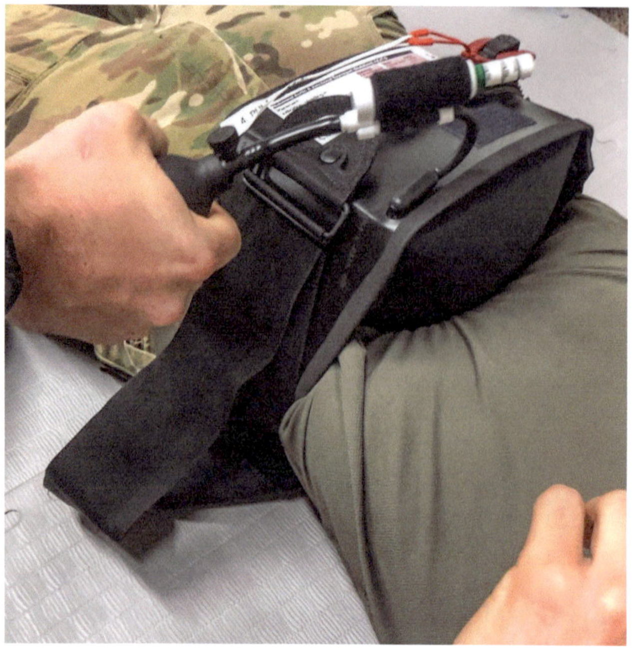

Fig. 34.2 Abdominal aortic tourniquet in training use. (S.Cowan, Personal File Photo)

Hemostatic Agents

Hemostatic agents are useful adjuncts that can aid in tamponade and accelerate hemostasis for accessible hemorrhagic injuries [68]. Despite the availability of many hemostatic agents, not all have applications in trauma resuscitation, due to practical and logistic limitations. Conceptually, hemostatic agents function through one or more of three main mechanisms: (1) mechanical tamponade or sealing, (2) concentration of clotting factors, and (3) initiating/accelerating the clotting cascade. These agents can be categorized into five general types: topical, chemical, physiologic, dressings, and adhesives. In trauma resuscitation, hemostatic dressings have the broadest applicability. The applicability of select agents in each category for use during trauma resuscitation is described below. The utilization of hemostatic agents should be viewed as an adjunct to effective pressure, packing, and surgical technique in order to control bleeding. These agents are ineffective stand-alone agents and should be used in conjunction with traditional hemorrhage control methods [69].

Topical Hemostatic Agents

Topical agents are further sub-categorized by agent or mechanism (see Table 34.2) [68]. Most topical agents are marketed and deployed for specific surgical indications and have limited use in trauma resuscitation outside of the operating room. However, some of the larger forms of mechanical agents, including porcine gelatin (e.g., Gelfoam) and oxidized regenerated cellulose (ORC) compounds (e.g., Surgicel), can be helpful for local control of non-massive hemorrhage. Of important note, ORC-based agents create a local acidic environment and are not compatible in conjunction with thrombin-based agents, which are denatured in the local acidity created by the ORC [70].

Chemical Hemostatics

Chemical hemostatics use a caustic agent such as silver nitrate to induce coagulation. The use of these agents is limited to minor, nuisance bleeding and are of limited clinical applicability in massive traumatic hemorrhage control [71].

Physiologic Hemostatics

Physiologic hemostatics aim to optimize or replace clotting factors through enhancing vasoconstriction at the site of bleeding, either systemically or locally. These can include topical epinephrine and topical tranexamic acid [72, 73].

Hemostatic Dressings

Hemostatic agents combine the advantages of various procoagulant mechanisms with a delivery method utilizing gauze packing technique. These are advantageous for non-operative hemorrhage control as they are packaged in convenient delivery systems, including gauze impregnation, expanding sponges, powder, and powder-directing applicators. Expanding sponges (e.g., XStat) function through rapidly expanding small sponges packed into a bleeding wound cavity, and the expansion mechanically tamponades bleeding [74]. Mineral agents utilizing zeolite absorb moisture, thus concentrating clotting factors at the site of application [75]. Kaolin agents promote clot formation through cascade activation and are delivered in powder or gauze form. These agents rely upon intrinsic clotting mechanisms and have reduced efficacy in coagulopathic states [76]. By contrast, the mucoadhesive dressing agents function through negative ionic charges, which bind to blood components at the site of injury, binding the dressing to the tissue, and as such, do not inherently rely on the functional clotting cascade for their performance and can be more effective in coagulopathic patients [77]. Of note, in cases with significant bleeding, these agents require tight packing to mechanically slow and/or tamponade the bleed temporarily plus application of manual pressure to maximize effectiveness. (Table 34.3)

A Note on Wound Packing

While packing for temporary hemorrhage control is well established for abdominal and pelvic hemorrhage in the operative setting, packing of extremity and junctional hemorrhage during trauma resuscitation outside the OR remains an underrated technique. The previously mentioned hemostatic dressings are useful adjuncts, but effective packing of an actively bleeding wound cavity remains a key skill for temporary control [78]. Recognition of this life-saving technique is highlighted by the inclusion of wound packing in the layperson trauma training course, Stop The Bleed™, devel-

Table 34.2 Select hemostatic agents and common areas of non-trauma use

Select topical hemostatic agents	
	Common non-trauma uses
Mechanical (passive) agents Bone wax Porcine Gelatin (e.g., Gelfoam, Surgifoam) Oxidized regenerated cellulose (e.g., Surgicel, WoundClot) Bovine collagen (e.g., Avitine) Polysaccharide spheres (e.g., arista, PerClot)	ENT, orthopedics General and colorectal procedures
Active agents Bovine thrombin Human pooled thrombin Recombinant thrombin.	Neurosurgery Cardiac surgery
Flowable agents Bovine Gelatin and human pooled thrombin (i.e., Flowseal) Porcine gelatin and human thrombin (i.e., Surgiflo)	Cardiac surgery Vascular surgery ENT surgery
Sealants Fibrin and thrombin combinations (i.e., Tisseel, Evicel, Hemopatch)	Vascular surgery Neurosurgery

Table 34.3 Select hemostatic dressings

Select hemostatic dressings
Mineral factor concentrators (zeolite)
Kaolin (combat gauze)
Chitosan (HemCon, Celox)
Expanding sponges (XStat)

oped with the American College of Surgeons Committee on Trauma [79]. Recent military combat experience has also shown a significant benefit of this temporizing skill [80]. Principles of effective packing include filling the cavity and packing it as tightly as possible. Once performed, firm pressure should be maintained for at least 10 minutes; this can potentially be reduced with the use of a hemostatic dressing as packing material [81]. A roll of simple gauze can be a powerful and inexpensive hemorrhage control tool. Videos demonstrating effective wound packing as per the Stop The Bleed™ approach are accessible online as both learning and teaching tools.

Intra-abdominal Foam

Intra-abdominal hemorrhage has traditionally been addressed via surgical and/or radiologic intervention. However, interest in temporizing and portable measures has led to the exploration of various intra-abdominal foams and compounds to arrest intra-abdominal bleeding [82, 83]. Initial research using these products has shown promise, improving survival from intra-abdominal hemorrhage in animal models [84]. A major challenge in advancing this technology is the subsequent need to remove the agent from the abdomen.

Several clinical trials are ongoing with products such as rescue foam and clot form [82]. These agents spread through the intra-abdominal cavity and stimulate the initiation of clotting in addition to providing mechanical tapenade. While not yet approved, this technology could theoretically shift the survival curve; previously non-survivable hemorrhage could be temporized to allow for transport and/or mobilization of resources required for definitive hemorrhage control [85]. Additional research in in vivo and clinical models is required.

Summary

Advancements in technologies have expanded the toolbox for hemorrhage control. Endovascular aortic control via REBOA has applications for trauma and non-trauma hemorrhage when appropriately introduced within a system. Other endovascular approaches, novel techniques, devices, and hemostatic agents are now part of the trauma resuscitationists' toolbox. Familiarity with a breadth of hemorrhage control options allows the trauma team to initiate hemorrhage control and mobilize appropriate resources to optimize patient care locally.

Key Points

- REBOA implementation within a healthcare and/or hospital system requires a thoughtful, multidisciplinary approach.
- Zone 1 aortic occlusion should be less than 30 minutes, and zone 3 aortic occlusion should be less than 60 minutes.
- Tourniquets are life-saving in field settings and have utility in select in-hospital indications.
- Novel devices exist for direct and indirect compression and control of hemorrhage for pelvic and junctional bleeding.
- Hemostatic agents can serve as adjuncts to direct pressure and packing for initial hemorrhage management.

References

1. Kauvar D, Lefering R, Wade C. Impact of hemorrhage on trauma outcome: an overview of epidemiology, clinical presentations, and therapeutic considerations. J Trauma. 2006;60(6 Suppl):S3–S11. https://doi.org/10.1097/01.ta.0000199961.02677.19.
2. Kelly J, Ritenour A, McLaughlin D, et al. Injury severity and causes of death from operation iraqi freedom and operation enduring freedom: 2003–2004 versus 2006. J Trauma. 2008;64(2 Suppl):S21–7. https://doi.org/10.1097/TA.0b013e318160b9fb.
3. Schreiber MA. The beginning of the end for damage control surgery. Br J Surg. 2012;99(S1):10–1. https://doi.org/10.1002/bjs.7773.
4. Klein MK, Tsihlis ND, Pritts TA, Kibbe MR. Emerging therapies for prehospital control of hemorrhage. J Surg Res. 2020;248:182–90. https://doi.org/10.1016/j.jss.2019.09.070.
5. Morrison JJ, Rasmussen TE. Noncompressible torso hemorrhage: a review with contemporary definitions and management strategies. Surg Clin North Am. 2012;92(4):843–58. https://doi.org/10.1016/j.suc.2012.05.002.
6. Holcomb J, Caruso J, McMullin N, et al. Causes of death in US special operations forces in the global war on terrorism: 2001-2004. US Army Med Dep J. 2007:24–37.
7. Moore LJ, Martin CD, Harvin JA, Wade CE, Holcomb JB. Resuscitative endovascular balloon occlusion of the aorta for control of noncompressible truncal hemorrhage in the abdomen and pelvis. Am J Surg. 2016;212(6):1222–30. https://doi.org/10.1016/j.amjsurg.2016.09.027.
8. HUGHES CW. Use of an intra-aortic balloon catheter tamponade for controlling intra-abdominal hemorrhage in man. Surgery. 1954;36(1):65–8.
9. Malina M, Holst J. Balloon control for ruptured AAAs: when and when not to use? J Cardiovasc Surg. 2014;55(2):161–7.
10. Rasmussen TE, Dubose JJ, Asensio JA, et al. Tourniquets, vascular shunts, and endovascular technologies: esoteric or essential? A report from the 2011 AAST military liaison panel. J Trauma Acute Care Surg. 2012;73(1):282–5. https://doi.org/10.1097/TA.0b013e3182569df4.
11. Villamaria CY, Eliason JL, Napolitano LM, Stansfield RB, Spencer JR, Rasmussen TE. Endovascular skills for trauma and

resuscitative surgery (ESTARS) course: curriculum development, content validation, and program assessment. J Trauma Acute Care Surg. 2014;76(4):929–36. https://doi.org/10.1097/TA.0000000000000164.
12. Teeter WA, Matsumoto J, Idoguchi K, et al. Smaller introducer sheaths for REBOA may be associated with fewer complications. J Trauma Acute Care Surg. 2016;81(6):1039–45. https://doi.org/10.1097/TA.0000000000001143.
13. Brenner ML, Moore LJ, DuBose JJ, et al. A clinical series of resuscitative endovascular balloon occlusion of the aorta for hemorrhage control and resuscitation. J Trauma Acute Care Surg. 2013;75(3):506–11. https://doi.org/10.1097/TA.0b013e31829e5416.
14. Matsumura Y, Matsumoto J, Kondo H, et al. Early arterial access for resuscitative endovascular balloon occlusion of the aorta is related to survival outcome in trauma. J Trauma Acute Care Surg. 2018;85(3):507–11. https://doi.org/10.1097/TA.0000000000002004.
15. Manzano-Nunez R, McGreevy D, Orlas CP, et al. Outcomes and management approaches of resuscitative endovascular balloon occlusion of the aorta based on the income of countries. World J Emerg Surg. 2020;15(1):1–57. https://doi.org/10.1186/s13017-020-00337-w.
16. Teeter W, Romagnoli A, Glaser J, et al. Resuscitative endovascular balloon occlusion of the aorta: pushing care forward. J Spec Oper Med. 2017;17(1):17–21.
17. Fisher AD, Teeter WA, Cordova CB, et al. The role I resuscitation team and resuscitative endovascular balloon occlusion of the aorta. J Spec Oper Med. 2017;17(2):65–73.
18. Sadek S, Lockey DJ, Lendrum R, Perkins Z, Price J, Davies GE. Resuscitative endovascular balloon occlusion of the aorta (REBOA) in the pre-hospital setting: an additional resuscitation option for uncontrolled catastrophic haemorrhage. Resuscitation. 2016;107:135–8. https://doi.org/10.1016/j.resuscitation.2016.06.029.
19. Lamhaut L, Qasim Z, Hutin A, et al. First description of successful use of zone 1 resuscitative endovascular balloon occlusion of the aorta in the prehospital setting. Resuscitation. 2018;133:e1–2. https://doi.org/10.1016/j.resuscitation.2018.07.027.
20. Vernamonti JP, Holcomb J, Mick NW, et al. 'Step up' approach to the application of REBOA technology in a rural trauma system. Trauma Surg Acute Care Open. 2019;4(1):e000335. https://doi.org/10.1136/tsaco-2019-000335.
21. Beldowicz BC, Galante JM. Resuscitative endovascular balloon occlusion of the aorta in inter-hospital transfers. J Endovasc Resuscit Trauma Manage. 2018;2(1):44. https://doi.org/10.26676/jevtm.v2i1.40.
22. Power A, Parekh A, Scallan O, et al. Size matters: first-in-human study of a novel 4 french REBOA device. Trauma Surg Acute Care Open. 2021;6(1):e000617. https://doi.org/10.1136/tsaco-2020-000617.
23. Brenner M, Hoehn M, Pasley J, Dubose J, Stein D, Scalea T. Basic endovascular skills for trauma course: bridging the gap between endovascular techniques and the acute care surgeon. J Trauma Acute Care Surg. 2014;77(2):286–91. https://doi.org/10.1097/TA.0000000000000310.
24. Basic endovascular skills for trauma (BEST©) course. American College of Surgeons Committee on Trauma; 2015.
25. Stannard A, Eliason JL, Rasmussen TE. Resuscitative endovascular balloon occlusion of the aorta (REBOA) as an adjunct for hemorrhagic shock. J Trauma. 2011;71(6):1869–72. https://doi.org/10.1097/TA.0b013e31823fe90c.
26. Romagnoli A, Teeter W, Pasley J, et al. Time to aortic occlusion: It's all about access. J Trauma Acute Care Surg. 2017;83(6):1161–4. https://doi.org/10.1097/TA.0000000000001665.
27. DuBose JJ, Scalea TM, Brenner M, et al. The AAST prospective aortic occlusion for resuscitation in trauma and acute care surgery (AORTA) registry: data on contemporary utilization and outcomes of aortic occlusion and resuscitative balloon occlusion of the aorta (REBOA). J Trauma Acute Care Surg. 2016;81(3):409–19. https://doi.org/10.1097/TA.0000000000001079.
28. Hilbert-Carius P, McGreevy D, Abu-Zidan FM, Hörer TM. Registry research group. Successfully REBOA performance: does medical specialty matter? International data from the ABOTrauma registry. World J Emerg Surgery. 2020;15(1):1–62. https://doi.org/10.1186/s13017-020-00342-z.
29. Osborn LA, Brenner ML, Prater SJ, Moore LJ. Resuscitative endovascular balloon occlusion of the aorta: current evidence. Open Access Emerg Med. 2019;11:29–38.
30. Zakaluzny SA, Beldowicz BC, Salcedo ES, DuBose JJ, Moore LJ, Brenner M. Guidelines for a system-wide multidisciplinary approach to institutional resuscitative endovascular balloon occlusion of the aorta implementation. J Trauma Acute Care Surg. 2019;86(2):337–43. https://doi.org/10.1097/TA.0000000000002138.
31. ER-REBOATM PLUS catheter quick reference guide. Prytime Medical.
32. Ogura T, Lefor AK, Nakamura M, Fujizuka K, Shiroto K, Nakano M. Ultrasound-guided resuscitative endovascular balloon occlusion of the aorta in the resuscitation area. J Emerg Med. 2017;52(5):715–22. https://doi.org/10.1016/j.jemermed.2017.01.014.
33. Bulger EM, Perina DG, Qasim Z, et al. Clinical use of resuscitative endovascular balloon occlusion of the aorta (REBOA) in civilian trauma systems in the USA, 2019: a joint statement from the american college of surgeons committee on trauma, the american college of emergency physicians, the national association of emergency medical services physicians and the national association of emergency medical technicians. Trauma Surg Acute Care Open. 2019;4(1):e000376. https://doi.org/10.1136/tsaco-2019-000376.
34. Morrison JJ, Morrison JJ, Galgon RE, et al. A systematic review of the use of resuscitative endovascular balloon occlusion of the aorta in the management of hemorrhagic shock. J Trauma Acute Care Surg. 2016;80(2):324–34. https://doi.org/10.1097/TA.0000000000000913.
35. van der Burg Boudewijn LS, Borger HTM, Eefting D, et al. Vascular access training for REBOA placement. J R Army Med Corps. 2019;165(3):147:147.
36. Borger van der Burg BLS, Kessel B, DuBose JJ, Hörer TM, Hoencamp R. Consensus on resuscitative endovascular balloon occlusion of the aorta: a first consensus paper using a delphi method. Injury. 2019;50(6):1186–91. https://doi.org/10.1016/j.injury.2019.04.024.
37. Parra MW, Ordoñez C, Rezende-Neto JB, Brenner ML, Rasmussen TE, Orlas C. Resuscitative endovascular balloon occlusion of the aorta consensus: the panamerican experience. Panamerican J Trauma Crit Care Emerg Surg. 2018;7(3):171–82. https://doi.org/10.5005/jp-journals-10030-1221.
38. Bradley NL, Leeper RJ, Roberts DJ, Ball CG, Beckett A, Engels P, Joos E, Khwaja K, Kirkpatrick A, Lampron J, Minor S, Parry N, Rezende Neto JB, Widder S, Ahmad N, Gomez D, Kim MJ, Murphy PB, Rice TJ, Vogt K. Resuscitative Endovascular Balloon Occlusion of the Aorta: a context-specific consensus statement from the Canadian Collaborative for Urgent Care Surgery (CANUCS). Can J Surg. 2022;65(3):310–6.
39. Bekdache O, Paradis T, Shen YBH, et al. Resuscitative endovascular balloon occlusion of the aorta (REBOA): a scoping review protocol concerning indications—advantages and challenges of implementation in traumatic non-compressible torso haemor-

rhage. BMJ Open. 2019;9(2):e027572. https://doi.org/10.1136/bmjopen-2018-027572.
40. Theodorou CM, Salcedo ES, DuBose JJ, Galante JM. Hate to burst your balloon: successful REBOA use takes more than a course. J Endovasc Resuscit Trauma Manage. 2020;4(1):21–9. https://doi.org/10.26676/jevtm.v4i1.106.
41. Russo RM, White JM, Baer DG. Partial resuscitative endovascular balloon occlusion of the aorta: a systematic review of the preclinical and clinical literature. J Surg Res. 2021 Jun;262:101–14. https://doi.org/10.1016/j.jss.2020.12.054.
42. DuBose JJ. How I do it partial resuscitative endovascular balloon occlusion of the aorta (P-REBOA). J Trauma Acute Care Surg. 2017;83(1):197–9. https://doi.org/10.1097/TA.0000000000001462.
43. Junior R, Marcelo AF, Feng CYD, Nguyen ATM, et al. The complications associated with resuscitative endovascular balloon occlusion of the aorta (REBOA). World J Emerg Surg. 2018;13(1):20. https://doi.org/10.1186/s13017-018-0181-6.
44. JOINT TRAUMA SYSTEM CLINICAL PRACTICE GUIDELINE. Resuscitative endovascular balloon occlusion of the aorta (REBOA) for hemorrhagic shock (CPG ID:38). https://jts.amedd.army.mil/assets/docs/cpgs/JTS_Clinical_Practice_Guidelines_(CPGs)/REBOA_%20Hemorrhagic_Shock_31_Mar_2020_ID38.pdf. Updated 2020.
45. Madurska MJ, McLenithan A, Scalea TM, Kundi R, White JM, Morrison JJ, DuBose JJ. A feasibility study of partial REBOA data in a high-volume trauma center. Eur J Trauma Emerg Surg. 2022;48(1):299–305. https://doi.org/10.1007/s00068-020-01561-4.
46. Kuckelman J, Derickson M, Barron M, et al. Efficacy of intermittent versus standard resuscitative endovascular balloon occlusion of the aorta in a lethal solid organ injury model. J Trauma Acute Care Surg. 2019;87(1):9–17. https://doi.org/10.1097/TA.0000000000002307.
47. Kuckelman JP, Barron M, Moe D, et al. Extending the golden hour for zone 1 resuscitative endovascular balloon occlusion of the aorta: improved survival and reperfusion injury with intermittent versus continuous resuscitative endovascular balloon occlusion of the aorta of the aorta in a porcine severe truncal hemorrhage model. J Trauma Acute Care Surg. 2018;85(2):318–26. https://doi.org/10.1097/TA.0000000000001964.
48. Johnson MA, Hoareau GL, Beyer CA, et al. Not ready for prime time: intermittent versus partial resuscitative endovascular balloon occlusion of the aorta for prolonged hemorrhage control in a highly lethal porcine injury model. J Trauma Acute Care Surg. 2020;88(2):298–304.
49. Wikström MB, Krantz J, Hörer TM, Nilsson KF. Resuscitative endovascular balloon occlusion of the inferior vena cava is made hemodynamically possible by concomitant endovascular balloon occlusion of the aorta-a porcine study. J Trauma Acute Care Surg. 2020;88(1):160–8.
50. Reynolds CL, Celio AC, Bridges LC, et al. REBOA for the IVC? Resuscitative balloon occlusion of the inferior vena cava (REBOVC) to abate massive hemorrhage in retrohepatic vena cava injuries. J Trauma Acute Care Surg. 2017;83(6):1041–6.
51. Sano H, Tsurukiri J, Hoshiai A, Oomura T, Tanaka Y, Ohta S. Resuscitative endovascular balloon occlusion of the aorta for uncontrollable nonvariceal upper gastrointestinal bleeding. World J Emerg Surg. 2016;11(1):20. https://doi.org/10.1186/s13017-016-0076-3.
52. Brenner M, Teeter W, Hoehn M, et al. Use of resuscitative endovascular balloon occlusion of the aorta for proximal aortic control in patients with severe hemorrhage and arrest. JAMA Surg. 2017;153(2):130–5. https://doi.org/10.1001/jamasurg.2017.3549.
53. Kragh J, John F, Swan KG, Smith DC, Mabry RL, Blackbourne LH. Review: historical review of emergency tourniquet use to stop bleeding. Am J Surg. 2012;203:242–52. https://doi.org/10.1016/j.amjsurg.2011.01.028.
54. Scerbo MH, Holcomb JB, Taub E, et al. The trauma center is too late: major limb trauma without a pre-hospital tourniquet has increased death from hemorrhagic shock. J Trauma Acute Care Surg. 2017;83(6):1165–72. https://doi.org/10.1097/TA.0000000000001666.
55. Passos E, Dingley B, Smith A, et al. Tourniquet use for peripheral vascular injuries in the civilian setting. Injury. 2014;45(3):573–7. https://doi.org/10.1016/j.injury.2013.11.031.
56. King DR, Larentzakis A, Ramly EP. Tourniquet use at the Boston marathon bombing: lost in translation. J Trauma Acute Care Surg. 2015;78(3):594–9. https://doi.org/10.1097/TA.0000000000000561.
57. Sharma JP, Salhotra R. Tourniquets in orthopedic surgery. Indian J Orthop. 2012;46(4):377–83. https://doi.org/10.4103/0019-5413.98824.
58. Kragh J, Baer D, Walters T. Extended (16-hour) tourniquet application after combat wounds: a case report and review of the current literature. J Orthop Trauma. 2007;21(4):274–8. https://doi.org/10.1097/BOT.0b013e3180437dd9.
59. Kragh J, John F., Dubick MA. Battlefield tourniquets: lessons learned in moving current care toward best care in an army medical department at war. USArmy Medical Department Journal; 2016, p. 29–36.
60. Callaway DW, MD, FACEP. Translating tactical combat casualty care lessons learned to the high-threat civilian setting: tactical emergency casualty care and the Hartford consensus. Wilderness Environ Med. 2017;28(2):S140–5.
61. Smith S, White J, Wanis KN, Beckett A, McAlister VC, Hilsden R. The effectiveness of junctional tourniquets: a systematic review and meta-analysis. J Trauma Acute Care Surg. 2019;86(3):532–9. https://doi.org/10.1097/TA.0000000000002159.
62. Douma MJ, Picard C, O'Dochartaigh D, Brindley PG. Proximal external aortic compression for life-threatening abdominal-pelvic and junctional hemorrhage: an ultrasonographic study in adult volunteers. Prehosp Emerg Care. 2019;23(4):538–42. https://doi.org/10.1080/10903127.2018.1532477.
63. Temporizing life-threatening abdominal-pelvic hemorrhage using proprietary devices, manual pressure, or a single knee: an integrative review of proximal external aortic compression and even "knee BOA". J Spec Oper Med. 2020;20(2):110–4.
64. Douma MJ, O'Dochartaigh D, Brindley PG. Bi-manual proximal external aortic compression after major abdominal-pelvic trauma and during ambulance transfer: a simulation study. Injury. 2016;48(1):26–31. https://doi.org/10.1016/j.injury.2016.11.003.
65. Mattias G, Andreas B. Reply to letter: Kheirabadi, et al. Long-term consequences of abdominal aortic and junctional tourniquet for hemorrhage control. J Trauma Acute Care Surg. 2019;87(3):741. https://doi.org/10.1097/TA.0000000000002361.
66. Rall JM, Ross JD, Clemens MS, Cox JM, Buckley TA, Morrison JJ. Hemodynamic effects of the abdominal aortic and junctional tourniquet in a hemorrhagic swine model. J Surg Res. 2017;212:159–66. https://doi.org/10.1016/j.jss.2017.01.020.
67. Handford C, Parker PJ. The potential use of the abdominal aortic junctional tourniquet® in a military population: a review of requirement, effectiveness, and usability. J Spec Oper Med. 2019;19(4):74–9.
68. Tompeck AJ, Gajdhar AUR, Dowling M, et al. A comprehensive review of topical hemostatic agents: the good, the bad, and the novel. J Trauma Acute Care Surg. 2020;88(1):e1–e21. https://doi.org/10.1097/TA.0000000000002508.
69. Chiara O, Cimbanassi S, Bellanova G, et al. A systematic review on the use of topical hemostats in trauma and emergency surgery. BMC Surg. 2018;18(1):68. https://doi.org/10.1186/s12893-018-0398-z.
70. Miller JM, Jackson DA, Collier CS. An investigation of the chemical reactions of oxidized regenerated cellulose. Exp Med Surg. 1961;19:196–201.

71. Howe N, Cherpelis B. Obtaining rapid and effective hemostasis: part I. Update and review of topical hemostatic agents. J Am Acad Dermatol. 2013;69(5):659.e1–659.e17. https://doi.org/10.1016/j.jaad.2013.07.014.
72. Palm MD, Altman JS. Topical hemostatic agents: a review. Dermatologic Surg. 2008;34(4):431–45. https://doi.org/10.1111/j.1524-4725.2007.34090.x.
73. Roberts I, Shakur H, Afolabi A, et al. The importance of early treatment with tranexamic acid in bleeding trauma patients: an exploratory analysis of the CRASH-2 randomised controlled trial. Lancet (British edition). 2011;377(9771):1096–1101.e2. https://doi.org/10.1016/S0140-6736(11)60278-X.
74. Warriner Z, Lam L, Matsushima K, et al. Initial evaluation of the efficacy and safety of in-hospital expandable hemostatic minisponge use in penetrating trauma. J Trauma Acute Care Surg. 2019;86(3):424–30. https://doi.org/10.1097/TA.0000000000002091.
75. Alam H, Chen Z, Jaskille A, et al. Application of a zeolite hemostatic agent achieves 100% survival in a lethal model of complex groin injury in swine. J Trauma. 2004;56(5):974–83. https://doi.org/10.1097/01.TA.0000127763.90890.31.
76. Boulton AJ, Lewis CT, Naumann DN, Midwinter MJ. Prehospital haemostatic dressings for trauma: a systematic review. Emerg Med J. 2018;35(7):449–57. https://doi.org/10.1136/emermed-2018-207523.
77. Khoshmohabat H, Paydar S, Kazemi HM, Dalfardi B. Overview of agents used for emergency hemostasis. Trauma Mon. 2016;21(1):e26023. https://doi.org/10.5812/traumamon.26023.
78. Picard C. Hemorrhage control, a fundamental skill: a review of direct pressure, dressings, wound packing and bandages for life-saving. Can J Emerg Nurs. 2020;40(2):26–8. https://doi.org/10.29173/cjen76.
79. Zwislewski A, Nanassy AD, Meyer LK, et al. Practice makes perfect: the impact of stop the bleed training on hemorrhage control knowledge, wound packing, and tourniquet application in the workplace. Injury. 2019;50(4):864–8. https://doi.org/10.1016/j.injury.2019.03.025.
80. Savage E, Forestier C, Withers N, Tien H, Pannell D. Tactical combat casualty care in the Canadian forces: lessons learned from the afghan war. Can J Surg. 2011;54:S118–23.
81. Pons P, Jacobs L. Save a life: What everyone should know to stop bleeding after an injury. Surg AC o(Ed) Google Sch 2016.
82. Peng HT. Hemostatic agents for prehospital hemorrhage control: a narrative review. Mil Med Res. 2020;7(1):13. https://doi.org/10.1186/s40779-020-00241-z.
83. Chang JC, Holloway BC, Zamisch M, Hepburn MJ, Ling GSF. ResQFoam for the treatment of non-compressible hemorrhage on the front line. Mil Med. 2015;180(9):932–3. https://doi.org/10.7205/MILMED-D-15-00049.
84. Peev MP, Rago A, Hwabejire JO, et al. Self-expanding foam for prehospital treatment of severe intra-abdominal hemorrhage: dose finding study. J Trauma Acute Care Surg. 2014;76(3):619–24. https://doi.org/10.1097/TA.0000000000000126.
85. Rago AP, Sharma U, Sims K, King DR. Conceptualized use of self-expanding foam to rescue special operators from abdominal exsanguination: percutaneous damage control for the forward deployed. J Spec Oper Med. 2015;15(3):39–45.

35 Interventional Radiology in Trauma

Andrew Kiraly, Kris Peet, and Jason Wong

What Is Interventional Radiology

Interventional radiology (IR) is the subspeciality of diagnostic radiology that specializes in performing minimally invasive image-guided procedures. Interventional radiologists (IRs) utilize the image interpretation skills developed from a foundation in diagnostic radiology to navigate difficult-to-access areas of the body percutaneously. The broad spectrum of procedures performed by IRs results in academic centers dividing into two broad domains: (1) body intervention and (2) neuro-intervention. Body interventionalists perform procedures below the thoracic inlet and exclude the spinal cord (but not necessarily the vertebra). Neuro-interventionalists perform procedures on the head, neck, and spinal cord. Broadly speaking, both domains of IR can be divided into vascular and non-vascular procedures. In smaller centers, IRs mainly focus on body procedures but can also perform some neuro IR procedures.

Non-vascular procedures, such as chest tubes, abscess drainage, and stent placement (e.g., biliary or renal), are common requests in the subacute trauma patient. However, in the acute trauma setting, intravascular procedures represent the bulk of IR consultations. It has previously been established that IR is an important part of a modern interdisciplinary trauma team [1, 2]. In this chapter, we will explore the role of IR on the trauma team by outlining the commonly performed procedures with the goal of fostering collaborative patient care and highlighting the willingness of IRs to engage in patient care.

A. Kiraly
Diagnostic Radiology Residency Program, University of Calgary, Calgary, AB, Canada
e-mail: agkiraly@ucalgary.ca

K. Peet
Working in Community Practice, Kamloops, BC, Canada

J. Wong (✉)
Cardiovascular and Interventional Radiology, Foothills Medical Centre, Cumming School of Medicine, University of Calgary, Calgary, AB, Canada
e-mail: jason.wong@ahs.ca

Diagnostic Imaging Workup

As imaging specialists, IRs are comfortable utilizing a broad range of imaging modalities to treat patients; however, in the initial work up of a trauma patient, computed tomography (CT) is the modality of choice due to its high sensitivity (especially with the use of specialized protocols), speed, and accessibility. The goal is to rapidly provide the multidisciplinary trauma team with actionable information for both medical and surgical intervention. In patients with high mechanisms of injury, a "trauma pan-scan" is a common request at our institution which includes non-contrast imaging of the head and cervical spine, followed by arterial phase intravenous contrast-enhanced images of the chest followed by portal venous phase images of the abdomen and pelvis. The thoracic and lumbar spine are extracted retrospectively from the chest, abdomen, and pelvis data. Injury-specific protocols, such as delayed nephrographic phase imaging for renal collecting system injuries or retrograde cystography for suspected bladder injuries with pelvic trauma, can be added to further increase sensitivity (CT scan in trauma is discussed further in Chaps. 46 and 47).

Rapid identification of hemodynamically significant hemorrhage is one of the initial findings to be excluded on a trauma CT. Hemorrhage characterization, including the location, source vessel, and estimation of the volume, is important for the multidisciplinary team to decide the most appropriate service for intervention. Interventional radiology consultation is warranted when bleeding is identified that does not require surgery or in areas where surgery may be difficult. Once an area of bleeding is identified that requires IR, angiography can be performed with the aim of embolization, thus stopping the bleed. Often, multiple bleeding sites are identified on CT, and these can all be treated in the same

L. Marshall Gillman, S. Widder (eds.), *Trauma Team Dynamics*, https://doi.org/10.1007/978-3-031-86312-7_35

setting. Empiric direct angiography is also occasionally performed if the stigmata of hemorrhage are identified on CT but an area of active extravasation is not identified as the sensitivity for small hemorrhage and pseudoaneurysms is higher than on CT [3].

Embolic Therapies

Endovascular embolic therapies are an alternative to surgical treatment for bleeding that is often safer and more effective [4]. Endovascular therapies can also manage bleeding in locations where traditional surgical management is challenging as these therapies can precisely target the site of bleeding, can assess for collateral perfusion, and are not limited by tight spaces [4]. Using real-time angiographic information throughout, the procedure is tailored to the patient, further reducing complications by super-selectively targeting only sites of active bleeding.

Embolic therapies are diverse, and selection of a specific therapy depends on multiple factors including: the size of the vessel to be occluded, how selective the anatomy and clinical situation allow the treatment to be, and whether the affected vessel can be sacrificed [4–6]. For example, specific territories of hepatic arterial supply may be embolized, due to dual supply of liver from both the portal venous system and the hepatic artery supply [4]. Other arteries, such as terminal splanchnic mesenteric territories supplying bowel, do not have collateral supply, and treatments must be focused (superselective) to avoid ischemia of unaffected tissue (i.e., non-target embolization) [4].

Anatomical factors such as vessel size and tortuosity may require the use of microcatheters for access, precluding larger devices, or the course of the catheter may be too tortuous to allow the passage of stiffer devices [4, 6]. In some cases, the need for expedient embolization may prevent taking the time to be completely super-selective [4].

All endovascular procedures including embolic therapies can have complications related to the access site, such as hematoma, pseudoaneurysm, or infection. Target organ complications must also be considered, including organ non-target embolization, end-organ sacrifice, or damage (such as bowel necrosis and bile leak) [4, 6]. Post-embolization syndrome is common when the embolized territory is large but is transient [4]. Post-embolization syndrome is characterized by pain, fever, increased white blood cell count, nausea, and vomiting.

For any embolization procedure, arterial access is the initial step. The femoral artery has been the most common site [5], but brachial or radial access is also often used, especially if anatomical or clinical considerations make femoral access less favorable [5, 7]. Access to the artery is obtained using Seldinger technique, and a vascular sheath is placed to secure access and prevent blood loss from the puncture site [4, 5]. Central arterial lines placed in the initial trauma assessment and resuscitation can be converted to hemostatic sheaths as appropriate to speed access and mitigate risks from puncture [4]. Less common, venous access may be required for embolization, such as pulmonary artery injuries.

Digital subtraction angiography (DSA) is performed usually through an inserted catheter early in the procedure to map the affected anatomy, to plan the approach, and as a baseline for comparison with DSA obtained post-embolization [4–6]. Once DSA has been done, appropriate catheters and microcatheters are used to select target branches for embolization [4, 6]. Catheters are available in a variety of shapes, lengths, and diameters, and guidewires are similarly diverse in diameter, stiffness, shape, and coating. The choice of catheters and wires is based on vascular territory and the anatomy involved [5, 6]. The precise territory to be embolized is selected based on the need for speed (critical bleeding) and precision (end-organs which are particularly sensitive to non-target embolization—i.e., bowel) [4, 6, 7]. In general, a super-selective technique decreases the risk of complications but is often limited by the time required and the relative instability of the patient [5, 7]. In all cases, the embolic agent is only delivered once the catheter or microcatheter is positioned as close to the target area as conditions allow. The specific embolic agent selected will depend on anatomical and clinical factors, as a wide variety of embolic agents and strategies exist.

Gelfoam

Gelfoam is a gelatin product refined from porcine skin [8]. which absorbs up to 45 times its own mass in water, and is often used due to its versatility. Gelfoam is typically sourced in sheets, which can be delivered intravascularly as pledgets of customizable sizes or prepared into a liquid slurry [4, 5, 8]. Preparation methods are diverse, but slurries are generally prepared using contrast media, in order to visualize the agent's progress into vessels under fluoroscopic monitoring [4, 6, 8]. Torpedo-like pledgets are useful for rapid hemostasis and are delivered directly through the catheter; however, a slurry preparation is a more commonly used format as it travels distally in arteries and can deliver more complete hemostasis (Fig. 35.1) [5, 6]. Gelfoam powder is also commercially available, which can be used to achieve maximal

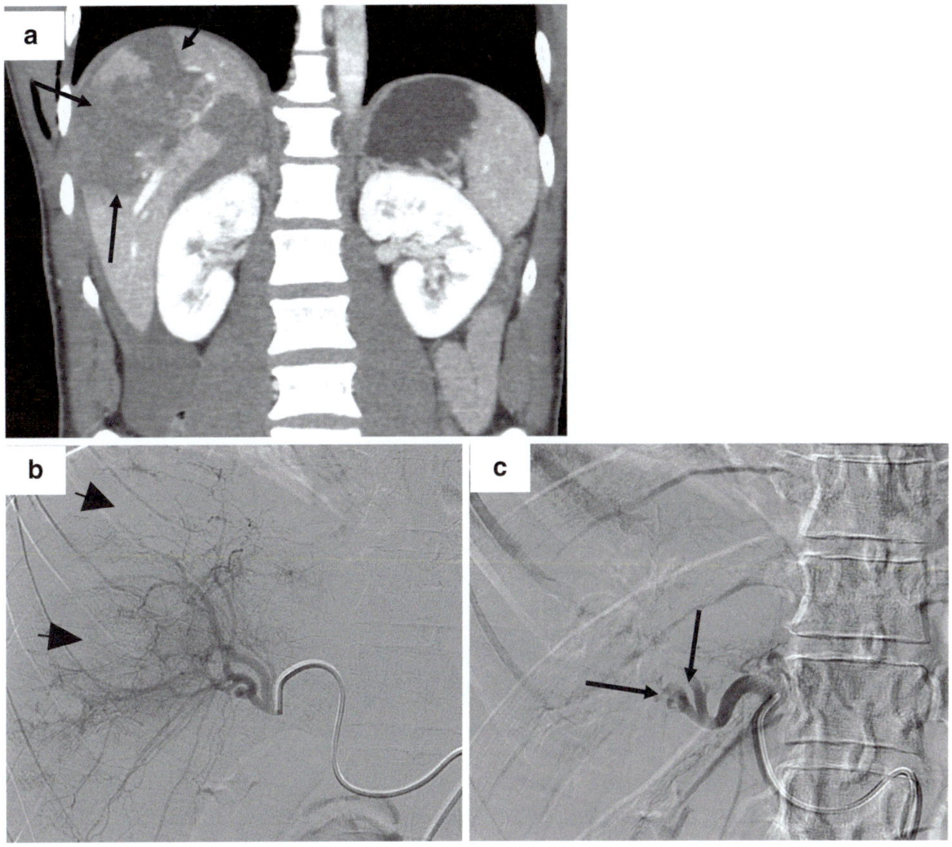

Fig. 35.1 A 37-year-old male pedestrian struck by a vehicle. (**a**) Coronal-enhanced CT demonstrating high-grade traumatic injury of the liver (irregular hypoattenuating regions within the liver; arrows) and (**b**) angiogram with corresponding regions of relative contrast hypoenhancement (arrows). (**c**) Truncated left and right hepatic arteries (arrowheads) demonstrating temporary occlusion of the main hepatic artery with a Gelfoam slurry

distal penetration, but the powder format is less commonly used due to significant increased complications including ulceration and non-target embolization [4–6, 8].

A major advantage of Gelfoam as an embolic agent is that it is considered “temporary” [5]. Expected durations for Gelfoam resorption vary depending on the method of delivery and the amount. Dense embolization can essentially be permanent [5], likely on the basis of a provoked inflammatory reaction [6]; however, more typical administrations of Gelfoam are resorbed in 3–16 weeks [8]. This non-permanent quality is most useful when the clinical conditions preclude a super-selective delivery.

Particles and Spheres

Direct occlusion of arteries can be performed with pre-manufactured polymer embolic agents available in a variety of pre-calibrated sizes. Most commonly, these embolic agents are made of polyvinyl alcohol, although other polymers and gelatin are also used [6]. As in Gelfoam, particle embolics are suspended in contrast media and administered through the catheter and travel distally with arterial blood flow, allowing for embolization of territories considerably more distal than catheters or even microcatheters can reach [6]. As particles are more homogenous in size than Gelfoam, more distal territories can be embolized; however, the ability to deliver particles distally results in the need to take additional care to prevent non-target embolization and significant downstream ischemia [6].

Coils and Plugs

Embolization coils are a precise method of rapid vessel occlusion that can be used when the catheter can be parked at the desired location of embolization [5]. Coils are particularly useful in the case of focal injuries or in cases where an entire arterial territory may be safely embolized (Fig. 35.2) [6]. Coils are generally metallic in construction [4], with either a predetermined shape and size, although entirely malleable coils can be used to fill larger spaces [4]. Structured framing coils with higher radial force are often used as an anchor point, with more malleable coils deployed after these, including coils with attached tiny prothrombotic fibers to fill the vessel lumen, leading to more rapid vessel occlusion [4]. Framing coils are

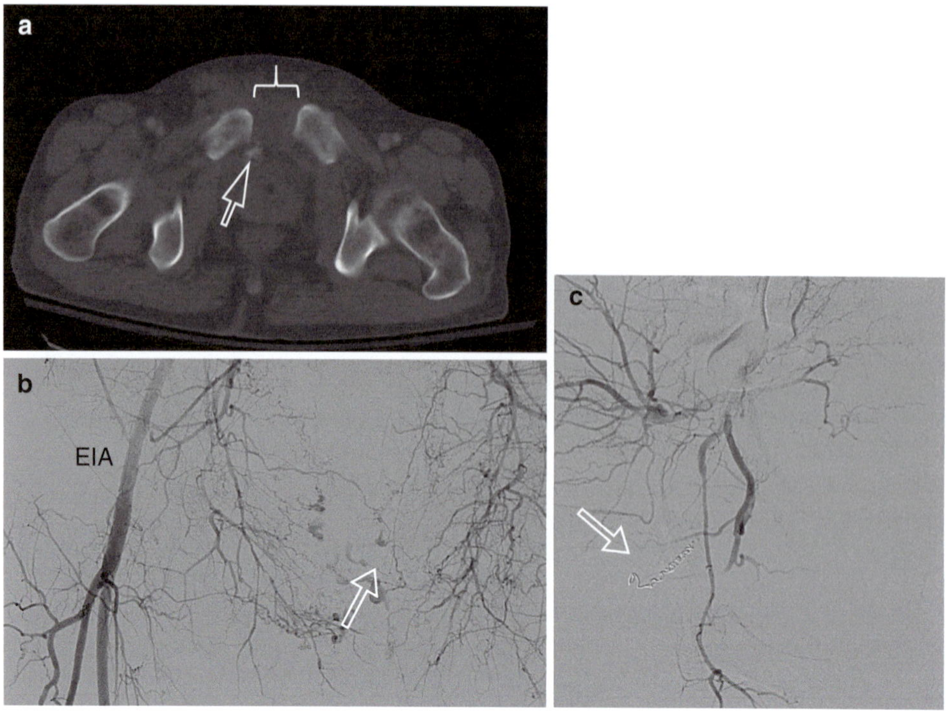

Fig. 35.2 (**a**) Patient with pelvic fractures (not shown) and pubic symphysis diastasis (caliper) with active extravasation of contrast on CT angiogram (open arrow). (**b**) Pseudoaneurysm arising from a deep pelvic branch on digital subtraction angiogram at the corresponding location from the CT (open arrow). (**c**) DSA post embolization demonstrating a coil pack within a pelvic artery (open arrow). EIA = external iliac artery, right

generally sized 10–20% larger than the target vessel diameter to ensure they become firmly seated [7]. Coils are available in sizes suitable for delivery through standard catheters (0.035″) or microcatheters (0.018″), allowing delivery into arterial branches [7]. Additional precision can be achieved by using newer "detachable" coils, which can be retrieved up to the point to final deployment, allowing for repositioning, and which are available in both 0.035″ and 0.018″ formats [7]. Detachable coils are particularly useful in areas with a high risk of coil migration, such as arteriovenous fistulas, pseudoaneurysms, and when embolizing a branch near its origin where adjacent branches must be preserved [1, 5].

Plugs are manufactured devices with three-dimensional structure that are used to rapidly occlude vessels (Fig. 35.3). The construction of plugs is varied and includes a collapsible metallic frame with or without a synthetic membrane which can occlude vessels immediately [6]. Appropriate plug selection/sizing requires consideration both of target artery diameter (measured from planning DSA images) in conjunction with the size of catheter or sheath system used to access the target vessel. Common manufacturer guidelines recommend oversizing the plug by 30–50% [9]. Older plugs needed to be deployed from larger diameter sheaths; newer products can be deployed from catheters (Amplatzer fourth generation) or even microcatheters (MVP). Despite the availability of microcatheter options, the inherent stiffness of the devices can limit their delivery through tortuous vessels, even when microcatheters can safely be delivered to the embolization target.

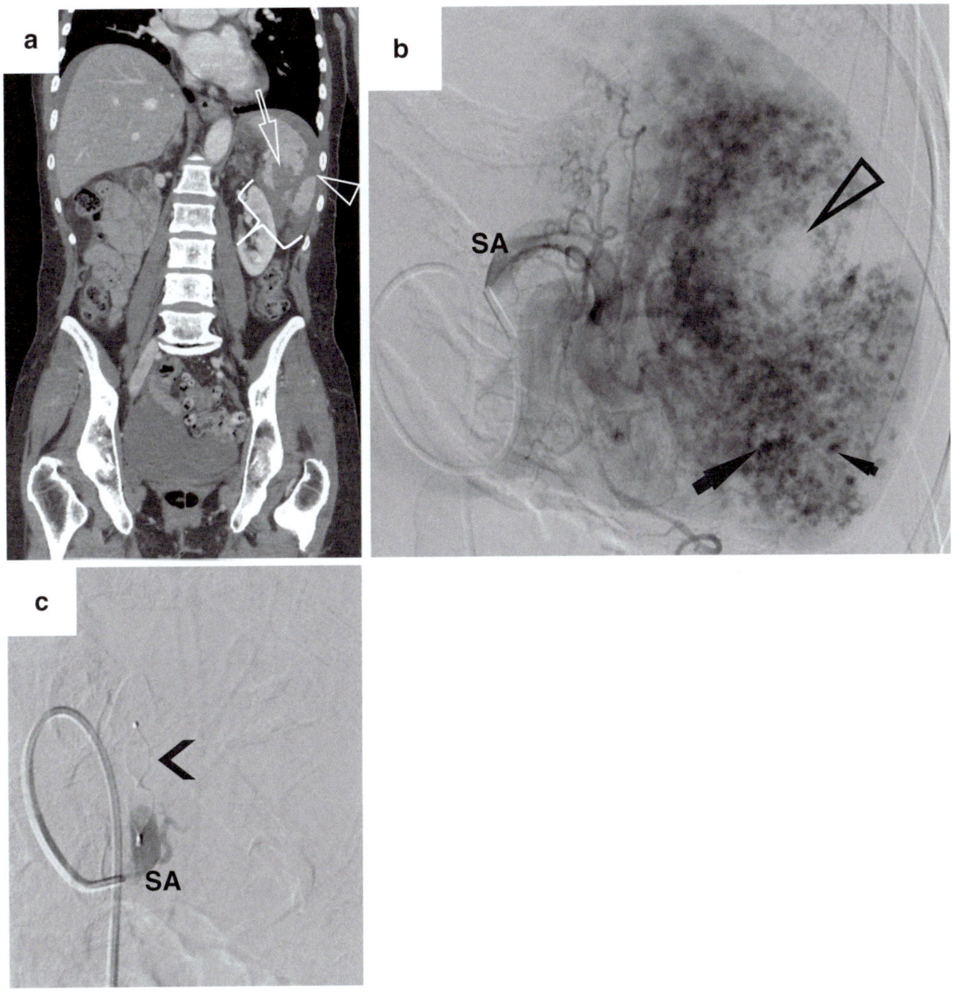

Fig. 35.3 (**a**) Coronal abdominal CT demonstrating traumatic American Association for the Surgery of Trauma (AAST) Grade 5 rupture of the spleen (regions of hypoenhancement; open white arrow) with extension to the splenic capsule (open arrow head) and surrounding perisplenic hematoma (caliper). (**b**) Corresponding DSA demonstrating numerous pseudoaneurysms (solid arrow heads) with perfusion defect representing the large region of capsular rupture (open arrowhead). (**c**) Early phase angiogram demonstrating Amplatzer plug in the splenic artery and complete downstream occlusion (solid chevron). SA splenic artery

Liquid Embolic and Sclerosant Agents

Sclerosing agents including absolute alcohol and sodium tetradecyl sulfate (STS) have been traditional tools for treating arteriovenous malformations (AVMs) and tumors; however, when low flow veins are the target for embolization, especially when the venous target is a network of vessels, sclerosants are a useful agent for embolization. Sclerosants function by causing direct endothelial damage inciting inflammation and fibrosis [6, 7]. These are used with due care as these low viscosity agents are free to travel anywhere delivered and can cause non-target embolization. For this reason, these agents are carefully used in high flow systems with occlusion balloons. In the case of STS, this agent is often administered as a foam prepared with iodinated contrast media. This preparation allows the foam to fill target vessels with a much lower risk of non-target embolization, and to be visualized under fluoroscopy [7]. Occasionally, absolute alcohol is used to sacrifice an entire organ, taking advantage of its propensity to travel distally from the point of administration [4, 6]. These agents are generally not used in the setting of trauma embolization.

Adhesive embolic agents are occasionally used to occlude vessels as they have a propensity to travel distally to the site of administration allowing for deployment in situations where the catheter cannot be advanced all the way to the target. However, this characteristic necessitates extreme care to avoid non-target embolization [4, 6]. The most commonly used agent is cyanoacrylate, which polymerizes upon contact with an ionic solution. This is delivered through a microcatheter after flushing the catheter with a non-ionic solution (D5W is typical), and the adhesive begins to polymerize on contact with the blood in the target vessel [6]. The microcatheter can be withdrawn when the appropriate amount of adhesive has been delivered [6].

A non-adhesive polymer option that can be used is Onyx™ (ethylene vinyl alcohol; Medtronic, USA). Like adhesives, Onyx™ polymerizes on contact with ionic solutions, occluding but not adhering to the vessel [6]. The non-adhesive nature decreases risk of the administration catheter becoming stuck within the vessel. An additional benefit of this agent is its higher viscosity, which can decrease (but not eliminate) non-target embolization [6].

Thrombin, obtained from bovine serum, can be used to directly stimulate thrombosis of contained systems, and is predominantly used in a contained space such as a pseudoaneurysm [7].

Mural Repair

All the embolization techniques described to this point have shared a common characteristic: they rely on sacrificing the vessel to be treated. Thus, they are not suitable when a vessel being treated *must* be preserved. In order to treat a vessel that must be preserved, such as the aorta, central arteries, or the major arteries of the extremities, covered stents are often used [4, 5, 10]. Covered stents are also used in the treatment of pseudoaneurysms when the anatomy is not favorable for coil embolization or thrombin therapy [7]. As with traditional stents, covered stents are constructed of a lattice of metal struts, which either self-expands based on metal memory, or is expanded in place using an angioplasty balloon (Figs. 35.4 and 35.5) [7]. Covered stents however feature an exclusive synthetic membrane which occludes flow into the covered branch or mural defect. Covered stents are deployed quickly and typically occlude the site of bleeding immediately with little chance of becoming displaced and occluding non-target vessels. As such, they are often used as the treatment of choice for large vessel injuries, such as in the aorta (Fig. 35.6) [11].

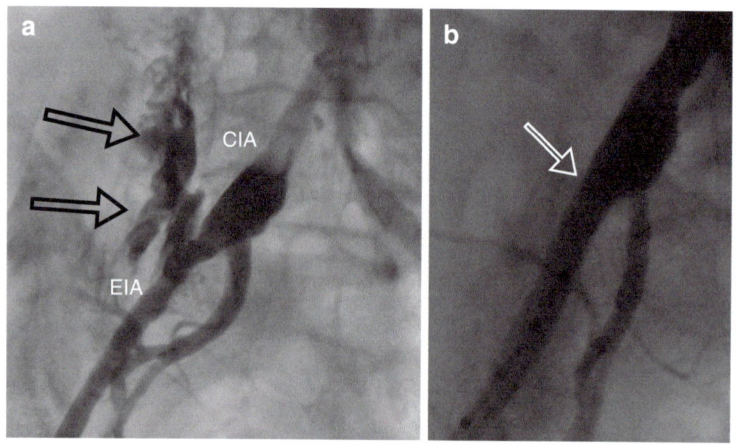

Fig. 35.4 (**a**) Iatrogenic injury of external iliac artery immediately peripheral to the bifurcation with brisk active contrast extravasation (arrows). (**b**) Covered stent within the external iliac with cessation of extravasation (open white arrow). CIA common iliac artery, EIA external iliac artery

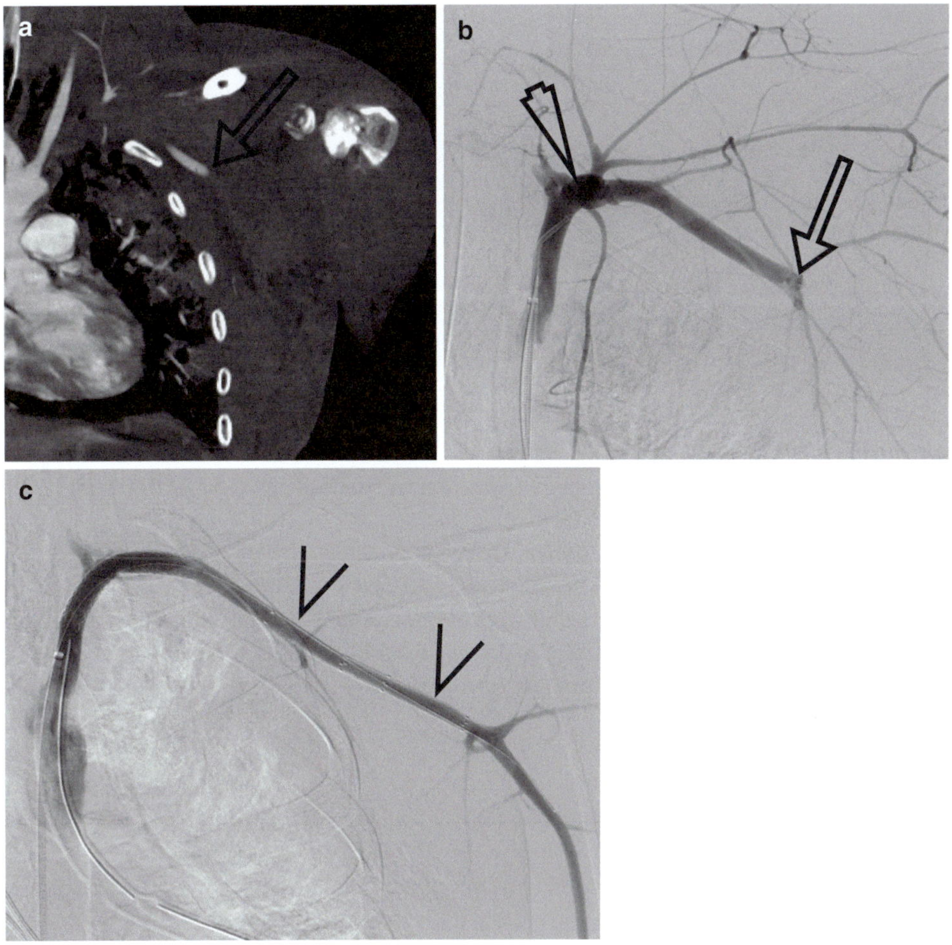

Fig. 35.5 (**a**) Coronal CTA demonstrating traumatic injury with resultant abrupt occlusion of the left subclavian artery (arrow). (**b**) Angiogram demonstrating proximal mural injury within the subclavian (focal luminal outpouching; arrowhead) and the abrupt occlusion of the axillary artery distally (arrow). (**c**) Subsequent angiogram demonstrating multiple covered stents in the subclavian and axillary arteries (solid arrow heads)

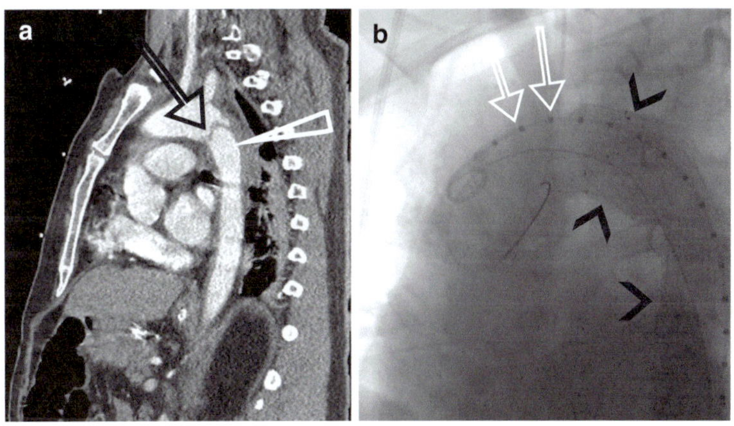

Fig. 35.6 (**a**) Sagittal CTA demonstrating mural injury of the proximal descending aortic arch (black arrow) with associated intramural hematoma (white arrowhead). (**b**) Fluoroscopic image demonstrating thoracic endovascular aortic repair (TEVAR; metal lattice between the black chevrons). Note the measuring pigtail catheter with radiopaque marking used to appropriately size the stent (white arrow)

Subacute Care of the Trauma Patient

Many routine procedures performed on all inpatients, including trauma patients, can be performed with image guidance at decreased risk. The use of ultrasound and fluoroscopic guidance, for example, reduces the risk of complications (pneumothorax, air embolism, arrhythmias, nerve damage, and arterial puncture) from 14% to 4% [12]. Given the number of such procedures performed, the use of image guidance results in a marked decrease in the absolute number of adverse events related to access.

Similarly, although the placement of thoracostomy tubes has been done using anatomic landmarks, the use of image guidance reduces the number of complications seen from placement (bleeding, infection, pneumothorax, extrapleural placement, or transgression of the diaphragm; Fig. 35.7)

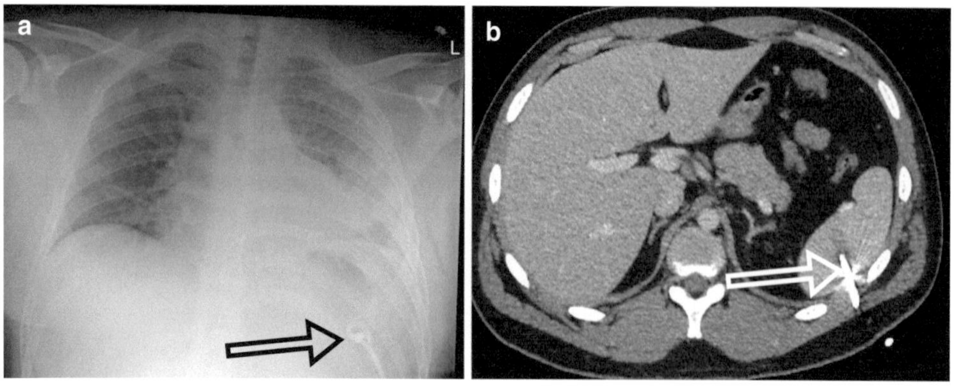

Fig. 35.7 (**a**) Chest radiograph post non-imaged guided percutaneous chest tube insertion demonstrating tube placement below the diaphragm (open black arrow) and (**b**) confirmation of malposition within the spleen (open white arrow)

[13]. Although the most common overall indication for pleural drainage is simple pleural effusion, trauma patients may have need of drainage of blood products, chyle, infected fluid, or GI contents, which increases complexity and the frequency of complications [13]. In particularly complex cases, CT guidance can be used [13]. Image guidance can also be used to assess and exchange blocked catheters, which is a common occurrence [13].

DVT and Pulmonary Embolism

Immobility is a major concern in the trauma patient, and abnormal thrombosis is common. When deep vein thrombosis (DVT) and pulmonary embolism (PE) are present, interventional radiology may be called on for additional treatment options over and above usual medical management.

While anticoagulation remains the first-line therapy for prophylaxis and treatment for DVT, immobile post-operative patients continue to have a relatively high incidence of DVT (up to 18%), and many of these go on to subsequently suffer from PE (up to 11%) [14]. Prophylactic placement of an IVC filter (Fig. 35.8) is often performed in such patients, although a definite advantage has not been demonstrated over optimized medical management [14]. A recently published retrospective meta-analysis demonstrated that prophylactic use of IVC filters in trauma patients reduce the risk of symptomatic PE; however, the rates of fatal PE were similar to the control group [15].

In the case of established DVT or PE, thrombolysis (using TPA, streptokinase, or other agents) can be directed to the target areas using catheter-directed administration of the medication, with the aim to maximize the concentration of the drug at the site of thrombosis [16]. When the burden of thrombus is particularly high, a variety of devices can be employed to disrupt and remove thrombus in both the deep veins and in the pulmonary arteries using mechanical force, vacuum, water jets, or a combination of these techniques (Fig. 35.9) [16].

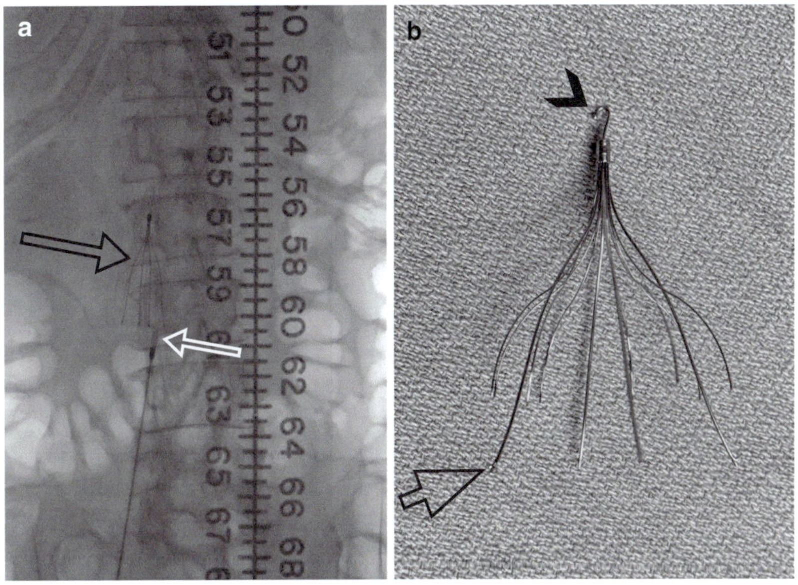

Fig. 35.8 (**a**) Fluoroscopic image acquired at the time of inferior vena cava insertion in a polytrauma patient from a right femoral vein approach. The deployed filter is seen (black arrow) prior to withdrawal of the insertion device (white arrow). (**b**) Cook Celect™ Platinum IVC filter showing primary struts with retention hooks (arrow head) and retrieval hook (chevron)

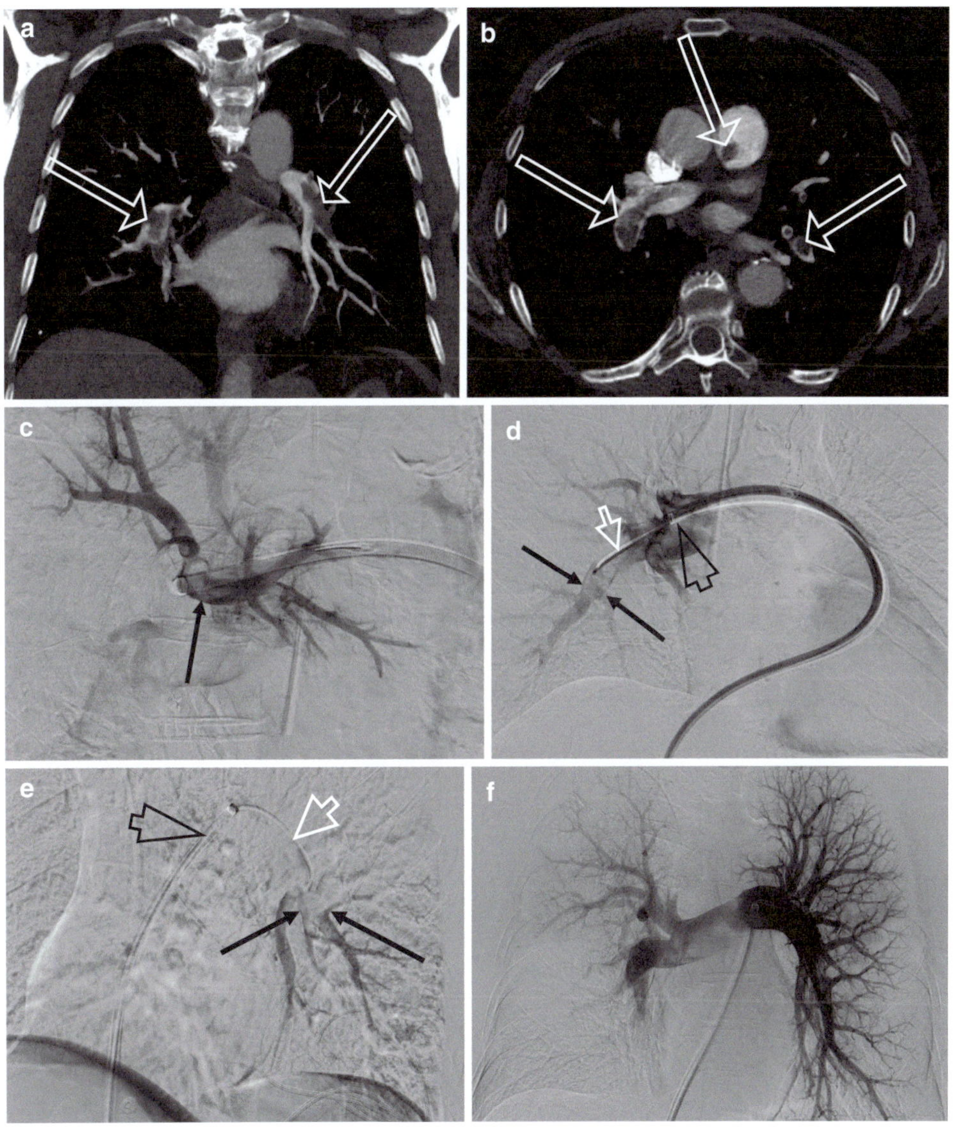

Fig. 35.9 (**a**) Coronal and (**b**) axial CT images demonstrating extensive thrombus within the right ventricle and extending into the right and left pulmonary arteries and segmental/ subsegmental arteries (open white arrows). (**c**) Angiographic images remonstrating filling defect within the pulmonary arteries (solid black arrow). (**d** and **e**) Penumbra Indigo® clot retrieval system with catheter (open black arrow heads) and separator device (open white arrow) removing clot (solid black arrows). (**f**) Post-thrombectomy image demonstrating clear pulmonary arteries

Summary of Safety Profiles

Traditionally, the minimally invasive image-guided procedures described in the chapter have been reserved for hemodynamically stable patients, while those patients requiring resuscitation or persistent instability were treated with surgical intervention [17]. However, recent retrospective studies have demonstrated positive results when comparing hospital survival in patients with both pelvic arterial injuries [17] and solid organ blunt trauma (spleen and liver) [17, 18]. Specifically, hemodynamically unstable patients who responded to initial resuscitation treated with embolization had equal in-hospital survival when compared to laparotomy [17, 18]. As interventional radiology continues to become further integrated into the trauma team, and therefore the initial management of trauma patients, new opportunities for optimizing the treatment of trauma patients will become available.

IR in the Interdisciplinary Team

The management of injured patients is a complex endeavor, engaging a varied team with complementary skills and capabilities [19]. The prompt use of multiple disciplines to manage the evolving needs of the patient leads to better outcomes, with outcomes exceeding the probability of survival predicted by the literature [2, 20]. As an integrated part of any diagnostic radiology department, interventional radiology provides a variety of technical skills and approaches, including both rapid and precise treatments for both acute concerns and those encountered in the convalescent period. Interventional radiologists are also proficient in the non-technical skills of "closed-loop communication" which is a major driver of the team-based approach [1, 2].

Key Points

- Interventional radiology is crucial in modern trauma care.
- IR's integration into trauma teams improves patient outcomes.
- CT imaging is the preferred modality for initial trauma workup.
- IR procedures include both vascular and non-vascular interventions.
- Embolization, using a variety of agents and devices, is a primary IR technique for managing hemorrhage.
- Non-vascular IR procedures reduce complication rates in subacute trauma care.

References

1. College A, of, S. Resources for optimal care of the injured patient: an update. Task force of the committee on trauma, American College of Surgeons. Bull Am Coll Surg. 1990;75:20–9.
2. Padia SA, et al. Society of interventional radiology position statement on endovascular intervention for trauma. J Vasc Interv Radiol. 2020;31:363–369.e2.
3. Hallinan J, Tan C, Pua U. The role of multidetector computed tomography versus digital subtraction angiography in triaging care and management in abdominopelvic trauma. SMEDJ. 2016;57:497–502.
4. Bauer JR, Ray CE. Transcatheter arterial embolization in the trauma patient: a review. Semin Interv Radiol. 2004;21:11–22.
5. Franco DF, Zangan SM. Interventional radiology in pelvic trauma. Semin Intervent Radiol. 2020;37:44–54.
6. Golzarian J, Siskin GP, Sharafuddin M, Mimura H, Coldwell DM. Embolization tools. In: Vascular embolotherapy; 2006. p. 15–33.
7. Lopera JE. Embolization in trauma: review of basic principles and techniques. Semin Intervent Radiol. 2021;38:18–33.
8. Abada HT, Golzarian J. Gelatine sponge particles: handling characteristics for endovascular use. Tech Vasc Interv Radiol. 2007;10:257–60.
9. Amplatzer Vascular Plug II (AVP II) - Sizing and Specs | Abbott. https://www.cardiovascular.abbott/us/en/hcp/products/peripheral-intervention/amplatzer-family-vascular-plugs/avp/avp-sizing-specs.html.
10. Bozlar U, et al. CT angiography of the upper extremity arterial system: part 1—anatomy, technique, and use in trauma patients. Am J Roentgenol. 2013;201:745–52.
11. Cullen E, Lantz E, Johnson CM, Young P. Traumatic aortic injury: CT findings, mimics, and therapeutic options. Cardiovascular Diagnosis and Therapy. 2014;4:238–44.
12. Brass P, Hellmich M, Kolodziej L, Schick G, Smith AF. Ultrasound guidance versus anatomical landmarks for subclavian or femoral vein catheterization. Cochrane Database Syst Rev. 2015;2018
13. Hogg J, et al. Tube Thoracostomy: a review for the interventional radiologist. Semin Interv Radiol. 2011;28:039–47.
14. Ho KM, et al. A multicenter trial of vena cava filters in severely injured patients. N Engl J Med. 2019;381:328–37.
15. Shariff M, Kumar A, Adalja D, Doshi R. Inferior vena cava filters reduce symptomatic but not fatal pulmonary emboli after major trauma: a meta-analysis with trial sequential analysis. Eur J Trauma Emerg Surg. 2021;47:1805–11.
16. Gregorio MAD, et al. Interventional radiology treatment for pulmonary embolism. World J Radiol. 2017;9:295.
17. Tuchayi AM, et al. Comparative effectiveness of pelvic arterial embolization versus laparotomy in adults with pelvic injuries: a National Trauma Data Bank analysis. Clin Imaging. 2022;86:75–82.
18. Aoki M, Abe T, Hagiwara S, Saitoh D, Oshima K. Embolization versus surgery for stabilized patients with solid organ injury. J Vasc Interv Radiol. 2021;32:1150–1155.e5.
19. Gillman LM, Brindley PG, Blaivas M, Widder S, Karakitsos D. Trauma team dynamics. J Crit Care. 2016;32:218–21.
20. Kataoka Y, et al. Hybrid treatment combining emergency surgery and intraoperative interventional radiology for severe trauma. Injury. 2016;47:59–63.

Communication and Leadership in the Operating Room

36

Thomas Blanks and Simon Denning

It goes without saying that whilst the operating room (OR) occupies a key aspect of the major trauma (MT) patients' journey, it must be placed in the wider context of their care and their journey through the hospital. Pre-hospital stabilisation, transfer to an MT centre (MTC) and ongoing resuscitation are all covered elsewhere in this book.

Exsanguination is a major component of pre-hospital and intra-hospital mortality [1] accounting for 33% of deaths. Damage control surgery (DCS) plays a critical role in the management of uncontrolled haemorrhage, and expedient transfer to the OR is, therefore, a core aspect of the patient's journey.

Communication within the OR represents a significant challenge, even without the time pressures of major traumatic injuries. The Canadian Institute for Health Information (2016) demonstrated that nearly one in ten surgical patients suffer complications as a result of error [2]. Leonard, Graham and Bonacum showed that communication failures are the most common cause of a series of outcomes—from errors, adverse events, to malpractice claims [3]. The three most frequently identified root causes of complications from surgery, as identified by The Joint Commission (2012) from 2010 through to 2011, were listed as human factors, leadership and communication [4]. The fact that these issues are represented in many developed healthcare environments demonstrates the ongoing challenge represented by this environment.

It is worth re-iterating that the principles of good communication and leadership remain as important in the OR as elsewhere. However, there are some specific challenges pertinent to the OR environment that the MT practitioner should be aware of as these have the potential to both positively and negatively impact patient care should they not be appreciated. Given the common themes of the solutions for these issues, we will start by discussing the specific barriers to effective communication and leadership before covering transferrable solutions.

1. Involvement of non-trauma specialist team members.
2. Hierarchy/responsibility gradients, including perceptions of such.
3. Specific environmental factors.

1. Involvement of non-trauma specialist team members

Given the unpredictable timing and nature of MT injuries, it is likely, on occasion, that allied healthcare practitioners (AHPs) who are not routinely exposed to MT will form a component of the surgical team. This may include theatre nurses, runners, anaesthetic nurses or anaesthesiologists and surgical sub-specialties. The situation may be further complicated by organisation and timing of shift patterns; depending on the time of the event, the trauma team may consist of members towards the end of their shift and others at the beginning. Handover of patients between team members changing shifts adds another element of risk [5].

Given that human performance is demonstrably reduced in unfamiliar and high-stress situations [6], it is vital to recognise that these team members may not be operating at peak performance, specifically regarding non-technical skills. Therefore, it is essential that the MT practitioner recognises a crucial aspect of leadership and teamwork—knowing the make-up and skill set of the team in attendance.

This step often begins long before the patient arrives in the operating room; the first time the trauma team gather as a unit will likely follow a trauma call "pre-alert", or even as the patient arrives in the emergency department. Whilst core elements of the team, including anaesthesiologists and surgeons, will stay with the patient throughout their trauma journey, many AHPs will come and go as the patient moves through the hospital. In the OR, the World Health Organization (WHO) safety checklist makes clear that team introductions should form a core part of the initial team

T. Blanks · S. Denning (✉)
Department of Anaesthesia, Queen's Medical Centre, Nottingham University Hospitals NHS Trust, Nottingham, UK
e-mail: thomas.blanks@nhs.net; simon.denning@nhs.net

L. Marshall Gillman, S. Widder (eds.), *Trauma Team Dynamics*, https://doi.org/10.1007/978-3-031-86312-7_36

briefing, and we would advocate for situational reports (sitreps) at key moments when the team changes, for example, when the patient leaves the emergency department or imaging department [7]. It is clear that the development of effective teams working in a stressful scenario begins with knowing who your team is made up of.

Each individual will have their own strengths and weaknesses, offering different values to the team. The importance of early recognition of skill sets within a team is consistently associated with high-performing teams outside of the healthcare environment [8]. However, an in-depth recognition of team roles and individual team proficiencies such as Belbin [9] is outside the realistic remit of, or the time available to, the MT practitioner; during clinical practice we must be more adaptable and explicit about practical skill sets. This applies to both leadership and followership.

2. Hierarchy and responsibility gradients

Within the OR environment, there are a broad range of professions represented—surgeons, anaesthesiologists, scrub practitioners and nurses and theatre support workers. In the context of MT, there is potentially a wider range of additional professionals such as interventional radiologists and major trauma specialists.

The presence of a perceived hierarchy is common both between these groups and within these groups (junior versus senior staff, for example), and these have a well-recognised impact on the overall effectiveness of any team [10]. The willingness of individuals to "speak out" when they perceive a harm incident occurring/pending is strongly associated with the hierarchy gradient within their team [11].

It is worth recognising that perceptions of hierarchy are mismatched between different professional groups. Consistently, nurses and physicians differ in their perceptions of how well or poorly their team is working and the impact of the culture within that team [12]. It is critical for the MT leader to recognise three fundamental principles relating to the hierarchy gradient and the involvement of multiple different professional teams in response to MT:

1. The MT leader may perceive their team culture differently to others within that team.
2. A positive team dynamic is fundamental to high performance in a stressful situation.
3. It is a requirement of high-quality leadership to ensure that an open and transparent system for reporting errors/harm situations is consistently and repeatedly reinforced through both word and action. Particularly as the team members may be rotating in and out of the team at frequent intervals.

It is also worth noting that leadership and hierarchy within the OR may be fluid, and there are numerous, often predictable, moments during surgical cases where leadership transfers to a more appropriate person. An obvious example being when the anaesthesiologist has safely induced anaesthesia and transfers leadership, within the OR, to the surgeon who may then proceed with the operation, and the team follows, usually, without any formal handover.

A full discussion around the creation of team climate, culture and flattening of hierarchy gradients is covered in more detail elsewhere however, there are several "quick wins" that can be readily implemented; for example, the utilisation of first names for all team members. This is a well-recognised approach, when modelled by a leader, that rapidly reduces hierarchy within a team and enables speaking up. Another example is that of the debrief. As an opportunity for the team to informally give feedback to one another about performance and reflections, it allows for the development of an ideal team culture. Managed properly, this is an excellent opportunity to flatten the hierarchy curve.

3. Specific environmental constraints

Practicalities of the OR impact on both non-verbal and verbal forms of communication; this creates a potential area for error if not adjusted for.

Non-verbal

Osborne-Smith and Hodgen [13] demonstrated that the wearing of surgical facemasks inhibits the interpretation of facial expressions, and it is evident that covering a significant proportion of the face will impact non-verbal communication.

This is only heightened in situations such as the SARS-Cov-2 pandemic and the widespread adoption of filtering facepieces class 3 (FFP 3) or N95 respirators and associated personal protective equipment (PPE) [14]. There is limited research pertaining to specific challenges to effective team-working in PPE; however, Hignett, Welsh and Banerjee [15] have shown that a wide range of human factors were perceived as impacted by staff—from communication through the task performance (both gross and fine motor). These issues were reported as affecting female members of staff more than male in conjunction with poorer fitting equipment. This is particularly pertinent to the OR as the majority of aerosol-generating procedures (AGPs) are performed here and subsequently the proliferation of PPE is particularly acute. It is the authors' experience that effective leadership and team-working are deeply affected by protracted working in PPE; from the physical impact of dehydration and discomfort, to the impact on verbal and non-verbal communication.

Verbal

The impact of PPE is also felt with verbal communication. Benitez, Guemes and Aranda et al. [16] have shown that, in surgical respondents from a widespread group of healthcare economies, 54% of respondents felt that PPE had affected intra-team communication. Also, in this study, it is of note that 48% of respondents reported that PPE had affected their decision-making processes. The reason for the impairment may be apparent; muffling of the voice by masks or noise interference from fans.

Wider Structural Perspective

With the development of Major Trauma Networks and the goal of treating a majority of trauma patients in Major Trauma Centres (MTC), there has been increasing focus on building and training trauma teams and MT specialists [17]. This begins with national oversight; designation of appropriate MTCs, publication of trauma guidelines and protocols [18]; and recommendations on team training and skills [19]. At an MTC level, the appointment of identifiable Major Trauma Team leaders and provision of a designated consultant available 24/7 allows for appropriate oversight and planning when major trauma occurs. Whilst MT leaders may often be surgeons, a multi-disciplinary group including anaesthesiologists, emergency physicians and intensive care consultants allows for assimilation and development of different leadership styles. With regular audit and service evaluation, the positives from each specialty leader can be rolled out to the team.

Naturally, trauma events are unpredictable, and a 24/7 MTC service is essential. OR teams should be maintained in readiness, with appropriate training, simulation, and day-to-day emergency work, where possible. MT Leaders should be able to communicate their plan effectively, along with any contingency plans and planning for post-operative destination, as the case progresses; adaptability is a key skill and relies on a low hierarchical gradient for the rapid transfer of information from the team to the team leader. However, planning and preparing for every single eventuality is a futile task in time-critical scenarios, and an awareness of potential task fixation should be maintained. Team leadership may need to be transferred as the patient moves to the OR, and this should be explicitly stated at the WHO briefing and during any appropriate sit-reps.

Allocation of tasks to each team member is an important step in identifying and utilising all resources available, yet this need not be left until the patient arrives. CRM training and planning may allow a proportion of this task management to be assigned ahead of time, with only those team members who are new or unfamiliar with the MT environment requiring more specific focus at the trauma team and WHO briefing.

Transferrable Solutions

Given the specific challenges covered so far, what tools are available to mitigate against them? It is important to recognise that although these challenges are intensified in the OR, they are not unique to it, and therefore, the solutions are also not unique to this environment.

In order to effectively lead an MT team, a clear and fundamental understanding of non-technical skills is critical. With respect to the OR, some readily implementable solutions exist to facilitate high-quality leadership and teamwork:

A. Teamwork

A great MT leader will understand the roles within the team and how to best utilise them. These might be standardised within a particular institution and training provided around this team structure. At the heart of the team ethos should be the understanding that the team can achieve more than any single individual when they work well together. This includes a positive response to feedback after events. Positive team culture allows for honest and constructive criticism whilst engendering a willingness to learn from mistakes. It is imperative that team members feel able to safely practice their skill sets.

Within the OR, there are many pre-defined roles, and the teams are well-versed in enacting those roles day-to-day. Training for major trauma/damage control surgery should focus on how those roles, and their communication and interaction with team leaders, pivot to provide the best care in time-critical situations.

Information is often shared in a more direct manner, and there must be less tolerance of ambiguity. Clear and concise communication is key when coordinating tasks within the team and passing information between team members.

The operating room should be notified as early as possible; in some centres, they are part of the trauma team activation, as to the arrival of an MT patient if operative intervention is anticipated. Potential operation, special equipment required and patient positioning are all important details to relay to the operating room team so that they can be adequately prepared. This sometimes requires the recruitment of additional team members, such as a perfusionist if cell salvage technology is required.

B. Communication

Communication strategies are critical to the clear exchange of information, and one of the most applicable strategies is that of closed-loop communication (CLC) as described by McIntyre and Salas [20]. In essence, this refers to a structured approach to communication whereby

- The sender initiates a message.
- The receiver interprets and acknowledges the message.
- The sender completes the loop by ensuring that the message was received as imparted.

Whilst it can seem laborious to document, in practice it is a much smoother process, for example:

Surgeon: "Size 10 blade please"
Scrub nurse: "Size 10 blade?"
Surgeon: "Correct, thank you"

This technique has seen widespread adoption throughout the military, aviation and healthcare industries [21]. There are multiple training packages for whole team training; however, this technique is valuable when employed during any time-critical situation. This aligns well with the requirement for simple, command-driven communication necessitated by the wearing of PPE.

C. Leadership

One critical tool for the MT leader is that of a brief [22]. Simply put, this pre-event strategy allows the building of a shared mental model and alignment of the team to short- and long-term goals. Within the OR, a short-term goal may be progression towards the next sit-rep, as covered above, with the long-term goal of completion of damage control surgery and transfer to the next area of ongoing care. It also allows the initiation of a team culture that facilitates safe teamwork—that of open, two-way communication and flat hierarchy where all can speak out if concerned.

It is inevitable that even the best-laid plan will come unstuck, as clinical events can rapidly outpace an existing plan. In this instance, the role of the situational report, sit-up or huddle is invaluable. These phrases describe a quick-fire opportunity for the team members and leader to reconfigure resources, allocate new tasks and refresh the mental model between the team.

Conclusion

In summary, there is an enormous challenge in transferring from one clinical environment to another, particularly when that environment includes some of the specific challenges that the OR entails. However, the authors are confident that the solutions for this environment are not uniquely difficult. These solutions will benefit the MT practitioner in all walks of their practice—be that the OR or beyond.

Key Points

1. Making explicit the unwritten behaviours to ensure group mental model sharing.
2. Flexibility of the leader role to pre-empt predictable task fixation.
3. Place of OR in wider context of trauma journey.

References

1. Cripps MW, Kutcher ME, Daley A, McCreery RC, Greenberg MD, Cachola LM, et al. Cause and timing of death in massively transfused trauma patients. J Trauma Acute Care Surg [Internet]. 2013 [cited 2021 Jan 31];75(2 SUPPL. 2):S255–S262. Available from: http://journals.lww.com/01586154-201308002-00026.
2. Measuring Patient Harm in Canadian Hospitals [Internet]. 2016 [cited 2021 Jan 31]. Available from: www.cihi.cacopyright@cihi.caISBN978-1-77109-514-3.
3. Leonard M. The human factor: the critical importance of effective teamwork and communication in providing safe care. Qual Saf Heal Care [Internet]. 2004 [cited 2021 Jan 31];13(suppl_1):i85–90. Available from: https://pubmed.ncbi.nlm.nih.gov/15465961/
4. NERC Improving Human Performance Sentinel Event Reporting, Analysis and prevention in healthcare Charles A. Mowll, FACHE, CSSBB Executive Vice President The Joint Commission. 2012.
5. Boet S, Djokhdem H, Leir SA, Théberge I, Mansour F, Etherington N. Association of intraoperative anaesthesia handovers with patient morbidity and mortality: a systematic review and meta-analysis [Internet]. Vol. 125, Br J Anaesth. Elsevier Ltd; 2020 [cited 2021 Jan 31]. p. 605–613. Available from: http://bjanaesthesia.org/article/S0007091220304657/fulltext.
6. Harvey A, Bandiera G, Nathens AB, LeBlanc VR. Impact of stress on resident performance in simulated trauma scenarios. J Trauma Acute Care Surg. 2012;72(2):497–503.
7. Arul GS, Pugh HEJ, Mercer SJ, Midwinter MJ. Human factors in decision making in major trauma in Camp Bastion, Afghanistan. Ann R Coll Surg Engl [Internet]. 2015 [cited 2021 Jan 31];97(4):262–8. Available from: /pmc/articles/PMC4473862/?report=abstract.
8. Chong E. Role balance and team development: a study of team role characteristics underlying high and low performing teams. 2007.

9. Dill DD. Management Teams: Why they succeed or fail Author: R. Meredith Belbin. Heinemann, 1981. R&D Manag [Internet]. 1982 [cited 2021 Jan 31];12(3):147–8. Available from: http://doi.wiley.com/10.1111/j.1467-9310.1982.tb00500.x.
10. Sacks GD, Shannon EM, Dawes AJ, Rollo JC, Nguyen DK, Russell MM, et al. Teamwork, communication and safety climate: a systematic review of interventions to improve surgical culture, vol. 24. BMJ Qual Safe. BMJ Publishing Group; 2015. p. 458–67.
11. Pattni N, Arzola C, Malavade A, Varmani S, Krimus L, Friedman Z. Challenging authority and speaking up in the operating room environment: a narrative synthesis [Internet]. Vol. 122, Br J Anaesth. Elsevier Ltd; 2019 [cited 2021 Jan 31]. p. 233–244. Available from: https://pubmed.ncbi.nlm.nih.gov/30686309/
12. Sexton JB, Holzmueller CG, Pronovost PJ, Thomas EJ, McFerran S, Nunes J, et al. Variation in caregiver perceptions of teamwork climate in labor and delivery units. J Perinatol [Internet]. 2006 [cited 2021 Jan 31];26(8):463–470. Available from: www.jcaho.org
13. Osborne-Smith L, Kyle Hodgen R. Communication in the operating room setting. Annu Rev Nurs Res [Internet]. 2017 [cited 2021 Jan 31];35(1):55–69. Available from: https://pubmed.ncbi.nlm.nih.gov/27935774/
14. (No Title) [Internet]. [cited 2021 Jan 31]. Available from: https://assets.publishing.service.gov.uk/government/uploads/system/uploads/attachment_data/file/954690/Infection_Prevention_and_Control_Guidance_January_2021.pdf
15. Hignett S, Welsh R, Banerjee J. Human factors issues of working in personal protective equipment during the COVID-19 pandemic. Anaesthesia [Internet]. 2021 [cited 2021 Jan 31];76(1):134–135. Available from: https://onlinelibrary.wiley.com/doi/10.1111/anae.15198
16. Yánez Benítez C, Güemes A, Aranda J, Ribeiro M, Ottolino P, Di Saverio S, et al. Impact of personal protective equipment on surgical performance during the COVID-19 pandemic. World J Surg [Internet]. 2020 [cited 2021 Jan 31];44(9):2842–2847. Available from: https://doi.org/10.1007/s00268-020-05648-2.
17. Moran CG, Lecky F, Bouamra O, Lawrence T, Edwards A, Woodford M, et al. Changing the system - major trauma patients and their outcomes in the NHS (England) 2008–17. EClinicalMedicine. 2018;2–3:13–21.
18. Overview | Major trauma: assessment and initial management | Guidance | NICE.
19. Overview | Major trauma: service delivery | Guidance | NICE.
20. McIntyre R, Salas E. McIntyre: Team effectiveness and decision making in organizations. 1995 [cited 2021 Jan 31];149–203. Available from: https://scholar.google.com/scholar_lookup?hl=en&publication_year=1995&author=+McIntyre%2C+R.M.author=+E.+Salasauthor=+R.A.+Guzzoauthor=+E.+Salas&title=Team+Effectiveness+and+Decision+Making+in+Organizations#d=gs_cit&u=%2Fscholar%3Fq%3Dinfo%3A1Vyq9yoh-SUJ%3Ascholar.google.com%2F%26output%3Dcite%26scirp%3D0%26hl%3Den.
21. Burke CS. How to turn a team of experts into an expert medical team: guidance from the aviation and military communities. Qual Saf Heal Care [Internet]. 2004 [cited 2021 Jan 31];13(suppl_1):i96–104. Available from: https://pubmed.ncbi.nlm.nih.gov/15465963/
22. TeamSTEPPS Fundamentals Course: Module 4. Leading Teams | Agency for Healthcare Research and Quality [Internet]. [cited 2021 Jan 31]. Available from: https://www.ahrq.gov/teamstepps/instructor/fundamentals/module4/slleadership.html#im6

Pain Management in the Trauma Patient

37

Javier Webar, Tom Hall, and Sebastian Layera

Introduction

In the midst of an unrelenting opioid epidemic in North America, as well as a climbing prevalence of chronic pain in the general population, the topic of pain management has received increasing attention in many different settings, including critical care and trauma medicine. The International Association for the Study of Pain (IASP) defines pain as an "unpleasant sensory and emotional experience associated with actual or potential tissue damage." Even though pain can be experienced differently by patients with similar conditions, inadequately treated pain has several predictable sequelae and potentially deleterious physiologic effects, mediated by neuroendocrine activation as well as activation of the sympathetic nervous system [1].

Acute pain is almost universally present in the trauma patient, being proportional to the severity of tissue damage [2]. The complexity of the trauma patient is often reflected in the recognized deficiency in pain management including failure to identify, acknowledge, and treat pain both in the prehospital and in-patient setting. This in turn contributes to the high prevalence of chronic pain observed in this population: more than 60% of patients still report moderate pain 1 year after a major trauma [3].

Pain Management and Clinical Outcomes

Up to 80% of critically ill trauma patients report moderate to severe pain during their hospitalization, and a similar proportion of them report their pain being treated inadequately throughout their stay in the intensive care unit [4]. In the acute setting, pain is a potent physiologic stimulus that can trigger a myriad of responses affecting virtually all major organ systems (Table 37.1). Pain can complicate medical management and has been shown to cause additional morbidity in the form of increased length of stay, delayed ambulation, and impaired pulmonary mechanics [5, 6].

Long-term sequelae have also been associated with severe and poorly managed pain during trauma hospitalization, including the higher prevalence of chronic pain, as well as major depression and posttraumatic stress disorder [7]. These outcomes may have long-lasting effects on quality of life and ability to return to work, despite the successful treatment of presenting injuries and absence of physical disability. Screening for psychological trauma should be pursued proactively and addressed early, reinforcing the value of a multidisciplinary acute pain team [8]. Chronic pain in particular acts as both a cause and consequence of psychiatric morbidity in this population. There is significant overlap in transitioning from acute to chronic pain in the posttraumatic and postsurgical setting, since most pathophysiologic changes stem from tissue injury. Similar risk factors predispose postoperative and trauma patients to chronic pain, such as the presence of thoracic trauma/surgery, major burns, spinal cord injury, preexisting chronic pain, preexisting anxiety and/or depression, and catastrophizing. Adequate pain control jumps out as one of the few potentially modifiable risk factors that could impact the development of chronic pain [9].

Table 37.1 Physiologic consequences of untreated severe pain [1]

System	Physiologic phenomena
Central nervous system	Agitation, delirium, insomnia
Cardiovascular system	Activation of the sympathetic nervous system leading to tachycardia and hypertension, resulting in an impaired oxygen delivery/consumption ratio
Respiratory system	Ventilation asynchrony potentially leading to high peak airway pressures
Gastrointestinal system	Delayed gastric emptying and increased GI secretions resulting in an overall increased risk of aspiration
Endocrine system	Activation of the renin-angiotensin-aldosterone system resulting in water and salt retention

J. Webar (✉) · T. Hall · S. Layera
Department of Anesthesiology, Perioperative and Pain Medicine, Health Science Center, University of Manitoba, Winnipeg, MB, Canada
e-mail: javier.webar@umanitoba.ca

L. Marshall Gillman, S. Widder (eds.), *Trauma Team Dynamics*, https://doi.org/10.1007/978-3-031-86312-7_37

Pain Assessment and Management

There are a multitude of tools for evaluation of analgesia aimed at sedated and ventilated trauma patients. These include the visual analog scale, behavioral pain scale, and critical pain observation scale. Their implementation, in conjunction with daily interruption of sedation in ventilated patients, have shown to reduce the duration of mechanical ventilation and ICU stay and lead to a decrease in the incidence of inadequately treated pain [10, 11]. In heavily sedated patients, sometimes it is necessary to use indirect signs of pain related to heightened sympathetic activity, such as hypertension, tachycardia, agitation, diaphoresis, and lacrimation.

Acknowledging the high prevalence of moderate-to-severe pain in trauma patients, it is preferable to be proactive during the initial phase of management. It can be reasonably assumed that both nociceptive and neuropathic pain components are present simultaneously in major trauma. Moreover, the identification of symptoms suggestive of neuropathic pain, such as spontaneous burning pain, paroxysmal pain, allodynia, paresthesia, painful numbness, or hyperalgesia, can be useful to guide specific therapy in an early and aggressive fashion with the goal of limiting the development of persistent pain syndromes after initial recovery [12].

Pharmacotherapy

Despite the proven effectiveness of multimodal analgesia in pain management, studies have found that many trauma patients receive intravenous opioids as the sole pain modality, which increases the risk of both side effects and inadequate pain control [13]. In major trauma, it is not infrequent for patients to display severe pain that cannot be adequately managed on opioids alone, which can be a clue as to the presence of a neuropathic component, frequently seen in complex trauma. Adhering to recommendations from the typical "pain ladder" medications, clinicians may be missing a crucial therapeutic target for relief. Beard and Wood published their approach to the complex polytrauma patient used to treat soldiers in Afghanistan [14]. In these cases, a neuropathic component is assumed a priori, and anti-neuropathic medication is started early. Specifically, anticonvulsants such as gabapentin and pregabalin, tricyclic antidepressant medications (TCA) such as amitriptyline or nortriptyline, and other adjuvants such as IV ketamine [15] and IV lidocaine [16] infusions (in a monitored setting such as ICU), and clonidine or dexmedetomidine which are also commonly used to address sedation and delirium. These medications are started in low doses but are accelerated in the young and otherwise healthy patients as the initial phase of shock subsides (See Table 37.2). As patients progress in the recovery process, most can stop antineuropathic medications. Those who have persistent neuropathic pain may require continuing these medications or pursue interventional modalities with a chronic pain specialist.

Table 37.2 Common adult analgesic drug doses

Drug	Dose range
Acetaminophen	500–1000 mg every 4–6 hrs. (max daily dose 4 gr)
Ibuprofen	200–400 mg every 6–8 hrs.
Celecoxib	100–200 mg BID
Hydromorphone IR	1–2 mg every 4–6 hrs. PRN
Hydromorphone CR	3 mg BID
Morphine CR	10–20 mg BID
Tramadol	50–100 mg every 4–6 hrs. PRN
Gabapentin[a]	Start 100 mg TID. Can increase after 4–7 days to 300 mg TID. Max dose 3600 mg in 24 hrs.
Pregabalin[a]	Start 50–75 mg BID. Can increase after 7 days to 100–150 mg BID. Max dose 600 mg in 24 hrs.
Ami- / Nortriptyline	Start 25 mg QHS. Can increase after 4–7 days to 50 mg QHS

[a]Dose needs correction in renal failure if GFR < 60 mL/min/1.73 m^2

There are several factors affecting drug's pharmacokinetics in the critically ill trauma patient due to different physiologic derangements such as acid-base balance alterations (increased free drug fractions), changes in compartment volumes due to shock, edema and/or fluid overload and altered splanchnic blood flow (reduction of liver-dependent metabolism) due to shock or high dose vasopressor use, as well as the potential for drug interactions in the setting of critical care polypharmacy. These changes in physiology make titration of drugs such as opioids and other sedatives paramount to avoid toxicity, as opposed to dosing regimens based solely on body weight.

Ultrasound-Guided Regional Analgesia for the Trauma Patient

With the advent of the ultrasound era, interventional pain management and regional anesthesia have been revolutionized thanks to numerous new procedures described in recent years. Epidural analgesia continues to be the "gold standard" for pain management in several scenarios but comes with disadvantages such as potential for hemodynamic compromise, increased risk of hemorrhagic complications in the coagulopathic patient, higher failure rate in the case of thoracic epidurals, the need for lateral decubitus positioning, as well as a cooperative patient, many of which can be avoided with the use of regional analgesic "nerve blocks" Peripheral nerve catheters can be maintained for longer compared to epidurals without significant risk of infection, and hemorrhagic complications are less frequent as well as threatening

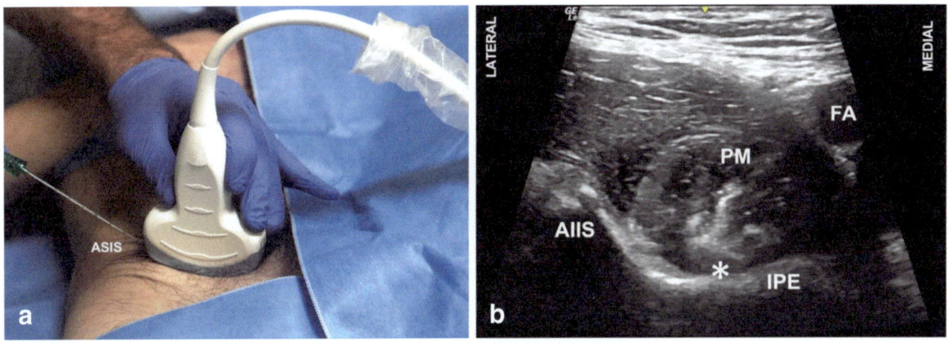

Fig. 37.1 PENG block. (a) Ultrasound probe position and needle approach. (b) Sonoanatomy. (AIIS: Anterior inferior iliac spine, PM: Psoas muscle, IPE: Iliopectineal eminence, FA: Femoral artery. Asterisk: Needle target)

[17]. Despite these assurances, practitioners and departments performing regional anesthesia techniques should be trained and equipped to deal with emergencies such as local anesthetic systemic toxicity (LAST), anaphylaxis, pneumothorax, intravascular injections, and brainstem anesthesia. In the trauma patient, preexisting hemodynamic instability, trauma coagulopathy, poor cooperation, and potential for masked compartment syndrome all must be weighed against the benefits of performing regional anesthesia, but their widespread use and growing record of safety underlines their positive risk-to-benefit ratio.

Following is a brief description of regional analgesic techniques that have been used effectively in the management of common injuries in the trauma patient. The performance of these techniques requires previous experience with ultrasound-guided regional analgesia as well as access to resuscitation equipment as per local or international guidelines [18].

PENG Block for Hip Fractures

Hip fractures are a major public health concern as they annually result in hospitalization for over 250,000 adults over the age of 65. Unfortunately, only 60% of patients return to walking post-surgery, and only 50% return to their baseline function. Pain presents a major impediment to recovery, and inadequately treated pain in hospital results in higher levels of delirium, increased length of stay, increased postoperative complications, and reduced function. Opioid analgesia is an effective option; however, it too comes with well-known side effects including nausea, constipation, respiratory depression, and delirium. Considering these barriers, the American Academy of Orthopedic Surgeons published practice guidelines with strong levels of evidence to support preoperative regional analgesia and the use of multimodal analgesia in the intra- and postoperative period. One such option is the pericapsular nerve group (PENG) block. First described in 2018 by Giron-Arango for use in patients with acute hip fractures, it has gained popularity and expanded use cases into perioperative care due to its efficacy and safety [19, 20].

Anatomy The anterior hip capsule is innervated by the femoral nerve (FN), obturator nerve (ON), and accessory obturator nerve (AON). Due to the prominence of these three nerves in the capsule, they are the target of the PENG block. Each of these nerves tracks toward the hip joint in the space between the inguinal ligament and the interior surface of the iliac bones. Relevant anatomic landmarks are the iliopsoas muscle and tendon, the femoral artery and femoral vein, the anterior inferior iliac spine (AIIS), and the iliopubic eminence (IPE).

Approach Most authors describe a lateral to medial approach (see Fig. 37.1) although it can be done out-of-plane as well. The goal is to direct the needle deep to the iliopsoas tendon and deposit 8–30 ml (most commonly 20 ml) of long-acting local anesthetic (L-bupivicaine, bupivicaine, or ropivicaine).

Advantages The PENG block is intended to be a motor-sparing block that produces significant reductions in pain scores, time to first opioid, and total opioid consumption in the hip fracture patient, when compared to other regional techniques such as the fascia iliaca compartment block [21].

While the original article describes preserved motor function in all five patients, Yu et al. describe two cases with quadricep weakness and inability to perform a straight leg raise [22]. They hypothesized that injection and spread too medially and cephalad resulted in a complete FN and ON block with resultant weakness. Furthermore, a large volume of local anesthetic may result in more cephalad spread and motor block.

Paravertebral Block

The paravertebral block and catheter is a well-established technique to provide prolonged unilateral analgesia and is beneficial in rib fracture management and thoracic surgery, with decreased adverse effects when compared with thoracic epidural analgesia [23]. The goal is to block the ventral and dorsal rami of the ipsilateral spinal nerves as they exit

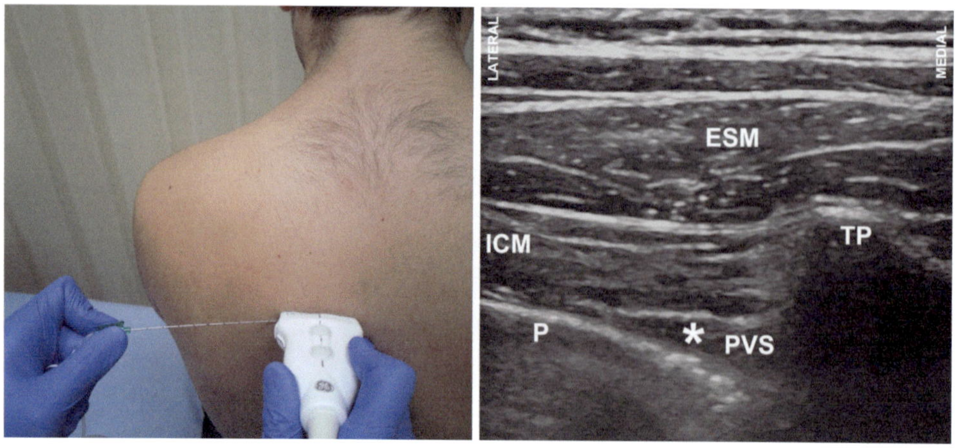

Fig. 37.2 Paravertebral block, transverse approach. (ICM: Intercostal muscle, ESM: Erector spinae muscle, PVS: Paravertebral space, TP: Transverse process, Asterisk: Needle target)

the vertebral foramen. The paravertebral space is a potential space bound medially by the vertebral body and intervertebral disc, anterolaterally by the parietal pleura and intercostal space, and posteriorly by the transverse process and superior costotransverse ligament.

This technique is often performed with a transverse probe orientation (see Fig. 37.2). The relevant landmarks are the lateral tip of the transverse process, the pleura with its characteristic sliding with respiratory motion, and the costotransverse ligament. The probe is then minimally slid caudally or cranially to visualize the pleura (Fig. 37.2), rather than the rib, creating a path for needle insertion that can be maintained throughout the block. Successful placement of the needle tip and injection of local anesthetic will result in the parietal pleura being pushed deeper as the pocket of LA expands.

Evidence In 2017, Yeying et al. published a prospective analysis of IV patient-controlled analgesia (PCA) versus paravertebral block and found significantly lower pain scores in the PVB group. Furthermore, respiratory indices such as PaO2 and FEV1/FVC were improved in the PVB group [24]. Respiratory improvements were also shown in a 2021 retrospective study of serratus anterior plane blocks, thoracic epidurals, and paravertebral blocks. They found a reduction in the rapid shallow breathing index (RSBI) for intubated patients immediately after receiving the nerve block [25]. In 2019, Womack et al. published a single-center retrospective analysis of 290 patients over a 4-year period which showed that PVB is a safe and effective analgesic strategy for rib fractures; however, it did not demonstrate a mortality benefit [26].

One of the pitfalls of paravertebral blocks and catheters is that they are subject to many of the same contraindications as epidurals in regard to catastrophic hemorrhagic complications affecting the spine in patients with bleeding diathesis [27]. To tackle this issue, several peripheral fascial plane blocks have been described to provide adequate blockade of nociceptive pathways in the trunk and abdomen, such as the serratus plane block, with inherently lower risk of bleeding complications. Despite the existence of multiple types of fascial plane blocks for rib fracture analgesia, robust literature is still lacking, and larger prospective studies are needed.

Serratus Plane Block

The SAPB is an ultrasound-guided block targeting the fascial plane between the latissimus dorsi muscle and the serratus anterior muscle, usually performed at the level of T5-T6 (see Fig. 37.3), targeting the lateral cutaneous branches of the intercostal nerves T2-T10, making a useful and safe technique for chest wall injuries including rib fractures and thoracotomy[25].

Evidence Beard et al. published a comparison of inspiratory volumes and mean change in pain scores comparing serratus anterior plane block to paravertebral block and thoracic epidurals. Across 354 patients, there was no difference in change of inspiratory volumes or mean change pain scores post block. Notably, 98% of patients reported severe pain prior to the block and only 34% percent post block, and there was no difference between groups [28]. Bhalla et al. demonstrated that SAPB was a viable alternative to thoracic epidural in the critical care setting for treatment of multiple rib fracture pain. This was demonstrated through measuring post block changes in RSBI and pain scores [25]. Overall, the SAPB provides another option for regional anesthesia in the management of traumatic rib fracture or other injuries affecting the chest, with the benefit of being able to be performed on a supine and sedated patient.

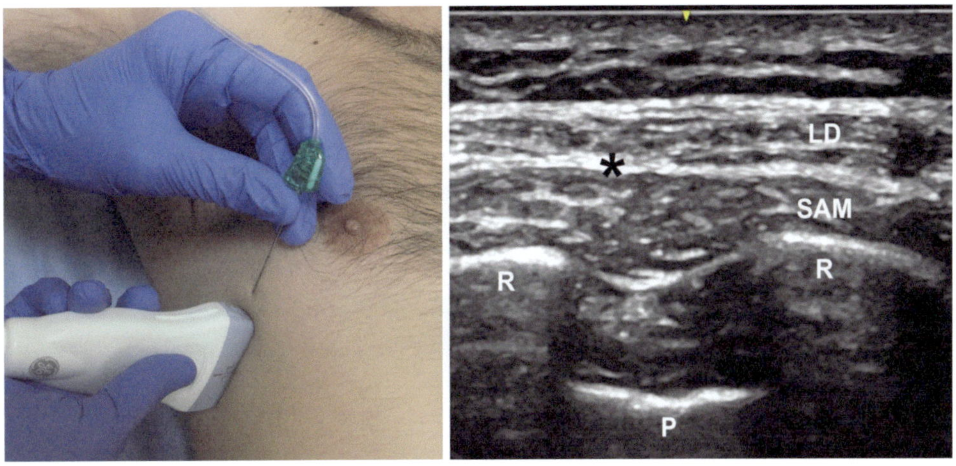

Fig. 37.3 Serratus plane block. (R: Rib, LD: Latissimus dorsi muscle, SAM: Serratus anterior muscle, P: Pleura, Asterisk: Needle target)

Transition to Practice: Rib Fracture Protocol

Rib fractures are present in 10% of all trauma patients and can lead to altered breathing mechanics, hypoventilation, and impaired gas exchange. Without adequate early management, high-risk patients are at risk of pneumonia and respiratory failure requiring mechanical ventilation. Elderly patients who sustain blunt chest trauma with rib fractures have twice the mortality and thoracic morbidity of younger patients with similar injuries. For each additional rib fracture in the elderly, the likelihood of mortality increases by 19% and the likelihood of pneumonia by 16%. High rates of disability and chronic pain are present in those who survive. It has been shown that implementation of a multidisciplinary management pathway that includes multimodal pain control and indications for surgical stabilization has been associated with improved outcomes [29].

At the author's institution, a rib fracture management protocol has recently been implemented to improve patient outcomes. The first step involves calculating a rib fracture score (see Fig. 37.4) to ensure proactive and aggressive analgesic management of patients at risk of severe pain and complications. The treatment algorithm is dynamic and requires pain score reassessment every 4 hours; therefore, if a patient continues to have severe pain despite the interventions appropriate to their initial screening, they are advanced to the next level for further analgesic management.

For those patients who begin in, or are advanced to level 3, an Acute Pain Service (APS) consultation is initiated to provide guidance regarding interventions such as a regional anesthesia (epidural for bilateral vs. PVB or SAB catheters for unilateral rib fractures) and ketamine or lidocaine infusions.

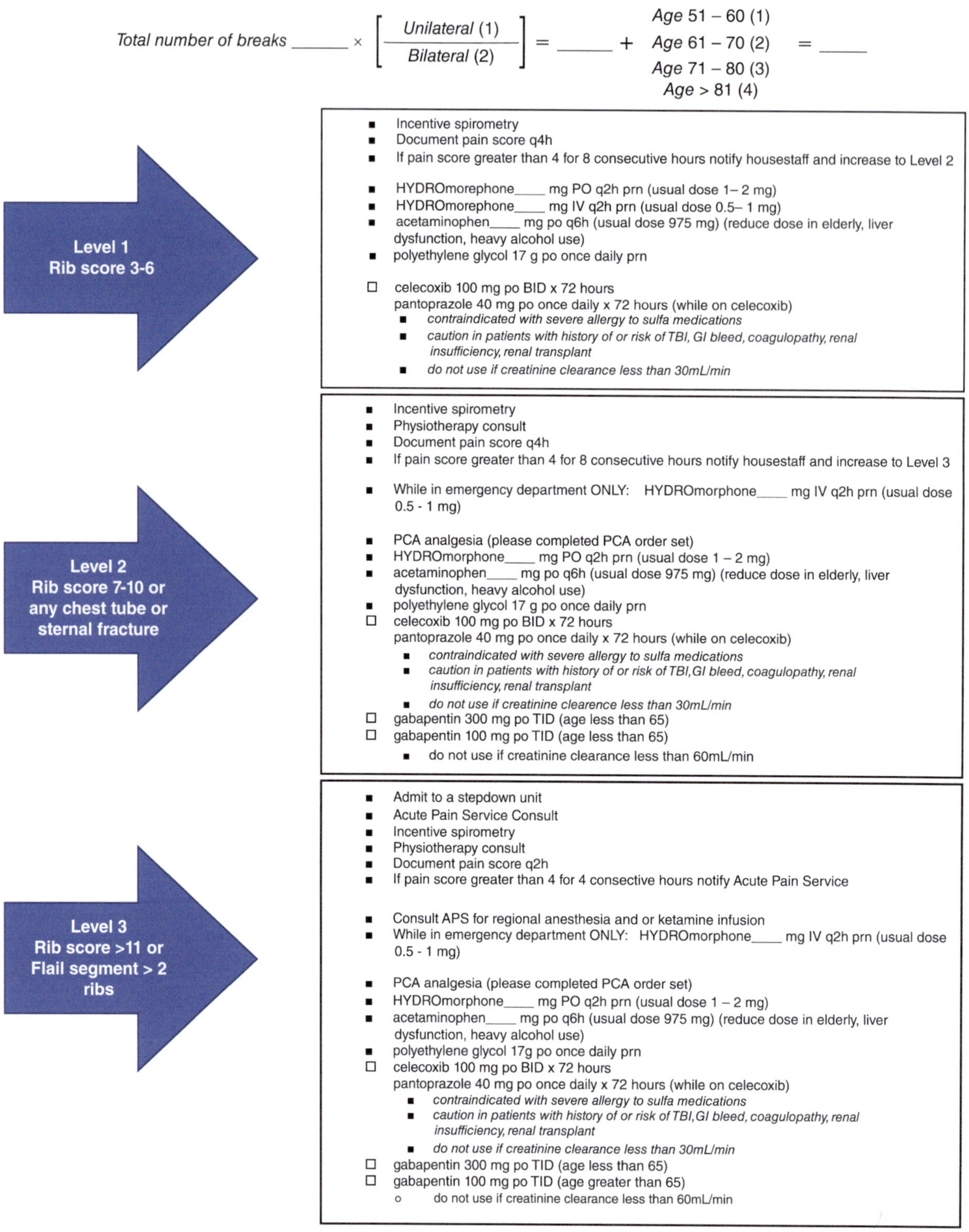

Fig. 37.4 Rib fracture pain management protocol (Health Science Center, Winnipeg Manitoba)

Key Points

- Up to 80% of critically ill trauma patients report moderate to severe pain during their hospitalization. Inadequate pain management in this population can lead to a myriad of complications both in the short and long term, including physiologic derangements, psychological morbidity, and development of chronic pain.
- Pain management should always be multimodal in nature, utilizing multiple pain modalities and pharmacologic agents aimed at targeting different pain receptors, as opposed to a high-dose opioid regimen.
- In patients with complex trauma, a neuropathic component of pain should be assumed a priori, and anti-neuropathic medication should be started early and scaled back as patient recovers.
- For injuries affecting the extremities, as well as rib fractures and surgical procedures, ultrasound-guided regional analgesia offers great pain relief with minimal risks. Peripheral nerve blocks, either single shot or continuous, have minimal hemodynamic impact and can be used safely even in coagulopathic patients.

References

1. Raja SN. Role of the sympathetic nervous system in acute pain and inflammation. Ann Med. 1995;27(2):241–6.
2. Berben SA, Meijs TH, van Dongen RT, van Vugt AB, Vloet LC, Mintjes-de Groot JJ, van Achterberg T. Pain prevalence and pain relief in trauma patients in the Accident & Emergency department. Injury. 2008;39(5):578–85. https://doi.org/10.1016/j.injury.2007.04.013.
3. Rivara FP, MacKenzie EJ, Jurkovich GJ, Nathens AB, Wang J, Scharfstein DO. Prevalence of pain in patients 1 year after major trauma. Arch Surg. 2008;143(3):282–7. https://doi.org/10.1001/archsurg.2007.61.
4. Stanik-Hutt JA, Soeken KL, Belcher AE, Fontaine DK, Gift AG. Pain experiences of traumatically injured patients in a critical care setting. Am J Crit Care. 2001;10:252–9.
5. Karamchandani K, Klick JC, Dougherty ML, Bonavia A, Allen SR, Carr ZJ. Pain management in trauma patients affected by the opioid epidemic: A narrative review. J Trauma Acute Care Surg. 2019;87(2):430–9. https://doi.org/10.1097/TA.0000000000002292.
6. Kehlet H, Holte K. Effect of postoperative analgesia on surgical outcome. Br J Anaesth. 2001;87(1):62–72. https://doi.org/10.1093/bja/87.1.62.
7. Shih RA, Schell TL, Hambarsoomian K, Belzberg H, Marshall GN. Prevalence of posttraumatic stress disorder and major depression after trauma center hospitalization. J Trauma. 2010;69(6):1560–6. https://doi.org/10.1097/TA.0b013e3181e59c05.
8. Visser E, Gosens T, Den Oudsten BL, De Vries J. The course, prediction, and treatment of acute and posttraumatic stress in trauma patients: A systematic review. J Trauma Acute Care Surg. 2017;82(6):1158–83. https://doi.org/10.1097/TA.0000000000001447.
9. Radresa O, Chauny JM, Lavigne G, Piette E, Paquet J, Daoust R. Current views on acute to chronic pain transition in post-traumatic patients: risk factors and potential for pre-emptive treatments. J Trauma Acute Care Surg. 2014;76(4):1142–50. https://doi.org/10.1097/TA.0000000000000188.
10. Payen JF, Chanques G, Mantz J, Hercule C, Auriant I, Leguillou JL, Binhas M, Genty C, Rolland C, Bosson JL. Current practices in sedation and analgesia for mechanically ventilated critically ill patients: A prospective multicenter patient- based study. Anesthesiology. 2007;106:687–95.
11. Payen JF, Bosson JL, Chanques G, Mantz J, Labarere J. DOLOREA Investigators. Pain assessment is associated with decreased duration of mechanical ventilation in the intensive care unit: a post Hoc analysis of the DOLOREA study. Anesthesiology. 2009;111(6):1308–16. https://doi.org/10.1097/ALN.0b013e3181c0d4f0.
12. Bennett MI, Attal N, Backonja MM, Baron R, Bouhassira D, Freynhagen R, Scholz J, Tölle TR, Wittchen HU, Jensen TS. Using screening tools to identify neuropathic pain. Pain. 2007;127(3):199–203. https://doi.org/10.1016/j.pain.2006.10.034.
13. Berben SA, Schoonhoven L, Meijs TH, van Vugt AB, van Grunsven PM. Prevalence and relief of pain in trauma patients in emergency medical services. Clin J Pain. 2011;27(7):587–92. https://doi.org/10.1097/AJP.0b013e3182169036.
14. Beard DJ, Wood P. Pain in complex trauma: lessons from Afghanistan. BJA Educ. 2015;15(4):207–12. https://doi.org/10.1093/bjaceaccp/mku035.
15. Schwenk ES, Viscusi ER, Buvanendran A, Hurley RW, Wasan AD, Narouze S, Bhatia A, Davis FN, Hooten WM, Cohen SP. Consensus Guidelines on the Use of Intravenous Ketamine Infusions for Acute Pain Management From the American Society of Regional Anesthesia and Pain Medicine, the American Academy of Pain Medicine, and the American Society of Anesthesiologists. Reg Anesth Pain Med. 2018;43(5):456–66. https://doi.org/10.1097/AAP.0000000000000806.
16. Eipe N, Gupta S, Penning JJBE. Intravenous lidocaine for acute pain: an evidence-based clinical update. BJA Educ. 2016;16(9):292–8.
17. Tsui BCH, et al. Practice advisory on the bleeding risks for peripheral nerve and interfascial plane blockade: evidence review and expert consensus. Can J Anaesth. 2019;66(11):1356–84. https://doi.org/10.1007/s12630-019-01466-w.
18. Mulroy MF, Weller RS, Liguori GA. A checklist for performing regional nerve blocks. Reg Anesth Pain Med. 2014;39(3):195–9. https://doi.org/10.1097/AAP.0000000000000075. Erratum in: Reg Anesth Pain Med. 2014 Jul-Aug;39(4):357.
19. Girón-Arango L, Peng PWH, Chin KJ, Brull R, Perlas A. Pericapsular Nerve Group (PENG) block for hip fracture. Reg Anesth Pain Med. 2018;43(8):859–63. https://doi.org/10.1097/AAP.0000000000000847.
20. Aliste J, Layera S, Bravo D, et al. Randomized comparison between pericapsular nerve group (PENG) block and suprainguinal fascia iliaca block for total hip arthroplasty. Reg Anesth Pain Med. Published Online First: 20 July 2021. https://doi.org/10.1136/rapm-2021-102997.
21. Mosaffa F, Taheri M, Manafi Rasi A, Samadpour H, Memary E, Mirkheshti A. Comparison of pericapsular nerve group (PENG) block with fascia iliaca compartment block (FICB) for pain control in hip fractures: A double-blind prospective randomized controlled clinical trial. Orthop Traumatol Surg Res. 2022;108(1):103135. https://doi.org/10.1016/j.otsr.2021.103135.
22. Yu HC, Moser JJ, Chu AY, Montgomery SH, Brown N, Endersby RVW. Inadvertent quadriceps weakness following the pericapsular nerve group (PENG) block. Reg Anesth Pain Med. 2019;44(5):611–3. https://doi.org/10.1136/rapm-2018-100354.

23. Yeung JH, Gates S, Naidu BV, Wilson MJ, Gao Smith F. Paravertebral block versus thoracic epidural for patients undergoing thoracotomy. Cochrane Database Syst Rev. 2016;2(2):CD009121. https://doi.org/10.1002/14651858.CD009121.pub2.
24. Yeying G, Liyong Y, Yuebo C, Yu Z, Guangao Y, Weihu M, Liujun Z. Thoracic paravertebral block versus intravenous patient-controlled analgesia for pain treatment in patients with multiple rib fractures. J Int Med Res. 2017;45(6):2085–91. https://doi.org/10.1177/0300060517710068. Epub 2017 Jun 21. PMID: 28635359; PMCID: PMC5805206.
25. Bhalla PI, Solomon S, Zhang R, Witt CE, Dagal A, Joffe AM. Comparison of serratus anterior plane block with epidural and paravertebral block in critically ill trauma patients with multiple rib fractures. Trauma Surg Acute Care Open. 2021;6(1):e000621. https://doi.org/10.1136/tsaco-2020-000621.
26. Womack J, Pearson JD, Walker IA, Stephens NM, Goodman BA. Safety, complications and clinical outcome after ultrasound-guided paravertebral catheter insertion for rib fracture analgesia: a single-centre retrospective observational study. Anaesthesia. 2019;74(5):594–601. https://doi.org/10.1111/anae.14580.
27. Association of Anaesthetists of Great Britain & Ireland; Obstetric Anaesthetists' Association; Regional Anaesthesia UK. Regional anaesthesia and patients with abnormalities of coagulation: the Association of Anaesthetists of Great Britain & Ireland The Obstetric Anaesthetists' Association Regional Anaesthesia UK. Anaesthesia. 2013;68(9):966–72. https://doi.org/10.1111/anae.12359.
28. Beard L, Hillermann C, Beard E, Millerchip S, Sachdeva R, Gao Smith F, Veenith T. Multicenter longitudinal cross-sectional study comparing effectiveness of serratus anterior plane, paravertebral and thoracic epidural for the analgesia of multiple rib fractures. Reg Anesth Pain Med. 2020;45(5):351–6. https://doi.org/10.1136/rapm-2019-101119. Epub 2020 Mar 11.
29. Witt CE, Bulger EM. Comprehensive approach to the management of the patient with multiple rib fractures: a review and introduction of a bundled rib fracture management protocol. Trauma Surg Acute Care Open. 2017;2(1):e000064. https://doi.org/10.1136/tsaco-2016-000064.

Trauma Resuscitation in the Health Information Technology Age

38

Digital Technology for Trauma Documentation, Situation Awareness, Decision Support, Performance Analytics, and Research

Jenna Kroeker, Barak Raguan, Olivia Hunter, Patricia Balmes, Larissa Roux, Harvey G. Hawes, and S. Morad Hameed

Trauma systems have often been at the forefront of innovation in healthcare. Advances such as damage control resuscitation, dedicated trauma units, trauma team dynamics, prehospital transport, regional inclusive trauma systems, and trauma education programs have been nothing short of transformational in their impact and influence. Successful innovation in trauma has always engaged deeply with complex challenges and matched those challenges with fresh perspectives from diverse fields.

Now, with the exponential growth in computing power and remarkable advancements in computer user interface design, modern trauma systems are on the brink of new transformational changes. Health information technology (HIT), encompassing the electronic collection, storage, processing, and exchange of health information [1], presents intriguing opportunities to revolutionize how trauma teams collaborate during resuscitations, approach decision-making, monitor and enhance their performance, and gain valuable insights for injury control and health policy.

This chapter will explore the exciting advances and future opportunities that HIT innovation can offer, from delivery of best practices at the bedside to controlling injury at the population level.

J. Kroeker
Department of Surgery, Maimonides Medical Center, New York, NY, USA

Section of Trauma and Acute Care Surgery, University of British Columbia, Vancouver, BC, Canada
e-mail: jdkroeke@ualberta.ca

B. Raguan
Section of Trauma and Acute Care Surgery, University of British Columbia, Vancouver, BC, Canada

Department of Surgery, Sheba Medical Center, Cel Hashomer, Tel Aviv, Israel

O. Hunter
Faculty of Medicine, University of British Columbia, Vancouver, BC, Canada

P. Balmes · H. G. Hawes
Section of Trauma and Acute Care Surgery, University of British Columbia, Vancouver, BC, Canada
e-mail: patricia.balmes@vch.ca; harvey.hawes@vch.ca

L. Roux
Primary Care and Population Health, Department of Medicine, Stanford Medicine, Stanford, CA, USA
e-mail: lroux@stanford.edu

S. Morad Hameed (✉)
Section of Trauma and Acute Care Surgery, University of British Columbia, Vancouver, BC, Canada

Primary Care and Population Health, Department of Medicine, Stanford Medicine, Stanford, CA, USA
e-mail: morad@stanford.edu

Current State of HIT in Trauma Care

Capturing point of care resuscitation data in digital form has the potential to unlock analytic strategies that could transform trauma teams' abilities to predict risk, make decisions under rapidly evolving conditions, and assess and improve performance. Paper records and flowsheets, despite their familiarity and their ease of use, especially in acute resuscitation, are not an effective conduit for the extremely rich data that arise from the point of trauma care. The widespread transition to electronic health records (EHRs) seen around the world offers the promise of digital data capture and data analysis.

Efforts to harness EHR data to support continuous quality improvement have shown some early successes. For example, Kannan and colleagues [2] generated specific clinical registries from a legacy EHR by implementing data collection

L. Marshall Gillman, S. Widder (eds.), *Trauma Team Dynamics*, https://doi.org/10.1007/978-3-031-86312-7_38

principles, developing data warehousing solutions, and employing agile development strategies. Within a year, they created 43 specialty chronic disease registries with hundreds of decision support tools, quality metrics, and dashboards to support process-mapping of care and continuous quality improvement [2]. However, to date, EHRs have not been widely adapted to support trauma systems optimization.

For this purpose, trauma systems continue to rely on trauma registries to inform performance improvement and to support clinical research. While these registries have been instrumental in trauma systems development for generations, their use in modern big data environments is limited by challenges such as data entry delays, limited configurability, and the absence of high-resolution data with precise time-stamping. Additionally, manual abstraction of health record data to populate trauma registries is costly and excludes resource-constrained centers from the benefits of conventional trauma systems quality improvement. Ideally, the next generation of HIT would combine the agility of paper documentation with the promise of digital data collection and rapid analysis while serving as an interoperable front end for conventional legacy EHRs.

HIT as an Engine for Trauma System Design Thinking

The utilization of modern health information technology tools could empower trauma systems to tap into vast amounts of multi-dimensional, high-resolution, time-stamped data generated throughout the patient care process. This wealth of information, made accessible through seamless flow through the digital ecosystem to intuitive user interfaces, serves as an engine for driving solutions across the entire spectrum of trauma care. From trauma resuscitations in the trauma bay to system-level injury prevention strategies, data can be harnessed to enhance patient outcomes and promote equity in healthcare.

Transforming insights from raw data (or even from sophisticated data analysis) to effective action that improves trauma system performance may require a critical intermediate step. Design thinking is an iterative and human-centered approach to problem-solving and innovation [3]. It emphasizes empathy, collaboration, and a deep understanding of user needs to generate creative and effective solutions [4, 5]. By employing design thinking, we can shift our focus from a technology-driven perspective to a user-centric mindset, ensuring that the solutions we develop truly address the needs and challenges of the people involved.

There are five key steps to the design thinking approach:

1. *Empathize*: Gain insight from individuals and systems affected by trauma care, such as patients, healthcare providers, and administrators. This involves actively listening, conducting observations, and engaging in meaningful conversations to gain insights into their experiences, pain points, and aspirations.
2. *Define the problem*: Reframe the problem by narrowing down the focus and identifying the core needs and opportunities for improvement based on insights gained from empathy.
3. *Ideate*: Generate a wide range of ideas and potential solutions to address the defined problem.
4. *Prototype*: Create low-fidelity prototypes of potential solutions and gather feedback from end-users and stakeholders.
5. *Test and iterate*: Foster a culture of continuous learning and improvement through iterative refinement of solutions, incorporating feedback and data analysis and adapting to evolving needs. This ensures that innovations remain effective and relevant over time.

Almost all of these steps would benefit from the collection of multidimensional, high-resolution data. By integrating high-resolution data into the design thinking process, trauma teams can measure the impact of their solutions and implement iterative improvements based on evidence. This iterative cycle of data analysis, solution refinement, and continuous learning ensures that solutions are responsive to the evolving needs of trauma care and can drive meaningful and sustained improvements in the trauma ecosystem.

The design thinking framework, powered by point of care data, can be applied to data flow and analyses at several scales: efficient and complete documentation and population of conventional EHRs, trauma team situation awareness, decision support in trauma resuscitation, trauma care quality improvement, trauma research, and trauma systems design, including injury prevention and access to high quality trauma care in highly integrated trauma networks (Fig. 38.1).

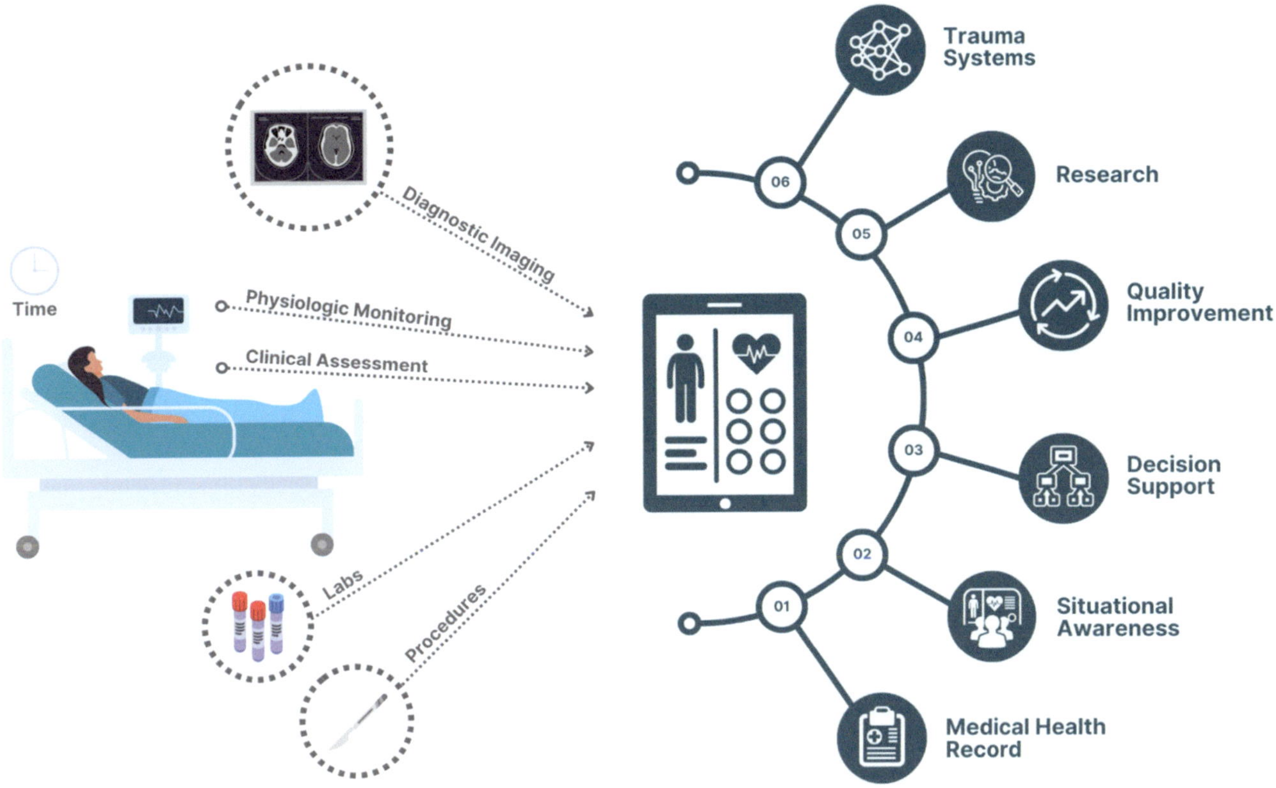

Fig. 38.1 Advances in HIT enable the integration of time-stamped, high-resolution data from numerous sources (i.e., multidimensional data) and the flow of that data to several tiers of analysis

Rapid and Complete Documentation

The major trauma patient medical record often requires input from multiple specialties and care providers along a complex and prolonged clinical pathway. Historically, this has led to inaccuracies in data entry and missing or lost data, even with the use of traditional electronic medical records [6, 7]. However, advances in HIT user interface design and mobility have enabled trauma teams to document right at the point of trauma resuscitation, and to create accurate, complete, and holistic patient electronic health records (EHRs). Numerous studies have validated the effectiveness of novel digital tools in improving documentation practices.

A pilot study at the Trauma Unit at Groote Schuur Hospital, University of Cape Town, demonstrated the successful implementation of an electronic trauma health record (eTHR) using mobile, iPad-based technology [8]. The transition from paper-based documentation to the eTHR resulted in higher documentation completion rates of trauma admission records, operative notes, and discharge summaries, along with increased provider satisfaction [8].

Similarly, the Craig Joint Theater Hospital in Afghanistan utilized the T6 Health Systems mobile application to improve their trauma documentation [9]. In a comparative study, the completeness and accuracy of data capture were evaluated by comparing T6 electronic records with handwritten documentation from the same trauma resuscitations. The study revealed an overall 13% increase in data capture compared to the gold standard paper resuscitation records, and a high accuracy rate of 96% with the electronic application [9]. This evidence supported the hypothesis that trauma-tailored electronic documentation applications, such as T6 Health Systems, can significantly enhance the completeness and accuracy of trauma documentation.

HIT, encompassing mobile applications and electronic records, enables the development of accurate, complete, and holistic patient EHRs in trauma care. The validation of these digital tools in real-world trauma settings underscores their potential to improve usable data capture, accessibility, and interoperability, with the potential to inform improved quality of patient care.

Situational Awareness: Overhead Dashboards in Trauma Resuscitation

Optimal patient outcomes in trauma resuscitation rely on seamless integration of multiple healthcare specialists and disciplines, all dependent on real-time data in a fast-paced and dynamic environment. Digital transformation brings forth the capability for multidisciplinary team members to share and access multidimensional data, contribute to shared mental models, and smooth the flow of resuscitation as data flows between user interfaces, monitors, labs and diagnostics, and overhead dashboards.

Studies in the field of cognitive science have revealed that the human brain possesses the highest capacity for processing visual information compared to other senses. In fact, it is estimated to be 10 times more efficient than touch and 100 times more efficient than hearing or smell [10]. Moreover, visual data is processed at such a remarkable speed and volume that a significant portion of this processing occurs subconsciously. This phenomenon, known as preattentive processing, plays a crucial role in reducing cognitive load, enabling us to effortlessly comprehend complex images by subconsciously organizing their components into a cohesive system. Consequently, through collaboration with cognitive psychologists and engineers, the application of visual cognition science has shown great promise in enhancing situational awareness within the healthcare domain.

To illustrate the potential benefits, Calder et al. conducted a study involving the implementation of an overhead visual dashboard that provided real-time updates on patient status during resuscitation simulations [11]. The participants in this study reported an increase in confidence levels and a reduction in stress during simulations. Furthermore, participants felt that the visual dashboard improved provider performance and facilitated smoother transitions in patient care. Similarly, Parush et al. (2017) showed how a visual dashboard improved teamwork (as measured by the Clinical Teamwork Scale), increased multidisciplinary discussion, and enhanced situational awareness (as measured by the Situational Awareness Global Assessment Technique tool) in resuscitation simulations [12]. Both studies suggest data visualization tools have the capacity to significantly improve team dynamics in real-life scenarios in the trauma bay.

T6 Health Systems, a mobile application specifically designed for the iPad to synchronize real-time data collection with trauma resuscitation workflows (as depicted in Fig. 38.2), offers options to display data on overhead dashboards, enhancing information accessibility and situational awareness (Fig. 38.3). This visual aid is designed to present real-time data in a way that reduces each practitioner's cognitive load, thereby allowing the trauma team to work together from a shared mental model. Ultimately, this technology enables a more synchronized and efficient approach to trauma resuscitation.

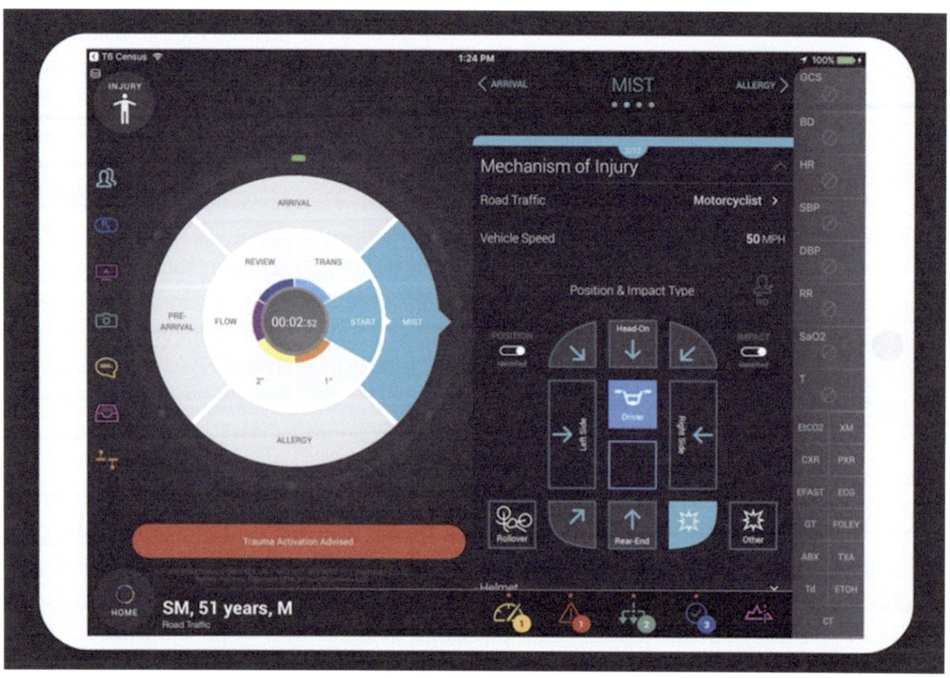

Fig. 38.2 Mobile, digital user interface configured to trauma workflows to support near real-time collection of resuscitation data. (Source: T6 Health Systems (used with permission))

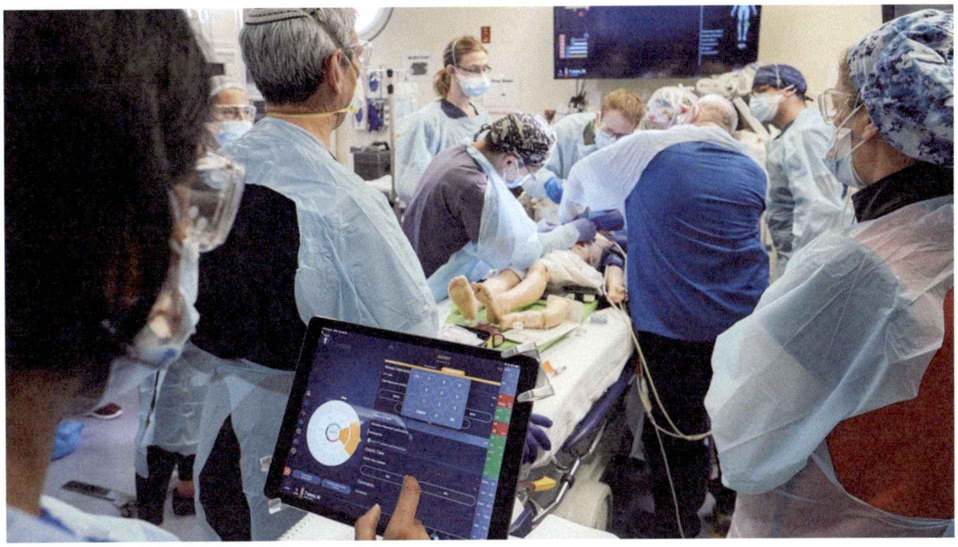

Fig. 38.3 T6 mobile application connected to overhead dashboard to enhance team situational awareness. (Source: Apple News (https://www.apple.com/newsroom/2021/11/veterans-use-apple-technology-to-revolutionize-trauma-medicine/))

Clinical Decision Support

The digital transformation of medical records enables context-based clinical decision support (CDS). CDS, including timely alerts, relevant clinical practice guidelines (CPGs), checklists, and risk scores, are triggered by incoming clinical assessments and offer tailored responses based on data inputs.

Integration of this digital technology in the trauma bay is already underway. For instance, a pilot study evaluating a digital decision support tool, called BloodNavigator, for massive transfusion during trauma resuscitation was found to be useful based on user feedback [13]. This tool featured a color display that changed based on the administered ratio of blood products, providing immediate visual feedback on adherence to evidence-based guidelines for blood product resuscitation.

Additionally, applications such as T6 offer customizable features that enable instant linkage to local clinical practice guidelines, checklists, and relevant risk scores when specific injury mechanisms are entered. For example, if a major blunt mechanism of injury is entered, the system will generate a suspected cervical spine injury clinical pathway with appropriate action items, such as ordering necessary imaging (Fig. 38.4). Whether CPGs or checklists are consulted or not, they bring tailored, evidence-based best practices to the bedside as a reference standard for teams working in stressful conditions under heavy time constraints.

Artificial intelligence and machine learning (AI/ML) have immense potential in enhancing clinical decision support in trauma care; however, they require high-resolution, time-stamped data that may not be readily available or accessible through conventional electronic health records (EHR) or registries to realize their full potential. A comprehensive review of AI/ML applications along the continuum of trauma care [14] showcased the promising capabilities of AI/ML in prognosticating critical care interventions and patient outcomes and informing patient trajectory. For instance, the Epic Deterioration Index (EDI), a machine learning tool, has been validated as effective in predicting mortality and unplanned ICU admission in trauma patients, achieving an impressive AUC of 0.98 [15]. Similarly, an algorithm utilizing vital signs, demographics, and Glasgow Coma Scale (GCS) achieved an AUC of 0.99 in determining the need for life-saving interventions upon emergency department (ED) presentation [16]. Moreover, utilization of AI/ML during the PROPPR trial, which collected rich data during the study period, revealed novel associations between hemostasis and time that were not discovered via conventional statistical analysis methods [17]. By integrating AI/ML into a comprehensive digital framework, as depicted in Fig. 38.5, its utility is amplified through unrestricted access to high-resolution data.

This integration allows for a more comprehensive assessment of all available clinical clues, accounting for variations in their importance over time, and revolutionizing decision-making. HIT capable of capturing and analyzing incoming high-resolution data at the point of care may make it possible to equip trauma teams with increasingly sophisticated AI/ML predictive analytics to support more effective clinical decision-making in rapidly evolving situations.

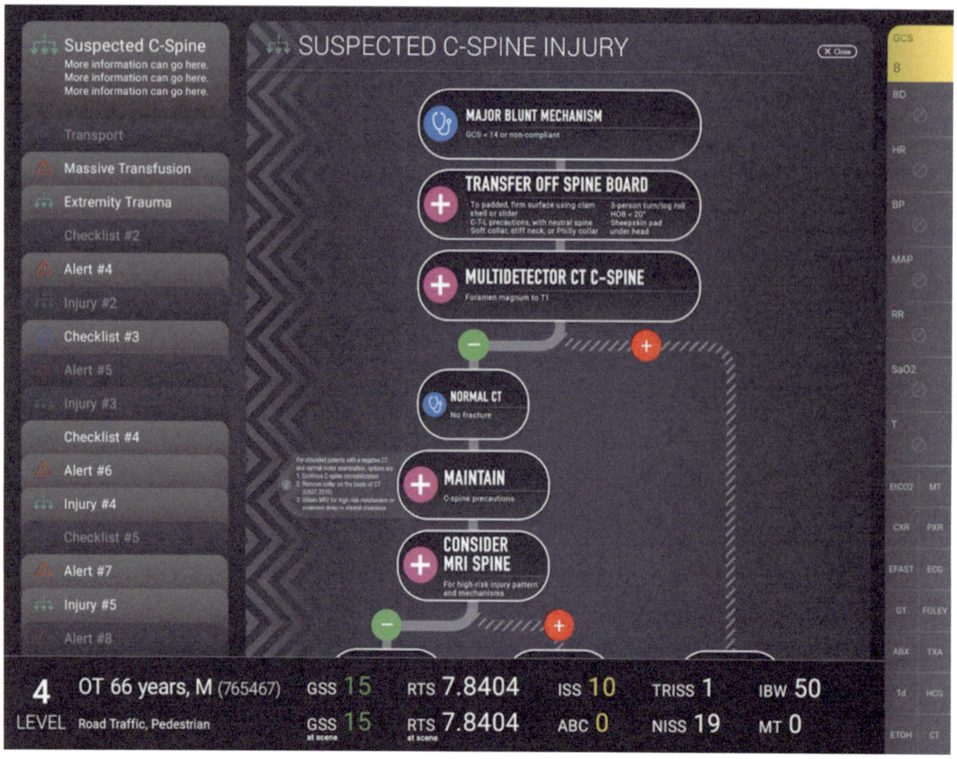

Fig. 38.4 T6 Dashboard displaying clinical practice guidelines in response to real-time data input. Here, input of a major blunt mechanism of injury triggered an institution-specific cervical spine injury pathway. (Source: T6 Health Systems (used with permission))

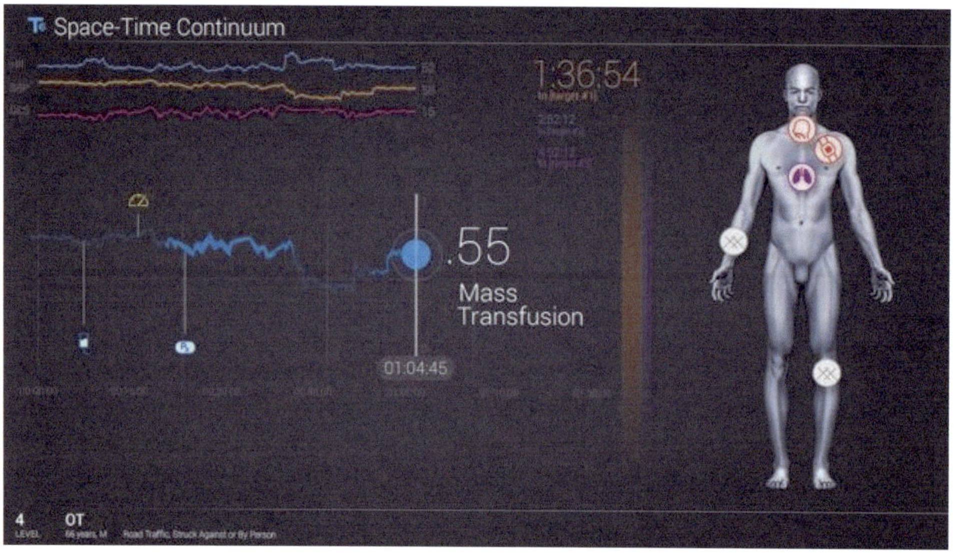

Fig. 38.5 Schematic of dashboard view demonstrating ongoing, real-time refinement of risk prediction (i.e., probability of massive transfusion) as new data accumulates over time, and data elements in the predictive AI/ML model undergo time-dependent changes in their clinical significance. (Source: T6 Health Systems (used with permission))

Quality Improvement

Utilizing digital tools, the collection and accessibility of high-resolution digital data along the continuum of trauma care enables tracking of specific actions performed during the care process and the instantaneous creation of process maps (Fig. 38.6).

Process mapping is a valuable tool in quality improvement efforts as it helps identify inefficiencies, bottlenecks, and variations in the care process. By visualizing the care pathway, healthcare teams can streamline workflows, reduce delays, and enhance overall efficiency. It also facilitates the identification of areas for standardization and the development of standardized protocols, ensuring consistent and high-quality care delivery, promoting patient safety, and reducing errors. For example, implementation of a hip fracture care pathway in response to patient process mapping improved patient throughput to operative intervention and complication identification [18].

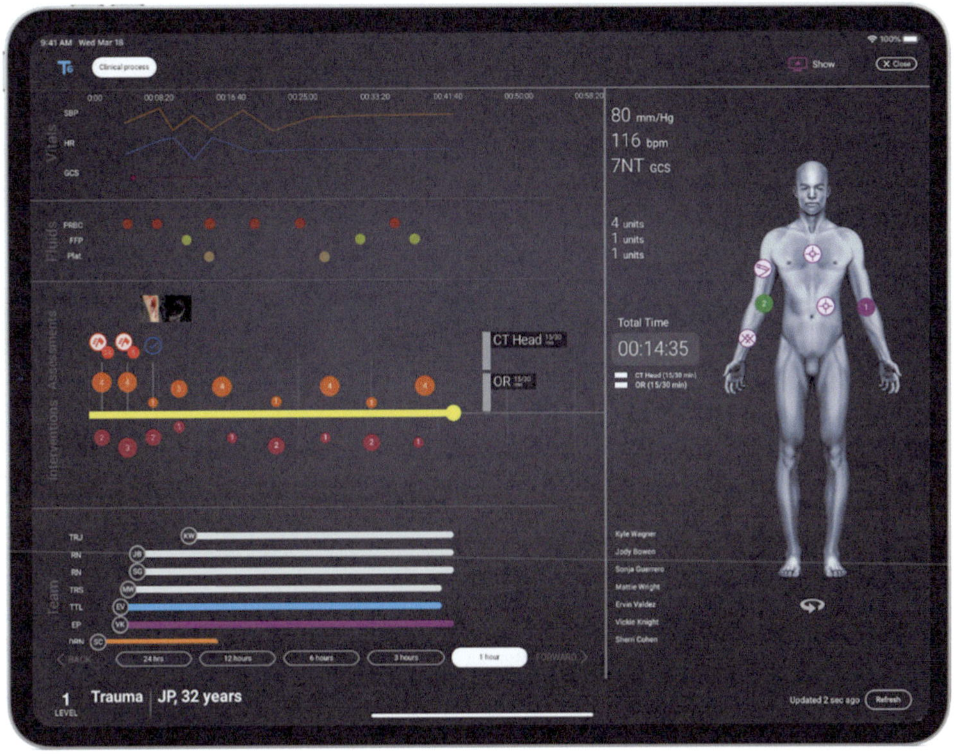

Fig. 38.6 Visualization of patient data along the space-time continuum facilitates tracking of specific actions during the care process and enables creation of process maps for quality improvement initiatives. (Source: T6 Health Systems (used with permission))

Moreover, process mapping serves as a foundation for value-based healthcare (VBHC) agendas. VBHC is a strategic healthcare delivery model that incorporates evidence-based medicine with patient-perceived value conferred by healthcare interventions [19]. Successful VBHC relies on high-resolution data for constant quality assessment, implementation of targeted interventions, monitoring of changes, and outcome measurement. This iterative approach allows for ongoing evaluation and refinement of care processes to continually improve patient outcomes and satisfaction. Developing HIT innovations has tapped potential in driving the adoption of VBHC initiatives in trauma centers. For example, the T6 application offers an automated framework that calculates personnel, equipment, supplies, and space costs, enabling time-driven activity-based costing (TDABC). This feature can measure the economic value of value-based healthcare initiatives by providing accurate cost assessments. However, additional research is required to validate the effectiveness of these types of digital tools in delivering these benefits.

Research

Digital transformation of the medical health record is revolutionizing trauma research by overcoming traditional barriers associated with data collection and analysis. Unlike conventional trauma registries built from traditional EHRs or paper charts, which lack configurability for efficient data retrieval and require substantial time and resources for creation and maintenance, digital data capture applications and advancements in data storage and exchange facilitate the seamless and instant creation of comprehensive, information-rich trauma databases.

A notable example of the power of digital technology in trauma research is the successful implementation of the electronic Trauma Health Record (eTHR) pilot in Groote Schuur Hospital, in Cape Town, South Africa [8]. Over the course of a year, the eTHR pilot generated an extensive dataset comprising more than 11, 000 trauma admissions, offering researchers valuable insights and opportunities for analyzing injury patterns, identifying trends, and evaluating clinical outcomes (Fig. 38.7) [20]. For instance, researchers were able to conduct in-depth analyses of a large cohort of 800+ patients with penetrating abdominal trauma to identify indicators predictive of successful nonoperative management [21]. These analyses were facilitated by leveraging the digital database created through the eTHR pilot project.

The success of the eTHR pilot exemplifies how digital technology can overcome barriers in injury surveillance and data collection for research purposes, even in resource-constrained settings. By enhancing the speed and ease of data retrieval and analysis, the eTHR pilot contributed to evidence-based decision-making and advancing trauma care practices. The transformative potential of mobile digital technology in trauma research is evident, as it improves the efficiency and effectiveness of research efforts in the field.

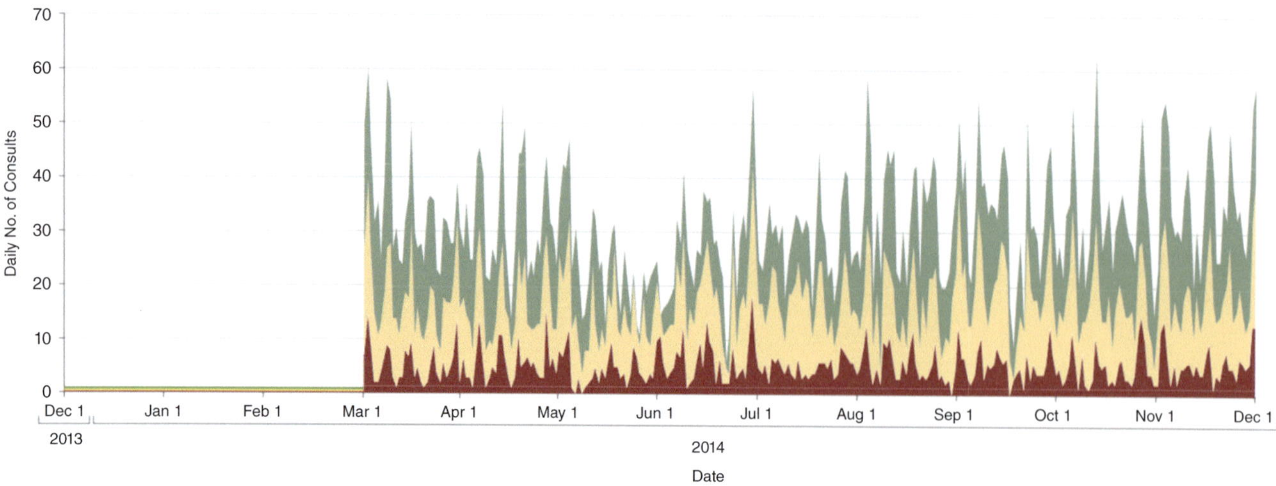

Fig. 38.7 Dashboard view of daily trauma center volumes showcasing the implementation of an iPad-based electronic trauma health record (eTHR) at a bustling South African trauma center. The eTHR facilitated the population of an electronic database, enabling data visualization, real-time reporting, and research-oriented data analysis. (Source: Authors original research, also published [Zargaran E, Spence R, Adolph L, Nicol A, Schuurman N, Navsaria P, Ramsey D, Hameed SM. Association Between Real-time Electronic Injury Surveillance Applications and Clinical Documentation and Data Acquisition in a South African Trauma Center. JAMA Surg. 2018 May 16;153 (5):e180087. doi: 10.1001/jamasurg.2018.0087. Epub 2018 May 16. PMID: 29541765; PMCID: PMC5875377.)

Trauma Systems

The pinnacle of data flow in trauma care is achieved when data captured through digital technology informs trauma systems performance improvement, including injury prevention strategies, trauma education, healthcare policy, and economics. This transformative opportunity lies in harnessing the continuously flowing data, leveraging analytics and data visualization strategies, and fusing creative innovations together to improve health equity.

One instance where digital technology is currently being utilized to address health equity by improving access to trauma care is through trauma education and mentoring. Using video-conferencing applications, trauma surgeons can provide remote guidance and instruction to non-surgeon physicians in performing critical procedures, such as a decompressive fasciotomy [22, 23]. Studies have demonstrated the effectiveness of telementoring in improving practitioner confidence and trauma team dynamics, paving the way for improving trauma patient outcomes in rural and resource-limited settings [22, 23]. The fusion of augmented reality (AR) technology with telementoring further elevates the potential of remote mentoring and guidance. For example, the United States military has explored its use for damage control procedures in battlefield situations where immediate access to a trauma surgeon may be challenging [24]. By using AR glasses and telestrated instructions, a remote surgeon can guide a nonsurgeon through critical procedures, effectively providing real-time support and guidance. AR telementoring allows participants to complete tasks with greater accuracy and fewer distractions, presenting exciting possibilities for future telementoring in real-life trauma scenarios [25]. Remote telementoring is discussed further in Chaps. 39 and 40.

While the above digital innovations have demonstrated positive impacts on a smaller scale, it is crucial to address the larger problem of the global burden of injury, which has gained international attention as a significant public health issue. Consensus among experts emphasizes two key factors for successful implementation of a global injury-prevention initiative using digital technology: (1) establishing seamless pathways for data linkage and analysis to enable real-time data flow to guide action in injury prevention and trauma care improvement/education, and (2) fostering strong partnerships among data scientists, health economists, data engineers, injury prevention workers, trauma clinicians, and policymakers to ensure analytical capacity keeps pace with the growing influx of data, leading to meaningful improvements in society's safety [26]. Currently, this goal of leveraging digital technology to address the global burden of injury has not been fully realized.

In an increasingly globalized world, the use of digital technology has the potential to shrink distances and open doors to new opportunities, addressing trauma system inequalities and inefficiencies.

Conclusion

We stand on the threshold of unprecedented transformations in healthcare propelled by digital technology. Looking ahead, we anticipate remarkable transformations in trauma care as advances in HIT drive innovations such as augmented reality (AR) with telementoring and the integration of AI/ML into clinical practice.

Advancements in data integration, mobile digital technology, and achieving both intraoperability (i.e., complete integration with existing electronic platforms within a hospital or healthcare setting) and interoperability (i.e., sharing a transfer of anonymized data sets between healthcare systems) will revolutionize trauma care and enable a collective global effort to reduce the burden of injury and improve trauma outcomes [26]. However, challenges such as generating incompatible data sets, ensuring privacy and data security, and carefully considering the potential harms and benefits of technology must be addressed to facilitate widespread adoption [26].

As we navigate this exciting journey, it is crucial to remember that technology is a tool, not a panacea, and that a deep understanding of the challenges in trauma care should guide our pursuit of innovative solutions. The integration of technology into clinical practice should be done thoughtfully so as to ensure solutions address the unique needs of patients, clinicians, and systems. By leveraging design thinking—an iterative process involving defining problems, ideating solutions, and continuous analysis to gain actionable insights—we can foster meaningful, transformative progress in the field of trauma. The future of trauma care is ours to shape with thoughtful and purposeful application of technology.

Key Points

- Advances in computing power, data storage, data analysis, and clinical informatics have created new opportunities for the evolution of trauma systems.
- Clinical data captured in near real time can be applied to clinical decision support and to enhance trauma team dynamics.
- Unprecedented access to high-resolution data can inform design thinking approaches to trauma systems quality improvement.
- High-quality data collected at the point of care holds the promise of driving more sophisticated analytic and risk prediction strategies for trauma care.
- Technological advances in telehealth can increase the reach and impact of trauma systems to rural and remote communities and vulnerable populations.

References

1. Office for Civil Rights (OCR). Health information technology. HHS.gov. Published May 7, 2008. https://www.hhs.gov/hipaa/for-professionals/special-topics/health-information-technology/index.html. Accessed 20 May 2023.
2. Kannan V, Fish JS, Mutz JM, Carrington AR, Lai K, Davis LS, et al. Rapid development of specialty population registries and quality measures from electronic health record data. An Agile Framework. Methods Inf Med. 2017;56(99):e74–83. https://doi.org/10.3414/ME16-02-0031.
3. Razzouk R, Shute V. What is design thinking and why is it important? Rev Educ Res. 2012;82(3):330–48. https://doi.org/10.3102/0034654312457429.
4. Roberts JP, Fisher TR, Trowbridge MJ, Bent C. A design thinking framework for healthcare management and innovation. Healthc (Amst). 2016;4(1):11–4. https://doi.org/10.1016/j.hjdsi.2015.12.002.
5. Lorusso L, Lee JH, Worden EA. Design thinking for healthcare: transliterating the creative problem-solving method into architectural practice. HERD. 2021;14(2):16–29. https://doi.org/10.1177/1937586721994228.
6. Kieffer JC, Thompson A, Elwell S, DePiero A. Comparison of paper and electronic documentation for trauma activations in a pediatric trauma center. Am J Emerg Med. 2021;50:719–23. https://doi.org/10.1016/j.ajem.2021.09.049.
7. Bilyeu P, Eastes L. Use of the electronic medical record for trauma resuscitations: how does this impact documentation completeness? J Trauma Nurs. 2013;20(3):166–8. https://doi.org/10.1097/JTN.0b013e3182a17195.
8. Zargaran E, Spence R, Adolph L, Nicol A, Schuurman N, Navsaria P, et al. Association between real-time electronic injury surveillance applications and clinical documentation and data acquisition in a South African Trauma Center. JAMA Surg. 2018;153(5):e180087. https://doi.org/10.1001/jamasurg.2018.0087.
9. Angotti LM, How RA, Barnack KR, Aden JK, Vitale DA, Folwell JS, et al. Electronic trauma resuscitation documentation and decision support using T6 Health Systems Mobile Application: a combat trauma center pilot program. J Trauma Acute Care Surg. 2020;89(6):1172–6. https://doi.org/10.1097/TA.0000000000002909.
10. Nørretranders T. The user illusion: Cutting consciousness down to size. 1991;467. https://psycnet.apa.org/fulltext/1998-07235-000.pdf
11. Calder LA, Bhandari A, Mastoras G, Day K, Momtahan K, Falconer M, et al. Healthcare providers' perceptions of a situational awareness display for emergency department resuscitation: a simulation qualitative study. Int J Qual Health Care. 2018;30(1):16–22. https://doi.org/10.1093/intqhc/mzx159.
12. Parush A, Mastoras G, Bhandari A, Momtahan K, Day K, Weitzman B, et al. Can teamwork and situational awareness (SA) in ED resuscitations be improved with a technological cognitive aid? Design and a pilot study of a team situation display. J Biomed Inform. 2017;76:154–61. https://doi.org/10.1016/j.jbi.2017.10.009.
13. Schmulevich D, Cacchione PZ, Holland S, Quinlan K, Hinkle A, Meador C, et al. Optimizing a decision support system for damage-control resuscitation using mixed methods human factors analysis.

J Trauma Acute Care Surg. 2021;91(2S Suppl 2):S154–61. https://doi.org/10.1097/TA.0000000000003224.
14. Hunter OF, Perry F, Salehi M, Bandurski H, Hubbard A, Ball CG, et al. Science fiction or clinical reality: a review of the applications of artificial intelligence along the continuum of trauma care. World J Emerg Surg. 2023;18(1):16. https://doi.org/10.1186/s13017-022-00469-1.
15. Mou Z, Godat LN, El-Kareh R, Berndtson AE, Doucet JJ, Costantini TW. Electronic health record machine learning model predicts trauma inpatient mortality in real time: a validation study. J Trauma Acute Care Surg. 2022;92(1):74–80. https://doi.org/10.1097/TA.0000000000003431.
16. Liu NT, Holcomb JB, Wade CE, Darrah MI, Salinas J. Utility of vital signs, heart rate variability and complexity, and machine learning for identifying the need for lifesaving interventions in trauma patients. Shock. 2014;42(2):108–14. https://doi.org/10.1097/SHK.0000000000000186.
17. Nguyen M, Pirracchio R, Kornblith LZ, Callcut R, Fox EE, Wade CE, et al. Dynamic impact of transfusion ratios on outcomes in severely injured patients: targeted machine learning analysis of the Pragmatic, Randomized Optimal Platelet and Plasma Ratios randomized clinical trial. J Trauma Acute Care Surg. 2020;89(3):505–13. https://doi.org/10.1097/TA.0000000000002819.
18. Sayeed Z, Anoushiravani A, El-Othmani M, Barinaga G, Sayeed Y, Cagle P Jr, et al. Implementation of a hip fracture care pathway using lean six sigma methodology in a level I trauma Center. J Am Acad Orthop Surg. 2018;26(24):881–93. https://doi.org/10.5435/JAAOS-D-16-00947.
19. Bae JM. Value-based medicine: concepts and application. Epidemiol Health. 2015;37:e2015014. https://doi.org/10.4178/epih/e2015014.
20. Spence RT, Zargaran E, Hameed SM, Navsaria P, Nicol A. Mobile health technology transforms injury severity scoring in South Africa. J Surg Res. 2016;204(2):384–92. https://doi.org/10.1016/j.jss.2016.05.021.
21. Sander A, Spence R, Ellsmere J, Hoogerboord M, Edu S, Nicol A, et al. Penetrating abdominal trauma in the era of selective conservatism: a prospective cohort study in a level 1 trauma center. Eur J Trauma Emerg Surg. 2022;48(2):881–9. https://doi.org/10.1007/s00068-020-01478-y.
22. Dawe P, Kirkpatrick A, Talbot M, Beckett A, Garraway N, Wong H, et al. Tele-mentored damage-control and emergency trauma surgery: a feasibility study using live-tissue models. Am J Surg. 2018;215(5):927–9. https://doi.org/10.1016/j.amjsurg.2018.01.016.
23. Hintz G, Haines V, Dawe P. Rural trauma telementoring: a pilot project. Can J Surg. 2022;65(5):E567–72. https://doi.org/10.1503/cjs.015020.
24. Harris TE, DeLellis SF, Heneghan JS, Buckman RF, Miller GT, Magee JH, et al. Augmented reality forward damage control procedures for nonsurgeons: a feasibility demonstration. Mil Med. 2020;185(Suppl 1):521–5. https://doi.org/10.1093/milmed/usz298.
25. Andersen D, Popescu V, Cabrera ME, Shanghavi A, Mullis B, Marley S, et al. An augmented reality-based approach for surgical telementoring in austere environments. Mil Med. 2017;182(S1):310–5. https://doi.org/10.7205/MILMED-D-16-00051.
26. Zargaran E, Adolph L, Schuurman N, Roux L, Ramsey D, Simons R, et al. A global agenda for electronic injury surveillance: Consensus statement from the Trauma Association of Canada, the Trauma Society of South Africa, and the Panamerican Trauma Society. J Trauma Acute Care Surg. 2016;80(1):168–70. https://doi.org/10.1097/TA.0000000000000880.

39 Telemedicine and Future Innovation

Corry J. Kucik, J. Jonas Carmichael, and William P. Mulvoy III

… and yet a true creator is necessity, which is the mother of our invention. (Plato, The Republic, Book II, 369c)

Introduction: The Need

Trauma remains a leading cause of death and disability throughout the world, including developed nations. Despite the rigorous construction of advanced trauma systems throughout the United States, regional differences persist and can be exacerbated by supply and geography constraints. Mismatches exist between the incidence of trauma throughout the United States and the number of traumatologists, Level 1 trauma centers, or even adequate community hospitals existing to service this need (Fig. 39.1). Due to multiple reasons (costs, inability to recruit and retain clinicians, rarity of certain types of trauma), there may never be a day that enough fully staffed and qualified centers will exist to enhance care in austere locations. Further, the "tyranny of distance" imposed not only on rural locations but also on special populations (e.g., correctional facilities, home health care settings, nursing homes, military populations overseas or at sea, cruise ship passengers) can never be fully alleviated by the construction of US trauma centers, exacerbating the shortfall all the more.

The Promise of Innovation and Telemedicine

Bridges to the future are needed not only to service this great need of trauma care, but perhaps, in time and with game-changing technologies, to prevent and obviate it. The use of the word "innovation" is common in medicine today, where everyone from startup companies to the boards of established companies ceaselessly searches to profit from the next "big thing" in medicine. Telemedicine, the delivery of health care and the exchange of health-care information across distances, holds particular promise in trauma care, particularly when existing limitations (supply, distance, etc.) render it either more acceptable than existing conventional services or indeed the only option available.

Telemedicine is defined by the Telemedicine Information Exchange (1997) as the "use of electronic signals to transfer medical data (photographs, x-ray images, audio, patient records, videoconferences, etc.) from one site to another via the Internet, Intranets, PCs, satellites, or videoconferencing telephone equipment in order to improve access to health care." According to the Telemedicine Report to Congress (1997), "telemedicine can mean access to health care where little had been available before. In emergency cases, this access can mean the difference between life and death. In particular, in those cases where fast medical response time and specialty care are needed, telemedicine availability can be critical. For example, a specialist at a North Carolina University Hospital was able to diagnose a rural patient's hairline spinal fracture at a distance, using telemedicine video imaging. The patient's life was saved because treatment was done on-site without physically transporting the patient to the specialist who was located a great distance away."

Telemedicine interactions are generally classified as either prerecorded (also called "store-and-forward") or real time (also called "synchronous"). In the former, information is acquired and stored before being sent to an expert for interpretation at some later time. E-mail is a common method of store-and-forward interaction today. In contrast, in real-time interactions, there is minimal appreciable delay between the information's collection, transmission, and display. Interactive communication between individuals at the sites is therefore possible. Videoconferencing is a common method of real-time interaction.

C. J. Kucik (✉)
Department of Anesthesiology and Pain Medicine, University of Washington School of Medicine, Seattle, WA, USA

J. J. Carmichael · W. P. Mulvoy III
Department of Anesthesiology, Division of Cardiac Anesthesiology and Critical Care Medicine, University of Florida College of Medicine, Gainesville, FL, USA
e-mail: wmulvoy@anest.ufl.edu

L. Marshall Gillman, S. Widder (eds.), *Trauma Team Dynamics*, https://doi.org/10.1007/978-3-031-86312-7_39

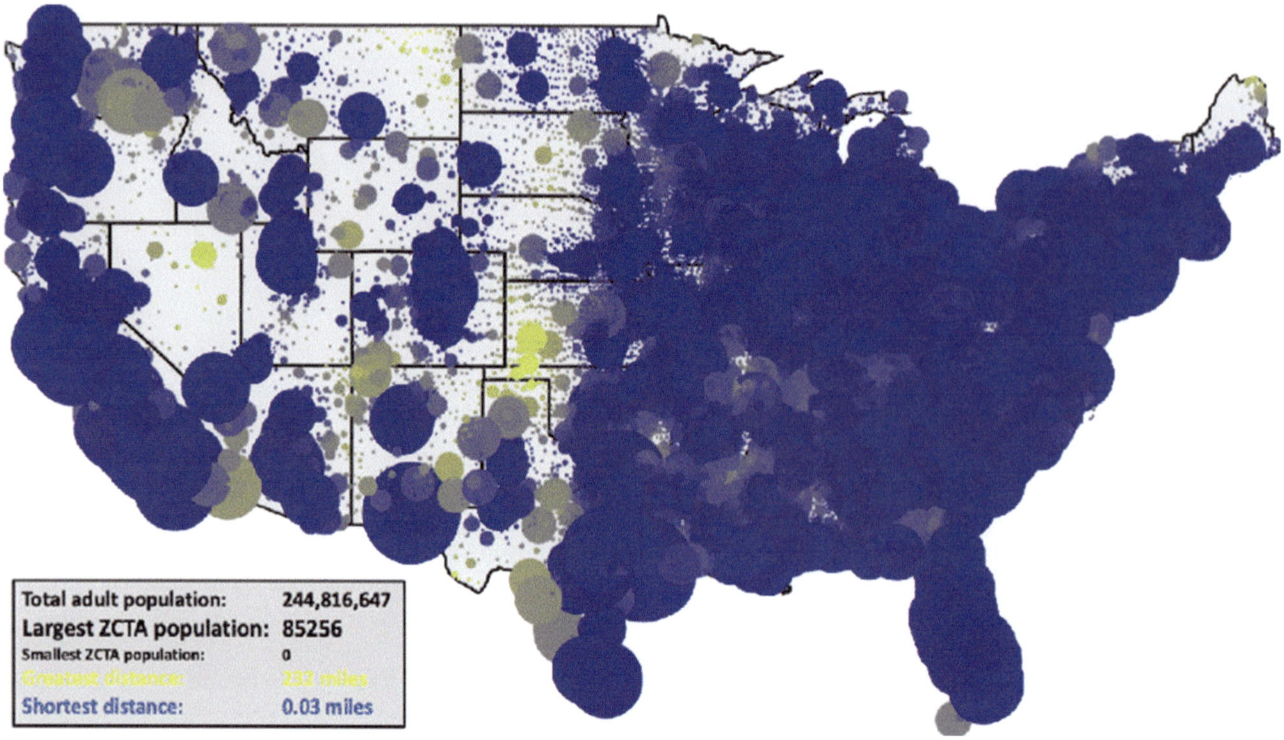

Fig. 39.1 Map of CONUS with relative population sizes and proximities to a civilian level 1 or level 2 trauma center. Every dot represents a single ZCTA. Smaller dots represent sparsely populated ZCTAs, whereas larger dots represent densely populated ZCTAs. Blue dots are relatively close to a civilian trauma center, whereas yellow dots are relatively distant. CONUS, continental USA; ZCTA, Zip Code Tabulation Area. Building trauma capability: using geospatial analysis to consider military treatment facilities for trauma center development—Scientific Figure on ResearchGate. (Available from: https://www.researchgate.net/figure/Map-of-CONUS-with-relative-population-sizes-and-proximities-to-a-civilian-level-1-or_fig 1_360816379 [accessed 26 Oct 2024])

The common thread for all telemedicine applications is that a client (e.g., patient or health-care worker) obtains advice or—as we will likely see in the future with haptics (tactile feedback technologies that recreate the sense of touch) and robotics—direct intervention from someone with more expertise, even when the parties are separated by space, time, or both.

History and Development

As human beings spread throughout every environment on the globe and even into space, the need for technology to push health care to the patient has followed. Telemedicine has thus developed into many different entities that at their core deliver information over great distances thus improving access to medical care. Describing its broad scope, Reid defines telemedicine as "the use of advanced telecommunications technologies to exchange health information and provide health care services across geographic, time, social, and cultural barriers" [1]. The need to overcome these varied barriers has driven the growth of telemedicine into multiple outlets and practices.

Telemedicine can be classified by the type of interaction between the client and health care expert in contrast with the content of the information being transmitted [2]. In "store and forward" telemedicine, the necessary information is compiled and then sent to an expert for evaluation later. There is an inherent delay in the interpretation of the data but access to advanced technologies aids the definitive care of the patient. Cardiology event monitors, diagnostic images, or expert e-mail consultation are examples of "store-and-forward" technologies. Real-time interactions allow an immediate assessment of the patient, data, and situation to expedite appropriate care with the remote assistance of a subject matter expert. One such example is simple audio feeds broadcast over various networks that provide first responders the ability to interact with Emergency Medicine physicians and appropriately triage patients to specialty centers. Tertiary care hospitals use networked programs to link with rural or suburban areas over high-speed lines or private point-to-point connections for telecommunication among providers. The information transmitted can range from text and audio to more sophisticated interactions such as images, video, or robotic interfaces that may allow a combination of several interfaces.

The term "telepresence" describes the ability of health care providers to interact in real time with telecommunication equipment, allowing for immediate feedback and assistance. Adapted for trauma, telepresence allows experienced trauma surgeons or critical care providers to bridge the experience and access gap to trauma care that may exist in rural settings [3]. Telemedicine serves as an interface for inter-hospital trauma care between echelons of care, in the pre-hospital setting to guide the care of first responders, or as a mobile system deployed to disaster settings [3].

In its simplest form, telemedicine began as a sort of public health service in the Middle Ages, where bonfires in Europe were lit to signal the spread of bubonic plague. Outside of simple mail service, the technology slowly developed until telegraphy was utilized in the 1800s by American Civil War surgeons to create casualty lists and request supplies. The telephone allowed further advances in the early twentieth century, ranging from simple communication to the transmission of heart sounds from an amplified stethoscope. A telepsychiatry program at the Nebraska Psychiatric Institute was developed by Dr. Cecil Wittson in the 1950s and expanded in the 1960s to encompass real-time consultation via closed-circuit television [4].

Early modern telemedicine is associated with another technological boon of the twentieth century—the National Aeronautics and Space Administration. NASA expanded on the telelinks that relayed biometric data collected from animals sent into space to develop the Integrated Medical and Behavioral Laboratories and Measurement Systems (IMBLMS) program in 1964. IMBLMS sought to move past simple monitoring to actual assistance of an astronaut in the delivery of self-aid or buddy-aid when a return from orbit was impractical [5]. This technology matured in a terrestrial form through a partnership between NASA, the Papago Indian Reservation, the Indian Health Service, and the Department of Health, Education, and Welfare with Arizona's Space Technology Applied to Rural Papago Advanced Health Care (STARPAHC). The service was provided from 1972 to 1975 and delivered health care in the underserved Papago Reservation through a van staffed by paramedics who broadcast data such as X-ray images over a two-way microwave transmission to physicians at the Public Health Service Hospital [6]. Given limitations in technology and timeliness of the care that could be provided, nearly all of these efforts focused on routine care.

In 1978, Dr. R Adams Cowley simulated a response to a crash of a DC-6 airplane wherein providers were able to transmit images of burn victims in real time via satellite to a burn unit in San Antonio and medical centers throughout the Washington DC area [7]. The use of satellites for medical support in disaster management was first seen during the coordination of international rescue assets after the Mexico City earthquake of 1985 [8]. Satellite transmission has become the mainstay of large data transmission, but its cost and large platform size often limit its wide-scale application. The expanded use of devices with access to broadband global area networks (BGAN) now allows for a portable communication device to provide telemedicine in areas devoid of local networks. Cost can still be an issue, though BGAN systems have the upload and download speeds to perform video teleconferencing in contrast to cheaper and very small aperture satellite systems. Used in multiple configurations, devices with BGAN connectivity have been used in remote settings such as rural Africa to provide real-time ultrasound interpretation [9]. The military has incorporated devices with BGAN connectivity to aid first responders in the triage and treatment of casualties [10]. In areas where the infrastructure exists, wireless cellular-based broadband has enabled a wide array of potential therapeutic interventions through the use of smartphones and laptops with applications to acquire, interpret, and transmit data. Modern trauma telemedicine and telepresence centers often use a combination of such systems to interact in prehospital and inter-hospital settings [3].

Outcomes

The use of telemedicine has amassed impressive evidence supporting its use as a reliable, reproducible technology feasible across multiple platforms and venues of care. Central to its utility is the ability to improve access to health care, but a significant cost advantage lies in its ability to improve the triage of trauma patients. Rogers et al. [11] in 2001 described a tele-trauma program in rural Vermont in an observational study evaluating the impact of a real-time telemedicine consult with a trauma surgeon and a community hospital emergency department. In 41 consultations consisting mostly of motor vehicle collisions (49%) and/or blunt trauma (95%), 31 were transferred to the tertiary care center, of which three cases were considered lifesaving. Patient disposition was the predominant query, and 15% of cases were kept at the referring facility. A total of 80% of providers surveyed felt that telemedicine improved patient care.

Duchesne et al. conducted a comparative analysis of outcomes before and after the introduction of telemedicine in the management of trauma patients treated at seven rural emergency departments in Mississippi, [12] demonstrating both improved rural evaluation and management. The hospitals utilized remote-controlled video cameras to evaluate the management of traumatically injured patients over 5 years, comparing 351 historical controls directly transferred to the trauma center with 463 virtual consults. Of the virtual consults, only 51 patients were triaged to the trauma center despite telemedicine patients having a higher injury severity score (18 vs. 10, $p < 0.001$), with no differences in patient age, sex, method of transportation, or mortality. An impressive difference in hospital cost was found between the groups (USD 1,126,683 versus 7,632,624, $p < 0.001$) suggesting that telemedicine significantly improved evaluation and management of rural trauma patients at reduced costs without significant changes in mortality.

In a retrospective analysis of one of the more robust telemedicine centers in the United States, Latifi et al. described their early experience of a telemedicine system involving five rural hospitals and a Level I trauma center in southern Arizona [13]. In a retrospective analysis of 59 tele-consults involving a mix of general surgery (41%) and trauma patients (59%), 29% of patients were held at their referring hospital for ongoing care while six tele-consults led to potentially lifesaving therapy. Reducing transfers saved an average of USD 19,698 per air transport or USD 2055 per ground transport, again suggesting that a telepresence can effectively improve trauma outcomes while reducing costs.

In a study of telemedicine for 70 burn patients, Saffle et al. described a 55.7% reduction in emergent transfers to a burn center compared with a historical cohort [14]. Ten patients were effectively discharged from their referral center's emergency department. In addition to the decreased transfers, this strategy allowed for more effective utilization of the increasingly limited resource of the modern burn center. Interestingly, estimates of burn sizes by burn center physicians correlated between telemedicine and direct inspection estimates, though both differed significantly from the estimates of the referring physician, suggesting not only a reduction in the over- or under-triage inherent in initial burn assessment but also the diagnostic integrity of the telemedicine system on a clinical variable likely to have significant impacts on care and patient outcome. Notably, the telemedicine interaction was also viewed favorably by both providers and patients.

In a Canadian evaluation using videoconferencing and the transfer of a real-time ultrasound information, Dyer et al. were able to observe and direct 20 acute, focused assessments with sonography for trauma (FAST) exams, identifying five cases of hemoperitoneum and two pneumothoraces, while also being able to provide feedback for the sonographer [15]. The ability of telepresence to fill the experience gap present in trauma care was again demonstrated when, using a video laryngoscope modified with a Wi-Fi module broadcasting over a telemedicine network, a physician specializing in airway management was able to assist a healthcare provider performing tracheal intubation in a remote hospital [16].

Developing a Telemedicine System

Multiple factors will inevitably surface to impede the easy implementation of a telemedicine program. Though an individual location's factors will vary widely, at a minimum, an institution considering adopting such an innovation should:

1. Develop a comprehensive business plan, to include information technology and administrative support at all hours if necessary.
2. Assess the need for administrative or structural changes required for its incorporation in the delivery of care.
3. Build infrastructure when necessary.
4. Encourage and provide funding for telemedicine development and research, often through the designation of promising and respected local champions.
5. Develop a plan for implementation (once clinical effectiveness and cost-effectiveness have been demonstrated).
6. Gain "buy-in" from all staff (physicians, nursing, information technology, administration, patient advocacy).
7. Create training, practice guidelines, credentialing, and continuing quality improvement mechanisms.
8. Address overarching and local ethical and medico-legal concerns.
9. Ensure the security of patient data under existing privacy regulations.
10. Integrate clinical staff (user) concerns into any engineering or technical changes.
11. Account for linguistic and literacy differences.
12. Be sensitive to particular technical and organizational factors, allowing for continuous reporting, disclosure, and full transparency.

Significant learning curves for the use of technology must be anticipated. Partnering with an existing telemedicine program may help to gain acceptance of new ideas through the careful application of lessons learned. Naturally, as with any new technology applied to a field with proud traditions (such as trauma care), reluctance to adopt new practices will need to be expected, appreciated, and managed through the careful accumulation of data and the politic presentation of new ideas.

The Future

"Moore's Law," the observation that computer processing speeds have doubled roughly every two years and will likely continue to do so for the foreseeable future, will further enable innovation in telemedicine to bridge the austerity-trauma divide. As internet and broadband communications improvements accumulate, the fidelity and reproducibility of telemedicine systems will lead to faster collaborations between clinicians, more efficient use of resources (including improved diversion amongst hospitals based on the availability of assets), cost savings throughout the spectrum of care, improved access to the electronic health record, and better patient outcomes, engagement, and even follow-up after discharge. Though there are several emerging technologies and ideas worth exploring, nearly all of their potential in contributing to augmented trauma care can be traced to improvements in computing power, speed, and integration.

While in some aspects it still may be considered the stuff of science fiction, telemedicine in its most developed state will compress or even negate the impositions and limitations of distance, rendering the recognized flow of "Point of Injury—Enroute Care—Emergency Department—Operating Room—Intensive Care Unit" distinctions obsolete. Integrated wearable or even implantable sensors [17] will instantly detect trauma in a particular patient, inform the echelons of care to initiate response and evacuation, and even, as in the case of certain designs of exoskeletons, either prevent certain traumas (as in the sense of a body armor function [18] or a haptic vibrating "early warning" system [19]) or initiate some form of self-aid (as in an exoskeleton with incorporated extremity tourniquets). Effective integrated sensors of this type are already being investigated by various militaries, and in the case of a mass casualty involving multiple injured soldiers, will even assist in triage, informing first responders even before their arrival on the scene of patient criticality and triage priority.

Once medical professionals arrive, several mobile diagnostic devices, miniaturized ultrasounds, and various other "apps" will augment their capabilities to diagnose and treat field trauma, including "Tricorder" devices solicited through such calls as the Nokia Sensing XCHALLENGE competition. Wearable integrated sensing and communications technologies such as the ULTRA-Vis [20] or the Google Glass and others will allow first responders and remote advanced practitioners to have instant decision support from trauma experts located anywhere in the world (or beyond), while at the hospital, such devices will contribute to more seamless integration of data or checklists in a real-time, hands-free "heads-up display" that a clinician will be able to utilize simultaneously, even while scrubbed into a procedure [21].

Remote diagnostics and therapeutics will be made even more accessible through the improvement in existing haptics technologies that transmit palpatory stimuli from the patient to a remote practitioner. While exoskeleton devices that provide tactile or auditory "early warning" are already in various stages of use in the military and can aid further in the prevention of trauma, further advances in such feedback modalities will continue to improve tactile sensation in remote robotic surgery. Though some skeptics may argue robotic surgery yields no better outcome than traditional surgery, [22] it is difficult to argue that remote robotic surgery is in any way inferior to receiving no treatment in those cases that no competent surgeon is on site to deliver care personally.

Although beyond the scope of this chapter, innovations in transportation and robotics deserve brief mention. Tremendous strides in communication and interconnectivity have drastically improved ground and aerial medical evacuation through better patient tracking, medical information sharing, and the integration of medical devices in various "flying ICU" configurations. Advanced device integration, already revolutionizing intensive care and patient safety, [23] can even allow remote monitoring of patients and adjustment of ventilators and medication pumps when medical attendants cannot be at the patient's bedside, as in fixed-wing takeoff and landing [24]. Nanotechnology applied to robotic surgery and embolic therapy is gaining acceptance, [25] while the self-driven car of today [26] will become the self-driven ambulance and self-flying helicopter of tomorrow. Robotic extraction systems [27] will expand the reach (and safety) of first responders, even obviating the need to put a person at risk to rescue a patient, just as unmanned underwater vehicles and robotic explosive ordnance devices have done, respectively, for human divers and bomb technicians.

Undergirding all these advances will be a powerful and ubiquitous network of data storage, decision support, additive manufacturing ("3D Printing"), and Artificial Intelligence aids that will be able to assist the clinician in determining courses of treatment based on best available evidence [28]. The additive manufacturing of today, which fashions surgical tools that more perfectly fits the surgeon's hand or which construct an implantable cranioplasty in alignment with the patient's native skull shape, will become the bioprinters [29] of tomorrow capable of "growing" tissues, and eventually, organs, from host cells. Remote computing will likewise allow for the completion of many tasks virtually, from interpreting a radiologic study remotely on a mobile device before patient arrival to ordering a study or writing that note one forgot to complete through a secure telework system at home.

But such network advances will not only help the clinician in addressing trauma, perhaps the greatest influence of technology will be in the realms of social media, crowdsourcing, the influencing of opinion, and the empowerment of the consumer toward healthy behaviors. Indeed, the traumatologist of the future may not only be able to care for victims of trauma more efficiently and effectively but will also play a role in steering them from harm, thereby preventing some from ever becoming patients in the first place.

Key Points

- Quality control is the process by which an organization reviews all the factors contributing to performing and production outcomes.
- Health care quality is defined as safe, effective, patient-centered, timely, efficient, and equitable criteria for health care and provider evaluation.
- Crew resource management is a methodology to effectively adapt team strategies, tools, and patient safety measures to ensure engagement of the trauma team and improve quality patient outcomes.
- Leadership is earned and adapted from historical shared experiences within the organization and team allowing for constructive open communications and corrections without reprisal.
- Team performance should be constantly evaluated and discussed to improve communication, effectiveness, and motivation of all members of the trauma team.

References

1. Reid J. A telemedicine primer: understanding the issues. Topeka KS: Innovative Medical Communications; 1996.
2. Craig J, Patterson V. Introduction to the practice of telemedicine. J Telemed Telecare. 2005;11(1):3–9.
3. Latifi R, Weinstein RS, Porter JM. Telemedicine and telepresence for trauma and emergency care management. Scand J Surg. 2007;96(4):281–9.
4. Benschoter RA, Wittson CL, Ingham CG. Teaching and consultation by television: I. Closed-circuit collaboration. J Hosp Commun Psychiatry. 1965;16:99–100.
5. National Aeronautics and Space Administration. NASA satellite aids in Mexico City rescue. NASA News; 1985. p. 85–133.
6. Bashshur R. Technology serves the people: technology serves the people: the story of a cooperative telemedicine project by NASA, the Indian Health Service, and the Papago people superintendent of documents. Washington, D.C.: US Government Printing Office; 1980. p. 110.
7. Maull K. The friendship airport disaster exercise: pioneering effort in trauma telemedicine. Eur Jour Med Research. 2002;7(supplement):48.
8. Houtchens BA. Telemedicine and international disaster response. Prehospital Disater Med. 1993;8:57–66.
9. Arbille P, Ayoub J, Kieffer V, et al. Abdominal and fetal echography tele-operated in several medical centres sites, from an expert center, using a robotic arm and telephone or satellite link. J Gravit Physiology. 2007;14(1):139–40.
10. Strode CA, Rubal BJ, Gerhardt RT, et al. Wireless and satellite transmission of prehospital focused abdominal sonography for trauma. Prehosp Emerg Care. 2003;7(3):375–9.
11. Rogers F, Ricci M, Shackford S, et al. The use of telemedicine for real-time video consultation between trauma center and community hospital in a rural setting improves early trauma care. Preliminary results. J Trauma. 2001;51(6):1037–1041A.
12. Duchesne JC, Kyle A, Simmons J, et al. Impact of telemedicine upon rural trauma care. J Trauma. 2008;64(1):92–7.
13. Latifi R, Hadeed GJ, Rhee PA, et al. Initial experiences and outcomes of telepresence in the management of trauma and emergency surgical patients. Am J Surg. 2009;198(6):905–10.
14. Saffle JR, Edelman L, Theurer L, et al. Telemedicine evaluation of acute burns is accurate and cost-effective. J Trauma. 2009;67(2):358–65.
15. Dyer D, Cusden J, Turner C, et al. The clinical and technical evaluation of a remote telementored telesonography system during the acute resuscitation and transfer of the injured patient. J Trauma. 2008;65(6):1209–16.
16. Sakles J, Mosier J, Hadeed G, et al. Telemedicine and telepresence for prehospital and remote hospital tracheal intubation using a GlideScope™ videolaryngoscope: a model for tele-intubation. Telemed J E Health. 2011;17(3):185–8.
17. Hodgetts TJ. The future character of military medicine. J R Army Med Corps. 2012 Sep;158(3):271–8.
18. Lewis EA, et al. The development and introduction of ballistic protection of the external genitalia and perineum. J R Army Med Corps. 2013 Mar;159(Suppl 1):i15–7.
19. Elliot LR, et al. Development of Tactile and Haptic Systems for U.S. Infantry Navigation and Communication, vol. 6771. Human Interface and the Management of Information, Interacting with Information Lecture Notes in Computer Science; 2011. p. 399–407.
20. Dent S. DARPA flaunts wearable display with Oculus-like head-tracking. May 22nd 2014, http://www.engadget.com/2014/05/22/darpa-ultra-vis-head-tracking/. Accessed 15 Sep 2014.
21. Viswanathan V. Is there a place for GoogleGlass in hospitals? The Atlantic, July 21, 2014.
22. Bochner BH, et al. A randomized trial of robot-assisted laparoscopic radical cystectomy. N Engl J Med. 2014;371:389–90.
23. Pronovost P. Re-engineering health care for safety and cost savings. http://armstronginstitute.blogs.hopkinsmedicine.org/2013/12/11/re-engineering-health-care-for-safety-and-cost-savings/. Accessed 20 Sep 2014.
24. Palmer RW. Integrated diagnostic and treatment devices for Enroute critical Care of Patients within theater. Combat Casualty Care Research Program, U.S. Army Medical Research and Materiel Command, Fort Detrick, Maryland; April 2010.
25. Hartgerink JD. Nanomedicine: new material stops bleeding in a hurry. Nat Nanotechnol. 2006;1:166–7.
26. Thrun S. Google's driverless car. Ted Talk, Ed (2011).
27. Tomoaki Y, et al. Improvements to the rescue robot quince toward future indoor surveillance missions in the Fukushima Daiichi nuclear power plant, vol. 92. Springer Tracts in Advanced Robotics; 2014. p. 19–32.
28. Watson D. From games shows. ITNOW, Summer. 2012;54(2):16–7.
29. Murphy S, Atala A. 3D bioprinting of tissues and organs. Nat Biotechnol. 2014;32:773–85.

Human Factors of Teleresuscitation and Telementoring

40

Lauren Hampton and Lawrence Marshall Gillman

Introduction

Telementoring in medicine refers to the remote guidance of a novice medical provider by an expert over distance [1]. The use of telementoring in medicine has become more commonplace as technology continues to provide new and improved ways of communicating all the way to the most remote corners of the globe [2, 3]. Telementoring from basic smartphone technology to augmented reality videoconferencing has been used to augment ultrasound assessment, trauma resuscitation, and advanced surgical procedures, despite thousands of miles of separation between experts and providers [4–12]. This chapter will focus on the ways telementoring can be applied to improve acute care wherever significant injuries, illness, or conflict occurs and regardless of whether the responder has any medical training. Despite its potential for far-forward lifesaving interventions, telementoring comes with additional interpersonal and communication challenges. Here we outline these challenges and identify strategies to overcome them. Overall, we believe that telementoring's potential will only be fully realized when technology is matched by teamwork, and procedural dexterity is matched by "verbal dexterity" [13].

L. Hampton
Departments of Surgery Section of General Surgery, University of Manitoba, Winnipeg, MB, Canada
e-mail: hamptonl@myumanitoba.ca

L. Marshall Gillman (✉)
Departments of Surgery Section of General Surgery, University of Manitoba, Winnipeg, MB, Canada

Internal Medicine Section of Critical Care, University of Manitoba, Winnipeg, MB, Canada
e-mail: Lawrence.Gillman@umanitoba.ca

Challenges

Communication in health care comes with many challenges, and even in-person interactions can be fraught with difficulty if there is a lack of understanding between the members of a team. Resuscitation over distance with a remote mentor brings additional challenges. Emotional stress may be amplified by isolation, lack of resources, and personal ties to the patient. Patient access in extreme environments may limit what can reasonably be achieved by the rescuer, who may even be injured themselves. Most importantly, we know that a lot of communication lies outside of what is said, and remote mentoring comes with a loss of non-verbal communication such as facial expressions or guiding the hands. While technology will play a role in bridging these gaps with videoconferencing, augmented reality, and telestration, there will be times when all you have is words, and optimizing communication is key.

Provider Stress

Imagine for a moment you are part of a six-person team deployed to the weather station in Resolute Bay, Nunavut, to conduct research on climate change. You and your colleagues all received advanced first-aid training before departure and have been working together for months in a close-knit unit. Now imagine one of your colleagues, and friend, is grievously injured with no hope of evacuation for hours, or even days. Are you stressed out yet? The reality of providing advanced interventions in the field is that they will be provided by people who are often near and dear to the patient. Fortunately, we know from a review of out-of-hospital cardiac arrests that emotional distress is not frequently a barrier to performing CPR, despite the victim being known to the provider. The most important limiting factors were physical barriers and the fitness of the rescuer to provide CPR [14]. Similarly, in a study of simulated remote damage-control surgery by non-physicians, participants had lower stress,

L. Marshall Gillman, S. Widder (eds.), *Trauma Team Dynamics*, https://doi.org/10.1007/978-3-031-86312-7_40

measured by a post-test survey and heart rate variability, than when they performed the same procedure without guidance [6, 15]. All of this means that you may be in a position to provide the right advice to the wrong situation if you do not know what it is like out there for the rescuer. Taking the time at the beginning of the interaction to establish the environment the rescuer is up against, whether they can safely access the patient and whether they are injured themselves, is imperative before delving into triage and resuscitation efforts.

Non-verbal Communication

Continuing the scenario above, imagine you need to insert a chest tube for a pneumothorax for the first time with no training. You've accepted the fact that you must plunge a knife into your friend and you are on speakerphone with a physician who is telling you to mark the fourth or fifth intercostal space between the mid and anterior axillary line. You have no idea what that means, and they can't point to the landmarks on the chest to show you. The loss of non-verbal communication is a challenging problem to overcome, and communication must be sufficiently robust to compensate [16]. Technological advancements such as video conferencing with telestration, augmented reality, and even remote-controlled robotics have all been used to virtually bring the remote mentor into the room to bridge this gap [2, 5, 7, 17]. While these are exciting options for remote-mentored surgery in controlled environments, it is imprudent to think that a robotic consultant will be available to each rural emergency room, army medic, or arctic expedition. The more likely scenario is a voice or video call from a commercially available smartphone, and the remote mentor must be ready to work within the confines of words and limited gestures. Standardized communication is one strategy a remote mentor can use to ensure they are conveying ideas in a way that is most likely to result in an effective action by the rescuer [14].

Standardized Communication

Communication is a vital medical skill and should be deliberate, in terms of both what is said and how it is understood and carried out [13, 18]. Telementoring is not equivalent to interacting face-to-face or conducting a typical telephone call. During telementoring, the mentor needs to convey indirectly not only data but also information and meaning. This then needs to translate rapidly into direct physical action, even though the provider is a relative novice, potentially scared, or both. Strategies that focus on standardized communication with concise language and short instructions appear to benefit both mentors and providers.

Strategy 1: Scripted Procedures

Most of what is known about telementoring comes from the world of dispatcher-directed CPR. While CPR is considerably simpler than a complex trauma resuscitation, the lessons learned from this more basic interaction provide principles that can be applied to more intricate scenarios. An excellent example is a study that found improvement in average chest compression depth when participants were instructed to "push as hard as you can" instead of "compress the chest 5 cm" [19]. Similarly, children have performed well with remotely mentored ultrasonography using simple "up," "down," "right," and "left" commands. In contrast, they were baffled by terms such as "parallel" and "rotate" [20]. Language choices are critical to a successful resuscitation and should not be left to chance in hopes that the mentor and provider understand one another. There may be value in preemptively scripting procedures, limiting the words said to critical steps in the correct order with avoidance of unnecessary jargon. Any script would require input from experts as well as from those who are going to carry out the instructions. Instructions might also need to be modified for language and educational levels. Those who work in dispatch already have experience giving instructions to a wide variety of recipients and would therefore be key contributors to modifications. Scripts would be "fit for task" only once validated by end-users and maintained through realistic ongoing simulations [14]. Work in this area is ongoing. Mentors who find themselves in this situation should break down these resuscitative procedures into equipment needed, identify the fundamental steps, and relay them in plain language to create a shared mental model between the provider and mentor. See Table 40.1 for an example script used to telementor novices through a tourniquet application.

Strategy 2: Structure Triage Tool

How many times have you hung up the phone after receiving a consult and thought, "I forgot to ask about X." Even experienced CPR dispatchers still failed to identify out-of-hospital cardiac arrests due to the omission of critical questions [14]. Out-of-hospital arrests are easier to identify and CPR is simpler to initiate than a complex multisystem trauma. The successful diagnosis of cardiac arrest has been improved by implementing standardized questions as part of the dispatcher's triage protocol. Patient handover is also a source of medical error due to poor communication between providers, and the SBAR (Situation-Background-Assessment-Recommendation) handover method has been shown to improve the transfer and retention of critical patient information to overcome communication errors. A structured approach to assessing a patient through telementored interactions is a logical extension of the ATLS algorithm and has

Table 40.1 Sample script for telementoring novices through tourniquet placement

I will walk you through putting on a tourniquet
Remove any clothing if possible so the tourniquet sits directly on the skin
Place the tourniquet around the limb four fingers above the wound
Insert the strap through the opening in the buckle
Grab the strap close to the buckle and tighten by pulling the strap against the buckle
While keeping it tight, velcro the extra strap back on itself
The tourniquet should now hold itself in place but it may still be bleeding
Now we're going to tighten the tourniquet
Twist the rod clockwise until the bleeding stops
Has it stopped?
IF NOT—Try to keep twisting the rod
IF YES—place the rod in the C-shaped hook beside it
Feed any extra band over the rod
Place the white velcro strap over top and write down the current time on the strap

the potential to ease the transfer of critical information, improve active listening, and simultaneously provide a means of documentation for a busy off-site trauma expert. While there is currently no standard triage tool available, those experienced in trauma management should transition to the deliberate use and documentation of these questions to improve communication and therefore patient outcomes.

Conclusions

Telementoring is becoming more common as medicine and technology improve worldwide. Optimization of the non-technical factors of telementoring must keep pace, and research and quality improvement efforts are essential. Communication strategies consisting of standard approaches, short, concise validated scripts using simple language, and systematic identification of available resources and barriers to success have the potential to improve the safety, efficacy, and overall experience for mentors and remote providers.

Key Points

- Telementoring in medicine refers to the remote guidance of a novice medical provider by an expert over a distance.
- Telementoring has proven to be a viable means of providing advanced medical care in remote or austere environments.
- Communication strategies consisting of standard approaches, short, concise and validated scripts using simple language, and systematic identification of available resources and barriers to success have the potential to improve the safety, efficacy, and overall experience for mentors and remote providers.

References

1. Gambadauro P, Torrejon R. The "tele" factor in surgery today and tomorrow: implications for surgical training and education. Surg Today. 2013;43:115–22.
2. Kirkpatrick AW, LaPorta A, Brien S, et al. Technical innovations that may facilitate real-time telementoring of damage control surgery in austere environments: a proof of concept comparative evaluation of the importance of surgical experience, telepresence, gravity and mentoring in the conduct of damage control laparotomies. Can JSurg. 2015;58(3 Suppl 3):S88.
3. Kirkpatrick AW. 2010 Trauma Association of Canada Presidential Address: Why the Trauma Association of Canada should care about space medicine. J Trauma. 2010;69:1313–22.
4. Ajami S, Lamoochi P. Use of telemedicine in disaster and remote places. J Educ Health Promot. 2014;3:26.
5. Cubano M, Poulose B, Talamini MA, et al. Long distance telementoring— a novel tool for laparoscopy aboard the USS Abraham Lincoln. Surg Endosc. 1999;13:673–8.
6. Kirkpatrick AW, McKee LJ, McBeth BP, et al. The Damage Control Surgery in Austere Environments Research Group (DCSAERG): a dynamic program to facilitate real-time telementoring/telediagnosis to address exsanguination in extreme and austere environments. J Trauma Acute Care Surg. 2017;83(Suppl 1):S156–63.
7. Nguyen N, Okrainec A, Anvari M, et al. Sleeve gastrectomy telementoring: a SAGES multi-institutional quality improvement initiative. Surg Endosc. 2018;32:682–7.
8. McBeth P, Crawford I, Tiruta C, et al. Help is in your pocket: the potential accuracy of smartphone- and laptop-based remotely guided resuscitative telesonography. Telemed J E Health. 2013;19:924–30.
9. Moore RG, Adams JB, Partin AW, et al. Telementoring of laparoscopic procedures: initial clinical experience. Surg Endosc. 1996;10:107.
10. Kirkpatrick AW, McKee I, McKee JL, et al. Remote just-in-time telementored trauma ultrasound: a double-factorial randomized controlled trial examining fluid detection and remote knobology control through an ultrasound graphic user interface display. Am J Surg. 2016;211:894–902.e1.
11. Lee Y, Kim C, Choi HJ, et al. A feasibility study of telementoring for identifying the appendix using smartphone-based telesonography. J Digit Imaging. 2017;30:148–55.
12. Dyer D, Cusden J, Turner C, et al. The clinical and technical evaluation of a remote telementored telesonography system during the acute resuscitation and transfer of the injured patient. J Trauma. 2008;65:1209.
13. Brindley PG, Reynolds SF. Improving verbal communication in critical care medicine. J Crit Care. 2011;26:155–9.
14. Hampton L, Brindley P, Kirkpatrick A, et al. Strategies to improve communication in telementoring in acute care coordination: a scoping review. Can J Surg. 2020;63(6):E569–77. Published 2020 Nov 30. https://doi.org/10.1503/cjs.015519.
15. Kirkpatrick AW, Tien TH, LaPorta EA, et al. The marriage of surgical simulation and telementoring for damage-control surgical training of operational first responders: a pilot study. J Trauma Acute Care Surg. 2015;79:741–7.
16. Wachs JP, Gomez G. Telementoring systems in the operating room: a new approach in medical training. Medicina (B Aires). 2013;73:539–42.
17. Budrionis A, Augestad K, Patel H, Bellika J. An evaluation framework for defining the contributions of telestration in surgical telementoring. Int J Med Res. 2013;2:e14. https://doi.org/10.2196/ijmr.2611.
18. Brindley PG, Cardinal P. Optimizing crisis resource management to improve patient safety and team performance: a handbook for all acute care health professionals. Ottawa: Royal College of Physicians and Surgeons; 2017. Available: https://www.royalcollege.ca/rcsite/documents/practice -performance-innovation/

optimizing-crisis-resource-management-improve-patient-safety-team-performance-e.pdf. Accessed 2020 Jan 15.
19. Mirza M, Brown TB, Saini D, et al. Instructions to "push as hard as you can" improve average chest compression depth in dispatcher assisted cardiopulmonary resuscitation. Resuscitation. 2008;79:97–102.
20. McBeth PB, Crawford I, Blaivas M, et al. Simple, almost anywhere, with almost anyone: remote low-cost telementored resuscitative lung ultrasound. J Trauma. 2011;71:1528–35.

Part IV

Specialized Trauma Populations

41 Trauma in Pregnancy

Alexandra Marseu, Michelle L. Morais, Lua R. Eiriksson, and Paul T. Engels

Introduction

Trauma is the leading cause of non-obstetric maternal death in pregnancy worldwide [1]. Trauma complicates 6–8% of all pregnancies [2], with 0.4% requiring hospitalization for the treatment of traumatic injuries [3], and 0.1% experiencing major trauma (injury severity score > 15) [4]. Unintentional trauma accounts for a large proportion of trauma in pregnancy, with motor vehicle collisions (MVCs) being the most common mechanism [5, 6]. Intentional trauma, most commonly domestic violence (DV) or intimate partner violence (IPV), is also associated with significant maternal and fetal morbidity [6] and is reported to occur in 4–8% of pregnancies [7], particularly clustering in the third trimester [8]. Blunt trauma (80%) predominates over penetrating trauma (20%) [9–11], with the latter resulting in perinatal mortality rates of up to 70% [12]. Compared to pregnancies unaffected by trauma, fetal demise at any gestational age is more common among trauma victims, and trauma is associated with a higher occurrence of neonatal death at any gestational age [13]. Leading mechanisms of fetal death related to trauma are MVCs (82%), firearm injuries (6%), and falls (3%), with 11% of cases involving concurrent maternal death [14]. Placental abruption is the leading cause of fetal death resulting from trauma, accounting for 50–70% of fetal losses related to trauma [15]. The next most common cause of trauma-associated fetal death is maternal death [15]. The leading causes of maternal death are head injury and hemorrhagic shock [16, 17]. Trauma patients also have an increased risk of obstetrical complications, whether trauma is severe or non-severe [18]; these include spontaneous abortion, preterm premature rupture of membranes, preterm labor, placental abruption, fetal-maternal hemorrhage, uterine rupture, fetal distress, maternal death, and stillbirth [9, 18, 19].

The management of the pregnant trauma patient may be complicated by delayed diagnoses of shock or hemorrhage due to minimal changes in vital signs secondary to physiologic changes of pregnancy, as well as challenges in the concurrent assessment of both the fetus and the mother. The prevailing principle is that fetal well-being is dependent on maternal status, such that optimal resuscitation of the mother will typically result in optimal resuscitation of the fetus, with consideration given to obstetrical complications that can compromise both mother and fetus.

Physiologic Changes of Pregnancy

Multiple organ systems undergo adaptation during pregnancy. The uterus remains intrapelvic until 12 weeks' gestation and subsequently rises out of the protection of the bony pelvis as it expands with the growing fetus. By 20 weeks, the uterus reaches the level of the umbilicus and is considered to be an abdominal organ; however, the fetus continues to be protected by a relatively large volume of amniotic fluid. It is during the third trimester when the now thin-walled uterus is at the greatest risk of penetration, rupture, and premature rupture of membranes [20]. The inelasticity of the placenta in comparison to the elastic uterus increases the risk of abruption when shearing forces are applied [21], and even cases of apparent minor blunt abdominal trauma may result in compromise or death [19]. The uterus and placenta receive 20% of the cardiac output in the third trimester, highlighting the urgency for assessment of the uterus during the primary survey. Due to the size and weight of the uterus, placement in

A. Marseu · P. T. Engels (✉)
Department of Obstetrics and Gynaecology, Division of Maternal Fetal Medicine, McMaster University, Hamilton, ON, Canada
e-mail: alexandra.marseu@medportal.ca; engelsp@mcmaster.ca

M. L. Morais
Departments of Surgery and Critical Care, McMaster University, Hamilton, ON, Canada
e-mail: moraism@mcmaster.ca

L. R. Eiriksson
Department of Obstetrics and Gynecology, McMaster University, Hamilton, ON, Canada
e-mail: eiriksson@hhsc.ca

L. Marshall Gillman, S. Widder (eds.), *Trauma Team Dynamics*, https://doi.org/10.1007/978-3-031-86312-7_41

the supine position results in compression of the inferior vena cava (IVC) and aorta, thereby negatively impacting cardiac output. Placing the patient in the left lateral decubitus position (log-rolled 4–6 inches or 15°), or manually displacing the uterus, will minimize iatrogenic hypotension and improve cardiac output [22, 23] while also improving fetal oxygenation [24]. This can be done while maintaining spine precautions.

A hypervolemic and hyperdynamic state is achieved during pregnancy to meet the metabolic demands of the mother and fetus. Total blood volume increases by up to 50% during pregnancy, with a greater increase in plasma volume compared to red cell mass, resulting in dilutional anemia [16]. Cardiac output increases up to 50% due to an increase in blood volume, a decrease in uterine and placental vascular resistance, and an increase in heart rate. While the placental vasculature is maximally dilated to facilitate fetal oxygenation, it is highly responsive to catecholamines, such that a stress response in the mother may result in diversion of blood from the uterus [20]. As such, blood pressure support with the administration of intravenous fluid and blood products is preferred over the use of vasopressors.

Maternal tidal volume and minute ventilation are increased, thought to be secondary to increased progesterone levels, with resultant hypocapnia and diminished buffering capacity. Elevation of the diaphragm contributes to a decreased residual volume and should be considered during placement of thoracostomy tubes in later pregnancy (where tube placement may be more appropriate in the fourth rather than fifth interspace). Penetrating injuries below the fourth intercostal space anteriorly, or the top of the scapula posteriorly, may result in intraabdominal injuries. Attention to respiratory status in the pregnant patient requires recognition of the increased oxygen demands placed by the fetus; early recognition of ventilatory failure despite apparent normal $PaCO_2$ values; and a high-risk airway secondary to upper airway edema, increased intra-abdominal pressures, decreased functional residual capacity, and delayed gastric emptying [20]. Supplemental oxygen should be administered without reservation to all pregnant trauma patients to maintain an $SpO_2 > 95\%$ or $PaO_2 > 70$ mmHg to improve the maternal-fetal oxygen diffusion gradient. Consideration should be given to early placement of a decompressive nasogastric tube to avoid aspiration. Because of increased upper airway edema, a tracheal tube of 0.5–1 mm diameter narrower than a nonpregnant woman of similar size should be used with preparation and backup for a difficult airway [25]. Early intubation should be considered if airway management or oxygenation concerns are anticipated [1].

Widening of the symphysis pubis (by 4–8 mm) [26] and sacroiliac joints may impede the interpretation of pelvic radiographs. Interpretation of chest radiographs is minimally affected by normal pregnancy. Possible normal findings include prominent pulmonary vasculature or a flattened left heart border (related to increased blood volume and cardiac output) and elevation of the diaphragm [27].

Due to pituitary enlargement, maternal hypovolemia may result in pituitary insufficiency secondary to pituitary necrosis in the setting of maternal hypovolemic shock. This may lead to long-term complications including hypothyroidism, adrenal insufficiency, and oligomenorrhea. A summary of

Table 41.1 Anatomic, physiology, and laboratory value changes during pregnancy

Parameter	Change in pregnancy
Heart rate	Baseline rate increased by 15 bpm
Blood pressure (systolic and diastolic)	Nadir of 15 mmHg below baseline by the end of the second trimester
Cardiac output	Increased by 1–1.5 L per minute over baseline
Total blood volume	Increased by 50% above normal
Red blood cell mass	Lesser increase compared to plasma volume resulting in dilutional anemia (lower hematocrit)
Respiration	Increased tidal volume and minute ventilation, with resultant hypocapnia and increased oxygen consumption
Lung volumes	Decreased residual volume (elevation of the diaphragm)
Gastrointestinal motility	Decreased small and large bowel motility
Gastrointestinal anatomy	Displacement of bowel into the upper abdomen
Musculoskeletal	Widening of symphysis pubis and sacroiliac joints
Fibrinogen	Increased (normal fibrinogen may hail the development of disseminated intravascular coagulation). >3.79 g/L (third trimester)
Pseudocholinesterase levels	Decreased (consider lower doses of succinylcholine during rapid sequence induction)
Airway	Increased mucosal engorgement of nasal and oral cavities
Hematocrit	32–42%
White blood cell count	5000—12,000/microL
Arterial pH	7.40–7.45
Bicarbonate	17–22 mEq/L
$PaCO_2$	25–30 mmHg

anatomic, physiologic, and laboratory value changes during pregnancy are presented in Table 41.1.

Shock in the Pregnant Patient

Due to the physiologic increase in intravascular volume, hemorrhage may initially be well compensated for in the pregnant trauma patient. It is typically only after significant blood loss that tachycardia and hypotension are encountered. At that point, however, catecholamine-induced maternal shunting of blood away from the uterus and placental vasculature will have deprived the fetus of vital perfusion, resulting in compromise. Maternal hypovolemic shock is associated with an 80% fetal mortality rate [28, 29]. Abnormal fetal lie (oblique or transverse), easy palpation of fetal parts, and/or inability to palpate the uterine fundus may suggest uterine rupture. Placental abruption is associated with vaginal bleeding, uterine tetany, and severe abdominal pain. Unfortunately, these clues to the presence of obstetrical causes of hemorrhage are not sufficiently sensitive (e.g., vaginal bleeding is absent in 30% of cases of placental abruption). An additional vital sign is therefore required in the assessment of shock in the pregnant trauma patient: the fetal heart rate (see Fetal Monitoring). Early fetal assessment should be performed during maternal stabilization, as fetal heart rate changes may be the first indicators of maternal hypovolemia and impending shock. Continuous fetal monitoring should be utilized where feasible, otherwise frequent intermittent monitoring is suggested. When using this approach, not only will resuscitation of the mother be improved, but also the risk of fetal complications, including fetal demise, will be decreased. Judgments regarding delivery for fetal indications should be based on mutual decision-making between the obstetric and trauma specialists, including patient input, to ensure that appropriate consideration is given regarding implications related to the mode of birth, outcomes related to prematurity, and other relevant points based on individual circumstances.

Distinct Aspects of the Pregnant Trauma Patient

While the management of thoracic and abdominal injuries during pregnancy differs little from the nonpregnant state, there are certain considerations unique to the pregnant trauma patient. All female trauma patients should be stratified as either potentially pregnant, pregnant at less than 23 weeks gestation, pregnant at greater than 23 weeks gestation, or perimortem. Fetal viability is achieved at approximately 23 weeks gestation, at which time maternal resuscitation and fetal assessment should take place concurrently. Gestational age (GA) and the estimated date of delivery (EDD)—or "due date"—are best calculated using a dating ultrasound performed between 7 and 12 weeks gestation [30]. If an ultrasound is not available, the EDD can be calculated using Naegele's rule: EDD = first day of last menstrual period (LMP)—3 months +7 days. To err on the side of fetal viability, if an accurate gestational age is not immediately known at the time of the patient's presentation, physical examination may be used as a surrogate indicator for an estimated GA of at least 20–24 weeks (Fig. 41.1). Initial evaluation of a reproductive-age woman should include a concise and focused obstetric and gynecologic history, ensuring universal pregnancy testing is performed [26]. In some instances, early pregnancy may be diagnosed during point-of-care ultrasound [30, 31].

A Kleihauer-Betke (KB) test should be performed in all pregnant trauma patients, regardless of Rh status, to identify significant fetal-maternal hemorrhage and guide anti-D immune globulin treatment in Rh(D)-negative women [32, 33]. All pregnant Rh(D)-negative trauma patients should receive anti-D immune globulin therapy due to the risk of fetal-maternal hemorrhage and subsequent alloimmunization. A standard dose of 300 micrograms is given, with additional doses pending results of the KB test, which quantifies the extent of fetal-maternal hemorrhage. The blood bank should be consulted for dose calculation, timing, and route of administration. There is no relationship between the severity of maternal injury and the incidence of fetal-maternal hemorrhage [21, 32], but a positive KB test has been associated with subsequent preterm labor after maternal trauma, with the extent of fetal-maternal hemorrhage correlating with the likelihood of preterm labor [32]. Fetal complications of fetal-maternal hemorrhage include neonatal anemia, cardiac arrhythmias, and fetal death [16]. In cases of significant fetal-maternal hemorrhage, fetal intrauterine transfusion may be required.

Preeclampsia is defined as preexisting or gestational hypertension, with new or worsening proteinuria, adverse conditions, or severe complications (Table 41.2) [34]. Adverse conditions are those that increase the risk of severe complications, and severe complications are those that warrant delivery [34]. Complications of preeclampsia may result in traumatic injuries, such as a motor vehicle collision secondary to visual impairment. Differentiating symptoms of preeclampsia from those of traumatic injury may, therefore, be difficult in such situations. An eclamptic seizure may mimic traumatic brain injury. Abdominal pain and placental abruption may result from preeclampsia or sustained blunt trauma. Coagulopathy may be caused by preeclampsia-induced disseminated intravascular coagulation or a consumptive process secondary to ongoing traumatic hemorrhage. In each scenario, the correct diagnosis is required to tailor and guide treatment.

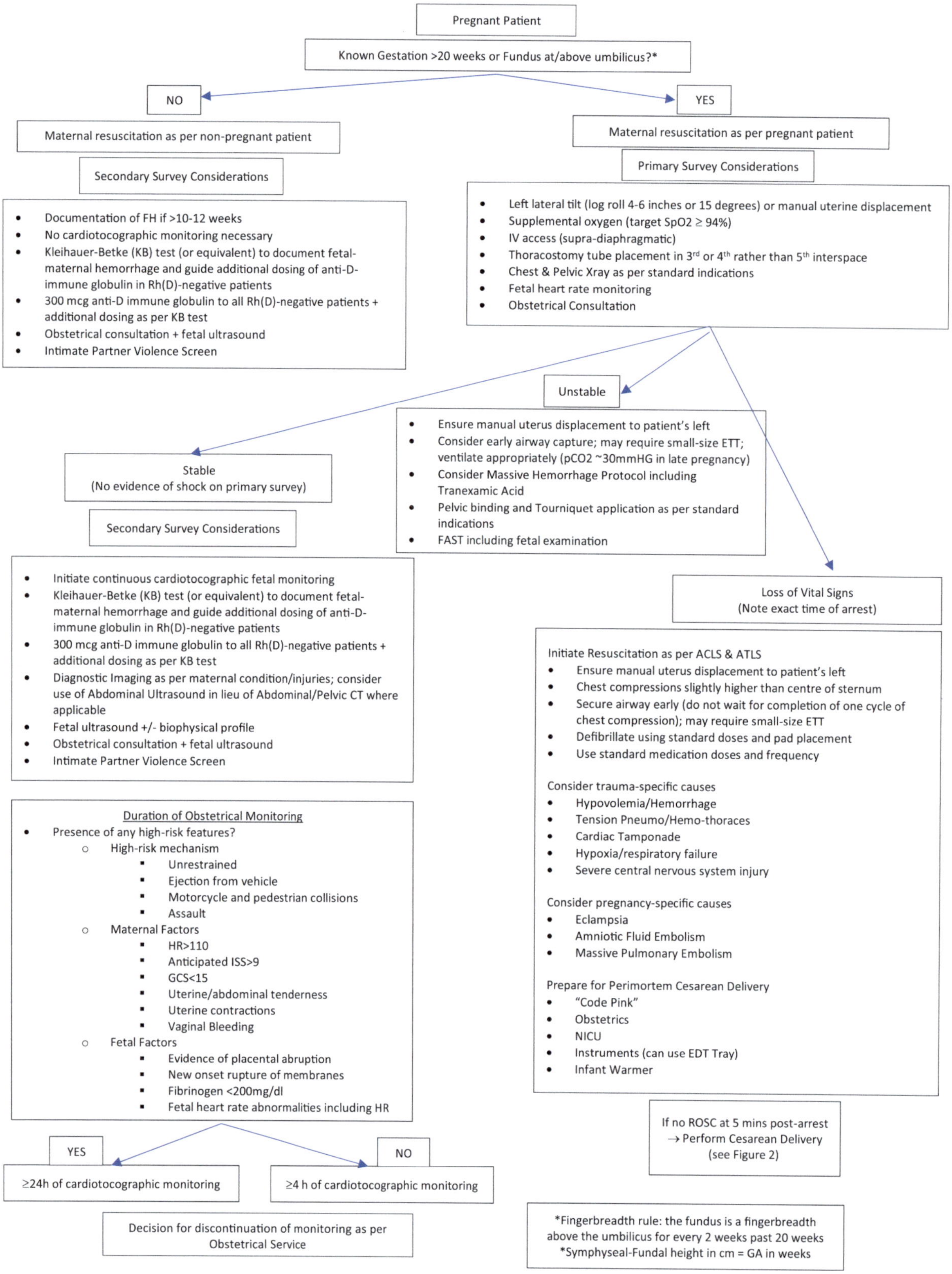

Fig. 41.1 Assessment and management of pregnant trauma patient. (Based on the content in Katz (2012) [73] and the American Heart Association (2020) [94]. ACLS advanced cardiac life support; CT computed tomography; EDT emergency department thoracotomy; ETT endotracheal tube; FAST Focussed Assessment with Sonography in Trauma; FH fetal heart tones; GA gestational age; GCS Glasgow coma scale; HR heart rate; ISS injury severity score; NICU neonatal intensive care unit; ROSC return of spontaneous circulation)

Table 41.2 Adverse conditions and severe complications associated with preeclampsia [34]

	Adverse conditions	Severe complications
Maternal conditions	Headache or visual symptoms Chest pain or dyspnea Nausea or vomiting Right upper quadrant or epigastric pain Oxygen saturation <97% Elevated WBC Count Elevated INR/aPTT Low platelet count Elevated serum creatinine Elevated serum uric acid Elevated serum AST, ALT, LDH or bilirubin Low plasma albumin	Eclampsia PRES Cortical blindness or retinal detachment Glasgow coma scale <13 Stroke, TIA Uncontrolled severe hypertension Oxygen saturation <90%, need for >50% oxygen for >1 h, intubation, pulmonary edema Need for inotropic support Myocardial ischemia or infarction Platelet count < 50 × 10^9/L Creatinine >150 microM with no previous renal disease Hepatic dysfunction (INR >2, without DIC or warfarin use) Hepatic hematoma or rupture
Fetal morbidity	Abnormal fetal heart rate Intrauterine growth restriction Oligohydramnios Absent/reversed end-diastolic flow by Doppler velocimetry	Abruption with evidence of maternal or fetal compromise Reverse ductus venosus A wave Stillbirth

PRES posterior reversible leukoencephalopathy syndrome; *TIA* transient ischemic attack; *WBC* white blood cell; *INR* international normalized ratio; *aPTT* activated partial thromboplastin time; *RUQ* right upper quadrant; *AST* aspartate aminotransferase; *ALT* alanine aminotransferase; *LDH* lactate dehydrogenase; *DIB* disseminated intravascular coagulation

A search should be made for conditions unique to the injured pregnant patient, such as blunt or penetrating uterine trauma, placental abruption, preterm labor, or premature rupture of membranes. Preterm labor complicates up to 5% of maternal traumas [21] and may be treated with tocolytics, such as nifedipine or indomethacin. Corticosteroids, such as betamethasone or dexamethasone, should be administered to women at 24 + 0 to 34 + 6 weeks' gestation who are at high risk for preterm birth in the next seven days (i.e., with preterm labor or premature rupture of membranes), to promote fetal lung maturity [35]. Those between 22 + 0 and 23 + 6 weeks gestation may be considered after appropriate counseling if early neonatal intensive care is planned [35]. However, if delivery is obstetrically indicated (i.e., significant placental abruption, fetal distress), it should not be delayed to achieve corticosteroid benefit.

A qualified surgeon and obstetrician should be consulted early in the evaluation of a pregnant trauma patient. In the setting of blunt trauma, splenic and retroperitoneal injuries are more common in pregnancy because of increased vascularity [16, 36], and pelvic fractures have been reported to cause direct fetal skull fractures or intracranial injuries [37–39]. In the setting of penetrating trauma, a trauma surgeon should be involved for consideration of surgical exploration to rule out bowel or diaphragmatic laceration [40, 41]. The pattern of anticipated injuries is modified by pregnancy: upper abdominal penetrating injuries are more likely to result in bowel injury due to cephalad displacement from the gravid uterus. There is decreased risk of visceral and retroperitoneal injury with lower abdominal penetrating injuries and non-operative management may be considered; however, there is higher occurrence of uterine and fetal injuries in such cases [41]. Diagnostic peritoneal lavage, if performed, should employ the open technique, above the uterine fundus [42]. Exploratory laparotomy is typically well tolerated and preferable to delayed diagnosis of intra-abdominal injuries but is associated with an increased risk of preterm labor [43]. Excessive uterine manipulation and maternal hypotension must be avoided. Careful consideration should be given to the need for Cesarean section, with the determination of fetal age, fetal maturity, and fetal well-being factored in the decision-making. Cesarean section will increase the intraoperative blood loss and operative time, while delayed recognition of fetal distress will increase the risk of perinatal loss [44]. Hysterotomy in the setting of an otherwise uninjured uterus may be necessary for adequate abdominal exploration or repair of identified injuries [20, 45]. If not required at the time of laparotomy, hysterotomy may be avoided in cases of fetal demise where induction of labor may be preferred [45].

Formal uterine and pelvic examination should be performed by the obstetrical team, if available, to evaluate for uterine contractions or tenderness, vaginal bleeding, rupture of membranes or cervical dilation in addition to evaluation for vaginal lacerations in the setting of pelvic fracture. Amniotic fluid can be identified by its alkaline pH and characteristic ferning pattern on microscopy. Cardiotocographic monitoring must be skillfully interpreted for fetal heart rate abnormalities. Venous thromboembolism prophylaxis should be provided in the form of low-molecular-weight heparin as per standard therapy. Obstetrical follow-up should be arranged to ensure identification and management of late complications since adverse obstetrical outcomes such as preterm delivery and low birth weight are increased in trauma patients [19, 46]. Screening for intimate partner violence is essential (Table 41.3).

Table 41.3 Partner violence screen [47–49]

1. Have you been kicked, hit, punched, or otherwise hurt by someone within the past year? If so, by whom?
2. Do you feel safe in your current relationship?
3. Is there a partner from a previous relationship who is making you feel unsafe now?

Fetal Monitoring

Continuous cardiotocographic fetal monitoring should be performed in all viable pregnancies (i.e., beyond 23–24-week gestation) since maternal hemodynamic parameters are not accurate predictors of fetal distress or risk of fetal loss [44, 50]. Cardiotocography will identify signs of placental abruption, fetal distress, and uterine contractions if monitored by a team member with experience in fetal heart rate interpretation. Care must be taken to distinguish the maternal versus fetal heart rate during monitoring. Continuous tachycardia, bradycardia, or repetitive decelerations may be indications for urgent delivery. Monitoring should continue throughout maternal resuscitation and continue for a minimum of 4–6 h in the absence of risk factors for fetal loss in an awake, asymptomatic patient. In the presence of risk factors or altered level of consciousness, monitoring should continue for ≥24 h [1] (Fig. 41.1) since the risk of immediate complications is increased in these patients [19]. Uterine rupture is strongly correlated with fetal mortality, the signs of which may be missed during the assessment of the mother alone [51]. Monitoring should be performed regardless of the apparent low severity and location of injuries sustained by the mother, as fetal compromise has been identified in up to 20% of cases of apparent minor injury [50, 52]. Placental abruption has been reported in 3% of cases of minor abdominal injuries and 40% of cases of severe blunt abdominal trauma where fetal mortality may be as high as 60% [51, 53]. Similarly, the symptoms of placental abruption may be minimal, depending on the location of retro-placental bleeding and the degree of placental detachment. Even ultrasound may fail to identify placental abruption in 50% of cases [54, 55]. Such adverse outcomes, however, are expected to manifest within 4–6 h [52] of presentation. In the presence of a reassuring fetal heart rate pattern for 4-6 h, in the absence of uterine contractions (<6 contractions per hour) at a gestational age of >20 weeks, the incidence of late fetal or maternal complications has been found to be minimal, and safe discharge following maternal clearance is supported in appropriately selected patients [51].

Radiology

The risk of fetal radiation exposure must be balanced with the benefit of radiographic investigations and/or image-guided procedures. It is impossible to reap the benefits of minimized radiation exposure unless one is alive to do so. It should be emphasized that the best initial treatment for the fetus is the provision of optimal resuscitation of the mother.

Imaging and investigations (including the use of iodinated contrast material) necessary to facilitate diagnosis and management of the injured pregnant patient are endorsed in guidelines published by the American College of Obstetricians and Gynecologists [55] and the American College of Radiology [56]. Consideration should be given to the degree of fetal radiation exposure in the selection of imaging modalities where a choice exists, and abdominal-pelvic lead shielding should be used where appropriate. Radiation levels should be kept as low as reasonably achievable and the use of specific dose-reduction techniques should be applied [57]. A medical physicist should be involved in the calculation of the actual fetal dose received, with prospective fetal dose estimatation accomplished via placement of dosimeters on the patient at the level of the uterus a useful adjunct [50].

Growth restriction, microcephaly, and intellectual disabilities are the most common adverse effects resulting from high-dose radiation exposure (Table 41.4) [55]. Fetal risks of anomalies, growth restriction, or spontaneous abortions are not increased with radiation exposure of less than 5 rad [1 rad = 10 mGy (milligray)] [55].

Table 41.5 lists estimated fetal exposure levels from common radiologic procedures. When tabulated using this data, a diagnostic imaging workup that includes chest and pelvic plain radiographic, extremity radiographs, and a "pan-scan" (CT of the head, cervical spine, single-phase CT chest/abdomen/pelvis including thoracolumbar spine) would not necessarily exceed the threshold of 5 rad. Indeed, Tien et al. [58] examined actual delivered radiation doses in trauma patients admitted to a Canadian Level 1 trauma center and found a mean dose of 2.27 rad with an average of 4.9 CT scans and 13.7 plain radiographs performed during their hospital stay. However, some modalities may expose the fetus to doses of radiation that exceed the safe limit, such as pelvic angiography and embolization in the setting of pelvic fracture. Such patients should be counseled appropriately by the obstetrical or perinatology service. The teratogenicity of radiation in pregnancy is most pronounced in the first trimester, highlighting the need for universal pregnancy testing in women of reproductive age [26, 59]. In addition, while no in vivo tests in animals have demonstrated mutagenic or teratogenic effects with low-osmolality contrast agents, there are no good studies in pregnant women and there are theoretical concerns of hypothyroidism developing in newborn infants [60]. Therefore, the American College of Radiology suggests that these agents should ideally be used in pregnancy only if (a) the information cannot be obtained without contrast administration or use of other imaging modalities, (b) the information will affect the care of the patient and/or fetus

Table 41.4 Effects of gestational age and radiation exposure [55]

Gestational period	*Potential effects*	*Estimated threshold radiation dose*
0–2 weeks post-fertilization (before implantation)	All-or-none effect (failure of implantation or no consequence)	50–100 mGy
2–8 weeks post-fertilization (organogenesis)	Congenital anomalies (skeleton, eyes, genitals) Growth restriction	200 mGy 200–250 mGy
Fetal period	*Potential effects*	*Estimated threshold radiation dose*
8–15 weeks	High risk of severe intellectual disability Lowered IQ Microcephaly	60–310 mGy 25 IQ-point loss per 1000 mGy 200 mGy
16–25 weeks	Low risk of severe intellectual disability	250–280 mGy

Table 41.5 Fetal absorbed dose from selected radiographic examinations

	Fetal absorbed dose		
Procedure	ACOG No. 723 [56]	McCollough et al. [93]	Wieseler et al. [57]
Plain radiographs			
Chest (AP and lateral)	0.0005–0.01 mGy	0.002 mGy	
Abdominal (single view)	0.1–3.0 mGy	1.0–3.0 mGy	
Extremities	< 0.001 mGy	< 0.001 mGy	
Cervical spine (AP and lateral)	< 0.001 mGy	< 0.001 mGy	
Thoracic spine (AP and lateral)	1.0–10 mGy	0.003 mGy	
Lumbar spine (AP and lateral)		1.0 mGy	
CT scans (single acquisition)			
Head	0.001–0.01 mGy	0	0.02 mGy
Chest (routine and for PE)	0.01–0.66 mGy	0.2 mGy	1.3 mGy
Abdomen	1.3–35 mGy	4.0 mGy	13.0 mGy
Abdomen and pelvis	< 1 mGy	25.0 mGy	11.0 mGy
Abdomen for stones (kidneys, ureters, bladder)		10.0 mGy 34.0 mGy	13.0 mGy
Angiography			
Angiography of aorta (chest through pelvis)			
CT pelvimetry			
Background fetal dose for 9 months of pregnancy	1.1–2.5 mGy	0.5–1.0 mGy	

Notes*:* A radiation shield is typically applied over the gravid abdomen when not in the imaging field although the effect is minimal
1 mGy = 0.1 rad.
<5 rad is generally accepted as a safe total fetal absorbed dose during pregnancy [55]
AP anteroposterior, *CT* computed tomography, *PE* pulmonary embolism

during the pregnancy, and (c) it is not prudent to wait until after the patient is no longer pregnant to obtain the information from the study. Obviously, most trauma imaging would satisfy these criteria.

Valuable information about the state of the fetus can be obtained from both plain radiographs as well as CT imaging. Plain radiograph findings such as the presence of extended fetal extremities, abnormal fetal position, or free intraperitoneal air can suggest a diagnosis of uterine rupture [26]. CT scan may identify placental abruption with both a sensitivity and negative predictive value of 100% when images are appropriately interpreted [61–63], with the degree of placental enhancement associated with the subsequent need for delivery [63]. Correlation of imaging and cardiotocographic findings may improve the specificity and positive predictive value of such scans and appropriately triage patients for further evaluation versus safe discharge.

Abdominal ultrasound, in general, is less sensitive for the detection of injuries in pregnant patients compared to non-pregnant patients; however, its specificity is preserved [64]. Focused Assessment with Sonography for Trauma (FAST) is used frequently in trauma patients to detect free fluid presumed to be due to hemoperitoneum and a sign of intra-abdominal injury. The finding of free fluid may be difficult to interpret in women of reproductive age, since free fluid may be associated with the menstrual cycle [65]. However, Hussain et al. demonstrated the presence of pelvic fluid in <7% of non-traumatically injured pregnant patients with a volume never exceeding a depth of 4 mm [66], thereby supporting the utility of FAST in this population.

Perimortem Cesarean Delivery In Trauma

Emergency hysterotomy, or perimortem Cesarean delivery (PCD), is the expeditious surgical delivery of a fetus while the mother is in a state of cardiac arrest. Historically, this was used as a procedure of last resort to attempt "fetal salvage" after failure of maternal resuscitation. In the 1980s, reports of maternal recovery after fetal delivery were published. Analysis by Katz and colleagues led to the "Four-Minute-Rule," whereby "Cesarean delivery should be begun within 4 min and the infant delivered within 5 min after maternal cardiac arrest" [67], the validity of which was reaffirmed in a follow-up study 20 years later [68]. Seventy percent of surviving infants were delivered within this time interval, while neonates delivered outside of the 5 min window were more likely to demonstrate neurological compromise [67]. Physiologically, evacuation of the gravid uterus has a number of beneficial maternal effects: it (1) alleviates IVC and aortic compression and thereby improves venous return; (2) allows for more mechanically effective CPR; and (3) allows redistribution of the low-resistance uterine blood flow to other organs [53, 68, 69]. The benefits of PCD therefore extend beyond the fetus and may positively impact the ability to successfully resuscitate the mother [68]. Following Cesarean section, cardiac output may increase by 30% and tissue perfusion requirements may significantly decrease, both thought to be advantageous in the setting of maternal resuscitation [70, 71]. See Fig. 41.2 for details on performing a PCD.

Specifically addressing the pregnant trauma patient, Morris et al. reviewed almost 115,000 trauma admissions from 1986 to 1994 at nine Level-1 US trauma centers [44]. They identified 441 pregnant women with 32 emergency Cesarean deliveries, with an overall maternal and fetal survival rate of 72% and 45%, respectively. Only three of these were true PCDs in the setting of maternal cardiac arrest. The authors found that a lack of pre-Cesarean fetal heart tones predicted 100% fetal mortality. Five deaths occurred when there were fetal heart rate tones, and the deaths were thought to be due to delayed recognition of fetal distress. The majority of these deaths were in women with mild to moderate injuries. The reliable exclusion of fetal heart tones in a busy trauma bay with a rapidly evolving clinical situation presents challenges. While the use of surgeon-performed trauma

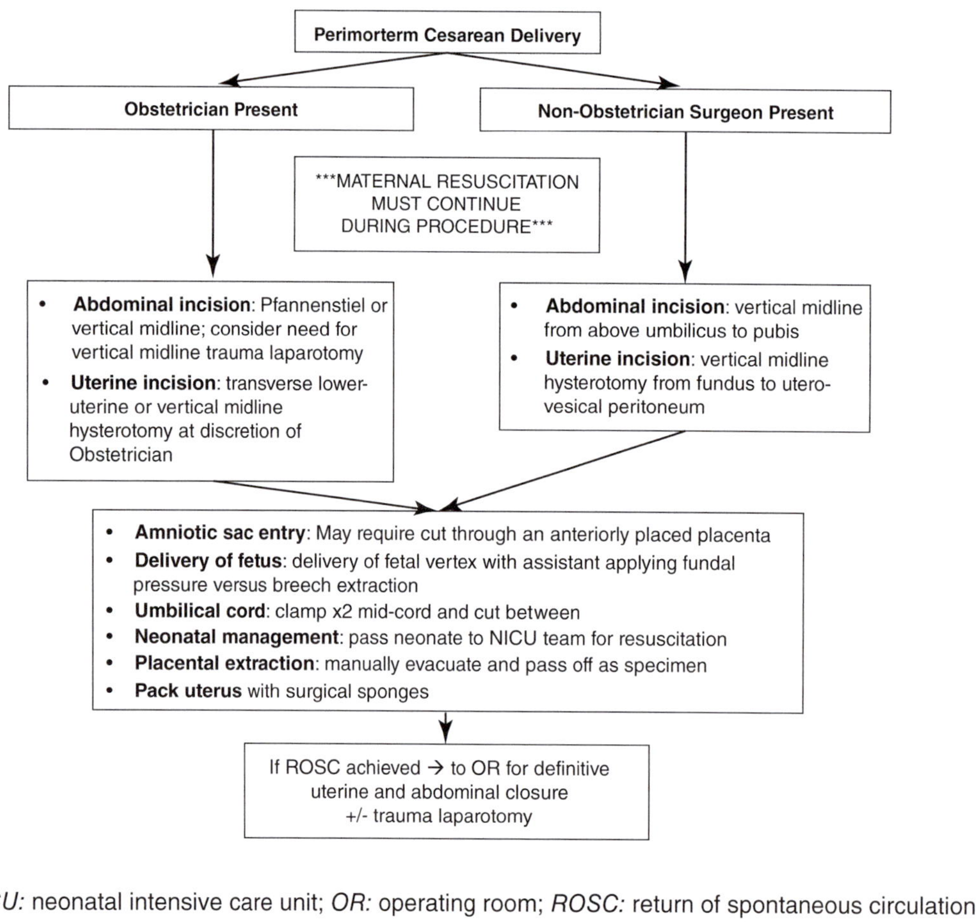

Fig. 41.2 Perimortem Cesarean delivery. (NICU neonatal intensive care unit; OR operating room; ROSC return of spontaneous circulation)

ultrasound to examine for fetal cardiac activity has been reported and suggested to supplant fetal heart tones in the setting of maternal collapse [72], the necessity of spending valuable time to confirm viability is questioned, given the potential for improved maternal resuscitation. Therefore, PCD is advocated irrespective of whether the viability of the fetus can be confirmed [73].

Currently, guidelines from the American Heart Association [74, 94], the European Resuscitation Council [75], and the Eastern Association for the Surgery of Trauma [76] include PCD as part of the treatment of a pregnant patient who has sustained a cardiac arrest. The successful use of PCD in pregnant trauma patients continues to be reported [77, 78].

Coordination of Specialties in the Trauma Bay

As discussed in others sections of this textbook, the trauma bay is often a complex and challenging environment and requires an effective team to optimally resuscitate a severely injured patient. The presence of a trauma patient who is also pregnant has the potential to amplify the stress of the situation and generate powerful emotional responses from the team members. Despite this, trauma evaluation and resuscitation must proceed systematically, with care coordinated by the Trauma Team Leader (TTL) between the trauma team and the obstetrical service.

Despite apparent minor injuries, pregnant patients may develop fetal complications. As such, all pregnant patients should be assessed by the obstetric service with appropriate monitoring and follow-up [76, 79]. Meanwhile, studies have shown that pregnancy itself as a sole criterion for trauma team activation (TTA) is not useful; standard physiologic, mechanistic, and anatomic activation criteria are sufficient to identify those patients requiring the response of the trauma team [79, 80]. A practical approach is that of TTA *only* when the patient meets standard institutional TTA criteria with the inclusion of the obstetric service in the TTA if the patient is known or suspected to have a gestational age of >20 weeks.

In response to the challenge of providing emergency obstetrical care, a number of programs and courses have been created including ALARM [81], MOET [82], ALSO [83], and MOREOB® [84]. The importance of interprofessional team function and use of crisis resource management skills are increasingly being recognized and incorporated into many of these programs. Indeed, the introduction of the MOET course in the Netherlands has been associated with an increased rate of perimortem Cesarean delivery in the setting of maternal cardiac arrest (a recommended procedure in this setting) [85]. The use of simulation is advocated to help improve the performance of obstetrical teams in such situations [73] and has been demonstrated to be effective [86–89]. The implementation of standardized institutional responses to obstetrical crises (e.g. "Code Pink") [90] with obstetric emergency teams contributes to the effective management of such crises on a hospital-wide basis [91, 92].

Optimal management of the severely injured pregnant trauma patient is dependent on the successful incorporation and integration of obstetrical services into the trauma team. Strategies to achieve this include the use of clear activation criteria, institutional obstetric emergency teams that can respond to the trauma venue, and multidisciplinary simulation-based team training.

Conclusions

Care of the traumatically injured female patient increases in complexity when she is also pregnant. While the majority of traumas do not result in severe injuries to the mother, they can result in significant and sometimes occult or delayed consequences to the fetus. Successful resuscitation and management of the pregnant trauma patient requires knowledge of and attention to pregnancy-specific physiologic changes and spectrum of potential injuries, and appropriate integration of obstetrical services into the trauma team with preparation for extreme cases that may require rapid obstetrical intervention. The management of any severely injured trauma patient requires careful coordination of a multidisciplinary team. There is no situation that more aptly demonstrates the necessity for a team approach than the management of trauma in pregnancy.

Key Points

- Physiologic adaptations to pregnancy result in a hyperdynamic and hypervolemic state which may be misleading in the trauma setting where blood pressure and heart rate do not reflect the degree of maternal hypovolemic shock.
- Normalcy of vital signs in the mother does not accurately reflect the status of the fetus, necessitating cardiotocographic monitoring for the early identification of obstetrical complications and fetal compromise.
- Fetal outcome is directly related to maternal outcome: maternal resuscitation and treatment are paramount.
- The presence of a fetus adds an additional layer of complexity in the care of injured pregnant patients, not only due to potential obstetrical complications but also due to the emotive aspect this may have on the trauma team.
- A multidisciplinary approach that includes obstetrics should be employed in the management of pregnant trauma patients.

References

1. SOGC Clinical Practice Guideline. No. 325, June 2015. Jain V, Chari R, Maslovitz S, Farine D. Guidelines for the management of a pregnant trauma patient. J Obstet Gynaecol Can. 2015;37(6):553–71.
2. Hill CC, Pickinpaugh J. Trauma and surgical emergencies in the obstetric patient. Surg Clin North Am. 2008;88:421–40.
3. Kuo C, Kamieson DJ, McPheeters ML, Meikle SF, Posner SF. Injury hospitalization of pregnant women in the United States, 2002. Am J Obstet Gynecol. 2007;196(2):161.
4. Sperry JL, Casey BM, McIntire DD, et al. Long-term foetal outcomes in pregnant trauma patients. Am J Surf. 2006;192:715–21.
5. Schiff MA, Holt VL, Daling JR. Maternal and infant outcomes after injury during pregnancy in Washington state from 1989 to 1997. J Trauma. 2002;53:939–45.
6. Mendez-Figueroa H, Dahlke JD, Vrees RA, Rouse DJ. Trauma in pregnancy: an updated systematic review. Am I Obstet Gynecol. 2013;209(1):1–10.
7. Gazmararian JA, Petersen R, Spitz AM, Goodwin MM, Saltzman LE, Marks JS. Violence and reproductive health: current knowledge and future research directions. Matern Child Health. 2000;4(2):79–84.
8. Stewart DR, Cecutti A. Physical abuse in pregnancy. CMAJ. 1993;149(90):1257–63.
9. El Kady D. Perinatal outcomes of traumatic injuries during pregnancy. Clin Obstet Gynecol. 2007;50(3):582–91.
10. Baerga-Varela Y, Zietlow SP, Bannon MP, Harmsen WS, Ilstrup DM. Trauma in pregnancy. Mayo Clin Proc. 2000;75:1243–8.
11. Warner MW, Salfinger SG, Rao S, Magann EF, Hall JC. Management of trauma during pregnancy. ANZ J Surg. 2004;74(3):125–8.
12. Petrone P, Talving P, Browder T, Teixeira PG, Fisher O, Lozornio A, Chan LS. Abdominal injuries in pregnancy: a 155- month study at two level 1 trauma centers. Injury. 2011;42:47–9.
13. Fabricant SP, Greiner KS, Caughey AB. Trauma in pregnancy and severe adverse perinatal outcomes. J Matern-fetal Neonatal Med. 2019; https://doi.org/10.1080/14767058.2019.1678129.
14. Weiss HB, Songer TJ, Fabio A. Fetal deaths related to maternal injury. JAMA. 2001;286(15):1863–8.
15. Brown S, Mozurkewich E. Trauma during pregnancy. Obstet Gyn Clin N Am. 2013;40(1):47–57.
16. Pearlman MD, Tintinalli JE, Lorenz RP. Blunt trauma during pregnancy. N Engl J Med. 1990;323:1609–13.
17. Knuppel RA, Hatangadi SB. Acute hypotension related to hemorrhage in the obstetric patient. Obstet Gynecol Clin N Am. 1995;22:111–29.
18. El Kady D, Gilbert WM, Anderson J, Danielsen B, Towner D, Smith LH. Trauma during pregnancy: an analysis of maternal and fetal outcomes in a large population. Am J Obstet Gynecol. 2004;190(6):1661–8.
19. Melamed N, Aviram A, Silver M, Peled Y, Wiznitzer A, Glezerman M, Yogev Y. Pregnancy course and outcome following blunt trauma. J Matern Fetal Neonatal Med. 2012;25(9):1612–7.
20. Weintraub AY, Leron E, Mazor M. The pathophysiology of trauma in pregnancy: a review. J Matern Fetal Neonatal Med. 2006;19(10):601–5.
21. Pearlman MD. Motor vehicle crashes, pregnancy loss and preterm labor. Int J Gynaecol Obstet. 1997;57:127–32.
22. Bamber JH, Dresner M. Aortocaval compression in pregnancy: the effect of changing the degree and direction of lateral tilt on maternal cardiac output. Anesth Analg. 2003;97:256–8.
23. Kundra P, Khanna S, Habeebullah S, Ravishankar M. Manual displacement of the uterus during caesarean section. Anesthesia. 2007;62:460–5.
24. Carbonne B, Benachi A, Leveque ML, Cabrol D, Papiernik E. Maternal position during labour: effects on fetal oxygen saturation measured by pulse oximetry. Obstet Gynecol. 1996;88:797–800.
25. Izci B, Vennelle M, Liston WA, Dundas KC, Calder AA, Douglas NJ. Sleep-disordered breathing and upper airway size in pregnancy and post-partum. Eur Respir J. 2006;27:321–7.
26. Advanced Trauma Life Support (ATLS). 9th ed. Chicago: American College of Surgeons; 2012.
27. Adamson D, Dhanjal M, Nelson-Piercy C. Heart disease in pregnancy. Oxford University Press; 2011.
28. Lavery JP, Staten-McCormick M. Management of moderate to severe trauma in pregnancy. Obstet Gynecol Clin N Am. 1995;22:69–90.
29. Corsi PR, Rasslan S, Bechelli de Oliveira L, Kronfly FS, Marinho VP. Trauma in pregnant women: analysis of maternal and fetal mortality. Injury. 1999;30(4):239–43.
30. SOGC Clinical Practice Guideline. No. 375, March 2019. Van den Hof MC, Smithies M, Nevo O, Oullet A. Clinical practice guideline on the use of first trimester ultrasound. J Obstet Gynaecol Can. 2019;41(3):388–95.
31. Bochicchio GV, Haan J, Scalea TM. Surgeon-performed focused assessment with sonography for trauma as an early screening tool for pregnancy after trauma. J Trauma. 2002;52:1125–8.
32. Muench MV, Baschat AA, Reddy UM, Mighty HE, Weiner CP, Scalea TM, et al. Kleihauer-Betke testing is important in all cases of maternal trauma. J Trauma. 2004;57:1094–8.
33. Pearlman MD, Tintinalli JE. Evaluation and treatment of the gravida and fetus following trauma during pregnancy. Obstet Gynecol Clin N Am. 1991;18:371–81.
34. SOGC Clinical Practice Guidelines. No. 307, May 2014. Magee LA, Pels A, Helewa M, Rey E, von Dadelszen P. Diagnosis, evaluation, and management of the hypertensive disorders of pregnancy: executive summary. J Obstet Gynaecol Can. 2014;36(5):416–38.

35. SOGC Clinical Practice Guidelines. No 364, September 2018. Skoll A, Boutin A, Bujold E, Burrows J, Crane J, Geary M, Jain V, Lacze-Masmonteil T, Liauw J, Mundle W, Murphy K, Wong S, Joseph KS. Antenatal corticosteroid therapy for improving neonatal outcomes. J Obstet Gynaecol Can. 2018;40(9):1219–39.
36. Van Hook JW. Trauma in pregnancy (obstetric emergencies). Clin Obstet Gynecol. 2002;45:414–24.
37. Bowdler N, Faix RG, Elkins T. Fetal skull fracture and brain injury after a maternal automobile accident. A case report. J Reprod Med. 1987;32:375–8.
38. Evrad JR, Sturner WQ, Murray EJ. Fetal skull fracture from an automobile accident. Am J Forensic Med Pathol. 1989;10:232–4.
39. Härtl R, Ko K. In utero skull fracture: case report. J Trauma. 1996;41:549–52.
40. Sakala EP, Kort DD. Management of stab wounds to the pregnant uterus: a case report and a review of the literature. Obstet Gynecol Surv. 1988;42:319–24.
41. Awwad JT, Azar GB, Seoud MA, Mroueh AM, Karam KS. High-velocity penetrating wounds of the gravid uterus: review of 16 years of civil war. Obstet Gynecol. 1994;83:259–64.
42. Nagy KK, Roberts RR, Joseph KT, Smith RF, An GC, Bohkari F, Barrett J. Experience with over 2500 diagnostic peritoneal lavages. Injury. 2000;31:479–82.
43. Visser BC, Glasgow RE, Mulvihill KK, Mulvihil SJ. Safety and timing of nonobstetrical abdominal surgery in pregnancy. Dig Surg. 2001;18:409–17.
44. Morris JA, Rosenbower TJ, Jurkovich GJ, Hoyt DB, Harviel JD, Knudson MM, et al. Infant survival after cesarean section for trauma. Ann Surg. 1996;223(5):481–91.
45. Moise KJ, Belfort MA. Damage control for the obstetric patient. Surg Clin North Am. 1997;77(4):835–52.
46. Sperry JL, Casey BM, McIntire DD, Minei JP, Gentilello LM, Shafi S. Long-term fetal outcomes in pregnant trauma patients. Am J Surg. 2006;192:715–21.
47. Feldhaus KM, Kozoil-McLain J, Amsbury HL, Nortom IM, Lowenstein SR, Abbott JT. Accuracy of 3 brief screening questions for detecting partner violence in the emergency department. JAMA. 1997;277(17):1357–61.
48. Helpern LR, Perciaccante VJ, Hayes C, Susarla S, Dodson TB. A protocol to diagnose intimate partner violence in the emergency department. J Trauma. 2006;60(5):1101–5.
49. MacMillan HL, Wathen C, Jamieson E, et al. Approaches to screening for intimate partner violence in health care settings: a randomized trial. JAMA. 2006;296(5):530–6.
50. Theodorou DA, Velmahos GC, Souter I, Chan LS, Vassiliu P, Tatevossian R, et al. Fetal death after trauma in pregnancy. Am Surg. 2000;66(9):809–12.
51. Brown HL. Trauma in pregnancy. Obstet Gynecol. 2009;114(1):147–60.
52. Curet MJ, Schermer CR, Demarest GB, Bieneik EJ, Curet LB. Predictors of outcome in trauma during pregnancy: identification of patients who can be monitored for less than 6 hours. J Trauma. 2000;49(1):18–24. Discussion 24-25
53. Henderson SO, Mallon WK. Trauma in pregnancy. Emerg Clin North Am. 1998;16:209–28.
54. Mirza FG, Devine PC, Gaddipati S. Trauma in pregnancy: a systematic approach. Am J Perinatol. 2010;27(7):579–86.
55. ACOG Committee on Obstetric Practice Opinion Number 723: Guidelines for diagnostic imaging during pregnancy and lactation. 130(4): 210–16. October 2017. Available from https://www.acog.org/-/media/project/acog/acogorg/clinical/files/committee-opinion/articles/2017/10/guidelines-for-diagnostic-imaging-during-pregnancy-and-lactation.pdf.
56. American College of Radiology-Society for Pediatric Radiology Practice Guideline for Imaging Pregnant or Potentially Pregnant Adolescents and Women with Ionizing Radiation. Practice guideline, revised 2018. Available from: https://www.acr.org/-/media/ACR/Files/Practice-Parameters/Pregnant-Pts.pdf.
57. Wieseler KM, Bhargava P, Kanal KM, Vaidya S, Stewart BK, Dighe MK. Imaging in pregnant patients: examination appropriateness. Radiographics. 2010;30:1215–33.
58. Tien HC, Tremblay LN, Rizoli SB, Gelberg J, Spencer F, Caldwell C, et al. Radiation exposure from diagnostic imaging in severely injured trauma patients. J Trauma. 2007;62(1):151–6.
59. Doll R, Wakeford R. Risk of childhood cancer from foetal irradiation. Br J Radiol. 1997;70:130–9.
60. American College of Radiology Committee on Drugs and Contrast Media. ACR Manual on Contrast Media, revised 2020. Available from: https://www.acr.org/-/media/ACR/Files/Clinical-Resources/Contrast_Media.pdf.
61. Wei SH, Helmy M, Cohen AJ. Ct evaluation of placental abruption in pregnant trauma patients. Emerg Radiol. 2009;16(5):365–73.
62. Manriquex M, Srinivas G, Bollepalli S, Britt L, Drachman D. Is computed tomography a reliable diagnostic modality in detecting placental injuries in the setting of acute trauma? Am J Obstet Gynecol. 2010;202(6):611.e1–5.
63. Kopelman TR, Berardoni NE, ManriquezM GD, Vail SJ, Pieri PG, et al. The ability of computed tomography to diagnose acute placental abruption in the trauma patient. J Trauma Acute Care Surg. 2013;74:236–41.
64. Richards JR, Ormsby EL, Romo MV, Gillen MA, McGahan JP. Blunt abdominal injury in the pregnant patient: detection with us. Radiology. 2004;233(2):473–0.
65. Koninckx PR, Renaer M, Brosens IA. Origin of peritoneal fluid in women: an ovarian exufation product. Br J Obstet Gynaecol. 1980;87(3):177–83.
66. Hussain ZJ, Figueroa R, Budorick NE. How much free fluid can a pregnant patient have? Assessment of pelvic free fluid in pregnant patients without antecedent trauma. J Trauma. 2011;70(6):1420–3.
67. Katz V, Dotters DJ, Droegemueller W. Perimortem cesarean delivery. Obstet Gynecol. 1986;68:571.
68. Katz V, Balderston K, DeFreest M. Perimortem cesarean delivery: were our assumptions correct? Am J Obstet Gynecol. 2005;192:1916–21.
69. Strong TH Jr, Lowe RA. Perimortem cesarean section. Am J Emerg Med. 1989;7:489–94.
70. Ueland K, Akamatsu TJ, Eng M, Bonica JJ, Hansen JM. Maternal cardiovascaular hemodynamics: VI. Cesarean section under epidural anesthesia without epinephrine. Am J Obstet Gynecol. 1972;114:775–80.
71. Page-Rodriguez A, Gonzalez-Sanchez JA. Perimortem cesarean section of twin pregnancy: case report and review of the literature. Acad Emerg Med. 1999;6:1072–4.
72. Phelan HA, Roller J, Minei JP. Perimortem cesarean section after utilization of surgeon-performed trauma ultrasound. J Trauma. 2008;64:E12–4.
73. Katz VL. Perimortem cesarean delivery: its role in maternal mortality. Semin Perinatol. 2012;36(1):68–72.
74. Jeejeebhoy FM, Zelop CM, Lipman S, Carvalho B, Joglar J, Mhyre JM, Katz VL, Lapinsky SE, Einav S, Warnes CA, Page RL, et al. Cardiac arrest in pregnancy: a scientific statement from the American Heart Association. Circulation. 2015;132(18):1747–73.
75. Truhlár A, Deakin CD, Soar J, Khalifa GEA, Alfonzo A, Bierens JJLM, et al. European Resuscitation Council Guidelines for Resuscitation 2015 Section 4: cardiac arrest in special circumstances. Resuscitation. 2015;95:148–201.
76. Barraco RD, Chiu WC, Clancy TV, Como JJ, Ebert JB, Hess W, et al. Practice management guidelines for the diagnosis and management of injury in the pregnant patient: the EAST Practice Management Guidelines Work Group. J Trauma. 2010;69:211–4.
77. Copobianco G, Balata A, Mannazzu MC, Oggiano R, Pinna Nossai L, Cherchi PL, et al. Perimortem cesarean delivery 30 min-

utes after a laboring patient jumped from a fourth-floor window: baby survives and is normal at age 4 years. Am J Obstet Gynecol. 2008;198(1):e15–6.
78. Guven S, Yazar A, Yakut K, Aydogan H, Erguven M, Avci E. Postmortem cesarean: report of our successful neonatal outcomes after severe trauma during pregnancy and review of the literature. J Matern Fetal Neonatal Med. 2012;25(7):1102–4.
79. Auforth R, Edhayan E, Dempath D. Should pregnancy be sole criterion for trauma code activation: a review of the trauma registry. Am J Surg. 2010;199(3):387–90.
80. Greene W, Robinson L, Rizzo AG, Sakran J, Hendershot K, Moore A, et al. Pregnancy is not a sufficient indicator for trauma team activation. J Trauma. 2007;63(3):550–5.
81. AdvancesinLabourandRiskManagement(ALARM).Availablefrom: http://sogc.org/events/advances-in-labour-andrisk-management/welcome/
82. Managing Obstetric Emergencies and Trauma (MOET). Advanced Life Support Group. Available from: http://www.alsg.org/uk/MOET
83. Advanced Life Support in Obstetrics (ALSO). Available from: http://www.aafp.org/about/initiatives/also.html
84. Managing Obstetrical Risk Efficiently (MOREOB.). Salus Global Corporation. Available: http://moreob.com
85. Dijkman A, Huisman CM, Smit M, Schutte JM, Zwart JJ, van Roosmalen JJ, et al. Cardiac arrest in pregnancy: increasing use of perimortem cesarean section due to emergency skills training? BJOG. 2010;117:282–7.
86. Daniels K, Lipman S, Harney K, Arafeh J, Druzin M. Use of simulation based team training for obstetric crises in resident education. Simul Healthc. 2008;3:154–60.
87. Robertson B, Schumacher L, Gosman G, Kanfer R, Kelley M, DeVita M. Simulation-based crisis team training for multidisciplinary obstetric providers. Simul Healthc. 2009;4:77–83.
88. Daniels K, Arafeh J, Clark A, Waller S, Druzin M, Chueh J. Prospective randomized trial of simulation versus didactic teaching for obstetrical emergencies. Simul Healthc. 2010;5:40–5.
89. Bradley NL, Innes K, Dakin C, Sawka A, Lakha N, Hameed SM. Multidisciplinary in-situ simulation to evalute a rare but high-risk process at a level 1 truam centres: the "Mega-Sim" approach. Can J Surg. 2018;61(5):357–60.
90. British Columbia Ministry of Health Services Policy Communique. Standardized Hospital Colour Codes. January 21, 2011. Available from: http://www.health.gov.bc.ca/emergency/pdf/standardizedhospital-colour-codes.pdf
91. Al Kadri HMF. Obstetric medical emergency teams are a step forward in maternal safety! J Emerg Trauma Shock. 2010;3(4):337–41.
92. Smith JA, Sosulski A, Eskander R, Moazzez A, Patel N, Putnam R, et al. Implementation of a multi-disciplinary perinatal emergerncy response team improves time to definitive obstetrical evaluation and fetal assessment. J Trauma Acute Care Surg. 2020;88:615–8.
93. McCollough CH, Schueler BA, Atwell TD, Braun NN, Regner DM, Brown DL, et al. Radiation exposure and pregnancy: when should we be concerned? Radiographics. 2007;27:909–18.
94. American Heart Association Guidelines for CPR and ECC. Available: https://cpr.heart.org/-/media/cpr-files/cpr-guidelines-files/highlights/hghlghts_2020_ecc_guidelines_english.pdf. Accessed 26 Jan 2021.

Medical Comorbidities and Trauma

42

Harvey G. Hawes and Renée-Anne Poirier

Introduction

According to the WHO, injuries account for 9% of global mortality and disable millions of people annually [1]. It is the infamous leading cause of death for age groups between 1 and 45 years old in the USA [2]. In Canada, unintentional injuries were the eighth leading cause of hospitalizations among all ages in 2018 and 2019 [3, 4]. The burden of trauma affects all age groups and carries a wide spectrum of impacts. From minor traumas with no long-term consequences to deadly injuries with a variety of long-term and short-term disabilities in between, the impact of the trauma pandemic is a significant public health issue.

As previously stated, all populations can be affected by trauma. ATLS makes special consideration for specific populations: pediatric, elderly, and pregnancy [5]. Even though these populations are usually well covered in most trauma textbooks, the specific considerations for comorbid patients are hard to find. Various studies have shown a link between the presence of preexisting medical conditions and an increase in trauma-related mortality. Thus, it is of the foremost importance to be aware of those specific conditions and their impact on the patient's management and outcomes. This chapter will provide an overview of the subject, starting with the definition and grading systems, then will detail the incidence of comorbidities in the trauma population and, finally, four main subjects will be discussed separately. We will cover some commonly seen trauma populations: obese patients, the aging population, psychiatric afflictions, and anticoagulated patients.

H. G. Hawes (✉)
Department of Surgery, Division of General Surgery, Section of Trauma Surgery, University of British Columbia, Vancouver, BC, Canada

R.-A. Poirier
Department of Surgery, Division of General Surgery, CIUSSS du Saguenay-Lac-Saint-Jean, Hôpital d'Alma, QC, Canada
e-mail: Renee-Anne.Poirier.med@ssss.gouv.qc.ca

Definition and Grading Systems

First and foremost, comorbidity is defined as "the presence of more than one distinct condition in an individual" [6]. Comorbidities affect patient outcomes, mortality, and overall health cost in all medical fields. In the context of trauma care, the word "comorbidity" usually implies that the injured person has an underlying disease that could impact his or her global management. Comorbidities have an impact on all phases of a trauma—the pre-injury, the injury, and the recovery phases. Those stages of injury will be detailed for all four main comorbidities listed above.

Many grading systems have been developed to try to quantify the burden of underlying disease. Most of those scores have general applications, but some are more specific to a particular field. For example, the ASA classification was developed in 1941 by Saklad et al. to try to predict the risk of perioperative mortality [7]. In trauma, many scores have been studied to evaluate the impact of comorbidities on patient outcomes. The most commonly used scoring system in trauma literature is the Charlson Index. Even though it is a well-known and validated score, it is not very user-friendly in the clinical setting of trauma where the fast pace of initial assessment and treatment doesn't always allow time for such a detailed score. Another score recently developed and studied in the trauma population is the comorbidity-polypharmacy score (CPS). It made its first appearance in the literature in 2011, and seems more accessible to trauma management, as it is a simple addition of the number of comorbidities and the number of pre-admission medications [8].

$$\text{Number of comorbidities} + \text{Number of pre-admission medications} = \text{CPS}$$

The CPS was validated in the trauma population and is a predictor of undertriage in elderly trauma patients [9]. A high CPS score was also shown to be a predictor of mortality in osteoporotic hip fractures and a predictor of 30-day readmission in trauma patients of 45 years and older [10, 11].

L. Marshall Gillman, S. Widder (eds.), *Trauma Team Dynamics*, https://doi.org/10.1007/978-3-031-86312-7_42

Hence, the CPS score seems to be the score of choice at the moment in trauma.

Obesity in Trauma

Obesity is a public health issue worldwide, particularly in developed countries. According to the WHO, in 2016, 39% of all adults in the world were overweight [12]. Globally, almost 2.3 billion children and adults are overweight. They also write that in the 2010s, 14 of the lowest-income countries faced a double burden of malnutrition (undernutrition and obesity) in different socio-economic cohorts. Those numbers reflect the global burden of this disease that is developing everywhere around the world. In the USA, the age-adjusted prevalence of obesity in adults was 42.4% in 2017–2018. It has been steadily increasing over the past decades [13]. In Canada, the prevalence of obesity is ranging from 23.1% to 40.2% depending on the province [14].

In the pre-injury phase, obesity seems to increase the risk of MVC-related injuries and mortality. In fact, a meta-analysis published in the *Asia-Pacific Journal of Public Health* in 2014 [15] showed a strong association between obesity and MVC-related fatalities and lower extremity fractures. Some injuries are now becoming classic affliction of the morbidly obese patients. For example, knee dislocation following ultralow velocity mechanism is now described for the morbidly obese population. An article published by Carr et al. in 2016 described the evaluation, management, and outcomes after this kind of injury [16]. It may go undetected considering the low-velocity mechanism and secondary consideration of knee pain in the polytrauma patient. Nevertheless, knee dislocation has a high risk for neurovascular injury, and a low threshold for detection is required to prompt emergent management in order to avoid limb compromise. On the other hand, there used to be a belief that obesity was protective for stab wounds to the torso. This has been invalidated by two recent studies showing no protective effect from obesity, neither in penetrating thoracoabdominal injuries nor in abdominal stab wounds. Their rates of therapeutic operations were equivalent in the obese and non-obese groups [17, 18]. So overall, there is no benefit in being overweight in trauma, it doesn't prevent severe injuries in penetrating trauma, and it even increases the risk of mortality from MVCs [15].

In the injury phase, obesity seems to bring its load of challenges in the transport, the diagnosis, and the in-hospital care of patients. Many barriers have been identified in the care of obese patients in trauma [19]. First, something as benign as transportation can be challenging because most ambulance gurneys can only carry up to 160 kg. Extrication of an obese patient can necessitate more manpower and special boards and equipment that are not quickly available in the regular setting. One could think that our hospitals are better equipped to care for morbidly obese people—after all, they represent a significant percentage of the population, but health care professionals face several obstacles in the care of those patients. In trauma, something as simple as putting reliable IV lines can become a challenge. The initial assessment and resuscitation can become a succession of difficulties. The airway should be expected to be difficult, by the anatomy of a large obstructive neck. Adequate ventilation can require the patient to have the head of the bed up to limit the restrictive syndrome caused by obesity. Chest tube insertion can be challenging in the presence of a thick layer of subcutaneous fat. An interesting case report published in 2011 described the insertion of a chest tube under direct vision, through an OptiView-type port in the operating room to ensure proper placement in the pleural cavity [20]. Their patient had a BMI of nearly 79 though, so even if it is an interesting technique, it is hardly applicable in the trauma bay. There is no literature on the rate of misplaced chest tubes in that population, but as that health issue grows, it would be very interesting to see a study on that. In the circulatory assessment, it can even be difficult to get a reliable blood pressure if the proper equipment is not available. A study published in 2019 showed that a regular cylindrical cuff can overestimate the blood pressure compared to an appropriate troncoconical cuff adapted for obese patients [21]. Another study published in the *British Journal of Nursing* showed a mean overestimation of 10 points when measurement of the blood pressure is taken on the forearm instead of a properly fitted upper arm cuff [22]. It shows the importance of using the proper equipment for these patients. Those studies have been done in healthy normovolemic patients, no data is available for obese patients in hemorrhagic shock. Even though the installation of invasive blood pressure monitoring is time-consuming compared to external monitoring, it could be a solution to overpass the issue of unreliable external measurements in the absence of reliable cuffs. Also, the reliability of the FAST exam decreases with a BMI over 35. It has been shown that the risk of an inaccurate FAST increases significantly with a BMI of 40 and more [23]. The reliability of other exams like CT scan hasn't been studied for trauma in obese patients.

In the recovery phase, many factors seem to impair the recovery of obese patients. For starters, there is good evidence suggesting that obesity increases the risk of mortality [24]. It also seems to significantly increase the risk of respiratory and infectious complications, deep venous thrombosis, and acute kidney injury [24]. Some of those results can be explained by the presence of concomitant chronic illness in obese persons, like diabetes, GERD, or sleep apnea. Regarding the risk of complications during operations, obese patients seem to have a higher risk for normally low-risk procedures. For example, a simple percutaneous tracheostomy in patients with a BMI over 27 was found to have a 43.8%

complication rate by Byhahn et al. in 2005. Those complications in obese patients were found to be severe in up to 9.6% of the cases [25].

In short, obesity has its loads of challenges in the trauma population. From the moment the injury occurs, until the person is back to his or her baseline functionality, the path to recovery is full of obstacles. Health care professionals and physicians need to be aware of them to improve the care of those patients.

Elderly Population

In 2019, there were over 703 million people aged 65 years and older in the world [26]. In Canada, the number of people over 65 years old is expected to increase by 68% between 2017 and 2037. The number of older elderly (more than 75 years old) is expected to double in that period [27]. The definition of geriatric trauma is somewhat controversial. Geriatric societies characterize their population as 65 years and older. Most trauma literature respects this cutoff when studying this population, but as the world population ages, this definition may be subject to change in the future. An objective way to evaluate the risk after a trauma in the geriatric population is to use a frailty index. There is evidence that frail patients have poorer outcomes [28]. The frail state seems to weigh more than the chronologic age in the outcomes of geriatric trauma. The Trauma-Specific Frailty Index (TSFI) is validated to predict unfavorable discharge disposition [29]. Its use can help prevent failed discharge by targeting which patients will need higher care for recovery. This index, as useful as it is, is quite complex with many variables. It takes into consideration comorbidities, dementia, ability to attend to daily activities, ability to mobilize, nutritional status, and attitude toward health conditions. It does not correlate with the age of the patients but was developed for patients 65 years and older. Its first aim was to predict discharge disposition in geriatric trauma patients. It is best integrated in a multidisciplinary approach, for long-term planning of discharge of the geriatric patient.

In the pre-injury phase, the older population is at risk for specific injuries. Labib et al. published an article in 2011 describing characteristics of geriatric trauma in a Montreal level 1 trauma center [30]. They found that nearly three-quarters of trauma in the older population was secondary to falls. MVCs and pedestrian injuries were the next most common mechanism with 12% of prevalence each. Penetrating injuries accounted for only 1% of their trauma mechanisms. These findings can be explained by several characteristics of the geriatric population. By advancing in age, people develop variate impairments of their basic function. For example, core strength, vivacity of reflexes, vision, balance, and judgment can be impaired with time. All those faculty losses can lead to falls or impaired driving abilities. They generally explain the special mechanisms of trauma in the elderly. For example, ladder-related injuries have been described in all age groups, but have a higher morbidity and mortality rate in the older population. A study published in *The Journal of Emergency Medicine* in August 2020 by Barbat et al. showed that about 25% of all ladder-related injuries were in patients aged 65 years and older. It has been targeted as a potentially very beneficial prevention program in the elderly population [31]. In general, elderly injuries happen at home. Oyetunj et al. described the distribution of elderly injuries mechanism, location, and demographics [32]. They conclude that 42% of injuries in elderly people happen in their own homes. The second most frequent location being the road, by motor vehicle crashes or pedestrians struck by vehicles. The fact that most elderly injuries happen in their own homes makes early intervention and screening in the community a good prevention measure in the pre-injury phase. Although studies of this type are not frequently seen in the trauma literature, the prevention of injuries in the elderly population is a trending subject and has the potential to reduce the burden on the healthcare systems.

In the injury phase, frail patients are known to have an increased inflammatory response [33]. This specific characteristic of the older population can explain in part poorer prognosis of several types of injuries. For instance, TBI in patients 60 years and older is more likely to cause permanent functional impairment [34]. This situation raises questions about futile care in the elderly population sustaining a traumatic injury. Even though this notion makes a lot of sense in the clinical setting, it is difficult to define and hard to study in an objective setting. Fleischman et al. published an article in 2012 in the *Journal of Trauma and Acute Care Surgery* defining futile care as an admission of more than 14 days associated with death within 7 days of discharge [35]. They evaluated the median cost in the "non-futile care" group to $33,373. It was significantly higher in the "futile care" group at $87,391. The exact definition of futile care in trauma is not commonly accepted. The one developed by Fleischman's study group is relevant for research purposes, but cannot be applied in real-life situations, as it is a retrospective judgment. This study has biases; nevertheless, it does necessitate a reflection on how aggressively we treat elderly trauma patients. The management of older patients should be tailored to their previously stated wishes, their baseline comorbidities, and their traumatic burden of injuries. Large trauma societies have advocated for aggressive initial management, even in the elderly population, as not every patient over the age of 65 years old has the same potential (or lack of potential) for recovery. EAST published a guideline in 2012 regarding the care of this age group [36]. They stated that aggressive initial management should be encouraged for the non-moribund patients and that the threshold for trauma team activations and multidisciplinary care should be lower in this population. Even though they advocate for aggressive initial therapy, they do take in consideration the notion of futile care in the following statement: "In patients 65 years of age and older with a GCS < 8, if substantial improvement in GCS is not realized within 72 h of injury, consideration should be given to limiting further aggressive therapeutic interventions". Hence, the management of the injury phase in the older population is a growing field of research, especially now that they are increasingly represented in the general trauma population. The literature about TBI in the elderly is evolving. Upcoming studies are looking at better scoring systems to predict outcomes in this population who are over-represented in the poor outcome category. For example, the eTBI Score shows promising results but has yet to be validated in large cohort studies [37].

Another frequent injury in the elderly population is fractures, mostly hip and rib fractures. Both have been studied extensively in the past few years. Hundreds of studies on the subject have been published in 2021 alone. Most outcomes studies show that aggressive early treatment of those conditions reduces the complication rate and mortality rate. Special units for seniors have shown improved outcomes for hip fracture admissions [38]. An article published in *Gerontology & Geriatric Medicine* in 2018 by Duran, Mazzurco, and Palmer showed that a specialized group of geriatricians helped with the care of the elderly who sustained a traumatic injury. Their most frequent interventions were transition of care and adjustment in medication [39]. Those specialized teams should be involved early in the care of elderly patients to prevent further complications during their hospital stay. The multidisciplinary approach seems beneficial in most geriatric trauma. For example, multimodal analgesia and multidisciplinary treatment pathways for rib fractures in older adults showed reduced rates of complications [40].

In the post-injury phase, the geriatric population needs more support for recovery. As discussed above, the TSFI can be used to plan which patient will need more assistance for discharge. Another aspect of the recovery phase concerns the prevention of injury recurrence. Considering falls are the most common mechanism, it is a good target for prevention programs. For example, a Japanese study from 2017 showed a significant decrease in fall recurrence after the implementation of a prevention program through senior centers in the community. They showed that even a single visit with a multidisciplinary team for assessment and counseling helped prevent falls in a total of 1863 elderly patients [41]. Those types of intervention are not only important for patients individually, but they are also very relevant on a societal level. Dieleman and al. published a cost-evaluation study in *JAMA* in 2016 and estimated that falls were the fourth most costly health problem in the USA [42]. Hence, having prevention programs has a potential benefit on an individual level as well as on an institutional level.

Psychiatric Comorbidities

Another population highly represented in trauma is the psychiatric patient. From substance use disorders to psychotic pathologies, including mood disorders and suicide attempts, a wide spectrum of psychiatric disorders are represented in the trauma population. A study performed in Los Angeles between 2008 and 2015 showed a prevalence of 11.5% for psychiatric illness in trauma admissions [43]. In the pre-injury phase, psychiatric disorders increase the risk of traumatic injuries compared to other disease processes. Psychiatric patients are over-represented in trauma admissions compared to general hospital admissions (44% vs 33%, $p < 0.01$) [44]. They present with self-harm injuries in 11.6% compared to 0.72% in the non-psychiatric patients [43].

In the injury phase, specific trauma mechanisms have been described in the psychiatric population. As stated above, self-harm is significantly more represented in this population compared to the general population. Trauma teams must be aware of those specificities to care properly for these patients. In fact, psychiatric comorbidities can have a significant impact on patients' recovery. For example, depression increases the complication rate in orthopedic polytrauma [45]. It was also shown that almost 50% of suicide attempts in men 70 years and older die in hospital from their attempt [46]. Those specifics of psychiatric illness in trauma patients have to be taken into consideration during the index admission. And even if the trauma is not due to the psychiatric condition, trauma teams should be aware of these comorbidities and consider it as any other physical illness during the admission. Chronic medication should be reordered and discharge follow up for those conditions should be planned throughout the hospital stay. The University of Florida Jacksonville's Department of Surgery developed an integrated model of care in 1995 for its inpatient trauma program. Since then it grew from one hired psychologist to at least two of them and a psychology post-doctoral resident. They address pre-existing psychiatric comorbidities and post-traumatic psychological issues. This Psychological Service Program (PSP) is part of the trauma multidisciplinary team; they are involved in all fields of recovery after trauma, from acute stress disorder to suicidal ideation/dangerousness, including post-TBI behavior issues, ethical considerations, and discharge planning. By integrating the PSP into their trauma program, they treat those mental health issues during the recovery of the patient, as aggressively as the physical issues. That way, they aim to prevent post-injury maladaptation which can be a risk factor for trauma recurrence [47].

The injury phase is also influenced when patients suffer from substance use disorders. The prevalence of accidental and violent injury in this population is significantly higher than in the general population. The most commonly used substance in the trauma population is alcohol, followed by cannabis and benzodiazepines. As expected, more patients are under the influence at nighttime and on the weekends [48]. Most studies about the association of substance use disorder and adverse outcomes in trauma often include only TBI patients. They are looking at the relationship between pre-injury use of drugs and in-hospital outcomes. A study published in 2016, based in Los Angeles, showed that benzodiazepines and opiates users had higher mortality rates when admitted after a trauma [49]. Physicians caring for these patients must be aware of this data to try and prevent complications in this population.

In the recovery phase, psychiatric pathologies and substance use disorders are over-represented in the homeless population [50], and it brings its load of challenges for discharge planning. Very little literature is available on discharge planning for the homeless trauma population. Social workers and psychiatric liaison teams should be involved early during admission to help prevent failed discharge. *The Lancet* published a series on homelessness in October 2014 that details the epidemiology of illnesses in the homeless population. They also suggest ways of improving care to the homeless population which can be applied to our trauma population. The most efficient programs combine housing provision with therapeutic intervention, for example, opioid replacement therapy or work therapy. Those programs reduce the recurrence of homelessness and the inappropriate use of the healthcare system. Mental health and social care programs that specialize in acute outreach after discharge seem to improve the sustainability of housing for the psychiatric homeless population during their transition to housing after a hospital admission [51]. Integrating these kinds of programs into trauma patient's discharge plans could potentially reduce failed discharges. This structure has not been studied in the trauma population specifically, but a study published in December 2020 by Shellito et al. showed the most common reasons for presentation to the emergency department after discharge of trauma patients were pain control and wound issues [52]. In an ideal world, those integrated programs would be available for vulnerable patients such as people with mental health, substance, or precarious housing issues. Targeting post-discharge trauma patients, the outreach team would need to be resourceful in various domains, including psychiatric crisis management, substance misuse counseling, wound assessment, and acute pain management.

Anticoagulated Patients

Many comorbidities can require blood thinners, but the anticoagulated state is more relevant to trauma care than the actual indication for it. That is why those individual medical conditions will not be discussed separately in this section. Instead, we will look at the overall key concepts of managing an anticoagulated patient.

Nowadays, several people use anticoagulation. In the USA in 2017, over four million people were using an oral anticoagulation [53] for various reasons. In trauma, this type of medication can be problematic and the management should be tailored to the medications used. It was controversial that the use of certain anticoagulation medications increased the risk of intracranial hemorrhage (ICH) in the pre-injury phase. Several recent articles address the question of risk associated with antiplatelet therapy, vitamin K antagonists, also called oral anticoagulants (OACs), and direct oral anticoagulants (DOACs) [54]. In the past, warfarin was the most commonly used OAC. It is hence the medication of comparison for any new anticoagulant. The largest study comparing adverse outcomes of OACs and DOACs is a systematic review and meta-analysis published in *Injury* in 2020 [55]. A total of 1,365,446 patients were pooled from 19 studies. As most studies previously demonstrated, this one showed that OACs increased the risk of mortality and the risk of ICH. DOACs did not. In fact, a post-hoc analysis on the ARISTOL trial published in *Blood* in 2017 showed that patients on Apixaban were 58% less likely to experience an intracranial hemorrhage compared to those on warfarin. The reduction of trauma-related bleeding was even higher with a 75% risk reduction. These studies support the widespread use of DOACs over OACs, even in the absence of reliable reversal agents because the data tend to show they have a better safety profile.

Main trauma societies published recent guidelines regarding the management of those medications in the trauma setting. The first step is to categorize the agent previously used by the patient (antiplatelets, warfarin, or DOACs). Secondly, it is foremost important to characterize the bleed (life-threatening hemorrhage, intracranial hemorrhage, or mild nonoperative bleed). Those two aspects of the initial evaluation will guide the indication for reversal. The EAST guidelines recommend the prompt evaluation of the coagulation profile in all patients using an anticoagulation medication [37]. They also recommend a head CT for elderly patients with a suspected TBI and anticoagulation reversal measures to be completed within 2 h of admission for patients with an intracranial hemorrhage. Evidence points to an improvement in the timely management of TBI patients with known use of warfarin after the implementation of a reversal protocol led by the nursing team [56]. Hence, a multidisciplinary management protocol should be considered in any high-volume trauma center.

Conclusion

In conclusion, several chronic conditions can affect outcomes after trauma. The four main conditions described above are commonly seen in trauma patients and they each bring their load of challenges. This review of recent literature on the subjects should help bring awareness on specific issues in those special populations. It certainly is a blooming field in the trauma literature and further studies should be done to continue improving the care of those patients.

Key Points

- Comorbidities impact all phases of trauma from injury prevention to rehabilitation.
- This is a rapidly growing subset of trauma patients.
- Definitions and validated grading systems are an active area of study in trauma care but will aid in research and guideline development.
- We discuss four common patient comorbidities that impact trauma outcomes and care pathways.

References

1. https://www.who.int/topics/injuries/en
2. https://www.cdc.gov/injury/images/lc-charts/leading_causes_of_death_by_age_group_2018_1100w850h.jpg
3. Yao X, Skinner R, McFaull S, Thompson W. At-a-glance—2015 injury deaths in Canada. Health Promot Chron Dis Prev Can. 2019;39(6/7 June/July):225–31. https://doi.org/10.24095/hpcdp.39.6/7.03
4. https://www.canada.ca/en/public-health/services/injury-prevention/facts-on-injury.html
5. *** ATLS Book reference***
6. Valderas JM, Starfield B, Sibbald B, Salisbury C, Roland M. Defining comorbidity: implications for understanding health and health services. Ann Fam Med. 2009;7(4):357–63. https://doi.org/10.1370/afm.983.
7. Mayhew D, Mendonca V, Murthy BVS. A review of ASA physical status—historical perspectives and modern developments. Anaesthesia. 2019;74:373–9. https://doi.org/10.1111/anae.14569.
8. Evans DC, Gerlach AT, Christy JM, et al. Pre-injury polypharmacy as a predictor of outcomes in trauma patients. Int J Crit Illn Inj Sci. 2011;1(2):104–9. https://doi.org/10.4103/2229-5151.84793.
9. Justiniano CF, Evans DC, Cook CH, Eiferman DS, Gerlach AT, Beery PR 2nd, Lindsey DE, Saum GE, Murphy CV, Miller SF, Papadimos TJ, Steinberg SM, Stawicki SP. Comorbidity-polypharmacy score: a novel adjunct in post-emergency department trauma triage. J Surg Res. 2013;181(1):16–9. https://doi.org/10.1016/j.jss.2012.05.042. Epub 2012 May 31. PMID: 22683074; PMCID: PMC3717608
10. Camur S, Celik H. Prediction of the mortality with comorbidity—polypharmacy score in the osteoporotic hip fractures. Acta Chir Orthop Traumatol Cechoslov. 2019;86(5):320–3. English. PMID: 31748105
11. Housley BC, Stawicki SP, Evans DC, Jones C. Comorbidity-polypharmacy score predicts readmission in older trauma patients. J Surg Res. 2015;199(1):237–43. https://doi.org/10.1016/j.jss.2015.05.014. Epub 2015 May 15. PMID: 26163329
12. https://www.who.int/news-room/fact-sheets/detail/obesity-and-overweight
13. https://www.cdc.gov/nchs/products/databriefs/db360.htm
14. https://www150.statcan.gc.ca/n1/en/pub/82-625-x/2019001/article/00005-eng.pdf?st=wWvQn2
15. Desapriya E, Giulia S, Subzwari S, Peiris DC, Turcotte K, Pike I, Sasges D, Hewapathirane DS. Does obesity increase the risk of injury or mortality in motor vehicle crashes? A systematic review and meta-analysis. Asia Pac J Public Health. 2014;26(5):447–60. https://doi.org/10.1177/1010539511430720. Epub 2011 Dec 20. PMID: 22186398
16. Carr JB, Werner BC, Miller MD, Gwathmey FW. Knee dislocation in the morbidly obese patient. J Knee Surg. 2016;29(4):278–86. https://doi.org/10.1055/s-0036-1571432. Epub 2016 Feb 2. PMID: 26838970
17. Hsiao V, Sim J, Zimmerman A, Stephen A. Obesity may not be protective in abdominal stab wounds. J Emerg Trauma Shock. 2019;12(3):168–72. https://doi.org/10.4103/JETS.JETS_41_18. PMID: 31543637; PMCID: PMC6735204
18. Nash N, Kimbrough CW, Mackowski M, Benns MV, Smith JW, Harbrecht BG, Bozeman M. Is obesity protective in thoracoabdominal penetrating trauma? Am Surg. 2019;85(1):34–8. PMID: 30760342
19. Koba P. Identifying obstacles for the obese trauma patient. J Trauma Nurs. 2016;23(1):45–8.
20. Schaefer GP, Pender J, Toschlog EA, Waibel BH, Cohen KC. Endoscopically-assisted tube thoracostomy placement in a super-morbidly obese patient with penetrating thoracoabdominal trauma. Am Surg. 2011;77(1):119–20. PMID: 21396324
21. Palatini P, Benetti E, Fania C, Saladini F. Only troncoconical cuffs can provide accurate blood pressure measurements in people with severe obesity. J Hypertens. 2019;37(1):37–41. https://doi.org/10.1097/HJH.0000000000001823. PMID: 29927843
22. Arnold A, McNaughton A. Accuracy of non-invasive blood pressure measurements in obese patients. Br J Nurs. 2018;27(1):35–40. https://doi.org/10.12968/bjon.2018.27.1.35. PMID: 29323991
23. Leichtle S, Lucas JW, Kim WC, Aboutanos M. Decreasing accuracy of the eFAST examination-another challenge due to morbid obesity. Am Surg. 2019;85(8):923–6. PMID: 31560313
24. Hatchimonji JS, Kaufman EJ, Vasquez CR, Shashaty MGS, Martin ND, Holena DN. Obesity is associated with mortality and complications after trauma: a state-wide cohort study. J Surg Res. 2020;247:14–20. https://doi.org/10.1016/j.jss.2019.10.047. Epub 2019 Dec 4. PMID: 31810640
25. Byhahn C, Lischke V, Meininger D, Halbig S, Westphal K. Peri-operative complications during percutaneous tracheostomy in obese patients. Anaesthesia. 2005;60(1):12–5. https://doi.org/10.1111/j.1365-2044.2004.03707.x. PMID: 15601266
26. https://www.un.org/en/development/desa/population/publications/pdf/ageing/WorldPopulationAgeing2019-Highlights.pdf
27. https://www.cihi.ca/en/infographic-canadas-seniors-population-outlook-uncharted-territory
28. Joseph B, Orouji Jokar T, Hassan A, Azim A, Mohler MJ, Kulvatunyou N, Siddiqi S, Phelan H, Fain M, Rhee P. Redefining the association between old age and poor outcomes after trauma: the impact of frailty syndrome. J Trauma Acute Care Surg. 2017;82(3):575–81. https://doi.org/10.1097/TA.0000000000001329. PMID: 28225741

29. Joseph B, Pandit V, Zangbar B, Kulvatunyou N, Tang A, O'Keeffe T, Green DJ, Vercruysse G, Fain MJ, Friese RS, Rhee P. Validating trauma-specific frailty index for geriatric trauma patients: a prospective analysis. J Am Coll Surg. 2014;219(1):10–17.e1. https://doi.org/10.1016/j.jamcollsurg.2014.03.020. Erratum in: J Am Coll Surg. 2016; 222(3):336. Epub 2014 Mar 19. PMID: 24952434
30. Glabib N, Nouh T, Winocour S, Deckelbaum D, Banici L, Fata P, Razek T, Khwaja K. Severely injured geriatric population: morbidity, mortality, and risk factors. J Trauma. 2011;71(6):1908–14. https://doi.org/10.1097/TA.0b013e31820989ed. PMID: 21537212
31. Barbat A, Partiali B, Oska S, Folbe A. Head, face, and neck fractures secondary to ladder-related injuries treated in United States emergency departments in 2009–2018. J Emerg Med. 2020;59(2):186–92. https://doi.org/10.1016/j.jemermed.2020.04.022. Epub 2020 Jun 16. PMID: 32561108
32. Oyetunji TA, Ong'uti SK, Bolorunduro OB, Gonzalez DO, Cornwell EE, Haider AH. Epidemiologic trend in elderly domestic injury. J Surg Res. 2012;173(2):206–11. https://doi.org/10.1016/j.jss.2011.05.003. Epub 2011 May 31. PMID: 21704329
33. Palmer J, Pandit V, Zeeshan M, Kulvatunyou N, Hamidi M, Hanna K, Fain M, Nikolich-Zugich J, Zakaria ER, Joseph B. The acute inflammatory response after trauma is heightened by frailty: a prospective evaluation of inflammatory and endocrine system alterations in frailty. J Trauma Acute Care Surg. 2019;87(1):54–60. https://doi.org/10.1097/TA.0000000000002229. PMID: 30768559
34. Livingston DH, Lavery RF, Mosenthal AC, Knudson MM, Lee S, Morabito D, Manley GT, Nathens A, Jurkovich G, Hoyt DB, Coimbra R. Recovery at one year following isolated traumatic brain injury: a Western trauma association prospective multicenter trial. J Trauma. 2005;59(6):1298–304; discussion 1304. https://doi.org/10.1097/01.ta.0000196002.03681.18. PMID: 16394900
35. Fleischman RJ, Mullins RJ, McConnell KJ, Hedges JR, Ma OJ, Newgard CD. Is futile care in the injured elderly an important target for cost savings? J Trauma Acute Care Surg. 2012;73(1):146–51. https://doi.org/10.1097/TA.0b013e318251f9aa. PMID: 22743384; PMCID: PMC3510698
36. Calland JF, Ingraham AM, Martin N, Marshall GT, Schulman CI, Stapleton T, Barraco RD. Eastern Association for the Surgery of trauma. Evaluation and management of geriatric trauma: an eastern Association for the Surgery of trauma practice management guideline. J Trauma Acute Care Surg. 2012;73(5 Suppl 4):S345–50. https://doi.org/10.1097/TA.0b013e318270191f. PMID: 23114492
37. Bobeff EJ, Fortuniak J, Bryszewski B, Wiśniewski K, Bryl M, Kwiecień K, Stawiski K, Jaskólski DJ. Mortality after traumatic brain injury in elderly patients: a new scoring system. World Neurosurg. 2019;128:e129–47. https://doi.org/10.1016/j.wneu.2019.04.060. Epub 2019 Apr 11. PMID: 30981800
38. Pablos-Hernández C, González-Ramírez A, da Casa C, Luis MM, García-Iglesias MA, Julián-Enriquez JM, Rodríguez-Sánchez E, Blanco JF. Time to surgery reduction in hip fracture patients on an integrated orthogeriatric unit: a comparative study of three healthcare models. Orthop Surg. 2020;12(2):457–62. https://doi.org/10.1111/os.12633. Epub 2020 Mar 13. PMID: 32167674; PMCID: PMC7189046
39. Duran SF, Mazzurco L, Palmer RM. Trauma consults by geriatricians: looking into the black box. Gerontol Geriatr Med. 2018;4:2333721418817668. https://doi.org/10.1177/2333721418817668. PMID: 30560148; PMCID: PMC6291867
40. Kelley KM, Burgess J, Weireter L, Novosel TJ, Parks K, Aseuga M, Collins J. Early use of a chest trauma protocol in elderly patients with rib fractures improves pulmonary outcomes. Am Surg. 2019;85(3):288–91. PMID: 30947776
41. Otaka Y, Morita M, Mimura T, Uzawa M, Liu M. Establishment of an appropriate fall prevention program: a community-based study. Geriatr Gerontol Int. 2017;17(7):1081–9. https://doi.org/10.1111/ggi.12831. Epub 2016 Aug 5. PMID: 27492888
42. Dieleman JL, Baral R, Birger M, Bui AL, Bulchis A, Chapin A, Hamavid H, Horst C, Johnson EK, Joseph J, Lavado R, Lomsadze L, Reynolds A, Squires E, Campbell M, DeCenso B, Dicker D, Flaxman AD, Gabert R, Highfill T, Naghavi M, Nightingale N, Templin T, Tobias MI, Vos T, Murray CJ. US spending on personal health care and public health, 1996–2013. JAMA. 2016;316(24):2627–46. https://doi.org/10.1001/jama.2016.16885. PMID: 28027366; PMCID: PMC5551483
43. Falsgraf E, Inaba K, de Roulet A, Johnson M, Benjamin E, Lam L, Matsushima K, Strumwasser A, Demetriades D. Outcomes after traumatic injury in patients with preexisting psychiatric illness. J Trauma Acute Care Surg. 2017;83(5):882–7. https://doi.org/10.1097/TA.0000000000001588. PMID: 28538629
44. Townsend LL, Esquivel MM, Uribe-Leitz T, Weiser TG, Maggio PM, Spain DA, Tennakoon L, Staudenmayer K. The prevalence of psychiatric diagnoses and associated mortality in hospitalized US trauma patients. J Surg Res. 2017;213:171–6. https://doi.org/10.1016/j.jss.2017.02.014. Epub 2017 Feb 23. PMID: 28601311
45. Weinberg DS, Narayanan AS, Boden KA, Breslin MA, Vallier HA. Psychiatric illness is common among patients with orthopaedic polytrauma and is linked with poor outcomes. J Bone Joint Surg Am. 2016;98(5):341–8. https://doi.org/10.2106/JBJS.15.00751. PMID: 26935455
46. Mathews EM, Woodward CJ, Musso MW, Jones GN. Suicide attempts presenting to trauma centers: trends across age groups using the National Trauma Data Bank. Am J Emerg Med. 2016;34(8):1620–4. https://doi.org/10.1016/j.ajem.2016.06.014. Epub 2016 Jun 7. PMID: 27321943
47. Silander NC, Chesire DJ, Scott KS. Psychological prophylaxis: an integrated psychological services program in trauma care. J Clin Psychol Med Settings. 2019;26(3):291–301. https://doi.org/10.1007/s10880-018-9586-3. PMID: 30341469
48. Bakke E, Bogstrand ST, Normann PT, Ekeberg Ø, Bachs L. Influence of alcohol and other substances of abuse at the time of injury among patients in a Norwegian emergency department. BMC Emerg Med. 2016;16(1):20. https://doi.org/10.1186/s12873-016-0085-2. PMID: 27277762; PMCID: PMC4898304
49. Cheng V, Inaba K, Johnson M, Byerly S, Jiang Y, Matsushima K, Haltmeier T, Benjamin E, Lam L, Demetriades D. The impact of pre-injury controlled substance use on clinical outcomes after trauma. J Trauma Acute Care Surg. 2016;81(5):913–20. https://doi.org/10.1097/TA.0000000000001229. PMID: 27537515; PMCID: PMC5074856
50. Fazel S, Khosla V, Doll H, Geddes J. The prevalence of mental disorders among the homeless in western countries: systematic review and meta-regression analysis. PLoS Med. 2008;5(12):e225. https://doi.org/10.1371/journal.pmed.0050225. PMID: 19053169; PMCID: PMC2592351
51. Hwang SW, Burns T. Health interventions for people who are homeless. Lancet. 2014;384(9953):1541–7. https://doi.org/10.1016/S0140-6736(14)61133-8. PMID: 25390579
52. Shellito AD, Sareh S, Hart HC, Keeley JA, Tung C, Neville AL, Putnam B, Kim DY. Trauma patients returning to the emergency department after discharge. Am J Surg. 2020;220(6):1492–7. https://doi.org/10.1016/j.amjsurg.2020.08.021. Epub 2020 Aug 29. PMID: 32921401
53. Colacci M, Tseng EK, Sacks CA, Fralick M. Oral anticoagulant utilization in the United States and United Kingdom. J Gen Intern Med. 2020;35(8):2505–7. https://doi.org/10.1007/s11606-020-05904-0. Epub 2020 Jun 8. PMID: 32514896; PMCID: PMC7403268
54. Kobayashi L, Barmparas G, Bosarge P, Brown CV, Bukur M, Carrick MM, Catalano RD, Holly-Nicolas J, Inaba K, Kaminski S, Klein AL, Kopelman T, Ley EJ, Martinez EM, Moore FO, Murry J, Nirula R, Paul D, Quick J, Rivera O, Schreiber M, Coimbra R. AAST multicenter prospective observational study of trauma patients on novel oral anticoagulants study group. Novel oral

anticoagulants and trauma: the results of a prospective American Association for the Surgery of Trauma Multi-Institutional Trial. J Trauma Acute Care Surg. 2017;82(5):827–35. https://doi.org/10.1097/TA.0000000000001414. PMID: 28431413

55. Lee ZX, Lim XT, Ang E, Hajibandeh S, Hajibandeh S. The effect of preinjury anticoagulation on mortality in trauma patients: a systematic review and meta-analysis. Injury. 2020;51(8):1705–13. https://doi.org/10.1016/j.injury.2020.06.010. Epub 2020 Jun 15. PMID: 32576378

56. Blackmore AR, Caputo LM, Bourg PW, Mains CW. Developing, implementing, and evaluating a nurse-driven rapid reversal protocol for patients with traumatic intracerebral hemorrhage in the presence of preinjury warfarin. J Trauma Nurs. 2016;23(3):138–43. https://doi.org/10.1097/JTN.0000000000000201. PMID: 27163221

Advanced Neuromonitoring for Moderate and Severe Traumatic Brain Injury

43

Carleen Batson, Logan Froese, Alwyn Gomez, Amanjyot Singh Sainbhi, and Frederick A. Zeiler

Introduction

Traumatic brain injury (TBI) is defined as damage to the brain's normal functioning caused by some form of external force, e.g., a blow to the head. The main causes of TBI are motor vehicle accidents (MVAs), falls, and assaults [1–3]. Globally, trauma-related disorders are the foremost cause of disability and second leading cause of death. Approximately sixty-nine million people around the world suffer a TBI each year, with the majority being mild (81%) and moderate (11%) in severity [4]. TBI costs 400 billion dollars (USD) annually worldwide, with mortality rates as high as 30–40% in the severe TBI cohorts [5]. Africa and Southeast Asia have the highest percentage of the annual global TBIs (both 56%) as a result of MVAs, while North America has the lowest (25%) [4]. However, the incidence of TBI per 100,000 people is greatest in North America (1299 cases, 95% CI 650–1947) and Europe (1012 cases, 95% CI 911–1113) and least in Africa (801 cases, 95% CI 732–871) and the Eastern Mediterranean (897 cases, 95% CI 771–1023) [4]. Numbers from low- and middle-income countries like Africa and the Eastern Mediterranean are estimates only due to poor reporting and poor-quality data [4].

Evaluating the demographic features of those suffering from TBI, we see a bimodal distribution of mainly the young and elderly, with the young cohort contributing to the major financial burden associated with TBI globally [1, 3]. TBI occurs on a spectrum of severity. Injury can be as mild as a concussion, or severe requiring intensive care unit (ICU) admission and management, which has a mortality of 30–40% [1, 6, 7].

The vast majority of globally reported cases of TBI are of mild severity. However, those with moderate and severe TBI, typically carry the highest degree of morbidity and mortality in TBI, leading to significant social and economic burden [1].

For the moderate and severe TBI populations, injury occurs in two main phases. First is the primary injury, defined as the structural damage to the brain occurring at the time of impact [6]. This type of injury is not modifiable by the treating clinical team and is the target of public awareness campaigns designed to reduce risky behaviors associated with TBI. This primary injury is followed by the secondary brain injury cascade. Secondary brain injury refers to the physiologic, metabolic, cellular, and molecular changes that occur during the acute phase after TBI, which lead to ongoing neural injury and cell death [6, 8]. This secondary brain injury includes, but is not limited to, impaired extracellular fluid homeostasis leading to elevated intracranial pressure, disrupted cerebral autoregulation, activation of pro-inflammatory cascades, generation of reactive oxygen species, shift to anaerobic metabolism and mitochondrial

C. Batson
Department of Anatomy and Cell Science, Rady Faculty of Health Sciences, University of Manitoba, Winnipeg, MB, Canada

L. Froese · A. S. Sainbhi
Department of Biomedical Engineering, Faculty of Engineering, University of Manitoba, Winnipeg, MB, Canada

A. Gomez
Department of Anatomy and Cell Science, Rady Faculty of Health Sciences, University of Manitoba, Winnipeg, MB, Canada

Department of Surgery, Section of Neurosurgery, Rady Faculty of Health Sciences, University of Manitoba, Winnipeg, MB, Canada
e-mail: gomeza35@myumanitoba.ca

F. A. Zeiler (✉)
Department of Anatomy and Cell Science, Rady Faculty of Health Sciences, University of Manitoba, Winnipeg, MB, Canada

Department of Biomedical Engineering, Faculty of Engineering, University of Manitoba, Winnipeg, MB, Canada

Department of Surgery, Section of Neurosurgery, Rady Faculty of Health Sciences, University of Manitoba, Winnipeg, MB, Canada

Centre on Aging, University of Manitoba, Winnipeg, MB, Canada

Department of Medicine, Division of Anaesthesia, Addenbrooke's Hospital, University of Cambridge, Cambridge, UK
e-mail: Frederick.zeiler@umantioba.ca

L. Marshall Gillman, S. Widder (eds.), *Trauma Team Dynamics*, https://doi.org/10.1007/978-3-031-86312-7_43

failure, and activation of cell death pathways [8–10]. Without intervention, secondary brain injury leads to substantial loss of neurological tissue and potentiates the morbidity and mortality seen in moderate and severe TBI [8–10].

Early and rapid intervention is critical to mitigate secondary brain injury. To facilitate rapid and pointed intervention directed at these secondary brain injury mechanisms, we have seen the development of guideline-based therapeutic approaches, such as those supported by the Brain Trauma Foundation (BTF) [11, 12]. Therapeutic intervention is further supported by continuous multi-modal assessments of various aspects of cerebral physiology at the bedside. Such advanced monitoring allows for early rapid detection of secondary brain insult, with continuous feedback regarding the therapeutic efficacy of interventions [11, 12]. This monitoring has advanced TBI care in recent years from guideline physiologic therapies to personalized medicine approaches in the intensive care unit (ICU) [3, 13, 14].

Acute-Phase Stabilization in Moderate/Severe TBI Care

Advanced Trauma Life Support (ATLS)—The Basics

Despite the presence of advanced monitoring techniques and interventions for moderate/severe TBI, the principles of acute-phase stabilization of the trauma patient still apply and take precedence at the beginning of care implementation. Advanced trauma life support (ATLS), common knowledge to most trauma care providers, comprises a set of guidelines via a primary and secondary survey in order to assess and manage patients who have suffered a traumatic injury [6, 15]. The basic premise of the primary survey is the ABCDE (Airway, Breathing, Circulation, Disability and Exposure/Environmental Control) of ATLS [15]. Routinely, most trauma patients have their vitals taken and are placed on a cardiac monitor, blood pressure monitor, and pulse oximeter in order to gather baseline information for management [15]. With sequentially addressing airway, breathing, and circulation during the primary survey, major contributors to secondary brain injury in the TBI patient, hypotension and hypoxia, are addressed. An additional and very important aspect of management in the field before arriving to the hospital is to ensure adequate immobilization of the head and neck in order to maintain cervical-spine alignment and to decrease the chance of any spinal cord injury secondary to any vertebral instability [6, 15]. This immobilization must be maintained throughout management where vertebral motion may arise, e.g., logrolls [15].

The disability section of the primary survey deals with the neurological status of a trauma patient [15]. Neurological status is assessed using various parameters like the Glasgow Coma Scale (GCS), pupillary status, blood glucose levels, and toxic substances levels [6, 15]. Neurological injuries are usually associated with decreased sensation, syncope, motor deficits, headache, aphasia, vital sign derangement, etc. Spinal cord injury can cause derangement in cardiovascular status, be refractory to fluid resuscitation, and can cause neurogenic shock [6, 8, 15]. Some patients may or may not require a CT scan of the head. The Canadian CT Head Injury/Trauma Rule assesses head injury status without imaging and identifies patients who do not require neurosurgical intervention. CT scan of the head and neck is warranted in a patient with neurological deficits providing they are stable enough to undergo this study. Based on the severity of trauma and findings, a patient may require transfer to a higher-level trauma center for more specialist care if the current facility is not able to provide the same [6, 15].

Advanced TBI Guideline-Based Care

Brain Trauma Foundation (BTF) guidelines are widely used in practice and aid in reduced mortality from moderate and severe traumatic brain injury (sTBI) [16]. It states that "in general a TBI patient with a poor neurological exam, abnormal CT of the brain and risk factors for secondary injury should be monitored" [17]. Invasive intracranial pressure (ICP) monitoring is done for TBI patients within the ICU; prolonged elevations are associated with poor patient outcomes [17]. The threshold for ICP treatment is 22 mmHg, with sustained periods of time spent above this threshold associated with poor global outcomes [17]. More recently, the Seattle International Severe Traumatic Brain Injury Consensus Conference (SIBICC) guidelines comprise tier zero to tier three management algorithms for sTBI [16]. Tier zero comprises basic care for an sTBI patient admitted to the ICU with an ICP monitor in place [16]. The aim is to stabilize the patient neurologically, e.g., manage intracranial hypertension, as the minimal cerebral perfusion pressure (CPP) threshold is 60 mmHg and the initial ICP threshold is 22 mmHg [16]. Tier 1–3 steps up management based on the severity of the situation [16]. We refer the interested reader to the BTF and SIBICC guidelines for more details surrounding the tiered management approaches for secondary brain injury mitigation [12, 16–18].

Acute Neuromonitoring Techniques in Moderate/Severe TBI

ICP and CPP—Invasive Monitoring and the Basics

The cornerstone of acute monitoring in moderate/severe TBI is ICP and CPP, as previously mentioned. ICP is the pressure exerted by the contents of an intact calvarium, i.e., brain tissue volume, blood, CSF, and any space-occupying lesion. ICP can be monitored invasively and noninvasively, with invasive techniques and external ventricular drains (EVDs) considered the "gold standard." The zero reference point for ICP is considered the foramen of Monro. The origins of ICP monitoring trace back to times when CT and MRI were unavailable. It aided with the detection of hematomas in postoperative patients, and the potential need for intervention could be signaled by increased values in postop recovery [17, 19]. Since then, ICP monitoring has been adopted for continuous bedside assessment in TBI care within the ICU, with the majority of current guideline targets and therapies based on ICP values, or derived measures such as CPP. BTF guidelines recommend ICP monitoring of patients admitted to the ICU with TBI and state that an ICP of ≥22 mmHg requires management [16, 17], as extensive literature documented the association between time spent above this ICP value and poor outcome at 6-months post-injury [17, 20].

Invasive methods for ICP monitoring include parenchymal devices (strain gauge monitors and fiber-optic-based pressure sensors) which can in theory be inserted anyplace in the cranial cavity (typically right frontal lobe), and external ventricular drains (EVD) inserted in the ventricular system, all used to assess liquid or tissue pressure within the cranium [17, 21]. Such techniques are considered the standard for ICP monitoring in TBI care. Table 43.1 provides an outline for each invasive and noninvasive monitoring technique, with advantages and disadvantages.

Aside from targeting ICP thresholds, we are also interested in maintaining cerebral blood flow (CBF) in TBI. Currently, we lack effective continuous bedside methods for objective CBF measurement. As such, we rely on potential surrogate metrics for CBF, with one such measure being CPP. CPP is thought to be the pressure within the brain that maintains CBF. In its simplistic form, CPP is defined as the difference between mean arterial pressure (MAP) and ICP. It is believed that low CPP causes low CBF which can cause harmful effects (ischemia and/or infarction) of the brain parenchyma as less oxygen and nutrients will reach the tissues [17]. Similarly, persistently high CPP is believed to be associated with cerebral hyperemia, break down of the blood-brain barrier, and potentially intracerebral hemorrhage. The gold standard for CPP measurement requires both invasive arterial blood pressure (ABP) and ICP measures [17, 20]. BTF guidelines recommend that CPP should be maintained between 60 mmHg and 70 mmHg, but some research works suggest a threshold of 70 mmHg and report unfavorable outcomes noted in patients with values below this number over time [17, 22]. Some controversy exists surrounding maintaining CPP above 70 mmHg, as historically the literature has linked this to unfavorable outcomes as a result of increased precapillary arteriolar pressure, capillary bed filtration pressures, cerebral edema, and even acute respiratory distress syndrome (ARDS) [17, 23]. However, recent literature suggests with advances in general cardiopulmonary care in the ICU, systemic complications of elevated CPP targets may not remain a substantial concern [23].

Noninvasive ICP/CPP Determination Methods

However, recent advances in transcranial ultrasonic techniques have led to the development of noninvasive methods including optic nerve sheath diameter (ONSD) ultrasound and transcranial Doppler (TCD) ICP estimations. First, for ONSD, it is thought that the subarachnoid space enclosing the optic nerve is continuous with the intracranial subarachnoid space, with pressure changes in the cranium causing similar changes in the optic nerve diameter due to stretching of the dural-based sheath [17]. The measured diameter is believed to approximate ICP [17]. Most studies have not clearly outlined what normal readings are, they suggest a cutoff of approximately 5 mm or less with readings exceeding that considered pathologic [17].

TCD was developed as a method of interrogating CBF through the basal cerebral arteries noninvasively [24]. By measuring cerebral blood flow velocity (CBFV) through these vessels, using the Doppler effect, CBF can be inferred so long as vessel caliber remains relatively constant. Shortly after its development, invasive studies in a non-TBI population found relatively good concordance with invasive CPP and those estimated by TCD [25]. This led to interest in developing TCD-based estimates of ICP and CPP in TBI patients [26–30]. Ultimately their conclusions were all similar. TCD was somewhat effective at identifying episodes of low CPP and high ICP but, regardless of the methodology used, estimates of ICP and CPP had too large a margin of error to effectively eliminate the need for invasive monitoring [29, 30]. TCD then, like ONSD, may have a place in guiding the management of TBI patients prior to the availability of invasive monitoring, such as in the pre-hospital setting [31].

Table 43.1 Summary of invasive and noninvasive ICP monitoring techniques

ICP monitoring techniques	Summary
Invasive	
Strain gauge	Location: Parenchyma, CSF compartments, or subdural space [17] Functioning: ICP changes cause sensors to bend. Helps approximate ICP Advantages: Easily inserted and easily manipulated Disadvantages: Risk of hemorrhage and infection, significant zero drift, and cannot re-zero once inserted [17]
Fiber optic	Location: Parenchyma Function: "Light is continuously transmitted through fiber optics to the probe tip. ICP changes lead to the deflection of a mirror in the tip, leading to varying light intensity reflected" [17]. Helps approximate ICP Advantages: Easily inserted compared to an EVD Disadvantages: Risk of hemorrhage and infection, significant zero drift and cannot re-zero once inserted [17]. Also, can be easily damaged by twisting/knotting
External ventricular drain (EVD)	Location: Ventricular CSF compartment Function: Manometer assesses fluid pressure. The foramen of Monro is considered the zero point [17] Advantages: "Gold standard" for ICP monitoring, can be re-zeroed at any time, used for CSF sampling, and can be used therapeutically Disadvantages: Insertion can be challenging and there is risk of infection and hemorrhage
Noninvasive	
Optic nerve sheath diameter (ONSD) ultrasound	Location: External Function: Optic nerve is covered with dura mater and therefore changes in ICP can be assessed via this method as it can cause stretching in optic nerve sheath. A cutoff of approximately 5 mm or less is considered normal ONSD; higher values are deemed abnormal Advantages: Noninvasive Disadvantages: Baseline normal non-pathologic ONSD varies from person to person, operator dependent, and may require invasive ICP monitoring [17]
TCD-based methods	Location: External Function: Mainly used to assess MCA flow velocity, and (in theory) can estimate ICP and CPP Advantages: Noninvasive Disadvantages: Lesions can interfere with recording, probe has to be repositioned every so often, and there is interoperator variability and low accuracy

CPP cerebral perfusion pressure, *CSF* cerebrospinal fluid, *EVD* external ventricular drain, *ICP* intracranial pressure, *MCA* middle cerebral artery, *ONSD* optic nerve sheath diameter, *TCD* transcranial Doppler

Advanced Invasive Techniques for Early Multi-modal Monitoring of Cerebral Physiology

In the following subsections, we will briefly overview common advanced invasive cerebral physiologic monitoring devices employed in TBI care within the acute phase. Such devices overviewed include brain tissue oxygen monitoring ($PbtO_2$), thermal diffusion CBF monitoring, and extracellular fluid chemistry through cerebral microdialysis. As these sub-sections only briefly introduce the techniques, we refer the interested reader to the referenced literature for more information if desired. Table 43.2 highlights the main points on these invasive techniques.

Brain Tissue Oxygen Monitoring ($PbtO_2$)

Parenchymal brain tissue oxygen ($PbtO_2$) was introduced as a means to potentially provide information regarding end-organ oxygen delivery in the brain. It is assessed by inserting an invasive parenchymal $PbtO_2$ probe, which analyzes the extracellular partial pressure of oxygen using a Clark electrode [17, 32]. This device provides continuous bedside extracellular oxygen values, updated every minute [32]. Normal threshold for intervention in TBI is considered 20 mmHg [17]. Recent literature supports a strong association between time spent below $PbtO_2$ of 20 mmHg and poor outcome at 6-month post-TBI [32]. Similarly, high $PbtO_2$ has been associated with poor outcomes in patients where mitochondrial failure is suspected, through cerebral microdialysis analysis, where high $PbtO_2$ with corresponding elevations in extracellular lactate:pyruvate ratios suggests failure of oxidative metabolism [17, 33]. This strong association with outcome in TBI has triggered phase II randomized control trial assessments of ICP versus ICP + $PbtO_2$-directed therapies in moderate/severe TBI patients [18, 32]. Such work has demonstrated the feasibility of implementing such combined therapeutic approaches and provides early support for ICP and $PbtO_2$ therapies leading to superior long-term outcomes over standard ICP-directed therapy alone [18, 32]. As such,

Table 43.2 Summary of invasive/noninvasive monitoring technique and role in TBI

Early multi-modal monitoring technique/ device	Summary	Role in TBI
Invasive techniques		
Brain tissue oxygen monitoring (Licox)	Assesses the extracellular partial pressure of oxygen within the brain parenchyma [39]. Normal threshold is 20 mmHg, values above or below 20 mmHg are linked to poor outcomes [17]	Monitors parenchymal partial pressure of oxygen
Continuous CBF monitoring (Hemedex/thermal diffusion probes)	Assesses power required to maintain a temperature difference between a proximal and distal TDF probe which is synonymous with CBF [58]. Levels thought to be normal are between 20–40 mL/100 g/min and 70–100 mL/100 g/min, values constantly below 20 mL/100 g/min and above 80–100 mL/100 g/min have been linked to poor outcome	Monitors CBF
Brain chemistry monitoring (cerebral microdialysis)	Assesses the following metabolites in the extracellular space: Glucose, lactate, pyruvate, glutamate, glycerol, sodium, and potassium [40]. Decreased levels of brain glucose and increased lactate:Pyruvate ratio have been linked to poor patient outcomes [40]	Monitors extracellular metabolites
Non-invasive techniques		
Transcranial Doppler (TCD)	Assesses the blood flow velocity through the cerebral vessels, with the MCA being the most commonly insonated vessel in TBI	Monitors MCA blood flow In theory can approximate ICP and CPP
Near-infrared spectroscopy (NIRS)	Involves the use of light between wavelengths of 700 and 1000 nm to monitor oxygenated hemoglobin, deoxygenated hemoglobin, and other derived regional brain oxygenation parameters [41]	Monitors frontal cerebral oxygen hemoglobin concentration Surrogate CBV marker
Electroencephalogram (EEG)	Assesses the electrical activity of the brain in TBI patients to detect secondary brain injury	Monitors brain electrical activity Auxiliary measure to assess brain death

CBF cerebral blood flow, *CBV* cerebral blood volume, *CPP* cerebral perfusion pressure, *EEG* electroencephalogram, ICP intracranial pressure, *MCA* middle cerebral artery, *mmHg* millimeters of Mercury, *NIRS* near-infrared spectroscopy, *nm* nanometers, *TBI* traumatic brain injury, *TDF* thermal diffusion flowmetry

phase III trials on ICP + $PbtO_2$-directed therapy are ongoing. Of note, SIBICC has also developed a management algorithm for patients with ICP and brain oxygen monitoring in situ. It comprises four types (A to D) where type A involves normal monitored values and types B to D involve abnormal values and their management [18].

Thermal Diffusion Cerebral Blood Flow Monitoring

In an attempt to avoid proxy measures of CBF, thermal diffusion flowmetry (TDF) probes have been developed to facilitate continuous bedside assessments of CBF. Such monitoring provides absolute measurements with a high temporal resolution, which can aid in the detection and prevention of secondary injury [34]. By this method, evidence suggests that continual high or low measures are linked to poor outcomes [34]. Commonly used TDF probes (Bowman Perfusion Monitor and Saber) function by evaluating the power needed to sustain a temperature difference between thermistors, which correlates to brain tissue blood flow [34, 35]. Probe placement can be on the cortical surface of interest (Saber) or placed in the brain tissue (Bowman Perfusion Monitor), typically the right frontal lobe concurrent with ICP monitor placement [34].

Although this method has been used for years in experimental models, and there is potential for it to be included in a multimodal monitoring regimen, there is no threshold agreed upon for this technique or an understanding of how to utilize this device for monitoring TBI patients [36]. Further, the consensus summary by the International Multidisciplinary Consensus Conference on Multimodality Monitoring provides little additional guidance regarding this matter [36]. Furthermore, some of the commercially available TDF probes are thought to assess blood flow "continuously," but in fact they require regular recalibration periods every 30 min to 2 h which takes about 2–5 min to complete and interrupts the recordings. CBF ranges considered normal by the TDF method range from 20–40 mL/100 g/min (lower threshold) to 70–100 mL/100 g/min (upper threshold), depending on if the TDF measurement was cortical or parenchymal [34, 37].

In theory, increasing CBF could be achieved by expanding plasma volume, inotropic support, and osmotic agents and lowering CBF achieved by hyperventilation and barbiturate coma [37]. Based on several small studies in adult TBI cohorts, it was noted that CBF continuously below 20 mL/100 g/min and above 80–100 mL/100 g/min (hyperemia) was linked to poor outcomes. Some probe-related complications that arose in some studies were CSF leak around the probe, meningitis, intracerebral abscess, and superficial soft tissue infection [37, 38]. Of note, the literature supports a positive correlation between changes in regional cerebral blood flow (rCBF) and $PbtO_2$, which is consistent with Xenon CT (Xe-CT) findings showing a positive correlation between brain tissue oxygen and regional blood flow [39]. Despite these promising findings, widespread adoption of this monitoring modality remains limited to leading academic neurotrauma centers globally.

Extracellular Brain Chemistry—Cerebral Microdialysis

Cerebral microdialysis done at the bedside serves as a means of invasively monitoring metabolites in the extracellular space via a semi-permeable intraparenchymal catheter which aids in avoiding metabolic derangements in TBI patients [40, 41]. Extracellular dialysate fluid is captured in microvials and processed typically by hour at the bedside for a panel of common analytes. This technique has mainly been described within the TBI population, and the information gained can be useful in guiding clinical therapy [10]. Main analytes processed at the bedside include glucose, lactate, pyruvate, glutamate, and glycerol. Decreased levels of brain glucose and increased lactate:pyruvate ratio can provide information on aerobic/anaerobic metabolism and oxidative mitochondrial function, with derangements in adult TBI patients linked to poor patient outcomes [10, 40, 42–44]. Glutamate, an excitatory neurotransmitter, provides information regarding potential excitotoxicity post-injury [9], whereas glycerol provides information regarding the degree of neural injury [10]. Given the cost and complexity of interpretation, cerebral microdialysis is another monitored modality in TBI relegated to leading academic neurotrauma units. However, with improvements in microfluidic chips, self-contained bedside microanalyzers are on the horizon, set to improve accessibility and cost associated with the technique.

Advanced Noninvasive Techniques for Early Multi-modal Monitoring of Cerebral Physiology

In the following subsections, we will briefly overview common advanced noninvasive cerebral physiologic monitoring devices employed in TBI care within the acute phase. Three such devices will be highlighted: TCD, near-infrared spectroscopy (NIRS), and continuous electroencephalogram (cEEG). As these subsections only briefly introduce the techniques, we refer the interested reader to the referenced literature for more information if desired. Table 43.2 provides highlights on these noninvasive techniques. Figure 43.1 provides an example of multi-modal cerebral physiologic monitoring using both invasive and noninvasive methods simultaneously.

Transcranial Doppler

As mentioned previously, TCD is a method of noninvasively measuring CBFV in the basal cerebral arteries [24]. In recent years, its adoption into neurointensive care units (NICU) has increased dramatically with one recent European study find-

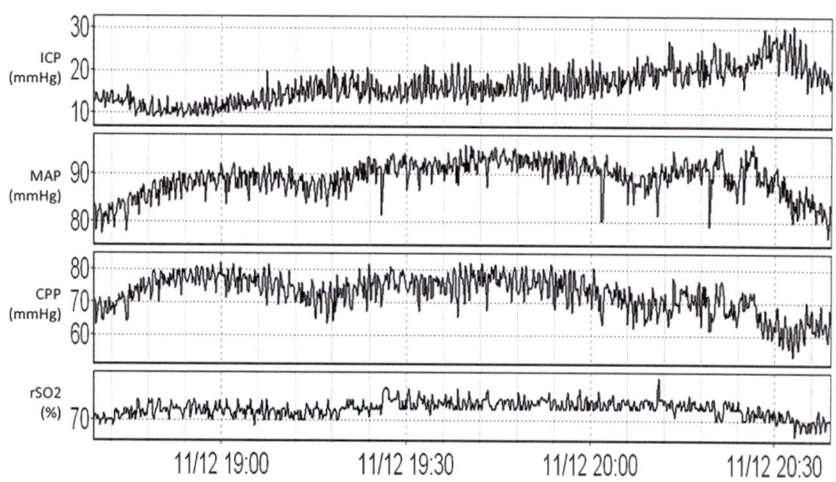

Fig. 43.1 Example of high-frequency multi-modal cerebral physiologic monitoring. *CPP* cerebral perfusion pressure, *ICP* intracranial pressure, *MAP* mean arterial pressure, *mmHg* millimeters of Mercury, rSO_2 regional cerebral oxygen saturations (Right Frontal Lobe), % percentage

ing it to be the second most common form of bedside intracranial monitoring behind only ICP monitoring [45]. Direct parameters measured by TCD include CBFV and the pulsatility index (PI) and have been found to be associated with global outcomes following TBI [46–50]. There has also been evidence linking episodes of reduced CBFV as measured with TCD and reduced $PbtO_2$ as measured by invasive monitors [51]. TCD has also been used as a robust method of identifying post-traumatic vasospasm at the bedside, which has independently been linked to poor outcomes [52]. Ultimately, TCD is limited by its need for expertise in order to both acquire consistent signals and interpret the data obtained.

Near-Infrared Spectroscopy

Near-infrared spectroscopy (NIRS) is a noninvasive technique utilized to monitor frontal cerebral oxygen hemoglobin concentration in TBI patients as a way of identifying brain tissue at risk for potential secondary injury [41]. It is used as a marker for pulsatile cerebral blood volume (CBV) [21]. Near-infrared (NIR) involves the use of wavelengths between 700 and 1000 nm on the electromagnetic spectrum, a range that allows signal penetration through tissues [41]. In neurocritical care, these spectrometers are usually used to measure the concentration of oxygenated hemoglobin (HbO) and deoxygenated hemoglobin (HHb) within the target tissue, to gain information on blood and oxygen supply [53]. Simpler NIRS equipment utilizes constant wave technology while newer versions utilize multi-distance techniques. They assess cerebral oxygenation status and newer versions are able to refine hemoglobin signals by removing interferences and thus purer results like total oxygen index (TOI) and total hemoglobin index (THI) are gained [53]. As opposed to other noninvasive neuromonitoring techniques, e.g., TCD-based methods, NIRS is not significantly impacted by interoperator variability [54] and can provide continuous multi-channel (typically bifrontal) assessments of regional cerebral oxygen saturations and oxy−/deoxyhemoglobin concentrations in the TBI patient. NIRS use in the TBI population can be challenged by signal issues related to injured extracranial tissue and intracranial lesions, but there has been improvement in the signal-to-noise ratio with newer multi-distance methods [41]. This technology is reasonably expensive but can provide long durations of uninterrupted intracranial oxygenated/deoxygenated cerebral blood flow volume (CBFV) surrogate measures, which can be used in concert with noninvasive arterial blood pressure (nABP) devices like the Finapres [21], to derive entirely noninvasive metrics of cerebrovascular reactivity (CVR). However, it must be acknowledged that arterial, venous, and capillary blood are assessed by NIRS in a portion of the cortex (typically frontal lobes), and recordings are affected by the degree of oxygen extraction [21].

Adult TBI literature for NIRS-based regional oxygen saturation supports an association between low regional saturations in the frontal lobes and poor functional outcomes after TBI [55]. Similarly, preliminary work with NIRS-based CVR metrics supports an association between impaired NIRS-derived CVR and poor outcomes in moderate/severe TBI [53]. Similarly, in theory, the device could be used for long-term follow-up, providing information on persistent cerebral physiologic dysfunction and long-term functional outcomes in TBI. Upcoming multi-center prospective trials on NIRS application in moderate/severe TBI are planned. It is expected that NIRS monitoring will become more standard in TBI bedside monitoring in the near future.

Continuous Electroencephalography (cEEG)

Continuous electroencephalography (cEEG) is a noninvasive means of monitoring the brain's electrical activity via superficial scalp electrodes. However, it must be acknowledged that the practice of placing the electrodes internally exists, where subdural paddles or parenchymal depth monitors can be inserted. Such invasive cEEG methods will not be discussed here, as they are primarily utilized for epilepsy monitoring and surgical intervention, not for TBI care [17]. Two types of cEEG existing for use with TBI patients in the neurointensive care unit (NICU) are the standard multi-channel and focal reduced channel [17]. In cases where regular epileptic specialists are unable to interpret the results, there are automatic signal detection algorithms accessible [56]. cEEG has been used in seizure detection, prognostication post-TBI, detection of ischemia, detection of spreading cortical depolarizations, and vasospasm post-aneurysmal subarachnoid hemorrhage [17]. Seizures after TBI are common, and early detection and treatment can prevent secondary brain injury [6]. This method has been used as an auxiliary test to assess brain death as it provides a comprehensive analysis of regional and global electrical activity [17, 57].

Derived Metrics for Continuous Physiologic Assessment

Aside from the raw physiologic measures provided by the above-mentioned core and advanced monitoring devices, much more can be obtained from the signal information provided. Advances in bedside data acquisition platforms and real-time signal processing have allowed us to derive additional, continuously updating, cerebral physiologic metrics in moderate/severe TBI care. In the subsections below, we will outline some of the main derived metrics that have demonstrated a strong association with outcomes in TBI, including cerebrovascular reactivity monitoring and cerebral compensatory reserve measures.

Cerebrovascular Reactivity Monitoring

Aside from derangements in ICP and CPP, recent work in bedside signal processing has afforded treating clinicians the ability to continuously measure aspects of cerebral autoregulation. Cerebral autoregulation is defined as the innate ability of the cerebral vessels to maintain constant CBF over a wide range of MAP or CPP, ensuring a steady state of oxygen and nutrient delivery to the brain [59]. In the injured state, cerebral autoregulation is known to be disrupted, leading to impaired or even absent autoregulation of CBF altogether.

By evaluating the relationship between slow-wave fluctuations in ICP (a surrogate for pulsatile CBV) and MAP (a driver for blood flow), one can provide some information regarding cerebrovascular responsiveness or reactivity [60]. This concept has led to the derivation of the pressure reactivity index (PRx) from the Pearson correlation between slow-wave vasogenic fluctuations in ICP and MAP [61]. This index is then updated every minute, providing real-time information regarding cerebrovascular reactivity, and potentially cerebral autoregulation. PRx has received validation as a measure of the autoregulatory curve in experimental animal models of intracranial hypertension and systemic arterial hypotension [62–64]. In its most simplistic interpretation, positive values of PRx indicate impaired autoregulation, while negative values denote intact autoregulation [65].

In the adult TBI literature, there exists numerous retrospective and prospective studies linking derangements in PRx and increased mortality and morbidity post-TBI [61, 65–68]. Thresholds for morbidity and mortality have been defined in multiple TBI populations [65, 67]. In addition, recent literature supports an association between impaired cerebrovascular reactivity and computed tomography (CT)-based contusion progression in the acute phase after TBI [69]. Further, evaluating the burden of physiologic derangements in TBI, recent work suggests that in the era of current guideline-based therapeutics, the majority of the acute phase physiology in moderate/severe TBI is dominated by impaired autoregulation, and not ICP, CPP, or $PbtO_2$ issues [70, 71]. These findings suggest that cerebrovascular reactivity monitoring may play a crucial future role in the monitoring and therapeutic intervention of the TBI patient.

Cerebral Compensatory Reserve

ICP alone provides only a small amount of information regarding the intracranial pressure dynamics after TBI. In an attempt to improve our ability to estimate how "tight" or "relaxed" the brain might be after injury, cerebral compensatory reserve metrics have been developed. By assessing the correlation between slow-wave vasogenic fluctuations in ICP and pulse amplitude of ICP (derived through Fourier decomposition of the ICP waveform), one in theory can produce an index of compliance or compensatory reserve [72]. The RAP (R—correlation, A—pulse amplitude of ICP, P—intracranial pressure) is derived through the moving Pearson correlation between slow-waves of ICP and pulse amplitude of ICP, updated every minute [19, 72–74]. This RAP measure varies from −1 to +1 and provides a continuous bedside assessment of cerebral compensatory reserve.

Though its use is not widespread, preliminary work supports its association with patient outcomes in TBI, with impaired compensatory reserve associated with increased mortality [19, 72, 74]. Similarly, impaired RAP values have been linked to diffuse intracranial injury patterns present on admission CT scans of the brain [72]. However, despite from initial promising results, much further work is required on RAP, with studies validating it as a true measure of compliance on the horizon (Fig. 43.2).

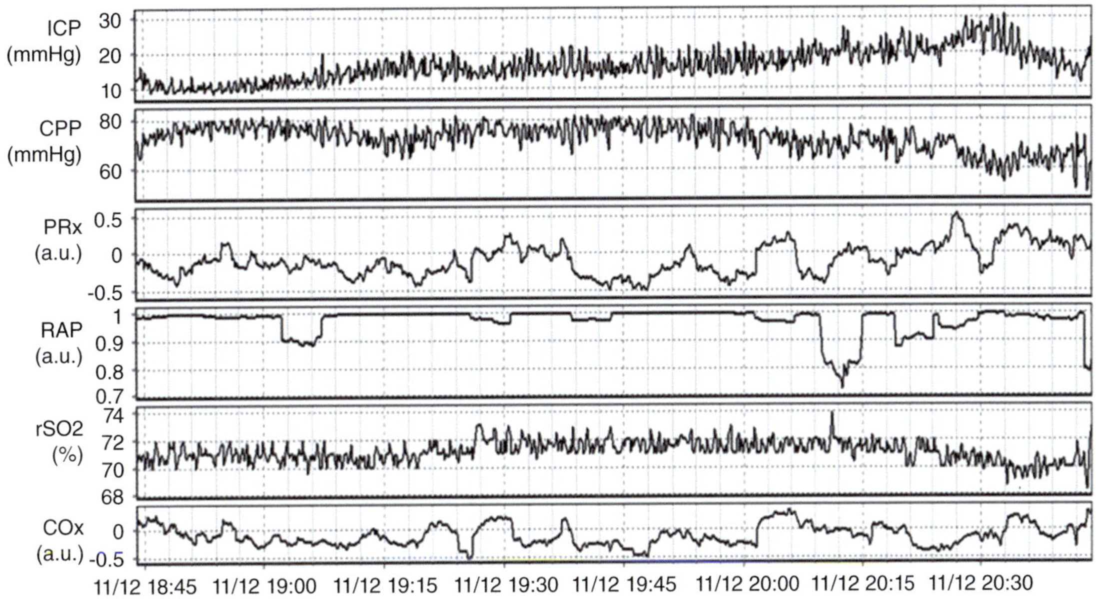

Fig. 43.2 Example of high-frequency multi-modal cerebral physiologic monitoring with advanced derived metrics—cerebrovascular reactivity and cerebral compensatory reserve. *a.u.* arbitrary units, *COx* cerebrovascular reactivity index using rSO_2 (correlation between slow-waves of rSO_2 and CPP), *CPP* cerebral perfusion pressure, *ICP* intracranial pressure, *MAP* mean arterial pressure, *mmHg* millimeters of Mercury, *PRx* pressure reactivity index (correlation between slow-wave vasogenic fluctuations in ICP and MAP), *RAP* cerebral compensatory reserve index (correlation (R) between slow-wave of pulse amplitude of ICP (A) and ICP (P)) rSO_2 regional cerebral oxygen saturations (Right Frontal Lobe), *%* percentage

Future Directions of Early Monitoring in Severe TBI

As outlined in the sections above, it is clear that there has been a massive expansion of advanced acute-phase monitoring for TBI patients. This has ushered in the era of multimodal monitoring (MMM) for the moderate/severe TBI patient, where numerous different/complimentary aspects of cerebral physiology are monitored and captured in real time at the bedside. This wealth of information has led to MMM consensus statements from major international critical care bodies and is slowly shifting the focus of acute TBI care from guideline-based approaches to individual personalized physiologic targets based on MMM information. In this final section, we will outline some of the main personalized physiologic approaches emerging in acute TBI care.

Optimal CPP (CPPopt) and Personalized CPP Targets

Recent multimodal monitoring (MMM) consensus statements have supported assessing cerebrovascular reactivity in severely ill TBI patients [75]. Given the strong association between cerebrovascular reactivity metrics, such as PRx, and patient outcome [61, 65–68, 76], there has been extensive exploration into how these metrics can be exploited to improve patient care and outcomes. Unfortunately, at this time, we do not have directed therapeutics at cerebrovascular reactivity, with recent multi-center data suggesting that current guideline-based treatments do not impact recorded PRx values [77, 78].

However, exploration of the relationship between PRx and CPP has demonstrated a reproducible parabolic relationship, where the minimum in this "U-shaped" curve represents the CPP value where PRx is the least deranged. This concept is referred to as the optimal CPP (CPPopt) [79, 80]. This CPPopt value can be derived from various windows of PRx and CPP data [14] and updated continuously at the bedside. Furthermore, CPPopt values vary from patient to patient, suggesting that the optimal CPP target is not the same between individuals. Finally, CPPopt values also vary over time within an individual patient, given changes in physiology and injury response mechanisms that occur during the acute phase after TBI [17]. Thus, the concept of CPPopt has ushered in the personalized physiologic target era for acute bedside care in TBI. Figure 43.3 provides an example of a CPPopt curve derived from PRx and CPP data.

Numerous retrospective single-center, [81] and recent prospective multi-center [82] data sets have confirmed that the time spent away from CPPopt during the acute phase of TBI care is directly associated with poor outcome at 6-month post-TBI. Furthermore, time spent away from CPPopt appears to be a stronger predictor of outcome, compared to time spent away from BTF guideline-based CPP targets.

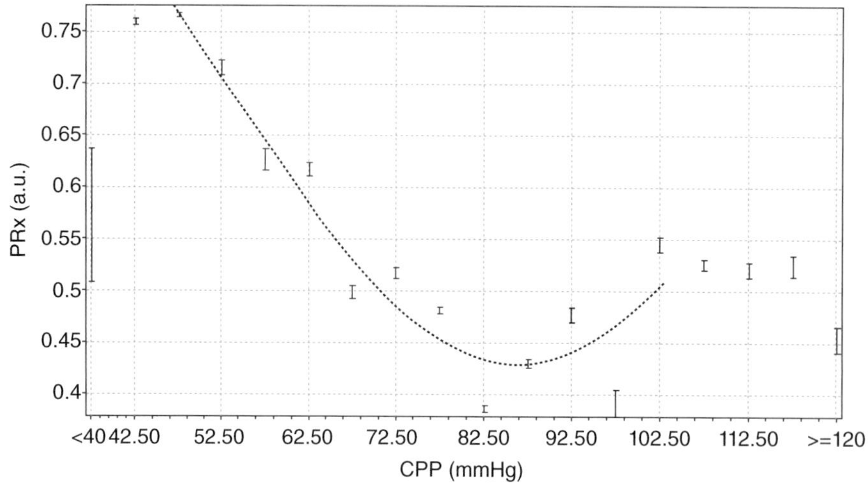

Fig. 43.3 Example of CPP optimum curve—4-hour window of data. *a.u.* arbitrary units, *CPP* cerebral perfusion pressure, *ICP* intracranial pressure, *MAP* mean arterial pressure, *mmHg* millimeters of Mercury, *PRx* pressure reactivity index (correlation between slow-wave vasogenic fluctuations in ICP and MAP). Figure depicts 4 h of data, with error-bar plotting of PRx vs. CPP. Error bars are generated for bins of CPP values (i.e., 5 mmHg bins of CPP). Then a parabolic curve is fit to the error-bar plot, with the minimum of the parabola demonstrating the CPP value with the most intact PRx (i.e., lowest PRx). This CPP value is the optimal CPP (i.e., CPPopt) for this individual patient, based on the prior 4 h of data. Note: the CPPopt here is outside of the guideline-defined CPP targets for acute TBI care

These critical findings have sparked a phase II randomized trial comparing BTF guideline-based CPP targets to CPPopt targets [14]. Phase III trials are already in the planning stage.

Individualized ICP Thresholds (iICP)

In line with individualized CPP targets, work has been conducted to explore the potential for personalized ICP thresholds in TBI. Again, given the literature supporting the importance of cerebrovascular reactivity and patient outcome in TBI, preliminary work into the relationship between ICP and PRx has been conducted [12, 83]. With the understanding that the PRx levels above +0.20 are considered grossly impaired cerebrovascular reactivity in TBI [65], evaluating the relationship between ICP and this PRx threshold of +0.20 has led to the possibility of generating individual ICP targets. The concept focuses on the ICP value, above which, PRx remains grossly impaired (i.e., above +0.20). This ICP value, in theory, would represent a patient's individual ICP (iICP) threshold. To date, only two studies have explored this concept, providing complimentary support for its potential [12, 83]. Approximately two-thirds of TBI patients displayed the ability to derive this iICP threshold, with iICP values often quite different from the suggested BTF guideline ICP threshold of 22 mmHg [12]. Both studies confirm that the time spent above iICP has a stronger association with mortality, compared to time spent above BTF guideline ICP thresholds [12]. However, one must be cautioned, as these results are still considered exploratory and very preliminary with much further work on the horizon required for both validation and improving the ability to continuously derive iICP targets at the bedside.

Integrating "Omics" into Acute Phase TBI Care—The Future

This chapter has mainly focused on advanced physiologic information and its value in the acute management of moderate/severe TBI patients. It is clear from the above sections that the "physiome" in acute TBI care is of critical importance in management. As we look into the future of acute TBI monitoring and care, it is expected that the physiome will be integrated with additional aspects of "omics" data at the bedside, facilitating ongoing transition into personalized therapeutic approaches [3, 8, 13, 84–88]. Such omics data is expected to take the form of integrated proteomic, genomic, and epigenomic information. Proteome data can be gleaned from serial serum CSF and microdialysis sampling. With the advances seen in multiplex immune-assays, numerous biomarkers can be readily obtained, including those pertaining to neural injury, [86] vascular/endothelial function and integrity [89], pro-inflammatory cytokine responses [8, 90, 91] and metabolic byproducts [9, 33, 92, 93]. Genomic information is expected to be rapidly provided through genome-wide association chips, allowing for simultaneous assessment of one million+ single nucleotide polymorphisms [3, 13, 85]. Similarly, advances in epigenetic techniques will lead to admission quantification of biological age based on methylation and histone methylation profiling.

This omics information provides the opportunity to improve both prognostication modeling in moderate/severe TBI care (physiome, proteome, genome, epigenome) and our ability to monitor treatment response (physiome and proteome), predict/sub-classify treatment responders (physiome, proteome, genome, epigenome), and uncover therapeutic pathways (physiome, proteome, and genome) [94, 95]. Such a wealth of information will require multidisciplinary teams of clinicians, epidemiologists, data scientists, statisticians, and biomedical engineers. It will also necessitate the utilization of complex machine learning and artificial intelligence techniques to aid in the interpretation of such large and continuously updating data sets. Preliminary advances in this field are being made by various multidisciplinary international collaborative efforts in Canada, [88] the USA, [96] and Europe [22, 76, 87, 97].

Conclusions

The acute-phase care of the moderate/severe TBI patient is complex, with increasing advances being made in cerebral physiologic monitoring. Current monitoring modalities allow for continuous bedside assessments of pressure-flow dynamics, oxygen delivery, metabolism, and electrophysiologic activity. Recent advances in cerebrovascular reactivity monitoring have led to the development of individual physiologic targets in acute TBI monitoring and care, ushering in the era of personalized medicine for TBI care. The future for acute TBI care will see further adoption of "omics" information for integrated real-time bedside updates on physiologic response to therapeutic measures, as well as the development of novel personalized treatments.

Key Points

- Recovery post-moderate/severe traumatic brain injury (TBI) is dependent on adherence to basic tenets of secondary neural injury detection and mitigation.
- Secondary neural injury after TBI takes multiple forms, including edema, neuroinflammation, impaired cerebral blood flow regulation, blood-brain barrier breakdown, metabolic dysfunction, and free radicle formation.
- Advanced cerebral physiologic monitoring of cerebral pressure flow, oxygen, and nutrient delivery during the acute phase of TBI care can be leveraged for early detection of secondary injury and subsequent intervention.
- Invasive and noninvasive multi-modal physiologic monitoring devices exist, providing both raw and derived metrics of cerebral physiology.
- Future care pathways for moderate/severe TBI will leverage such monitoring for the derivation of personalized cerebral physiologic targets, with the goal of neural tissue preservation.

Acknowledgments FAZ receives research support from the Manitoba Public Insurance (MPI) Neuroscience/TBI Research Endowment, the Health Sciences Centre Foundation Winnipeg, the United States National Institutes of Health (NIH) through the National Institute of Neurological Disorders and Stroke (NINDS) (Grant #: R03NS114335-01), the Canadian Institutes of Health Research (CIHR) (Grant #: 432061), the Canada Foundation for Innovation (CFI) (Project #: 38583), Research Manitoba (Grant #: 3906), the University of Manitoba VPRI Research Investment Fund (RIF), the University of Manitoba Centre on Aging, and the University of Manitoba Rudy Falk Clinician-Scientist Professorship.

LF is supported through the University of Manitoba (Department of Surgery GFT Research Grant) and the University of Manitoba Office of Research Services (ORS) (University Research Grant Program (URGP)).

CB is supported through the Centre on Aging Fellowship at the University of Manitoba.

AG is supported through the University of Manitoba Clinician Investigator Program.

Disclosures The authors have nothing to disclose.

References

1. Maas AI, Menon DK. Integrated approaches to paediatric neurocritical care in traumatic brain injury. Lancet Neurol [Internet] [cited 2020 Nov 17]. 2013;12(1):26–8. Available from: https://linkinghub.elsevier.com/retrieve/pii/S1474442212702727
2. Feigin VL, Theadom A, Barker-Collo S, Starkey NJ, McPherson K, Kahan M, et al. Incidence of traumatic brain injury in New Zealand: a population-based study. Lancet Neurol [Internet]. [cited 2020 Nov 17]. 2013;12(1):53–64. Available from: https://linkinghub.elsevier.com/retrieve/pii/S1474442212702624
3. Zeiler FA, Thelin EP, Donnelly J, Stevens AR, Smielewski P, Czosnyka M, et al. Genetic drivers of cerebral blood flow dysfunction in TBI: a speculative synthesis. Nat Rev Neurol [Internet]. 2019;15(1):25–39. [cited 2020 Sep 26]. Available from: http://www.nature.com/articles/s41582-018-0105-9
4. Dewan MC, Rattani A, Gupta S, Baticulon RE, Hung Y-C, Punchak M, et al. Estimating the global incidence of traumatic brain injury. J Neurosurg [Internet]. [cited 2020 Nov 10]. 2019;130(4):1080–97. Available from: https://thejns.org/view/journals/j-neurosurg/130/4/article-p1080.xml
5. Trauma brain injury fact sheet.pdf.
6. Rosenfeld JV, Maas AI, Bragge P, Morganti-Kossmann MC, Manley GT, Gruen RL. Early management of severe traumatic brain injury. The Lancet [Internet]. [cited 2020 Nov 17]. 2012;380(9847):1088–98. Available from: https://linkinghub.elsevier.com/retrieve/pii/S0140673612608642
7. Carney N, Totten AM, O'Reilly C, Ullman JS, Hawryluk GWJ, Bell MJ, et al. Guidelines for the management of severe traumatic brain injury, Fourth Edition. Neurosurgery [Internet]. [cited 2020 Nov 17]. 2017;80(1):6–15. Available from: https://academic.oup.com/neurosurgery/article/80/1/6/2585042
8. Thelin EP, Tajsic T, Zeiler FA, Menon DK, Hutchinson PJA, Carpenter KLH, et al. Monitoring the neuroinflammatory response following acute brain injury. Front Neurol. 2017;8:351.
9. Stovell MG, Yan J-L, Sleigh A, Mada MO, Carpenter TA, Hutchinson PJA, et al. Assessing metabolism and injury in acute human traumatic brain injury with magnetic resonance spectroscopy: current and future applications. Front Neurol. 2017;8:426.

10. Timofeev I, Carpenter KLH, Nortje J, Al-Rawi PG, O'Connell MT, Czosnyka M, et al. Cerebral extracellular chemistry and outcome following traumatic brain injury: a microdialysis study of 223 patients. Brain. 2011;134(Pt 2):484–94.
11. Hasen M, Almojuela A, Zeiler FA. Autonomic dysfunction and associations with functional and neurophysiological outcome in moderate/severe traumatic brain injury: a scoping review. J Neurotrauma [Internet]. [cited 2020 Sep 26]. 2019;36(10):1491–504. Available from: https://www.liebertpub.com/doi/10.1089/neu.2018.6073
12. Lazaridis C, DeSantis SM, Smielewski P, Menon DK, Hutchinson P, Pickard JD, et al. Patient-specific thresholds of intracranial pressure in severe traumatic brain injury. J Neurosurg. 2014;120(4):893–900.
13. Zeiler FA, McFadyen C, Newcombe VFJ, Synnot A, Donoghue EL, Ripatti S, et al. Genetic influences on patient-oriented outcomes in traumatic brain injury: a living systematic review of non-apolipoprotein E single-nucleotide polymorphisms. J Neurotrauma. 2019;38:1107.
14. Beqiri E, Smielewski P, Robba C, Czosnyka M, Cabeleira MT, Tas J, et al. Feasibility of individualised severe traumatic brain injury management using an automated assessment of optimal cerebral perfusion pressure: the COGiTATE phase II study protocol. BMJ Open. 2019;9(9):e030727.
15. James D, Pennardt AM. Trauma care principles. In: StatPearls [Internet]. Treasure Island: StatPearls Publishing; 2020. [cited 2020 Oct 3]. Available from: http://www.ncbi.nlm.nih.gov/books/NBK547757/.
16. Hawryluk GWJ, Aguilera S, Buki A, Bulger E, Citerio G, Cooper DJ, et al. A management algorithm for patients with intracranial pressure monitoring: the Seattle International Severe Traumatic Brain Injury Consensus Conference (SIBICC). Intensive Care Med [Internet]. 2019;45(12):1783–94. [cited 2020 Oct 3]. Available from: http://link.springer.com/10.1007/s00134-019-05805-9
17. Zeiler FA, Czosnyka M. Monitoring in neurotrauma. In p. 24.
18. Chesnut R, Aguilera S, Buki A, Bulger E, Citerio G, Cooper DJ, et al. A management algorithm for adult patients with both brain oxygen and intracranial pressure monitoring: the Seattle International Severe Traumatic Brain Injury Consensus Conference (SIBICC). Intensive Care Med. 2020;46(5):919–29.
19. Zeiler FA, Ercole A, Cabeleira M, Beqiri E, Zoerle T, Carbonara M, et al. Compensatory-reserve-weighted intracranial pressure versus intracranial pressure for outcome association in adult traumatic brain injury: a CENTER-TBI validation study. Acta Neurochir. 2019;161(7):1275–84.
20. Hasen M, Gomez A, Froese L, Dian J, Raj R, Thelin EP, et al. Alternative continuous intracranial pressure-derived cerebrovascular reactivity metrics in traumatic brain injury: a scoping overview. Acta Neurochir [Internet]. [cited 2020 Sep 26]. 2020;162(7):1647–62. Available from: http://link.springer.com/10.1007/s00701-020-04378-7
21. Gomez A, Dian J, Zeiler FA. Continuous and entirely non-invasive method for cerebrovascular reactivity assessment: technique and implications. J Clin Monit Comput [Internet]. 2020. [cited 2020 Sep 26]; Available from: http://link.springer.com/10.1007/s10877-020-00472-4;35:307.
22. Güiza F, Meyfroidt G, Piper I, Citerio G, Chambers I, Enblad P, et al. Cerebral perfusion pressure insults and associations with outcome in adult traumatic brain injury. J Neurotrauma. 2017;34(16):2425–31.
23. Thiara S, Griesdale DE, Henderson WR, Sekhon MS. Effect of cerebral perfusion pressure on acute respiratory distress syndrome. Can J Neurol Sci. 2018;45(3):313–9.
24. Aaslid R, Markwalder T-M, Nornes H. Noninvasive transcranial Doppler ultrasound recording of flow velocity in basal cerebral arteries. J Neurosurg [Internet] [cited 2020 Nov 18]. 1982;57(6):769–74. Available from: https://thejns.org/view/journals/j-neurosurg/57/6/article-p769.xml
25. Aaslid R. The Doppler principle applied to measurement of blood flow velocity in cerebral arteries. In: Aaslid R, editor. Transcranial Doppler Sonography [Internet]. Vienna: Springer Vienna; [cited 2020 Nov 18]; 1986. p. 22–38. Available from: http://link.springer.com/10.1007/978-3-7091-8864-4_3.
26. Goraj B, Rifkinson-Mann S, Leslie DR, Lansen TA, Kasoff SS, Tenner MS. Correlation of intracranial pressure and transcranial doppler resistive index after head trauma. AJNR Am J Neuroradiol. 1994;15:1333.
27. Kashif FM, Verghese GC, Novak V, Czosnyka M, Heldt T. Model-based noninvasive estimation of intracranial pressure from cerebral blood flow velocity and arterial pressure. Sci Transl Med [Internet]. [cited 2020 Nov 18]. 2012;4(129):129ra44–4. Available from: https://stm.sciencemag.org/lookup/doi/10.1126/scitranslmed.3003249
28. Zweifel C, Czosnyka M, Carrera E, de Riva N, Pickard JD, Smielewski P. Reliability of the blood flow velocity Pulsatility index for assessment of intracranial and cerebral perfusion pressures in head-injured patients. Neurosurgery [Internet]. [cited 2020 Nov 18]. 2012;71(4):853–61. Available from: https://academic.oup.com/neurosurgery/article/71/4/853/2594044
29. Cardim D, Robba C, Bohdanowicz M, Donnelly J, Cabella B, Liu X, et al. Non-invasive monitoring of intracranial pressure using transcranial Doppler ultrasonography: is it possible? Neurocrit Care [Internet]. [cited 2020 Nov 18]. 2016;25(3):473–91. Available from: http://link.springer.com/10.1007/s12028-016-0258-6
30. Czosnyka M, Kirkpatrick PJ. Cerebral perfusion pressure in head-injured patients: a noninvasive assessment using transcranial Doppler ultrasonography. J Neurosurg. 1998;88:7.
31. Tazarourte K, Atchabahian A, Tourtier J-P, David J-S, Ract C, Savary D, et al. Pre-hospital transcranial Doppler in severe traumatic brain injury: a pilot study: pre-hospital transcranial Doppler. Acta Anaesthesiologica Scandinavica [Internet]. [cited 2020 Nov 18] 2011;55(4):422–428. Available from: http://doi.wiley.com/10.1111/j.1399-6576.2010.02372.x
32. Okonkwo DO, Shutter LA, Moore C, Temkin NR, Puccio AM, Madden CJ, et al. Brain oxygen optimization in severe traumatic brain injury phase-II: a phase II randomized trial. Crit Care Med. 2017;45(11):1907–14.
33. Zeiler FA, Thelin EP, Helmy A, Czosnyka M, Hutchinson PJA, Menon DK. A systematic review of cerebral microdialysis and outcomes in TBI: relationships to patient functional outcome, neurophysiologic measures, and tissue outcome. Acta Neurochir [Internet]. [cited 2020 Sep 26]. 2017;159(12):2245–73. Available from: http://link.springer.com/10.1007/s00701-017-3338-2
34. Mathieu F, Khellaf A, Thelin EP, Zeiler FA. Continuous thermal diffusion-based cerebral blood flow monitoring in adult traumatic brain injury: a scoping systematic review. J Neurotrauma [Internet]. [cited 2020 Sep 26]. 2019;36(11):1707–23. Available from: https://www.liebertpub.com/doi/10.1089/neu.2018.6309
35. Rosenthal G, Sanchez-Mejia RO, Phan N, Hemphill JC, Martin C, Manley GT. Incorporating a parenchymal thermal diffusion cerebral blood flow probe in bedside assessment of cerebral autoregulation and vasoreactivity in patients with severe traumatic brain injury. J Neurosurg. 2011;114(1):62–70.
36. Le Roux P, Menon DK, Citerio G, Vespa P, Bader MK, Brophy GM, et al. Consensus summary statement of the International Multidisciplinary Consensus Conference on Multimodality Monitoring in Neurocritical Care: a statement for healthcare professionals from the Neurocritical Care Society and the European Society of Intensive Care Medicine. Neurocrit Care. 2014;21(Suppl 2):S1–26.
37. Dickman CA, Carter LP, Baldwin HZ, Harrington T, Tallman D. Continuous regional cerebral blood flow monitoring in acute craniocerebral trauma. Neurosurgery. 1991;28(3):467–72.

38. Schröder ML, Muizelaar JP. Monitoring of regional cerebral blood flow (CBF) in acute head injury by thermal diffusion. In: Unterberg AW, Schneider G-H, Lanksch WR, editors. Monitoring of cerebral blood flow and metabolism in intensive care [internet], vol. 59. Vienna: Springer Vienna; [cited 2020 Nov 18]; 1993. p. 47–9. Available from: http://link.springer.com/10.1007/978-3-7091-9302-0_8.
39. Valadka AB, Hlatky R, Furuya Y, Robertson CS. Brain Tissue P02: Correlation with Cerebral Blood Flow: 2.
40. Hutchinson PJ, Jalloh I, Helmy A, Carpenter KLH, Rostami E, Bellander B-M, et al. Consensus statement from the 2014 International Microdialysis Forum. Intensive Care Med. 2015;41(9):1517–28.
41. Mathieu F, Khellaf A, Ku JC, Donnelly J, Thelin EP, Zeiler FA. Continuous near-infrared spectroscopy monitoring in adult traumatic brain injury: a systematic review. J Neurosurg Anesthesiol [Internet] [cited 2020 Sep 26]. 2020;32(4):288–99. Available from: https://journals.lww.com/10.1097/ANA.0000000000000620
42. Oddo M, Schmidt JM, Carrera E, Badjatia N, Connolly ES, Presciutti M, et al. Impact of tight glycemic control on cerebral glucose metabolism after severe brain injury: a microdialysis study. Crit Care Med. 2008;36(12):3233–8.
43. Stein NR, McArthur DL, Etchepare M, Vespa PM. Early cerebral metabolic crisis after TBI influences outcome despite adequate hemodynamic resuscitation. Neurocrit Care. 2012;17(1):49–57.
44. Vespa PM, McArthur D, O'Phelan K, Glenn T, Etchepare M, Kelly D, et al. Persistently low extracellular glucose correlates with poor outcome 6 months after human traumatic brain injury despite a lack of increased lactate: a microdialysis study. J Cereb Blood Flow Metab. 2003;23(7):865–77.
45. Wijayatilake DS, Talati C, Panchatsharam S. The monitoring and Management of Severe Traumatic Brain Injury in the United Kingdom: is there a consensus? J Neurosurg Anesthesiol [Internet] [cited 2020 Nov 18]. 2015;27(3):241–5. Available from: http://journals.lww.com/00008506-201507000-00007
46. van Santbrink H, Schouten JW, Steyerberg EW, Avezaat CJJ, Maas AIR. Serial Transcranial Doppler Measurements in Traumatic Brain Injury with Special Focus on the Early Posttraumatic Period: 9.
47. Zurynski YA, Dorsch NWC, Fearnside MR. Incidence and effects of increased cerebral blood flow velocity after severe head injury: a transcranial Doppler ultrasound study II. Effect of vasospasm and hyperemia on outcome. J Neurol Sci [Internet]. [cited 2020 Nov 18]. 1995;134(1–2):41–6. Available from: https://linkinghub.elsevier.com/retrieve/pii/0022510X9500178X
48. Chan K-H, Miller JD, Dearden NM, Andrews PJD, Midgley S. The effect of changes in cerebral perfusion pressure upon middle cerebral artery blood flow velocity and jugular bulb venous oxygen saturation after severe brain injury. J Neurosurg [Internet]. [cited 2020 Nov 18]. 1992;77(1):55–61. Available from: https://thejns.org/view/journals/j-neurosurg/77/1/article-p55.xml
49. Moreno JA, Mesalles E, Gener J, Tomasa A, Ley A, Roca J, et al. Evaluating the outcome of severe head injury with transcranial Doppler ultrasonography. Neurosurg Focus. 2000;8(1):e8.
50. Fatima N, Shuaib A, Chughtai TS, Ayyad A, Saqqur M. The role of transcranial Doppler in traumatic brain injury: a systemic review and meta-analysis. Asian J Neurosurg. 2019;14(3):626–33.
51. Sokoloff C, Williamson D, Serri K, Albert M, Odier C, Charbonney E, et al. Clinical usefulness of transcranial Doppler as a screening tool for early cerebral hypoxic episodes in patients with moderate and severe traumatic brain injury. Neurocrit Care. 2020;32(2):486–91.
52. Ziegler D, Cravens G, Angles G, Gandhi R, Cho P. Use of transcranial Doppler in patients with severe traumatic brain injury. Crit Care [Internet]. [cited 2020 Nov 18]. 2010;14(Suppl 1):P292. Available from: http://ccforum.biomedcentral.com/articles/10.1186/cc8524
53. Zweifel C, Castellani G, Czosnyka M, Helmy A, Manktelow A, Carrera E, et al. Noninvasive monitoring of cerebrovascular reactivity with near infrared spectroscopy in head-injured patients. J Neurotrauma [Internet]. [cited 2020 Nov 18]. 2010;27(11):1951–8. Available from: http://www.liebertpub.com/doi/10.1089/neu.2010.1388
54. Weatherall A, Skowno J, Lansdown A, Lupton T, Garner A. Feasibility of cerebral near-infrared spectroscopy monitoring in the pre-hospital environment. Acta Anaesthesiol Scand. 2012;56(2):172–7.
55. Storm C, Leithner C, Krannich A, Wutzler A, Ploner CJ, Trenkmann L. Regional cerebral oxygen saturation after cardiac arrest in 60 patients—A prospective outcome study. 2014;5
56. Alotaiby T, El-Samie FEA, Alshebeili SA, Ahmad I. A review of channel selection algorithms for EEG signal processing. EURASIP J Adv Signal Process [Internet]. [cited 2020 Nov 19]. 2015, 2015;(1):66. Available from: https://asp-eurasipjournals.springeropen.com/articles/10.1186/s13634-015-0251-9
57. Guideline Three: Minimum Technical Standards for EEG Recording in Suspected Cerebral Death. J Clin Neurophysiol [Internet]. [cited 2020 Nov 19]. 1986;3:12–7. Available from: http://journals.lww.com/00004691-198610001-00004
58. Tackla R, Hinzman JM, Foreman B, Magner M, Andaluz N, Hartings JA. Assessment of cerebrovascular autoregulation using regional cerebral blood flow in surgically managed brain trauma patients. Neurocrit Care [Internet]. [cited 2020 Nov 19]. 2015;23(3):339–46. Available from: http://link.springer.com/10.1007/s12028-015-0146-5
59. Lassen NA. Regulation of cerebral circulation. Acta Anaesthesiol Scand Suppl. 1971;45:78–80.
60. Sánchez-Porras R, Santos E, Czosnyka M, Zheng Z, Unterberg AW, Sakowitz OW. 'Long' pressure reactivity index (L-PRx) as a measure of autoregulation correlates with outcome in traumatic brain injury patients. Acta Neurochir [Internet]. [cited 2020 Nov 19]. 2012;154(9):1575–81. Available from: http://link.springer.com/10.1007/s00701-012-1423-0
61. Czosnyka M, Smielewski P, Kirkpatrick P, Laing RJ, Menon D, Pickard JD. Continuous assessment of the cerebral vasomotor reactivity in head injury. Neurosurgery [Internet]. [cited 2020 Nov 17]. 1997;41(1):11–9. Available from: https://academic.oup.com/neurosurgery/article/41/1/11/2859060
62. Brady KM, Lee JK, Kibler KK, Easley RB, Koehler RC, Shaffner DH. Continuous measurement of autoregulation by spontaneous fluctuations in cerebral perfusion pressure: comparison of 3 methods. Stroke. 2008;39(9):2531–7.
63. Zeiler FA, Donnelly J, Calviello L, Lee JK, Smielewski P, Brady K, et al. Validation of pressure reactivity and pulse amplitude indices against the lower limit of autoregulation, part I: experimental intracranial hypertension. J Neurotrauma. 2018;35(23):2803–11.
64. Zeiler FA, Lee JK, Smielewski P, Czosnyka M, Brady K. Validation of intracranial pressure-derived cerebrovascular reactivity indices against the lower limit of autoregulation, part II: experimental model of arterial hypotension. J Neurotrauma. 2018;35(23):2812–9.
65. Sorrentino E, Diedler J, Kasprowicz M, Budohoski KP, Haubrich C, Smielewski P, et al. Critical thresholds for cerebrovascular reactivity after traumatic brain injury. Neurocrit Care. 2012;16(2):258–66.
66. Donnelly J, Czosnyka M, Adams H, Cardim D, Kolias AG, Zeiler FA, et al. Twenty-five years of intracranial pressure monitoring after severe traumatic brain injury: a retrospective, single-center analysis. Neurosurgery. 2019;85(1):E75–82.
67. Zeiler FA, Donnelly J, Smielewski P, Menon DK, Hutchinson PJ, Czosnyka M. Critical thresholds of intracranial pressure-derived continuous cerebrovascular reactivity indices for outcome prediction in noncraniectomized patients with traumatic brain injury. J Neurotrauma. 2018;35(10):1107–15.

68. Zeiler FA, Ercole A, Beqiri E, Cabeleira M, Thelin EP, Stocchetti N, et al. Association between cerebrovascular reactivity monitoring and mortality is preserved when adjusting for baseline admission characteristics in adult traumatic brain injury: a CENTER-TBI study. J Neurotrauma. 2020;37(10):1233–41.
69. Mathieu F, Zeiler FA, Ercole A, Monteiro M, Kamnitsas K, Glocker B, et al. Relationship between measures of cerebrovascular reactivity and intracranial lesion progression in acute traumatic brain injury patients: a CENTER-TBI study. J Neurotrauma. 2020;37(13):1556–65.
70. Zeiler FA, Beqiri E, Cabeleira M, Hutchinson PJ, Stocchetti N, Menon DK, et al. Brain tissue oxygen and cerebrovascular reactivity in traumatic brain injury: a collaborative European NeuroTrauma effectiveness research in traumatic brain injury exploratory analysis of insult burden. J Neurotrauma. 2020;37(17):1854–63.
71. Zeiler FA, Ercole A, Cabeleira M, Stocchetti N, Hutchinson PJ, Smielewski P, et al. Descriptive analysis of low versus elevated intracranial pressure on cerebral physiology in adult traumatic brain injury: a CENTER-TBI exploratory study. Acta Neurochir. 2020;162(11):2695–706.
72. Zeiler FA, Kim D-J, Cabeleira M, Calviello L, Smielewski P, Czosnyka M. Impaired cerebral compensatory reserve is associated with admission imaging characteristics of diffuse insult in traumatic brain injury. Acta Neurochir. 2018;160(12):2277–87.
73. Kim D-J, Czosnyka Z, Keong N, Radolovich DK, Smielewski P, Sutcliffe MPF, et al. Index of cerebrospinal compensatory reserve in hydrocephalus. Neurosurgery. 2009;64(3):494–501. discussion 501–502
74. Calviello L, Donnelly J, Cardim D, Robba C, Zeiler FA, Smielewski P, et al. Compensatory-reserve-weighted intracranial pressure and its association with outcome after traumatic brain injury. Neurocrit Care. 2018;28(2):212–20.
75. Le Roux P, Menon DK, Citerio G, Vespa P, Bader MK, Brophy G, et al. The international multidisciplinary consensus conference on multimodality monitoring in neurocritical care: evidentiary tables: a statement for healthcare professionals from the Neurocritical Care Society and the European Society of Intensive Care Medicine. Neurocrit Care. 2014;21(Suppl 2):S297–361.
76. Bennis FC, Teeuwen B, Zeiler FA, Elting JW, van der Naalt J, Bonizzi P, et al. Improving prediction of favourable outcome after 6 months in patients with severe traumatic brain injury using physiological cerebral parameters in a multivariable logistic regression model. Neurocrit Care. 2020;33(2):542–51.
77. Zeiler FA, Ercole A, Beqiri E, Cabeleira M, Aries M, Zoerle T, et al. Cerebrovascular reactivity is not associated with therapeutic intensity in adult traumatic brain injury: a CENTER-TBI analysis. Acta Neurochir. 2019;161(9):1955–64.
78. Froese L, Batson C, Gomez A, Dian J, Zeiler FA. The limited impact of current therapeutic interventions on cerebrovascular reactivity in traumatic brain injury: a narrative overview. Neurocrit Care. 2020;34:325.
79. Aries MJH, Czosnyka M, Budohoski KP, Steiner LA, Lavinio A, Kolias AG, et al. Continuous determination of optimal cerebral perfusion pressure in traumatic brain injury. Crit Care Med. 2012;40(8):2456–63.
80. Steiner LA, Czosnyka M, Piechnik SK, Smielewski P, Chatfield D, Menon DK, et al. Continuous monitoring of cerebrovascular pressure reactivity allows determination of optimal cerebral perfusion pressure in patients with traumatic brain injury. Crit Care Med. 2002;30(4):733–8.
81. Needham E, McFadyen C, Newcombe V, Synnot AJ, Czosnyka M, Menon D. Cerebral perfusion pressure targets individualized to pressure-reactivity index in moderate to severe traumatic brain injury: a systematic review. J Neurotrauma. 2017;34(5):963–70.
82. Zeiler FA, Ercole A, Cabeleira M, Carbonara M, Stocchetti N, Menon DK, et al. Comparison of performance of different optimal cerebral perfusion pressure parameters for outcome prediction in adult traumatic brain injury: a collaborative European NeuroTrauma effectiveness research in traumatic brain injury (CENTER-TBI) study. J Neurotrauma. 2019;36(10):1505–17.
83. Zeiler FA, Ercole A, Cabeleira M, Beqiri E, Zoerle T, Carbonara M, et al. Patient-specific ICP epidemiologic thresholds in adult traumatic brain injury: a CENTER-TBI validation study. J Neurosurg Anesthesiol. 2019 Jun;18:28.
84. Zeiler FA, Ercole A, Czosnyka M, Smielewski P, Hawryluk G, Hutchinson PJA, et al. Continuous cerebrovascular reactivity monitoring in moderate/severe traumatic brain injury: a narrative review of advances in neurocritical care. Brit J Anaesthesia [Internet]. [cited 2020 Sep 26]. 2020;124(4):440–53. Available from: https://linkinghub.elsevier.com/retrieve/pii/S0007091219309663
85. McFadyen CA, Zeiler FA, Newcombe V, Synnot A, Steyerberg E, Gruen RL, et al. Apolipoprotein E4 polymorphism and outcomes from traumatic brain injury: a living systematic review and meta-analysis. J Neurotrauma. 2019;17
86. Thelin EP, Zeiler FA, Ercole A, Mondello S, Büki A, Bellander B-M, et al. Serial sampling of serum protein biomarkers for monitoring human traumatic brain injury dynamics: a systematic review. Front Neurol. 2017;8:300.
87. Maas AIR, Menon DK, Steyerberg EW, Citerio G, Lecky F, Manley GT, et al. Collaborative European NeuroTrauma effectiveness research in traumatic brain injury (CENTER-TBI): a prospective longitudinal observational study. Neurosurgery. 2015;76(1):67–80.
88. Bernard F, Gallagher C, Griesdale D, Kramer A, Sekhon M, Zeiler FA. The CAnadian high-resolution traumatic brain injury (CAHR-TBI) research collaborative. Can J Neurol Sci. 2020;47(4):551–6.
89. Guilfoyle MR, Carpenter KLH, Helmy A, Pickard JD, Menon DK, Hutchinson PJA. Matrix metalloproteinase expression in contusional traumatic brain injury: a paired microdialysis study. J Neurotrauma. 2015;32(20):1553–9.
90. Zeiler FA, Thelin EP, Czosnyka M, Hutchinson PJ, Menon DK, Helmy A. Cerebrospinal fluid and microdialysis cytokines in severe traumatic brain injury: a scoping systematic review. Front Neurol. 2017;8:331.
91. Needham EJ, Helmy A, Zanier ER, Jones JL, Coles AJ, Menon DK. The immunological response to traumatic brain injury. J Neuroimmunol. 2019;332:112–25.
92. Killen MJ, Giorgi-Coll S, Helmy A, Hutchinson PJ, Carpenter KL. Metabolism and inflammation: implications for traumatic brain injury therapeutics. Expert Rev Neurother. 2019;19(3):227–42.
93. Orešič M, Posti JP, Kamstrup-Nielsen MH, Takala RSK, Lingsma HF, Mattila I, et al. Human serum metabolites associate with severity and patient outcomes in traumatic brain injury. EBioMedicine. 2016;12:118–26.
94. Helmy A, Guilfoyle MR, Carpenter KLH, Pickard JD, Menon DK, Hutchinson PJ. Recombinant human interleukin-1 receptor antagonist promotes M1 microglia biased cytokines and chemokines following human traumatic brain injury. J Cereb Blood Flow Metab. 2016;36(8):1434–48.
95. Thelin EP, Carpenter KLH, Hutchinson PJ, Helmy A. Microdialysis monitoring in clinical traumatic brain injury and its role in neuroprotective drug development. AAPS J. 2017;19(2):367–76.
96. Yue JK, Vassar MJ, Lingsma HF, Cooper SR, Okonkwo DO, Valadka AB, et al. Transforming research and clinical knowledge in traumatic brain injury pilot: multicenter implementation of the common data elements for traumatic brain injury. J Neurotrauma. 2013;30(22):1831–44.
97. Thelin EP, Raj R, Bellander B-M, Nelson D, Piippo-Karjalainen A, Siironen J, et al. Comparison of high versus low frequency cerebral physiology for cerebrovascular reactivity assessment in traumatic brain injury: a multi-center pilot study. J Clin Monit Comput. 2020;34(5):971–94.

Part V

Emergency Ultrasound and Trauma Imaging

Basic Trauma Ultrasound

44

Markus Ziesmann, Andrew W. Kirkpatrick, and Lawrence Marshall Gillman

Introduction

During the assessment of an acutely unstable trauma patient, favor is given to rapid investigations which will expedite definitive care. In conjunction with the chest and pelvis X-rays, the Focused Assessment with Sonography for Trauma, or FAST, is perhaps the most readily available diagnostic tool that is capable of changing the management of that patient. This role had historically been fulfilled by Diagnostic Peritoneal Lavage (DPL), but the quicker, noninvasive FAST scan has replaced DPL as the standard of care. Point-of-care ultrasound examination can be performed quickly, can expedite decision-making, and can diagnose surgical injuries faster, facilitating more rapid transition to the operating theatre.

The goal of the FAST exam is to identify free fluid in the abdomen or around the pericardium. It is not possible to differentiate on FAST between blood, urine, amniotic fluid, or GI contents, but in the context of a hemodynamically unstable trauma victim, it is presumed that any free fluid represents intraabdominal hemorrhage, and thus any exam revealing free fluid is a positive test. Notably, any of the mentioned non-bloody fluids found in an unstable patient would also represent a surgical diagnosis and, therefore, the goal of FAST is to diagnose free fluid, not blood. The extended FAST (E-FAST) includes the addition of ultrasonography of the thorax to look for pneumothoraces and is discussed further in Chap. 45: Trauma Ultrasound: Beyond the FAST Exam.

M. Ziesmann (✉) · L. Marshall Gillman
Health Sciences Centre, Winnipeg, MB, Canada
e-mail: mziesmann2@hsc.mb.ca; lawrence.gillman@umanitoba.ca

A. W. Kirkpatrick
Trauma Services, Foothills Hospital, Calgary, AB, Canada
e-mail: Andrew.Kirkpatrick@albertahealthservices.ca

The FAST Examination

Technique

Because most patients will be subject to spine mobility limitations at the time of the FAST exam, positioning simply requires a supine patient with a table parallel to the floor. The examination of all four sites may be performed in any order, so long as all four sites are imaged systematically and accurately. Some sonographers prefer to start the exam with the pericardial view which will allow for calibration of the device's gain setting based on intra-cardiac blood. Others advocate starting the exam in the right upper quadrant, as this is the region most likely to yield positive findings. Regardless of the order of exams, approaching the exam in a systematic and organized way is necessary to both learn the techniques and ensure that nothing is overlooked. Examination of the thorax if proceeding to an E-FAST exam occurs after the conventional FAST is complete.

The FAST exam is performed using a low frequency (2.5 to 5 MHz) curvilinear or phased array probe which will allow for adequate depth of visualization during the study. In brief, the ultrasound device creates images based on the detection of reflected sound waves such that dense tissue appears bright white and non-echogenic tissue appears dark black on the ultrasound's display. The exam may be made more difficult by the presence of obesity, gas-distended viscera, subcutaneous emphysema, or COPD [1], and the presence of preexisting ascites makes the exam uninterpretable. An inverse relationship exists between the depth of penetration and resolution of the scan; patients with a large body habitus may be difficult to investigate.

The pericardium is examined in the subxiphoid view using the liver as an acoustic window. The pericardium forms a potential space around the heart, sometimes containing a trivial amount of fluid that would not be detected on FAST (Fig. 44.1). Any anechoic fluid seen within this space therefore represents a positive study and a presumed diagnosis of hemopericardium. One common mistake in evaluating the

L. Marshall Gillman, S. Widder (eds.), *Trauma Team Dynamics*, https://doi.org/10.1007/978-3-031-86312-7_44

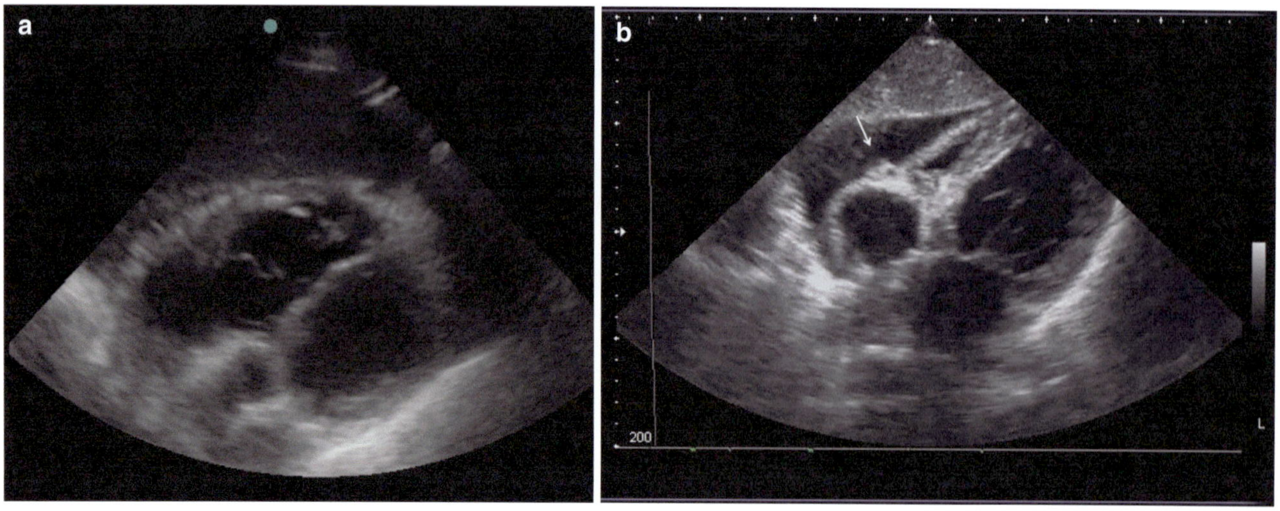

Fig. 44.1 Pericardial view of the FAST exam - Image a shows a normal pericardium with no fluid, while image b shows a positive pericardial FAST with fluid indicated by the arrow

pericardium is to declare a positive study after mistaking epicardial fat for free fluid; an epicardial fat pad is adherent to the cardiac tissue and will move with the cardiac contractions. A false negative pericardial FAST exam may result from a large rent in the pericardium decompressing hemopericardium into the pleural space rather than developing a cardiac tamponade; considering the pericardial FAST in context with other clinical signs is important.

If the sonographer cannot obtain satisfactory views in the subxiphoid plane, a left parasternal approach may be attempted. The probe should be placed immediately to the left of the sternum at the fourth or fifth intercostal space, initially with the probe marker to the patient's right. After obtaining a view of the heart, the probe can be rotated with the marker toward the right shoulder and then the left shoulder, for long-axis and short-axis views respectively. This technique may be preferred in patients with significant obesity.

The view of the right upper quadrant also uses the liver as a sonographic window. The probe is placed on the patient between the anterior and mid-axillary line, positioning the probe in the eighth to eleventh intercostal space, parallel to the ribs. Angle the probe counter-clockwise to minimize rib shadows if necessary. The probe indicator should be oriented toward the patient's head. Proper examination of the right upper quadrant should visualize the liver edge, the inferior pole of the right kidney, and Morison's Pouch (the potential space between the liver and the right kidney, or the hepatorenal space) (Fig. 44.2). Landmarking Morison's Pouch may be made easier by identifying the bright white Gerota's fascia of the kidneys posteriorly. No single probe orientation will adequately visualize all of these landmarks and thus sweeping of the probe, moving the probe superiorly or inferiorly, and/or angling cephalad and caudad may be required. An awake and responsive patient may be coached on controlling their breathing to allow adequate visualization. Visualization of an anechoic (black) stripe between the liver and kidney or near the tip of the liver is considered a positive exam.

Proceeding in a clockwise manner to the left upper quadrant, the spleen is used as a sonographic window and the probe is placed on the posterior axillary line at the eighth or ninth intercostal space. Again, the probe indicator is pointed toward the patient's head and the probe may need to be rotated to minimize rib shadows. Examining the left upper quadrant requires visualization of the subphrenic and perisplenic spaces and the left kidney (Fig. 44.3). The probe must be systematically swept, moved, or angled to visualize all three spaces. Anechoic (black) blood may be seen between the spleen and kidney or often above the spleen and just under the diaphragm with either of these findings being considered a positive test.

Finally, the pelvic view is obtained by using the bladder as a sonographic window (Fig. 44.4). While we describe this as a pelvis view, the view obtained is actually the inferior abdomen; the anatomic pelvis is a retroperitoneal location, and the FAST does not function well at finding retroperitoneal fluid. A good pelvic view is dependent on a full bladder, as an empty bladder limits the ability to detect small amounts of free fluid. In patients with a urinary catheter inserted, the examiner may clamp this catheter or instill up to 200 cc of warm isotonic fluid to optimize the study. The pelvic view is obtained with a sagittal probe orientation, again orienting the marker toward the patient's head. The probe is swept from right to left or vice versa, paying attention to the retrovesicular space in males and the retro-uterine space in females for the presence of anechoic (black) free fluid. As before the presence of anechoic fluid is considered a positive finding. The probe is then turned to a transverse orientation and the pelvis reexamined.

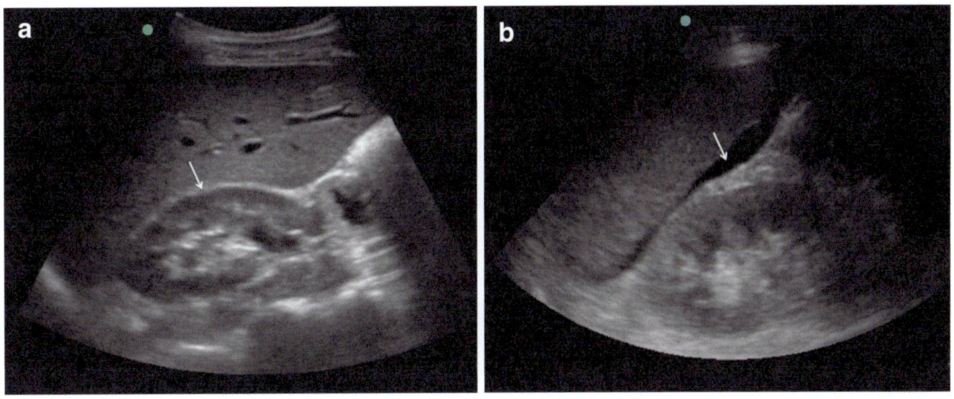

Fig. 44.2 Right upper quadrant (RUQ) view of the FAST exam - Image a shows a normal RUQ view with no fluid in the hepatorenal space (arrow), while image b shows a positive RUQ FAST with fluid indicated by the arrow

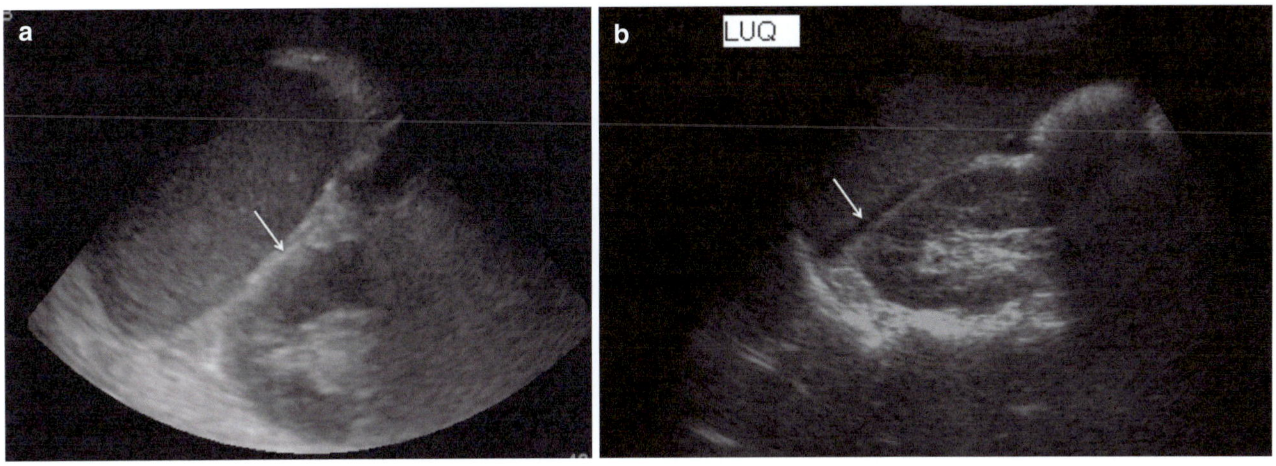

Fig. 44.3 Left upper quadrant (LUQ) view of the FAST exam - Image a shows a normal LUQ view with no fluid in the splenorenal space (arrow), while image b shows a positive LUQ FAST with fluid indicated by the arrow

A positive FAST is one that demonstrates *any* free fluid *any*where. Even if some views are incomplete, the presence of even a single positive view renders the exam positive. A negative FAST is one that demonstrates *no* fluid *every*where; all four sites must be adequately and completely imaged without positive findings. If any view of any space is not adequately visualized, but the visualized spaces are negative, the exam must be scored "indeterminate" and the patient will require further investigation.

Uses

Blunt Abdominal Trauma

FAST is best studied in the context of blunt abdominal trauma. The Sonographic Outcomes Assessment Program (SOAP) trial was a prospective randomized study that concluded that FAST offered significant benefits including a 64% reduced time to operative intervention, decreased numbers of computed tomography (CT) scans, a 27% decrease in length of hospital stay, fewer complications, and a significant cost savings [2]. Investigation with FAST has been shown to significantly change management plans in 33% of applications, including a 28% reduction in CT scans, and an 89% reduction in DPL performance [3].

One review compared the FAST to various examinations and investigations in blunt trauma patients, concluding that a positive FAST is better at detecting intra-abdominal injuries than exam findings of rebound tenderness, seatbelt signs, hypotension, abdominal distention, and guarding and also was better than adjunct investigations including reported base deficits, deranged liver enzymes, anemia, or an abnormal chest X-ray. The presence of free intraperitoneal fluid on bedside ultrasonography corresponds to a likelihood ratio of 30 that there is indeed an intraabdominal injury [4].

Perhaps the biggest advantage that FAST provides a Trauma Team Leader is its ready availability as a bedside tool. In circumstances of hemodynamic instability which would normally preclude CT scanning, the sensitivity of FAST is greatly increased. The sensitivity of ultrasound in the hypotensive trauma population approaches 100% [5, 6]. In an unstable patient, sonographic examinations can be completed in 2–4 min [5, 7, 8]. Up to 90% of patients with massive hemoperitoneum may be identified by examining only Morison's Pouch [6], with a mean examination time in one study of only 19 s for patients with positive findings [5].

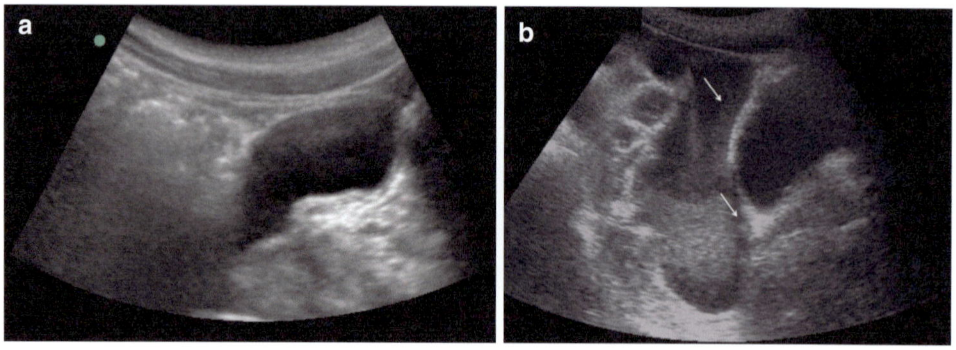

Fig. 44.4 Pelvic view of the FAST exam - Image a shows a normal pelvic view with no fluid, while image b shows a positive pelvic FAST with fluid indicated by the arrow

The point-of-care nature of the FAST exam facilitates repeat exams where necessary. When confronted by a negative examination and no immediate indication for surgery, definitive diagnostic testing (usually with a CT scan) is usually the next step. In scenarios where a CT scan is not available, such as a mass casualty scenario or in a resource-limited clinical setting, repeating the FAST exam can be considered. With time—and thus, in a bleeding patient, an increased volume of intraperitoneal free fluid—sensitivity of the exam increases. Repeat examination may be useful in assessing GI injuries that are poorly detected by FAST, increasing the sensitivity from 38% to 85% when repeated in 12–24 h in one study [9].

While FAST is most often associated with level 1 trauma centers, the exam may have a role in triaging patients either prehospital or from peripheral centers to centers of definitive care. A patient requiring transfer to a trauma center with a positive FAST exam may be considered for transport directly to an operating theater which can be prepared in advance of the patient's arrival. In regions with access to prehospital FAST, time in the emergency room is reduced, with shorter door-to-CT and door-to-OR times [10, 11] while preserving a high reported sensitivity and sensitivity of the exam [12].

After considering the evidence, we are left with the conclusion that FAST in the blunt trauma population requires an assessment of hemodynamic stability as a decision point. As we will discuss in the "Limitations" section, in the patient who is hemodynamically stable, other diagnostic modalities may yield more definitive diagnoses and subsequent management. FAST has replaced diagnostic peritoneal lavage and, like DPL [13], FAST serves to alter management only in the unstable patient. In a hypotensive population after blunt abdominal trauma, FAST was able to identify 97% of patients with surgical injuries; in a subset of patients too unstable to undergo CT scanning, 64% of patients with a positive FAST had surgical injuries, whereas zero patients with a negative FAST had surgical injuries [14].

In summary, in the blunt trauma population, FAST changes management only in the unstable population. In the stable population, FAST may have limited use as part of the ATLS Circulation assessment, for reassessment of a dynamically changing patient, in austere or resource-limited environments, and potentially for the triaging of inbound patients referred from non-trauma centers.

Penetrating Trauma

The role of FAST in penetrating injuries is somewhat lessened, as hollow organ injury does not necessarily present with massive hemoperitoneum and thus FAST is less sensitive in this population [15]. One particularly useful application, however, is to confirm or rule out massive hemoperitoneum in cases of junctional injuries for the purposes of surgical planning about which body cavity contains the primary problem [16].

The most significant application of FAST in the penetrating trauma population is to rule out cardiac injuries. Though much of the evidence is derived from small studies, the sensitivity of FAST to pericardial blood after penetrating chest trauma consistently approaches 100% [17–19]. Of patients with a positive pericardial FAST, surgical intervention is the next step [17]. In patients with a high clinical suspicion of cardiac injury, examination is rapid, with a mean time to examine the pericardium of under one minute [20]. The FAST exam shows some ability to discriminate survivable versus non-survivable patients presenting with trauma-induced cardiac arrest, for the purposes of triaging candidacy for a resuscitative thoracotomy. In patients with traumatic arrest and cardiac standstill on FAST, resuscitative thoracotomy may be futile [21].

Limitations

The major limitations of FAST studies all pertain to its primary purpose: to detect free fluid. The purpose, in other words, is not to definitively diagnose all possible injuries. When considering the evidence surrounding the use of FAST exams, it is important to consider the outcome variables for a given study. Outcomes of "agreement with findings at laparotomy" or "agreement with CT scanning" invariably demonstrate low sensitivity. CT scanning is far more sensitive for any injury that does not produce significant amounts of free fluid, such as hollow organ injury, retroperitoneal injury, or solid organ injury with minimal blood loss. The goal of a FAST exam is singular: to identify free fluid contributing to hemodynamic instability. Thus, when interpreting the data for or against the use of FAST, one must bear in mind the outcomes against which it is compared.

Critics of the FAST exam note that it is a poor single test for diagnosing the presence of an abdominal visceral injury. Using CT as a reference standard, we know that 34% of patients with known visceral injuries have no appreciable hemoperitoneum [22]. Studies comparing FAST to CT scan or laparotomy findings have reported sensitivities ranging from 41% to 94% [23–27]. When specifically considering sensitivity for hemoperitoneum, FAST has a sensitivity of 91%, considerably better than its sensitivity for detecting all injuries (69%) [26].

Because we know that ultrasound may not detect all injuries, a negative FAST in a clinically deteriorating patient requires further investigation or exploration. False-negative FAST exams—that is, studies failing to detect free fluid despite the presence of intraabdominal injury—often result in clinical deterioration of the patient. A large proportion of false-negative FAST patients require operative intervention [16, 23, 24, 28, 29] with false-negative rates of 1.7–6.1% in blunt trauma [23, 24. 28] and 9–29% in penetrating trauma [16, 29, 30] reported. Therefore, while a negative FAST may be reassuring, further clinical deterioration *always* mandates further investigations. Notably, patients with severe pelvic fractures are one known cohort at increased risk of false-negative exams [31], and up to 19% of true-positive exams in this population represent uroperitoneum rather than hemoperitoneum [32]. Whenever possible, hemodynamically stable patients without indications for urgent interventions should be investigated with cross-sectional imaging to rule out missed injuries.

The smallest amount of free fluid detectable by FAST exam varies by the location of the exam and the origin of the fluid. For pelvic-originating free fluid to be visible in the left upper quadrant for example, the fluid must have tracked up the right paracolic gutter, through the right upper quadrant and to the left upper quadrant, implying a significant volume of fluid even if the actual observed amount is quite small. Over 600 cc of pelvic fluid is required before it can be detected in the right upper quadrant [29], but in contrast, trace physiologic free fluid, ranging from 5 to 20 cc, is occasionally identified on pelvis views which may contribute to false-positives [30]. In female patients, fluid isolated to the anatomic cul-de-sac (Pouch of Douglas) is of traumatic origin only 1.8% of the time, whereas 57.7% of patients with upper-quadrant free fluid have injuries [32]. A small amount of visualized fluid does not necessarily represent a small amount of bleeding and, therefore, the scoring of the FAST exam is categorical and not quantitative and must be interpreted in a clinical context of the patient's stability.

The FAST exam remains somewhat controversial in a pediatric patient population, with mixed study results reported. The FAST exam does have moderate to high sensitivity and specificity in hemodynamically unstable pediatric blunt abdominal trauma patients, and does correlate positively with a need for surgical intervention; however, a high sensitivity was only achieved in this population by delaying FAST performance for several hours, which undermines the goal of using FAST to make rapid triage and treatment decisions [33]. Like in adult patients, the routine use of FAST exams in stable pediatric patients is not supported by evidence and demonstrates no benefit as measured by ER length of stay, missed injuries, or cost of care [34].

Finally, all ultrasound investigations are limited by operator abilities. Because FAST, like all ultrasound techniques, depends on a single individual to perform the exam and interpret the results—typically in real time—the quality of the test depends both on the operator's technical ability to capture images and also on the operator's ability to interpret them. Thus, there are two main areas in which an individual operator's success rate may be negatively impacted.

One study investigating operator dependence assessed resident physicians and attending physicians in their reviews of pre-recorded pericardial ultrasounds in penetrating trauma patients. Substantial differences in diagnostic specificity were found between residents and attending physicians (67% vs. 90%) and those self-reporting minimal versus large experience with the ultrasound technique (65% vs. 93%) [35]. Evidence of operator dependence also exists for the detection of hemoperitoneum. One attempt at assessing the FAST learning curve found that novice sonographers have error rates of 17% with incomplete exam rates of 25%; after completing twenty-five studies, both rates decreased to 5% [36]. The optimum number of studies needed to certify competence in FAST performance has not been defined with consensus, and credentialing requirements vary around the globe and by certifying organization.

Summary

The FAST examination is a powerful tool that can potentially change patient management when used as part of a trauma resuscitation. The exam is rapid, provides management-changing information, does not significantly delay other tests or resuscitative efforts, and does not harm the patient when performed without significant delay. A positive FAST examination is an indication of laparotomy in the unstable patient. Negative examinations, which risk possible missed injuries, should always be followed with further investigations such as CT scanning in the stable population. Negative FAST investigations in the unstable trauma patient should prompt a rapid reassessment of the ATLS primary survey, but ultimately persistent hemodynamic instability may be an indication for exploratory surgery regardless of FAST results, recognizing that user experience, training, and exam limitations may contribute to false-negative studies.

Rapid interpretation of FAST results allows the Trauma Team Leader to assess the patient's immediate needs and may reduce delays to operative interventions, costs, and adverse outcomes.

Key Points

- Ultrasound is an important tool in the resuscitation of trauma patients; it is an adjunct to, not a replacement of, existing standards of resuscitation such as the clinical exam or ATLS surveys.
- A negative FAST exam is one where all four regions are thoroughly imaged and no fluid is seen; an indeterminate exam is one where all four regions cannot be adequately imaged.
- Any free fluid in any quadrant, even in an otherwise indeterminate exam, is a positive FAST exam.
- The sensitivity of ultrasound is diminished by inexperienced operators, obesity, COPD, excessive bowel gas, and some associated injuries; a negative exam in an unstable patient is *not* reassuring and warrants further investigation.

References

1. Boulanger BR, Brenneman FD, Kirkpatrick AW, McLellan BA, Nathens AB. The indeterminate abdominal sonogram in multisystem blunt trauma. JTACS. 1998;45(1):52–6.
2. Melniker LA, Leibner E, McKenney MG, Lopez P, Briggs WM, Mancuso CA. Randomized controlled clinical trial of point-of-care limited ultrasonography for trauma in the emergency department: the first sonography outcomes assessment program trial. Ann Emerg Med. 2006;48(3):227–35.
3. Ollerton JE, Sugrue M, Balogh Z, D'Amours SK, Giles A, Wyllie P. Prospective study to evaluate the influence of FAST on trauma patient management. JTACS. 2006;60(4):785–91.
4. Nishijima DK, Simel SL, Wisner DH, Holmes JF. Does this adult patient have a blunt intra-abdominal injury? JAMA. 2012;307(14):1517–27.
5. Wherrett LJ, Boulanger BR, McLellan BA, Brenneman FD, Rizoli SB, Culhane J, Hamilton P. Hypotension after blunt abdominal trauma: the role of emergent abdominal sonography in surgical triage. JTACS. 1996;41(5):815–20.
6. Rozycki GS, Ballard RB, von Feliciano D, Schmidt JA, Pennington SD. Surgeon-performed ultrasound for truncal injuries. Ann Surg. 1998;228(4):557–67.
7. Thomas B, Falcone RE, Vasquez D, Santanello S, Townsend M, Hockenberry S, Innes J, Wanamaker SB. Ultrasound evaluation of blunt abdominal trauma: program implementation, initial experience, and learning curve. JTACS. 1997;42(3):384–90.
8. Ma OJ, Mateer JR, Ogata M, Kefer MP, Wittmann D, Aprahamian C. Prospective analysis of a rapid trauma ultrasound examination performed by emergency physicians. JTACS. 1995;38(6):879–85.
9. Mohammadi A, Ghasemi-rad M. Evaluation of gastrointestinal injury in blunt abdominal trauma "FAST is not reliable": the role of repeated ultrasonography. World J Emerg Surg. 2012;7(1):2–6.
10. Lucas B, Hempel D, Otto R, Brenner F, Stier M, Marzi I, Breitkreutz R, Walcher F. Prehospital FAST reduces time to admission and operative treatment: a prospective, randomized, multicenter trial. Eur J Trauma Emerg Surg. 2021;48:2701.
11. Gamberini L, Tartaglione M, Giugni A, Alban L, Allegri D, Coniglio C, Lupi C, Chiarini V, Mazzoli CA, Heusch-Lazzeri E, Tugnoli G, Gordini G. The role of prehospital ultrasound in reducing time to definitive care in abdominal trauma patients with moderate to severe liver and spleen injuries. Injury. 2022;53(5):1587–95.
12. van der Weide L, Popal Z, Terra M, Schwarte LA, Ket JCF, Kooij FO, Exadaktylos AK, Zuidema WP, Giannakopolous GF. Prehospital ultrasound in the management of trauma patients: systematic review of the literature. Injury. 2022;50(12):2167–75.
13. McKenney M, Lentz K, Nunez D, Sosa JL, Sleeman D, Axelrad A, Martin L, Kirton O, Oldham C. Can ultrasound replace diagnostic peritoneal lavage in the assessment of blunt trauma? JTACS. 1994;37(3):439–41.
14. Farahmand N, Sirlin CB, Brown MA, Shragg GP, Fortlage D, Hoyt DB, Casola G. Hypotensive patients with blunt abdominal trauma: performance of screening US. Radiology. 2005;235(2):436–43.
15. Quinn AC, Sinert R. What is the utility of the focused assessment with sonography in trauma (FAST) exam in penetrating torso trauma? Injury. 2011;42(5):482–7.
16. Boulanger BR, Kearney PA, Tsuei B, Ochoa JB. The routine use of sonography in penetrating torso injury is beneficial. JTACS. 2001;51(2):320–5.
17. Tayal VS, Beatty MA, Marx JA, Tomaszewski CA, Thomason MH. FAST (focused assessment with sonography in trauma) accurate for cardiac and intraperitoneal injury in penetrating anterior chest trauma. J Ultrasound Med. 2004;23(4):467–72.
18. Varin DS, Ringburg AN, van Lieshout EM, Patka P, Schipper IB. Accuracy of conventional imaging of penetrating torso injuries in the trauma resuscitation room. Eur J Emerg Med. 2009;16(6):305–11.
19. Rozycki GS, Feliciano DV, Ochsner MG, Knudson MM, Hoyt DB, Davis F, Hammerman D, Figueredo V, Harviel JD, Han DC, Schmidt JA. The role of ultrasound in patients with possible penetrating cardiac wounds: a prospective multicenter study. JTACS. 1999;46(4):551–2.
20. Rozycki GS, Feliciano DV, Schmidt JA, Cushman JG, Sisley AC, Ingram W, Ansley JD. The role of surgeon-performed ultrasound in patients with possible cardiac wounds. Ann Surg. 1996;223(6):737–44.
21. Inaba K, Chouliaras K, Zakaluzny S, Swadron S, Mailhot T, Seif D, Teixeira P, Sivrikoz E, Ives C, Barmparas G, Koronakis N, Demetriades D. FAST ultrasound examination as a predictor of outcomes after resuscitative thoracotomy. Ann Surg. 2015;262(3):512–8.
22. Shanmuganathan K, Mirvis SE, Sherbourne CD, Chiu WC, Rodriguez A. Hemoperitoneum as the sole indicator of abdominal visceral injuries: a potential limitation of screening abdominal US for trauma. Radiology. 1999;212(2):423–30.
23. Natarajan B, Gupta PK, Prateek K, Gupta MD, Cemaj S, Sorensen M, Hatzoudis GI, Amor FR. FAST scan: is it worth doing in hemodynamically stable blunt trauma patients? Surgery. 2010;148(4):695–701.
24. Miller MT, Pasquale MD, Bromberg WJ, Wasser TE, Cox J. Not so FAST. JTACS. 2003;54(1):59–60.
25. McGahan JP, Rose J, Coates TL, Wisner DH, Newberry P. Use of ultrasound in the patient with acute abdominal trauma. Journal of Ultrasound Medicine. 1997;16(10):653–62.
26. Tso P, Rodriguez A, Cooper C, Militello P, Mirvis S, Badellino MM, Br B, Foss FA Jr, Hinson DM, Mighty HE. Sonography in

blunt abdominal trauma: a preliminary progress report. JTACS. 1992;33(1):39–43.
27. Lingawi SS, Buckley AR. Focused abdominal US in patients with trauma. Radiology. 2000;217(2):426–9.
28. Dolich MO, McKenny MG, Varela JE, Compton RP, McKenney KL, Cohn SM. 2576 ultrasounds for blunt abdominal trauma. JTACS. 2001;50(1):108–12.
29. Udobi KF, Rodriguez A, Chiu WC, Scalea TM. Role of ultrasonography in penetrating abdominal trauma: a prospective clinical study. JTACS. 2001;50(3):475–9.
30. Soffer D, McKenny MG, Cohn S, Garcia-Roca R, Namias N, Schulman C, Lynn M, Lopez P. A prospective evaluation of ultrasonography for the diagnosis of penetrating trauma. JTACS. 2004;56(5):953–9.
31. Hoffman L, Pierce D, Puumala S. Clinical predictors of injuries not identified by focused abdominal sonogram for trauma (FAST) examinations. J Emerg Med. 2009;36(3):271–9.
32. Tayal VS, Nielsen A, Jones AE, Thomason MH, Kellam J, Norton HJ. Accuracy of trauma ultrasound in major pelvic injury. JTACS. 2006;61(6)1453:1457.
33. Long MK, Vohra MK, Bonnette A, Vega Parra PD, Miller SK, Ayub E, Wang HE, Cardenas-Turanzas M, Gordon R, Ugalde IT, Allukian M, Smith HE. Focused assessment with sonography for trauma in predicting early surgical intervention in hemodynamically unstable children with blunt abdominal trauma. JACEP. 2022;3(1):emp2.12650:e12650.
34. Holmes JF, Kelley KM, Wootton-Gorges SL, Utter GH, Abramson LP, Rose JS, Tancredi DJ, Kuppermann N. Effect of abdominal ultrasound on clinical care, outcomes, and resource use among children with blunt torso trauma. JAMA. 2017;317(22):2290–6.
35. Blaivas M, DeBehnke D, Phelan MB. Potential errors in the diagnosis of pericardial effusion on trauma ultrasound for penetrating injuries. Acad Emerg Med. 2000;7(11):1261–6.
36. Shackford SR, Rogers FB, Osler TM, Trabulsy ME, Clauss DW, Vane DW. Focused abdominal sonogram for trama: the learning curve of nonradiologist clinicians in detecting Hemoperitoneum. JTACS. 1999;46(4):553–62.

Trauma Ultrasound: Beyond the FAST Examination

45

Michael Blaivas, Ashot E. Sargsyan, and Dimitrios Karakitsos

Introduction

Ultrasound in the evaluation of the trauma patient has moved far beyond the simple search for free fluid in the abdomen as a marker of intra-peritoneal hemorrhage from solid organ injury. The modern clinician evaluating and treating a trauma patient employs ultrasound to search not only for blood in the abdomen but also detect solid organ injury as well as trauma to the chest, head, and extremities. In fact, as ultrasound use grows by clinicians and they become familiar with more advanced musculoskeletal and vascular applications, a more extensive evaluation with ultrasound will become the norm rather than the exception. In this chapter, we focus on advanced trauma ultrasound applications.

Trauma Ultrasound Development

The basis of advanced trauma ultrasound is still the original FAST application. Its history dates back to the 1980s and it was used successfully with good reliability by German trauma surgeons [1–3]. In time, the FAST examination migrated to North America where, despite competing with computed tomography, it spread widely among trauma surgeons and emergency physicians who used it to evaluate first blunt and then penetrating trauma patients. Eventually, it replaced the diagnostic peritoneal lavage (DPL) [4, 5] except for certain rare circumstances (DPL and its current role are discussed further in Chap. 33). While initially compared to clinical outcomes in Germany, which yielded extremely high sensitivity and specificity, the FAST examination revealed potential pitfalls when compared to computed tomography. These included missed liver and splenic injuries which did not hemorrhage into the peritoneal cavity [6–9].

Initially excluded from the patient group evaluated with a FAST examination, penetrating cardiac injuries have been well studied in trauma patients, and without question, ultrasound can deliver rapid and critical diagnosis when it reveals the presence of pericardial effusion [10, 11]. Further, impending hemodynamic compromise may be diagnosed when evidence of early tamponade is suspected due to right atrial and ventricular free wall movement or collapse. An early study by Plummer documented the impact of cardiac ultrasound as part of the FAST examination in averting patient deaths from unsuspected pericardial effusion and tamponade [11]. The authors noted a decrease from 50% to 0% mortality in patients when comparing those presenting prior to ultrasound use and after. Rozycki performed a large-scale study of trauma surgeons evaluating for pericardial effusion in cases of penetrating trauma [10]. The investigators reported that trauma surgeons accurately diagnosed pericardial effusions from penetrating cardiac injury.

Despite the large number of studies from radiology, trauma surgery, and emergency medicine researchers, there was a paucity of data that utilizing ultrasound in the care of the traumatized patient improved outcomes and decreased cost or mortality. A study by Melniker et al., despite its small size, accurately documented the impact of the FAST examination on traumatized patient care [12]. The authors found that time to operative care was 64% less for patients receiving a FAST exam compared to control patients who did not. FAST patients underwent fewer CTs with an odds ratio of 0.16. They also spent 27% fewer days in hospital and had fewer complications (odds ratio 0.16). Finally, of critical importance for the modern health care economies, FAST patients had lower hospital charges that were 35% less compared to control or non-FAST patients.

M. Blaivas (✉) · D. Karakitsos
Department of Emergency Medicine, School of Medicine, University of South Carolina, Columbia, SC, USA
e-mail: mike@blaivas.org

A. E. Sargsyan
Wyle Science, Technology & Engineering Group/NASA Bioastronautics, Houston, TX, USA
e-mail: Ashot.Sargsyan@us.kbr.com

L. Marshall Gillman, S. Widder (eds.), *Trauma Team Dynamics*, https://doi.org/10.1007/978-3-031-86312-7_45

The FAST Examination in Critical Review

The FAST has seen its fair share of controversy with questions about sensitivity, specificity, as well as utility in the modern computed tomography-driven trauma assessment [13, 14]. A Cochrane review of trauma ultrasound in 2013 evaluated the impact of the FAST examination on trauma patient outcomes [15]. Despite the poorly performed study, it raised important questions about ultrasound in abdominal trauma and suggested not only that better-designed studies are needed but also there is a requirement for more research documenting the impact of ultrasound in abdominal trauma.

In addition, various non-trauma pathologies such as preexisting ascites, acute intra-abdominal infections with and without gastrointestinal perforation, cancer perforations, and sterile serositis (e.g., from familial Mediterranean fever or connective tissue disease) may result in the acute or subacute accumulation of liquid matter in the abdominal cavity, which in turn may render the patient FAST-positive. Many of these fluid collections will be small or even trace fluid amounts and ascites from liver cirrhosis are often found with particular findings allowing identification as to the underlying cause. Despite this, interpretation of FAST findings should always be performed with caution by physicians and in the clinical context of the individual case scenario. Rapid, sterile fluid sampling, either via formal DPL or via a simpler diagnostic peritoneal aspirate (DPA), may be still useful in this setting.

Ultrasound Equipment and Settings

The standard ultrasound equipment required for a FAST examination is quite simple as much of the latter can be performed with just one transducer. The curved abdominal transducer with a frequency range of 2 to 5 MHz is commonly utilized; however, it is severely limited in cardiac imaging, and a phased array or micro-convex transducer may be needed in patients who are obese or have other co-morbidities [16]. Ideally, the operator will have a modern ultrasound machine with good imaging capability and adequate penetration for the rapidly growing proportion of obese patients in the developed world. A machine that allows rapid, one-touch changes in ultrasound transducer selection is important. Additionally, the optimal ultrasound unit not only requires a short boot-up time (less than 15 s), but also the time required for a new transducer to be ready to scan upon switching has to be very short (less than 5 s). Documentation capability is critical and digital video loops should be stored on the machine. Ideally, there would be capability to annotate and export loops for later review and integration into the medical record. A micro-convex transducer has a narrow footprint allowing easier cardiac imaging, especially if the traditional subxiphoid window does not yield adequate results. However, it also provides worse resolution for the abdominal portion of the examination when compared to a typical curved abdominal transducer. Thus, many established programs and experienced individuals prefer to have more than one transducer at their disposal including a curved abdominal and phased array.

Additional Ultrasound Applications in Trauma

Additional Equipment and Views

The additional applications involved in trauma ultrasound examination essentially mandate a linear array transducer. While a curved array can be used as well as a micro-convex or phased array, most sonographers will quickly grow frustrated with the image resolution and difficulty in interpretation. The linear array transducer will allow for required high resolution in the near field of several applications. Apart from two-dimensional imaging, the application of various other modes such as M-mode, color, and power Doppler is important.

Pleural Effusion

The simplest extension of the basic FAST is the additional view acquired while examining the right and left upper quadrants. As mentioned previously, a focused look at the dome of the liver, spleen, and diaphragms is a critical portion of the modern FAST examination. That same view affords the ability to detect fluid in the right or left hemithorax. Studies suggest as little as 25 cc of fluid may be detected [17]. While the clinical significance of such a small collection is questionable, the ability to detect fluid more accurately than plane radiograph is an important tool [18]. Fluid will appear as anechoic, or dark, with the typical stipulation that coagulating blood will be more echogenic. The lung may be seen moving in the fluid (Fig. 45.1). Best imaged with a phased array transducer when scanning through ribs posteriorly, most sonographers simply

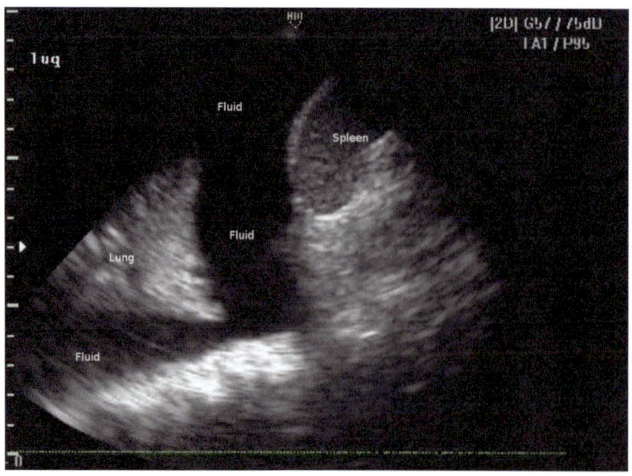

Fig. 45.1 Dark or anechoic fluid surrounds the relatively echogenic lung

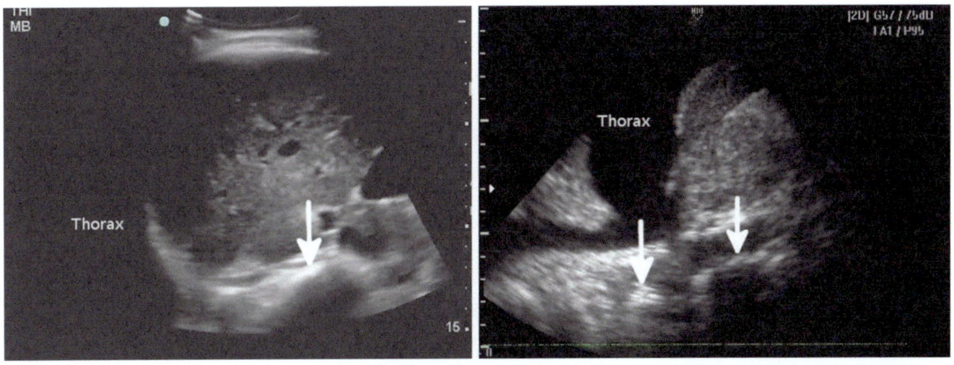

Fig. 45.2 The left image shows an ultrasound with no fluid in the chest; the spine seems to end at the diaphragm and cannot be traced further (arrow). The right image shows a collection of fluid in the chest, with the spine continuing above the diaphragm (arrows)

pan their curved abdominal transducer ultrasound beam more cephalad and make sure to include the diaphragm on both the left and right sides. A helpful sign that brings the novice's attention to fluid in the chest is looking for the spine above the diaphragm [19]. Typically not noted without a good acoustic window, which is provided by fluid in the chest, it is an obvious sign that fluid is present in the chest (Fig. 45.2). This is more important than ever because modern equipment can eliminate echoes typically seen above the diaphragm to such an extent as to leave a dark, anechoic area above the hemidiaphragm when no fluid is present. The volume of an effusion can even be roughly estimated using one of several simple methods [20, 21]. A hemothorax can be followed for changes in size and moderate increases should be obvious.

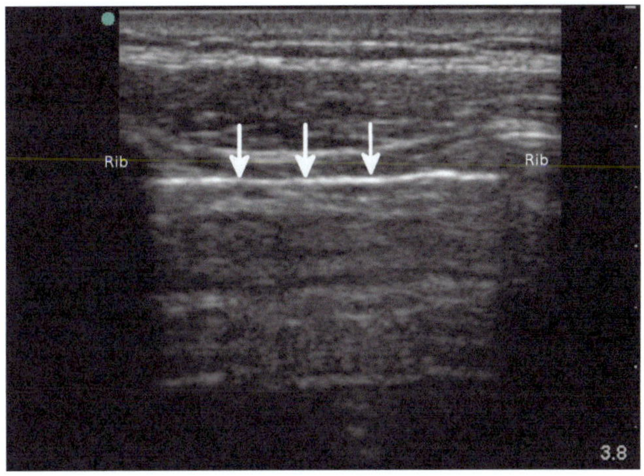

Fig. 45.3 The white line (arrows) in between the ribs is the pleural line, the visceral and parietal pleura cannot be distinguished

Pneumothorax

One of the most popular and clinically useful advanced trauma ultrasound applications is the detection and exclusion of pneumothorax. The basis for this application is that ultrasound can detect the back-and-forth movement of the visceral and parietal pleura occurring during lung expansion and contraction, something that should be present in spontaneously breathing and ventilated patients. While ultrasound does not detail lung parenchyma in the healthy lung, it does show the pleural line, without distinguishing visceral from parietal pleura (Fig. 45.3). In order to visualize the movement of the layers past each other, known as the Sliding Lung Sign (SLS), both the visceral and parietal pleura must be imaged. However, when air is present between the layers as in the case of a pneumothorax, it blocks diagnostic ultrasound from imaging the visceral pleura since medical ultrasound is not transmitted through air [22, 23]. Thus, when air is present between the visceral and parietal pleura, ultrasound shows loss of the sliding lung sign. Confirmation of lung sliding can be verified using M- Mode. The area under investigation, between the ribs shadows, is centered in the screen, while M-Mode is initiated after aligning the vertical line through the area in question. The "Barcode sign" or "stratosphere sign" is the appearance of parallel horizontal lines extending through the entire field in view, which indicates the lack of normal motion of an inflated lung on M-mode (Fig. 45.4). While lack of Lung Sliding is not specific to pneumothorax, the presence of Lung Sliding sign effectively rules out pneumothorax at the intercostal locations under the applied ultrasound probe. The sensitivity and specificity of this sign have varied significantly in multiple studies. Reported values have ranged from 40 to 99% and 60 to 100% for sensitivity and specificity, respectively [24–28].

The lung ultrasound examination was traditionally performed using a rudimentary micro-convex transducer [29]. However, modern lung ultrasound for evaluation of pneumothorax is best performed using a high-resolution linear ultrasound transducer. Such a transducer allows high-resolution imaging of the pleural interface and enables the sonographer to detect subtle sliding of the pleural surfaces. Improved imaging can lead to higher confidence when such movement is absent, a problem with earlier ultrasound probes. In the trauma patient, the intra-thoracic air will seek the least gravitationally dependent area in the chest. Therefore, if the patient is supine, it should be in the anterior chest. Both sides of the chest should be evaluated. The ultrasound transducer is placed in a sagittal orientation with the indicator pointed

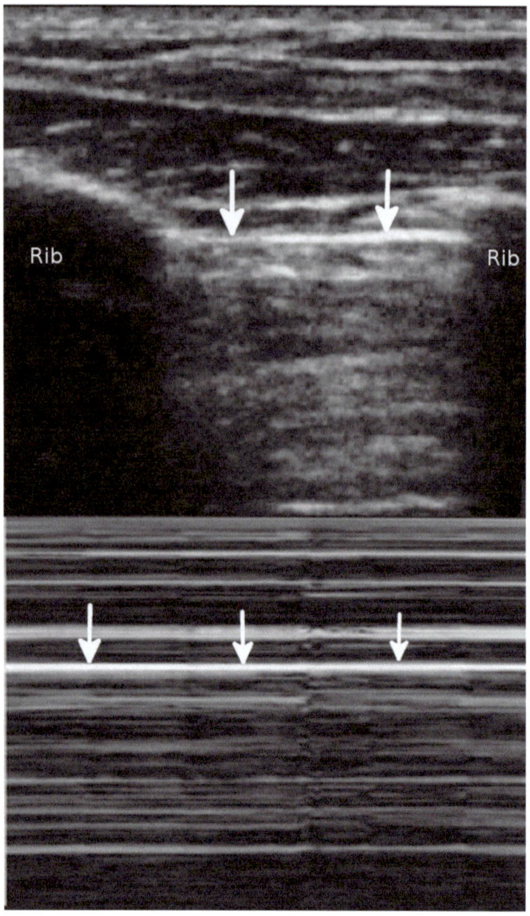

Fig. 45.4 The stratosphere or barcode sign. No movement occurs above or below the pleural line on the m-mode tracing as signified by the identical appearance above and below the pleural line (arrows). This occurs as a result of the pneumothorax preventing visualization of the visceral pleura

cephalad. This allows one to use ribs as an anatomic landmark (Fig. 45.5). This is important since multiple tissue lines may be present that simulate a pleural line and could be confusing. The pleural line will be just deep to the ribs as noted. In the normal lung, it will be seen moving back and forth, typically disappearing under the bony ribs. This movement will be timed to respirations, not the heart rate. When the lung sliding appears to be stunted, but still present (sometimes described as shimmering), and is timed to the heart rate, it is likely a lung pulse [30]. The lung pulse occurs when no pneumothorax is present to introduce air between the visceral and parietal pleura. However, if the lung is not ventilated, such as in a misplaced endotracheal tube, the pleural line will appear to pulse, not moving significantly, in time with the heart. The identification of a lung pulse can be coupled with simple deductive reasoning to decide if a main stem or esophageal intubation is present. If seen unilaterally, a lung pulse should indicate ipsilateral main stem bronchus intubation or obstruction such as mucous plugging [31].

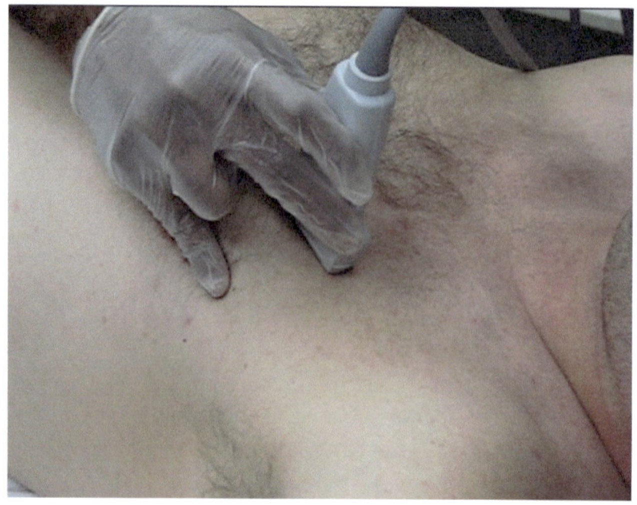

Fig. 45.5 The ultrasound transducer is in a cephalad orientation resulting in a sagittal scanning plane

Absence bilaterally suggests an esophageal intubation or tracheal obstruction. Appropriate correction such as slowly pulling back the endotracheal tube in a main-stem intubation can be tracked in real time by observing the disappearance of a unilateral lung pulse as the tube is pulled back.

While pleural line sliding may be absent not only in cases of pneumothorax, given a clinical setting where PTX is high in the differential, an absent SLS may be critical for clinical decision-making. Pathologic processes that may eliminate the SLS also include pneumonia, COPD (especially in the case of bullae formation), and others. A near pathognomonic finding for PTX is the lung point [32]. The lung point is literally the intersection of normal lungs with free intra-thoracic air or PTX. Additionally, other artifacts from the pleura such as echogenic B lines may be seen sliding in and out as the normal lung moves in and out of view [32]. While several pitfalls with this finding can be seen including the edge of the heart, diaphragm, and contused lung, careful scanning and awareness of nearby anatomy makes this sign almost 100% specific [33]. It is important to note that as a PTX increases in size, the lung point will become more lateral and posterior in a supine patient and then disappear completely as no visceral pleura can be seen contacting the parietal pleura anywhere along the thoracic wall (Fig. 45.6).

Resuscitation and Volume Status

Adding a view of the inferior vena cava to the cardiac assessment allows the operator to assess patient volume status and potential rates of blood loss [34–38]. While not without controversy, since the IVC diameter and collapsibility is a well-proven monitor of volume status in its extremes (such as significant collapse or greater than 2 cm dilation with no

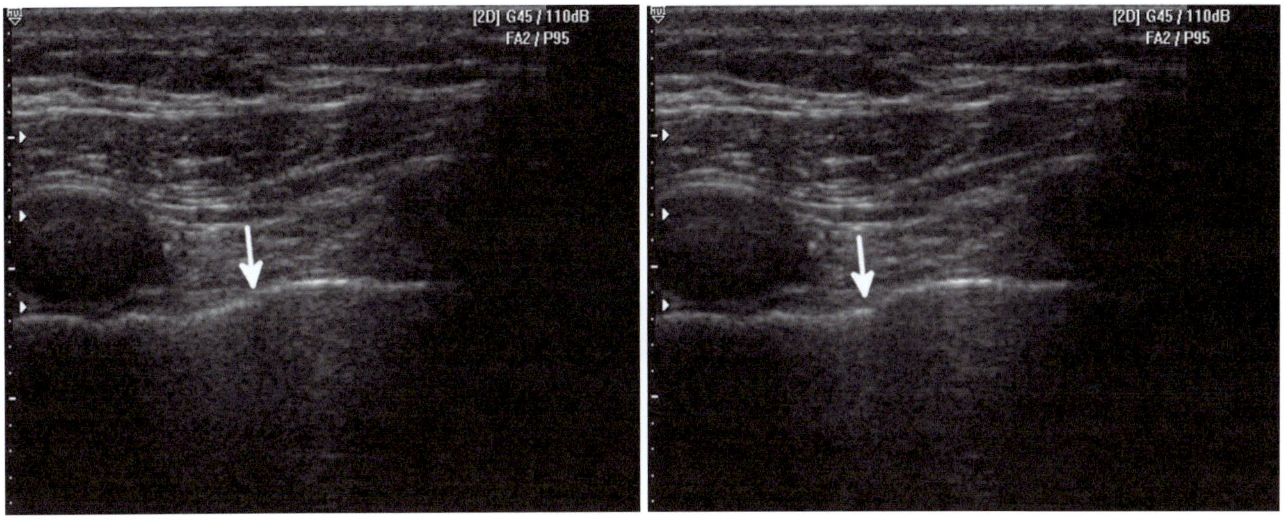

Fig. 45.6 A lung point is demonstrated, with pleural sliding and aerated lung on the left side of the screen and the beginning of the pneumothorax or intra-pleural air on the right. The left image lung point is in a different location than the right image (arrow depicts the leading edge). The lung point location changes with respiration

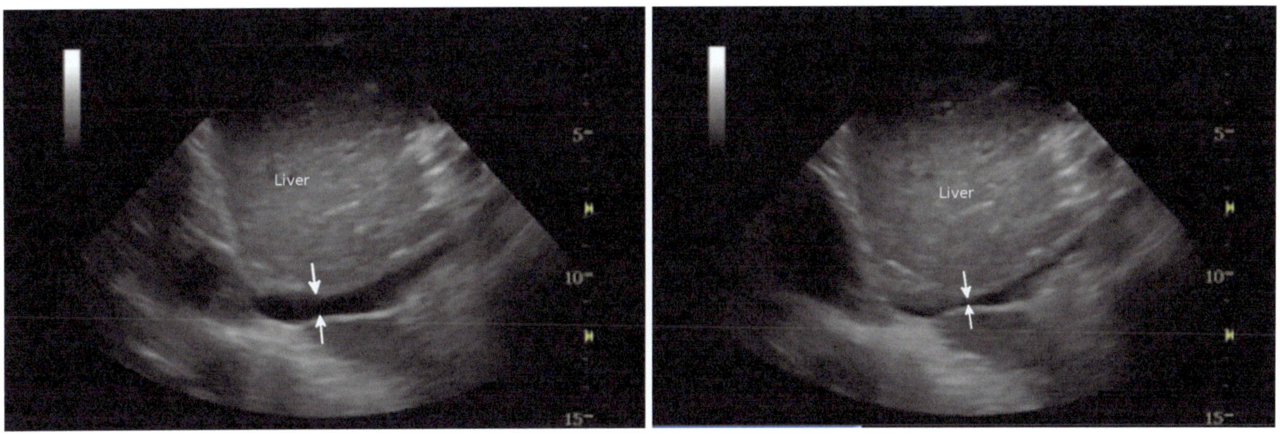

Fig. 45.7 The left image shows an IVC prior to a normal inspiration; it does not appear significantly collapsed (arrows). The right image shows significant collapse of the IVC with respiration. With deep breath, the IVC could not be visualized due to flattening

variation), it is a reasonable adjunct in the trauma patient. Studies of dehydrated or volume-depleted patients have shown that an IVC that collapses completely with normal respiration is an indicator of low intra-vascular volume and also low central venous pressure (Fig. 45.7). Conversely, a dilated, non-varying IVC that is greater than 2 cm in diameter measured 2 cm distal to the confluence of the hepatic veins into the IVC, suggests fluid overload and increased central venous pressures. In trauma patients, it is the flat, completely collapsing IVC that is likely to be of greatest concern. This is especially useful in cases where blood loss may be suspected but cannot be proven in an unstable patient. One study suggested that as little as 450cc of blood removed over 5 min may be detected by serial IVC measurements [38]. However, other studies have called this into question [39]. None of the studies, either pro or con, have had the power to settle the argument [40]. However, the principle is potentially useful. One should be cautious, however, as this assessment may become less accurate in patients on positive pressure ventilation as the elevated intra-thoracic pressures may mask the IVC variability.

Musculoskeletal Ultrasound

In terms of clinical logistics, our research group has recently launched the holistic approach (HOLA) concept of critical care ultrasound (CCU) imaging. We have envisioned HOLA-CCU as part of the patient examination by a clinician to visualize all or any parts of the body, tissues, organs, and systems in their live, anatomically, and functionally interconnected state and in the context of the whole patient's clinical circumstances [40]. In that sense, any ultrasound view obtained through the skin contains some information about soft tissues. While serving as imaging window and anatomical reference structures in focused techniques (e.g., the chest wall in lung scanning), soft tissues themselves are often a primary target (e.g., in extremity injury). This is particularly true regarding musculoskeletal (MSK) ultrasound scanning [41, 42]. Ultrasound in MSK evaluation is well established and not surprisingly has been adopted for trauma patient evaluation as well. High-resolution ultrasound imaging through the use of linear array transducers allows a detailed look at the cortex of long bones, ribs, and other structures. Since nearly all fractures should involve some sort of cortical disruption, a highly magnified look at the cortex is ideal for detecting fractures. In trauma cases, some of the long bones sought may be quite deep, and curved abdominal transducers may need to be utilized to image the femur, especially in large patients. Already present at the patient's bedside, ultrasound allows detection of fractures such as the one seen here in the femoral shaft of a motor vehicle accident patient (Fig. 45.8).

Bony cortex is seen as a bright echogenic line, typically linear. The ultrasound examination should be performed in at least two orthogonal planes as with any organ of interest. Especially with bones such as the radius and ulna, one axis may appear grossly normal, while the orthogonal one shows a step off, suggesting a fracture that can be investigated more closely. Typically a long bone is imaged in its longitudinal and transverse axes. In the short axis, a long bone such as the humerus or femur will be curved while the tibia will relatively flat. The key is to focus on any cortical disruptions. The operator must take the patient's age into account and avoid mistaking growth plate regions for fractures. One of the single most useful aspects of MSK ultrasound is that a normal comparison is almost always readily available in the form of the contralateral limb or side of the torso.

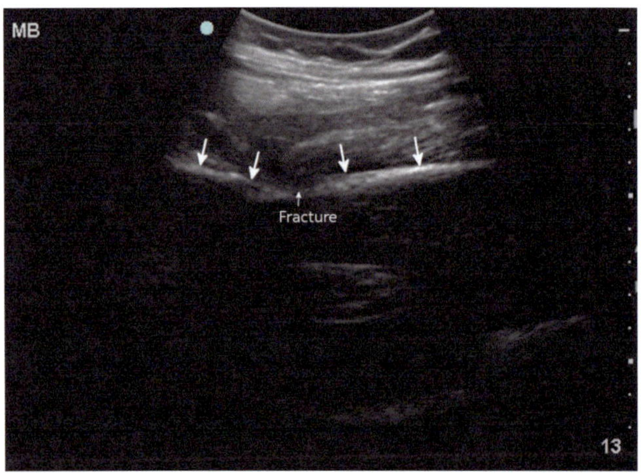

Fig. 45.8 A disruption is seen in the cortical continuity of the femur in this femoral shaft fracture. Notice the change in the angle (arrows) of the femoral shaft

Apart from bone pathology, ultrasound has the potential to detect muscle, tendon, and soft tissue pathology in trauma victims. Acute muscle contusion and hemorrhage appear hyperechoic, while later stages of injury exhibit mixed patterns. Partial or complete musculotendinous tears with or without retraction are usually obvious. Intramuscular hematomas may later evolve into seromas or intramuscular cysts (anechoic fluid collections) that may require aspiration or surgical drainage. Hypoechoic muscular swelling with architectural disorganization may be observed in traumatic rhabdomyolysis.

In crush injuries, ultrasound can assist in critical decision-making and have extremity and life-saving significance, since a buildup of pressure within the fascial compartment disrupts tissue perfusion (compartment syndrome) with dire consequences unless fasciotomy is emergently performed. An advanced HOLA protocol in extremity crush injuries could include assessment of (a) the shape and structure of all the fascial compartments (looking for outward convexity of the normally flat fascial partitions between compartments), fractures, tears, hematomas, and hypoechoic areas of potential fluid collection or necrosis); (b) color and pulsed-wave Doppler monitoring of the vessels within the compartment and the main artery feeding the compartment; (c) renal imaging (monitoring of size/volume, renal arterial spectral Doppler, and parenchymal differentiation); and (d) search for free abdominal fluid if the thigh and pelvis areas are involved.

Head Trauma

Ultrasound in head trauma offers surprising utility. The same MSK applications described above apply to the skull, and remarkable detail can be noted such as small disruptions in the smooth bony cortex. Any disruption in the cortex or step-off may be a skull fracture line. Evaluation in two orthogonal planes will help better define the area in question. Suture lines have a potential for confusion, but some practice scanning the normal skull will help the sonologist become familiar with their appearance. Additionally, most skull fractures will be associated with an overlying soft tissue hematoma [43]. In children, suture lines, especially partially closed ones and fontanels, may present additional challenges. However, known anatomic locations and the ability to trace the suture line and evaluate any skull fractures in two orthogonal planes allow one to differentiate between a traumatic injury and normal anatomy. Facial fractures can also be detected using a linear array transducer but require more experience. Again, the sonologist looks for cortical disruptions of facial bones and compares the injured and uninjured sides whenever possible. The ultrasound literature contains studies documenting ultrasound's high accuracy in the evaluation of the sinuses and blood-filled sinuses and orbital air, and a multitude of other injuries can be diagnosed with sufficient skill [44–46].

There is additional utility to ultrasound in estimating and tracking intracranial pressure (ICP). While direct visualization of brain injury in the adult is rarely possible with ultrasound, a secondary marker of significant (although sometimes still non-operative) brain injury is elevation in the ICP. When significant brain injury results from trauma, it is typically associated with some level of elevation in ICP. With a large intracranial hemorrhage, this may be a marked elevation, while with a smaller one, the elevation is relatively minor. Dating back to the 1960s, researchers realized the spinal fluid bathing the optic nerve inside the optic nerve sheath communicated directly with the ventricles [47]. Any rise in ICP from the ventricles was noted almost instantaneously in the optic nerve sheath. Being a distensible structure, the sheath dilates in a somewhat predictable fashion. Multiple studies have evaluated the utility of measuring the optic nerve sheath diameter (ONSD) in trauma and other patients [48]. The main challenges are careful technique and inter-operator reliability. Due to the relatively small-size changes involved, precise measurements are required. However, a recent meta-analysis suggested that ONSD measurement had utility in predicting elevated ICP and in trauma suggesting intracranial injury [49]. While CT may be the common test of choice in most trauma setting, it is not ubiquitously available in all locations and is very expensive. During transport and for serial monitoring, ONSD measurement through ocular ultrasound holds considerable promise and utility in the right clinical context until other technologies are developed that are also noninvasive, affordable, but largely user-independent.

To perform an ONSD measurement, a linear ultrasound transducer is the probe of choice and the scan is performed through a closed lid. Both eyes should be scanned when possible for comparison. A large amount of gel is placed in the orbit for good coupling and also to avoid any pressure on the eye. In the ideal technique, the ultrasound screen will show an obvious anechoic stripe at the top of the screen signifying the presence of gel between the transducer and eyelid. While sophisticated equipment may be able to measure some transmission of pressure through ultrasound gel, it is not of any physical significance. Sterile gel can be used and is widely available in small lubricant packets in clinical settings. Wiping off the gel has to occur with great care to avoid pressing on the globe if ocular injury is suspected or noted on ultrasound. As an aside, ultrasound is superb at detecting several ocular injuries such as lens displacement, globe rupture, retinal detachments, and vitreous bleeding. However, the optic nerve is the goal of this examination and is visualized just posterior to the globe. The ideal for simple measurement of the ONSD is to obtain a clear image of the optic nerve as it travels posterior from the globe. Measured at approximately 3 mm posterior to the globe, the internal diameter should be obtained several times and averaged (Fig. 45.9). A meta-analysis suggested that using a cutoff value around 5.8 mm may be reasonable [49]. Our group has recently suggested new quality criteria for sonographic ONSD measurements which are summarized below:

- ONSD measurement should not be made through the lens.
- Sonographic differentiation between the nerve proper and the arachnoid (CSF space) must be obvious.
- The outer border of the arachnoid must be identifiable for actual ONSD measurement; clear, well-focused images must thus allow confident measurement of the inner diameter of the dural sheath.
- Ideal views of the optic nerve demonstrate the point of its penetration into the globe.
- Good views offer opportunities for additional information potentially useful with growing experience, such as tortuosity of the nerve, hypo-echogenicity of the arachnoid, and its irregularity due to distention of CSF-containing "cells."
- Correct standardized measurements: since the most distensible portion of the sheath is at the 3–4 mm distance from the vitreo-retinal interface, measurements should be performed at this level in a direction perpendicular to the axis of the nerve. In extreme gaze deviations, this may be difficult to achieve due to the acute angle between the nerve axis and the posterior wall of the globe.

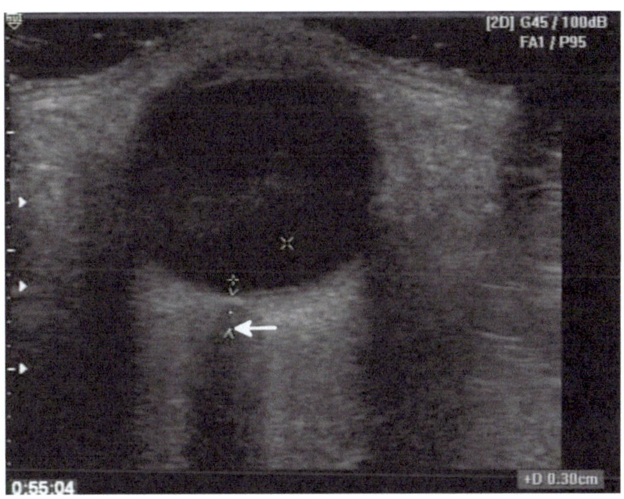

Fig. 45.9 A normal optic nerve sheath diameter is seen. The transverse measurement should be taken at a location 3 mm posterior to the globe (arrow)

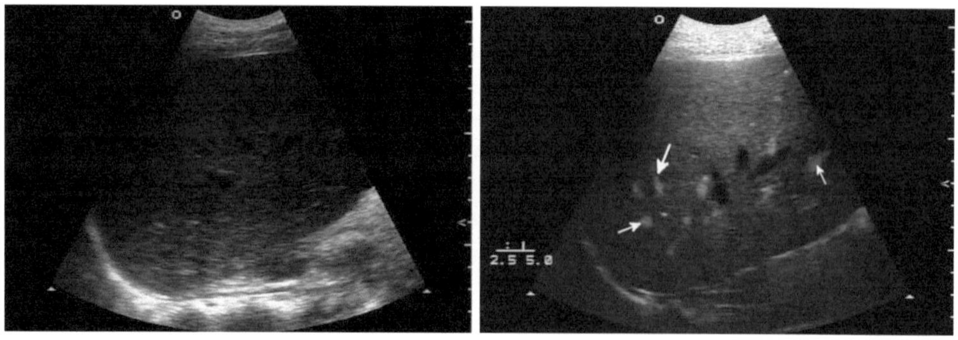

Fig. 45.10 Contrast material is seen appearing in the liver on the right image (arrows). Prior to contrast administration, the liver on the left lacked the glow provided by the intravenous contrast agent

- It is highly recommended to measure ONSD bilaterally and in more than one image frame.
- For ONSD trend monitoring, the previous record with images must be reviewed to ensure similar views and measurement techniques [50].

Contrast-Enhanced Ultrasound

One of the most significant limitations of trauma ultrasound is a relative insensitivity to solid organ injury detection when free fluid in the abdomen is absent. While such liver and spleen fractures may not be as immediately threatening, they do pose potential for morbidity and even mortality and should not go undetected. Ultrasound contrast, while still not approved for use in the United States for body imaging, is widely used in the rest of the world. Studies have indicated that trauma team members can rapidly perform FAST examinations with ultrasound contrast use, and one dose of agent may last long enough for the examination to be completed. The contrast could be seen even with a rudimentary ultrasound machine. More recent literature has suggested an impressive sensitivity and specificity of ultrasound for solid organ detection when used with contrast. While still lagging behind the gold standard of computed tomography, contrast-enhanced ultrasound is much less expensive and delivers no ionizing radiation.

Although contrast agents vary in their length of effect and phases, in general, the liver and spleen appear to glow actively after contrast agent injection (Fig. 45.10). An area of hematoma or lack of active perfusion is outlined by surrounding contrast-enhanced tissue. Similarly, active bleeding may be denoted by a concentration or pooling of contrast agents in some cases. Delayed phases of some contrast agents as they are being absorbed by cells in the liver or spleen may further outline the area of hematoma or even active bleeding. One group from Italy reported a sensitivity of 91.4% and a specificity of 100% in a group of 32 traumatized patients, stating that it was almost as sensitive as CT [51]. Clearly, the future for contrast-enhanced trauma ultrasound is potentially bright and appears to be largely unwritten. With the increased realization of the dangers of medical ionizing radiation from CT and this technologies overuse and expense to health care systems, contrast ultrasound will likely see further development and utilization.

Future Directions in Trauma Ultrasound

It is likely that the future of trauma ultrasound will heavily involve the utilization of not only contrast agent as suggested above but also three-dimensional imaging. Several studies have suggested the utility of 3D ultrasound imaging in trauma. When applied to other disease processes, 3D ultrasound has revolutionized pelvic organ evaluation as well as studies of the liver. Vascular ultrasound is benefiting from 3D technology, and other sectors of ultrasound are likely to follow. The ability to image an organ or section of the organ in three dimensions is critical in the overall evaluation of its architecture and function. By utilizing this technology, the severity of injury or size of a hematoma in a liver may be better detailed, the tract and damage from a projectile in a leg may be traced, and the potential for damage to nearby vital structures may be fully appreciated.

Conclusions

Advanced trauma ultrasound applications allow the clinician to evaluate for more pathology than ever thought possible when the FAST examination was first created. In fact, it is evolving into a head-to-toe focused diagnostic imaging evaluation. In the future, trauma ultrasound is likely to further be enhanced by newly developed and upcoming technology. The expansion beyond the basic FAST is inevitable, given the multiple challenges health care systems face around the world and the efficiency and accuracy ultrasound presents at the patients' bedside.

Key Notes

- The FAST examination lacks sensitivity for solid organ injury without intra-peritoneal hemorrhage.
- Evaluation for blood in the thorax is a simple modification of the typical FAST examination.
- A linear transducer is important for the evaluation of long bone injury, pneumothorax, and elevation in intracranial pressure.
- Sonologists should practice and become familiar with advanced techniques before attempting these applications on actual trauma patients as several require additional experience and expertise.
- Technical advances in other ultrasound fields continue to filter down into trauma ultrasound and expand its utility including through contrast-enhanced evaluation of solid organ injury and three-dimensional evaluation of hemorrhage.

References

1. Wening JV. Evaluation of ultrasound, lavage, and computed tomography in blunt abdominal trauma. Surg Endosc. 1989;3(3):152–8.
2. Grüessner R, Mentges B, Düber C, Rückert K, Rothmund M. Sonography versus peritoneal lavage in blunt abdominal trauma. J Trauma. 1989;29(2):242–4.
3. Hoffmann R, Nerlich M, Muggia-Sullam M, Pohlemann T, Wippermann B, Regel G, Tscherne H. Blunt abdominal trauma in cases of multiple trauma evaluated by ultrasonography: a prospective analysis of 291 patients. J Trauma. 1992;32(4):452–8.
4. Bhan C, Forshaw MJ, Bew DP, Kapadia YK. Diagnostic peritoneal lavage and ultrasonography for blunt abdominal trauma: attitudes and training of current general surgical trainees. Eur J Emerg Med. 2007;14(4):212–5.
5. Chak Wah K, Wai Man C, Janet Yuen Ha W, Lai V, Kit Shing John W. Evolving frontiers in severe polytrauma management – refining the essential principles. Malays J Med Sci. 2013;20(1):1–12.
6. Natarajan B, Gupta PK, Cemaj S, Sorensen M, Hatzoudis GI, Forse RA. FAST scan: is it worth doing in hemodynamically stable blunt trauma patients? Surgery. 2010;148(4):695–700.
7. Schnüriger B, Kilz J, Inderbitzin D, Schafer M, Kickuth R, Luginbühl M, Candinas D, Exadaktylos AK, Zimmermann H. The accuracy of FAST in relation to grade of solid organ injuries: a retrospective analysis of 226 trauma patients with liver or splenic lesion. BMC Med Imaging. 2009;9:3. https://doi.org/10.1186/1471-2342-9-3.
8. Kirkpatrick AW, Sirois M, Laupland KB, Goldstein L, Brown DR, Simons RK, Dulchavsky S, Boulanger BR. Prospective evaluation of hand-held focused abdominal sonography for trauma (FAST) in blunt abdominal trauma. Can J Surg. 2005;48(6):453–60.
9. Coley BD, Mutabagani KH, Martin LC, Zumberge N, Cooney DR, Caniano DA, Besner GE, Groner JI, Shiels WE 2nd. Focused abdominal sonography for trauma (FAST) in children with blunt abdominal trauma. J Trauma. 2000;48(5):902–6.
10. Plummer D, Brunette D, Asinger R, Ruiz E. Emergency department echocardiography improves outcome in penetrating cardiac injury. Ann Emerg Med. 1992;21(6):709–12.
11. Rozycki GS, Feliciano DV, Ochsner MG, Knudson MM, Hoyt DB, Davis F, Hammerman D, Figueredo V, Harviel JD, Han DC, Schmidt JA. The role of ultrasound in patients with possible penetrating cardiac wounds: a prospective multicenter study. J Trauma. 1999;46(4):543–51.
12. Melniker LA, Leibner E, McKenney MG, Lopez P, Briggs WM, Mancuso CA. Randomized controlled clinical trial of point-of-care, limited ultrasonography for trauma in the emergency department: the first sonography outcomes assessment program trial. Ann Emerg Med. 2006;48(3):227–35.
13. Vassiliadis J, Edwards R, Larcos G, Hitos K. Focused assessment with sonography for trauma patients by clinicians: initial experience and results. Emerg Med (Fremantle). 2003;15(1):42–8.
14. McGahan JP, Rose J, Coates TL, Wisner DH, Newberry P. Use of ultrasonography in the patient with acute abdominal trauma. J Ultrasound Med. 1997;16(10):653–62.
15. Stengel D, Bauwens K, Rademacher G, Ekkernkamp A, Güthoff C. Emergency ultrasound-based algorithms for diagnosing blunt abdominal trauma. Cochrane Database Syst Rev. 2013;7:CD004446.
16. Finkelhor RS, Moallem M, Bahler RC. Characteristics and impact of obesity on the outpatient echocardiography laboratory. Am J Cardiol. 2006;97(7):1082–4.
17. Lichtenstein DA. Ultrasound in the management of thoracic disease. Crit Care Med. 2007;35(5 Suppl):S250–61.
18. Ma OJ, Mateer JR. Trauma ultrasound examination versus chest radiography in the detection of hemothorax. Ann Emerg Med. 1997;29(3):312–5.
19. Tirado A, Wu T, Noble VE, Huang C, Lewiss RE, Martin JA, Murphy MC, Sivitz A, Cohen SG. Ultrasound-guided procedures in the emergency department-diagnostic and therapeutic asset. Emerg Med Clin North Am. 2013;31(1):117–49.
20. Balik M, Plasil P, Waldauf P, Pazout J, Fric M, Otahal M, Pachl J. Ultrasound estimation of volume of pleural fluid in mechanically ventilated patients. Intensive Care Med. 2006;32(2):318–21.
21. Usta E, Mustafi M, Ziemer G. Ultrasound estimation of volume of postoperative pleural effusion in cardiac surgery patients. Interact Cardiovasc Thorac Surg. 2010;10(2):204–7.
22. Lichtenstein DA, Mezière G, Lascols N, Biderman P, Courret JP, Gepner A, Goldstein I, Tenoudji-Cohen M. Ultrasound diagnosis of occult pneumothorax. Crit Care Med. 2005;33(6):1231–8.
23. Volpicelli G, Elbarbary M, Blaivas M, Lichtenstein DA, Mathis G, Kirkpatrick AW, Melniker L, Gargani L, Noble VE, Via G, Dean A, Tsung JW, Soldati G, Copetti R, Bouhemad B, Reissig A, Agricola E, Rouby JJ, Arbelot C, Liteplo A, Sargsyan A, Silva F, Hoppmann R, Breitkreutz R, Seibel A, Neri L, Storti E, Petrovic T, International Liaison Committee on Lung Ultrasound (ILC-LUS) for International Consensus Conference on Lung Ultrasound (ICC-LUS). International evidence-based recommendations for point-of-care lung ultrasound. Intensive Care Med. 2012;38(4):577–91.
24. Ku BS, Fields JM, Carr B, Everett WW, Gracias VH, Dean AJ. Clinician-performed beside ultrasound for the diagnosis of traumatic pneumothorax. West J Emerg Med. 2013;14(2):103–8.
25. Blaivas M, Lyon M, Duggal S. A prospective comparison of supine chest radiography and bedside ultrasound for the diagnosis of traumatic pneumothorax. Acad Emerg Med. 2005;12(9):844–9.
26. Rowan KR, Kirkpatrick AW, Liu D, Forkheim KE, Mayo JR, Nicolaou S. Traumatic pneumothorax detection with thoracic US: correlation with chest radiography and CT – initial experience. Radiology. 2002;225(1):210–4.
27. Lichtenstein D, Mezière G, Biderman P, Gepner A. The "lung point": an ultrasound sign specific to pneumothorax. Intensive Care Med. 2000;26(10):1434–40.
28. Lichtenstein D, Mezière G, Biderman P, Gepner A. The comet-tail artifact: an ultrasound sign ruling out pneumothorax. Intensive Care Med. 1999;25(4):383–8.
29. Lichtenstein DA, Menu Y. A bedside ultrasound sign ruling out pneumothorax in the critically ill. Chest. 1995;108(5):1345–8.

30. Lichtenstein DA, Lascols N, Prin S, Mezière G. The "lung pulse": an early ultrasound sign of complete atelectasis. Intensive Care Med. 2003;29(12):2187–92.
31. Blaivas M, Tsung JW. Point-of-care sonographic detection of left endobronchial main stem intubation and obstruction versus endotracheal intubation. J Ultrasound Med. 2008;27(5):785–9.
32. Lichtenstein D. FALLS-protocol: lung ultrasound in hemodynamic assessment of shock. Heart Lung Vessel. 2013;5(3):142–7.
33. Gillman LM, Alkadi A, Kirkpatrick AW. The "pseudo-lung point" sign: all focal respiratory coupled alternating pleural patterns are not diagnostic of a pneumothorax. J Trauma. 2009;67(3):672–3.
34. Zengin S, Al B, Genc S, Yildirim C, Ercan S, Dogan M, Altunbas G. Role of inferior vena cava and right ventricular diameter in assessment of volume status: a comparative study: ultrasound and hypovolemia. Am J Emerg Med. 2013;31(5):763–7.
35. Thanakitcharu P, Charoenwut M, Siriwiwatanakul N. Inferior vena cava diameter and collapsibility index: a practical non-invasive evaluation of intravascular fluid volume in critically-ill patients. J Med Assoc Thai. 2013;96(Suppl 3):S14–22.
36. Anderson KL, Jenq KY, Fields JM, Panebianco NL, Dean AJ. Diagnosing heart failure among acutely dyspneic patients with cardiac, inferior vena cava, and lung ultrasonography. Am J Emerg Med. 2013;31(8):1208–14.
37. Akkaya A, Yesilaras M, Aksay E, Sever M, Atilla OD. The interrater reliability of ultrasound imaging of the inferior vena cava performed by emergency residents. Am J Emerg Med. 2013;31(10):1509–11.
38. Lyon M, Blaivas M, Brannam L. Sonographic measurement of the inferior vena cava as a marker of blood loss. Am J Emerg Med. 2005;23(1):45–50.
39. Juhl-Olsen P, Vistisen ST, Christiansen LK, Rasmussen LA, Frederiksen CA, Sloth E. Ultrasound of the inferior vena cava does not predict hemodynamic response to early hemorrhage. J Emerg Med. 2013;45(4):592–7.
40. Sargsyan A, Blaivas M, Lumb P, Karakitsos D. Fundamentals. In: Lumb, Karakitsos, editors. Critical care ultrasound. Elsevier; 2014.
41. Sargsyan A, et al. Soft tissue, musculoskeletal system and miscellaneous targets. In: Lumb, Karakitsos, editors. Critical care ultrasound. Elsevier; 2014.
42. Akilli B, Bayir A, Kara F, Ak A, Cander B. Inferior vena cava diameter as a marker of early hemorrhagic shock: a comparative study. Ulus Travma Acil Cerrahi Derg. 2010;16(2):113–8.
43. Rabiner JE, Friedman LM, Khine H, Avner JR, Tsung JW. Accuracy of point-of-care ultrasound for diagnosis of skull fractures in children. Pediatrics. 2013;131(6):e1757–64.
44. Lichtenstein D, Biderman P, Mezière G, Gepner A. The "sinusogram", a real-time ultrasound sign of maxillary sinusitis. Intensive Care Med. 1998;24(10):1057–61.
45. McIlrath ST, Blaivas M, Lyon M. Diagnosis of periorbital gas on ocular ultrasound after facial trauma. Am J Emerg Med. 2005;23(4):517–20.
46. Friedrich RE, Heiland M, Bartel-Friedrich S. Potentials of ultrasound in the diagnosis of midfacial fractures. Clin Oral Investig. 2003;7(4):226–9.
47. Hayreh SS. Pathogenesis of edema of the optic disc. Die Ophthalmol. 1968;24:289–411.
48. Dubourg J, Messerer M, Karakitsos D, Rajajee V, Antonsen E, Javouhey E, Cammarata A, Cotton M, Daniel RT, Denaro C, Douzinas E, Dubost C, Berhouma M, Kassai B, Rabilloud M, Gullo A, Hamlat A, Kouraklis G, Mannanici G, Marill K, Merceron S, Poularas J, Ristagno G, Noble V, Shah S, Kimberly H, Cammarata G, Moretti R, Geeraerts T. Individual patient data systematic review and meta-analysis of optic nerve sheath diameter ultrasonography for detecting raised intracranial pressure: protocol of the ONSD research group. Syst Rev. 2013;2:62. https://doi.org/10.1186/2046-4053-2-62.
49. Dubourg J, Javouhey E, Geeraerts T, Messerer M, Kassai B. Ultrasonography of optic nerve sheath diameter for detection of raised intracranial pressure: a systematic review and meta-analysis. Intensive Care Med. 2011;37(7):1059–68. https://doi.org/10.1007/s00134-011-2224-2.
50. Sargsyan A, Blaivas M, Geeraerts T, Karakitsos. Ocular ultrasound in the intensive care unit. In: Lumb, Karakitsos, editors. Critical care ultrasound. Elsevier; 2014.
51. Valentino M, Serra C, Zironi G, De Luca C, Pavlica P, Barozzi L. Blunt abdominal trauma: emergency contrast-enhanced sonography for detection of solid organ injuries. AJR Am J Roentgenol. 2006;186(5):1361–7.

Imaging in the Stable Trauma Patient

46

Bradley S. Moffat and Neil G. Parry

Abbreviations

ABC	Airway, breathing, circulation
AP	Anteroposterior
ATLS	Advanced trauma life support
c-spine	Cervical spine
E-FAST	Extended focused assessment by sonography in trauma
EMS	Emergency medical services
FAST	Focused assessment by sonography in trauma

Introduction

The hemodynamically stable trauma patient affords the trauma team valuable time to consider a variety of treatment adjuncts. Such patients are excellent candidates for a wide arsenal of imaging modalities; however, thoughtful planning of the types and sequence of imaging tests can minimize the time spent in uncontrolled environments and facilitate transition to definitive care.

When considering appropriate imaging studies for any trauma patient, the most important question to ask is: "Is this patient hemodynamically stable?" Any patient showing signs of significant tachycardia, hypotension, or any other Airway, Breathing, Circulation (ABC) concern should not leave the trauma bay for imaging purposes and should never be sent to the CT scanner. Being in the CT suite or in transit can be very challenging if the patient deteriorates or needs ongoing aggressive resuscitation.

B. S. Moffat
Department of Surgery, Schulich School of Medicine and Dentistry, Western University, London, ON, Canada

N. G. Parry (✉)
Departments of Surgery and Medicine, Schulich School of Medicine and Dentistry, Western University, London, ON, Canada
e-mail: neil.parry@lhsc.on.ca

In this chapter, we will review the imaging modalities available for stable trauma patients. Further, we will discuss strategies for a smooth and efficient transition from the trauma bay to the imaging suite and finally to definitive care.

Imaging Modalities

Plain X-ray

Plain film X-rays confer a major advantage over many other modalities in that they are portable, can easily be performed in the trauma bay, and are relatively inexpensive and widely available compared to other imaging modalities. Many trauma bays are equipped with ceiling-mounted X-ray systems which eliminate the need for bulky portable equipment. Plain film X-rays are an important adjunct to the Advanced Trauma Life Support (ATLS) primary survey and include an anteroposterior (AP) chest, AP pelvis, and occasionally lateral cervical spine (c-spine) [1].

The chest X-ray is a critical imaging study for all trauma patients. Certain key findings mandate treatment prior to leaving the trauma bay. Patients with a clinically significant hemo- or pneumothorax should have a chest tube inserted prior to leaving the trauma bay as these injuries can worsen rapidly (Fig. 46.1). With intubated patients, the chest film is also helpful to confirm adequate endotracheal tube position prior to transport; however, it is important to remember that a chest X-ray cannot differentiate between esophageal or tracheal intubation. Ultrasound can also play a key role in diagnosing and ruling out hemo- or pneumothorax. Additionally, ultrasound can reliably detect esophageal intubation and main stem intubation at the bedside, in real time.

The pelvic film must be performed if there is clinical concern for a pelvic fracture, if there is any suggestion of hemodynamic instability, or if the patient is not going for CT imaging (Fig. 46.2). With a clinically stable pelvis, it is sometimes omitted if the patient is hemodynamically stable and going for CT. With the clinically unstable pelvis, a

L. Marshall Gillman, S. Widder (eds.), *Trauma Team Dynamics*, https://doi.org/10.1007/978-3-031-86312-7_46

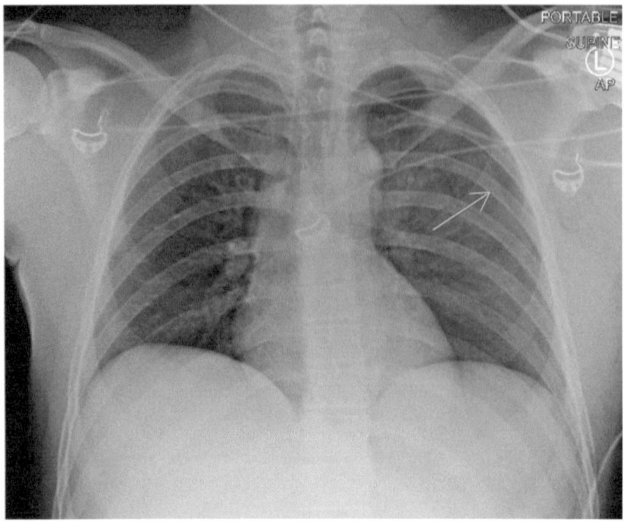

Fig. 46.1 AP chest X-ray— yellow arrow indicating left pneumothorax

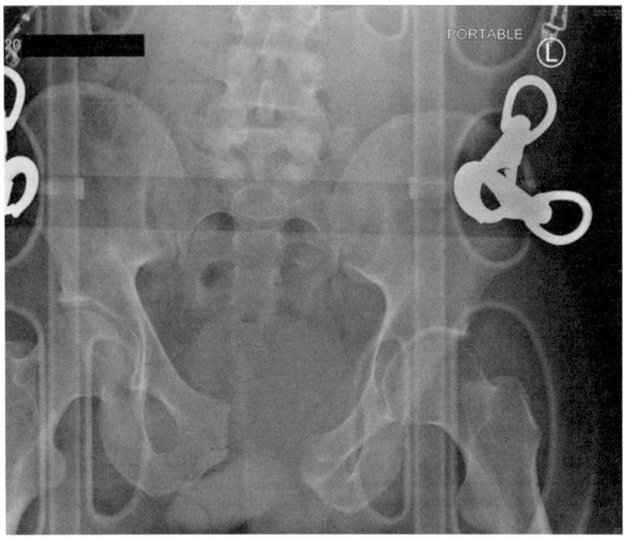

Fig. 46.2 AP pelvis X-ray—open book pelvic fracture

binder should be applied and a pelvic film should be obtained prior to leaving the trauma bay.

The lateral c-spine plain film has been largely replaced by CT [2]. Even in centers where CT is not available, lateral c-spine films alone are often insufficient to clear c-spine precautions and may miss up to 55% of injuries [3]. However, in select alert patients, c-spine precautions may be cleared clinically using a tool such as the Canadian C-Spine Rules [4] (Fig. 46.3). Most patients with a significant mechanism of injury will go on to have a CT c-spine and hence the plain film is not necessary. The cervical collar must therefore remain on until the c-spine has been cleared.

Extremity films may be considered as adjuncts to the ATLS secondary survey as they can often guide the urgency of orthopedic intervention(s) [1]. With limb-threatening orthopedic injuries, pre- and post-reduction films may be necessary prior to leaving the trauma bay. Extremity films may also be helpful in guiding the astute trauma practitioner to add extremity CT scans for injuries in which the orthopedics or vascular teams may require them (such as injuries involving major joints or diminished pulse distal to the fracture). This can help eliminate the need for additional trips to the radiology suite after the patient reaches definitive care; however, timely transit to CT should not be delayed in favor of getting extremity films.

Focused Assessment with Sonography in Trauma (FAST)

As outlined in the preceding chapters, the FAST exam has become a critical adjunct to the ATLS primary survey [1, 5–7]. While the primary function of the FAST exam is to exclude hemoperitoneum and hemopericardium in the unstable patient, it remains a mandatory adjunct in the stable patient as well. Stable patients with a positive abdominal FAST should still proceed to CT scan. However, if a patient with a positive FAST becomes unstable after leaving the trauma bay, they can be quickly rerouted to the operating room for definitive management (Fig. 46.4). On the other hand, stable patients with a positive pericardial FAST should most likely proceed directly to the operating room.

Many trauma providers are facile with the extended FAST (E-FAST) exam. In addition to the four abdominal views, the E-FAST includes bilateral assessment for pneumothorax and hemothorax. Like the standard FAST, the primary utility of the E-FAST is to guide chest intervention in the unstable trauma patient. The E-FAST views can still be a helpful tool in the stable trauma patient where the clinical exam is equivocal, and the chest X-ray is either delayed or equivocal. An important consideration to the use of E-FAST in the stable patient is its high specificity; that is, the E-FAST may detect small volumes of air or fluid which are not apparent on chest X-ray [8]. Such occult injuries in stable patients are often managed conservatively, and hence chest tube placement may not be required.

Computed Tomography (CT) Scan

CT is the mainstay imaging modality for the stable trauma patient and careful consideration should be given to each body area which may require CT imaging. Once the primary and secondary surveys are complete, the patient may be prepared to travel to the CT suite. Mechanism of injury and physical exam findings generally dictate which areas should be further imaged with CT. However, certain injuries warrant special mention.

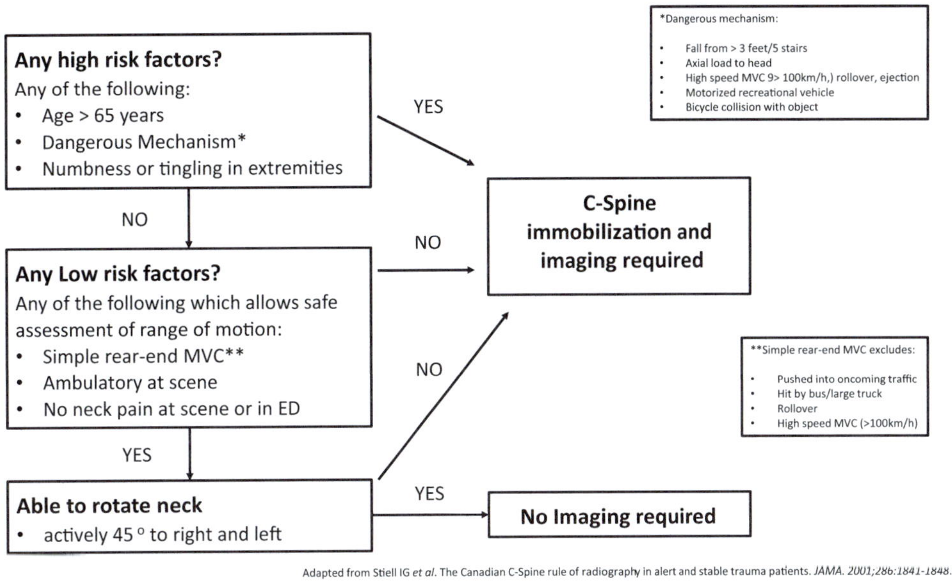

Fig. 46.3 Canadian C-spine rule

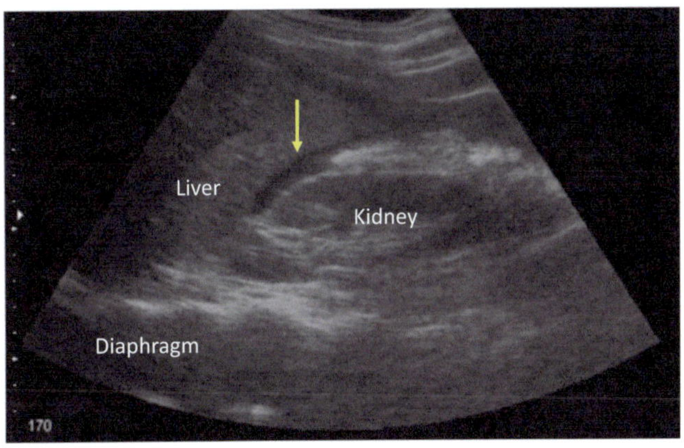

Fig. 46.4 Positive Focused Assessment with Sonography in Trauma (FAST)—fluid in the right upper quadrant

Much like with c-spine, the Canadian CT Head Rule helps determine who requires a CT head with a clinically minor head injury and mechanism [9] (Fig. 46.5). All patients with moderate to severe brain injury (GCS <13) require CT imaging.

CT angiogram (CTA) of the chest has become the gold standard to diagnose blunt thoracic aortic injury. This injury can be highly lethal and should be suspected with any patient involved in a sudden acceleration-deceleration type injury (e.g., head-on collision or fall from significant height).

CT angiogram of the neck is being used more frequently to screen for blunt cerebrovascular injury (BCVI). Historically, it was felt that BCVI occurred in less than 1% of all major traumas; however, recent evidence suggests that it occurs in up to 5% of all major traumas and that delayed or missed diagnosis increases mortality [10–12]. Many authors now recommend screening for BCVI in major blunt polytrauma patients [13–15].

Trauma CT scans of the thorax, abdomen, and pelvis require intravenous contrast but not oral contrast (Fig. 46.6). Good arterial phase images are essential to identify major vascular injuries (e.g., blunt aortic injury) and solid organ injuries (parenchymal as well as contrast extravasation and/or pseudoaneurysm). Delayed films for venous phase or to evaluate urinary tract injuries may also be very helpful. Most stable trauma patients with abdominal pain and/or a positive FAST should undergo CT imaging of abdomen and pelvis. Phases of scanning will be discussed further in the following chapter.

Many trauma patients undergo a "pan-scan" or "trauma-scan" which includes CT head, c-spine, chest, abdomen, and pelvis. Early data suggested that there was a distinct survival benefit to patients who undergo pan-scan; however, the largest randomized control trial failed to detect any difference in mortality [16–18]. CT pan-scans can detect additional injuries, up to 40%, of which 20% are clinically significant when compared to selective imaging [19–21]. This method also allows one to radiographically examine the entire spine. Prior to ordering a pan-scan, one must consider the long-term effects of undue radiation exposure versus the risk of missing a significant injury. Although this topic remains somewhat controversial, CT pan-scans are frequently used and should be considered for blunt polytrauma patients with significant mechanism of injury and/or decreased level of consciousness.

Stable patients without obvious need for surgery (e.g., peritonitis, evisceration) sustaining penetrating trauma are also candidates for more selective imaging. Consideration must be given to the possible path of the missile, and all body cavities at risk should be included if CT imaging is sought [22]. Hemodynamically stable penetrating wounds to the neck without hard signs for surgical exploration (e.g.,

Fig. 46.5 Canadian CT-head rule

CT Head is required for patients with suspected minor head injuries (witnessed loss of consciousness, definitive amnesia or witnessed disorientation with GCS 13-15) and with ANY one of the following:

High Risk (for neurologic intervention):

- GCS <15 2 h after injury
- Suspected open or depressed skull fracture
- Signs of basal skull fracture (hempotympanum, "raccoon eyes", Battle sign, CSF otorrhea/rinorrhea
- Vomiting > 2 episodes
- Age > 65

Medium risk (for brain injury on CT)

- Amnesia > 30 mins before impact
- Dangerous mechanism (pedestrian struck by vehicle, ejected from vehicle, Fall > 3 feet or five stairs)

Adapted from Stiell IG *et al.* The Canadian CT Head Rule for patients with minor head injury. *Lancet. 2001;357:1391-1396.*

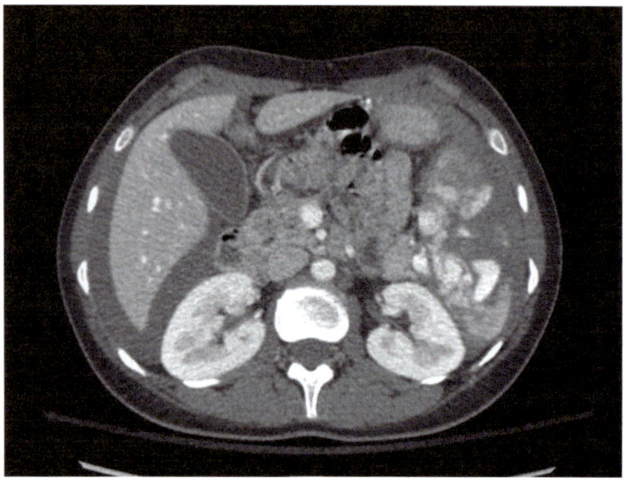

Fig. 46.6 CT abdomen— demonstrates hemoperitoneum (blood around the liver and spleen) due to a major splenic injury

impending loss of airway, active bleeding, expanding hematoma, hemoptysis, subcutaneous emphysema) are triaged based on clinical exam and contrast-enhanced CT [23].

There are several approaches to the stable patient with penetrating thoracoabdominal trauma; some of which are dictated by the mechanism of the injury (e.g., stab versus gunshot). Any injury to the thoracoabdominal junction needs to be evaluated for diaphragmatic injury. While CT technology is improving the radiographic detection rate, laparoscopic or thoracoscopic evaluation of the diaphragm is usually warranted [24, 25]. Stab wounds to the anterior abdomen do not require CT scans and can generally be managed by serial physical examination [26]. Penetrating injuries to the flank should undergo triple contrast CT scan (IV, oral, and rectal contrast) as serial exams may miss retroperitoneal injury [22]. CT imaging may be warranted in blunt or penetrating extremity trauma based on clinical exam, and contrast studies are often helpful to exclude major peripheral vascular injury.

The trauma practitioner is tasked with weighing the benefits of CT imaging against the potential risks of radiation exposure. The average radiation exposure for a single trauma pan-scan is about 31 millisieverts (a standard CT head is about 1.7 millisieverts) [27]. The use of CT in the pediatric population warrants extra caution as it has been associated with increased cancer risk, especially in young children [28]. While the CT pan-scan provides invaluable information, consideration should always be given to cumulative radiation exposure, especially in the younger patient. Imaging in the pregnant patient also requires specific considerations which are discussed in detail in Chap. 41.

Other Modalities

Magnetic resonance imaging (MRI) is used in trauma but more often after the patient has already been admitted to hospital. Acutely, however, it may be used in the assessment and evaluation of spinal cord injuries. MRI is also helpful to aid with diagnosis and prognostication of traumatic brain injuries.

Critical Thinking

There are a variety of important considerations when planning a trip to the imaging suite with a stable trauma patient (Fig. 46.7). Careful planning and clear communication are key to ensuring a smooth process.

A chest X-ray and a FAST exam should be performed on all trauma patients before they leave the trauma bay. Calling for the X-ray technician early will avoid delays waiting for plain films to be obtained. Likewise, having an ultrasound machine and a certified FAST user close at hand is a must.

If an inter-facility transfer is anticipated, advanced imaging (such as CT) should be kept to a minimum. The appropriate land or air emergency medical services (EMS) personnel should be contacted as soon as a transport decision is made such that delays in waiting for their arrival are minimal. Bear in mind that CT scans performed at your hospital may not be transferable to the receiving facility, may not use the same protocols, and, as such, often end up being repeated when the

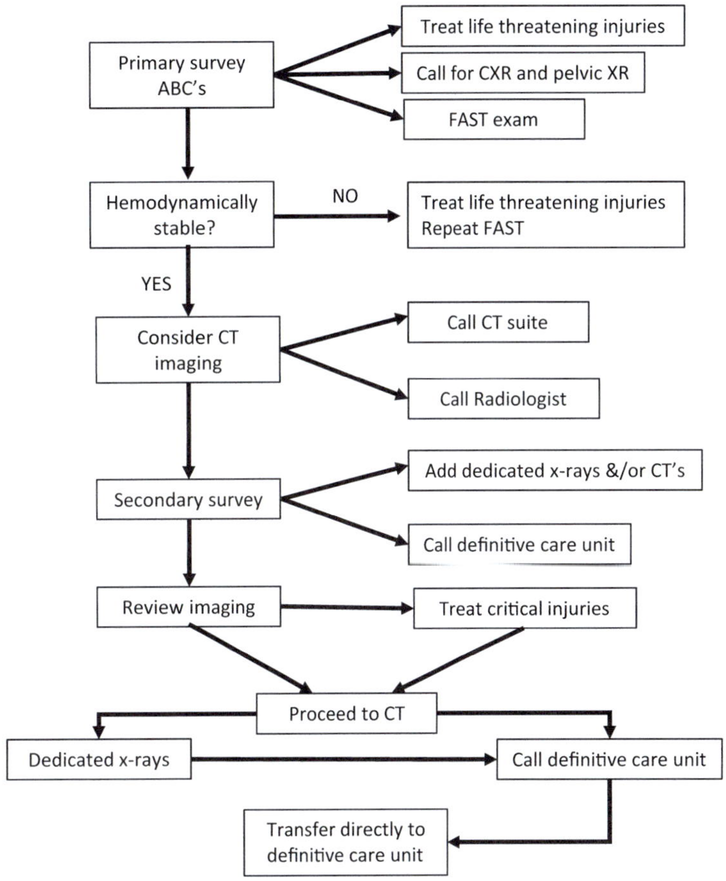

Fig. 46.7 Algorithm for imaging the stable trauma patient

patient arrives [29]. Hence, scanning prior to transfer may expose the patient to additional radiation and/or delays in transfer. Only consider scans which may alter your management prior to, or during transfer.

Upon completion of the primary survey in a stable patient, the trauma practitioner should start considering which CT scans may be required. As soon as this decision is made, the trauma team leader should immediately be in communication with the CT suite to notify them and find out when they can accept the patient.

Once CT has been notified, the FAST exam and the plain film X-rays should be in progress or already be available. These studies should be carefully examined for any injuries which may need to be treated prior to leaving the trauma bay (such as a pneumothorax). The secondary survey should also be completed at this point.

It is important to anticipate additional CT scans that may be needed based on specific injury patterns. For example, if there is significant facial trauma on clinical exam, adding a dedicated CT face to the initial trauma scans will save an additional trip to the scanner later. Another common example is fractures involving major joints which often require CT imaging prior to operative intervention. Clear and early communication with consulting services can also help plan such adjunctive imaging.

Before leaving for the scanner, it is important to ensure you have the appropriate transfer equipment. Be sure to bring standard resuscitation equipment as well as any analgesic and sedating medications you may need. At a minimum, a physician (ideally the trauma team leader) and a nurse should accompany the patient at all times until they reach definitive care. If the patient is intubated, a respiratory therapist should also stay with the patient at all times.

Another important consideration before leaving the trauma bay for the CT suite is where the patient will go after their scans. If the patient is being admitted, the trauma team leader should decide what level of care is required as soon as possible. It is critical to give the floor, observation unit, or intensive care unit as much notice as possible to ensure a bed is available and staffed. Frequent communication with those in charge of these beds is important. The goal should be to transfer the patient from the trauma bay to the scanner and then directly to definitive care. This avoids unnecessary time spent in transit and in the ER and further minimizes the time spent in uncontrolled environments. After the bed request is made, it is helpful to touch base when leaving the trauma bay to the CT suite, and again when leaving the CT suite to ensure the bed is prepared and the definitive care team is ready to transfer care as soon as the patient arrives.

Key Points

- Always ask: "Is this patient stable?" If not, do not transfer them to the CT scanner.
- Ensure all trauma patients have a chest X-ray and FAST exam done prior to leaving for the scanner and act on any injuries which could progress.
- CT scan with a low threshold for pan-scan is the modality of choice for most stable, blunt trauma patients.
- Carefully consider which scans are needed urgently and anticipate additional scans which may be required by consulting services.
- Communicate early and clearly with the CT suite and the definitive care unit to ensure a smooth transit for the patient.

When caring for the stable trauma patient, astute planning and a smooth transfer from the trauma bay, through the imaging department and finally to definitive care will improve patient care and maximize efficiency.

References

1. American College of Surgeons Committee on Trauma. Advanced trauma life support. 10th ed. Chicago: American College of Surgeons; 2018.
2. Walters BC, Hadley MN, Hurlbert RJ, Aarabi B, Dhall SS, Gelb DE, et al. Guidelines for the management of acute cervical spine and spinal cord injuries: 2013 update. Neurosurgery. 2013;60(Suppl 1):82–91.
3. Mathen R, Inaba K, Munera F, Teixeira PG, Rivas L, McKenney M, et al. Prospective evaluation of multislice computed tomography versus plain radiographic cervical spine clearance in trauma patients. J Trauma. 2007;62(6):1427–31.
4. Stiell IG, Wells GA, Vandemheen KL, Clement CM, Lesiuk H, De Maio VJ, et al. The Canadian C-spine rule for radiography in alert and stable trauma patients. JAMA. 2001;286(15):1841–8.
5. Rozycki GS, Ballard RB, Feliciano DV, Schmidt JA, Pennington SD. Surgeon-performed ultrasound for the assessment of truncal injuries: lessons learned from 1540 patients. Ann Surg. 1998;228(4):557–67.
6. Rozycki GS. Abdominal ultrasonography in trauma. Surg Clin North Am. 1995;75(2):175–91.
7. Rozycki GS, Ochsner MG, Schmidt JA, Frankel HL, Davis TP, Wang D, et al. A prospective study of surgeon-performed ultrasound as the primary adjuvant modality for injured patient assessment. J Trauma. 1995;39(3):492–8; discussion 498–500.
8. Nandipati KC, Allamaneni S, Kakarla R, Wong A, Richards N, Satterfield J, et al. Extended focused assessment with sonography for trauma (EFAST) in the diagnosis of pneumothorax: experience at a community based level I trauma center. Injury. 2011;42(5):511–4.
9. Stiell IG, Wells GA, Vandemheen K, Clement C, Lesiuk H, Laupacis A, et al. The Canadian CT Head Rule for patients with minor head injury. Lancet. 2001;357(9266):1391–6.
10. Murphy PB, Severance S, Holler E, Menard L, Savage S, Zarvur BL. Treatment of asymptomatic blunt cerebrovascular injury (BCVI): a systematic review. Trauma Surg Acute Care Open. 2021;6:e000668.
11. Hundersmarck D, Slooff WBM, Homans JF, van der Vliet QMJ, Moayeri N, Hietbrink F, de Borst GJ, Oner FC, Mujis SPJ, Leenan LPH. Blunt cerebrovascular injury: incidence and long-term follow-up. Eur J Trauma Emerg Surg. 2021;47(1):161–70.
12. Esnault P, Cardniale M, Boret H, D'Aranda E, Moncriol A, Bordes J, Prunet B, Joubert C, Dagain A, Goutorbe P, Kaiser E, Meaudre E. Blunt cerebrovascular injuries in severe traumatic brain injury: incidence, risk factors and evolution. J Neurosurg. 2017;127:16–22.
13. Kim DY, Biffl W, Bokhari F, Brakenridge S, Chao E, Claridge J, Fraser D, Jawa R, Kasotakis G, Kerwin A, Khan U, Kurek S, Plurad D, Robinson B, Stassen N, Tesoriero R, Yorkgitis B, Como JJ. Evaluation and management of blunt cerebrovascular injury: a practice management guideline from the Eastern Association for the Surgery of Trauma. J Trauma Acute Care Surg. 2020;88(6):875–87.
14. Leichtle SW, Banerjee D, Schrader R, Torres B, Jayaraman S, Rodas E, Broering B, Aboutanos MB. Blunt cerebrovascular injury: the case for universal screening. J Trauma Acute Care Surg. 2020;89(5):880–6.
15. Müther M, Sporns PB, Hanning U, Düsing H, Hartensuer R, Raschke M, Schwake M, Stummer W, Glasgow S. Diagnostic accuracy of different clinical screening criteria for blunt cerebrovascular injuries compared with liberal state of the art computed tomography angiography in major trauma. J Trauma Acute Care Surg. 2020;88(6):789–95.
16. Saltzherr TP, Goslings JC, Multidisciplinary REACT 2 Study Group. Effect on survival of whole-body CT during trauma resuscitation. Lancet. 2009;374(9685):198; author reply 198–9.
17. Sierink JC, Treskes K, Edwards MJ, Beuker BJ, Den Hartog D, Hohmann J, Dijkgraaf MG, Luitse JS, Beenen LF, Hollmann MW, Goslings JC. Immediate total-body CT scanning versus conventional imaging and selective CT scanning in patients with severe trauma (REACT-2): a randomized controlled trial. Lancet. 2016;388:673–83.
18. Chidambaram S, Goh EL, Khan MA. A meta-analysis of the efficacy of whole-body computed tomography imaging in the management of trauma and injury. Injury. 2017;48(8):1784–93.
19. Salim A, Sangthong B, Martin M, Brown C, Plurad D, Demetriades D. Whole body imaging in blunt multisystem trauma patients without obvious signs of injury: results of a prospective study. Arch Surg. 2006;141(5):468–73; discussion 473–5.
20. Tillou A, Gupta M, Baraff LJ, Schriger DL, Hoffman JR, Hiatt JR, et al. Is the use of pan-computed tomography for blunt trauma justified? A prospective evaluation. J Trauma. 2009;67(4):779–87.
21. Lang P, Kulla M, Kerwagen F, Lefering R, Friemert B, Palm HG. The role of whole-body computed tomography in the diagnosis of thoracic injuries in severely injured patients – a retrospective multi-centre study based on the registry of the German trauma society (TraumaRegister DGU). Scand J Trauma Resusc Emerg Med. 2017;25(1):82.
22. Chiu WC, Shanmuganathan K, Mirvis SE, Scalea TM. Determining the need for laparotomy in penetrating torso trauma: a prospective study using triple-contrast enhanced abdominopelvic computed tomography. J Trauma. 2001;51(5):860–8; discussion 868–9.
23. Inaba K, Branco BC, Menaker J, Scalea TM, Crane S, DuBose JJ, et al. Evaluation of multidetector computed tomography for penetrating neck injury: a prospective multicenter study. J Trauma Acute Care Surg. 2012;72(3):576–83; discussion 583–4; quiz 803–4.
24. Stein DM, York GB, Boswell S, Shanmuganathan K, Haan JM, Scalea TM. Accuracy of computed tomography (CT) scan in the detection of penetrating diaphragm injury. J Trauma. 2007;63(3):538–43.
25. Berg RJ, Karamanos E, Inaba K, Okoye O, Teixeira PG, Demetriades D. The persistent diagnostic challenge of tho-

racoabdominal stab wounds. J Trauma Acute Care Surg. 2014;76:418–23.
26. Biffl WL, Kaups KL, Pham TN, Rowell SE, Jjurkovitch GJ, Burlew CC, Elterman J, Moore E. Validating the Western Trauma Association algorithm for managing patients with anterior abdominal stab wounds: a Western Trauma Association multicenter trial. J Trauma Acute Care Surg. 2011;71:1494–502.
27. Sharma OP, Oswanski MF, Sidhu R, Krugh K, Culler AS, Spangler M, et al. Analysis of radiation exposure in trauma patients at a level I trauma center. J Emerg Med. 2011;41(6):640–8.
28. Miglioretti DL, Johnson E, Williams A, Greenlee RT, Weinmann S, Solberg LI, et al. The use of computed tomography in pediatrics and the associated radiation exposure and estimated cancer risk. JAMA Pediatr. 2013;167(8):700–7.
29. Moore HB, Loomis SB, Destigter KK, Mann-Gow T, Dorf L, Streeter MH, et al. Airway, breathing, computed tomographic scanning: duplicate computed tomographic imaging after transfer to trauma center. J Trauma Acute Care Surg. 2013;74(3):813–7.

Advanced Considerations in Cross-Sectional Imaging in Trauma

47

Signy Holmes

Introduction

CT and MRI have progressed dramatically since the early days of cross-sectional imaging and continue to advance. While the radiologist should ideally serve as the ultimate resource for determining the next best step in imaging for a given trauma patient, several advances permit more general approaches for common questions in trauma imaging.

Once the decision has been made to proceed to cross-sectional imaging, there are various considerations to optimize CT protocol selection for any particular patient. There are also a number of options for problem-solving around questions remaining after initial imaging, which integrate additional techniques and modalities. This chapter is intended to review several of these techniques and the contexts in which they may prove most helpful in guiding decision-making during trauma resuscitation.

Initial Trauma CT Protocol

Many of the considerations in initial imaging of the hemodynamically stable trauma patient have already been reviewed (see Chap. 46). With increased capabilities of modern CT scanners, however, the question of which body parts to image is now supplemented by the ancillary question of how best to image those regions. The overall guiding principles in both questions must include gathering enough information to guide appropriate management, mitigating unnecessary exposure to ionizing radiation, and minimizing harm related to iodinated contrast administration.

S. Holmes (✉)
Department of Radiology, University of Manitoba, Winnipeg, MB, Canada
e-mail: sholmes@hsc.mb.ca

Iodinated Contrast Administration

Iodinated contrast can be critical for detection and characterization of injury as well as road mapping for potential transcatheter therapy by Interventional Radiology. The principal risks of iodinated contrast material administration fall either under nephrotoxicity or under allergic and allergic-like reactions. Recently updated guidelines have deemphasized the nephrotoxic risks of iodinated contrast in underlying renal dysfunction [1]. Contrast-induced nephropathy is not uncommon in trauma patients with incidence in some cohorts reported as high as 14.7% but has not been demonstrated to contribute significantly to morbidity or mortality when controlling for confounding factors [2, 3]. Therefore, while the decision to proceed with contrast-enhanced imaging in patients with known or suspected renal disease should be based on the level of concern for significant injury and on discussion with the radiology department, intravenous contrast is almost always warranted when clinical concern for significant injury is high. Similar principles should guide the decision whether to delay imaging for results of serum measurement of renal function [4]. Of note, the total volume of iodinated contrast material administered is directly associated with risk of contrast-induced nephropathy [5]. Repeated contrast administration should therefore be avoided where possible and optimal imaging strategies used the first time.

Up to 1 in 2500 patients may develop a severe and potentially life-threatening reaction to injection of iodinated contrast [6, 7]. The strongest predictor of these reactions is history of previous reactions, with re-exposure rates of reaction reported at 31.1% in the absence of premedication [8]. Hemodynamically stable trauma patients with known history of allergic-type reaction to iodinated contrast and low to intermediate suspicion for significant injury may undergo premedication prior to imaging. While this will potentially delay initial cross-sectional imaging, emergency premedication protocols can be administered where risks of incomplete CT imaging outweigh the risks of breakthrough reaction [9]. The protocol we use at our institution includes methylpred-

L. Marshall Gillman, S. Widder (eds.), *Trauma Team Dynamics*, https://doi.org/10.1007/978-3-031-86312-7_47

nisolone 40 mg IV or hydrocortisone 200 mg IV 4 h before the scan followed by diphenhydramine 50 mg IV 1 h before. Premedication is not required in patients with a history of mild reaction [8].

Planning an Initial CT Protocol

As previously noted in Chapter 46, most widely utilized trauma protocols include noncontrast imaging of the brain and cervical spine as well as contrast-enhanced imaging of the chest, abdomen, and pelvis. Selective imaging may be appropriate in penetrating injury and in some cases of blunt trauma in younger patients more vulnerable to lifetime risk of radiation-induced cancers but has been found to result in only minimal decreases in radiation exposure (20.6 vs. 20.9 mSv) and may result in delayed imaging as well as missed injuries [10, 11].

Imaging of the chest and abdomen should be timed for peak arterial enhancement in order to optimize vascular assessment. In the chest, there is very little downside to obtaining only arterial phase images. In the abdomen and pelvis, multiple phases may be required for adequate detection and characterization of injury. For example, identification and accurate classification of splenic injury is of great importance given trends towards nonoperative management and need for angioembolization [12]. Arterial phase imaging is required to roadmap vascular supply and identify small bleeds, while the background spleen enhances with sufficient homogeneity to allow detection of small lacerations only later in the portal venous phase. Comparison of both phases is required in many cases to differentiate active bleeds from pseudoaneurysms (Fig. 47.1).

Some trauma protocols include both arterial phase and portal venous phase imaging of the entire abdomen and pelvis. To reduce total radiation dose, the total craniocaudad extent of imaging in either phase could be reduced, although this carries its own risk of missed or incompletely characterized injuries. In particular, if an institution does not routinely include arterial phase imaging of the lower abdomen and pelvis, the radiology department should be informed of any major penetrating abdominopelvic trauma, particularly gunshot injury, and of suspected pelvic fracture or unstable pelvis to ensure caudal extension of the arterial phase. Potential renal injuries also merit extension of arterial phase imaging as accessory renal arteries can arise anywhere from the abdominal aorta. Additional delayed phases may be indicated in the setting of suspected renal or bladder injury, further discussed below.

Arterial phase imaging of the neck is indicated in the case of penetrating injury or in suspected blunt cerebrovascular injury (BCVI). This may be included routinely in cases of high clinical suspicion, added following on-table review of noncontrast imaging of the cervical spine for fracture, or if necessary performed as a separate follow-up examination requiring an additional contrast bolus.

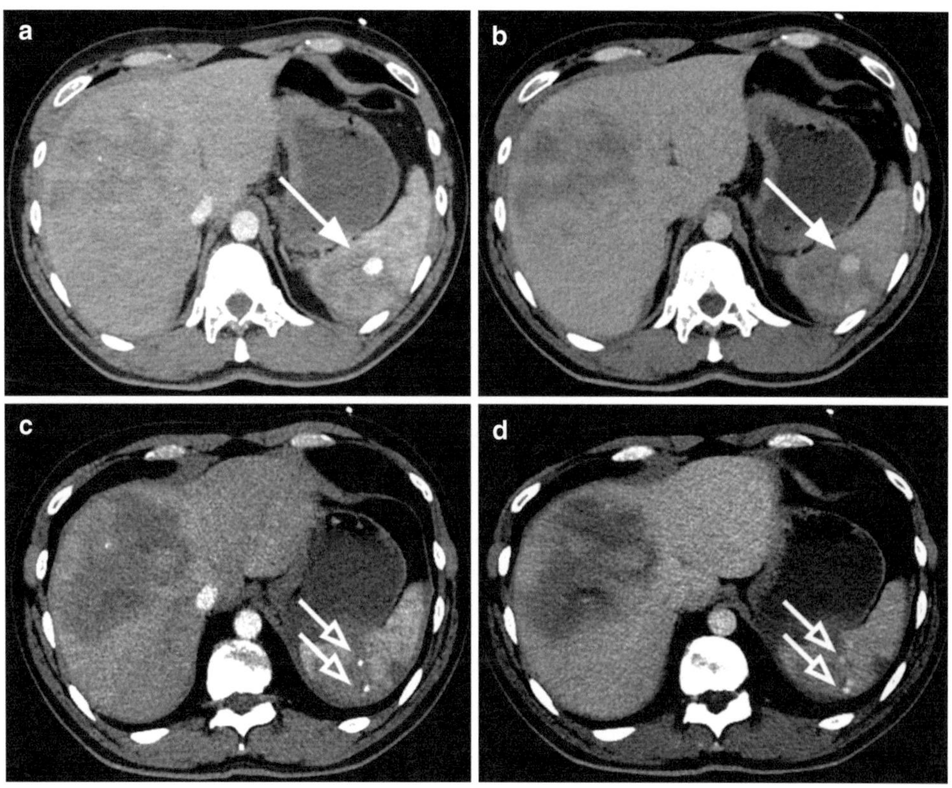

Fig. 47.1 Multiphase imaging in MVC trauma. A round focus of extraluminal contrast on arterial phase imaging through the spleen (closed arrow, **a**) is unaltered in morphology on portal venous phase imaging (closed arrow, **b**) compatible with a pseudoaneurysm. Smaller foci higher in the spleen in the same patient (open arrows) are punctate on arterial phase imaging (**c**) and demonstrate blooming on portal venous phase imaging (**d**) compatible with areas of active arterial extravasation. The patient underwent nonoperative management with transarterial embolization. Extensive liver lacerations were also present in this case

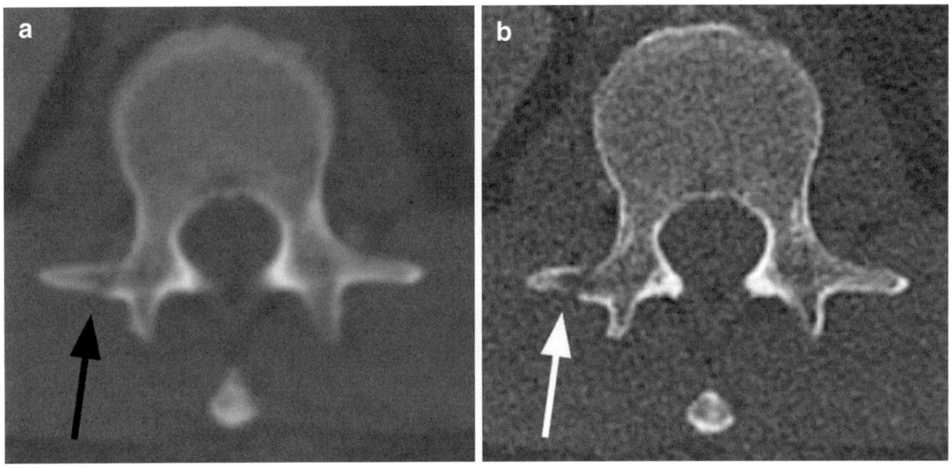

Fig. 47.2 Subtle fracture in MVC trauma. A nondisplaced right L1 transverse process fracture which could easily be overlooked or interpreted as artifact on 5 mm soft tissue algorithm reconstructions (black arrow, **a**) is much more apparent on 1.25 mm bone algorithm reconstruction (white arrow, **b**)

CT angio runoff imaging of the lower extremities may be included as clinically indicated. CT angio of the upper extremities can also be performed at the time of initial CT but may require repositioning of the patient. Detection and characterization of upper or lower fractures, including imaging for preoperative planning, can often be performed at the time of initial CT, and may or may not mandate CT angio depending on clinical neurovascular status. 3D reformatted images generated from these studies can assist in preoperative planning.

To reduce the total volume of administered contrast and time on the table, the number of full contrast boluses administered should be limited where possible. Depending on specific scanner parameters, there may be restrictions to the craniocaudad extent of adequate arterial phase imaging that can be obtained with a single contrast bolus. This is of particular importance given the increasing role of nonoperative management by Interventional Radiology, which often requires administration of significant volumes of iodinated contrast but also requires good vascular road mapping for procedure planning. This again emphasizes the importance of good communication with the radiology department to ensure all areas of concern are adequately imaged at the time of initial CT.

Incorporating appropriate reformations into a baseline trauma protocol or requesting these early in the imaging process can prevent delays in diagnosis of subtle injury. For example, diaphragmatic injuries may be apparent only on multiplanar reformatted images. A dedicated CT of the facial bones should be added to initial imaging where clinically appropriate. While a CT of the chest, abdomen, and pelvis includes the entire thoracolumbar spine and sacrum, subtle fractures may not be apparent without appropriate reformations (Fig. 47.2). Imaging of the spine should be reviewed with soft tissue and bone reformats in multiple planes, typically at a thickness of no less than 1.25 mm [13].

Oral and rectal contrast can also be considered either as part of a baseline trauma protocol or for specific clinical scenarios to better delineate potential bowel injury. While some centers routinely administer oral and rectal contrast as part of their baseline trauma protocol (so-called triple-contrast CT), others selectively administer rectal contrast only in penetrating flank injuries or as a problem-solving tool after initial imaging [14]. There are no randomized controlled studies comparing single-contrast CT with rectal contrast in the detection of bowel injury, although single-contrast CT has been found to have comparable accuracy to triple-contrast CT, and leakage of enteric contrast material is a relatively insensitive marker for bowel injury seen in only 15–29% of cases [15]. Workflow and potential delays in imaging related to enteric contrast administration must also be taken into consideration. Ultimately, in the absence of definitive evidence one way or the other, local factors and preferences should guide protocol selection in these cases.

Approaches to Advanced Workup

After initial cross-sectional imaging there may be additional diagnostic questions. Some of these will be raised by findings on the initial imaging, as in equivocal findings of bowel or pancreatic ductal injury. Others may be clinical, as in the case of suspected spinal cord injury with no vertebral fracture or dislocation identified on initial CT. Finally, there are sometimes questions remaining after initial intervention, whether invasive or noninvasive. Our discussion of this final category will be limited in scope, as these questions only rarely fall under the umbrella of acute trauma management.

Adjunct CT Series Based on Initial CT Findings

Injury to the renal collecting system, ureters, or bladder may be best characterized with delayed CT urography imaging. First, the potential injury must be identified either based on clinical factors such as hematuria or unstable pelvic fracture or by initial imaging review by the radiologist. Delayed imaging is preferred for assessment of the renal collecting systems and ureters, however, may not lead to sufficient bladder distension to rule out bladder injury. Retrograde CT or fluoroscopic cystography is performed via Foley catheter, where the bladder is distended to a minimum of 300 cc, which is required for reliable assessment [16] (Fig. 47.3). It should be noted that delayed imaging will be ineffective for assessment of the urinary tracts in the setting of severe renal impairment due to lack of contrast excretion by the kidneys.

While CT angio imaging of the neck is clearly indicated in penetrating neck trauma, blunt cerebrovascular injury (BCVI) is an increasingly recognized, potentially devastating entity that is important to identify and treat early to reduce the risk of complicating stroke [17]. As mentioned above, CT angio may be performed in initial patient imaging when there are clinical risk factors for BCVI including high energy mechanism, displaced midface, complex skull fracture, or near hanging. In other cases, risk of BCVI may not be recognized until initial noncontrast CT of the cervical spine is complete. In these cases, either following on-table or other preliminary review of the images by the radiologist, CT angio carotids should be added where and when patient stability permits. The two most widely applied sets of guidelines for BCVI screening are the Western Trauma Association/modified Denver (WTA) recommendations and the Eastern Association for the Surgery of Trauma (EAST) guidelines, which differ slightly in which categories of cervical spine fracture and/or ligamentous injury merit screening [18, 19]. The more conservative WTA recommendations would advise BCVI screening in all cervical spine fractures, subluxations, and confirmed ligamentous injuries.

Emergency Trauma MRI

Assessment of the pregnant trauma patient presents unique challenges covered elsewhere (Chapter 41). Initial imaging workup should minimize radiation exposure where possible, but not at the expense of the immediate safety of the mother or fetus. Accordingly in major trauma, the same initial CT protocol as in a nonpregnant patient is almost always the most appropriate first step in imaging. One entity unique to pregnancy which may be equivocal on initial CT is placental abruption. The heterogeneous appearance of the mature placenta can mimic the appearance of partial abruption, in which case either ultrasound or MRI can be used for further characterization in the stable mother and fetus. MRI is the more sensitive and specific modality for retroplacental hemorrhage [20].

MRI may have a limited role in characterization of suspected abdominal injuries. Pancreatic transections and lacerations involving the main duct often require surgical repair but can be subtle on initial imaging [21]. Short interval follow-up pancreatic protocol CT in 24–48 h is recommended in appropriate equivocal cases, but magnetic resonance cholangiopancreatography (MRCP) can be used as an alternative for shorter interval problem-solving. Bile duct injuries can also be well demonstrated by MRI, typically after initial trauma management, particularly with the use of hepatobiliary contrast agents which can more precisely localize active or contained bile leaks [22].

CT is the primary modality for assessment of patients meeting criteria for spinal imaging [23]. However, MRI offers markedly improved sensitivity for soft tissue ligamentous injury. Positive MRI findings in the absence of CT findings rarely require surgical intervention, so MRI is not routinely undertaken as part of the initial trauma imaging workup. However, this modality can serve as a highly useful adjunct in settings including persistent pain and/or neurologic defects with negative CT or advanced degenerative change on CT, unexaminable patients, for operative planning in the mechanically unstable spine, or in other significant injury on CT [23, 24]. This typically does not require administration of gadolinium-based contrast.

Noncontrast head CT permits identification of pathologies requiring intervention but lacks assessment of underlying perfusion status and poorly visualizes underlying posttraumatic parenchymal changes. CT perfusion imaging

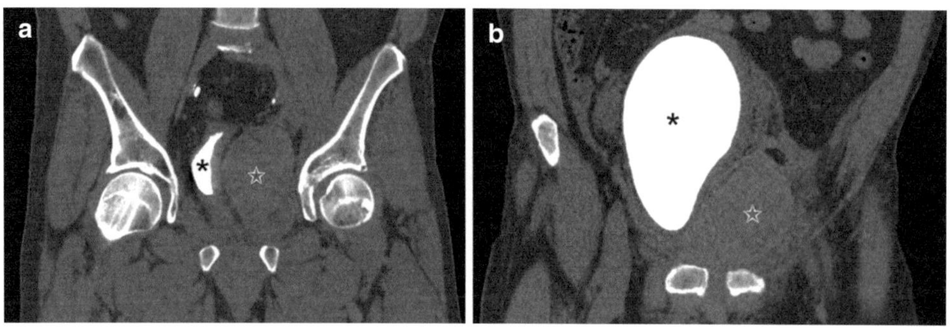

Fig. 47.3 Assessment for bladder injury in the setting of pelvic hematoma. Initial CT cystogram performed using a delayed urography technique following intravenous contrast injection (**a**) demonstrates good bladder opacification (*) but poor distension. A repeat examination was performed with retrograde contrast administration via an indwelling Foley catheter and demonstrates sufficient bladder distension to exclude leak (**b**). Adjacent fluid and hematoma (☆) can obscure or mimic leaks when cystography is not included in the imaging workup

or MRI brain, with or without perfusion imaging, can typically be deferred until after resuscitation and initial management of concurrent injuries, but at some centers rapid noncontrast MRI brain is now being trialed for initial imaging in certain settings including severe closed head trauma in the pediatric population and may in the future expand into more general usage [25].

Finally, MRI can be an appropriate adjunct in the stable patient with contraindications to iodinated contrast administration and equivocal findings on non-contrast CT. These situations arise relatively infrequently, however, and should be discussed with the radiologist to optimize workup.

Considerations Guiding Advanced Cross-Sectional Imaging

Patients can always be returned for follow-up imaging after a period of observation or after either operative or nonoperative management. Imaging should never lead to delays in ongoing care of the acute trauma patient. Advances in cross-sectional imaging and the availability of problem-solving tools do not mandate that all imaging options be exhausted prior to definitive management. Adjunct tools including CT cystography, BCVI screening, and MRI for suspected biliary or pancreatic ductal injury may be performed as part of initial imaging workup in a stable patient but may also be appropriate to defer in the setting of other significant injury. Clinical factors remain the most important guide to the next best step for a given patient.

Advanced Techniques in Trauma Imaging

Beyond considerations of general CT protocol selection and of appropriate supplementation with MRI, there are several techniques which can be pursued to optimize cross-sectional imaging in the setting of trauma.

ECG-gated thoracic CT is a broad term encompassing multiple techniques for reducing motion artifact which may obscure or mimic cardiac and aortic root injury. Where available, this tool can be utilized either for immediate characterization of suspected injury or for short-term follow-up of nonoperatively managed injury. ECG-gated CT also improves detection of coronary artery lacerations and subtle pericardial injury [26].

Dual-energy CT (DECT) is an emerging area of interest in trauma imaging, with broad potential applications [27, 28]. This technique involves acquisition of data both at high and low kilovolt peaks, allowing differentiation and quantification of materials with different X-ray absorption behaviors. Iodine selective imaging renders areas of abnormal bowel wall enhancement and subtle solid organ parenchymal injury more apparent. Virtual noncontrast images can increase conspicuity of hemorrhage, including bowel wall hemorrhage. Calcium subtraction from bone, particularly vertebral bodies, is a promising alternative to MRI for identifying marrow edema in the settings of microfracture and in age indeterminate fractures [29]. Virtual monoenergetic images can be used to reduce artifact from hardware, from equipment external to the patient, and from bullet or shrapnel fragments (Fig. 47.4).

Split bolus single pass CT was developed in an attempt to reduce radiation exposure resulting from multiphase imaging. This technique consists of two or three sequential boluses of intravenous contrast followed by a single CT acquisition of the chest, abdomen, and pelvis reflecting a combination of arterial and portal venous phases, plus or minus a urinary excretory phase. Subjective image quality and diagnostic accuracy for abdominal injuries are quite promising, but there remain concerns in the assessment of splenic parenchyma, which can appear heterogeneous, and in the characterization of areas of active extravasation particularly within the pelvis [30]. Accordingly, acceptance of this technique remains site-specific.

Trajectory analysis can serve as an important tool in the assessment of penetrating abdominal and pelvic trauma. This consists of double-obliqued reformatted imaging based on entry and exit wound sites to identify potential sites of subtle injury along the tract (Fig. 47.5) [31]. Trajectory analysis can provide valuable information by drawing attention to injuries which might otherwise have been overlooked, particularly in the setting of complex polytrauma, and by confirming suspected artifacts are outside the path of potential injury. This technique has been found to have similar accuracy with improved sensitivity when compared to enteric contrast in the detection of colorectal injury [32].

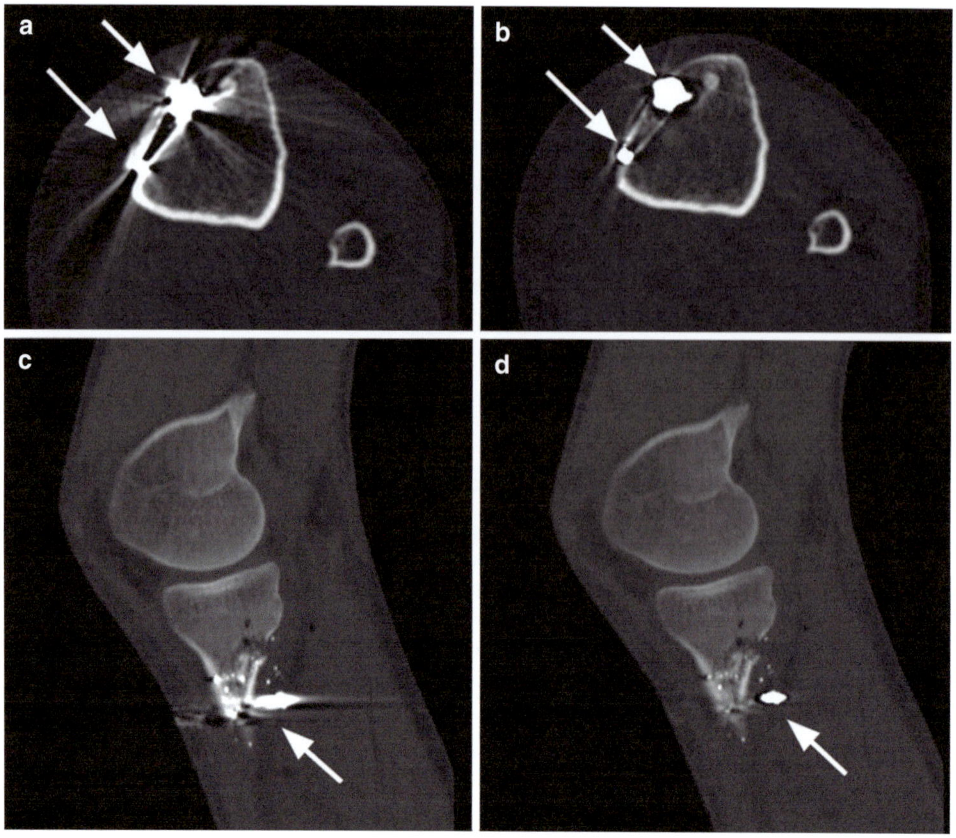

Fig. 47.4 DECT for metal artifact reduction in gunshot injury of the lower extremity with multiple bullet fragments (white arrows). Axial (**a** and **b**) and sagittal (**c** and **d**) imaging demonstrating improved image quality when comparing baseline images (**a** and **c**) to images following application of metal artifact reduction (**b** and **d**) using dual-energy CT

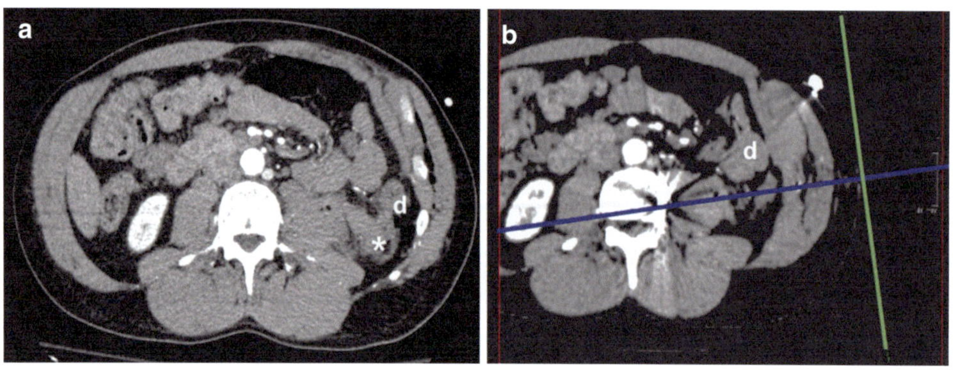

Fig. 47.5 Trajectory analysis in gunshot injury of the abdomen. Axial images (**a**) demonstrate blood products (*) in the retroperitoneum tracking adjacent to the descending colon (d), raising concern for colonic injury. Multioblique reformatted trajectory analysis (**b**) shows a bullet tract away from the descending colon. Absence of colonic injury was confirmed at laparotomy

Key Points

- The radiologist remains the principal resource for determining how advanced cross-sectional imaging may benefit either a general institutional protocol or an individual patient.
- Modern CT and MRI scanners allow a range of methods for problem-solving based either on clinical findings or initial CT findings. Good communication between the trauma team and the radiologist and prompt review of the initial CT are therefore critical.
- The increasing role of Interventional Radiology and nonoperative management mandates both accurate detection and characterization of significant injuries and good vascular road mapping.
- New and emerging cross-sectional techniques for initial trauma imaging including DECT and trajectory analysis are variably accessible and may lack high-level evidence at this stage in their development but can provide valuable information when integrated appropriately.

References

1. Davenport MS, Perazella MA, Yee J, Dillman JR, Fine D, McDonald RJ, Rodby RA, Wang CL, Weinreb JC. Use of intravenous iodinated contrast media in patients with kidney disease: consensus statements from the American College of Radiology and the National Kidney Foundation. Radiology. 2020;294(3):660–8.
2. Bashir AA, Kong V, Skinner D, Bruce J, Laing G, Brysiewicz P, Clarke D. Contrast-induced nephropathy following CT scan for trauma is not rare and is associated with increased mortality in South African trauma patients. Eur J Trauma Emerg Surg. 2019;45(6):1129–35.
3. Kelemen JA, Kaserer A, Jensen KO, Stein P, Seifert B, Simmen HP, Spahn DR, Pape HC, Neuhaus V. Prevalence and outcome of contrast-induced nephropathy in major trauma patients. Eur J Trauma Emerg Surg. 2020:1–7.
4. Pantel H, Stensland KD, Hashim J, Rosenblatt M. Is measurement of renal function necessary for all trauma patients before iodinated contrast administration? Emerg Radiol. 2017;24(5):541–6.
5. Gurm HS, Dixon SR, Smith DE, Share D, Lalonde T, Greenbaum A, Moscucci M. BMC2 (Blue Cross Blue Shield of Michigan Cardiovascular Consortium) Registry. Renal function-based contrast dosing to define safe limits of radiographic contrast media in patients undergoing percutaneous coronary interventions. J Am Coll Cardiol. 2011;58(9):907–14.
6. Bush WH, Segal AJ. Recognition and treatment of acute contrast reactions. Appl Radiol. 2009 Dec;38:16–21.
7. Iyer RS, Schopp JG, Swanson JO, Thapa MM, Phillips GS. Safety essentials: acute reactions to iodinated contrast media. Can Assoc Radiol J. 2013 Aug;64(3):193–9.
8. Huynh K, Baghdanian AH, Baghdanian AA, Sun DS, Kolli KP, Zagoria RJ. Updated guidelines for intravenous contrast use for CT and MRI. Emerg Radiol. 2020;27(2):115–26.
9. ACR Committee on Drugs and Contrast Media. ACR manual on contrast media, Version 7. 2010;5–6, 20–1.
10. Sierink JC, Treskes K, Edwards MJ, Beuker BJ, den Hartog D, Hohmann J, Dijkgraaf MG, Luitse JS, Beenen LF, Hollmann MW, Goslings JC. REACT-2 study group. Immediate total-body CT scanning versus conventional imaging and selective CT scanning in patients with severe trauma (REACT-2): a randomised controlled trial. Lancet. 2016;388(10045):673–83.
11. Salim A, Sangthong B, Martin M, Brown C, Plurad D, Demetriades D. Whole body imaging in blunt multisystem trauma patients without obvious signs of injury: results of a prospective study. Arch Surg. 2006;141(5):468–73. discussion 473–5
12. Coccolini F, Montori G, Catena F, Kluger Y, Biffl W, Moore EE, et al. Splenic trauma: WSES classification and guidelines for adult and pediatric patients. World J Emerg Surg. 2017;12:40.
13. Jo AS, Wilseck Z, Manganaro MS, Ibrahim M. Essentials of spine trauma imaging: radiographs, CT, and MRI. Semin Ultrasound CT MR. 2018;39(6):532–50.
14. Ozimok CJ, Mellnick VM, Patlas MN. An international survey to assess use of oral and rectal contrast in CT protocols for penetrating torso trauma. Emerg Radiol. 2019;26(2):117–21.
15. Jawad H, Raptis C, Mintz A, Schuerer D, Mellnick V. Single-contrast CT for detecting bowel injuries in penetrating abdomino-pelvic trauma. AJR Am J Roentgenol. 2018;210(4):761–5.
16. Dane B, Baxter AB, Bernstein MP. Imaging genitourinary trauma. Radiol Clin North Am. 2017;55(2):321–35.
17. Rutman AM, Vranic JE, Mossa-Basha M. Imaging and management of blunt cerebrovascular injury. Radiographics. 2018;38(2):542–63.
18. Biffl WL, Cothren CC, Moore EE, et al. Western Trauma Association critical decisions in trauma: screening for and treatment of blunt cerebrovascular injuries. J Trauma. 2009;67(6):1150–3.
19. Bromberg WJ, Collier BC, Diebel LN, et al. Blunt cerebrovascular injury practice management guidelines: the Eastern Association for the Surgery of Trauma. J Trauma. 2010;68(2):471–7.
20. Fadl SA, Linnau KF, Dighe MK. Placental abruption and hemorrhage-review of imaging appearance. Emerg Radiol. 2019;26(1):87–97.
21. Heiken JP, Katz DS, Menu Y. Chapter 13: Emergency radiology of the abdomen and pelvis: imaging of the non-traumatic and traumatic acute abdomen. In: Hodler J, Kubik-Huch RA, von Schulthess GK, editors. Diseases of the abdomen and pelvis 2018–2021: diagnostic imaging – IDKD book [Internet]. Cham: Springer; 2018.
22. LeBedis CA, Bates DDB, Soto JA. Iatrogenic, blunt, and penetrating trauma to the biliary tract. Abdom Radiol (NY). 2017;42(1):28–45.
23. Theocharopoulos G, Chatzakis JD. Is radiography justified for the evaluation of patients presenting with cervical spine trauma? Med Phys. 2009;36(10):4461–70.
24. Yelamarthy PKK, Chhabra HS, Vaksha V, Agarwal Y, Agarwal A, Das K, Erli HJ, Bapat M, Singh R, Gautam D, Tandon R, Balamurali G, Rajan S. Radiological protocol in spinal trauma: literature review and Spinal Cord Society position statement. Eur Spine J. 2020;29(6):1197–211.
25. Smith LGF, Milliron E, Ho ML, Hu HH, Rusin J, Leonard J, Sribnick EA. Advanced neuroimaging in traumatic brain injury: an overview. Neurosurg Focus. 2019;47(6):E17.
26. Gosavi S, Tyroch AH, Mukherjee D. Cardiac trauma. Angiology. 2016;67(10):896–901.
27. Wortman JR, Uyeda JW, Fulwadhva UP, Sodickson AD. Dual-energy CT for abdominal and pelvic trauma. Radiographics. 2018;38(2):586–602.
28. Hamid S, Nicolaou S, Khosa F, Andrews G, Murray N, Abdellatif W, Qamar SR. Dual-energy CT: a paradigm shift in acute traumatic abdomen. Can Assoc Radiol J. 2020;71(3):371–87.
29. Suh CH, Yun SJ, Jin W, Lee SH, Park SY, Ryu CW. Diagnostic performance of dual-energy CT for the detection of bone marrow oedema: a systematic review and meta-analysis. Eur Radiol. 2018;28(10):4182–94.
30. Jeavons C, Hacking C, Beenen LF, Gunn ML. A review of split-bolus single-pass CT in the assessment of trauma patients. Emerg Radiol. 2018;25(4):367–74.
31. Sodagari F, Katz DS, Menias CO, Moshiri M, Pellerito JS, Mustafa A, Revzin MV. Imaging evaluation of abdominopelvic gunshot trauma. Radiographics. 2020;40(6):1766–88.
32. Dreizin D, Boscak AR, Anstadt MJ, Tirada N, Chiu WC, Munera F, Bodanapally UK, Hornick M, Stein DM. Penetrating colorectal injuries: diagnostic performance of multidetector CT with trajectography. Radiology. 2016;281(3):749–62.

Part VI

Tactical Emergency and Disaster Medicine

Disaster Medicine

48

Michelangelo Bortolin and Gregory R. Ciottone

Abbreviations

CBRN	Chemical, Biologic, Radiological, and Nuclear
COVID-19	Coronavirus Disease 2019
CWA	Chemical-Warfare Agents
EMS	Emergency Medical Services
EOP	Emergency Operations Plan
HIV	*Human Immunodeficiency Virus*
HVA	Hazard and Vulnerabilities Assessments
IAP	Incident Action Plan
IC	Incident Commander
ICS	Incident Command System
PTS	Posttraumatic Stress
SARS	Severe Acute Respiratory Syndrome
SOP	Standard Operating Procedures

Disasters include natural events like the Australian bushfire (2020) and the COVID-19 pandemic (2019–2020); intentional events like the terrorist attacks in Paris (2015), Nice (2016), and Vienna (2020); and accidental man-made events like the August 2020 Beirut explosion and demonstrate the ubiquitous nature of such devastating incidents.

Disaster is defined as any event that causes "A serious disruption of the functioning of a community or a society involving widespread human, material, economic or environmental losses and impacts, which exceeds the ability of the affected community or society to cope using its own resources" [1].

Considering that any number of different events can strike a population at any time, there is no place on earth completely immune to disasters. However, communities must be able to mitigate against and be prepared to respond to these situations, in short, be resilient to disaster.

Disaster Medicine was created as a broad specialty grounded in Emergency Medicine but also utilizing the skill sets of other surgical and medical specialties, in combination with the systems supported by Disaster Management, which applies organizational, management, and leadership knowledge to mitigate, prepare, and respond to these events. For example, during an earthquake several specialties are involved in the response and immediate care of the victims: emergency physicians, surgeons, anesthesiologists, and orthopedics; however, other subspecialties are also required in the ongoing care of victims. These include nephrologists to treat acute renal failure related to crush syndrome, and in the days following the event, primary care, psychosocial, and rehabilitation specialties for continued care. These medical and surgical specialists are only able to perform their roles under the umbrella of Disaster Management. Without being enabled by the logistics and operations capabilities seen in a large-scale disaster response, these specialists would not be functional. The global experience of the COVID-19 pandemic has emphasized how Disaster Medicine is a broad specialty that requires specific knowledge from different fields, including epidemiology, virology, emergency medicine, critical care, public health, statistics, respiratory medicine, leadership, and crisis management.

Natural or Man-made Disaster

Disasters are typically categorized as being from natural or man-made events. Natural disasters such as floods, tsunamis, and earthquakes typically have a more extensive impact on

M. Bortolin (✉)
BIDMC Fellowship in Disaster Medicine, Boston, MA, USA

CRIMEDIM - Center for Research and Training in Disaster Medicine, Humanitarian Aid, and Global Health, UPO - University of Eastern Piedmont, Novara, Italy;
http://www.disasterfellowship.org

G. R. Ciottone
BIDMC Fellowship in Disaster Medicine, Boston, MA, USA

Harvard Medical School, Boston, MA, USA

Harvard T.H. Chan School of Public Health, Boston, MA, USA
e-mail: gciotton@bidmc.harvard.edu;
http://www.disasterfellowship.org

L. Marshall Gillman, S. Widder (eds.), *Trauma Team Dynamics*, https://doi.org/10.1007/978-3-031-86312-7_48

population centers, causing more disruption. The 2020 Australian bushfire crisis killed at least 25 people, destroyed 2000 homes, and burned more than 15.6 million acres [2]. Hurricane Katrina in 2005 ravaged Louisiana, Mississippi, Alabama, and Florida causing death, numerous casualties, mass evacuations, and broad societal disruptions.

Natural disasters also include epidemics and pandemics. In the past, influenza, cholera, bubonic plague, and other diseases affected entire nations causing millions of casualties. Today the entire world has gained firsthand experience with a pandemic's effect on populations and economies. The COVID-19 pandemic has changed how everyone lives through the implementation of non-pharmaceutical interventions (NPI). However, the consequences have not been the same everywhere. Some countries have been more devastated by COVID-19 than others, whether because of incompetence, indifference, or ill luck [3], highlighting the importance of Disaster Medicine to enhance resiliency. Another viral pandemic that has resulted in differences in transmission and death rate, particularly in developing countries, is Human Immunodeficiency Virus (HIV). It is estimated that since its emergence in the early 1980s, HIV has caused more than 33 million deaths around the world, further demonstrating that an estimated 97% of natural disaster-related deaths occur in developing countries (World Bank, 2000–2001) [4].

Man-made disaster is defined as any event that is caused by the activity of human beings. Explosions, building collapses, civil wars, and radiation accidents are some examples. The collapse of the Hyatt Regency Hotel in Kansas City in 1981 is one such example. Investigations found that the cause of the collapse was due to an engineering problem. There were more than one hundred deaths and more than two hundred casualties from that disaster.

The transportation industry is commonly involved in incidents that cause large numbers of injured and deaths. In 1998, a high-speed train derailed in Eschede, Germany, causing 101 fatalities. Other industrial sectors, such as the chemical industry, have also been involved in man-made catastrophes. In December 1983 in Bhopal, India, more than half a million people were exposed to methyl isocyanate. In the immediate phase after the leak almost 10,000 people died. The Indian Government has calculated that this event has caused over the years almost 600,000 casualties due to lingering effects of the chemical exposures. The ammonium nitrate explosion in Beirut in August 2020 caused more than 170 deaths, 6,500 injuries, and left an estimated 300,000 people homeless.

The 9/11/2001 terrorist attack in New York and the Oklahoma City bombing (1995) are intentional man-made disasters. It is important to recognize and underline that disasters can also result from war, and conflict zones, as well as economic and social policies, particularly in developing countries [5]. The Syrian civil war arose in 2011 and has caused more than 400,000 deaths and 5.5 million refugees since 2013 [6].

The Disaster's Cycle

Disasters and the response to them follow a pattern called the Disaster Cycle, which is defined in four phases: mitigation and prevention, preparedness and planning, response, and recovery.

Mitigation and prevention involve measures designed either to prevent hazards from occurring or to lessen the effects of the disasters [7]. These measures involve multiple different agencies and commissions, for example, policymakers introduce regulations regarding the storage, transportation, and disposal of chemical substances. Another example of mitigation is to empower a public health system to monitor and conduct surveillance for infectious diseases and at the same time introduce rules regarding health screening at the borders. The importance of the mitigation phase is to avoid disaster or to reduce the impact on the population.

It becomes clear if we compare the 2010 earthquake in Haiti, with a magnitude of 7.0, and similar earthquakes in Japan where despite the same magnitude the number of dead and injured was much more limited. The effects of a disaster are often dependent on the underlying conditions of the area affected. For decades Japan has introduced strict building codes that follow seismic regulations. Nevertheless, it is not possible to fully mitigate against all disaster events. For instance, the 2011 earthquake in the Pacific Ocean produced a tsunami that hit the east coast of Japan and caused severe damage, in particular a failure of the nuclear plant in Fukushima, with release of radiation that affected the local community.

The preparedness and planning phase includes activities that occur on an ongoing basis, in advance of any potential incident. Preparedness involves an integrated combination of assessment, planning, procedures and protocols, training and exercises, personnel qualifications, licensure, and certification and should undergo regular evaluation and revision [8]. The first step of preparedness is defining what events are more likely to strike and how well prepared the community is for them. The Hazard Vulnerability Analysis (HVA) is a way to objectively risk-stratify those hazards that are more likely to strike a given community. The HVA takes into account different events: natural, man-made, and CBRN (Chemical, Biologic, Radiological, and Nuclear), among others. The output from an HVA prioritizes the risks to which a population is most susceptible and should therefore be prepared for. After the HVA, it is possible to then establish Standard Operating Procedures (SOP) and the Emergency Operations Plan (EOP) for the community or hospital. It is a good rule that the EOP adopts an all-hazards approach to preparedness, with annexes and appendices specific for every type of probable event [9].

An important part of the preparedness phase is training. In particular, every healthcare professional must be trained when to activate disaster response and their own specific roles and responsibilities within the framework of the response. The drills commonly used are tabletop and full-scale exercises. They are important also to identify shortfalls, bottlenecks, and gaps in the EOP. The staff should take part in the training and the EOP should be tested, reviewed, and updated at least once per year.

Response is the phase in which agencies and sections with responsibility to deploy to disasters activate their emergency response plan as a result of specific threats or situations and can incorporate local, regional, and federal response agencies [10]. The response is conducted through a collaboration between several agencies and must be flexible and adaptable for any type of event.

It is important to immediately establish a response framework with a unified command structure that establishes a chain of command and control and coordinates the resources, in terms of staff, stuff, and space. The Incident Command System (ICS) provides a structure to enable agencies with different legal, jurisdictional, and functional responsibilities to coordinate, plan, and interact effectively on scene [11]. The medical response is provided at the scene by the Emergency Medical Services (EMS), with triage, treatment, and transport to the hospitals, which plays a crucial role in the immediate phase of the response to disaster. The response must be quick and effective, on-scene as well as in the determination of hospital destinations for every patient, to guarantee an appropriate standard of care and to avoid bottlenecks and congestion at hospitals. Rarely, EMS is able to triage, treat, and transport every single patient from the scene. More often some casualties reach the closest hospital on their own, giving rise to disruption in the chain of triage and to the hospital. The ability of a healthcare system to suddenly expand its capacity beyond normal services to meet the increased demand for qualified medical staff and services during a large-scale event is defined as "surge capacity" [12]. The surge capacity depends on the features of the healthcare system, but also by an effective EOP and training level of the staff.

The post-impact period revolves around disaster recovery in which the goal is to eliminate impairment caused by a disaster and rebuild communities and infrastructures [13]. This phase involves several agencies and may be long-lasting, ranging from weeks to years. People affected by a catastrophic disaster often face a long recovery phase. Survivors of the September 11, 2001, terrorist attacks on the Twin Towers not only had immediate treatment in the field and in the hospitals that day, but their treatment has continued for years. The majority of people exposed to disasters do well; however, some individuals develop psychiatric disorders, distress, or risky behaviors such as an increase in alcohol or tobacco use [14]. The Department of Health and Human Services spent months and years addressing this following the 9/11 attacks and has gone on to provide healthcare, both physical and mental, to those who were, and continue to be, affected and in need [15]. The recovery phase often also involves rescue workers as their exposure to the traumatic event can have a severe impact on their mental health. Studies confirm that rescue workers are prone to have diseases or documented behavioral health disturbances during and following events. For example, several articles describe how the acute and prolonged exposures were both associated with a large burden of asthma and posttraumatic stress (PTS) symptoms years after the 9/11 attack. In addition, the suicides of a prominent New York City emergency physician and a nurse in Italy, both of whom had been on the frontlines of the COVID-19 response, are tragic indicators of the traumatic events incurred by many healthcare workers during disasters [16].

Incident Command System

During an incident the response must be effective and efficient. To achieve this, and thereby ensure that the best care possible is rendered to victims, it is fundamental to have a well-prepared and organized system. The Incident Command System (ICS) is a standardized, on-scene, all-hazard incident management system and allows its users to adopt an integrated organizational structure to match the complexities and demands of single or multiple incidents without being hindered by jurisdictional boundaries [17].

The ICS was developed in the 1970s in California to manage, command, and control fire brigades during their operations to extinguish wildfires. It was then adopted by EMS and other agencies, as well as endorsed by the U.S. Department of Homeland Security as a fundamental element of incident management.

The ICS is used for all events and is modified depending on the size of the incident. Its goal is to manage and resolve the incident with an efficient use of resources while protecting all persons involved. The ICS is a modular and flexible organizational system that can be standardized for multiple uses. The ICS is modified according to the size and complexity of the incident, specificity of the hazard, environment affected by the incident, the incident planning process, and incident objectives (ICS expansion and contraction) [18].

The ICS establishes an Incident Commander (IC), who is in charge of all the activities regarding the incident; a chain of command; and unified command between the agencies. The priorities of the IC are three: the safety of the casualties and the rescue team, incident stabilization, and property preservation. Every incident must have an Incident Action Plan (IAP) that establishes incident goals, operational period objectives, set activities, and the response strategy defined by the IC during response planning [19].

The IC manages and carries out their responsibilities with three features of command that are important for every role within the framework of the ICS: the chain of command, the unity of command, and the span of control. The chain of command is a key part of the ICS and is defined as a structure with a clear line of authority. The unity of command infers that every responder knows without question who their supervisor is. Span of control describes the typically 6–7 people a supervisor directly leads.

During a disaster, it is extremely important to establish a Unified Command, because it enables all responsible agencies to manage and coordinate an incident together by establishing a common approach and a single IAP. It permits the integration of staffing and shared facilities, with everyone having the same objectives and not replicating efforts [20].

The IAP describes activities, responsibilities, and communication procedures. This system is fundamental to avoid confusion and lack of communication. Adequate and redundant communication systems are very important during the response to disaster. It is essential that the ICS uses common terminology and integrated communications among agencies and establishes precise ways of communication. The communication systems should be: interoperable between agencies; reliable to function in the context of any kind of emergency; portable, built on standardized radio technologies, protocols, and frequencies; scalable as the needs of the incident dictate; resilient to perform despite damaged or lost infrastructure; and redundant to enable use of alternate communication methods when primary systems go out [21].

The ICS is supported by a command staff that includes a safety manager, a liaison officer, and a public information officer. It is organized into four sections which support the ICS: operation, planning, logistics, and finance/administration. The operation section is in charge of managing all activities on the scene including fire brigades, EMS, and all agencies required for the incident. The planning section is responsible for drafting the IAP; receiving, assimilating, and sharing information; and tracking all resources. The logistics section provides the required equipment and facilities and supports personnel with food and water. The finance/administration section provides funding, tracks all costs, and manages contracts.

These sections, like the ICS, are modular organizations and can be further expanded into: units (the organizational element with functional responsibility for specific incident planning, logistics, or finance/administration activity), divisions (only for the operations section and used to divide an incident geographically), groups (only for operation section and established to divide the incident management structure into functional areas), and branches (used when the number of divisions or groups exceeds the span of control and can be either geographical or functional for major aspects of incident operations) [22].

Triage

The word triage is derived from the French word "trier" that literally means "to categorize, or to sort." The concept of triage was proposed for the first time by Baron Dominique Jean Larrey, Surgeon in Chief to Napoleon's Imperial Guard in the eighteenth century. The innovation of Baron Larrey was that he was the first to implement the idea of treating the sickest first and evacuating them to the most appropriate care facility in priority order, thereby maximizing the use of available resources for optimal patient benefit, and aiming for a minimum time to definitive treatment [23].

The most commonly used disaster triage system places casualties into four classes: black (expectant), red (immediate priority), yellow (delayed priority), or green (minor priority), depending on the severity of the injuries. When sorting casualties, it is important to give immediate medical care to critical patients that have a chance of survival with prompt, advanced treatment. In less critical patients, and patients who are so severely injured that they have very little chance of survival, treatment is delayed. The goal is to provide the greatest good for the greatest number of patients, forcing the triage officer to decide whether the chance of a patient surviving is so low in comparison to the burden such care would place on the medical system that the patient must be consigned to the "expectant" category (dying; little or no treatment) [24]. Triage will be discussed further in Chapter 49.

The concept of triage must be seen in a wider context and is composed of the following elements: rapid evaluation of all disaster victims; assessment of the nature and severity of the injuries and its consequences on the vital functions of the casualties, categorization of the casualties, resuscitation, stabilization for transport, distribution, and evacuation of the casualties [25]. Triage is a quick and dynamic process. This means that it must be repeated often and at every moment in which a new healthcare professional takes control of a patient. For example, during transport, upon arrival at the hospital, or if there is a suspicion that the state of the patient has changed.

One concern in disaster triage is the possible use of chemical or radiation weapons in a terrorist attack. The recent use of chemical weapons (CW) on civilian populations, as seen in the Syrian civil war and in assassination attempts in the United Kingdom, Malaysia, and Russia, has increased that concern. This has demonstrated the importance of a new system of triage to use for these CW attacks to quickly differentiate and recognize among classes of agents and implement the correct therapy decontamination protocols.

Gregory Ciottone has proposed a flowchart for toxidrome-based rapid identification of chemical warfare agent classes. This acute-phase triage system first addresses the initial suspicion at the scene of a CW release and then differentiates based on toxidromes (signs and symptoms), such as respiratory noise, bradypnea or apnea, gasping, collapse, seizures, sedation, confusion, miosis or mydriasis, dry skin, elevated temperature, pain, and skin blistering. This novel triage system can quickly differentiate between nerve agent, asphyxiant, opioid agent, anesthetic agent, anticholinergic agent, vesicant, caustic or riot-control agent, central or peripheral-compartment (large-airway or small-airway) pulmonary agent, and botulinum toxin. The Ciottone triage system for chemical weapons attack ensures safety of the responders in the field and reduces the time-to-treat for the casualties of these horrific incidents [26].

"Second Hit" Phenomenon

The "second hit" is a classic tactic and pattern seen in terrorist attacks. It is defined as a second intentional incident following the first event, with the goal of striking first responders who are on scene. Typically, it is a second explosion close to the scene and often more powerful than the first detonation, with the intention of creating casualties and attracting responders to the scene and then striking them with a larger secondary detonation. This achieves the goal of a terrorist attack: to cause additional chaos thereby delaying the response and causing great physical and psychological impact on the populations and on the rescuers.

An example of this was the terrorist attack in 2002, in Bali. Two bombs detonated within a short period of time. The first was concealed in a vest worn by a suicide bomber. The second charge was in a minivan about 15 meters away when the first explosion happened. The force of the car bomb was enormous [27].

Terrorist attacks are very challenging and difficult to manage, because they are designed to create loss of life, disruption of the agencies involved in the response, and instill fear in the population.

The Israeli response system is very seasoned to terrorist attacks and has specific guidelines and protocols in case of attack to avoid damage from a "second hit." Traditionally, medical teams do not enter the scene of the explosion until it is deemed safe by police or army personnel. With many of the terrorist attacks in Israel, a secondary explosion or bomb is set off timed to cause additional injuries to the emergency personnel and bystanders responding to the primary event. However, because time is critical, often EMS does not wait for such security clearance and attempts to rapidly remove the casualties from the immediate vicinity of the initial event. The only medical care given before this initial evacuation is external hemorrhage control [28]. They apply the "scoop and run" approach on the scene (minimal resuscitation on the scene and immediate transportation to the trauma center) to clear the casualties from the area of the event and minimize the risk to the rescuers. Therefore, in the case of a terrorist attack, it is imperative to maintain the role of the Incident Commander, the coordination between the agencies, and the training of the rescuers to guarantee the safety of all the workers involved in the response.

The August 2020 port explosion in Beirut at an ammonium nitrate storage facility with inadequate safety measures, although not due to a terrorist attack, has shown a "second hit" phenomenon. The fire brigade was dispatched to the scene to put out a fire and a few minutes later there was a first explosion and, seconds later, a second more substantial explosion. This event can substantially change the standard operating procedures for rescuers in fires and explosions. Even if the event is not caused by a terroristic attack: a "scoop and run" approach, minimizing time and number of rescuers on scene, seems a safer strategy.

Conclusions

Disaster Medicine is a broad specialty that integrates the medical response to disaster with the systems of disaster management. The Disaster Cycle is defined in four phases including (1) mitigation and prevention, (2) preparedness and planning, (3) response, and (4) recovery.

Key Points

- Disaster is defined as any event that causes serious disruption of society which exceeds the ability of the affected community to cope using its own resources.
- Disasters are usually categorized as natural or man-made, and response to all follows the same pattern, called the Disaster Cycle and defined in four phases: mitigation and prevention, preparedness and planning, response, and recovery.
- The Incident Command System (ICS) is a standardized and modular organization for on-scene, all-hazard incident management and allows its users to adopt an integrated organizational structure to match the complexities and demands of single or multiple incidents.
- The word triage means "to categorize or to sort." The purpose of triage in a disaster event is to cata-

log the casualties with respect to the severity of injuries. Sorting casualties is important to provide emergent medical care to those critical patients that have the highest chance of survival with the goal of doing the greatest good for the greatest number of patients.

- The "second hit" phenomenon is a classic tactic and a pattern of terrorist attacks. It is defined as a second incident following the first event that is designed to strike the first responders who are on scene. The August 2020 port explosion in Beirut can substantially change the standard operating procedures for rescuers in the case of fire and explosions, even if the event is not a terrorist attack. A "scoop and run" approach that may minimize the time and number of rescuers on scene may be a safer strategy.

References

1. The United Nations Office for Disaster Risk Reduction, Terminology, [Internet]. 2013. Available from http://www.unisdr.org/we/inform/terminology. Last accessed 5 Nov 2020.
2. https://www.dosomething.org/us/articles/2020-australian-bushfire-crisis?&utm_source=twitter&utm_medium=social&utm_campaign=australian-bushfire-crisis. Last accessed 5 Nov 2020.
3. https://www.ft.com/content/9b8223bb-c5e4-4c11-944d-94ff5d33a909. Last accessed 5 Nov 2020.
4. Bendimerad F "Disaster Risk Reduction and Sustainable Development," World Bank Seminar on The Role of Local Governments in Reducing the Risk of Disasters, Held in Istanbul, Turkey, 28 April – 2 May 2003, World Bank, Washington, DC.
5. Harding S. Man-made disaster and development – the case of Iraq. Int Soc Work. 50(3):295–306.
6. United Nations High Commissioner for Refugees, Stories From Syrian Refugees [Internet]. 2020. Available from https://data2.unhcr.org/en/situations/syria. Last accessed 5 Nov 2020.
7. World Health Organization. Community Emergency Preparedness: a manual for managers and policy-makers. WHO; 1999. p. 12.
8. U.S. Department of Homeland Security, National Incident Management System (NIMS) December 2008, p. 7. Available from http://www.fema.gov/pdf/emergency/nims/NIMS_core.pdf
9. U.S. Federal Emergency Management Agency "Guide for All-Hazard Emergency Operations Planning" September 1996, p. 2–11. Available from http://www.cdc.gov/nceh/ehs/Docs/State_and_Local_Guide_101_HEOP.pdf. Last accessed 5 Nov 2020.
10. Lee CY, Riley JM. Chapter 2: Public health and disasters. In: Ciottone GR, editor. Disaster medicine. 3rd ed. Mosby; 2006. p. 8.
11. U.S. Department of Homeland Security National Response, National Response Framework (NRF) January 2008, p. 10. Available from http://www.fema.gov/pdf/emergency/nrf/nrf-core.pdf
12. Bey T, Koenig KL, Barbisch DF, Das Konzept von. „Surge Capacity" im Katastrophenfall Notfall Rettungsmed 2007, p. 1–5
13. Kano M, Wood MM, Siegel JM, Bourque LB. Disaster research and epidemiology. In: Koenig KL, Schultz CH, editors. Koenig and Schultz's disaster medicine: comprehensive principles and practices. Cambridge University Press; 2010. p. 8.
14. Ursano RJ, Fullerton CS, Weisaeth L, Raphael B. Chapter 1: Individual and community responses to disasters. In: Textbook of disaster psychiatry. Cambridge University Press; 2007. p. 8.
15. Agwunobi JO, Testimony before the Committee on Oversight and Government Subcommittee on Government Management, Organization and Procurement United States House of Representatives, on 9/11 Health Effects: HHS's Monitoring and Treatment of Responders.
16. Benham TL, Hart A, Bortolin M, Court M, Groves J, Kraus A, Newbury B, Voskanyan A, Yogman M, AlHajjaj F, AlMalki Y, Alossaimi B, Awoniyi O, Bardeesi A, Cattamanchi S, Edwards B, Hernandex A, Issa F, Manners P, Molloy M, Romney D, Weiner D, Ciottone GR. Preparing for the second surge: preventing post-traumatic stress disorder and building resilience for healthcare workers in the face of COVID-19. Disaster Medicine and Public Health Preparedness; 2020. p. 1–14. https://doi.org/10.1017/dmp.2020.371.
17. U.S. Federal Emergency Management Agency "ICS-100.A: Introduction to ICS EMI Course Number: IS100" Student Manual Version 2008, U.S. Department of Homeland Security Unit, 2, p. 2–4.
18. U.S. Federal Emergency Management Agency "ICS-200: Single Resources and Initial Action Incidents" EMI Course Number: IS200 Instructor Guide Version 2.0 April 2008 December 2008, Unit 6, p. 6.
19. U.S. Department of Health & Human Services, Office of the Assistant Secretary for preparadness and Response. What Is An Incident Action Plan? [Internet] 2013. Available from http://www.phe.gov/Preparedness/planning/mscc/handbook/pages/appendixc.aspx. Last accessed 5 Nov 2020.
20. U.S. Federal Emergency Management Agency "ICS-300 Intermediate ICS for Expanding" Student Manual April 2012, Unit 1, p. 1.20.
21. U.S. Federal Emergency Management Agency "IS-700.A: National Incident Management System, An Introduction" Student Manual January 2009, Unit 4, p. 4.9.
22. U.S. Federal Emergency Management Agency "Introduction to the Incident Command System (ICS 100) Student Manual August 2010.
23. Robertson-Steel I. Evolution of triage systems. Emerg Med J. 2006;23(2):154–5.
24. Burstein JL. Mostly dead: can science help with disaster triage? Ann Emerg Med. 2009;54(3):431. https://doi.org/10.1016/j.annemergmed.2009.02.012.
25. Debacker M. "Triage" [unpublished lecture notes] Università del Piemonte Orientale Vercelli (Italy) and Vrije Universiteit Brussel (Belgium) Lecture given during the European Master in Disaster Medicine (EMDM) 2008.
26. Ciottone GR. Toxidrome recognition in chemical-weapons attacks. N Engl J Med. 2018;378(17):1611–20. https://doi.org/10.1056/NEJMra1705224.
27. Swedish Defense Research Agency, Unit for Emergency Preparedness, Committee for Disaster Medicine Studies. The terror attack on Bali, 2002. Kamedo report 89.
28. Singer AJ, Singer AH, Halperin P, Kaspi G, Assaf J. Medical lessons from terror attacks in Israel. J Emerg Med. 2007;32(1):87–92.

The Multi-casualty Trauma

49

Daniel Roizblatt, Amin Madani, Tarek Razek, and Kosar Khwaja

Introduction

Multi-casualty trauma following unexpected natural and human-made disasters creates major stress on receiving hospitals and regional trauma systems as local emergency services attempt to treat multiple seriously injured victims simultaneously. However, the strain of a multi-casualty trauma event remains within the confines of an institution's surge capacity to adequately manage all patients. This is in contrast to "mass-casualty trauma" (MCT), where the required resources exceed the surge capacity of a single institution and at times the trauma system as a whole. Therefore, it is the availability of local and regional resources to the event, and not the absolute number of victims, that differentiates a *multi-casualty trauma* from a *mass-casualty trauma*. Timely and effective coordination of all available resources at the local and regional level is critical when attempting to manage the varying number of patients in such events.

The purpose of this chapter is to discuss principles of triage during MCT, describe the various components of the response team and their roles during such events, and discuss the role of simulation training to prepare healthcare personnel for unexpected MCT.

D. Roizblatt
Department of Surgery, McGill University Health Centre, Montreal, QC, Canada

Department Trauma Surgery, Montreal General Hospital, Montreal, QC, Canada
e-mail: droizblatt@hts.cl

A. Madani
Department of Surgery, McGill University Health Centre, Montreal, QC, Canada
e-mail: amin.madani@mail.mcgill.ca

T. Razek · K. Khwaja (✉)
McGill University Health Centre, Montreal, QC, Canada
e-mail: tarek.razek@mcgill.ca; kosar.khwaja@mcgill.ca

Historical Perspective

While MCT has existed for centuries, priority of care was often given to patients depending on rank, socioeconomic status, and specific nationalities, without taking into account the severity of injuries [1]. As outlined in the previous chapter, it was not until Baron Dominique Jean Larrey, Surgeon-in-Chief of Napoleon's Imperial Guard, and the French Service de Santé coined the term "triage" (meaning "to sort") and began to systematically organize the care of patients during MCT [2]. Larrey's triage system, along with his horse-pulled ambulances, allowed him to treat patients according to the severity of their injuries, similar to principles used in today's modern triage systems.

Ethical Issues in Multiple Casualty Trauma

Healthcare workers are often confronted with ethical dilemmas while managing an MCT. Oftentimes, first responders who arrive at the scene place their own lives at risk while attempting to help victims. Hostile environments include urban zones in the aftermath of natural disasters (such as earthquakes and hurricanes), where buildings are still at risk of collapsing, or a district that has suffered terrorist bombings and is at risk of subsequent explosions. For instance, during the 9/11 attack, 343 firefighters lost their lives while attempting to rescue victims [3]. The duty to treat and to put oneself in harm's way during disasters often contradicts one's duty to themselves [4].

Another ethical issue commonly associated with MCT is determining which patients receive priority care. Under normal circumstances, triage in the emergency department prioritizes which patients receive care first. When multiple casualties are involved however, not every patient may receive immediate medical attention [5]. This requires good judgment by healthcare personnel to make decisions which are not always easy to make. Resource allocation is often done in the context of three key principles [6]:

L. Marshall Gillman, S. Widder (eds.), *Trauma Team Dynamics*, https://doi.org/10.1007/978-3-031-86312-7_49

1. Utilitarianism—"the greatest good for the greatest number"
2. Principle of equal chances—"first come, first served"
3. Egalitarianism—"those most in need should receive"

Utilitarianism normally takes precedence over other principles in MCT, since the primary goal is to treat the greatest number of victims in the best possible way. Often, the response team needs to make difficult and timely decisions regarding the allocation of resources to a patient depending on their "salvageability." Personnel in charge of triage should therefore be cognizant of the utilitarian principle governing MCT in order to avoid any interference with a systematic and effective resource-allocation protocol.

Prehospital Management

Triage

Triage, a fundamental concept in the management of MCT, involves sorting the wounded according to the severity of their injuries and assigning treatment priorities in the context of available resources for a relatively large patient load. This is a paradigm shift compared to normal circumstances, where an assumption is made that adequate resources are available for everyone.

In a typical MCT, it is estimated that 10–15% of victims will sustain severe injuries, while the remainder will suffer mild to moderate traumas [7]. The primary objective of the triage process is to identify the subset of victims who are both severely injured and salvageable and transfer them to a trauma center in a timely fashion. Identifying this priority group can be quite challenging. Due to the number of patients presenting simultaneously during MCT, rather than focusing on each injured patient individually, personnel in charge of triage focus their attention on the entire injured population [8]. Both severity of injuries and degree of salvageability of patients should be taken into consideration when deciding how to allocate resources, with the aim of saving as many lives as possible. Other factors that should be taken into consideration include the total number and nature of the wounded, the geographic location, available facilities and personnel, lines of evacuation, and transport duration. To assist with objective decision-making, several triage tools have been developed.

The process of triage is not a single event. Instead it is continuous and patients are consistently reevaluated. It is imperative that decisions be respected with optimal teamwork and communication. The triage process can be categorized as follows:

- *Primary triage* is performed at the scene of the event, normally by paramedics or first responders.
- *Secondary triage* is performed at the facility where patients are transferred, typically at the entrance of the emergency department by the most experienced healthcare professional, usually an experienced surgeon or emergency physician. Based on the level of care required, injury severity of the patient, and the resources available, the patient is moved to a predesignated area where further appropriate care is provided.
- *Tertiary triage* is performed by surgeons, emergency physicians, anesthesiologists, or intensive care physicians in order to determine where in the hospital the patient should be transferred. The intensive care unit (ICU), operating room, radiology suite, and a designated "minor" care area are some of the most common destinations. Based on available human resources and severity of injuries, the following are done: vital signs measurements, intravenous line placement, initial resuscitation, administration of antibiotics and tetanus vaccine, obtaining blood work, and preparation for transfer.

Ultrasound (Focused Assessment with Sonography in Trauma (FAST) or "extended" FAST) can be an effective tool that may help during tertiary triage. Use of ultrasonography in a mass casualty scenario was described by Sharkisian et al. following the 1988 American earthquake. More recently, the use of FAST in multiple casualty scenarios was described in a retrospective Israeli study that showed that FAST enabled immediate triage of casualties to laparotomy, CT, or clinical observation, with a positive predictive value of 88.2%, negative predictive value of 94.1%, and accuracy of 93.1% [9, 10].

Effective triage should be accompanied with a simple patient identification system that is unambiguous and understandable by all healthcare personnel. Each patient should be tagged with a visible triage card containing their demographics, medical assessment, and triage allocation (Fig. 49.1).

Despite timely triage efforts, there exists the possibility of patients either receiving less than the level of care required to treat their injuries (under-triage) or receiving more than the level of care required (over-triage) leading to inappropriate utilization of limited resources (e.g., transportation, beds, imaging modalities). A less than 5% under-triage rate and less than 50% over-triage is generally acceptable [11].

Because triage decisions can be difficult and at times emotionally challenging for healthcare personnel, the triage officer should be someone of authority, well-respected, and not only knowledgeable of patterns of injury but also must have a very clear understanding of all resources available at any given time.

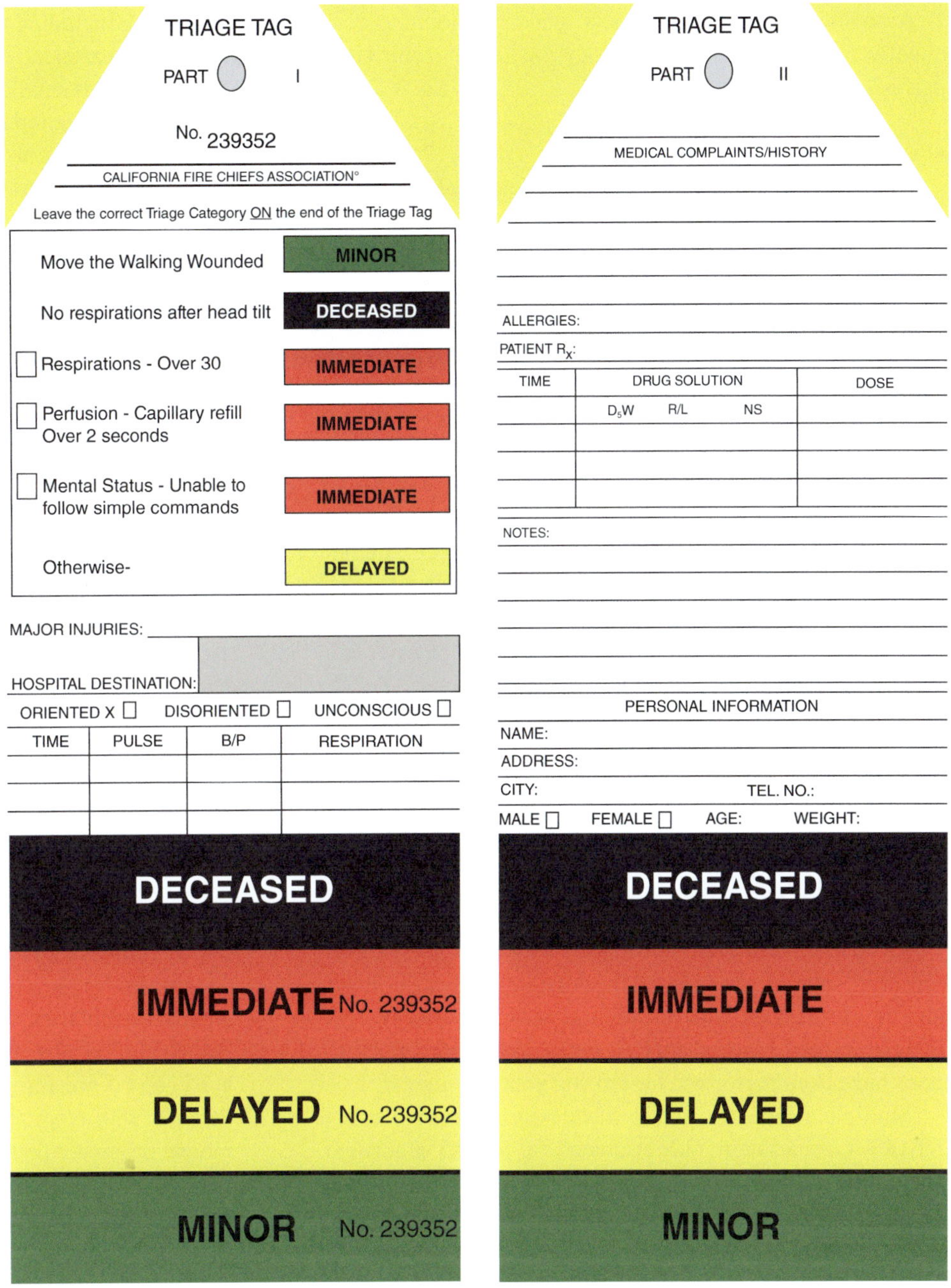

TRIAGE TAG
PART I
No. 239352
CALIFORNIA FIRE CHIEFS ASSOCIATION®
Leave the correct Triage Category ON the end of the Triage Tag

Move the Walking Wounded	MINOR
No respirations after head tilt	DECEASED
☐ Respirations - Over 30	IMMEDIATE
☐ Perfusion - Capillary refill Over 2 seconds	IMMEDIATE
☐ Mental Status - Unable to follow simple commands	IMMEDIATE
Otherwise-	DELAYED

MAJOR INJURIES:
HOSPITAL DESTINATION:
ORIENTED X ☐ DISORIENTED ☐ UNCONSCIOUS ☐

TIME	PULSE	B/P	RESPIRATION

DECEASED
IMMEDIATE No. 239352
DELAYED No. 239352
MINOR No. 239352

TRIAGE TAG
PART II
MEDICAL COMPLAINTS/HISTORY
ALLERGIES:
PATIENT R_x:

TIME	DRUG SOLUTION	DOSE
	D_5W R/L NS	

NOTES:

PERSONAL INFORMATION
NAME:
ADDRESS:
CITY: TEL. NO.:
MALE ☐ FEMALE ☐ AGE: WEIGHT:

DECEASED
IMMEDIATE
DELAYED
MINOR

Fig. 49.1 Multi-casualty trauma patient identification and triage tag utilizing a color code to indicate the level of care needed based on the Simple Triage and Rapid Treatment (START) system. Reprinted with permission from the California Fire Chiefs Association

"START" System for Triage

In order to assist with the on-scene primary triage process, several tools have been developed to allow for a timely and objective decision-making. This includes the Simple Triage And Rapid Treatment (START) system, initially created in 1983 by the Newport Beach Fire Department in California. This system is easy to use and focuses on patient physiology, providing a rapid assessment for each patient which lasts no more than 30 s. Using the START protocol therefore permits very few rescuers to rapidly triage a large number of patients, which is invaluable for multi- and mass-casualty traumas.

Patients are initially designated a color depicting the level of care needed (Fig. 49.1):

- Red: immediate care
- Yellow: delayed care
- Green: ambulatory care
- Black: deceased

Initially, walking patients are identified, tagged as green (i.e., ambulatory care), and directed to a designated area for detailed assessment and treatment. Ambulatory care patients can also assist first responders.

Assessment for nonambulatory patients should subsequently focus on patient physiology, including respiration, perfusion, and mental status.

- *Respiration*:
  - Patients who do not breathe spontaneously despite opening the airway manually are designated as black (i.e., deceased).
  - If patients breathe spontaneously at a respiratory rate greater than 30 per minute, or initiate spontaneous breaths after the airway is opened manually, they are designated as red (i.e., immediate care).
  - Patients with spontaneous respiration at a rate less than 30 per minute should undergo perfusion assessment.
- *Perfusion*:
  - Patients with either absent radial pulse or capillary refill longer than 2 s are designated as red (i.e., immediate care).
  - If both radial pulse is present and capillary refill is less than 2 s, the patient's mental status should be assessed.
- *Mental status*:
  - Patients who cannot follow simple commands, are unconscious, or have altered mental status are tagged as red (i.e., immediate care).
  - All other patients, whose respiration, perfusion, and mental status are nonremarkable, are tagged as yellow (i.e., delayed care).

Red patients require immediate care and should be transferred as soon as possible, after addressing either an upper airway obstruction or controlling obvious hemorrhage. Patients tagged black should be reevaluated once interventions have been performed for red and yellow patients.

Multiple validation studies have been performed using START. Gebhart et al. [12] evaluated the START algorithm on trauma patients, showing strong efficacy. An important point to highlight is that patients tagged as black during multi-casualty traumas may receive a level of care that is very different than if that same patient were to arrive to the emergency room on any other day. For instance, a patient without spontaneous breathing after a trauma typically requires a definitive airway (normally with endotracheal tube intubation). When the START protocol is activated, this same patient might be tagged as black and thus considered unsalvageable. Several authorities have suggested that, given resources are overextended and not overwhelmed in multi-casualty trauma, patients have more access to definitive care compared to mass-casualty traumas. The use of the START tool should therefore be discouraged in these situations to avoid under-triaging patients. Other triage methods have been introduced, including the Sacco Triage Method (STM) and the Fire Department of New York (FDNY) method. While triage methods should focus on predicting clinical priority, most studies comparing triage tools have instead focused on their ability to predict mortality [13]. Further studies will be required to determine which tools are most appropriate during multi-casualty traumas.

Pediatric Considerations

In MCT, special considerations during triage should be given to the pediatric population. The JumpSTART algorithm is used to triage children under 8 years old (this algorithm can be retrieved online from http://www.jumpstarttriage.com/uploads/Combined_Algorithm.pdf).

Children who can walk independently are designated as green and subsequently undergo a secondary triage. Similar to the adults START algorithm, all other patients are evaluated based on their physiologic status, including their breathing, perfusion, and mental status.

- *Breathing*:
  - If patient is apneic or has irregular breathing, the airway is opened manually. Patients in whom spontaneous respirations resume are designated as red (i.e., immediate care). If spontaneous respirations do not resume *and* patients do not have a palpable radial pulse, they are designated as black (i.e., deceased).
  - Apneic patients with a palpable pulse should receive five rescue breaths. If apnea persists, they are tagged black, and if breathing resumes, red.
  - Patients with respiratory rate either less than 15 per minute or greater than 45 per minute are designated as red, while those between 15 and 45 per minute should undergo perfusion assessment.
- *Perfusion*:
  - Patients with either absent radial pulse or capillary refill longer than 2 s are designated as red (i.e., immediate care).
  - If both radial pulse is present and capillary refill is less than 2 s, the patient's mental status should be assessed.
- *Mental status*:
  - Assessed using the AVPU (Alert, Response to verbal stimulus, Pain, Unresponsive patient) scale.
  - Patients who inappropriately respond to pain or are unresponsive are tagged as red (i.e., immediate care).
  - Patients who are alert or responsive to verbal commands or pain are tagged as yellow (i.e., delayed care).

Patient Transportation and Allocation Within the Trauma System

Following the initial primary triage, patients are transferred to an appropriate hospital for definitive management. Although lines of evacuation can be predetermined for disaster events leading to multi-casualty trauma, they often need to be established during the disaster itself. For instance, after natural disasters such as earthquakes or hurricanes, roads can be entirely destroyed, creating significant and unanticipated challenges when attempting to evacuate and transport victims.

Appropriate allocation of patients to different trauma centers is an important part of multi-casualty trauma management. All available healthcare facilities within a reasonable distance from the event, including level 2 trauma centers and community hospitals, should be utilized by the dispatch team. This strategy will avoid overcrowding level 1 trauma centers. On the other hand, underutilization of level 1 trauma centers should also be avoided. Gill et al. compared their trauma system's response to two multi-casualty trauma train crash disasters which occurred in 2005 and 2008. Post-crash analysis after the initial 2005 event showed that most victims were transferred to local community hospitals while trauma centers were underutilized. Improving the system by which patients were allocated to various regional institutions based on injury severity and needs demonstrated an improvement in the distribution of victims in the subsequent 2008 train crash [14]. Novel computer-based models to support patient allocation have recently been developed, which take into account variables such as road traffic, hospital capacity, and hospital capabilities [15]. A thorough understanding of one's regional trauma system and consistent communication among all personnel involved in trauma care is necessary to provide effective and timely patient care.

Independent predictors of evacuation to dedicated trauma centers include being the hospital closest to the event, evacuation within 10 min of the event, and having a patient requiring urgent care in the ambulance [16]. Ideally, patients with more severe injuries should be transferred to level 1 trauma centers where they can receive definitive care, instead of the nearest hospital. Transferring these patients to a level 2 trauma center will only delay definitive care. Conversely, patients who have sustained less severe injuries should be transferred to level 2 or 3 trauma centers, where they can be adequately treated for their injuries. This will prevent overcrowding level 1 trauma centers with patients who can receive satisfactory care elsewhere.

Intrahospital Management

Although first responders have initiated primary triage at the scene of the disaster, resources within each hospital should begin to be mobilized immediately in preparation for the patient load and surge capacity of their facility. Resources include anesthesiology, intensive care unit (ICU), operating room, trauma team, emergency department, and blood bank personnel, as well as the availability of beds, resuscitation equipment, imaging modalities, transportation, and communication systems. The hospital incident commander should be working with senior hospital administration to help manage resources in an effective manner.

Secondary triage takes place at the emergency department entrance by a designated triage officer. The triage officer should be consistently receiving feedback from the field units regarding the expected patient load, as well as from in-hospital staff to determine the conditions within the hospital. This two-way feedback allows the triage officer to manage available resources effectively. The triage area should be equipped with essentials such as stretchers, blankets, dressings, intravenous fluids, plasma expanders, respiratory support equipment, and other equipment normally used in the trauma bay.

Far less literature exists on how to triage patients following multi-casualty traumas once they pass through a trauma center's doors, compared to prehospital triage. At our institution, following the Dawson College shooting in 2006, triage was done using a combined anatomic and physiologic classification based on the location of the injury and signs of physiologic instability [17].

- Green: stable walking wounded
- Yellow: complex extremity wounds needing neurovascular assessment
- Red: thoracoabdominal injuries and patients with hemodynamic instability
- Black: gunshot injury to the head

The city of Montreal suffered three multiple shooting incidents over the last 20 years. The last of such events occurred at the Dawson College in downtown Montreal with 15 victims, 11 of which were transferred to a level 1 trauma center. Analysis of the event revealed that hospital capacity was sufficient for all patients to receive adequate care, including accommodation of five more operating rooms and ten more ICU admissions, with no in-hospital mortalities. This system of anatomic and physiologic classification proved to be an effective system for in-hospital triage at a trauma center to assign patients rapidly to appropriate care.

During the multiple casualty event of the Dawson shooting, the Montreal General Hospital was fortunate to have many individuals available to assist (including physicians, nurses, orderlies, allied-health workers, medical students, and others). If not managed appropriately, this can lead to overcrowding of healthcare personnel and inefficient care. While it is important to take advantage of all manpower available, this should be done in an organized fashion, directed by the appropriate leadership. Teams consisting of one surgeon, house staff, and nursing were created to tend to each victim arriving following the school shooting in 2006.

Transfer Corridors

Access to hospital emergency services, for both trauma and nontrauma patients, should be limited to one entrance at the ambulance arrival zone. All admitted patients should have an identification tag, similar to the one given during primary triage, with their name or a given number to assist with management and reassessment. Official hospital registration typically occurs at later stages.

Patients in the emergency department prior to the multi-casualty trauma should be transferred to an adjacent zone, with predesignated physicians, paramedics, and nurses. These patients can continue to receive necessary care, while attempts are made to either discharge or transfer them to the appropriate ward or to another hospital if possible. Furthermore, daily emergencies unrelated to the multi-casualty trauma, such as cardiac arrests, surgical emergencies, and obstetrical emergencies, should be diverted to other secondary nontrauma hospitals.

Blood Bank

Blood banks play an important role during a multi-casualty trauma. Although the blood banks of trauma centers are able to cope with multi-casualty trauma depending on the number of casualties, it is important to have a surge capacity to respond to such events. When all casualties are taken into account, some authors describe the need for on average 1.3 units of red blood cells and 1.0 units of component per patient [18]. With many patients needing transfusion at the same time, efforts should be made in patient identification to avoid mistransfusions; use of wristbands, barcode tagging, or other devices can help to avoid this problem [19]. Protocols should also include how to manage the large number of blood donors that may arrive after an event, wanting to donate blood. After the 9/11 attack, in spite of collecting 500,000 units of blood after an American Red Cross appeal, many of the collected units were analyzed and categorized as nonusable [20]. This highlights the importance of maintaining a high standard of quality control with donated blood despite the possible immediate need of large amount of blood products to respond to a disaster.

Staff-Recalling Systems

The hospital should have an organized system to allow timely contact of essential staff to assist with multi-casualty trauma. Any situation involving breakdown of communication infrastructure (i.e., when natural disasters occur, or disasters occurring during the night or on weekends when staff are not in-house) makes it difficult to recall essential personnel. Regular updating of contact information, testing, and analysis of responses to simulated disaster alerts should be done periodically [21]. Each hospital should also have a tested communication system that best suits its needs, using pagers, mobile phones, or other devices.

Intensivists and Anesthesiologists

Intensivists and anesthesiologists are important resources and play important roles alongside surgeons and emergency physicians during a response to multi-casualty trauma, by having the capacity to manage severely injured patients with advanced resuscitation skill and equipment (such as mechanical ventilators).

Forward deployment systems, involving the use of one anesthesiologist to provide continuity of care for each patient, have been shown to be effective [22]. After initial assessment by the trauma team, the anesthesiologist can accompany the patient throughout other levels of care, including the trauma bay, radiology suites, and operating room if needed. If the patient is taken to the operating room, the anesthesiologist has a thorough understanding of the patient, which is especially useful when multiple specialties are needed at different stages in the operating room. This model has the advantage of keeping the surgeons in the emergency department to assess and manage incoming patients or proceeding directly to the operating room for patients who need immediate surgery.

In multi-casualty trauma, ICUs are typically one of the first resources to be saturated. Under normal circumstances, they are fully occupied with critically ill patients, making it difficult to maintain a high surge capacity. It has been reported that 4.7% of multi-casualty trauma patients will require ICU admission, 73% of which will require mechanical ventilation [23]. Intensivists should be actively involved in multi-casualty trauma, having direct communication with the hospital incident commander, trauma team leaders, and anesthesiologist in charge to effectively manage ICU beds, ensuring the required number of beds are liberated for incoming patients.

The use of ICU resources across the region is an important component in any disaster response planning. During the 2006 Dawson College shooting in Montreal, the ICU at the level 1 trauma center immediately initiated protocols to transfer hemodynamically stable patients already in the ICU (both medical and surgical patients) to nontrauma center ICUs to liberate capacity to accommodate incoming victims.

Finally, it is important to have a clear inventory of all potential places within the institution, outside of the ICU, where critically ill ventilated patients can be accommodated as surge capacity. Such areas may include postoperative recovery rooms, post-procedure recovery rooms, coronary care units, and even procedure rooms such as day surgery and interventional cardiac suites.

Training, Simulations, and Preparing for MCT

The use of simulation has recently gained significant momentum, allowing trainees to learn in a controlled environment free of any adverse consequences to patients, reach proficiency faster, and improve overall performance. The recent Boston marathon bombing is a great example of how the use of simulation and drills prior to the event can help prepare the response team for multi-casualty trauma. Although three patients were killed that day, all three died before reaching the hospital. The effectiveness of the response to this tragedy has been largely ascribed to the deliberate preparatory actions that were taken prior to this event, leading to rapid response of first responders, field triage, and delivery of care in trauma centers [24]. For instance, in 2002, the city of Boston simulated a large-scale disaster drill, with one of their main hospitals receiving 72 simulated patients (compared to the 39 casualties during the marathon bombing). During the following years, 73 exercises were performed, including communications and power failure drills, and a mass casualty bombing drill in 2010. Apart from drills, the city also analyzed multi-casualty trauma events occurring in other cities and initiated trauma team training with physicians, nurses, and administrative personnel. The use of simulated drills, including all personnel involved in a multi-casualty trauma, improved the performance of the response team on the day of the bombing. Having training assessments helps communications and triage performance [25] and tests how the system is working and its pitfalls. The use of large-scale simulations is resource-intensive and challenging. However, done periodically, it allows us to test various levels of the response to multi-casualty traumas, while having a disaster committee identify and improve weaknesses. It is important to recognize that simulation is crucial not only for front-line healthcare workers but for every component of the system, including law enforcement, hospital administrators, patient transport, patient attendants, housekeeping, equipment/supply replenishment personnel, and even food services.

Debriefing

Once all patients have been transferred to the hospital and initial treatment plans have been provided, debriefing allows the entire team to be updated on the situation—both in and out of the hospital. Meeting with the team after the initial chaos also provides a sense of unity and helps to reorganize available resources. After the Montreal 2006 Dawson College shooting, the overall performance of our trauma center and system was reviewed via numerous multidisciplinary team debriefings. These debriefings and a careful review of each case revealed areas of strength and weakness that may prove to be useful to trauma centers that may have to deal with such unfortunate events in the future.

Last but not least, debriefing should also center on the psychosocial aspects, including posttraumatic stress disorder (PTSD), that can be suffered by the medical teams and emergency medical service personnel. As described by Lubin et al., healthcare personnel should receive constant training on how to cope with these situations and have the appropriate psychosocial support following an event [26].

Conclusions

Multi-casualty trauma is thankfully a rare occurrence in most trauma systems. Nonetheless, adequate preparation, training, and simulation are essential for all those involved. A well-structured system can help mitigate the intense chaos and confusion that undoubtedly accompanies these events and can ultimately lead to better outcomes for all injured patients.

Key Points

- Multi-casualty traumas following unexpected natural and human-made disasters create major stress on receiving hospitals and regional trauma systems.
- Timely and effective coordination of all available resources, including those in the prehospital and intrahospital settings, is critical when attempting to cope with the patient load.
- Effective and objective triage is paramount in multi-casualty trauma.
- Institutions should be familiar with their surge capacity.
- Adequate preparation allows for an effective and coordinated response to unexpected multi-casualty trauma.

References

1. Skandalakis PN, Lainas P, Zoras O, Skandalakis JE, Mirilas P. "To afford the wounded speedy assistance": Dominique Jean Larrey and Napoleon. World J Surg. 2006;30(8):1392–9.
2. Robertson-Steel I. Evolution of triage systems. Emerg Med J. 2006;23(2):154–5.
3. penta. PDFlib PLOP: PDF linearization, optimization, protection-page inserted by evaluation version. www.pdflib.com-sales@pdflib.com. 2014:1–3.
4. Iserson KV, Heine CE, Larkin GL, Moskop JC, Baruch J, Aswegan AL. Fight or flight: the ethics of emergency physician disaster response. Ann Emerg Med. 2008;51(4):345–53.
5. Merin O, Ash N, Levy G, Schwaber MJ, Kreiss Y. The Israeli field hospital in Haiti – ethical dilemmas in early disaster response. N Engl J Med. 2010;362(11):e38.
6. http://www.ceep.ca/resources/Disaster-Triage-Allocation-Resources.pdf. Accessed 23 Jan 2014.
7. Hirshberg A, Holcomb JB, Mattox KL. Hospital trauma care in multiple-casualty incidents: a critical view. Ann Emerg Med. 2001;37(6):647–52.
8. Frykberg ER. Triage: principles and practice. Scand J Surg. 2005;94(4):272–8.
9. Sarkisian AE. Sonographic screening of mass casualties for abdominal and renal injuries following the 1988 Armenian earthquake. J Trauma. 1991;31(2):247–50.
10. Beck-Razi N. The utility of focused assessment with sonography for trauma as a triage tool in multiple-casualty incidents during the Second Lebanon War. J Ultrasound Med. 2007;26:1149–56.
11. Lavoie A, Emond M, Moore L, Camden S, Liberman M. Evaluation of the Prehospital Index, presence of high-velocity impact and judgment of emergency medical technicians as criteria for trauma triage. CJEM. 2010;12(2):111–8.
12. Gebhart ME, Pence R. START triage: does it work? Disaster Manag Response. 2007;5(3):68–73.
13. Kilner TM, Brace SJ, Cooke MW, Stallard N, Bleetman A, Perkins GD. In "big bang" major incidents do triage tools accurately predict clinical priority? A systematic review of the literature. Injury. 2011;42(5):460–8.
14. Cryer HG, Hiatt JR, Eckstein M, Chidester C, Raby S, Ernst TG, et al. Improved trauma system multicasualty incident response: comparison of two train crash disasters. J Trauma. 2010;68(4):783–9.
15. Amram O, Schuurman N, Hedley N, Hameed SM. A web-based model to support patient-to-hospital allocation in mass casualty incidents. J Trauma Acute Care Surg. 2012;72(5):1323–8.
16. Einav S, Feigenberg Z, Weissman C, Zaichik D, Caspi G, Kotler D, et al. Evacuation priorities in mass casualty terror-related events. Ann Surg. 2004;239(3):304–10.
17. Spicer J, Razek T, Fata P, Bernardin B, Gursahaney A, Mulder D, et al. "In-hospital triage of a mass casualty incident following a school shooting in a Canadian regional trauma system", Trauma Association of Canada (TAC) Halifax. Can J Surg. 2010;53
18. Shinar E, Manny N. Use of blood and blood products in disasters-background paper; 2014. 18.
19. Dann EJ, Bonstein L, Arbov L, Kornberg A, Rahimi-Levene N. Blood bank protocols for large-scale civilian casualty events: experience from terrorist bombing in Israel. Transfus Med. 2007;17(2):135–9.
20. Schmidt PJ. Blood and disaster – supply and demand. N Engl J Med. 2002;346(8):617–20.
21. Epstein RH, Ekbatani A, Kaplan J, Shechter R, Grunwald Z. Development of a staff recall system for mass casualty incidents using cell phone text messaging. Anesth Analg. 2010;110(3):871–8.
22. Shamir MY, Weiss YG, Willner D, Mintz Y, Bloom AI, Weiss Y, et al. Multiple casualty terror events: the anesthesiologist's perspective. Anesth Analg. 2004;98(6):1746–52. Table of contents
23. Avidan V, Hersch M, Spira RM, Einav S, Goldberg S, Schecter W. Civilian hospital response to a mass casualty event: the role of the intensive care unit. J Trauma. 2007;62(5):1234–9.
24. Walls RM, Zinner MJ. The Boston marathon response. JAMA. 2013;309(23):2441.
25. Glow SD, Colucci VJ, Allington DR, Noonan CW, Hall EC. Managing multiple-casualty incidents: a rural medical preparedness training assessment. Prehosp Disaster Med. 2013;28(04):334–41.
26. Lubin G, Sids C, Vishne T, Shochat T, Ostfield Y, Shmushkevitz M. Acute stress disorder and post-traumatic stress disorder among medical personnel in Judea and Samaria areas in the years 2000–2003. Mil Med. 2007;172(4):376–8.

Critical Incident Team Dynamics and Logistics

50

Jeremy W. Cannon, Jose L. Pascual, and Lewis J. Kaplan

Introduction

The interplay of internal coordination and member cohesion with the extrinsic forces of chaos, stress, and unpredictability underscores the need to understand and develop high-functioning teams to support success during critical incidents [1]. This concept is termed critical incident team dynamics and enjoys substantial overlap with team logistics. The successful functioning of teams that perform in high-stress and unpredictable environments with unpredictable timing (critical incident team) hinges on training so that requisite skills are developed and enhanced. Performance is continually assessed and improved, thus establishing a competency-based hierarchy that can function within a fluid environment. The methods by which to assemble, select, train, and review such teams rest on scientifically sound principles that form the thrust of this chapter's exploration. This chapter provides a readily understandable and deployable blueprint for team administrators, liaisons, leaders, as well as members.

Crew Resource Management (CRM)

As discussed in Part I of this text, the goal of CRM is to ensure the success of teams by reducing human error [2, 3]. A formal approach to team development is essential since the unexpected will occur, and for trauma teams as well as law enforcement agencies, failure to operate efficiently can lead to loss of life as well as substantial and potentially avoidable morbidity [4]. CRM works to control human factors to the greatest degree possible to remove their influence from the calculus of success. Teams that benefit from CRM are those that operate in environments where unknown external forces continually and adversely impact plans during their execution. For instance, airline crews, firefighters, oil riggers, and, pertinent to this book, police and healthcare workers often employ CRM methodology when developing service lines [5].

Another hallmark of CRM is establishing a culture of safety where all team members, regardless of rank or tenure, are empowered to voice concerns and engage in process improvement. Essential elements include promoting situational awareness, problem identification, decision-making for problem resolution, effective and equitable workload distribution, time management, and conflict resolution (a learned skill that relies on courtesy, respect, and trust) [6, 7]. The above processes help define the atmospheric tone of the organization, a feature that strongly influences the likelihood that individual members will feel comfortable enough to challenge the status quo in search of excellence. CRM works if it is embedded in the organizational structure, inaugurated with each and every project and task, iterative in nature, as well as modified and improved using hard data [8]. Prime examples of the successful application of these principles may be found in the airline industry or military special operations teams [9–11]. In each example, the organization is continually improved by empowered individuals whose goal is continual process improvement as failure is indeed not an option. Crisis is the crucible whereby the success of CRM is measured.

Characteristics of Crises

Critical incidents qualify as crises since they are emotionally charged, stressful, and unanticipated events that presage abrupt and often undesired change. Many events represent critical incidents including natural disasters (hurricanes, floods, etc.), mechanical disasters (plane

J. W. Cannon · J. L. Pascual · L. J. Kaplan (✉)
Perelman School of Medicine, University of Pennsylvania, Department of Surgery, Division of Trauma, Surgical Critical Care and Emergency Surgery, Philadelphia, PA, USA

Corporal Michael J Crescenz VAMC, Surgical Services, Philadelphia, PA, USA
e-mail: Jeremy.Cannon@pennmedicine.upenn.edu; Jose.Pascual@pennmedicine.upenn.edu; Lewis.Kaplan@pennmedicine.upenn.edu

L. Marshall Gillman, S. Widder (eds.), *Trauma Team Dynamics*, https://doi.org/10.1007/978-3-031-86312-7_50

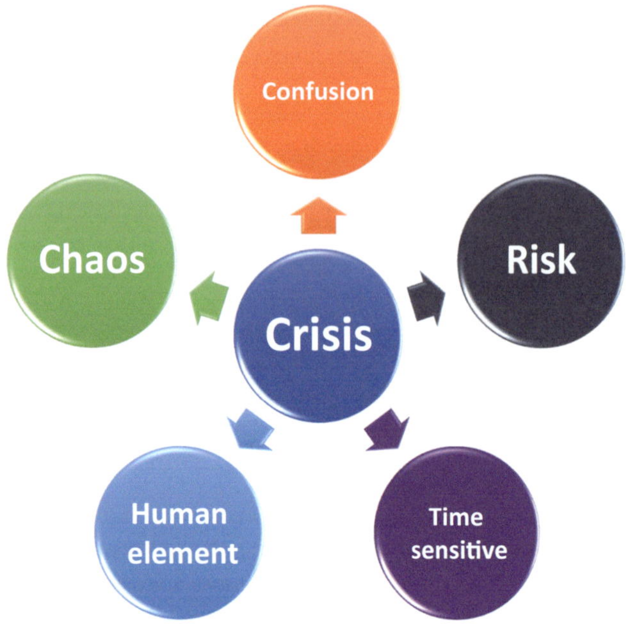

Fig. 50.1 Crisis characteristics

crashes, bridge collapses, etc.), and civilian police-related events. Wars have some features of critical incidents but are differentiated by having a slower pace toward change and are more, rather than less, anticipated. Crises that erupt within wars, on the other hand, occur in an episodic and unpredictable fashion and benefit from appropriate team training. Examples include improvised explosive device detonations and sniper attacks that occur in an unanticipatable cadence and tempo. Crises are different from conflicts in that conflicts represent the opposition of two different wills rather than physical events. Understanding the five hallmarks of crises helps optimize successful management strategies (Fig. 50.1).

First, confusion is a hallmark of crisis in that there is information and plan disarray, since crises are unclear in nature and course. Confusion impedes obtaining useful and timely information regarding current events. Second, all crises are imbued with risk which may oppose decisive action. Third, since crises are unexpected, they represent a unique and transient concatenation of circumstances, individuals, and locations, establishing a time sensitivity to their solution. When the crisis involves individuals, the crisis may be characterized as time competitive in that the commander needs to maintain the initiative to reach a rapid and successful resolution. Fourth, even when individuals are not the focus of the crisis, there is a human element centered about the responders and victims that must be acknowledged both during and after the crisis is resolved. Fifth, tactical crises powerfully tend to degenerate toward chaos. Effective teams that are integrated into highly functional systems provide the main mechanism to resolve, but not prevent, critical incidents.

Key Elements of Team Dynamics

Even great leaders cannot craft a superb team if the membership is not up to the task. Member selection is therefore a key event. There is no single metric that will allow a leader to select ideal team members, but a montage of metrics may be ideal [12]. Performance metrics that highlight dedication, drive, and aptitude combined with a relevant physical fitness assessment may enable optimal member selection for high-speed teams such as SWAT teams [13]. The Cooper Institute Fitness Assessment is a commonly used instrument that has been validated as a predictor of a police officer's ability to complete patrol duties [14]. However, it is less rigorous than measures employed by US Military Special Operations Teams during member selection and performance review. The latter is a key element that is often overlooked, especially in low-activity (i.e., infrequent SWAT team callouts) regions with dually tasked individuals (patrol officer and SWAT operator, firefighter and urban search and rescue operator, etc.) [15]. Instead, iterative assessment is required for team membership. Military special operations teams have the benefit of continual assessment during deployments as well as between deployment training sessions. Indeed, fitness is part of the job description, and time is allotted for fitness maintenance; no such time is generally allotted for civilian special response team members, and such activities are generally not funded. Fitness maintenance or development is therefore the shared responsibility of the team leader and team members.

Command and Control

The notion of command overlaps with the concept of control. It is useful to distinguish the two as they are not necessarily embodied in the same individual. Command identifies that the individual can (by virtue of their position, power, and authority) compel compliance. Control implies that the individual is providing direction but cannot compel adherence to their plan. Control is enabled by persuasion, influence, and example. Both command and control are inextricably intertwined in critical incidents. Indeed, command is said to have delegated authority, while control is said to represent perceived authority (Fig. 50.1). Military parlance denotes the two as C2.

Team commanders may be selected on the basis of perceived or demonstrated skill in related or unrelated domains. Real-world experience (immersive, direct) is always preferable to tenure-based (inferred) experience [16, 17]. Commanders and team leaders need to maintain the initiative during critical incidents in order to direct the interrelated events necessary for resolution. This task is enabled by crafting an effective command and control architecture.

Command and Control Architecture

Since critical incidents are temporary, command and control architecture is similarly temporary. Embracing the need to have a single command entity, such temporary architecture should be explicitly constructed to be directed by a single entity. Such constructs may be typified by Emerging Multi-Organizational Networks (EMON) which consist of task-oriented and mission-specific collaborations of individuals and resources [18, 19]. EMON structure defines lines of authority (effectively but not necessarily equitably), distributes power, and efficiently allocates resources for critical incident resolution. EMON resources may be broadly grouped into the following eight domains:

1. Selecting common technology platforms and across-team procedures
2. Developing modular teams and responses
3. Establishing the required elements for a unified command structure
4. Advance planning for every major and predictable type of critical incident the team might face, as well as recovery planning for initial plan failure or inefficacy during an incident
5. Defining the maximum number of supervised individuals
6. Identifying critical incident relevant facilities
7. Developing resource management plans for all teams
8. Articulating an integrated communication system

Communication systems pose a unique challenge to EMON structure as crisis events often involve disparate elements and must integrate different communication systems and protocols. The most effective team is likely to fail if unique assets are unable to communicate in a timely and effective fashion. One such example is the Area Command Team (ACT) concept of the LA County Sheriff's office. Following the 1992 Los Angeles riots, the LA County Sheriff's Department completed an in-depth review process that evaluated the logistics behind their successful and unsuccessful resource management that laid the foundation for modern management paradigms. The ACT concept has articulated structures that parallel how SWAT teams function today. Those structures include a central command with linked field command coupled with teams that have independent operational authority in response to conflict exigencies that depart from the anticipated course. Such a structure is readily adapted to non-police command team structures as well. Effective ACTs require resources to be funded and allocated for team use.

Resources

Resource management includes acquisition, cataloging, maintenance, revision, funding, allocation, mobilization, and deployment of needed elements in a fashion designed to swiftly resolve the critical incident. Therefore, resource management includes not only material but human resources. Since critical incidents often span more than one responder type (i.e., police, SWAT, EMS, fire), a system for resource management is essential. Resources can be housed at a single depot location or mobilized from various staging locations as needed. Both approaches work and the selection of the most appropriate method should be influenced by local dynamics. An oft underappreciated aspect of resource management is team member development [10]. This includes ongoing skills maintenance training as well as advanced training of existing members. Recruitment, education, and development of new members for force augmentation and succession planning are critical for ongoing competence and success. Regular review of all of the above elements helps teams and their administrators determine how best to manage teams and their resources.

Review Process Including Logistics

Developing and maintaining a review process that evaluates team construction, resource allocation, and coordination within an agency as well as with other agencies should be distinct from the review process that evaluates team performance during critical incident deployment. The first relates to funding and the mechanics of relationship development, while the latter addresses real-world implementation of what the former has put in place. An essential element of the review process is to identify gaps in logistics for critical incident response and coordination. A templated approach to the review will support a regular process and should identify elements that are missing or deficient in number or extent, as well as those that are ideal. Best practices that may be exported to other agencies should be identified and considered for dissemination at multiple levels. Agency templates should broadly overlap across general domains (Fig. 50.2). The domains may include, but are not limited to:

1. Commander, leader(s), and team members (number, training, and capabilities)
2. Tools and equipment
3. Communication (equipment and protocols) and mobile platforms
4. Computer and information technology infrastructure and architecture
5. Intelligence gathering/analysis and dissemination
6. Training time and scope

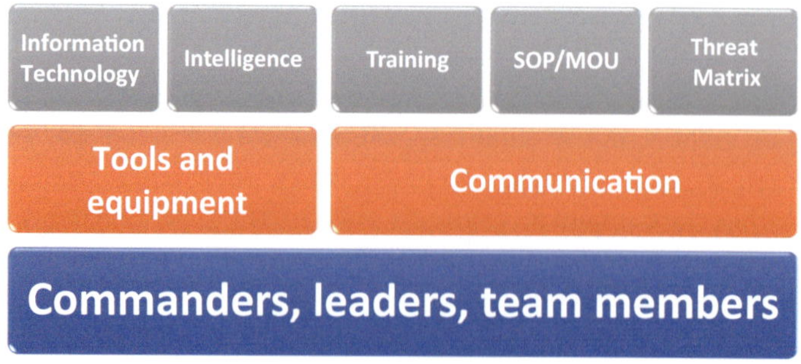

Fig. 50.2 Agency template domains

7. Standard operating procedures and memoranda of understanding with relevant agencies, policies, and protocols
8. Threat matrix-driven team deployment triggers and succession planning

The review process and logistical evaluation optimize strategy and resource allocation to ensure that essential elements are available and accessible during critical incidents.

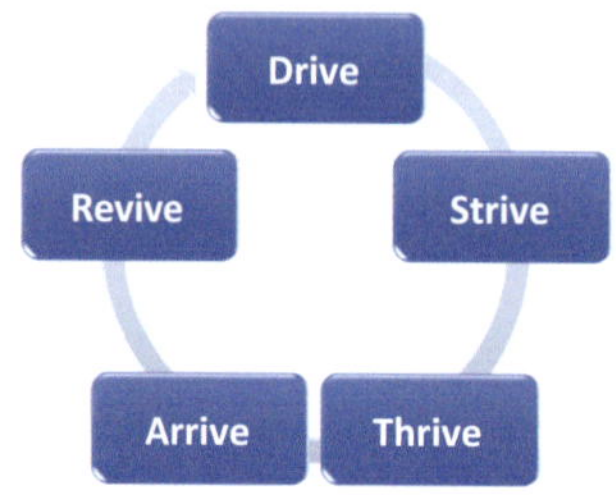

Fig. 50.3 Team life cycle

Transactive Memory

Transactive memory is a characteristic of successful teams that results from iterative training with the team as a whole [20]. Each team member understands their role as well as that of the other team members. Integrated training exploits the expertise of each team member and makes it clear to the other members of the team. An external reviewer might note smooth performance without significant need for communication to address challenges. Such observations characterize special operations teams that continually practice, train, and deploy together. Civilian teams rarely do so to such a degree, and many elements that are mobilized during a critical incident are accustomed to working alone rather than as part of a dynamic team (i.e., patrol officer who is the first responder to an active shooter scenario). Thus, the cultivation of transactive memory must be a fundamental goal of team training throughout the life cycle of a team.

Life Cycle of Teams

Teams are characterized by standard time frames during their lifespan (Fig. 50.3). Prior to the team's creation, there is a perceived need for such a team that may be termed the "drive" for team creation. Without such a need, the driving force for team assembly is notably less focused, leading to a team that is diffuse in targeting and broad in scope. Lack of focus may compromise training and utilization leading to a team that is ill equipped to address the mission at hand. Once assembled, critical incident response teams "strive" to achieve a high level of performance that is task oriented and mission specific. It would not be appropriate for a SWAT team to prepare for firefighting, for example. Once assembled, trained, and deployed, teams "thrive" and refine their membership, skills, and capabilities. It is during this period that teams refine their mission. Some teams expand and others contract depending on local need and capability. Having done so, teams achieve a level of competency and may be characterized as having "arrived," demonstrating organization that reflects a competency-based hierarchy. After a period of time and without a new drive, teams may atrophy, losing the crispness of their skill sets and decreasing the rate of new skill acquisition. Such events may reflect the aging of team members, lack of utilization as the original drive has been eliminated or decayed, or leadership failure as well as a host of other influences including deficient funding for training.

Team salvage hinges on entering a phase of "revival," relying on a new entry into the life cycle demonstrated in Fig. 50.3. Such driving forces often represent changes in the threat matrix or dynamic, changing environmental demographics, shifts in leadership priorities, as well as new team leadership or membership. One way to help support team dynamics is to evolve a stepwise plan for team management that addresses team building, performance, and debriefing (Fig. 50.4).

Team Building (Before)

Team building is both an internal and external process. The internal aspect involves progressive team training for different scenarios so that team members become facile at their

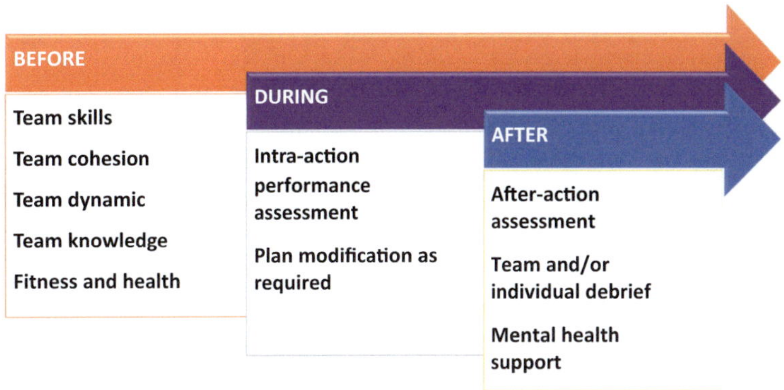

Fig. 50.4 Stepped plan for team management

tasks and are prepared to address the spectrum of challenges that they might face. Besides supporting the development of transactive memory, teams also develop an esprit de corps, especially in teams where members are directly responsible for each other's lives [21]. Accordingly, a sense of personal responsibility characterizes well-functioning teams. These intense relationships generally do not occur within disparate teams. Nonetheless, specialty teams should prepare to interface and work with other teams, rendering team building an external process as well. Regional exercises that bring disparate teams together and drive EMON evolution followed by a performance review support this goal. City-wide mock disaster exercises are prime examples of this kind of team building. Since details are easily lost, trained observers as well as digital recording of events for post hoc critique might identify otherwise unappreciated opportunities for performance improvement.

Team Performance (During)

Military actions frequently benefit from real-time digital oversight via satellite imagery, drone-based feed, as well as fixed or mobile digital feed. Recorded actions, environmental elements, verbal cues and directives, and reactions may be integrated with pre-action and intra-action intelligence as one method of evaluating team and commander performance. Other methods exist, and the selected method should reflect the available resources. Non-military critical incidents were previously generally bereft of such imaging and integrated data. More recently, the rapid rise of dashboard cameras, bystander video imaging, as well as the increasingly ubiquitous traffic and store security cameras may allow for a piecemeal approach to critical incident team performance reconstruction. While urban locales often demonstrate a greater density of digital surveillance tools, suburban and rural settings have fewer coverage gaps than in prior years. Regardless of locale, planning for intra-incident team performance evaluation tools should be included in resource management planning.

Additionally, critical incident managers can team with media outlets to obtain data such as wide-angle helicopter footage or multi-angle imaging. Such relationships also allow managers to restrict the flow of information back to the general public, where perpetrators of a crime might access it. Such was the case during hostage negotiations that occurred in January 2013. In this widely televised negotiation of the release of a 5-year-old boy from a bunker, the FBI Hostage Rescue Team used information to build a full-scale bunker model. The model was then analyzed and accessed multiple times via various techniques in full scale to best plan the breach and rescue. With excellent data flow control, all of this was done in close proximity to the bunker and remained unbeknownst to the kidnapper; the victim was successfully rescued several days later.

Team Debrief (After)

Post hoc review is a cornerstone of performance improvement and quality assessment. Improvements in individual performance, team coordination, information flow, communication resources, resource management, command decision-making, initiative maintenance, as well as interagency coordination rely on post hoc reviews [22]. Obtaining perspectives from individual team members, the on-scene team leader, and the command post is ideal as it provides a broader perspective on performance. It is essential that reviews are nonjudgmental. This encourages accurate and honest evaluation and insight into process improvement. Additionally, a key element in maintaining a longitudinal perspective is accurate documentation of elements that are beneficial, those that are merely acceptable—and equally important—those that hinder plan execution [23]. Such a log is also useful in identifying evidence-based interventions targeted to improve focused performance areas. This information will be important to administrators who will be funding the interventions. More importantly, such a log creates a matrix of capabilities that have been developed. Clear identification of the review process leader encourages ownership of the review, improves the utility of the process, and supports operator development. Frequently, more intensive training follows in the wake of after-action analysis. Of course, ensuring sufficient time for training is an element that should be managed under team building and resource management, but unique needs for focused training may arise.

The above process is even more important when the performance issue embraces interagency coordination and dynamics. Such improvements may require ironing out new relationships—in particular—command architecture. Regardless, changes should be recorded and may be codified into a standard operating procedure (SOP) or a memorandum of understanding (MOU). Train derailments are an event that brings multiple agencies together to address a disaster whether it involves retail products, flammables such as oil or gas, or people as was the case in 2015 in Philadelphia [24, 25]. With the panoply of responding agencies, and even when the National Incident Management System is utilized, different agencies may have different priorities [26]. Different priorities may flow from divergent views on causation and on-scene risk. A train derailment could be viewed as the result of human error, environmental challenges such as track debris, or as the result of targeted violent extremism. The lack of clarity may disable clear lines of leadership for interagency coordination. This can lead to counterproductive decisions including transporting bluntly injured patients by law enforcement vehicle instead of ground or air ambulance. While police transport is highly prized to rapidly transport victims of penetrating trauma, bluntly injured patients may not enjoy similar benefits and may even suffer harm [27]. Unmanaged spine injury, displaced fractures, and the like may be unfavorably managed during police transport—even if the goal is rapid scene clearance and rapid access to definitive care. Regardless of which elements need to be improved, human elements that impact individual responder performance must be accounted for and actively managed [5].

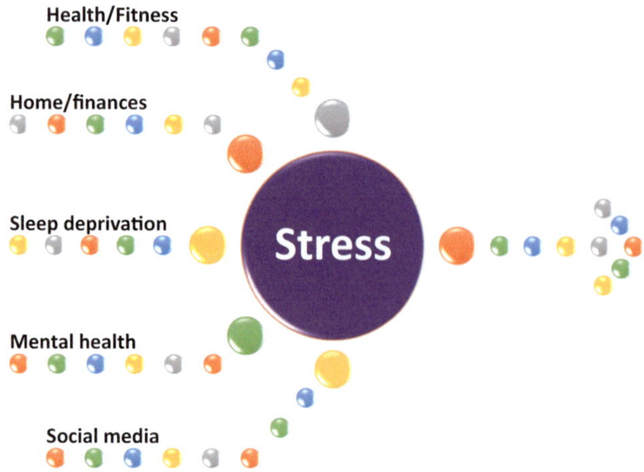

Fig. 50.5 Stressors that impact stability and performance

Stressors to Be Managed (Fig. 50.5)

Health

Health assessment and maintenance are important in keeping team members on the job and capable of performing their duties. Each agency utilizes screening health evaluations of new hires. Often, the ongoing health maintenance is less stringent than the initial assessment [14, 15]. It is unclear if more intense health recertification would translate into outcome benefit, but considering regular maintenance for critical incident response teams seems intuitively appropriate. There are few teams with embedded physicians, but those teams might enjoy enhanced health maintenance compared to teams without physician teammates. Of note, certain health conditions preclude participation on a critical incident response team including, but not limited to: active coronary artery disease, seizures, diabetes, poorly controlled asthma, active anticoagulation, clinically severe obesity, unrepaired cataracts, and psychiatric illness [28]. Health maintenance is increasingly important as team members become older, especially in civilian domains where critical incident response team members are likely dually tasked with primary patrol, canine, or detective duties. Such duties are generally less physically demanding than the responsibilities of the activated critical response team, potentially impeding fitness maintenance and enhancement.

Fitness

Fitness differs from health in that it is the measure of physical capability rather than the overall well-being of organ systems individually and in concert with one another. As mentioned previously, the Cooper Institute Fitness Assessment is the most commonly used measure of civilian police fitness. Its application to critical incident teams is limited in that it overlooks the unique aspects of these teams such as the additional weight of body armor, medical equipment, firearms, ammunition, and other tools, including communication, entry, and surveillance gear that must be transported over uneven surfaces [29]. Just as important is the impact of the extreme stress associated with these situations on the ability to perform physical tasks.

Maintaining a high level of fitness helps support the ability to perform well, recover after burst energy expenditure, and enable a stable shooting platform as needed. Indeed, fitness may be utilized as part of an agglomerated approach to member selection and maintenance. Such a paradigm has been crafted using iterative aerobic and strength assessment sequences both with and without duty gear and job-relevant task assessments. Such assessments have been demonstrated to correlate well with job performance for a regional SWAT team in the USA. Fitness may be significantly impacted by diverse elements including sleep deprivation.

Sleep Deprivation and Fatigue

No condition may be more insidious than cumulative sleep deprivation. Once acquired, the effects remain even after obtaining an appropriate amount of sleep thereafter. A plethora of untoward effects accrue from sleep deprivation including, but not limited to:

1. Inability to focus or concentrate
2. Micro sleep events
3. Lack of impulse control
4. Anger
5. Depression
6. Compromised motor skills
7. Reduced tolerance and ineffective coping skills
8. Cardiovascular disease
9. Weight gain and reduced endurance
10. Impaired judgment

As a result, high-risk occupations such as airline pilots and truck drivers have established safety limits for wakeful hours on the job. Even medical trainees must work within an hour-limited paradigm. Sleep deprivation has been linked with disruptive physician behavior as well as burnout and disordered personal relationships [30, 31]. There is no reason to believe that sleep deprivation would not have similar effects on critical incident response personnel [32]. Therefore, it is reasonable to establish a sleep deprivation awareness program as well as embedding the notion that sleep deprivation may render one unfit to serve on a critical incident response team if it is identified [33]. The commander of the team must craft and enforce a surveillance program to ensure safe and effective team performance. It is possible that team medics or physicians might strengthen the awareness of sleep deprivation and help to police the team from such problems. In particular, lengthy operations that occur without the benefit of mutual aid from neighboring teams accelerate the risk of creating sleep deprivation and fatigue in the deployed members of a single team. Therefore, resource management is essential in ensuring that there are appropriate substitution plans to mitigate against sleep deprivation and fatigue.

Home and Family

This domain is perhaps the most difficult to manage as personal issues escape the control of resource management. Additionally, stressors in personal life are often intimately related to factors such as fatigue and time management. The impact of family illness, family discord, as well as financial stressors cannot be overstated as they may have broad effects including sleep deprivation, loss of focus and concentration, diminished tolerance, and frayed temper control and anger. It has been suggested that these factors are associated with diminished performance and impaired interpersonal relations, particularly when several stressors are found in combination. Unmitigated home stressors are strongly linked to maladaptive solutions including alcohol and illicit substance misuse and abuse.

Alcohol, Illicit Substances, and Mental Health

Substance abuse is a well-documented problem throughout the membership of teams faced with fluid and high-stress scenarios, as well as individuals faced with the ravages of dysfunctional dynamics including poverty, domestic violence, interpersonal violence, and drug-related culture and behavior. Depression and anxiety coexist and thrive in the daily reinforcement of failed social (police, social service, child welfare, etc.) interventions. As a result, law enforcement personnel are particularly vulnerable to these influences, as are social workers, EMS providers, and individuals working in the Emergency Department regardless of discipline. Education is a useful step to combat this process but must be coupled with surveillance and intervention elements to prevent maladaptive behavior. Multiple screening tools are available but often perform less well than the candid observations of well-meaning team members [13]. A robust employee assistance program is invaluable in this regard, as is the iterative feedback from invested team leadership and membership. In particular, suicide has arisen as an epidemic in the LEO and first responder communities [34].

Stress and the Pyramid of Complexity

One method of understanding stress is to visualize it as a pyramid. In this regard, the critical incident itself forms the base, upon which all other stressors will rest. The next tier is the team, the essential elements of which have been covered above. The third tier is the community in which the team finds itself and is shaped by the community's attitudes toward team members and their mission. A well-regarded and well-funded team will be less stressed by its interaction with the community compared to one in which the teams' presence is regarded as intrusive, unwanted, and unsupported. The culture of the police environment is tied to both internal and external forces including hierarchy, monetary investments, commitment to education, and support in terms of hours trained and resources allocated. The local government structure support of the agency is also linked to its success and regard.

The critical incident team also participates in image building in that interactions with community members, local leaders, and media outlets shape the way that the team is perceived. Political issues top the pyramid and serve as the "sharp, pointy end" of the stress climate. Even when everything goes as well as one could hope, the political spin can substantially alter how the process, conduct, and outcome of a particular critical incident are viewed. It is essential that the politics be kept at arm's length from the team and their mission. Political issues are optimally handled by the upper reaches of administration instead of the deployed team or its commander. The commander is a key figure in negotiating pre-incident relationships with other agencies.

Interagency Collaboration

The success of local critical response teams is in part dependent on healthy relationships with state, regional, and federal agencies. Fusion centers provide key information to a variety of agencies throughout the country in an effort to streamline the response to violent extremism and reduce its occurrence. It is not uncommon to need to interact with the National Guard, Federal Bureau of Investigation, Alcohol Tobacco and Firearms, Department of Homeland Security, US Marshalls, and others even within a low-activity locale. Therefore, roles, responsibilities, and communication lanes are ideally established by protocol prior to a critical incident or joint task force undertaking. Doing so reduces the likelihood of error, injury, and even loss of life. Members of the aforementioned agencies are trained operators. As such, they share many similarities with the members of a local team. Interagency preparedness underpinned the success of events like that of the Orlando, Florida Pulse nightclub shooting [35, 36]. Orlando is a city that works on preparedness on a regular basis, driven in part, by the location of a popular vacation destination within the region (Disneyworld). Therefore, the disaster brought together team members who were highly trained and who anticipated working together. Bystanders, on the other hand, are in general not so well trained and do not practice working in tandem with skilled operators.

Bystanders

Nonetheless, the untrained bystander plays an increasingly prominent role in critical incident response [37]. However, these spontaneous responders fall outside of the paradigm of crew resource management and team dynamics as they do not participate in any aspect thereof. The frequency and impact of bystander efforts are underscored by the Boston Marathon Bombing of 2013. Initial rescue efforts were undertaken by bystanders in advance of trained rescue crews [38]. The Centers for Disease Control and Prevention as well as the Federal Emergency Management Agency have recognized the impact and efforts of bystanders in critical incidents. Accordingly, these agencies have developed bystander training tools to better prepare for critical incident participation in advance of trained team arrival, especially where team arrival will be delayed or nearly impossible due to local geography or weather concerns (i.e., rural sites, mountain locales, etc.).

Therefore, trained operators of multiple specialties will need to determine how best to interact with engaged bystanders to optimize bystander assistance. Specific training may be required to best use this resource, while the nation works toward establishing a culture of competence in the setting of critical incident response. Despite the wide availability of tourniquets and procoagulant gauze to the public, most episodes of mass casualty from firearm violence—exemplified by the Orlando, Florida Pulse Nightclub shootings—deliver patients to the hospital without such hemorrhage control devices in place [39]. Community preparation to store and have such supplies readily available at "soft targets" that are generally easily accessible have limited to no security and limited protective measures is one option to explore to enhance survival from potentially lethal hemorrhage [40]. Soft targets would include—but are not limited to—malls, schools, theme parks, sporting arenas, transportation hubs, and hospitals. Many hospitals preposition such life-saving supplies across multiple floors and locations. Critical incident team integration into facility safety preparation underscores this kind of approach to equipment and tool logistic supply and deployment.

Emergency Medical Services/Tactical EMS

Durable changes in the thinking behind how best to position and utilize trained medics and physicians who are embedded in critical incident response teams have moved medical providers closer to—and sometimes into—the hot zone or inner perimeter. Previously, providers were commonly positioned outside of the threat zones. This ensured their safety and separated team members based on the type and degree of their training. Recently, medical providers have been integrated into critical response teams where they largely remained unarmed [41]. In the wake of the well-publicized active shooter events in schools, malls, and other locales, bringing a trained provider to an injured individual who cannot be extricated may be lifesaving.

The tenets of Tactical Combat Casualty Care (TCCC) provide guidance on what kinds of lifesaving activities are appropriate when under fire, as well as when out of the line

Table 50.1 Phase interventions

Phase / interventions
Care under fire
Threat elimination, tourniquet application, temporary hemorrhage control including procoagulant gauze packing, airway intervention generally deferred until tactical field care
Tactical field care
Airway control, additional hemorrhage control, fluid resuscitation including intraosseous line insertion
Combat casualty evacuation care
Tube thoracostomy insertion, continued fluid resuscitation, NO wound repair, supplemental oxygen administration (if/when available)

Adapted from Garbarino and Magnavita [30]

of fire (Table 50.1) [41]. To provide medical care in high-stress and low-resource settings, the provider must be a valued team member as their life is in the hands of the operators that escort the provider to an injured team member, victim, or suspect. A detailed exploration of these issues may be found elsewhere, as it is outside of the scope of this chapter [42–44]. Nonetheless, like bystanders, teams must develop specific methods of interacting with, and embracing, medical support that follows them into dangerous territory to preserve life.

Overlap with Pandemic Preparedness

The recent pandemic has brought challenges in healthcare as well as public health and public safety [45]. The tensions that were noted during periods of lockdown seemed fueled by local and national politics and were exacerbated by mixed messaging around mask use, therapeutics, and vaccines. Public unrest, riots, and accelerated firearm violence established a dangerous and protracted period for law enforcement, especially in the wake of wide laypress coverage of civilian deaths involving LEOs [46]. It was clear that individual agencies were not sufficiently prepared nor resourced for widespread riots such as those in Portland [47], nor encampments such as that of Seattle's now disbanded autonomous zone [48]. Agencies were surprised at the difficulties they encountered despite resources, training, and prior successes in responding to local crises.

There is a parallel to be found with COVID-19 preparedness in the medical community. Even exceptionally well-resourced quaternary facilities were readily overwhelmed and, given the rate of use of equipment, subsequently under-resourced for surge needs. The lessons learned in determining how to respond to such a vast surge and for such a protracted period of time can readily translate to the LEO community as well. Since agencies were overwhelmed, the situations that can lead to that specific state should be incorporated into training and preparedness planning. It is in this space that virtual or augmented reality as well as computer-based simulation scenario evolution can be particularly useful but must be informed by data. The current experience provides that data to establish models and enable outcome changes in response to step-by-step decision-making [49]. Such an approach has been undertaken in fashioning war games involving the nuclear arsenal. It seems like adapting an iterative approach to medical or LEO decision-making and asset utilization is logical and appropriate. Moreover, performance within a simulation scenario aids in team development and skill set acquisition to support outcome excellence.

Conclusions

Team dynamics are both complex and straightforward. Scientific principles allow one to understand the complex interplay of forces that may enhance or degrade crew resource management. Dedicated efforts at team building, performance review, and performance improvement serve as the basis for enhancing team dynamics. However, a skillful leader who is empowered with both command and control is required to craft a culture of safety and competence. Careful planning for contingencies and difficult scenarios, as well as interaction with other agencies—including untrained or partially trained bystanders—helps underpin team success. However, even the most careful planning will fail if it rests upon a dysfunctional team. Therefore, improving team capabilities, competencies, fitness, health, and interpersonal dynamics is the linchpin that holds together all components of the successful critical incident team.

Key Points

- Understanding critical incident response dynamics and logistics is enabled by a scientific approach to each element.
- Command, control, and communication are key elements that are required for successful critical incident leadership.
- An iterative process evaluating team dynamics and logistics before, during, and after incident response is essential in supporting continued team performance improvement.
- Individual team member management dovetails with team performance.

- Interagency coordination should be specifically planned, tested, and critiqued to optimize performance and help ensure a successful resolution upon team deployment.
- There are valuable lessons to learn from agency coordination that flows from the recent integration of medical resources to address the COVID-19 pandemic.

References

1. Grubb AR, Brown SJ, Hall P, Bowen E. The self-perceived successful hostage and crisis negotiator profile: a qualitative assessment of negotiator competencies. Police Pract Res. 2019;20(4):321–42.
2. Cooper GE, White MD, Lauber JK. Resource management on the flightdeck: proceedings of a NASA/Industry Workshop. Moffett Field: NASA—Ames Research Center; 1980. NASA Conference Publication No. CP-2120.
3. Kanki BG, Anca J, Chidester TR, editors. Crew resource management. Academic Press; 2019.
4. Home – Mission Critical Team Institute (missioncti.com). Accessed 21 Feb 2021.
5. Wakeman D, Langham MR Jr. Creating a safer operating room: groups, team dynamics and crew resource management principles. Sem Pediatr Surg. 2018;27(2):107–13. WB Saunders.
6. Kayser JB, Kaplan LJ. Conflict management in the ICU. Crit Care Med. 2020;48(9):1349–57.
7. Royce CS, Hayes MM, Schwartzstein RM. Teaching critical thinking: a case for instruction in cognitive biases to reduce diagnostic errors and improve patient safety. Acad Med. 2019;94(2):187–94.
8. Franco I, Sweeney RE, Marks JA, McLaughlin C, Henry M, Yaport MA, Arriaga AF. Crisis resource management and interdisciplinary team training. In: Comprehensive healthcare simulation: anesthesiology. Cham: Springer; 2020. p. 47–60.
9. Hagemann V, Kluge A, Greve J. Measuring the effects of team resource management training for the fire service. Proc Hum Fact Ergonom Soc Annu Meet. 2012;56(1):2442–6.
10. Nullmeyer RT, Spiker VA. The importance of crew resource management behaviors in mission performance: implications for training evaluation. Mil Psychol. 2003;15(1):77.
11. Havinga J, De Boer RJ, Rae A, Dekker SW. How did crew resource management take-off outside of the cockpit? A systematic review of how crew resource management training is conceptualised and evaluated for non-pilots. Safety. 2017;3(4):26.
12. Young AT, Hennington C, Eggleston D. US SWAT operator experience, personality, cognitive-emotion regulation and decision-making style. Policing Int J. 2018;41:247.
13. Super JT. A survey of pre-employment psychological evaluation tests and procedures. J Police Crim Psychol. 2006;21(2):83–7.
14. Marins EF, David GB, Del Vecchio FB. Characterization of the physical fitness of police officers: a systematic review. J Strength Cond Res. 2019;33(10):2860–74.
15. Marins E, Crespo P, Rombaldi A, Del Vecchio F. Occupational physical fitness tests for police officers-a narrative review. TSAC Rep. 2018;50:26–34.
16. van der Haar S, Koeslag-Kreunen M, Euwe E, Segers M. Team leader structuring for team effectiveness and team learning in command-and-control teams. Small Group Res. 2017;48(2):215–48.
17. Yurii P, Serhii A. Training of strategic leader as an investment in the reform of the military command and control system. Strateg Priorities. 2017;45(4):141–6.
18. Heal S. Planning (Emerging Multi-Organizational Networks—EMONs). Tact Edge. 1999;17(1):62.
19. Bunker R, Heal S. Splitting an EMON. Tact Edge. 2008;26(4):58–60.
20. Wang Y, Huang Q, Davison RM, Yang F. Effect of transactive memory systems on team performance mediated by knowledge transfer. Int J Inf Manag. 2018;41:65–79.
21. Super JF, Betts TK, Keller H, Humphreys JR. Simulation game outcomes: a multilevel examination of knowledge sharing norms, transactive memory systems, and individual learning goal orientations. Simul Gaming. 2020;51(6):830–58.
22. Gilfoyle E, Koot DA, Annear JC, Bhanji F, Cheng A, Duff JP, Grant VJ, St George-Hyslop CE, Delaloye NJ, Kotsakis A, McCoy CD. Improved clinical performance and teamwork of pediatric interprofessional resuscitation teams with a simulation-based educational intervention. Pediatr Crit Care Med. 2017;18(2):e62–9.
23. Mission Critical Team Institute | Coleman@missioncti.com. Accessed 21 Feb 2021.
24. Amtrak train crash survivors describe chaos in Philadelphia – CBS News. Accessed 21 Feb 2021.
25. 3 Things fire chiefs and firefighters need to know about train derailment responses (firerescue1.com). Accessed 21 Feb 2021.
26. National Incident Management System | FEMA.gov. Accessed 21 Feb 2021.
27. Winter E, Hynes AM, Shultz K, Holena DN, Malhotra NR, Cannon JW. Association of police transport with survival among patients with penetrating trauma in Philadelphia, Pennsylvania. JAMA Netw Open. 2021;4(1):e2034868.
28. Dawes JJ, Lindsay K, Bero J, Elder C, Kornhauser C, Holmes R. Physical fitness characteristics of high vs. low performers on an occupationally specific physical agility test for patrol officers. J Strength Cond Res. 2017;31(10):2808–15.
29. Violanti JM, Ma CC, Fekedulegn D, Andrew ME, Gu JK, Hartley TA, Charles LE, Burchfiel CM. Associations between body fat percentage and fitness among police officers: a statewide study. Saf Health Work. 2017;8(1):36–41.
30. Garbarino S, Magnavita N. Sleep problems are a strong predictor of stress-related metabolic changes in police officers. A prospective study. PLoS One. 2019;14(10):e0224259.
31. Freeman D, Sheaves B, Waite F, Harvey AG, Harrison PJ. Sleep disturbance and psychiatric disorders. Lancet Psychiatry. 2020;7(7):628–37.
32. Taylor Y, Merat N, Jamson S. The effects of fatigue on cognitive performance in police officers and staff during a forward rotating shift pattern. Saf Health Work. 2019;10(1):67–74.
33. Dugan K. Recognizing and mitigating fatigue caused by sleep deprivation: a command perspective. Tact Edge. 2012;30(1):14–21.
34. Roberts KA. Correlates of law enforcement suicide in the United States: a comparison with army and firefighter suicides using data from the national violent death reporting system. Police Pract Res. 2019;20(1):64–76.
35. Melmer P, Carlin M, Castater CA, Koganti D, Hurst SD, Tracy BM, Grant AA, Williams K, Smith RN, Dente CJ, Sciarretta JD. Mass casualty shootings and emergency preparedness: a multidisciplinary approach for an unpredictable event. J Multidiscip Healthc. 2019;12:1013.
36. Smith CP, Cheatham ML, Safcsak K, Emrani H, Ibrahim JA, Gregg M, Eubanks WS, Lube MW, Havron WS, Levy MS. Injury characteristics of the Pulse Nightclub shooting: lessons for mass casualty incident preparation. J Trauma Acute Care Surg. 2020;88(3):372–8.
37. Haider AH, Haut ER, Velmahos GC. Converting bystanders to immediate responders: we need to start in high school or before. JAMA Surg. 2017;152(10):909–10.
38. Walls RM, Zinner MJ. The Boston marathon response: why did it work so well? JAMA. 2013;309(23):2441–2.

39. Smith ER, Shapiro G, Sarani B. Fatal wounding pattern and causes of potentially preventable death following the pulse night club shooting event. Prehosp Emerg Care. 2018;22(6):662–8.
40. US DHS ST-CP Security Overview. 2018. www.dhs.gov.
41. Butler FK, Holcomb JB, Shackelford S, Barbabella S, Bailey JA, Baker JB, Cap AP, Conklin CC, Cunningham CW, Davis M, DeLellis SM. Advanced resuscitative care in tactical combat casualty care: TCCC guidelines change 18-01: 14 October 2018. J Spec Oper Med Peer Rev J SOF Med Prof. 2018;18(4):37–55.
42. Heiskell LE, Carmona RH. Tactical Emergency Medical Services: an emerging subspecialty of emergency medicine. Ann Emerg Med. 1994;23(4):778–85.
43. Chaudhuri R, Jamali AM, Tang N. Tactical emergency medical support. In: Operational and medical management of explosive and blast incidents. Cham: Springer; 2020. p. 245–53.
44. Stiles CM, Cook C, Sztajnkrycer MD. A descriptive analysis of tactical casualty care interventions performed by law enforcement personnel in the state of Wisconsin, 2010-2015. Prehosp Disaster Med. 2017;32(3):284–8.
45. Hartley DM, Perencevich EN. Public health interventions for COVID-19: emerging evidence and implications for an evolving public health crisis. JAMA. 2020;323(19):1908–9.
46. Van Dijcke D, Wright AL. Using mobile device traces to improve near-real time data collection during the George Floyd Protests. 7 June 2020. Available at SSRN: https://ssrn.com/abstract=3621731 or https://doi.org/10.2139/ssrn.3621731.
47. den Heyer G. Police response to riots. Springer International Publishing; 2020.
48. Miller RW. CHAZ, a 'no Cop Co-Op': here's what Seattle's Capitol Hill Autonomous Zone looks like. USA Today, 12 June 2020.
49. Vu L. Bringing out the science of war games. 7 May 2019. https://engineering.berkeley.edu/2019/05/bringing-out-science-war-games. Accessed 16 Feb 2021.

Terrorism and Urban Trauma

51

Jose L. Pascual, Jeremy W. Cannon, and Lewis J. Kaplan

Introduction

The last few decades have witnessed a fundamental shift in how the public, law enforcement, government agencies, and the military plan to address terrorism as well as urban trauma. Previously, terrorism and urban trauma were considered distinct entities. Terrorism in particular, was an event that primarily occurred outside of North America, most notably affecting certain countries in the European Union, the Middle East, and areas of South America plagued by the opium trade and religious extremism as well. The historic events of 9/11 revamped those perceptions and painted terrorism and urban trauma onto the same canvas. Currently, urban trauma principally—but not exclusively—occurs in large densely populated cities and in zones with depressed socioeconomics. Nonetheless, the culture of urban intentional violent injury has crafted its own set of norms that impact multiple forms of media—including most notably social media (SoMe)—and has shifted interpersonal dynamics and social behavioral expectations [1].

Terrorism—or violent extremism—has similarly exploded and encompasses a vast array of forms and has an expanding set of drivers [2]. Soft targets such as schools, malls, movie theaters, transportation hubs, and hospitals are well-publicized sites of violent extremism [3]. Hospital assaults are well tracked by the World Health Organization on a yearly basis [4]. The overlap of soft target assault and urban intentional violent injury has welded urban trauma and terrorism together in important ways [5–8]. Other forms of terrorism include cyber-terrorism, identity theft, and random interpersonal violence that follows a dictated form such as "knockouts" that have occurred on public transportation and urban sidewalks or iPhone thefts known as "apple picking" by roving gangs on bicycles and scooters [9]. Together, terrorism, regardless of specific form, and urban trauma have the potential to craft an interwoven culture of fear, - a goal that underpins terrorist activities in all forms.

J. L. Pascual · J. W. Cannon · L. J. Kaplan (✉)
Perelman School of Medicine, University of Pennsylvania, Department of Surgery, Division of Trauma, Surgical Critical Care and Emergency Surgery, Philadelphia, PA, USA

Corporal Michael J Crescenz VAMC, Surgical Services, Philadelphia, PA, USA
e-mail: Jose.Pascual@pennmedicine.upenn.edu; Jeremy.Cannon@pennmedicine.upenn.edu; Lewis.Kaplan@pennmedicine.upenn.edu

Forms of Terrorism and Urban Trauma

Mass casualty scenarios often typify thinking about terrorist events whether domestic or international. However, most terrorist-driven mass casualty events result in large numbers of dead individuals with far fewer individuals with serious injury requiring inpatient hospital care. Instead, there are large numbers who require Emergency Department care with 9/11 serving as a prime example [10]. Mass shootings, on the other hand, like the events of 1 October in Las Vegas, Nevada, result in large numbers of victims who require inpatient as well as ED care. Such events lead to substantial health system stress that was in part mitigated by using existing approaches to disaster management [11]. Natural disasters, including typhoons and earthquakes, have a more balanced injury profile that tends to overwhelm medical care facility capacity and engender logistical difficulties in enhancing disaster site capabilities. Examples include those that struck Haiti, as well as the southern USA during hurricanes Irene and Sandy [12–14]. Individual terror attacks, including those derived from autonomous "cells" are characterized by high mortality at the epicenter, but decreased mortality with increased need for care with increasing distance from the attack's origin. Numerous examples are found throughout the history of Israel, and more recently in Belgium, Iraq, Afghanistan, and Nigeria with a notable increase in female suicide bombers [15–18].

Regardless of the precise nature of a terrorist attack, mass panic accompanied by civil and financial disruption are other consequences that compound the loss of life [19]. Such

L. Marshall Gillman, S. Widder (eds.), *Trauma Team Dynamics*, https://doi.org/10.1007/978-3-031-86312-7_51

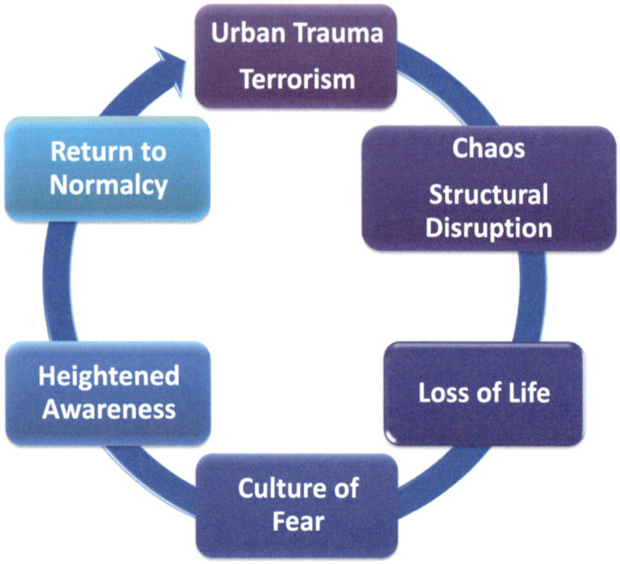
Urban Trauma
Terrorism
Chaos
Structural Disruption
Loss of Life
Culture of Fear
Heightened Awareness
Return to Normalcy

Fig. 51.1 Trauma/terror cycle

events foment a culture of fear initially characterized by heightened awareness followed by a gradual return to normalcy—a cycle that inadvertently readies the system for the next event (Fig. 51.1) [2]. The loss of vigilance as normalcy returns provides a weakness that may be exploited to reinitiate the cycle. Most urban trauma does not aim to create widespread unrest but nonetheless feeds into a similar cycle. On the other hand, the recent protest-related violence focused on individuals who died after Police contact appeared designed to disrupt normal activities throughout the entire country [20]. Rioting gripped the USA throughout 2020 including marches, property destruction, looting, and firebombing including Molotov cocktail-style incendiary devices [21]. Accordingly, both medical and law enforcement domains have evolved and adapted to respond to preserve life, limit damage, and maintain or restore peace. The evolution of medical and law enforcement responses is driven in part by the kinds of injuries that individuals and groups may sustain.

Injuries and Injury Patterns

Urban trauma in population dense settings is often typified by penetrating trauma that includes firearm and edged weapon injuries. Nonetheless, most urban trauma centers evaluate and care for more patients with blunt, rather than penetrating, injury. Individuals injured in falls, motor vehicle (including motorcycle) crashes, and vehicle-pedestrian collisions often form the majority of patients cared for at a regional resource facility. Combined penetrating and blunt injury in the same patient is uncommon. Scene transport patient flow is augmented by transfer after stabilization at a less well-resourced medical facility as part of patient care within a tiered trauma network.

Unlike urban trauma, terrorism often leads to both penetrating and blunt injury in the same patient [22]. This circumstance derives from the increased use of devices such as vests, backpacks, and other canisters packed with explosives as well as metal projectiles. Explosive agents such as C4 (cyclotrimethylene trinitramine) or Semtex (RDX-research department explosive, an explosive nitroamine, and PETN-pentaerythritol tetranitrate) are more commonly used in small devices and may be detected by technology used in current Explosive Trace Detection systems [23, 24]. Larger explosives including weaponized vehicles (aka suicide vehicles) may be packed with fertilizer as well as diesel fuel such as in the 1995 Oklahoma City bombing. Vehicle bombs using other explosives have been deployed and at multiple sites during the Global War on Terror (GWOT), and throughout the Mexican Cartel conflicts [25, 26]. The magnitude of vehicle bomb detonations creates shrapnel from damaged structures as well as the vehicle in which the explosive was delivered. Such explosives lead to penetrating injury within the blast zone and blast effect within the blast radius; individuals may be thrown into stationary objects or mobile objects may be explosively moved into individuals [22].

Improvised Explosive Device

Improvised Explosive Devices (IEDs) are a unique category of explosive that became commonplace during GWOT. Often placed in roadways, and underneath or within obstructions that need to be cleared to permit passage, IEDs are particularly devastating to those dismounted. Early troop transport vehicles provided little occupant protection from IEDs. Service members often suffered both penetrating and blunt injury from driving over an IED. The Mine-Resistant Ambush Protected (MRAP) vehicle shields occupants and provides substantial protection from penetrating injury related to IEDs, rocket-propelled grenades, other explosive devices, and small arms fire [27]. Blunt injuries persist, especially the dismounted injury complex (aka. deck slap lesion) [28]. The civilian parallel is the Lenco BearCat G3 which is an armored vehicle suitable for use by federal and civilian law enforcement and is especially ideal for Special Weapons and Tactics teams [29]. No vehicle provides ideal protection against blunt forces that flow from explosive device detonation.

Blast Effect

Blast effect is a concussive injury derived from blast pressure measured in pounds per square inch (psi) during the rapid overpressure phase of the explosion [22, 30]. For example an overpressure of 1 psi leads to a maximum wind speed of 38 mph while overpressure of 10 psi creates wind up to 294 mph leading to severe damage to concrete structures and death in the majority of individuals exposed to the overpressure wave (www.cdc.gov/niosh/docket/archive/NIOSH-125/125-Explosionsand refugeChambers.pdf). While military organizations are well acquainted with such injuries, civilian law enforcement and EMS may benefit from specific preparation including focused education, training, and resource management (see Chap. 50). The 2013 Boston Marathon bombing underscored the need for such training [31, 32].

Chemical, Biological, Radiological, Nuclear, and Explosive (CBRN-E)

Terror-related mechanisms of injury may be housed within a framework of Chemical, Biological, Radiological, Nuclear, and Explosive (CBRN-E); explosives including firearm-related penetrating injury are discussed above [33]. Of the CBRN four, the Chemical and Radiological appeared more readily acquirable and deployable by terrorist organizations due to the seemingly more limited availability of biologic agents such as weaponized anthrax, smallpox, or other viruses in comparison to nerve agents or radioactive materials [34]. The nuclear arsenal is tightly controlled and falls under the control of nation states rather than terrorist organizations. Nerve agents such as Sarin gas have been previously deployed in Japan and Syria, while to date, no radioactive "dirty bomb" has been detonated [35]. Unfortunately, CBRN-E terrorism may be initially difficult to detect (other than a bomb or lethal gas explosion) and result in the unprotected exposure of first responders who are unaware of the exposure hazard [36, 37]. Nonetheless, in the event of a CBRN-E terrorist attack, the availability of appropriate personal protective gear is critical to protect first responders who arrive to evacuate and care for the victims of the incident.

Microbe biohazard protection is provided by the appropriate Biohazard gear (Biohazard Level I–IV suits) while chemical and biologic protection is provided by gear including the military Mission-Oriented Protective Posture suits (MOPP suits 0–4) [38]. The availability of higher level gear may be limited outside of special facilities. High-level suits are not commonly available even at major medical facilities, including regional resource trauma centers. Accordingly, a close working relationship with local federal and military resources is essential in bringing suitably trained and garbed individuals to an event site. Little, if any, nuclear radiation protective gear is readily available outside of specialized agencies and their designated protective details such as those at the Lawrence Livermore National Laboratory (https://www.llnl.gov) or investigative and decontamination crews from the Nuclear Regulatory Commission (www.nrc.gov) and the National Nuclear Security Administration (www.nnsa.doe.gov). Regardless of attack type, CBRN-E events create fear of another attack and lead to the notion that there is no safe refuge. Indeed, a primary goal of terrorism is to perpetuate a culture of fear [39].

Paradigm Shifts in Terrorism

The 9/11 attack on US soil launched a major change in US policy as terror firmly landed in North America, initiating the Global War on Terror [20]. Instead of supplanting a country's governmental infrastructure, or unseating its political leadership to establish new rule, or driving out an invading force, terrorism shifted to coordinated attacks performed by small teams of terrorists as well as independent attacks initiated by autonomous cells [40]. While structures were destroyed, the primary impact was on people and their view of government. The small units termed "cells" operate both as part of a coordinated structure and independently [15]. Some may be in place for a short period of time prior to their specified activity, while others may remain dormant for long periods of time and are dubbed "sleeper cells" [15]. Thus, terrorist activities became personally focused instead of government or country focused.

The rise of social media (SoMe) and the widespread use of digital platforms as communication tools and enablers of daily activity—such as the sharing of medical information (and disinformation) during the COVID-19 pandemic in a global fashion—has afforded multiple opportunities for cyber-terrorism [41, 42]. Such activities span network disruption and identity theft, lead to organization member recruitment, and have resulted in an expansive need for law enforcement capabilities including cybersurveillance and cyberprotection [43, 44]. Even small police departments support electronic expertise in crime solving and therefore complement cyber policing that is performed by federal agencies including the National Security Agency, the Federal Bureau of Investigation (FBI), and international agencies that include the Central Intelligence Agency. Education efforts to improve cybersecurity competency are available through public (FBI)-private (citizen) partnerships such as InfraGard that work to protect US Critical Infrastructure [InfraGard. Partnership for Protection. https://www.infragard.org/; accessed March 7, 2021]. Critical Infrastructure protection is a national imperative, while episodic violent extremism is a local crisis.

Domestic terror events such as the Texas belltower shootings that occurred in 1966 spurred the formation of Special Weapons and Tactics (SWAT) teams. Since the 1970s, the number of SWAT teams has nearly doubled. Such teams respond to urban and suburban terror events spanning—but not limited to—barricaded hostage/suspect, riots, gang warfare, dignitary protection, and high-risk warrant service. US rioting during 2020 was interwoven with the SARS-CoV-2 pandemic as well as political uncertainty in an election year; SWAT teams prominently featured in local city responses. Driving the development, training, and outfitting of local SWAT teams is the need to respond to the changing demographic and advanced, high-powered equipment of perpetrators of violent crimes. Suspects and organized criminal elements have ready access to body armor and high-performance weapons as a result of military surplus obtained both legally and illegally. Additionally, increasing numbers of perpetrators of violent crime may have served as members of the armed forces, and received specific weapon and tactical training [45]. Therefore, local police departments need to be able to respond to a host of different events forcing a metamorphosis from community-based policing to a threat matrix-based response [46]. The transition has often been termed the "militarization" of local police forces and is typified by the inclusion of military-relevant firearms, body armor, communications gear, training tactics, sound and light diversionary devices, and uparmored vehicles such as the Lenco BearCat, or the militarily deployed MRAP as noted earlier. More relevant is the articulation of multi-jurisdictional teams whose need is driven by the rising frequency of SWAT or Special Response Team (SRT) activations whose intensity is unsupportable in isolation by smaller towns [47]. Shared resources, akin to mutual aid policies, help distribute manpower demands, resource-related finances, and oversight and after-action evaluation responsibilities.

Similarly, instead of standard community policing where apprehending criminals constitutes approximately 10% of total police work, departments increasingly devote time and resources to elements that address active shooter and mass casualty scenarios.[24] Medical threat intelligence and biohazard training—especially in the wake of COVID-19—is especially important as well [48]. Furthermore, and in a fashion parallel to that of the military, police officers are increasingly trained in self- and buddy-aid using concepts and tactics borrowed from the Tactical Combat Casualty Care (TCCC) approach initially advocated by the Naval Special Warfare command. Recognizing that the patrol officer is likely to be the first responder to urban trauma or terror acts, this officer's capabilities need to be enhanced and reinforced to increase the likely survival of the officer and those whose lives the officer has sworn to protect.

Such needs have also driven increased interagency collaboration with other law enforcement agencies including but not limited to State Police, US Marshalls, Alcohol-Tobacco-Firearms, Drug Enforcement Agency, FBI, US Secret Service, and the National Guard. Local teams such as those devoted to urban search and rescue also excel when inter-agency collaboration works smoothly [49]. Since communication is key to such activities, the USA has developed Fusion Centers under the aegis of the Department of Homeland Security that are designed to funnel key and actionable intelligence to appropriate agencies within a specified territorial domain designed to disrupt potential or validated terrorist threats [50]. Integrated domains include state, local, tribal, and territorial as well as private sector partners (www.dhs.gov/state-and-major-urban-area-fusion-centers). Such communication is key in protecting and preserving national security by establishing and improving an information-sharing environment to help counter violent extremism. The previously mentioned InfraGard public-private partnership also serves as a portal for information channeling to relevant agencies. In turn, members serve as subject matter experts for agencies and reflect the benefits of a partnership structure.

Anti-police Violence

The last few years have been marked by mounting anti-law enforcement sentiment within certain groups. Triggered by the deaths of minorities during or after arrest or warrant search, and spread across a multiplicity of digital platforms, protests and anti-police rhetoric captured the nation's focus. The premeditated assassination of law enforcement officers is a readily identifiable sequel of such events [51–53]. More durable impacts include enhanced scrutiny of police activity by those outside of the law enforcement community and swift assignation of culpability by the public when there is a police action inquiry that is spread across SoMe. Perhaps the most devastating effects are on law enforcement officer morale, stress, and perhaps on-scene judgment. As explored in the chapter on Critical Incident Team Dynamics, demoralization and stress exert maladaptive psychologic and physical health impacts that may degrade officer capability and efficiency but may also lead to suicide [54]. An overlap with on-scene judgment may lead to hesitancy in engaging due to fear of censure or inquiry. Critical incidents may then progress unimpeded, become intervened upon too late, or may result in officer or bystander injury or death. Guilt over failing to meet performance standards may lead to depression and suicide as well.

Collectively, it is a precarious time to serve in law enforcement, and the rich tradition of publically "serving and protecting" has been under assault. The Seattle Autonomous Zone is a prime example of how anti-police actions have undervalued the dedication and sacrifice of those who put their lives on the line on a daily basis [55]. Instead of having individuals flee the scene of large gatherings such as parties that are prohibited during the pandemic, arriving police officers are met with wanton property destruction and seemingly anti-police violence [56]. National attempts, some of which have been successful, to reduce, limit, or otherwise "defund" local law enforcement budgets are anticipated to further hamper effective policing as urban trauma and violent extremism continue to escalate [57]. In one such city—Portland, Oregon—law enforcement officers are reportedly leaving policing in larger numbers than can be accounted for by attrition or phase of career [58]. From a public health perspective, the intensity and longevity of anti-police actions and public proclamations appear to condone violence toward those sworn to uphold the law. These actions raise serious concerns regarding the desirability of policing as a career goal, perhaps even in families that have given rise to generations of law enforcement officers or military operatives. Law enforcement is not the only sector that has undergone significant change in structure and focus as substantial changes have also impacted EMS.

Changes in Emergency Medical Systems Structure

Medical care as part of an organized trauma system began in the 1970s and continues to be refined today. In general, urban Emergency Medical Services combine ground and rotary wing air ambulance transport into a working network that embraces support from both the local Fire Department and the local Police Department. Rural trauma systems may enfold aid from other agencies including the US National Park Service (www.nps.gov) and in Canada, the Royal Canadian Mounted Police (www.rcmp-grc.gc.ca). Of necessity, the EMS response to urban violence is reactive in nature rather than preemptive. Nonetheless, despite the close working relationship with local law enforcement, only few areas of crossover have blossomed that leverage the capabilities of EMS in combination with those of law enforcement.

The prevalence of urban violence supports police officers as medical first responders. Indeed, during periods of lockdown and socio-political unrest, urban trauma centers noted a substantial increase in intentional violent injury and a later increase in motor vehicle collisions (automobile and motorcycle) [59]. As they are often first on scene compared to EMS workers, police officers are in a unique position to render aid. First Aid and STOP-The-Bleed techniques have been advocated as key elements to teach law enforcement officers since the Hartford Consensus Conference in 2013 [60]. Penetrance, and funding, however, in both large and small cities across the USA has been more variable, especially in comparison to military medical and special operations domains [61]. Accordingly, rather than spending time rendering immediate healthcare, police in a few urban cities engage in primary transport to the local trauma center with excellent results noted for those with penetrating injury [62]. This practice stands in stark contrast to on-scene care that is common outside of the USA, as well as EMS-based transport with *en route* care that is more typical for US prehospital practice. While police transport appears effective for episodic violence victim rescue when the threat has been neutralized, a different solution is required when threat suppression or elimination has yet to be accomplished.

One approach to care is Tactical EMS, a concept spawned in the military, and in particular, in Special Operations forces where one individual embraces both operator and medic roles [63]. This uniquely and dually trained operator provides immediate and skilled life-sustaining emergency care to an injured combatant rather than needing to await evacuation to a higher echelon of care. While a superb concept, such an individual seems more difficult to task in the civilian domain where issues such as divided loyalty (which role at which time) as well as skills maintenance and certification (medic and police officer) are particularly problematic. Instead, at least in US practice, the medic and police officer roles are generally shouldered by separate individuals. Previously, EMS care during a SWAT or Special Response team activation (call-out) for a barricaded suspect/hostage would await threat elimination and scene clearance for on-scene care and extrication of a wounded individual from within the inner perimeter or "hot" zone (Fig. 51.2).

Based on the work of individuals such as Richard Carmona, MD, a former US Army Medic and former Surgeon General, medics embedded in US SWAT teams have flourished. Such medics train with the SWAT teams and are viewed as integral members, but are tasked with medical care, not room clearing or suspect apprehension. Given the tenor and pace of active shooter scenarios starting with the Columbine, CO, school shootings in 1999, former US President Barack Obama provided strong support to send medics into the warm zone to effect rapid care of injured individuals [64]. As mass casualty events have escalated in

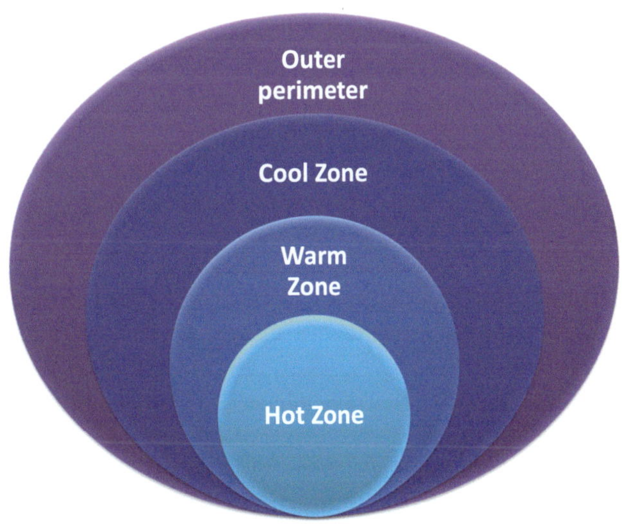

Fig. 51.2 Zone schematic

number and frequency, the role and need for embedded medics has also blossomed, as has the need for public space (soft target) preparation for acute life-threatening injury care [65]. Indeed, the role and efficacy of tactical EMS teams were highlighted in the aftermath of the Tree of Life Synagogue shootings in Pittsburgh, PA [66].

Physician involvement in Tactical EMS (TEMS) is principally limited to providing medical command for the tactical team medics, rather than direct participation. Furthermore, the vast majority of physicians involved in TEMS in the USA are primarily trained in Emergency Medicine; only a handful of surgeons participate in TEMS. However, the majority of TEMS-embedded surgeons involved do so as integrated tactical team members, deploy with the team and provide on-scene medical care as well as medical command. Such physicians are equipped with gear nearly identical to the SWAT operators but generally trade firearms for medical equipment. Bearing the added weight of body armor, communications gear, and medical necessities can present a significant physical challenge, leading to robust physical fitness requirements for the interested individual [67]. The ethics of placing a physician in such a role has been extensively explored [68].

An embedded physician parallels the military structure of some far-forward teams with on-scene physician support such as has been utilized by the US and the Israeli militaries [69, 70]. Moreover, once a physician integrates with a SWAT team, the opportunities for influencing care across the entire Police Department abound. Importantly, such influences may change medical preparedness for both urban violent injury, acts of terrorism, or routine patrol encountered medical emergencies, especially those involving hemorrhage. Such examples may include changing the medical kits that populate mobile police platforms to ones that include tourniquets, personal protective gear, and procoagulant dressings. Implicit in such a change is that there is appropriate training to enable gear deployment and use in a safe and effective fashion. In many ways, non-law enforcement members of the local community may have already done so in the form of "go bags" and immediate care gear that is secured in their personal vehicles.

Other innovations that impact the medical and law enforcement response to high-risk crises include thermal mapping devices to detect the position and number of individuals who are not visible behind a wall, as well as a remotely controlled mobile explosive delivery device (i.e., drone). The latter was deployed to great effect during the July 2016 Dallas police officer shooting crisis [71]. Such devices can eliminate an active threat while shielding officers from life-threatening threats such as high-velocity projectiles or explosives. Other mobile platforms such as those offered by Callyo or Boston Robotics can provide video as well as audio at a remove helping keep officers out of the line of fire while supporting communication and data acquisition [72, 73].

Improved Community Preparedness

In many ways, civilians are moving toward embracing a culture of competence. Such mobility is spurred on by terror events such as those of the 2013 Boston Marathon bombing where community aid was key to preserving the lives of many of the injured. Community training and resource management enhance bystander willingness to participate in events where they may sustain injury while offering aid. Relatedly, lay-person transport of the injured to area facilities was a life-saving event in the Las Vegas shooting of 1 October [74]. Indeed, organizations such as the American Red Cross and the Canadian Red Cross have a host of training courses designed to improve an individual's ability to provide self or buddy care. A readily downloadable app serves as an immediate guide for most major medical emergencies if instruction or immediate aid is unavailable including step-by-step instructions as needed [75]. The US Federal Emergency Management Agency has articulated bystander emergency preparedness training to improve the ability of lay responders to participate in disaster care [76]. Certainly, wilderness exploration and the related organizations have championed "Wilderness Medicine" courses that teach advanced aid skills [77]. The ready availability of tactical load-out bags, EMS bags, personal protective equipment, and hemorrhage control aids (including tourniquets and procoagulant dressings) enables the competent civilian bystander to be ready to render aid in an on-demand fashion be it at a motor vehicle crash, a drive-by shooting, or a terrorist attack [78]. In an extreme fashion, movements such as the so-called Doomsday Preppers may have enhanced medical gear including gas masks, providing both enhanced medical capabilities and providing increased protection from standard SWAT techniques that utilize chemical irritant gas to deny the suspect protected space. The widespread availability of body armor, including shirts, backpacks, and standard vests, has important implications for preparedness, but also for law enforcement, EMS, and federal agency response to violent extremism, urban trauma, and disasters.

During or in the immediate aftermath of a disaster, blood component therapy is often in short supply. While some trauma centers are using whole blood for acute trauma resuscitations, the majority of transfusion occurs as individual components [79]. The military "buddy transfusion" approach for life-threatening hemorrhage is key when separated from well-resourced blood banks and blood suppliers. A similar approach is being explored for mass casualty responses [80]. Unfortunately, the outpouring of blood donors "on-demand" after an act of terrorism and poorly coordinated acute blood drives lead to both short-term waste and longer-term shortages. For example, after the 1 October shootings in Las Vegas, large numbers of acute blood donations led to a 17% unnecessary excess in donated blood units [81]. These authors advocated for improved oversight of blood collection during disaster care. The 2015 Paris attacks illustrated the life-saving role of transfusion support in the early administration of blood products (within the first 6 hours) for critically injured patients [82]. However, like the Las Vegas experience, these authors did not advocate for bolstering the immediate stockpile in an acute, on-demand fashion, but rather endorsed enhanced efficiency at mobilizing existing blood supplies to the bedside. Thus, community engagement and ongoing research to bolster blood product inventories in an ongoing fashion—rather than only on-demand—represents a key aspect of preparedness for violent acts of extremism.

Conclusions

Urban trauma and terrorism share a wide variety of overlapping features that impact how law enforcement and EMS prepare for and respond to emergencies. The changing threat matrix has driven significant changes in policing from a community-based approach to a threat-based posture. Key events including the Global War on Terror, access to military-grade weaponry and surplus gear, as well as global connectivity via social media have revamped the landscape of both urban trauma and activity designed to thwart violent extremism. Interagency synergy hinges on communication and the timely distribution of actionable intelligence but at present still relegates most law enforcement and EMS activity to reacting to established events rather than being able to preempt events. Integration of medics and physicians into a TEMS approach may enhance outcomes for injured individuals, as may police transport of victims of penetrating trauma. Community preparedness and bystander involvement help to shape a culture of competence. Both EMS and law enforcement will need to determine how best to effectively train, utilize, and interact with engaged bystanders during the response to urban trauma or terrorism.

Key Points

1. Urban trauma and violent extremism share broad areas of overlap with regard to their impact on social structure and preparedness.
2. Terrorism paradigms have shifted to small units that are difficult to preempt.
3. EMS and law enforcement both benefit from including medically trained personnel in rapid response teams.
4. EMS and law enforcement will need to proactively prepare to interact with trained bystanders.

References

1. Duncombe C. Social media and the visibility of horrific violence. Int Aff. 2020;96(3):609–29.
2. Vergani M, Iqbal M, Ilbahar E, Barton G. The three Ps of radicalization: push, pull and personal. A systematic scoping review of the scientific evidence about radicalization into violent extremism. Stud Conflict Terrorism. 2020;43(10):854.
3. US DHS ST-CP Security Overview 2018. www.dhs.gov. Accessed 3 Mar 2021.
4. Surveillance System for Attacks on Healthcare (SSA). SSA Home | Index (who.int). Accessed 3 Mar 2021.
5. Galhotra S. Domestic terror: are we doing enough to combat the threat from within? 2012. http://www.cnn.com/2012/16/us/domestic-terrorism/.
6. Jacobs LM, Wade DS, McSwain NE, et al. The Hartford Consensus: THREAT, a medical disaster preparedness concept. J Am Coll Surg. 2013;217:947–53.
7. Elster EA, Butler FK, Rasmussen TE. Implications of combat casualty care for mass casualty events. JAMA J Am Med Assoc. 2013;310:475–6.
8. Dishman C. The leaderless nexus: When crime and terror converge. Stud Conflict Terrorism. 2005;28:237–52.
9. Three "knockout attacks" reported in Philadelphia area. CBS Philly. 2013. http://philadelphia.cbslocal.com/2013/11/20/three-knockout-game-attacks-reported-in-philadelphia-area/.
10. Alper HE, Yu S, Stellman SD, Brackbill RM. Injury, intense dust exposure, and chronic disease among survivors of the World Trade Center terrorist attacks of September 11, 2001. Inj Epidemiol. 2017;4(1):1–10.
11. Kuhls DA, Fildes JJ, Johnson M, Dort SD, Jacobs LM, Eastman AE, Winchell RJ, Stewart RM. Southern Nevada Trauma System uses proven techniques to save lives after 1 October shooting. Bull Am Coll Surg. 2018;103(3):39–45.
12. Zanotti L. Cacophonies of aid, failed state building and NGOs in Haiti: setting the stage for disaster, envisioning the future. Third World Q. 2010;31:755–71.
13. Degennaro V Jr, Degennaro V Sr, Ginzburg E. Haiti's dilemma: how to incorporate foreign health professionals to assist in short-term recovery while capacity building for the future. J Public Health. 2011;33:459–61.
14. Perlman L, Waltman S, Irene as teacher. Lessons learned combating East Coast hurricane apply elsewhere. Mod Healthc. 2011;41:18.
15. Torres-Soriano MR. How do terrorists choose their targets for an attack? The view from inside an independent cell. Terror Polit Violence. 2019;33:1–5.
16. Galehan J. Instruments of violence: female suicide bombers of Boko Haram. Int J Law Crime Justice. 2019;58:113–23.
17. Alakoc BP. Competing to kill: terrorist organizations versus lone wolf terrorists. Terror Polit Violence. 2017;29(3):509–32.
18. Adini B, Peleg K. On constant alert: lessons to be learned from Israel's emergency response to mass-casualty terrorism incidents. Health Aff. 2013;32:2179–85.
19. Burnham G. Suicide attacks--the rationale and consequences. Lancet. 2011;378:855–7.
20. Valentine R, Valentine D, Valentine JL. Relationship of George Floyd protests to increases in COVID-19 cases using event study methodology. J Public Health. 2020;42(4):696–7.
21. Britannica's 2020 year in review. Social revolution: the year to be counted. Protests and Riots in 2020 – Year In Review | Encyclopaedia Britannica. Accessed 4 Mar 2021.
22. DePalma RG, Burris DG, Champion HR, Hodgson MJ. Blast injuries. N Engl J Med. 2005;352:1335–42.

23. Liscouski R, McGann W. The evolving challenges for explosive threat detection in the aviation sector and beyond. CTC Sentinel. 2016;9(5):1–6.
24. Gates JD, Arabian S, Biddinger P, Blansfield J, Burke P, Chung S, Fischer J, Friedman F, Gervasini A, Goralnick E, Gupta A. The initial response to the Boston marathon bombing: lessons learned to prepare for the next disaster. Ann Surg. 2014;260(6):960.
25. Oklahoma City Bombing. History. Oklahoma City Bombing — FBI. Accessed 4 Mar 2021.
26. Shvetsov A, Shvetsova S, Kozyrev VA, Spharov VA, Sheremet NM. The "car-bomb" as a terrorist tool at metro stations, railway terminals and airports. J Transp Secur. 2017;10(1):31–43.
27. Mine Resistant Ambush Protected Vehicles (MRAP). United States Army Acquisition Support Center. Mine Resistant Ambush Protected Vehicles (MRAP) – USAASC (army.mil). Accessed 4 Mar 2021.
28. Balazs GC, Polfer EM, Brelin AM, Gordon WT. High seas to high explosives: the evolution of calcaneus fracture management in the military. Mil Med. 2014;179(11):1228–35.
29. BearCat G3. Lenco armored vehicles. BearCat G3 – Lenco Armored Vehicles. Accessed 4 Mar 2021.
30. Mayorga MA. The pathology of primary blast overpressure injury. Toxicology. 1997;121:17–28.
31. Biddinger PD, Baggish A, Harrington L, d'Hemecourt P, Hooley J, Jones J, Kue R, Troyanos C, Dyer KS. Be prepared—the Boston Marathon and mass-casualty events. N Engl J Med. 2013;368(21):1958–60.
32. Goralnick E, Van Trimpont F, Carli P. Preparing for the next terrorism attack: lessons from Paris, Brussels, and Boston. JAMA Surg. 2017;152(5):419–20.
33. Coleman CN, Bader JL, Koerner JF, Hrdina C, Cliffer KD, Hick JL, James JJ, Mansoura MK, Livinski AA, Nystrom SV, DiCarlo-Cohen A. Chemical, biological, radiological, nuclear, and explosive (CBRNE) science and the CBRNE science medical operations science support expert (CMOSSE). Disaster Med Public Health Prep. 2019;13(5–6):995.
34. Rossodivita A, Rizzardini G, Gismondo MR, Villa GF, Picco C, Zoli A. CBRNE Preparedness. Metropolis the first Italian non conventional biological drill. Prehosp Disaster Med. 2017;32(S1):S6.
35. Tokyo subway attack of 1995 | Facts, Background, & AUM Shinrikyo | Britannica. Accessed 21 Feb 2021.
36. Razak S, Hignett S, Barnes J. Emergency department response to chemical, biological, radiological, nuclear, and explosive events: a systematic review. Prehosp Disaster Med. 2018;33(5):543–9.
37. Romney DA. Chemical, biological, radiological, or nuclear event (CBRNE): prehospital and hospital management. In: Operational and medical management of explosive and blast incidents. Cham: Springer; 2020. p. 569–82.
38. Madigan ML. HAZMAT guide for first responders. CRC Press; 2017.
39. Godefroidt A, Langer A. How fear drives us apart: explaining the relationship between terrorism and social trust. Terror Polit Violence. 2020;32(7):1482–505.
40. Bouhana N, Malthaner S, Schuurman B, Lindekilde L, Thornton A, Gill P. Lone-actor terrorism: radicalisation, attack planning and execution. In: The Routledge handbook of terrorism and counterterrorism. London: Routledge; 2017.
41. Pollett S, Rivers C. Social media and the new world of scientific communication during the COVID-19 pandemic. Clin Infect Dis. 2020;71(16):2184–6.
42. O'Connor C, Murphy M. Going viral: doctors must tackle fake news in the COVID-19 pandemic. BMJ. 2020;369:m1587. https://doi.org/10.1136/bmj.m1587.
43. Hu M. From the national surveillance state to the cybersurveillance state. Annu Rev Law Soc Sci. 2017;13:161–80.
44. Matania E, Yoffe L, Goldstein T. Structuring the national cyber defence: in evolution towards a Central Cyber Authority. J Cyber Policy. 2017;2(1):16–25.
45. Gruenewald J, Chermak S, Freilich JD. Distinguishing "loner" attacks from other domestic extremist violence. A comparison of far-right homicide incident and offender characteristics. Criminol Public Policy. 2013;12:65–91.
46. McGhee S. Mass casualty shooting events across America: examining how organizational cultures adapt to emerging patterns from the homeland security perspective. In: Homeland security cultures: enhancing values while fostering resilience. Rowman & Littlefield; 2018. p. 165.
47. Coleman W. Rationalization of a Regional SWAT Team. The Bill Blackwood Law Enforcement Management Institute of Texas. 2019. Rationalization of a Regional SWAT Team (tdl.org). Accessed 7 Mar 2021.
48. Laufs J, Waseem Z. Policing in pandemics: a systematic review and best practices for police response to COVID-19. Int J Disaster Risk Reduct. 2020;51:101812.
49. Duggan J Jr. The New York City Urban Search and Rescue Team (NY-TF1): a case study of interagency effectiveness. Monterey: Naval Postgraduate School; 2011.
50. http://www.dhs.gov/state-and-major-urban-area-fusion-centers. 2014. Website. Accessed 1/20/2014.
51. Benson TG. Federal murder charges filed in assassination of Philadelphia police officer. Breaking 911, 10 Dec 2020. Federal Murder Charges Filed in Assassination of Philadelphia Police Officer – Breaking911. Accessed 14 Mar 2021.
52. Haworth J, Pereira I, Katersky A, Margolin J. NYPD cops shot in the Bronx in 2 separate 'assassination' incidents, 1 suspect in custody. ABC News, 9 Feb 2020. NYPD cops shot in the Bronx in 2 separate 'assassination' incidents, 1 suspect in custody – ABC News (go.com). Accessed 14 Mar 2021.
53. Morrow WJ, Vickovic SG, Shjarback JA. Motivation to enter the police profession in the post-Ferguson era: an exploratory analysis of procedural justice. Crim Justice Stud. 2020;51:1–21.
54. Violanti JM, Steege A. Law enforcement worker suicide: an updated national assessment. Policing Int J. 2020;44:18.
55. Miller RW. CHAZ, a 'no Cop Co-Op': here's what Seattle's Capitol Hill Autonomous Zone looks like. USA Today, 12 June 2020.
56. Mastrangelo D. Officers responding to massive party in Boulder assaulted. The Hill, 7 Mar 2021. Officers responding to massive party in Boulder assaulted (msn.com). Accessed 7 Mar 2021.
57. Chiarello R. Oregon mayor slams 'culture of criminality' in Portland amid riots: 'this is defund the police'. FOX News, 1 Feb 2021. Oregon mayor slams 'culture of criminality' in Portland amid riots: 'This is defund the police' | Fox News. Accessed 7 Mar 2021.
58. Devlin B. REPORT: cops quitting at "unprecedented" number in Portland. The Daily Caller, 23 Dec 2020. REPORT: Cops Quitting At 'Unprecedented' Numbers In Portland | The Daily Caller. Accessed 7 Mar 2021.
59. Abdallah HO, Zhao C, Kaufman E, Hatchimonji J, Swendiman RA, Kaplan LJ, Seamon M, Schwab CW, Pascual JL. Increased firearm injury during the COVID-19 pandemic: a hidden urban burden. J Am Coll Surg. 2020;232:159.
60. Jacobs LM, McSwain NE Jr, Rotondo MF, Wade D, Fabbri W, Eastman AL, Butler FK Jr, Sinclair J. Improving survival from active shooter events: the Hartford Consensus. J Trauma Acute Care Surg. 2013;74(6):1399–400.
61. Walker P, Martin N, Allen S, Pascual J, Kaplan LJ. Critical care preparedness in law enforcement: tales of two types of cities. J Trauma Acute Care Surg. 2016;81(4):775–9.
62. Winter E, Hynes AM, Shultz K, Holena DN, Malhotra NR, Cannon JW. Association of police transport with survival among patients with penetrating trauma in Philadelphia, Pennsylvania. JAMA Netw Open. 2021;4(1):e2034868.

63. Heiskell LE, Carmona RH. Tactical emergency medical services: an emerging subspecialty of emergency medicine. Ann Emerg Med. 1994;23:778–85.
64. http://www.NYTimes.com/2013/12/08/us/in-mass-attacks-new-advice-lets-medics-rush-in.html?hp. Website. 2014. Accessed 1/20/2014.
65. Goolsby C, Strauss-Riggs K, Rozenfeld M, Charlton N, Goralnick E, Peleg K, Levy MJ, Davis T, Hurst N. Equipping public spaces to facilitate rapid point-of-injury hemorrhage control after mass casualty. Am J Public Health. 2019;109(2):236–41.
66. Tobias AZ, Roth RN, Weiss LS, Murray K, Yealy DM. Tree of Life Synagogue Shooting in Pittsburgh: preparedness, prehospital care, and lessons learned. West J Emerg Med. 2020;21(2):374.
67. Kaplan LJ, Glenn K, Cantele A, et al. Tactical team operator evaluation: a paradigm for iterative team member assessment. Tactical Edge. 2013;Summer:40–6.
68. Kaplan LJ, Siegel M, Eastman A, et al. Ethical considerations in embedding a surgeon in a military or civilian tactical team. Prehosp Disaster Med. 2012;27:1–6.
69. Campbell K, Naumann DN, Remick K, Wright C. Damage control resuscitation and surgery for Indigenous combat casualties: a prospective observational study. BMJ Mil Health. 2021;167(1):18–22.
70. Malgras B, Aoun O, Pauleau G, Boddaert G, Hornez E, Dulou R, Delmas JM, Haen P, Laversanne S, Crambert A, Balandraud P. Deployment of the Surgical Life-saving Module (SLM) in 2017: lessons learned in setting up and training operational surgical units. Injury. 2019;50(5):1133–7.
71. Donaghue E. Dallas shooting: experts say use of bomb robot a "first". CBS News, 8 July 2016. Dallas shooting: Experts say use of bomb robot to kill police shooting suspect a "first" – CBS News. Accessed 14 Mar 2021.
72. Crisis Negotiation. Callyo enhances safety in high risk negotiations. Callyo. Crisis and Hostage Negotiations – Callyo. Accessed 14 Mar 2021.
73. Spires J. NTPD's Spot robot dog arrives at the scene of a home invasion. DroneDJ, 26 Feb 2021. NYPD's Spot robot dog arrives at the scene of a home invasion – DroneDJ. Accessed 14 Mar 2021.
74. Klauer KM. Emergency physician and victim share experiences from Las Vegas mass shooting. ACEPNow, 11 Feb 2018. Emergency Physician and Victim Share Experiences from Las Vegas Mass Shooting – ACEP Now. Accessed 14 Mar 2021.
75. American Red Cross. Mobile apps. Mobile Apps | American Red Cross. Accessed 14 Mar 2021.
76. National Preparedness. FEMA. National Preparedness | FEMA.gov. Accessed 14 Mar 2021.
77. Burdick TE. Wilderness event medicine: planning for mass gatherings in remote areas. Travel Med Infect Dis. 2005;3:249–58.
78. Hatfill SJ, MaJMO MD. Immediate bystander aid in blast and ballistic trauma. J Am Phys Surg. 2013;18:101–4.
79. Hazelton JP, Cannon JW, Zatorski C, Roman JS, Moore SA, Young AJ, Subramanian M, Guzman JF, Fogt F, Moran A, Gaughan J, Seamon MJ, Porter J. Cold-stored whole blood: a better method of trauma resuscitation? J Trauma Acute Care Surg. 2019;87(5):1035–41. https://doi.org/10.1097/TA.0000000000002471. PMID: 31389912.
80. Holcomb JB, et al. Civilian walking blood bank emergency preparedness plan. Transfusion. 2021;61:S313.
81. Lozada MJ, Cai S, Li M, Davidson SL, Nix J, Ramsey G. The Las Vegas mass shooting: an analysis of blood component administration and blood bank donations. J Trauma Acute Care Surg. 2019;86(1):128–33.
82. Martinez T, François A, Pouget T, Carli P, Lapostolle F, Gauss T, Hamada SR, Langlois M, Yordanov Y, Féral-Pierssens AL, Woloch A, Ogereau C, Gayat E, Attias A, Pateron D, Castier Y, Ludes B, Dolla E, Tourtier JP, Riou B, Raux M, Ausset S, TRAUMABASE group. Blood product needs and transfusion timelines for the multisite massive Paris 2015 terrorist attack: a retrospective analysis. J Trauma Acute Care Surg. 2020;89(3):496–504.

Tactical Emergency Medicine, Procedures and Point-of-Care Evaluation in Austere Environments

52

Michael Blaivas, Ashot E. Sargsyan, and Dimitrios Karakitsos

Introduction

Most physicians never experience the practice of medicine outside the hospital, emergency department (ED), or the office clinic setting. Some physicians will spend time on ground or rotary wing ambulances where capability is significantly limited over the broad scope of the ED and trauma bay. However, most modern ambulances and especially air ambulances have electrical power, EKG (electrocardiogram), and ventilator capability as well as defibrillation, suction, and many other pieces of equipment that allow the well-trained emergency providers to complete an array of critical, lifesaving procedures. eFAST (Extended Focused Assessment with Sonography in Trauma) available via a new generation of highly portable ultrasound machines is a cornerstone of trauma imaging evaluation by methods other than plain X-ray, computed tomography (CT), angiography, or magnetic resonance imaging (MRI).

Hospital-based clinicians are typically surprised by the varied procedures performed with equipment carried in a physician's backpack with a Special Weapons And Tactics (SWAT) team aided by the use of a portable ultrasound machine. Not only are many of the same procedures performed in the ED or trauma bay possible in the field, but accurate diagnosis of potentially life-threatening or life-threatening injuries such as pneumothorax, hemothorax, main stem bronchial intubation, head injury, and others are possible in the most remote locations. Although there is evidence to support a scoop-and-run approach for trauma patients in typical settings, these studies are not applied well to a situation where evacuation is unsafe such as a combat zone, or impossible due to remoteness or inaccessibility of the setting [1–5]. In such cases, intubation and ventilation, placement of thoracostomy tubes, and other procedures are hours to days off and may have to be performed on-site.

Austere and Tactical Environment Emergency Medicine

The austere and tactical emergency medicine environments are typically similar but not synonymous. One tends to assume that in most tactical situations organized help is readily at hand and standing by. However, in some similarity to an austere setting, the tactical emergency physician may be deployed with a SWAT team seeking an active shooter in a modern office building of a large city, and have no access for hours to equipment or gear other than what they carry on their back. While most SWAT team members carry gear in addition to their body armor and helmets, such as gas masks, they are not weighed down as much as a tactical physician who carries a large amount of medical equipment on his/her back (Fig. 52.1). Despite the encumbrance a large heavy bag provides, it is necessary for the tactical emergency physician to perform their job. In many cases, tactical physicians are armed only with side arms and do not carry long guns. They are tasked with protecting their patients who may be victims, SWAT team members, or even suspects but are typically not the first to enter a building.

Physicians performing emergency care in a non-tactical, austere setting still benefit from a well-stocked equipment bag. Not wearing body armor, helmet, or other tactical gear saves weight and may allow the physician to carry additional medical supplies. As opposed to a tactical deployment, a physician providing care in the austere environment may be much further away from potential evacuation and medical

M. Blaivas (✉)
University of South Carolina, School of Medicine, Columbia, SC, USA

University of South Carolina School of Medicine, Department of Emergency Medicine, St Francis Hospital, Columbus, Georgia
e-mail: mike@blaivas.org

A. E. Sargsyan
Wyle Science, Technology & Engineering Group/NASA Bioastronautics, Houston, TX, USA

D. Karakitsos
University of South Carolina, School of Medicine, Columbia, SC, USA

L. Marshall Gillman, S. Widder (eds.), *Trauma Team Dynamics*, https://doi.org/10.1007/978-3-031-86312-7_52

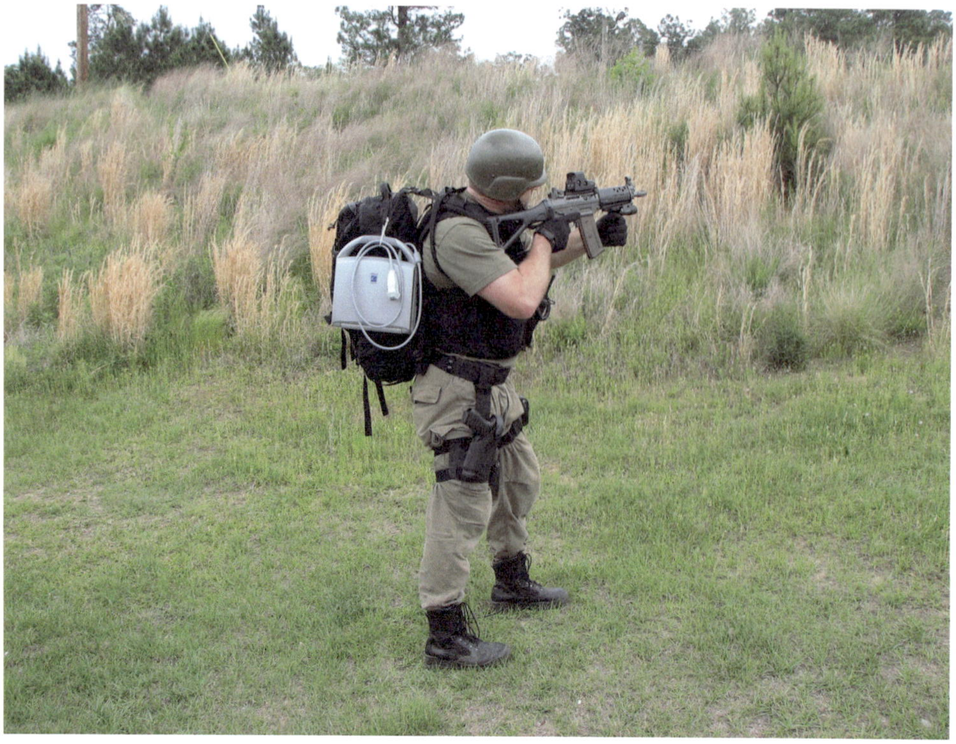

Fig. 52.1 A tactical emergency physician equipped with a medical pack, portable ultrasound machine, body armor, and weaponry

help and be required to care for their patients not just for hours but days. Prolonged care without evacuation is most likely to happen in a remote expedition setting, and patients may have to be cared for through recovery and continuation of the expedition.

Equipment for the Tactical and Austere Environment

Although it is still unrealistic to carry a laboratory analyzer in the physician's bag, some point-of-care testing consisting of small analyzers using cartridges could be transported. Such tests typically evaluate cardiac-related processes such as troponin and beta natriuretic peptide, but other additional testing such as electrolytes may also be available. For a physician traveling to an austere environment such equipment may be desirable, especially if members of the group are older and/or have existing illnesses. Such portable blood analyzers are less likely to benefit the tactical physician on a deployment or rendition. Equipment recharging capability may be available by employing one of a host of over-the-counter solar recharging kits often capable of slowly charging batteries in portable devices. One piece of equipment that provides broad diagnostic imaging capability is found more and more frequently in tactical and austere settings [6–10]. As Fig. 52.1 shows, the portable ultrasound machine has its place in tactical medicine as well as in austere environments.

The remainder of the gear focuses on critical procedures and traumatic injury care. Since blunt trauma is always a risk, the equipment bag should include a cervical collar and splinting material, the latter of which could be of the inflatable variety. Almost like an athletic trainer, tape and bandages are important to have. In reality, one would bring much of the trauma bay if room allowed. Equipment trays take up too much space, but essential sterile pieces can be brought. Chest tubes, typically two, suture equipment, and a stapler are essential. Clotting material such as a lava rock product is imperative along with tactical tourniquets for hemorrhage control. Compression devices to occlude the abdominal aorta or ipsilateral common iliac artery may be lifesaving in cases of inguinal wounds where hemorrhage cannot be adequately controlled with local compression [11, 12].

Intubation equipment is likely to be limited to one handle and one or two blades as well as several endotracheal tubes. A cricothyrotomy kit is essential, as well as a bag valve mask valve apparatus. Suction is typically limited to a large syringe and rubber tube to suction the mouth and airway if absolutely needed.

Medications are essential, including intravenous fluids, but providers are unlikely to have more than one or two doses of any medicine, and carrying more than one or at most two liters of fluid may significantly weigh down the medical bag. Antibiotics are more critical for longer expeditions and a large portion of the pack may have to be devoted to a variety of antibiotics, anti-parasitics, and anti-fungals, depending on the destination. Antibiotics carried would include broad-spectrum drugs in states not requiring refrigeration. Coverage would typically include skin, bowel pathogens, urinary tract, and pulmonary tract pathogens. Realistically, a handful of antibiotics such as a third-generation cephalosporin, a broad-spectrum fluoroquinolone, and a lincosamide can be used to cover a broad swatch of bacterial illnesses encountered. Tactical physicians will have few antibiotics, mostly in the case of open fractures and deep penetrating wounds providing coverage for skin and bowel pathogens. These would be given when immediate evacuation is impossible such as in a relatively remote area or when the area may remain unsecured for a prolonged period of time, limiting Emergency Medical Services (EMS) or aircraft access. Essential medications include paralytics and sedatives along with standard Advanced Cardiac Life Support (ACLS) medications such as epinephrine, atropine, and others. Pain medications are likely to be required with penetrating wounds and blast injuries as well as blunt trauma.

Procedures

Procedures such as intubation, thoracostomy tube placement, and peripheral and central line placement are performed in much the same way one would in a trauma bay or ICU setting. Intraosseus (IO) access can be a rapid, albeit a very temporizing measure to obtain access. The inherent vulnerability of an IO line to unknown dislodgement is exaggerated in the field where the patient may be moved rapidly and roughly due to terrain, weather, or even gunfire. However, no backup is likely to be available, and other than portable ultrasound, no follow-up imaging to confirm either chest or endotracheal tube placement. Pain control may be required in either tactical settings or austere environments; in either case, capabilities to provide long-term pain management are likely to be limited. In some cases nerve blocks may be ideal in dealing with significant extremity injury, especially in settings when evacuation is likely to be delayed.

Procedures are likely to be performed in less than satisfactory conditions and improvisation may be required. An example is a resuscitation during a SWAT team deployment in Columbia County, Georgia, in 2006. A SWAT team containing two tactical physicians entered a house of an armed barricaded suspect. Upon entry the suspect produced a handgun and shot himself in the left anterior chest. The suspect was in impending respiratory arrest but continued to struggle and resist assessment and treatment within the confines of his small bedroom. A peripheral IV was established and the patient was given etomidate and succinylcholine. However, during the struggle the IV infiltrated and he did not receive the medications. Additional saline for dilution of the succinylcholine was unavailable and the physicians mixed the last dose of etomidate with the powdered succinylcholine. The medication was injected directly into the suspected femoral vein due to the failure of another IV line. The patient was bagged and rapidly intubated. Auscultation, however, revealed no breath sounds in the left chest even after endotracheal tube withdrawal. The patient's chest was needled and physicians proceeded to place a thoracostomy tube. The equipment bag had been overturned and bedsheets mixed with the equipment. Additionally, electrical power was cut during the raid, and procedures were performed under illumination of the SWAT team weapon's lights. Clamps for blunt dissection to the ribs and penetration into the thoracic cavity could not be located. After scalpel incision the physician placing the chest tube was forced to bluntly dissect with his thumb through the soft tissue and was able to penetrate through the chest wall, releasing a large amount of air. The chest tube was inserted but no needle drivers could be located to suture the chest tube in place. A utility tool borrowed from a SWAT team member was used to complete suturing. A latex glove with a finger cut distally was taped at the end of the tube to act as a Heimlich valve. A large quantity of chlorhexidine was available and used extensively during the procedure. The patient was later airlifted and survived to discharge. He required no surgical intervention during his stay in the hospital.

This example serves to highlight the need for improvisation in tactical and remote conditions. Such improvisation especially critical in combat zones where patients may have to be treated rapidly and moved to a more secure location.

Assessment and Testing

Performing point-of-care laboratory testing during prolonged expeditions may be possible in some cases. For most, the physical examination is the major assessment tool. Even more than in the hospital environment, the tactical physician is likely to have a first-hand understanding of the limitations of the physical examination, the accuracy of which is being questioned more than ever [13]. Patients may be severely injured and unconscious or be in loud environments or unsecured locations. It may be necessary to maintain a covert position and the use of lighting at night might be too risky. The portable ultrasound machine is an ideal all-purpose diagnostic tool and an extension of the physical exam. The tactical physician will typically use eFAST applications to search for free fluid, cardiac injury, pneumothorax, and signs of head or vascular injury. In the austere environment of an expedition, the physician may encounter general medical complaints and be required to image the gallbladder, bowel, and pelvis among others. The tactical physician is not immune to such requirements either. During a large-scale drug raid in 2005, a tactical physician performed not only several trauma-related examinations but a lung examination diagnosing pulmonary edema in one bystander, as well as an abdominal ultrasound examination revealing a large left adnexal mass that later turned out to be an ectopic pregnancy in another bystander. These assessments were necessitated due to the remote rural location of the raid and the large curtained-off area that took time to secure.

Conclusions

Tactical and austere medicine both provide a wide variety of potentially critical ill patient scenarios. The critical difference is the need for a physician to be prepared for combat in the former. Many of the same procedures performed in a modern trauma bay or ED may be performed at the patient's side in combat or remote areas. With limited backup and evacuation options such procedures may be life-saving. Improvisation is critical, and the use of the only imaging technology available from a pocket or backpack, the portable ultrasound unit, greatly enhances the providers' capabilities and accuracy. With proper training and preparedness, the tactical and austere medicine provider will serve a critical role in patient care and in turn be rewarded with a unique work experience few participate in.

Key Notes

- Most procedures available in the trauma bay may be required in the field.
- Prepare with intubation and resuscitation medications and fluid.
- Few diagnostic tests are available.
- Portable ultrasound greatly enhances the providers' diagnostic and therapeutic capabilities.
- Improvisation and use of available tools can help overcome limitations in the field.

References

1. Solomon SD, Saldana F. Point-of-care ultrasound in medical education–stop listening and look. N Engl J Med. 2014;370(12):1083–5.
2. Rainer TH, Houlihan KP, Robertson CE, Beard D, Henry JM, Gordon MW. An evaluation of paramedic activities in prehospital trauma care. Injury. 1997;28(9–10):623–7.
3. Di Bartolomeo S, Sanson G, Nardi G, Michelutto V, Scian F. HEMS vs. Ground-BLS care in traumatic cardiac arrest. Prehosp Emerg Care. 2005;9:79–84.
4. Davis DP, Peay J, Serrano JA, Buono C, Vilke GM, Sise MJ, Kennedy F, Eastman AB, Velky T, Hoyt DB. The impact of aeromedical response to patients with moderate to severe traumatic brain injury. Ann Emerg Med. 2005;46:115–22.
5. Ryynänen OP, Iirola T, Reitala J, Pälve H, Malmivaara A. Is advanced life support better than basic life support in prehospital care? A systematic review. Injury. 2013;44(5):634–8.
6. Blaivas M, Kuhn W, Reynolds B, Brannam L. Change in differential diagnosis and patient management with the use of portable ultrasound in a remote setting. Wilderness Environ Med. 2005;16(1):38–41.
7. Shorter M, Macias DJ. Portable handheld ultrasound in austere environments: use in the Haiti disaster. Prehosp Disaster Med. 2012;27(2):172–7.
8. Whelan L, Justice W, Goodloe JM, Dixon JD, Thomas SH. Trauma ultrasound in civilian tactical medicine. Emerg Med Int. 2012;2012:781570.
9. Gay DA, Ritchie JV, Perry JN, Horne S. Ultrasound of penetrating ocular injury in a combat environment. Clin Radiol. 2013;68(1):82–4.
10. Nations JA, Browning RF. Battlefield applications for handheld ultrasound. Ultrasound Q. 2011;27(3):171–6.
11. Blaivas M, Shiver S, Lyon M, Adhikari S. Control of hemorrhage in critical femoral or inguinal penetrating wounds–an ultrasound evaluation. Prehosp Disaster Med. 2006;21(6):379–82.
12. Lyon M, Shiver SA, Greenfield EM, Reynolds BZ, Lerner EB, Wedmore IS, Schwartz RB. Use of a novel abdominal aortic tourniquet to reduce or eliminate flow in the common femoral artery in human subjects. J Trauma Acute Care Surg. 2012;73(2 Suppl 1):S103–5.
13. Wipf JE, Lipsky BA, Hirschmann JV, et al. Diagnosing pneumonia by physical examination: relevant or relic? Arch Intern Med. 1999;159:1082–7.

An Introduction to Tactical Medicine Concepts

53

Military and Law Enforcement Medical Considerations

William Guse, Shaun Cowan, Andrew Beckett, and Kenji Inaba

Introduction

Tactical medicine can be defined as medicine practiced in direct support of military or law enforcement operations. This typically applies only during tactical operations, however includes aspects such as supporting the team in training, training the team in self-aid, medical mission planning, and acting as a medical intelligence source operations.

Tactical medicine grew from research and the recognition that past clinical practice guidelines were not preventing combat deaths. In 1984, Col. Bellamy released his pivotal paper: "The Causes of Death in Conventional Land Warfare: Implications for Combat Casualty Care Research." His longitudinal retrospective research into combat casualties and causes of death in WW2, Korea, and Vietnam demonstrated a trend of preventable deaths; 9% of casualties exsanguinated from wounds to the extremities, 5% died from tension pneumothorax, and 1% suffocated from airway obstruction [1]. While law enforcement and military medical operations have significant differences in injury patterns, variable operational assets, and mission priorities, the last decade has demonstrated lessons and experience of both law enforcement and military medical care that can be adapted and applied between the two broad areas of tactical medical operations. These lessons and experience create valuable synergy; however, it remains important to be critical of dogma and implement medical intervention and care based on environment-specific evidence when available and with carefully applied expert consensus when evidence is scarce.

W. Guse
Royal Canadian Medical Service, Canadian Armed Forces, Ottawa, ON, Canada

S. Cowan (✉)
Departments of Surgery and Critical Care, University of Alberta, Edmonton, AB, Canada
e-mail: cowan@ualberta.ca

A. Beckett
Royal Canadian Medical Service, Canadian Armed Forces, Ottawa, ON, Canada

Department of Surgery, University of Toronto, Toronto, ON, Canada
e-mail: andrew.beckett@forces.gc.ca

K. Inaba
University of Southern California, Los Angeles, CA, USA
e-mail: Kenji.Inaba@med.usc.edu

Military Tactical Medicine: A Recent History

In 1996, Butler et al. released the first Tactical Combat Casualty Care (TCCC) guidance. These recommendations were based upon 2 years of research sponsored by the United States Special Operations Command (USSOCOM). These guidelines recommended a scenario-based approach to casualty care, divided into specific phases, within a special operations environment. Each phase had specific skills and interventions recommended, established on the unique and dynamic realities of combat. This approach to tactical medicine was calculated to treat preventable deaths effectively, while maintaining the safety of the care provider and, further, not jeopardizing mission success. Interventions and recommendations were conceived with the understanding of the austere environment, adverse lighting, environmental factors, limited supplies and assistance, multiple casualty events, and specific evacuation platforms that make up this particular operational environment [2].

In 2001, the Committee on Tactical Combat Casualty Care was established to examine new equipment, procedures, and interventions to integrate within TCCC Guidelines. As a pan-service mission, the committee's members include: medics, pararescue, special operations, and physicians to ensure a realistic and relevant approach to tactical medicine. The committee meets regularly to

L. Marshall Gillman, S. Widder (eds.), *Trauma Team Dynamics*, https://doi.org/10.1007/978-3-031-86312-7_53

update guidelines on current research and practice [3]. The TCCC Guidelines are reviewed quarterly and updated as required, in association with the Joint Trauma System (JTS), which ensures evidence-based practice guidelines [4]. The TCCC guidelines have also been part of the Prehospital Trauma Life Support (PHTLS) manual and program since their Fourth Edition publication. PHTLS now publishes a specific military edition of their manual centering on the more in-depth nuances of TCCC [5]. "The trauma care recommendations found in the Prehospital Trauma Life Support Manual carry the endorsement of the American College of Surgeons' Committee on Trauma and the National Association of EMTs, making TCCC the first set of battlefield trauma care guidelines to have earned this dual endorsement" [6]. Tactical Combat Casualty Care has been adopted by the ABCA (America, Britain, Canada, Australia, and New Zealand militaries) and the majority of NATO [6].

The success of Tactical Combat Casualty Care has been undeniable. Both the 75th Ranger Regiment and the Canadian Armed Forces have reported an incidence of 100% application of life-saving interventions in combat (Fig. 53.1). These units have experienced greater casualty survival rates than others in recent conflicts [7, 8].

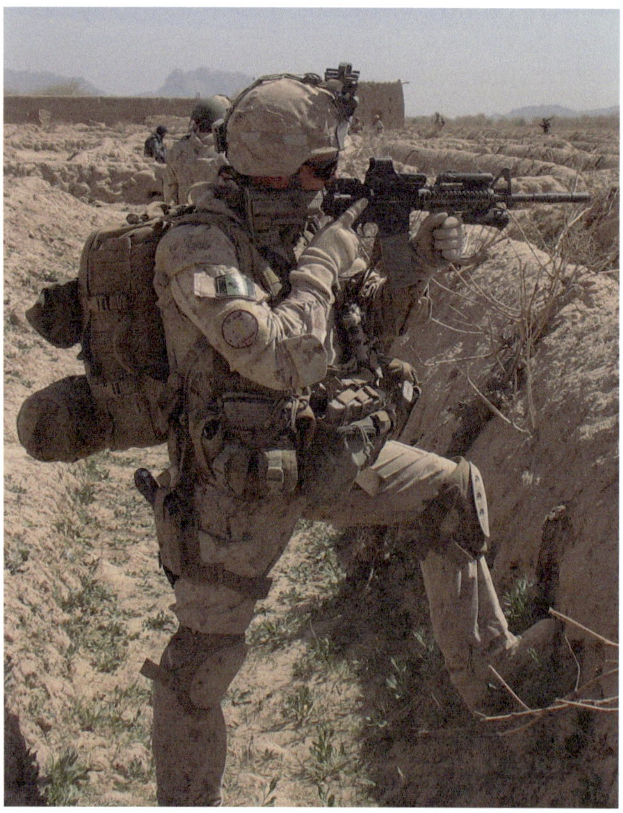

Fig. 53.1 A Canadian Forces Medic on patrol, equipped for dismounted medical care. (File photo, W. Guse)

Law Enforcement Medicine: A Recent History

While military forces around the world have long recognized the need for medical support on the battlefield dating back to Napoleon and earlier, where early triage and evacuation concepts originated, the close support of law enforcement operations by medical support personnel is new by comparison [9]. The civil environment of the United States in the 1960s saw the development of SWAT or tactical teams to counter increasing civilian violence; however, most traditional models used civilian ambulances staged in a cold (green) zone and were not initially integrated into forward operations [10].

Early integration of medical provider integration within police tactical operations occurred in Los Angeles County in the early 1970s, thanks to the recognition and advocacy by Cpt. Kolman and Cdr Rasmunoff with the Los Angeles Sheriff's Department, where EMTs were integrated within the tactical teams within the county. Concurrently, a similar model evolved in Tucson, Arizona, with the Pima County Sheriff's Department under the direction of Dr. Carmona [11]. With the early experiences of these teams to guide discussions, in 1989, conference proceedings discussed standardization of tactical emergency medical support (TEMS) in the USA. Law enforcement community and annual representation of TEMS within the tactical law enforcement community evolved [12, 13]. This culminated in a position paper by the National Tactical Operators Association, formally establishing TEMS as a component of police tactical operations in the USA in 1993 [14]. In 2001, the National Association of EMS Physicians endorsed the TEMS concept through their own position paper recognizing the need for specialized tactical medical providers in law enforcement operations [15].

The above is a brief overview of several key historical points in the development of TEMS. Many others have contributed to the development and growth of tactical medical support systems over the past three decades since the original NTOA position paper and formalization of TEMS standards and utilization. The concurrent domestic experiences of these units, coupled with the lessons learned from military special forces medical support have resulted in synergistic growth in TEMS utilization, as well as the recognition of specialized training and experience needed for these medical providers in law enforcement operations. Bridging these synergistic relationships between military and law enforcement medical elements and promoting research in these areas, the Special Operations Medical Association (SOMA) brings a formal collective body of shared experience and research [16]. Training and experience are needed in a multitude of spheres to develop a competent and reliable tactical medical operator. Team tactics, weapons and less lethal munition knowledge, tactical communications, hazardous materials safety, and many other aspects comprise the tactical training required; however, this is only but a single pillar in developing an individual tactical medical operator. Training and experience in the unique aspects of medical care in hostile and austere environments, remote assessment and medicine across the barricade, medical intelligence, sports medicine, and leadership are also critical elements beyond civilian EMS or medicine training required for a well-trained tactical medical operator.

An Approach to Tactical Medicine

Much like the doctrine of Advanced Trauma Life Support (ATLS) programs gives an approach for civilian trauma care, the phases of care in tactical medicine, including an algorithmic approach within each phase, guide appropriate care as dictated by the environment and tactical situation. Similar to planning for a thoracotomy in the radiology department is not optimal, obtaining vascular access or placing a patient in spinal motion restriction in the middle of a tactical situation or kinetic operation are equally, if not more egregious, errors in medical decision-making. An often repeated dictum of tactical medicine outlines that good medicine often equates to bad tactics, and good tactics may not allow the best medicine to be practiced at the time. The understanding of this intricate balance is a key skill, which any medical provider in a tactical environment must master in order to allow sound critical thinking and safe decision-making in a dynamic tactical environment.

Tactical operations fall into two categories primarily, upon meeting engagement or planned operations. An example of met engagement is the police officer who comes under fire during a traffic stop or a unit of soldiers who trigger an Improvised Explosive Device (IED) while on routine patrol. Resources available during this type of incident are limited to individual or small unit organic skills and supplies. Planned operations, by comparison, include the following examples: a Law Enforcement tactical team raiding a known criminal location with prior reconnaissance or surveillance, a Special Operations team boarding a target ship underway, or an Army combat team conducting an organized counter-insurgency sweep. Since these operations are planned, rehearsed, and executed with a command and control structure, greater assets are available to the operators on the ground as well as pre-stage assets, including medical and evacuation planning and assets.

Phases of Care

In most common doctrine, tactical medicine is divided into three phases of care. The first phase occurs when an active threat is still ongoing. This is commonly referred to, within military circles, as Care Under Fire. It is abbreviated as CuF. Law Enforcement teams may use different terms, such as Direct Threat Care (DTC). DTC can also be defined by operational zones. These zones include cold (green), warm (yellow), and hot (red) zones, with CuF being comparable to the hot (red) zone. An example of this includes an active gun fight or a planned assault on an objective. In the CuF phase of care, the best medicine is prevention of additional casualties and rapid control of exsanguinating hemorrhages, primarily, tourniquet application. The doctrine of this phase of care centers around winning the fight and eliminating the threat to prevent additional casualties. Self-extraction of conscious, capable wounded casualties, self-application of tourniquets, and then in specific circumstances, application of tourniquets to casualty are the only medical treatments included in this phase of care.

Tactical field care (TFC) is the second phase of care, referenced in Law Enforcement, as Indirect Threat Care (ITC), the yellow zone, or the warm zone. This phase is when the majority of field medicine occurs. Conceptually, a threat still exists, although it's either controlled, not active, or sufficient hard cover exists, while medical treatments are being rendered. In order to provide security, control, and efficient use of resources, casualties are collocated in a Casualty Collection Point or CCP. Casualties will likely be moved to this location using drags, carries, and improvised means. In a military setting, the majority of care done before the casualty is moved to the CCP is completed by soldiers or troops specially trained in Tactical Combat Casualty Care. Once moved to the CCP, this may be the first time that they are treated by a medic. Depending on the law enforcement agency and operational structure, arrival at a CCP may be the first time that casualties will be seen by a medical professional as well. A paramedic, doctor, or both could be in place depending on the team structure and source of medical support members. Regardless of team structure, in military or law enforcement settings, Tactical Field Care is the care provided in active areas of operation when the threat is controlled, often to variable degrees, resulting in dynamic and nuanced shifts between care under fire and TFC approaches. The response to the Boston Marathon Bombing is an excellent example of Indirect Threat Care within a civilian setting, where the attacks and injuries had occurred, but the threat of additional bombs or attacks was not contained while medical care was being provided.

Tactical Evacuation Care (TEC) is the third phase of care and includes the medical therapies and treatment modalities rendered during the evacuation of a casualty from the point of injury to some level of medical treatment facility. Remember, in an austere military setting, this phase allows more medical assets, both advanced equipment and advanced providers, access to the patient depending on the evacuation platform. Helicopters and armored ambulances are reliable platforms in most military scenarios. In a Law Enforcement operation, this is simply referred to as Evacuation Care. According to the triage done onsite, Advanced Life Support Paramedics in traditional wheeled ambulances or helicopter transport can be brought into play at this time with evacuation to an appropriate trauma center.

In cases of delayed evacuation, austere environments, or immature operational settings, a fourth phase of care comes into play. Prolonged Field Care is now being considered a fourth phase of care, where the evaluation phase is delayed for tactical, geographical, or limited resource reasons. The general concepts in prolonged field care mirror many of the principles associated with wilderness medicine, critical care medical, and nursing care.

The MARCHE Algorithm Approach

Combat injuries historically attribute 9% of casualties exsanguinated from wounds to the extremities, 5% died from tension pneumothorax, and 1% expired second to airway obstruction discussed above [1]. The MARCHE algorithm (Table 53.1) was initially set up to address Col. Bellamy's report on preventable deaths rapidly with follow on stabilization and precautionary interventions implemented later in the protocol [2]. As the tactics, techniques, and technology of tactical medicine evolved, the MARCHE algorithm continues to be updated by governing bodies based on best practices and novel medical devices [3, 17]. Programs such as the American College of Surgeons "Stop the Bleed" program have simplified protocols for the trauma layman but maintain the principles of MARCHE [17, 18].

During CuF or DTC, the only indicated interventions include tourniquets and, when feasible, recovery position, dependent upon the tactical situation. Extremity hemorrhage and simple airway interventions are the only acts safe enough to be performed rapidly in active combat [17].

There are tactical considerations and actions a tactical medic must undertake outside the MARCHE algorithm that must be performed prior to any medical intervention. The first consideration is securing a safe location to collect and treat casualties. This was discussed previously as the establishment of a Casualty Collection Point. Casualties with an altered mental status must be disarmed for the safety of providers. Additionally, communications, lighting, and explosive equipment on these casualties must be either removed or turned off to further secure casualty, provider, and team safety and security. Triaging casualties as they enter the CCP should be completed rapidly to identify those that most urgently need and to organize the CCP for efficient follow on care.

Table 53.1 MARCHE approach to tactical field care (TFC) and common interventions

Tactical medicine: MARCHE approach to casualty management	
	Interventions
M—Massive hemorrhage	Tourniquets Wound packing Hemostatic gauze packing Junctional tourniquets
A—Airway	Positioning Basic airway adjuncts Supraglottic airway Surgical Airway
R—Respirations	Chest seals Needle, finger, and tube thoracostomy Positive pressure ventilation
C—Circulation	Non-massive bleeding control Vascular access Blood and fluid resuscitation Tranexamic acid Pelvic binder
H—Hypothermia and head injury	Cooling prevention Active warming Hypoxia and hypotension prevention Hypertonic saline
E—Eyes & everything else	Monitoring and documentation Pain management Antibiotics Secondary survey Management of other wounds Nursing care

Massive Hemorrhage Management ("M")

Tourniquets

Traditional methods of direct and indirect pressure are used as a temporizing measure in MARCHE. The preferred method of gaining hemorrhage control for extremity injuries is tourniquets, with windlass and ratchet styles of tourniquet preferred. Elastic-based tourniquets are not recommended [19, 20]. It is recommended that commercially available tourniquets be used rather than improvised tourniquets (Fig. 53.2). Studies have demonstrated that non-windlass improvised tourniquets fail to control extremity hemorrhage in 99% of tests consistently. While windlass improvised tourniquets are more effective in controlling extremity hemorrhage, there is still a 32% failure rate [21, 22].

Wound Packing

For ballistic or blast injuries with deep wound tracts or junctional injuries (i.e., groin or axillary injuries), wound packing is recommended to gain direct pressure along the wound tract. The packed wound should then be covered with a pressure bandage or closed with a hemostatic clamp [20]. Effective wound packing is a key hemorrhage control skill for tactical medical providers and is critical to effective use of most hemostatic dressings.

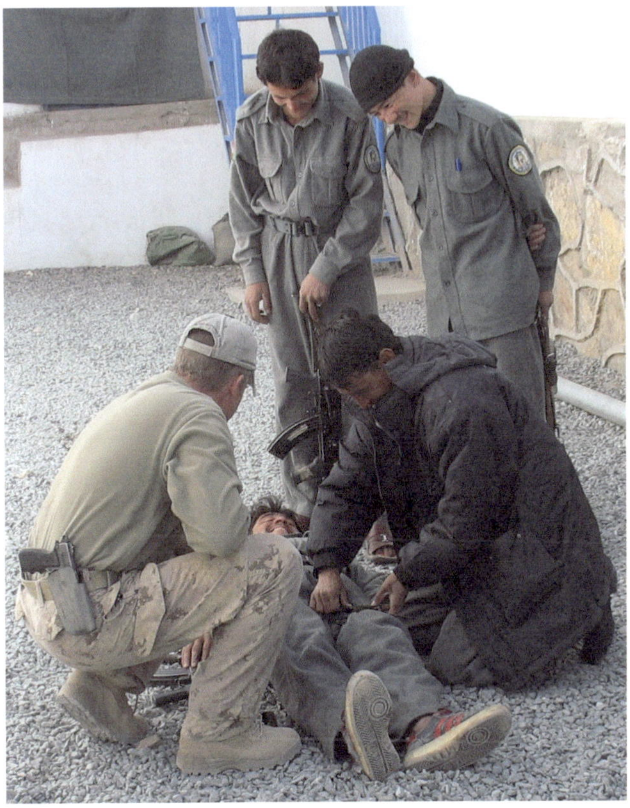

Fig. 53.2 Tourniquet training with coalition forces. (File photo, W. Guse)

Hemostatic Dressings

With uncontrollable hemorrhage in wounds not amenable to a tourniquet, there are a few options available. Hemostatic packing materials, such as QuikClot Combat Gauze, Celox Rapid, or HemCon ChitoGauze, can be used to gain control. While they have different mechanisms of action, they are generally applied using wound packing with gauze [23]. While lab data is favorable for the use of these agents for massive hemorrhage control, there is a lack of human data supporting use of hemostatic agents over regular gauze appropriately packed for bleeding control. Direct clinical translation of this data has not been studied, and given the dynamic and diverse environments, users and injury patterns, may never be well studied. The use of hemostatic dressings in tactical environments is nonetheless widespread but should be considered for use with consideration to cost, expiry, and frequency of use [24].

Junctional Tourniquets

Junctional Tourniquets, such as Abdominal Aortic and Junctional Tourniquet, Junctional Emergency Treatment Tool, and SAM Junctional Tourniquet, can be used to gain hemorrhage control. Junctional tourniquets have been demonstrated to be simple and effective with the ability to be applied rapidly in multiple studies [25, 26]. They are, however, cost-prohibitive and require additional training and ongoing skill practice for effective and rapid use.

Airway Management ("A")

Once massive hemorrhage is controlled, at least temporarily, focus shifts to the airway. In conscious casualties that can follow directions, simple positioning can be used to manage the airway. Positioning can also be used as a temporizing measure for casualties prior to the use of airway adjuncts. The lateral recumbent position commonly referred to as recovery position for unconscious casualties or sitting or tripod position for chest trauma or maxillofacial injuries has been used effectively and is often a position of comfort for these patients. A high index of suspicion is required for any casualties with blast exposure or enclosed space fires as the airway can rapidly deteriorate due to edema from superheated gas exposure.

Limiting airway intervention to basic adjuncts is preferred in the tactical environment. Simple manual airway techniques including a chin lift or jaw thrust maneuvers to allow inspection, manual sweeps of oral pharynx and suctioning, when tactically feasible, are the initial standard of care. The routine use of orotracheal intubation is not feasible in an operational environment when considering adverse lighting, equipment required, monitoring, and provider skill fade. For unconscious casualties with no impending airway collapse, the nasopharyngeal airway (NPA) is recommended as it is well tolerated and requires little monitoring [3]. With casualties with impending airway collapse, supraglottic airways are the next step, when tactically feasible, for their ability to be inserted blindly and simplicity of insertion facilitate rapid airway management. Any supraglottic airway that uses an air-filled cuff needs to be constantly monitored to avoid overpressurization and ensure continued placement, especially in the context of pressure changes in aircraft evacuation or changes in altitude. The CoTCCC specifically names the I-gel™ as the preferred supraglottic airway. The gel-filled cuff is simple to use, decreases the requirement for monitoring, and avoids the dangers of cuff over-inflation [27].

In the event of failure of the aforementioned interventions, the surgical airway is the next recommended intervention when appropriately trained providers are available. An open surgical technique, with or without bougie, is preferred in the austere environment. This procedure relies upon tactile guidance and landmarks, allowing use in low or no light conditions. There are multiple prefabricated kits available on the market or a trimmed 6.0 ET tube can serve as an improvised cricothyrotomy tube. Early use of the awake surgical airway is recommended in patients with severe maxillofacial trauma and casualties with signs of inhalation injuries. This can be facilitated via local and transtracheal administration of local anesthetic [28].

All casualties with airway adjuncts or surgical airways should be monitored using pulse oximetry to ensure adequate oxygenation and end-tidal carbon dioxide monitoring via colorimetric, or ideally, capnographic devices. The use of supplemental oxygen is best deferred to the evacuation phase for a number of reasons. Operators involved in tactical operations, as a rule, are very healthy individuals and, therefore, have a large physiological reserve. Delivery of oxygen (DO_2) is a function of cardiac output (CO), hemoglobin (Hb), and its saturation (SaO_2) and, to a much lesser extent, dissolved in plasma (PaO_2).

$$DO_2 = CO \times \left(1.39 \times [Hb] \times SaO_2 + \left(0.003 \times PaO_2\right)\right)$$

By maintaining hemostasis, cardiac output is stabilized which has a direct effect on arterial oxygen concentrations. Aggressive hemorrhage control and IV blood products are most effective in maintaining adequate perfusion in these patients. Additionally, oxygen tanks are explosive if penetrated by projectiles, a real risk in combat environments. It would be akin to carrying a bomb on one's back. The current technology for miniaturized oxygen concentrator is not robust enough for an operational environment.

In both law enforcement and military settings, supplemental oxygen should be available on evacuation platforms. Supplemental oxygen is recommended during the evacuation phase, especially when at high altitude or aerial platforms are used [29].

Respiration ("R")

Any penetrating injury to the thorax should be covered by a vented chest seal. A non-vented chest seal can be used as an alternative but carries an increased risk of developing into tension pneumothorax [30, 31]. In some cases, maintaining an open thorax may be prudent to avoid tensioning the thorax; monitor and "burp" the chest as required. Due to the unpredictable wound tracts of ballistic injuries, it is generally accepted that any wound from the umbilicus and superior should be managed as though there is thoracic involvement. For multiple penetrating chest injuries, the vented chest seal should be applied to the largest defect, and occlusive dressings are appropriate for the remaining wounds [27].

In ballistic or blast injuries, maintain a high index of suspicion for tension pneumothorax. Severe/gradual respiratory distress or tachypnea, unilateral decreased or absent breath sounds, decreased O_2 saturation of less than 90%, shock or cardiac arrest without obviously fatal wounds are the well-known symptoms. However, it can be as insidious as progressively worsening mental status in a seemingly uninjured casualty after a blast exposure [27].

Casualties with suspected tension pneumothorax should be decompressed using a 10–14 gauge 3.25″ catheter unit at either the fifth intercostal space on the anterior axillary line or the traditional second intercostal space in the midclavicular line by a trained provider [32, 33]. Additionally, for advanced trained providers, a simple finger thoracostomy can be used on the fifth intercostal space on the anterior axillary line [34–37]. A traditional tube thoracostomy can be completed in TFC/ITC as well, with a simple duckbill one-way valve (Heimlich valve) inserted on the distal end of the chest tube to prevent air reentry and promote one-way flow out of the thorax. During the evacuation phase, an appropriate drainage management system should be attached. For casualties with severe torso trauma or blast injury and vital signs absent (VSA), a protocol for triage of potentially salvageable patients should be established, considering signs of life such as pupil response and downtime. A protocoled set of actions including bilateral thoracic decompression is recommended before discontinuing treatment [27].

Circulation ("C")

Management of circulatory insult includes assessment and control of any non-massive bleeding, vascular access, fluid resuscitation, and reassessment of previously placed tourniquets. Suspicion of occult bleeding into the pelvis, abdomen, thorax, and long bones should be considered in unstable patients without overt bleeding or continued instability despite external hemorrhage control and with pneumothorax ruled out. A high index of suspicion should be maintained for any casualty with a mechanism of injury (MOI) that includes blast exposure, blunt force trauma, and penetrating trauma to the pelvic region. Changes in mental status, tachycardia, or pain are often the only reliable indicators of underlying injury in austere conditions. Rapid application of a pelvic binder is indicated for any suspected pelvic fracture based upon mechanism alone, or in conjunction with clinical findings [38]. Improvised pelvic binding using casualties trousers has been shown to be effective [39, 40]. Splint all fractures while maintaining the distal pulse. Folding traction splits are available that can maintain traction as required. Traction provides both hemorrhage control and pain management.

Vascular Access

Continually assess for signs of shock while securing large bore intravenous access early for the administration of analgesia, antibiotics, other drugs, and possible fluid resuscitation. The use of intraosseous access is recommended when peripheral intravenous attempts fail or injuries preclude upper extremity IV sites. Intraosseous has been used with great success in tactical environments for many years [17]. While the intravenous route is preferred, blood transfusion can be administered through intraosseous access with high flow rates [27, 41–43]. Central line access is technically difficult and equipment intensive and should be reserved for use in more controlled environments.

Fluid and Hemostatic Resuscitation

Fluid resuscitation has undergone drastic change in military medicine and has prompted a shift in practice in domestic trauma care as well. Early tactical medicine practice employed large volume crystalloid resuscitation, which we now know was a major source of coagulopathy and mortality [44]. The evolution of fluid resuscitation then moved to starch-based colloids, thought to give longer duration of intravascular expansion and lower weight as hypertonic solutions allowed for reduced volumes required for similar effect. 250 ml of hypertonic saline and dextran (HSD), for example, has similar vascular expansion to a liter of crystalloid [45, 46]. For the tactical medic, this was appealing from a logistical perspective which meant carrying less weight in IV fluid. The military experience between 2000 and 2010 fueled a body of evidence to move away from these harmful interventions, and this area of trauma care continues to rapidly evolve [47].

Crystalloid

The use of crystalloid fluid should be recognized as harmful in most trauma patients. Exceptions include burn resuscitation and head injury management but need to be considered and weighed for risk and benefit in multisystem trauma patients including these mechanisms.

When logistics limit fluid access to only crystalloid products, a focus should be placed on minimal fluid for desired effect, and recognizing that patients with active bleeding have worse outcomes when compared to fluid-restricted approaches [3, 44]. Crystalloid infusion should be limited to volume expansion to achieve a perfusing blood pressure, in limited volume [48]. Ideally, some level of blood product, as discussed in the next section, should be employed in all tactical medical trauma care for fluid resuscitation.

Blood and Products

Replacement of lost fluid (blood) in trauma has been shown to be best replaced by equivalent fluid, thus, replacement with whole blood [49–51]. This has logistical complexity in traditional medicine and is compounded in tactical medical environments. Small, specialized military units employ field donation and transfusion of fresh whole blood using a buddy transfusion approach. The use of cold-stored low-titer whole blood simplifies the field use of whole blood by eliminating the donor portion of the procedure from the workflow of the combat medic and expedites administration when indicated [52]. The logistics of both fresh and cold-stored whole blood remain a significant limitation for widespread use of blood in tactical environments. 1:1:1 or 1:1 component replacement is thought to be the next best option but still carries logistical and distribution challenges [53, 54]. Current evidence suggests in the absence of blood access, dried plasma may be the best option in tactical settings. Table 53.2 provides the most recent approach for tactical field care fluid resuscitation. Field resuscitation should target improved LOC, a palpable pulse, and/or systolic blood pressure of 80–90 mmHg or <90 mmHg with suspected or confirmed head injury [27].

Table 53.2 Preferred resuscitation fluids in tactical field care

Fluid resuscitation in tactical field care	
Not in shock	IV fluids not indicated Oral rehydration
Shock present Weak or absent radial pulse and/or altered LOC (shock)	(Order of preference) 1. whole Blood 2. Plasma, RBCs, and platelets (1:1:1) 3. Plasma and RBCs (1:1) 4. RBCs only 5. Dried, liquid, or thawed plasma only 6. Lactated ringers or plasma-lyte A crystalloid

Hemostatic Resuscitation

The evidence in support of tranexamic acid in hemostasis, particularly in the context of massive blood transfusion during resuscitation, has been well documented. TXA is known to be more effective when given early, less than an hour after injury. Field administration of TXA will ensure that casualties are treated within that window [55–57]. Recent studies have pointed to its successful use in traumatic brain injuries and should be considered in these casualties [58]. Early administration in trauma patients is indicated in the tactical environment during tactical field care via the intravenous or intraosseous routes.

Tourniquet Re-assessment

During the circulatory assessment, reassess applied tourniquets for effectiveness and the need for re-tightening. Due to fluid shifts in the limb compartment under tourniquet, they may need to be re-tightened to ensure efficacy. Inspect the wounds on tourniqueted extremities, especially in cases where the tourniquet was applied during CuF or DTC. Due to the tactical situation, a limb may have been tourniqueted with an otherwise manageable, compressible injury. If the tourniquet has been in place for less than 2 hours, these injuries could be converted from tourniquet to other methods of hemorrhage control, including wound packing, hemostatics, and pressure dressings, as the tactical situation or evacuation times allow. Do not attempt tourniquet conversion in the field setting if the tourniquet has been in place for more than 6 hours, signs of shock are present, or if close monitoring for re-bleeding is not possible. Never remove a tourniquet in cases of, partial or complete, traumatic amputations outside of the OR [19]. While there have been case studies of successful outcomes with extended tourniquet application times, it is generally accepted that the window evacuation for casualties with a tourniquet applied is 2 hours [59].

Hypothermia Prevention/Head Injury ("H")

Hypothermia Management

Aggressive hypothermia management is a cornerstone of trauma care and is of paramount importance in austere medicine. Even in the hot climates of Iraq and Afghanistan, casualties become hypothermic, especially when exposed to higher altitudes and onboard evacuation platforms. The more severely injured casualty is at greater risk of hypothermia, and an associated increase in mortality and increases the incidence of trauma-induced coagulopathies [60]. The body loses heat through four primary means: evaporation, radiation, conduction, and convection. Hypothermia management should be a combination of active and passive measures to combat these heat loss avenues. Examples of passive measures include, but are not limited to: early use of a litter (conduction), windproof emergency blankets (radiation and convection), removing blood-soaked clothes, and drying the casualty while packaging (evaporation). Active measures are the use of rewarming blankets and warm fluids. There are a multitude of well-thought-out active rewarming kits available; even a simple wool blanket can suffice in Prolonged Field Care. Aggressive hypothermia management is effective to disrupting the "Lethal Triad" [27, 61–64]. Strategies to avoid hypothermia and its treatments are discussed further.

Traumatic Brain Injury

In recent conflicts, the asymmetrical threat of improvised explosive devices (IEDs) has grown in prevalence; the incidence of traumatic brain injury (TBI) has increased as well, with mild TBIs being the most common in large cohort studies [65]. Casualties with a suspected TBI with oxygen saturation below 90% should be administered oxygen as soon as it is available and tactically feasible. TBI casualties are an exception for crystalloid fluid resuscitation in field settings where blood is not available. In these patients, maintaining a target of 90 mmHg systolic blood pressure or palpable radial pulse is recommended [66]. The use of Ringer's Lactate is associated with decreased mortality over normal saline [67]. Casualties that present with a severe or worsening TBI, pupillary dilation, and decreasing mental status, a 250 ml bolus of 3% hypertonic saline is indicated. HSD is preferred over mannitol in TFC/ITC as it avoids the diuretic effects which are more difficult to manage in an operational setting [66, 68]. Hyperventilation (targeting end-tidal CO_2 between 30 and 35 mmHg or a ventilatory rate of 16 when capnometry is unavailable) should be used as a temporizing measure only when there are observable signs of cerebral herniation [66]. In law enforcement and for paramedics responding to intentional mass casualty events, such as the Boston Marathon Bombing, the military experiences with IEDs and TBIs should be considered.

Eyes and Everything Else ("E")

This portion of the MARCH approach catches the remaining goals and interventions the tactical medical provider should consider. Getting this far in the treatment algorithm will be dependent upon the environment, number and severity of casualties, and time with the patient.

Eye Injuries

While the use of ballistic-rated glasses and goggles has significantly reduced globe injuries, these injuries remain a source of morbidity [69, 70], and there remains a reasonable threat of open globe injuries in any combat environment. Treatment in the field should include a baseline visual acuity test, a rigid shield type dressing, and early prophylaxis with an appropriate antibiotic if transport is prolonged. In civilian emergency care, both eyes are usually dressed to avoid ocular movement increasing damage. This may not be appropriate in a tactical setting as the patient then becomes completely dependent upon others in a dangerous environment.

Monitoring and Vital Signs

At this stage of care, regular monitoring of vitals and interventions should be started. Tactical medical operators will be limited in their diagnostic equipment. Most will have a pulse oximeter, stethoscope, and blood pressure cuff [6]. However, the background sounds of operations may preclude the effective use of hearing-based diagnostic equipment. More tactile and visual techniques can be used in those cases, such as the presence of distal pulses and mental status assessment to assess end-organ perfusion. All injuries, interventions, time of interventions, and results of intervention need to be documented [27].

Analgesia

Pain management is addressed in a tiered system. In a military setting, casualties with minor injuries who can still fight may need to remain engaged or be used for security of the casualty collection point (CCP). A 1 gram dose of acetaminophen in conjunction with an appropriate oral antibiotic is all that is indicated. For patients with moderate injuries that cannot remain operational and are not exhibiting the signs of shock or respiratory distress, oral transmucosal fentanyl citrate lozenges (OTFC) have become the standard of care in many military medical units. OTFC has demonstrated excellent efficacy in recent conflicts and when administered with the lozenge taped to the patient's thumb, has a self-limiting administration. For patients in severe pain, ketamine is used both for pain management and sedation. Sedation should be considered prior to invasive procedures, securing the airway, and if the casualty is a danger to themselves or operational success. The use of benzodiazepines is not routinely used in a field environment. They should be considered in sedation and violent patient interventions (a law enforcement consideration). Naloxone should be included in any pain management plan for management of both overdose and iatrogenic overadministration. As in many other settings, pain is often undermanaged in austere settings [71–73].

Secondary Survey

A full secondary survey should be completed, time permitting. Fractures, not splinted already, should be splinted, and distal perfusion reassessed and documented. Burns should be assessed using the Rule of Tens. The Rule of Tens is simply the Rule of Nines rounded up to the nearest percent and is easier in a chaotic environment. Burns should be dressed with a dry sterile dressing. Fluid resuscitation using Ringer's Lactate or other balanced crystalloid should be initiated accordingly guided by the modified Parkland formula [74, 75]. Abdominal eviscerations should be reduced into the abdominal cavity to protect viability and maximize splanchnic circulation [27]. If the evisceration cannot be reduced, the eviscerated organs should be covered and secured with moist sterile dressings or a water impermeable non-adhesive material. All minor wounds should be inspected and dressed. All findings and interventions should be added to the current documentation.

Antibiotic Administration

With the rates of open orthopedic trauma in tactical operations and the realities of unhealthy, austere environments where they are conducted, prophylactic antibiotic administration, based on local flora, should be considered in any tactical medicine plan. The current CoTCCC guidelines recommend that all open combat wounds receive point-of-wounding prophylaxis. When the environment, wound modalities, and delayed time to care are considered, this is a prudent response [76–80]. In a law enforcement setting with rapid evacuation and less austere conditions available, this will require the input of the physician in a medical director role. However, vast areas of North America where law enforcement conducts operations would still be considered austere and have extended evacuation times. Prudent stewardship of antibiotics is important but not all law enforcement operations take place in urban areas.

Prolonged Field Care

Prolonged field care includes nursing and critical care interventions beyond the interventions discussed previously in tactical field care and following the MARCHE algorithmic approach. Situations where evacuation is delayed, the need for ongoing management of critical trauma patients can occur in both military and law enforcement settings and need to be a consideration in medical planning. Remote and telemedicine support care be a significant force multiplier in extending critical care far forward, where expert guidance can be directed where tactical medical providers may require consultation. For teams where the threat of prolonged evacuation is high, additional training, planning, and equipment are required [81].

Medical Equipment in Tactical Medical Care

The medical interventions reviewed herein require significant logistical and equipment investment. Especially in a mass-casualty event, the tactical medical provider's medical kit can be quickly exhausted [82]. By contrast, the tactical medical provider can quickly become overloaded with equipment, impeding their ability to move and work effectively. Layered positioning of medical supplies is advantageous in planning for casualties and can ensure the medical providers are not overloaded, while also ensuring required equipment is available when needed. Each operator or team member should carry basic medical equipment including tourniquet, packing gauze and bandage, and chest seal in an individual first aid kit (IFAK) [83].

The tactical medical provider kit can then be focused on carrying advanced procedure equipment in a first-line medical bag, in addition to a second-line treatment bag or various mission-specific kits or components tailored to different missions and medical threats [84, 85]. Additional equipment for re-supply or mass-casualty or disaster events can be pre-positioned in team vehicles or other pre-planned caches. Careful consideration to medical bag packing needs to be considered as weight and space are at a premium. Consideration for multi-use items and reducing redundancy where able are strategies to minimize the medic load. As noted above, spreading kit among the team also expands the supplies available, while keeping the medical provider light and agile in order to function well.

Drone technology has evolved rapidly, and drone use for equipment deployment for supplies, medications, or just-in-time blood product delivery is within operational reach with this technology [86].

Less-Lethal and Chemical Munitions

The injury patterns, decontamination, and management associated with less-lethal impact and energy weapons and chemical agents require a subset of knowledge for the tactical medical provider. These devices and agents are commonly employed in law enforcement, and weaponized chemicals and biologic agents pose threats in both military and law enforcement operations. Understanding energy weapons such as the Taser™, various types and sizes of impact projectiles, distraction devices, oleoresin capsicum spray, and CS gas which are commonly employed in tactical operations is important [87, 88] (Fig. 53.3).

Chemical, biological, radiological, nuclear, and explosive (CBRNE) weapon effects and associated medical man-

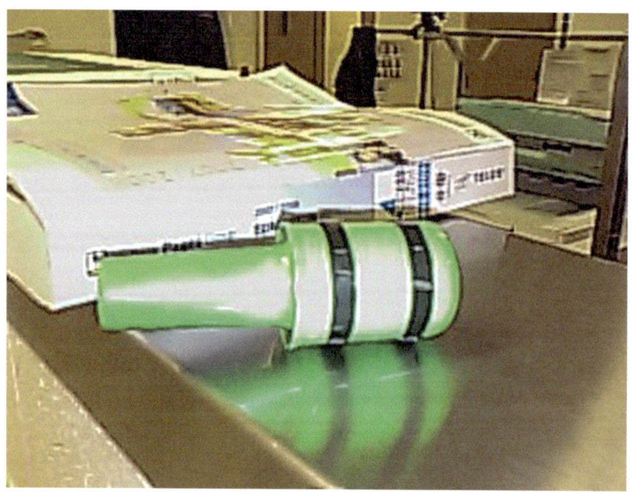

Fig. 53.3 40 mm less-lethal projectile baton. (File photo, S. Cowan)

agement present yet another specialized area of knowledge the tactical medical provider should be versed in. The breadth of this topic is vast and will be covered further in Chaps. 56 and 57 [89, 90].

Environmental and Operational Differences: TCCC Versus TECC

Military Tactical Combat Casualty Care is conducted in non-permissive or semi-permissive austere environments and primarily involves treatment of young, fit operators with minimal comorbidities. Military humanitarian missions can quickly become a tactical medicine situation with attacks on NGOs being commonplace. Depending on the enemy, the use of CBRNE agents may complicate the battlespace further.

The Geneva Convention (GC) allows military medics, persons tasked to medical units and evacuation platforms to be armed for self-defense, the defense of their casualties, and defense of the medical unit, if required [91]. In recent conflicts, asymmetrical threats are not signatories to the GC and have been specifically targeting medical personnel and facilities [92]. Military Medics are embedded with combat units and in many instances come under fire (self-defense) and move forward with their engaged units. An armed medic can participate, if required, in protecting themselves but runs the risk of being actively engaged and may be unable to move to render aid to casualties. An unarmed medic, by contrast, could be a hindrance to a unit engaged in active combat requiring a guardian from the embedded unit.

Tactical Emergency Casualty Care is conducted in permissive and semi-permissive environments. Operations can be non-austere and austere depending on the region of the country. TECC casualties include the general population with all the variances in age ranges, infant, pediatric, adult, and geriatric, with all the expected comorbidities and physiological conditions. Due to the permissive nature of these operations, follow on medical assets and evacuation to definitive trauma care are more readily available (Fig. 53.4). Active shooter and intentional mass casualty events do occur. In these specific incidences, TECC providers would typically advance and position themselves similar to military medics [93].

Law enforcement teams can have armed providers, unarmed providers, or a combination in their resources. Many times, armed tactical medical operators are sworn officers or constables with specialty medical training. In some agencies, specific paramedics are recruited and trained in tactics and firearms and then added to the team. In other agencies, unarmed medics are used and staged in the Yellow or Warm Zone and brought forward when the objective is secured. These teams should train their non-medical operators to the TECC First Responder standard to provide Red or Hot Zone Care for the possibility of a protracted operation. Training physicians and advanced care paramedics to give solid medical direction and advice over communications is an excellent tool to mitigate liability in protracted or austere operations.

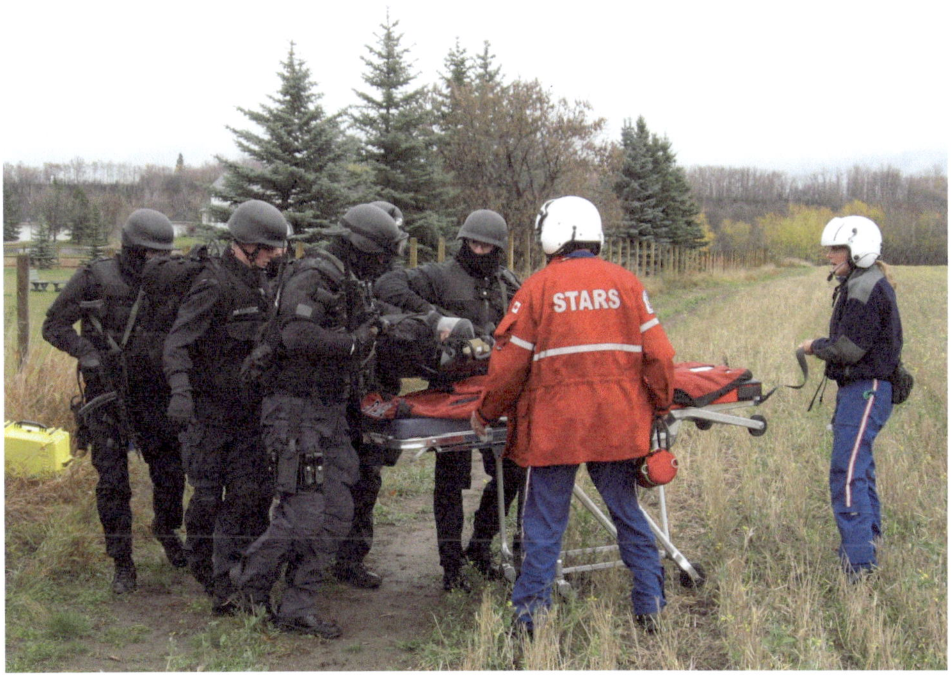

Fig. 53.4 Handover of a trauma patient in a law enforcement tactical simulation. (File photo: S. Cowan)

There are distinct differences between law enforcement and military operations. Unfortunately, with asymmetrical threats of the last decade, the lines have blurred and there can be significant overlap. The differences between TCCC and TECC need to be balanced by any physician tasked as LE medical director or any military physician.

Summary

Tactical medicine combined the dynamic and hazardous environments of military and law enforcement operations with the complexity of modern trauma care. Simply practicing in-hospital style medicine in these environments is dangerous and requires the tactical medical provider to balance the requirements of the operation and tactical environment with the medical needs of patients during operations. Initial and ongoing individual and team training and experience in this nuanced field of trauma care have been demonstrated to improve outcomes and have become a standard of care.

Key Points

- Tactical medicine is not simply transferring traditional trauma care into a law enforcement or military environment.
- Tactical medicine is driven by environmental constraints and requires an understanding of evidence from conflict-related injury research.
- Training to safely provide tactical medicine is broad and multifaceted.
- Specific interventions, approached in an algorithmic fashion, must be tailored to the incidence of injury and environment.

References

1. Bellamy RF. The causes of death in conventional land warfare: implications for combat casualty care research. Mil Med. 1984;149(2):55–62. https://www.ncbi.nlm.nih.gov/pubmed/6427656. https://doi.org/10.1093/milmed/149.2.55.
2. Butler FK, Haymann J, Butler EG. Tactical combat casualty care in special operations. Mil Med. 1996;161(suppl_1):3–16. https://www.ncbi.nlm.nih.gov/pubmed/8772308. https://doi.org/10.1093/milmed/161.suppl_1.3.
3. Butler FK, Holcomb JB, Giebner SD, McSwain NE, Bagian J. Tactical combat casualty care 2007: evolving concepts and battlefield experience. Mil Med. 2007;172(Supplement 1):S1–S19. http://www.ingentaconnect.com/content/amsus/zmm/2007/00000172/A00101s1/art00001. https://doi.org/10.7205/MILMED.172.Supplement_1.1.
4. https://Deployedmedicine.com/market/11/content/40.
5. 76–PreHospital trauma life support (PHTLS) 8th edition (military) manuals. FedBizOpps. 2015.
6. Butler J, Frank K, Blackbourne LH. Battlefield trauma care then and now: a decade of tactical combat casualty care. J Trauma Acute Care Surg. 2012;73(6 Suppl 5):S395–402. https://www.ncbi.nlm.nih.gov/pubmed/23192061. https://doi.org/10.1097/TA.0b013e3182754850.
7. Kotwal RS, Montgomery HR, Kotwal BM, et al. Eliminating preventable death on the battlefield. Archi Surg (Chicago 1960). 2011;146(12):1350–8. https://doi.org/10.1001/archsurg.2011.213.
8. Pannell D, Brisebois R, Talbot M, et al. Causes of death in Canadian forces members deployed to Afghanistan and implications on tactical combat casualty care provision. J Trauma. 2011;71(5 Suppl 1, Canadian Forces Operational Medicine Supplement):S401–7. http://ovidsp.ovid.com/ovidweb.cgi?T=JS&NEWS=n&CSC=Y&PAGE=fulltext&D=ovft&AN=00005373-201111001-00004. https://doi.org/10.1097/TA.0b013e318232e53f.
9. Grissinger JW. The development of military medicine. Bull N Y Acad Med (1925). 1927;3(5):301–56. https://www.ncbi.nlm.nih.gov/pubmed/19311570.
10. Rinnert KJ, Hall WL. Tactical emergency medical support. Emerg Med Clin North Am. 2002;20(4):929–52. https://doi.org/10.1016/S0733-8627(02)00036-6.
11. Carmona RH. The history and evolution of tactical emergency medical support and its impact on public safety. Top Emerg Med. 2003;25(4):277. https://search.proquest.com/docview/203346442.
12. Rasumoff D. EMS at tactical law enforcement operations seminar a success. Tact Edge J. 1989;(Fall 1989):25–9.
13. Carmona RH, Brennann K. Review of the national conference on tactical emergency medical support. Tact Edge. 1990;(Summer 1990):7–11.
14. NTOA, National Tactical Officers Association. Position statement on the inclusion of physicians in tactical law enforcement operations in the USA. Tact Edge J. 1994;12:86.
15. Heck JJ, Pierluisi G. Law enforcement special operations medical support. Prehosp Emerg Care. 2001;5(4):403–6. https://www.ncbi.nlm.nih.gov/pubmed/11642594.
16. Llewellyn CH. The antecedents of tactical emergency medical support: a personal perspective. Top Emerg Med. 2003;25(4):274. https://search.proquest.com/docview/203372510.
17. Savage E, Forestier C, Withers N, Tien H, Pannell D. Tactical combat casualty care in the Canadian forces: lessons learned from the Afghan war. Can J Surg. 2011;54:S118–23.
18. Goolsby C, Jacobs L, Hunt RC, et al. Stop the bleed education consortium: education program content and delivery recommendations. J Trauma Acute Care Surg. 2018;84(1):205–10. https://www.ncbi.nlm.nih.gov/pubmed/29077676. https://doi.org/10.1097/TA.0000000000001732.
19. Montgomery HR, Hammesfahr R, Fisher AD, et al. 2019 recommended limb tourniquets in tactical combat casualty care. J Spec Oper Med. 2019;19(4):27–50. https://www.ncbi.nlm.nih.gov/pubmed/31910470.
20. St John AE, Wang X, Lim EB, Chien D, Stern SA, White NJ. Effects of rapid wound sealing on survival and blood loss in a swine model of lethal junctional arterial hemorrhage. J Trauma Acute Care Surg. 2015;79(2):256–62. https://www.ncbi.nlm.nih.gov/pubmed/26218694. https://doi.org/10.1097/TA.0000000000000746.
21. King DR, Larentzakis A, Ramly EP. Tourniquet use at the Boston marathon bombing: lost in translation. J Trauma Acute Care Surg. 2015;78(3):594–9. https://www.ncbi.nlm.nih.gov/pubmed/25710432. https://doi.org/10.1097/TA.0000000000000561.
22. Altamirano MP, Kragh JF Jr, Aden JK 3rd, Dubick MA. Role of the windlass in improvised tourniquet use on a manikin hemorrhage model. J Spec Oper Med. 2015;15(2):42–6. https://www.ncbi.nlm.nih.gov/pubmed/26125163.

23. Rall JM, Cox JM, Songer AG, Cestero RF, Ross JD. Comparison of novel hemostatic dressings with QuikClot combat gauze in a standardized swine model of uncontrolled hemorrhage. J Trauma Acute Care Surg. 2013;75(2 Suppl 2):S150–6. https://www.ncbi.nlm.nih.gov/pubmed/23883900. https://doi.org/10.1097/TA.0b013e318299d909.
24. Charlton NP, Swain JM, Brozek JL, et al. Control of severe, life-threatening external bleeding in the out-of-hospital setting: a systematic review. Prehosp Emerg Care. 2020;ahead-of-print:1–33. http://www.tandfonline.com/doi/abs/10.1080/10903127.2020.1743801.
25. Smith S, White J, Wanis KN, Beckett A, McAlister VC, Hilsden R. The effectiveness of junctional tourniquets: a systematic review and meta-analysis. J Trauma Acute Care Surg. 2019;86(3):532–9. https://www.ncbi.nlm.nih.gov/pubmed/30507857. https://doi.org/10.1097/TA.0000000000002159.
26. Kragh JF, Kotwal RS, Cap AP, et al. Performance of junctional tourniquets in normal human volunteers. Prehosp Emerg Care. 2015;19(3):391–8. http://www.tandfonline.com/doi/abs/10.3109/10903127.2014.980478.
27. Drew B, Montgomery HR, Butler J, Frank K. Tactical combat casualty care (TCCC) guidelines for medical personnel: 05 November 2020. J Spec Oper Med. 2020;20(4):144–51. https://www.ncbi.nlm.nih.gov/pubmed/33320328.
28. Mabry RL, Kharod CU, Bennett BL. Awake cricothyrotomy: a novel approach to the surgical airway in the tactical setting. Wilderness Environ Med. 2017;28(2):S61–8.
29. Grissom C, Weaver L, Clemmer T, Morris A. Theoretical advantage of oxygen treatment for combat casualties during medical evacuation at high altitude. J Trauma. 2006;61(2):461–7. http://ovidsp.ovid.com/ovidweb.cgi?T=JS&NEWS=n&CSC=Y&PAGE=fulltext&D=ovft&AN=00005373-200608000-00035. https://doi.org/10.1097/01.ta.0000221699.71596.9d.
30. Kheirabadi BS, Terrazas IB, Koller A, et al. Vented versus unvented chest seals for treatment of pneumothorax and prevention of tension pneumothorax in a swine model. J Trauma Acute Care Surg. 2013;75(1):150–6.
31. Kotora Jr JG, Henao J, Littlejohn LF, Kircher S. Vented chest seals for prevention of tension pneumothorax in a communicating pneumothorax. J Emerg Med. 2013;45(5):686–94. https://www.clinicalkey.es/playcontent/1-s2.0-S0736467913005076. https://doi.org/10.1016/j.jemermed.2013.05.011.
32. Goodman DM. Radiologic evaluation of alternative sites for needle decompression of tension pneumothorax. JAMA: J Am Med Assoc. 2012;308(19):1958. https://search.proquest.com/docview/1233077814.
33. Inaba K, Karamanos E, Skiada D, et al. Cadaveric comparison of the optimal site for needle decompression of tension pneumothorax by prehospital care providers. J Trauma Acute Care Surg. 2015;79(6):1044–8. https://www.ncbi.nlm.nih.gov/pubmed/26488319. https://doi.org/10.1097/TA.0000000000000849.
34. Jodie P, Kerstin H. BET1: pre-hospital finger thoracostomy in patients with traumatic cardiac arrest. Emerg Med J: EMJ. 2017;34(6):417–8. https://doi.org/10.1136/emermed-2017-206808.1.
35. Hannon L, St Clair T, Smith K, et al. Finger thoracostomy in patients with chest trauma performed by paramedics on a helicopter emergency medical service. Emerg Med Australas. 2020;32(4):650–6. https://onlinelibrary.wiley.com/doi/abs/10.1111/1742-6723.13549.
36. Jodie P, Kerstin H. BET 2: pre-hospital finger thoracostomy in patients with chest trauma. Emerg Med J: EMJ. 2017;34(6):419. https://doi.org/10.1136/emermed-2017-206808.2.
37. Menzies D, O'Neill S, Leonard J, Butcher P, Creevy P, Irwin D. Advanced paramedic delivered finger thoracostomy. Irish J Paramed. 2018;3(2). https://explore.openaire.eu/search/publication?articleId=doajarticles::718486de14e535c1653093e8051aa86a. https://doi.org/10.32378/ijp.v3i2.129.
38. Parker WJ, Despain RW, Delgado A, et al. Pelvic binder utilization in combat casualties: does it matter? Am Surg. 2020;86(7):873–7. https://journals.sagepub.com/doi/full/10.1177/0003134820939928.
39. Loftus A, Morris R, Friedmann Y, Pallister I, Parker P. Combat trousers as effective improvised pelvic binders a comparative cadaveric study. J Spec Oper Med. 2017;17(3):35–9. https://www.ncbi.nlm.nih.gov/pubmed/28910465.
40. Nunn T, Cosker TDA, Bose D, Pallister I. Immediate application of improvised pelvic binder as first step in extended resuscitation from life-threatening hypovolaemic shock in conscious patients with unstable pelvic injuries. Injury. 2006;38(1):125–8. https://www.clinicalkey.es/playcontent/1-s2.0-S0020138306003974. https://doi.org/10.1016/j.injury.2006.06.026.
41. Savell S, Mora AG, Perez CA, Bebarta VS, Maddry MJK. En route intraosseous access performed in the combat setting. Am J Disaster Med. 2016;11(4):225–31. https://www.ncbi.nlm.nih.gov/pubmed/28140436. https://doi.org/10.5055/ajdm.2016.0243.
42. Bjerkvig CK, Fosse TK, Apelseth TO, et al. Emergency sternal intraosseous access for warm fresh whole blood transfusion in damage control resuscitation. J Trauma Acute Care Surg. 2018;84(6S Suppl 1):S120–4. https://www.ncbi.nlm.nih.gov/pubmed/29462086. https://doi.org/10.1097/TA.0000000000001850.
43. Burgert JM. Intraosseous vascular access in disasters and mass casualty events: a review of the literature. Am J Disaster Med. 2016;11(3):149–66. https://www.ncbi.nlm.nih.gov/pubmed/28134414. https://doi.org/10.5055/ajdm.2016.0235.
44. Kasotakis G, Sideris A, Yang Y, et al. Aggressive early crystalloid resuscitation adversely affects outcomes in adult blunt trauma patients: an analysis of the glue grant database. J Trauma Acute Care Surg. 2013;74(5):1215–22. https://www.ncbi.nlm.nih.gov/pubmed/23609270. https://doi.org/10.1097/TA.0b013e3182826e13.
45. Bickell WH, Bruttig SP, Millnamow GA, O'Benar J, Wade CE. Use of hypertonic saline/dextran versus lactated ringer's solution as a resuscitation fluid after uncontrolled aortic hemorrhage in anesthetized swine. Ann Emerg Med. 1992;21(9):1077–85. https://doi.org/10.1016/S0196-0644(05)80648-1.
46. Kramer GC, Perron PR, Lindsey DC, et al. Small-volume resuscitation with hypertonic saline dextran solution. Surgery. 1986;100(2):239–47. https://www.ncbi.nlm.nih.gov/pubmed/2426818.
47. Cap AP, Pidcoke HF, Spinella P, et al. Damage control resuscitation. Mil Med. 2018;183(suppl_2):36–43. https://www.ncbi.nlm.nih.gov/pubmed/30189070. https://doi.org/10.1093/milmed/usy112.
48. Bennett B, Wedmore I, Butler F. Tactical combat casualty care: transitioning battlefield lessons learned to other austere environments. Wilderness Environ Med. 2017;28(2):S3–4. https://www.clinicalkey.es/playcontent/1-s2.0-S1080603217300066. https://doi.org/10.1016/j.wem.2017.01.003.
49. Holcomb JB, Tilley BC, Baraniuk S, et al. Transfusion of plasma, platelets, and red blood cells in a 1:1:1 vs a 1:1:2 ratio and mortality in patients with severe trauma: the PROPPR randomized clinical trial. JAMA: J Am Med Assoc. 2015;313(5):471–82. https://doi.org/10.1001/jama.2015.12.
50. Cordova CB, Cap AP, Spinella PC. Fresh whole blood transfusion for a combat casualty in austere combat environment. J Spec Oper Med. 2014;14(1):9–12. https://www.ncbi.nlm.nih.gov/pubmed/24604433.
51. Spinella P, Perkins J, Grathwohl K, Beekley A, Holcomb J. Warm fresh whole blood is independently associated with improved survival for patients with combat-related traumatic injuries. J Trauma. 2009;66(4 Suppl):S69–76. http://ovidsp.ovid.com/ovidweb.cgi?T=JS&NEWS=n&CSC=Y&PAGE=fulltext&D=ovft

&AN=00005373-200904001-00008. https://doi.org/10.1097/TA.0b013e31819d85fb.

52. Zhu CS, Pokorny DM, Eastridge BJ, et al. Give the trauma patient what they bleed, when and where they need it: establishing a comprehensive regional system of resuscitation based on patient need utilizing cold-stored, low-titer O+ whole blood. Transfusion (Philadelphia, PA). 2019;59(S2):1429–38. https://onlinelibrary.wiley.com/doi/abs/10.1111/trf.15264.
53. Butler FK, Blackbourne LH, Gross K. The combat medic aid bag: 2025. CoTCCC top 10 recommended battlefield trauma care research, development, and evaluation priorities for 2015. J Spec Oper Med. 2015;15(4):7–19. https://www.ncbi.nlm.nih.gov/pubmed/26630091.
54. Holcomb JB, Donathan DP, Cotton BA, et al. Prehospital transfusion of plasma and red blood cells in trauma patients. Prehosp Emerg Care. 2015;19(1):1–9. http://www.tandfonline.com/doi/abs/10.3109/10903127.2014.923077.
55. Morrison JJ, Dubose JJ, Rasmussen TE, Midwinter MJ. Military application of tranexamic acid in trauma emergency resuscitation (MATTERs) study. Arch Surg (Chicago 1960). 2012;147(2):113–9. https://doi.org/10.1001/archsurg.2011.287.
56. Roberts I, Shakur H, Afolabi A, et al. The importance of early treatment with tranexamic acid in bleeding trauma patients: an exploratory analysis of the CRASH-2 randomised controlled trial. Lancet (British Edition). 2011;377(9771):1096–1101.e2. https://www.clinicalkey.es/playcontent/1-s2.0-S014067361160278X. https://doi.org/10.1016/S0140-6736(11)60278-X.
57. Shakur H, Roberts I, Bautista R, et al. Effects of tranexamic acid on death, vascular occlusive events, and blood transfusion in trauma patients with significant haemorrhage (CRASH-2): a randomised, placebo-controlled trial. Lancet (British Edition). 2010;376(9734):23–32. https://www.clinicalkey.es/playcontent/1-s2.0-S0140673610608355. https://doi.org/10.1016/S0140-6736(10)60835-5.
58. Brenner A, Belli A, Chaudhri R, et al. Understanding the neuroprotective effect of tranexamic acid: an exploratory analysis of the CRASH-3 randomised trial. Crit Care (London, England). 2020;24(1):1–560. https://search.proquest.com/docview/2461842505. https://doi.org/10.1186/s13054-020-03243-4.
59. Kragh J, Baer D, Walters T. Extended (16-hour) tourniquet application after combat wounds: a case report and review of the current literature. J Orthop Trauma. 2007;21(4):274–8. http://ovidsp.ovid.com/ovidweb.cgi?T=JS&NEWS=n&CSC=Y&PAGE=fulltext&D=ovft&AN=00005131-200704000-00009. https://doi.org/10.1097/BOT.0b013e3180437dd9.
60. Fisher AD, April MD, Schauer SG. An analysis of the incidence of hypothermia in casualties presenting to emergency departments in Iraq and Afghanistan. Am J Emerg Med. 2020;38(11):2343–6. https://doi.org/10.1016/j.ajem.2019.11.050.
61. Bennett BL, Holcomb JB. Battlefield trauma-induced hypothermia: transitioning the preferred method of casualty rewarming. Wilderness Environ Med. 2017;28(2):S82–9. https://www.clinicalkey.es/playcontent/1-s2.0-S1080603217300972. https://doi.org/10.1016/j.wem.2017.03.010.
62. Schauer SG, April MD, Hill GJ, Naylor JF, Borgman MA, De Lorenzo RA. Prehospital interventions performed on pediatric trauma patients in Iraq and Afghanistan. Prehosp Emerg Care. 2018;22(5):624–9. http://www.tandfonline.com/doi/abs/10.1080/10903127.2018.1439130.
63. Husum H, Olsen T, Murad M, Heng YV, Wisborg T, Gilbert M. Preventing post-injury hypothermia during prolonged prehospital evacuation. Prehosp Disaster Med. 2002;17(1):23–6. https://doi.org/10.1017/S1049023X00000078.
64. Lier H, Krep H, Schroeder S, Stuber F. Preconditions of hemostasis in trauma: a review. the influence of acidosis, hypocalcemia, anemia, and hypothermia on functional hemostasis in trauma. J Trauma. 2008;65(4):951–60. https://www.ncbi.nlm.nih.gov/pubmed/18849817. https://doi.org/10.1097/TA.0b013e318187e15b.
65. Eskridge SL, Macera CA, Galarneau MR, et al. Injuries from combat explosions in Iraq: injury type, location, and severity. Injury. 2012;43(10):1678–82. https://www.clinicalkey.es/playcontent/1-s2.0-S0020138312002288. https://doi.org/10.1016/j.injury.2012.05.027.
66. Otten EJ, Dorlac WC. Managing traumatic brain injury: translating military guidelines to the wilderness. Wilderness Environ Med. 2017;28(2):S117–23. https://www.clinicalkey.es/playcontent/1-s2.0-S1080603217300935. https://doi.org/10.1016/j.wem.2017.02.008.
67. Rowell SE, Fair KA, Barbosa RR, et al. The impact of prehospital administration of lactated ringer's solution versus normal saline in patients with traumatic brain injury. J Neurotrauma. 2016;33(11):154–1059. https://www.liebertpub.com/doi/abs/10.1089/neu.2014.3478.
68. Pinto F, Capone-Neto A, Prist R, e Silva M, Poli-de-Figueiredo L. Volume replacement with lactated ringer's or 3% hypertonic saline solution during combined experimental hemorrhagic shock and traumatic brain injury. J Trauma. 2006;60(4):758–64. http://ovidsp.ovid.com/ovidweb.cgi?T=JS&NEWS=n&CSC=Y&PAGE=fulltext&D=ovft&AN=00005373-200604000-00008. https://doi.org/10.1097/01.ta.0000214581.89316.73.
69. Thomas R, McManus J, Johnson A, Mayer P, Wade C, Holcomb J. Ocular injury reduction from ocular protection use in current combat operations. J Trauma. 2009;66(4 Suppl):S99–S103. http://ovidsp.ovid.com/ovidweb.cgi?T=JS&NEWS=n&CSC=Y&PAGE=fulltext&D=ovft&AN=00005373-200904001-00012. https://doi.org/10.1097/TA.0b013e31819d8695.
70. Cockerham KP, Zumhagen L, Cockerham GC, et al. Closed-eye ocular injuries in the Iraq and Afghanistan wars. N Engl J Med. 2011;364(22):2172–3. https://doi.org/10.1056/NEJMc1010683.
71. Schauer SG, Robinson JB, Mabry RL, Howard JT. Battlefield analgesia: TCCC guidelines are not being followed. J Spec Oper Med. 2015;15(1):85–9. https://www.ncbi.nlm.nih.gov/pubmed/25770803.
72. Wedmore IS, Kotwal RS, McManus JG, et al. Safety and efficacy of oral transmucosal fentanyl citrate for prehospital pain control on the battlefield. J Trauma Acute Care Surg. 2012;73(6 Suppl 5):S490–5. https://www.ncbi.nlm.nih.gov/pubmed/23192075. https://doi.org/10.1097/TA.0b013e3182754674.
73. Aronoff GM, Brennan MJ, Pritchard DD, Ginsberg B. Evidence-based oral transmucosal fentanyl citrate (OTFC®) dosing guidelines. Pain Med (Malden, MA). 2005;6(4):305–14. https://onlinelibrary.wiley.com/doi/abs/10.1111/j.1526-4637.2005.00045.x.
74. Chung KK, Salinas J, Renz EM, et al. Simple derivation of the initial fluid rate for the resuscitation of severely burned adult combat casualties: in silico validation of the rule of 10. J Trauma. 2010;69(1 Suppl):S49–54. http://ovidsp.ovid.com/ovidweb.cgi?T=JS&NEWS=n&CSC=Y&PAGE=fulltext&D=ovft&AN=00005373-201007001-00008. https://doi.org/10.1097/TA.0b013e3181e425f1.
75. Ennis J, Chung K, Renz E, et al. Joint theater trauma system implementation of burn resuscitation guidelines improves outcomes in severely burned military casualties. J Trauma. 2008;64(2 Suppl):S146–52. http://ovidsp.ovid.com/ovidweb.cgi?T=JS&NEWS=n&CSC=Y&PAGE=fulltext&D=ovft&AN=00005373-200802001-00022. https://doi.org/10.1097/TA.0b013e318160b44c.
76. Roddy E, Patterson JT, Kandemir U. Delay of antibiotic administration greater than 2 hours predicts surgical site infection in open fractures. Injury. 2020;51(9):1999–2003. https://doi.org/10.1016/j.injury.2020.04.031.

77. Murray CK. Field wound care: prophylactic antibiotics. Wilderness Environ Med. 2017;28(2):S90–S102. https://www.clinicalkey.es/playcontent/1-s2.0-S1080603217300029. https://doi.org/10.1016/j.wem.2016.12.009.
78. Murray C. Epidemiology of infections associated with combat-related injuries in Iraq and Afghanistan. J Trauma. 2008;64(3 Suppl):S232–8. http://ovidsp.ovid.com/ovidweb.cgi?T=JS&NEWS=n&CSC=Y&PAGE=fulltext&D=ovft&AN=00005373-200803001-00005. https://doi.org/10.1097/TA.0b013e318163c3f5.
79. Hospenthal DR, Murray CK, Andersen RC, et al. Guidelines for the prevention of infections associated with combat-related injuries: 2011 update: endorsed by the Infectious Diseases Society of America and the Surgical Infection Society. J Trauma. 2011;71(2 Suppl 2, Prevention of infections associated with combat-related injuries: clinical practice guidelines update):S210–34. http://ovidsp.ovid.com/ovidweb.cgi?T=JS&NEWS=n&CSC=Y&PAGE=fulltext&D=ovft&AN=00005373-201108002-00003. https://doi.org/10.1097/TA.0b013e318227ac4b.
80. Eastridge B, Jenkins D, Flaherty S, Schiller H, Holcomb J. Trauma system development in a theater of war: experiences from operation Iraqi freedom and operation enduring freedom. J Trauma. 2006;61(6):1366–73. http://ovidsp.ovid.com/ovidweb.cgi?T=JS&NEWS=n&CSC=Y&PAGE=fulltext&D=ovft&AN=00005373-200612000-00011. https://doi.org/10.1097/01.ta.0000245894.78941.90.
81. Joint Trauma System. The Department of Defense Center of Excellence for Trauma, clincal practice guidelines. https://jts.amedd.army.mil/index.cfm/PI_CPGs/cpgs.
82. Schauer SG, Naylor JF, Uhaa N, April MD, De Lorenzo RA. An inventory of the combat medics' aid bag. J Spec Oper Med. 2020;20(1):61–4. https://www.ncbi.nlm.nih.gov/pubmed/32203608.
83. Young JB, Galante JM, Sena MJ. Operator training and TEMS support: a survey of unit leaders in northern and central California. J Spec Oper Med. 2013;13(3):92–7. https://www.ncbi.nlm.nih.gov/pubmed/24048997.
84. Geers D. Special operations individual medical equipment part 2 – the in-use and survival medical kits. J Spec Oper Med. 2010;10(1):3–15. https://www.ncbi.nlm.nih.gov/pubmed/20306410.
85. Geers D. Special operations individual medical equipment: part I--the major trauma kit. J Spec Oper Med. 2009;9(4):43–52. https://www.ncbi.nlm.nih.gov/pubmed/20112648.
86. Mesar T, Lessig A, King DR. Use of drone technology for delivery of medical supplies during prolonged field care. J Spec Oper Med. 2018;18(4):34–5. https://www.ncbi.nlm.nih.gov/pubmed/30566722.
87. Dobrowolski A, Moore S. Less lethal weapons and their impact on patient care. Top Emerg Med. 2005;27(1):44.
88. Haar RJ, Iacopino V, Ranadive N, Dandu M, Weiser SD. Death, injury and disability from kinetic impact projectiles in crowd-control settings: a systematic review. BMJ Open. 2017;7(12):e018154. https://doi.org/10.1136/bmjopen-2017-018154.
89. Strain JW 2nd. CBRNE TC3: a hybrid approach to casualty care in the CBRNE environment. J Spec Oper Med. 2013;13(2):44–53. https://www.ncbi.nlm.nih.gov/pubmed/23817878.
90. Baker DJ. CBRNE trauma: a unified approach to clinical management. Prehosp Disaster Med. 2010;25(S1):S5. https://doi.org/10.1017/S1049023X00021804.
91. International Red Cross. Customary international humanitarian law – practice relating to rule 25. Medical Personnel. https://ihl-databases.icrc.org/customary-ihl/eng/docs/v2_rul_rule25_sectionb.
92. US National Counterterrorism Center – Joint Counterterrorism Assessment Team. Counterterrorism guide for public safety personnel. https://www.dni.gov/nctc/jcat/index.html.
93. Callaway, DW. Translating tactical combat casualty care lessons learned to the high-threat civilian setting: tactical emergency casualty care and the Hartford consensus. Wilderness Environ Med. 2017;28(2):S140–5. https://www.clinicalkey.es/playcontent/1-s2.0-S1080603216302885. https://doi.org/10.1016/j.wem.2016.11.008.

Hypothermia and the Trauma Team

54

Susan Marjorie Roberts, Sean Lynch, Dean Gubler, and Anthony J. LaPorta

Introduction

Normal human body temperature is thermoregulated in the range of 36.4–37.5 °C [1, 2]. Significant changes to the core body temperature can lead to potentially fatal systemic effects. Hypothermia can occur as a consequence of traumatic injury and can be influenced by predisposing risk factors, including care provided by the medical team [3, 4]. Attention to preventing hypothermia is critical throughout all phases of trauma care. Hypothermia is common in severely injured patients, but further decrease in temperature can be prevented by the trauma team taking certain pertinent actions [1]. It is critical to effectively manage hypothermia, due to hypothermia's relationship to worsening coagulopathy and effect on organ function. The trauma team must be able to both recognize and treat hypothermia to decrease the associated morbidity and mortality and increase the patient's likelihood of survival [5].

Hypothermia

Definition

The 2018 Advanced Trauma Life Support (ATLS) guidelines define hypothermia as any core body temperature less than 35 °C [1]. Without any associated traumatic injury, hypothermia can further be divided into mild hypothermia at 35–32 °C, moderate hypothermia at 32–28 °C, and severe hypothermia <28 °C. With traumatic injury the classifications of hypothermia are modified: mild hypothermia at 36 °C, moderate hypothermia at 36–32 °C, and severe hypothermia <32 °C. Trauma patients are more susceptible to hypothermia, and it can be detrimental to these patients.

Diagnosing hypothermia requires measurement of the core body temperature. Special thermometers capable of reading low temperatures are necessary to diagnose moderate and severe hypothermia. Temperatures can vary according to location, perfusion, and ambient temperature [3]. Locations to measure temperature include forehead, mouth, esophageal, ear, pulmonary artery (most reliable), axillary, and rectal. In situations where core body temperatures are difficult to measure, such as in the rescue zone, hypothermia can be staged according to clinical signs based on the Swiss staging system [6]. The Swiss system divides hypothermia into grades with corresponding correlation to estimated core body temperature. Mild hypothermia is grade 1 (35–32 °C) and is associated with a conscious patient who is shivering. Moderate hypothermia is grade 2 (32–28 °C) and is associated with a drowsy patient who is not shivering. Grave hypothermia is grade 3 (28–24 °C) and is associated with an unconscious patient who still has vital signs. Deep hypothermia is grade 4 (24–13.7 °C) and irreversible hypothermia is grade 5 (13.7–<9 °C).

Prevalence of Hypothermia After Trauma

Accurately determining the prevalence of hypothermia after traumatic injury can be difficult due to variations in methods of recording core body temperature, variable accuracy of measurement tools, inconsistent documentation, and variability of cut-off levels for hypothermia classes [3]. Hypothermia occurs more frequently in severely injured patients, such as trauma patients (30–50%). Hypothermia, a component in the lethal triad (or more recently lethal diamond), can progress to increased mortality and organ failure [1].

Etiology

Many factors are involved in a patient developing hypothermia after a traumatic injury [3]. Significant risk factors for

S. M. Roberts (✉) · S. Lynch · D. Gubler · A. J. LaPorta
Rocky Vista University College of Osteopathic Medicine, Englewood, CO, USA
e-mail: dgubler@rvu.edu

L. Marshall Gillman, S. Widder (eds.), *Trauma Team Dynamics*, https://doi.org/10.1007/978-3-031-86312-7_54

hypothermia include severity of injury, environmental conditions, and medical care provided by EMS. All phases of trauma care should be analyzed to minimize the cause or worsening of hypothermia by the trauma team.

Several patient factors influence the likelihood of a patient developing hypothermia. Risk of hypothermia is increased in patients with less muscle and fat, due to decreased ability of fat to insulate [4]. Medical conditions can increase the likelihood of developing hypothermia if they interfere with thermoregulation or total body heat production. Such conditions include hypoglycemia and low caloric intake that decrease the shivering response and heat production and chronic skin conditions and burns that increase total body heat loss. Additionally, decreased activity and alcohol or drug use causing vasodilation can interfere with a patient's ability to conserve heat [1]. Age, young and old, can also predispose to hypothermia. Children are susceptible due to increased body surface area to body mass, increased metabolic rate, and small amount of subcutaneous tissue. Older adults are susceptible due to loss of subcutaneous fat, nutritional deficiencies, and chronic medical conditions that impair the body's ability to maintain heat production.

Common hospital factors that exacerbate hypothermia for trauma patients include exposure for examination, administration of room temperature fluids, medications that affect the body's ability to thermoregulate, hypovolemia, and cavitary exposure during surgery [3].

Pathophysiology

Trauma-induced shock leads to anaerobic metabolism, which results in reduced ATP synthesis and decreased hydrolysis of ATP to ADP, ultimately decreasing heat production [3]. When the body is exposed to cold temperature, in order to preserve core body temperature, the body's initial response is peripheral vasoconstriction [4]. This allows the blood to be more centrally located, therefore decreasing heat loss to the environment. Impairment in the threshold for vasoconstriction may occur after trauma [3]. Trauma patients have decreased heat production as a result of low perfusion of muscles and might experience heat loss through radiation, conduction, or evaporation through exposed body cavities if they require surgery.

Signs of Hypothermia

Signs of hypothermia can be broken into different categories based on body temperature, although there is no specific cut-off temperature where one event may occur. Effects of hypothermia are influenced by many factors, including age, comorbidities, and associated injuries. Signs of mild hypothermia (35–32 °C) include increased shivering and muscle tone, cool skin due to vasoconstriction, and social withdrawal [1, 3, 4]. Moderate hypothermia (32–28 °C) characteristics include cessation of shivering, confusion, apathy, slurred speech, loss of fine motor skills, and loss of consciousness. Severe hypothermia (<28 °C) signs consist of severe bradycardia, dilated pupils, hypotension, cardiac conduction abnormalities, loss of deep tendon reflexes and voluntary motion, decreased or cessation of respiratory rate, and cardiac arrest. The risk of cardiac arrest increases as the core body temperature decreases below 32 °C and is increasingly common below 28 °C. Heart rate and blood pressure can be variable for hypothermic patients, and absence of respiratory and cardiac activity is not uncommon for hypothermic patients who eventually recover. Since hypothermic patients can have severely depressed respiratory rate and heart rate, the trauma team must carefully assess the patient to avoid missing signs of respiratory or cardiac activity.

Systemic Manifestations of Hypothermia

Hypothermia leads to many systemic consequences and impairs the normal function of organs. Cardiac effects include reduction of cardiac output and cardiac conduction abnormalities (ventricular fibrillation, more common below 28 °C, and asystole below 25 °C). Nonspecific EKG changes occur and include J (Osborn) waves (upward deflection after the QRS complex [1]), bradycardia, atrial fibrillation with slow ventricular response, and prolongation of PR, QRS, and QT intervals [7]. Additional cardiovascular effects include vasoconstriction and hypotension with low organ flow status [6]. Nervous system effects include behavioral changes, disorientation, amnesia, apathy, ataxia, dysarthria, pupil dilation, pupil nonreactivity, and decreased or absent reflexes. Respiratory consequences include bradypnea and respiratory acidosis. Endocrine responses include an initial increase in the stress hormones of cortisol, catecholamines, and thyroxin to increase metabolic rate to maintain core body temperature. These mechanisms cease to be effective with the progression of hypothermia.

Lethal Triad (Diamond) Component

The lethal triad consists of acidosis, hypothermia, and coagulopathy and is associated with high mortality [3]. The recent change to lethal diamond also adds hypocalcemia. Recent changes in trauma resuscitation for patients with hemorrhagic shock involve moving away from crystalloid resuscitation and towards "Damage Control Resuscitation" (DCR) [1]. This method involves a restrictive use of crystalloid fluids and early administration of balanced ratios of packed red blood cells, fresh frozen plasma, and platelets (1:1:1). This approach interrupts the lethal triad and has been associated with improved outcomes in severely injured patients. Hypothermia, acidosis, hypocalcemia and coagulopathy all interact with one another in a vicious cycle worsening the coagulopathy. The goal of DCR is to avoid the start of the cycle or to reverse its progression [8]. Hypothermia and acidosis are generally corrected with resuscitation, while coagulopathy is harder to correct. Coagulopathy is exacerbated by excessive crystalloid administration, hypothermia impairs the clotting cascade, and metabolic acidosis in trauma patients occurs from hypoperfusion due to massive blood loss and impairs clotting enzyme activities [9]. Commonly in severe trauma, the combination of acidosis, hypothermia, and hypotension worsens due to ongoing bleeding [8]. This then exacerbates the patient's shock, including worsening acidosis and hypothermia, thus leading to a vicious cycle of the lethal triad components.

Influence of Hypothermia on Coagulation

Traumatic injury is a leading cause of death, and uncontrolled bleeding from coagulation defects is one of the leading causes of potentially preventable mortality [9]. The lethal triad components are important contributors to coagulation defects after trauma. In a bleeding trauma patient, impaired hemostasis occurs as a result of disproportionally impaired coagulation, anti-coagulation, and fibrinolysis. Trauma-induced coagulopathy (TIC) is primarily due to blood loss from injury, hemodilution from crystalloid administration, and development of hypothermia and acidosis. Hypothermic patients have a prolonged PT and PTT, which are independently associated with increased blood transfusion and higher mortality. Thromboelastography (TEG) is a test of whole blood coagulation and provides information on speed of clot formation and growth, clot strength, and whether the clot is maintained or broken down [10]. TEG can differentiate the mechanism of coagulopathy and guide blood product administration [11].

Fibrinolysis occurs as a result of tissue factor exposure after trauma, through a pathway coagulation factor consumption [9]. Traumatic injury and shock-related hypoperfusion are the two most important initiators of early coagulopathy after trauma. In the resuscitation phase, metabolic acidosis and hypothermia can develop alongside hemodilution from resuscitative fluids; this further impairs the existing coagulopathy from the traumatic injury. Acidosis inhibits thrombin generation and propagation and increases fibrinogen degradation, and hypothermia inhibits thrombin generation and impairs fibrinogen synthesis [8]. Hypothermia decreases enzymatic activity of clotting factors and impairs platelet aggregation, resulting in hypo-coagulation [1, 3].

Several days after the traumatic event and TIC, there is a transition from hypo-coagulation to hyper-coagulation [9]. Systemic levels of cytokines (IL-1, IL-6, and TNF [12]) increase, leading to endothelial cell activation (with cytokines and thrombin), resulting in a gradual transition of endothelial cell phenotype from antithrombotic to prothrombotic. Activation of the endothelial cells downregulates thrombomodulin and fibrinolysis, and fibrinogen levels increase [9]. Overall, a prothrombotic environment develops and puts the patient at risk for thrombotic events, often requiring heparin or other anticoagulant medications.

Treatment

Identifying hypothermia is the first step in management and appropriate treatment. All members of the trauma team should be aware of the classic clinical presenting signs of hypothermia and be able to identify hypothermia when present. Diligent screening for core body temperature should be performed initially and throughout management in order to detect, prevent, and treat further temperature loss [3]. Aggressive measures should be taken to prevent loss of body heat and increase the core body temperature [1]. Hypothermia can be present on initial presentation, or it can develop secondary to progressing injury or iatrogenically.

Prior to hospital arrival, the treatment care team should focus on improving the patient's core body temperature. In order to prevent heat loss, the patient should be removed from the cold environment, have wet clothing removed, and be covered with warm blankets or an external warming device. This will prevent further temperature loss in the trauma resuscitation area while the patient undergoes further evaluation and treatment. Utilization of blood warmers in the trauma resuscitation area is critical for resuscitation, as the most efficient method to prevent hypothermia for patients receiving substantial amounts of crystalloid and blood is by warming the products before infusion. Popular fluid infusers include the Belmont and Level 1, which both allow for infusing large amounts of warmed fluids.

Methods of Rewarming

There are various warming modalities for a hypothermic patient, and the appropriate technique is selected based on core body temperature, clinical condition, available resources, and the experience of the trauma team [1]. From least to most invasive, the modalities are passive external rewarming, active external rewarming, and active internal rewarming. Generally, the modalities selected for a particular patient are correlated with that patient's degree of hypothermia: passive external rewarming for mild hypothermia

(35–32 °C), active external rewarming for moderate hypothermia (32–28 °C), and active internal rewarming for severe hypothermia (<28 °C) [4]. Passive rewarming involves placing the patient in an environment that reduces heat loss and relies on the patient's intrinsic thermoregulatory mechanisms to generate heat. Active rewarming involves supplying additional sources of heat energy to the patient [1]. Passive rewarming is utilized for mild hypothermia, while active rewarming is utilized for moderate and severe hypothermia.

Passive external warming techniques consist of removal of cold, wet clothing with replacement of dry clothing and blankets, and transfer from a cold environment to a warm environment. The temperature in the trauma resuscitation area should be increased to maintain a warm ambient temperature and minimize body heat loss.

Active external rewarming involves insulation with heating pads, external convection heaters like heat lamps, thermal caps, warm packs to areas of high vascular flow, warm blankets, and external devices such as a Bair Hugger or other warmed forced-air blankets.

Active internal rewarming includes warmed IV fluids and blood products, heated humidified oxygen or air, warm fluid lavage through nasogastric tubes for intragastric, urinary bladder irrigation, chest tubes for thoracic lavage, peritoneal lavage, and extracorporeal blood warming. Massive transfusions have been associated with marked hypothermia and elevated risk of cardiac arrest [13]. Studies have shown a decrease in core body temperature of 0.5–1.0 °C after transfusion of 500 mL of cold blood [14]. Crystalloid solutions should be warmed to 39 °C before administration. Various extracorporeal rewarming methods exist and yield rapid rewarming (1.5–10° per hour) but are more difficult to manage. Implementing these various and often simultaneous rewarming techniques requires attention and effort from all team members. Organization and communication between the team must be maintained to ensure adequate rewarming.

Afterdrop

Afterdrop is a phenomenon observed after rewarming has started in a hypothermic patient, most commonly moderate to severe hypothermia, that consists of an additional decrease in core body temperature once rewarming has been initiated [6]. External rewarming causes peripheral vasodilation and return to the heart of cold peripheral blood with acidemia accumulated from the extremities. Afterdrop can trigger severe hypotension or lethal arrhythmias such as ventricular fibrillation.

Cardiac Arrest and Role of CPR

Hypothermic cardiac arrest includes ventricular fibrillation, ventricular tachycardia without pulse, pulseless electrical activity, and asystole. Cardiac irritability begins around 33 °C [1], and when the core body temperature of an injured patient decreases 1.3 °C, the probability of adverse cardiac events increases twofold [14]. Clinical presentation of severely hypothermic patients is challenging to distinguish from clinical signs of death, including absence of pulse, respiration, or consciousness and with dilated or nonreactive pupils and muscle rigidity [15]. This overlap necessitates critical attention from team members during the exam. These patients should be resuscitated and treated aggressively, as many dysrhythmias will correct with rewarming alone [7].

Hypothermic patients often require prolonged, high-quality CPR, and cardiac activity should be continuously monitored [6]. Defibrillation is the best method to treat lethal arrhythmias or cardiac arrest. Cardiac arrhythmias often don't respond to defibrillation until core body temperature is greater than 30 °C. Cardiac drugs and defibrillation are generally ineffective in the presence of acidosis, hypoxia, and hypothermia. As such, these methods should be delayed until the patient's core body temperature is at least 28–30 °C [1].

Resuscitation Progression

During rewarming, the patient's temperature should be taken repeatedly to identify if the temperature is decreasing, indicating the need for a different or more aggressive warming technique. Coagulopathy may develop or worsen in hypothermic patients; monitor for this complication early since it is difficult to reverse. Lab tests can help monitor rewarming process, with poor prognosis indicators consisting of hyperkalemia, hypernatremia, and elevated ammonia and lactate [16]. Recommended key factors in guiding treatment include level of consciousness, intensity of shivering, and hemodynamic stability [6].

The well known saying for hypothermia exists: "You're not dead until you're warm and dead." It's necessary to fully rewarm hypothermic patients before pronouncing death [4]. Resuscitation should be continued in a hypothermic patient until the core body temperature is greater than 30–32 °C, and there are still no signs of apparent life [7].

Prognosis

Several retrospective studies have shown an independent relationship between mortality and hypothermia after trauma [3]. It has been proposed that the mortality prediction related to hypothermia is likely in co-existence with acidosis and coagulopathy. Hypothermic fatalities in general had a lower average body temperature, higher injury severity score, and increased blood transfusion requirement. Increased morbidity associated with hypothermia includes a higher risk for organ dysfunction and risk factor for surgical site infections in trauma laparotomies.

Team Dynamics

Effect on Trauma Team Dynamics

The purpose of a trauma team is to provide advanced simultaneous care from various specialties to severely injured patients [5]. Trauma teams have been shown to improve survival rates for severely injured patients, through reduction of resuscitation time and reduced time to CT scan, ED discharge, and OR. Similar to other trauma cases, hypothermic patients require the same concepts, organization, and fluidity that make trauma teams so effective. Important team dynamics that have been specifically identified for hypothermia situations include closed-loop communication and a healthcare team with clear definition of roles [16].

The initial phase of hospital care in the trauma resuscitation area is where most preventable problems occur [5]. Common problems include errors or delays in diagnosis or treatment and failing to perform diagnostic or therapeutic measures at the appropriate time with the right frequency or in the proper order. Additional problems include unfamiliarity with the trauma scenario, disorganization of the team, and failure to prioritize complexity of issues. These problems can be addressed by formal teaching and simulations for trauma team members to familiarize them with recognizing and managing hypothermic patients.

Hypothermia in a severely injured patient is a highly demanding clinical challenge, due to effect of injury severity and associated bleeding complications that is often found in these patients [17]. Team members should be knowledgeable about common pitfalls associated with treating hypothermia, so they can try to avoid or more quickly mitigate them. Some common pitfalls include excessive exposure of the patient, failure to infuse warm blood and fluids, and failure to activate the Massive Transfusion Protocol (MTP) quickly. In order to limit exposure, the patient should immediately be covered with external warming devices such as a Bair hugger. Fluid warmers such as Belmont or Level 1 should be available, nearby, and properly functioning for immediate use. Trauma teams should be aware of the lethal triad and activate the MTP as soon as possible. Education and established protocols for the trauma team surrounding these common pitfalls are essential to improve care.

For hypothermic patients, it's important that they are transported to a hospital that has the appropriate treatment capabilities. Mortality decreases if the patient is brought to a hospital with specialized trauma services, especially if completed in less than 60 minutes [16]. Proper notification and hand-off from the prehospital team to the hospital team is also important. The prehospital team should ensure that the hospital team is aware of the incoming hypothermic patient, the patient status, and current interventions to improve efficiency of care.

Effect on Resuscitation

Steps to caring for a hypothermic patient involve: prioritizing ABCDE, appropriately measuring the core body temperature, applying appropriate rewarming techniques, and managing complications of hypothermia such as arrhythmias. In the primary survey, the trauma team should be aware of the potential for severely decreased respiratory rates and pulse. The trauma team should be mindful of the potential for arrhythmias or cardiac arrest and attach the patient to a cardiac monitor or defibrillator. Trauma team members should be aware of common complications of hypothermia, such as the lethal triad. It's important to recognize which rewarming techniques are most practical with the timing of the initial assessment, such as less invasive techniques started while the patient is still being assessed. Monitoring the patient during rewarming with repeating core body temperature measurements, secondary surveys, and complications is critical to assess rewarming progress and further interventions. The trauma team should be aware that resuscitation may take several hours in a hypothermic patient. Knowing the sequence of treatment events for the care of hypothermic patients is important for the trauma team to know and be efficient [18]. This can be practiced through simulations to improve familiarity and efficiency for trauma teams.

Conclusion

To prevent mortality in hypothermic patients, it's essential for team members to be attentive to hypothermia as part of the lethal triad and other complications of hypothermia. It is imperative that the trauma team recognize hypothermia and aggressively address it to improve outcomes.

Key Points

1. Hypothermia is best managed by prevention, so prevention should be emphasized.
2. The lethal triad consists of hypothermia, acidosis, and coagulopathy. Hypothermia worsens coagulopathy, and in a trauma patient causes hypocoagulation initially and shifts to hyper-coagulation after several days.
3. Rewarming techniques for hypothermia are categorized into passive external rewarming, active external rewarming, and active internal rewarming. Techniques are utilized based on severity of hypothermia.
4. Trauma team dynamics play an essential role in the successful outcome of a hypothermic patient, particularly in recognizing the hypothermia and the sequence of management.

References

1. Stewart RM. ATLS: advanced trauma life support student course manual. 10th ed. Chicago: American College of Surgeons; 2018.
2. Gjeraa K, Moller TP, Ostergaard D. Efficacy of simulation-based trauma team training of non-technical skills: a systematic review. Acta Anaesthesiol Scand. 2014;58:775–87.
3. Soreide K. Clinical and translational aspects of hypothermia in major trauma patients: from pathophysiology to prevention, prognosis and potential preservation. Injury. 2014;45:647–54.
4. Fudge J. Preventing and managing hypothermia and frostbite injury. Sport Health. 2016;8(2):133–9.
5. Georgiou A, Lockey DJ. The performance and assessment of hospital trauma teams. Scand J Trauma Resusc Emerg Med. 2010;18:66.
6. Avellanas Chavala ML, Ayala Gallardo M, Soteras Martinez I, Subirats BE. Management of accidental hypothermia: a narrative review. Med Intensiva. 2019;43(9):556–68.
7. McCullough L, Arora S. Diagnosis and treatment of hypothermia. Am Fam Physician. 2004;70(12):2325–32.
8. Samuels JM, Moore HB, Moore EE. Damage control resuscitation. Chirurgia. 2017;112(5):514–23.
9. Martini WZ. Coagulation complications following trauma. Mil Med Res. 2016;3:35.
10. Gentilello LM, Pierson DJ. "Damage control" approach to trauma surgery. Am J Respir Crit Care Med. 2001;163(3):604–7.
11. Jeger V, Zimmermann H, Exadaktylos AK. The role of thromboelastography in multiple trauma. Emerg Med Int. 2011;2011:895674.
12. Grignani G, Maiolo A. Cytokines and hemostasis. Haematologica. 2000;85:967–72.
13. Horosz B, Malec-Milewska M. Methods to prevent intraoperative hypothermia. Anaesthesiol Intensive Ther. 2014;46(2):96–100.
14. Wei C, Yu Y, Chen Y, Wei Y, Ni X. Impact of warming blood transfusion and infusion toward cerebral oxygen metabolism and cognitive recovery in the perioperative period of elderly knee replacement. J Orthop Surg Res. 2014;9:8.
15. Zhou F, Jong R, Heroux A, Dubrowski A. Hypothermia in a rural setting: an emergency medicine simulation scenario. Cureus. 2017;9(12):e1998.
16. Hilmo J, Naesheim T, Gilbert M. "Nobody is dead until warm and dead": prolonged resuscitation is warranted in arrested hypothermic victims also in remote areas – a retrospective study from northern Norway. Resuscitation. 2014;85:1204–11.
17. Kirkpatrick AW, Chun R, Brown R, Simons RK. Hypothermia and the trauma patient. Can J Surg. 1999;42(5):333–43.
18. Jensen KO, Jensen JM, Sprengel K. Practicability of avoiding hypothermia in resuscitation room phase in severely injured patients. J Med Eng Technol. 2015;39(4):223–5.

Burns

55

Adam Padalko, Rae Paulene Spiwak,
and Sarvesh Logsetty

Burns are devastating injuries that result in significant short-term and long-term impact. They are non-discriminatory in their incidence, however are overrepresented in marginalized populations [1]. Their care requires specialized knowledge in acute management, surgical techniques, inpatient and outpatient care, and extensive long-term multidisciplinary involvement by a trained burn care team. This chapter will discuss initial management, a team-based approach to recovery and burn prevention, with an emphasis on appropriate resource utilization.

Incidence

Burns are the fourth most common type of trauma worldwide [2]. According to Statistics Canada, an average of 110 Canadians died yearly from burns, and ten times that number were admitted to hospital for fire-related injury [3]. Fortunately, advancements in acute management and burn care have decreased the mortality rate, with less than 4% of burns admitted to burn centers proving to be fatal [4]. A low mortality rate emphasizes the growing importance of post-burn recovery and long-term follow-up with psychosocial support and resources and a specialized multidisciplinary burn care team.

Etiology

Thermal injuries (flame/scald) are the most common cause of burn injury; however, chemicals, electricity, or cold may also result in burn injuries. Table 55.1 outlines unique causes of burn injuries, as well as important considerations with each.

A. Padalko
Department of Family Medicine, Max Rady College of Medicine, Rady Faculty of Health Sciences, University of Manitoba, Winnipeg, MB, Canada
e-mail: umpadala@myumanitoba.ca

R. P. Spiwak
Department of Surgery, Max Rady College of Medicine, Rady Faculty of Health Sciences, University of Manitoba, Winnipeg, MB, Canada
e-mail: Rae.Spiwak@umanitoba.ca

S. Logsetty (✉)
Department of Surgery, Psychiatry, Children's Health, Max Rady College of Medicine, Rady Faculty of Health Sciences, University of Manitoba, Winnipeg, MB, Canada
e-mail: Logsetty@umanitoba.ca

L. Marshall Gillman, S. Widder (eds.), *Trauma Team Dynamics*, https://doi.org/10.1007/978-3-031-86312-7_55

Table 55.1 Cellular mechanism, treatment, and clinical pearls relating to burn mechanisms

Etiology	Mechanism	Treatment	Clinical pearls
Chemical	Acidic—Coagulation necrosis Alkali—Liquefaction necrosis	Limit duration of contact Flush with warm water for 20–30 min Obtain information from Material Safety Data Sheet regarding systemic toxicity	Do not attempt to neutralize chemical, may cause exothermic reaction and further tissue damage Remove powders before irrigating
Electrical	When tissue conducts electricity, the heat generated causes thermal injury to tissue in addition to direct electrical damage	May require timely fasciotomies to prevent compartment syndrome Ensure EKG monitor and indwelling bladder catheter in addition to acute burn care Volume resuscitation to prevent acute renal failure in those with myoglobinuria	Normal overlying tissue may co-exist with deep muscle necrosis, maintain a high degree of clinical suspicion
Cold	Ice crystal formation in tissue, microvascular occlusion, and tissue anoxia	Place injured area in circulating water at 38–40 °C until thawed Be wary of reperfusion syndrome, which may occur on rewarming (characterized by acidosis, hyperkalemia, local edema)	Avoid dry heat for reperfusion as injury is often insensate and risking further thermal injury

Prognosis

Major predictors of mortality in burn injuries include age, total body surface area (TBSA), and presence of an inhalation injury [5, 6]. The Baux score allows timely estimation of the chance of mortality secondary to burn injury using age and % TBSA. Revision of the Baux score includes the presence of an inhalation injury to modify mortality risk.

$$Baux\ Score = TBSA + Age$$

$$Modified\ Baux\ Score = TBSA + Age + 17^{*}(Inhalation\ injury)$$

Recent literature has evaluated the utility of the modified Baux score compared with alternative prediction models (Baux, APACHE II, Smith, Ryan, ABSI score) [7, 8]. The modified Baux score remains an accurate and efficient way of predicting mortality in burn survivors [9]. While the Baux/Revised Baux scores remain valid prediction models of burn-related mortality, this is not a 1:1 relationship. The improvements in care mean that the Baux scores at which mortality is estimated to be 50% has moved up to 110 and the Baux score at which 100% mortality is predicted is 160 [10].

Initial Management: "ABCDE" Approach

Initial management of burn injuries is critical to limit the extent of the burn injury, stabilize the patient, and appropriately triage for further management. It is important to obtain information regarding the event as early as possible. Burns can be associated with other forms of traumatic injury. This can be an obvious association, such as in a motor vehicle/airplane crash or less obvious as in a house fire where a propane tank exploded. As standard trauma practice, a primary survey is indicated in the acute setting. Using a structured approach ensures consistency and efficiency: airway, breathing, circulation, disability, and exposure. The major difference in burn injury compared to other traumatic injuries is the response to injury is directly linked to the inflammatory response to the burn. This link to inflammation means that some of the life-threatening sequelae may take time to evolve and should be considered in managing the acute burn injury.

The Airway must be evaluated immediately to assess for an inhalation injury or edema from direct thermal injury. Evaluate the oropharynx with any degree of clinical suspicion for compromise. Maintain a low threshold for initiation of endotracheal intubation, especially in those with >40% TBSA burn injuries or co-occurring inhalation injury. Be aware that there is a synergistic rise in inflammatory response when an integumentary burn occurs combined with inhalation injury [11]. This increased inflammation results in increased fluid resuscitation requirements and subsequent formation of edema.

Breathing concerns are often the result of smoke inhalation-related hypoxia, carbon monoxide poisoning, or the consequences of chemical and particulate injury to the lung parenchyma. Prompt supplemental oxygen is warranted. A chest escharotomy should be considered if the patient has a significant full-thickness burn injury that restricts chest wall motion impeding ventilation and oxygenation. One should suspect carbon monoxide poisoning with burns that occur in a closed space or if there is an altered level of consciousness. Diagnosis is confirmed with measurement of carboxyhemoglobin levels (HbCO). Treat carbon monoxide poisoning with high-flow 100% oxygen via non-rebreathing mask if not intubated. The role of Hyperbaric Oxygen (HBO) therapy is controversial. A randomized controlled trial by Weaver et al. suggests [12] that there may be long-term cognitive benefit from HBO; however, a significant portion of the population studied had low carboxyhemoglobin levels raising questions about the applicability of the findings. In addition, availability of a readily accessible hyperbaric chamber and limitations on the ability to safely monitor and resuscitate a multi-injured patient while in most chambers significantly limit its potential application.

Parenchymal smoke inhalation injury results from smoke particulate and chemical matter settling in distal bronchioles, causing inflammation and diminished clearance and increasing inflammation and risk of pneumonia. History of exposure to smoke in a closed space for an extended period of time should increase suspicion of inhalation injury. Chest radiograph and arterial blood gas determination are initial steps of evaluation. Treatment requires supportive management; height of the bed should be elevated 30 degrees to decrease neck and chest wall edema. Prophylactic intubation should be considered in those with an associated significant burn injury (>40% TBSA) in co-occurrence with an inhalation injury. Controlled laboratory studies have shown that under-resuscitating these individuals does not minimize the edema and may worsen the overall response [13].

Circulating volume needs to be maintained to counteract the ongoing losses secondary to capillary leak due to inflammation. Failure to replace fluids has the potential to compromise end-organ perfusion and lead to burn shock. Resuscitation fluid should be initiated in all deep partial or full-thickness injuries greater than 20% TBSA. The endpoint of resuscitation is to maintain adequate perfusion; most frequently assessed through hourly urine output. Choosing Wisely Canada recommends against the routine use of fluid administration in burns <15% TBSA [14]. Oral fluids and maintenance therapy are appropriate for minor burns. Clinical correlation is recommended. Two large-caliber intravenous lines in the upper extremities are the preferred method of administration for warmed isotonic crystalloid solution, such as Ringer's Lactate. Central venous access or intraosseous infusion may be a second option. Note that large-volume resuscitation with normal saline is not recommended due to the possibility of hyperchloremic metabolic acidosis.

The American Burn Association: Advanced Burn Life Support (ABLS) course recommends calculating the burn resuscitation with 2 cc/kg/%TBSA and titrating to a urine output of 0.5 cc/kg/%TBSA in adults and 1 cc/kg/%TBSA in children [15].

$$2\,mL\ RL \times patient\ weight\left(kg\right) \times \%TBSA\ of\ deep\ partial\ and\ full\ thickness\ burns\ half\ administered\ in\ the\ first\ eight\ hours.$$

An indwelling catheter must be placed for monitoring urine output and assessment of organ perfusion, with a target of 0.5 mL/kg/h for adults. Children <30 kg require a maintenance fluid of D5W + ½ NS IV in addition to parkland with the goal urine output of 1 ml/kg/h for children 1–2 years old, and 2 mL/kg/h for children <1 year old. Dramatic changes in fluid rate should be avoided, instead, adjust fluid rate of fluids at 10–20% maximum each hour to titrate to optimal urine output. Patients should be monitored with electrocardiography for any cardiac rhythm disturbances, as these may be a sign of hypoxia or electrolyte disturbances [15]. Patients with co-existing either acute or chronic renal insufficiency make resuscitation and monitoring that much more complex. In these populations alternate endpoints for resuscitation must be considered including central venous pressures, pulse pressure variability, serial base deficit, and lactate levels, among others. There is currently no evidence to support the use of colloids (e.g., albumin) during early resuscitation. The role of albumin in later resuscitation is controversial with some retrospective data suggesting that the resuscitation fluid given can be decreased with the use of albumin after 18–24 h [16]. There has not been an effect on mortality observed with the use of albumin.

Disability refers to neurologic status and gross deformities. Level of consciousness may be assessed through neurological exam. Findings of altered level of consciousness may indicate smoke inhalation, carbon monoxide toxicity, substance abuse, hypoxia, exacerbation of secondary medical conditions, or excessive anesthesia. A thorough secondary survey with complete history is helpful to discriminate the cause. Be cautious with burn-injured persons with altered consciousness who have limited history; they should be assessed for other physical trauma (i.e., closed head injury).

Anesthesia should be adequate to alleviate patient pain intolerance; however, Choosing Wisely Canada recommends that opioids be co-administrated with adjunctive agents such as acetaminophen and NSAIDs. Daily reassessment is needed to minimize opioid overuse. In addition, neuropathic pharmacotherapy and physical and psychological interventions should be optimized [14]. If NSAIDs are used, remember to use adequate gastric ulcer prophylaxis, and consider avoiding if there is a recent history of ulcers.

Exposure of the patient is necessary to delineate the extent of burn injury and assess for any co-occurring injuries. Clothing should be removed to stop the burning process, and patients should be warmed to minimize losses.

A thorough secondary survey should be used to complete a full medical history and physical exam to evaluate the injury. Physical exam findings noted should include extent of the burned skin (% TBSA), depth of the injury, anatomic location, and evidence of other non-burn injuries.

Classification

Classification of burn injuries is based on the depth, as outlined in Table 55.2. Depth of burn depends on etiology, temperature of offending agent, contact time, and skin thickness. Sensation can be an important physical exam finding to history, and burn depth is important to guiding wound care and evaluating the utility of surgical management.

Table 55.2 Classification of burn injuries

	Affected layers	Characteristics
Superficial	Epidermis	Erythematous, Painful Sensate Does NOT blister
Superficial partial	Epidermis and papillary dermis	Moist, blistered, homogenously pink Hypersensitive Blanchable
Deep partial	Epidermis, papillary, and reticular dermis	Dryer, red Non blanchable Insensate to light touch
Full thickness	Epidermis and all layers of dermis	Leathery, waxy, gray coloration Painless, dry, pale

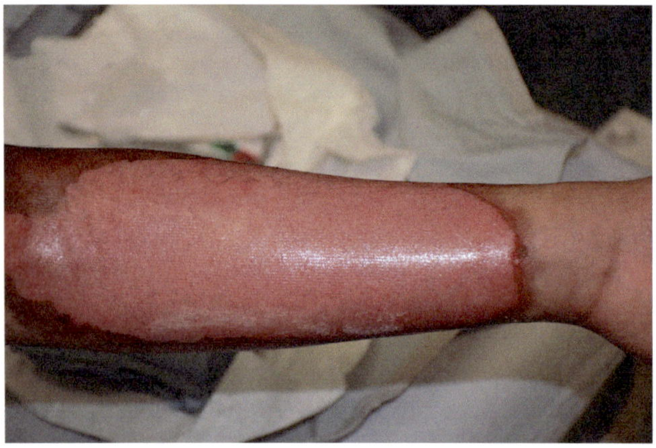

Fig. 55.1 Superficial partial thickness

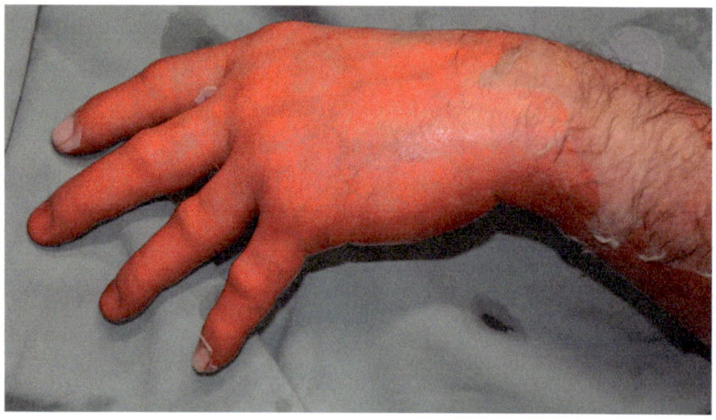

Fig. 55.2 Deep partial thickness.Deep partial thickness (**a**). Note: the non-blanching erythema (Fig. 55.2)

Superficial partial thickness (Fig. 55.1):

Full thickness (Fig. 55.4)

Estimation of partial- and full-thickness burn injury is done using percentage of Total Body Surface Area (TBSA) and the "Rule of 9's." This allows the adult body to be anatomically split into areas that represent TBSA percentages in fractions of 9's. Smaller burn injuries or those extending beyond anatomical zones may be estimated with the "Palm" method, where the patient's volar hand surface with digits extended but together represents 1% TBSA of burn injury. Children are proportionally different than adults, with proportionately larger heads and smaller lower extremities. Burn extent in children should be estimated using the "Palm" method.

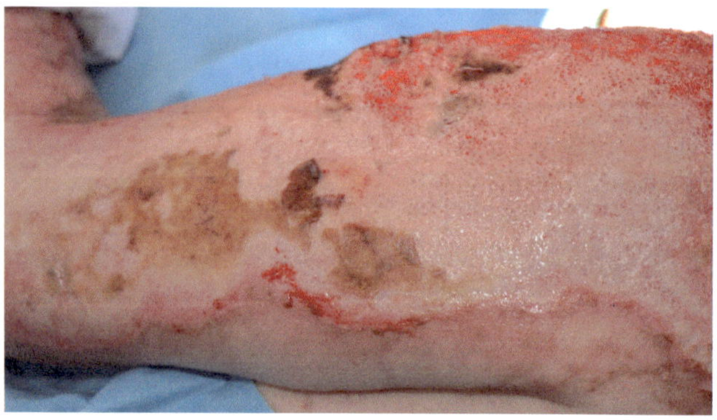

Fig. 55.3 Deep partial thickness (**b**). Note the mixed pictures, with central areas of near full thickness (Fig. 55.3)

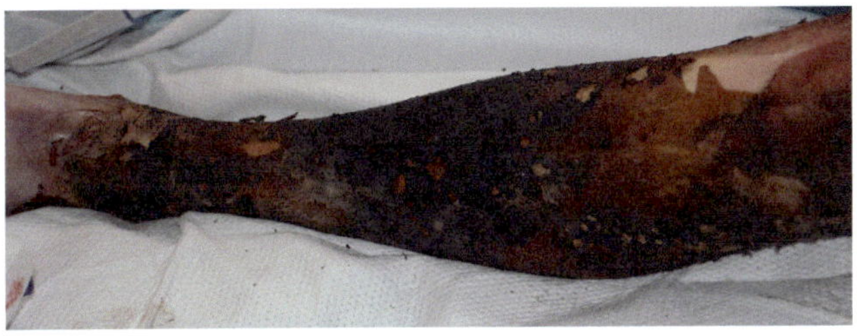

Fig. 55.4 Full thickness

Admission

Admission should be considered for burn injuries that are:

- Significant (>10% TBSA) partial thickness
- Full thickness of sufficient size to require surgery
- Sensitive areas (face, hands, feet, perineum, or genitals)
- Special etiology (electrical, chemical, tar)
- Immunocompromised or co-morbid patients (require specialized medical, rehabilitation, or psychosocial care)

Choosing Wisely Canada has outlined a set of recommendations to encourage mindful use of resources when outlining admission orders and treating burn injuries. First, early systemic antibiotics should not be administered prophylactically, as this encourages growth of antimicrobial-resistant organisms which can limit antimicrobial dressings at a later time [14]. Wound swabs and antibiotics should be used when suspicious of a wound infection. Next, correcting hypoalbuminemia is not recommended, as this is often the normal result of the hypermetabolism, protein loss, and impaired synthesis associated with the burn injury. Instead, diet and nutrition should be optimized. Lastly, patients should not have routine blood work or chest radiographs unless these will be critical in guiding clinical management. Daily reassessment should be performed to examine the necessity of these orders [14].

Dressings

Burn wound care aims to protect the injury, promote a moist environment for burn wound healing, and prevent infections. Topical antimicrobials in conjunction with non-adherent dressings are standard [17].

Superficial burn wounds do not require antimicrobial dressings as the protective skin layer has not been compromised. For deeper wounds while waiting for the wound to demarcate, antimicrobial dressings are recommended. These dressings can consist of topical antibiotic ointments or silver-containing dressings. Superficial partial requires antimicrobial treatment with a non-adherent dressing, such as polysporin ™ with an adaptic™ dressing.

Deeper burn injuries may require excision/grafting. In the interim [17], it should be noted that not all silver dressings are equally effective in antimicrobial activity [18]; the dressing chosen should be discussed with the regional burn center.

Nutrition

Burn injuries result in a hypermetabolic response and associated insulin resistance [19]. Energy requirements increase in proportion with TBSA of burn injury [20]. With larger burns patients may require more than 30 Kcal/Kg/day of total energy and 2.5 grams/Kg/day of protein. Inadequate nutrition has been associated with impaired wound healing and increased length of stay [19]. Burns <20% TBSA should be placed on a high protein, high energy diet with a daily multivitamin. Burns >20% require high protein tube feeds, a daily multivitamin, vitamin C, and zinc. In addition, frail elderly patients or those with bilateral hand burns may also require tube feeds. Metabolic carts can help calculate caloric requirements in large burns and multi-injured patients.

Multidisciplinary Recovery

Survivors of burn injury face a prolonged and difficult recovery. Immediate post-injury challenges include adequate resuscitation, pain management, adapting to physical disfigurement, regaining function, and managing co-morbid conditions. Long-term challenges include physical rehabilitation, social reintegration, developing healthy coping mechanisms, being connected with community, and financial supports [21, 22].

Rehabilitation with physical and occupational therapy prevents physical dysfunction and reduction of muscle mass and leads to improved functional recovery [23]. Early consultation is recommended for assessment and timely decisions regarding splints, exercises, and contracture risk with burn anatomy.

Recent literature outlines the underutilization of mental health screening and connection with psychosocial resources in Canadian burn centers [24]. Survivors of burn injuries have higher rates of mental disorders, substance abuse, suicide attempt, and physical illness after burn injury [21]. Consultation with psychiatric services familiar with burn survivors and routine screening for mental health risk factors are indicated in burn survivors.

Burn injuries are known to be overrepresented in those with adverse social determinants and psychosocial obstacles [25]. Connection of these individuals with appropriate resources should be considered, which may necessitate the involvement of social work familiar with community supports.

Variable accessibility and timing of resources in the post-burn setting may lead to significant differences in physical and psychosocial outcomes based on geography [24, 26]. Standardized burn treatment across regions is needed to optimize recovery and decrease long-term consequences of burn injury. Routine burn care educational sessions may be beneficial to review up-to-date treatment recommendations [27], coordinate specialized burn care between disciplines, and standardize burn treatment to optimize patient outcomes. The dissemination of advanced burn care knowledge to the burn team can be facilitated effectively using multidisciplinary burn journal clubs, with each discipline leading discussion of an article of interest [27].

High-Risk Populations and Prevention

Burns are a preventable injury. Risk of sustaining a burn injury is heavily influenced by environment and social determinants of health [25]. Recent literature has identified a number of social determinants of health that are associated with an increased risk of burn injury in Canadian children. Children from a low family income, from families receiving income assistance, in foster care, or born to a teen mother were all seen to increased risk of burn injury [25]. Identifying populations at an increased risk of burn injury enables personalization and targeting of burn prevention programs to those that would benefit most.

Active prevention methods, such as burn prevention programs, have been shown to decrease incidence of burn injury [28, 29]. Initiating prevention programs in low-income areas would provide the most benefit.

Summary

Burns are a preventable injury with significant sequelae. The most common cause of burn injury depends on age groups but is predominantly flame related, except in the younger and older ages in whom scalds become common. The physiologic effects of burn injury are directly related to the inflammatory response to injury. The physiologic response may be evident immediately or take time to evolve. The response to the cutaneous burn injury is compounded by the presence of inhalation injury. Smoke inhalation can result in not only airway injury but also systemic toxicity through agents such as carbon monoxide. The inflammatory response causes capillary leakage requiring fluid resuscitation. The most common formula used is the Parkland formula. The endpoint of the resuscitation is adequate tissue perfusion as measured by urine output in most situations. Under-resuscitation has been shown to worsen the inflammatory response. Prophylactic systemic antibiotics are not indicated, but topical antibiotic dressings should be used. Early consultation with the regional burn center is advised for any larger or deeper burns, burns from unusual etiologies, and burns affecting specialized body parts. Through ongoing education and dissemination of advanced multidisciplinary burn care the mortality from burn injuries has improved dramatically. Future work is needed to identify optimal treatment pathways and to improve the psychosocial outcomes from burn injury.

Key Points

- Burn injuries are complex and may benefit from a team-based approach.
- Initial management of burns can benefit from the ABCDE approach (Airway, Breathing, Circulating, Disability, Exposure).
- Burn patients benefit from a high protein/caloric diet due to significant hypermetabolic drive.
- Understanding social determinants of health that may place individuals at increased risk of future burn injury may be useful for targeted burn prevention programs.

References

1. Padalko A, Cristall N, Gawaziuk JP, Logsetty S. Social complexity and risk for pediatric burn injury: a systematic review. J Burn Care Res. 2019;40:478–99. https://doi.org/10.1093/jbcr/irz059.
2. Peck MD. Epidemiology of burns throughout the world. Part I: distribution and risk factors. Burns. 2011;37:1087–100. https://doi.org/10.1016/j.burns.2011.06.005.
3. Parachute Canada – some stats 2021. http://www.parachutecanada.org/child-injury-prevention/item/burns-and-scalds-prevention. Accessed 10 May 2021.
4. American Burn Association. Burn incidence fact sheet; n.d.
5. Ryan CM, Schoenfeld DA, Thorpe WP, Sheridan RL, Cassem EH, Tompkins RG. Objective estimates of the probability of death from burn injuries. N Engl J Med. 1998;338:362–6. https://doi.org/10.1056/nejm199802053380604.
6. Jeschke MG, van Baar ME, Choudhry MA, Chung KK, Gibran NS, Logsetty S. Burn injury. Nat Rev Dis Prim. 2020;6:11. https://doi.org/10.1038/s41572-020-0145-5.
7. Osler T, Glance LG, Hosmer DW. Simplified estimates of the probability of death after burn injuries: extending and updating the baux score. J Trauma. 2010;68:690–7. https://doi.org/10.1097/TA.0b013e3181c453b3.
8. Dokter J, Meijs J, Oen IMMH, Van Baar ME, Van Der Vlies CH, Boxma H. External validation of the revised Baux score for the prediction of mortality in patients with acute burn injury. J Trauma Acute Care Surg. 2014;76:840–5. https://doi.org/10.1097/TA.0000000000000124.
9. Haigas B, Bay C, Foster K. A comparison of injury scoring systems in predicting burn mortality. Ann Burns Fire Disasters. 2018;31:89–93.
10. Roberts G, Lloyd M, Parker M, Martin R, Philp B, Shelley O, et al. The Baux score is dead. Long live the Baux score: a 27-year retrospective cohort study of mortality at a regional burns service. J Trauma Acute Care Surg. 2012;72:251–6. https://doi.org/10.1097/TA.0b013e31824052bb.

11. Matsumoto N, Noda H, Nakazawa H, Traber LD, Herndon DN, Traber DL. The sequence of injury determines the degree of lung damage in both inhalation and thermal injuries. Shock. 1994;1:166–70. https://doi.org/10.1097/00024382-199403000-00002.
12. Weaver LK, Hopkins RO, Chan KJ, Churchill S, Elliott CG, Clemmer TP, et al. Hyperbaric oxygen for acute carbon monoxide poisoning. N Engl J Med. 2002;347:1057–67. https://doi.org/10.1056/NEJMoa013121.
13. Herndon DN, Traber DL, Traber LD. The effect of resuscitation on inhalation injury. Surgery. 1986;100:248–51.
14. Choosing Wisely. Twenty things physicians and patients should question; 2019. https://www.choosingwisely.org/wp-content/uploads/2015/02/AAFP-20-things-List_Updated101119.pdf.
15. American Burn Association. Advanced burn life support course. Provider manual 2018 update; 2018.
16. Eljaiek R, Heylbroeck C, Dubois MJ. Albumin administration for fluid resuscitation in burn patients: a systematic review and meta-analysis. Burns. 2017;43:17–24. https://doi.org/10.1016/j.burns.2016.08.001.
17. Carta T, Gawaziuk JPP, Diaz-Abele J, Liu S, Jeschke M, Logsetty S. Properties of an ideal burn dressing: a survey of burn survivors and front-line burn healthcare providers. Burns. 2018;45:364. https://doi.org/10.1016/j.burns.2018.09.021.
18. Ross JA, Allan N, Olson M, Schatz C, Nation PN, Gawaziuk JP, et al. Comparison of the efficacy of silver-based antimicrobial burn dressings in a porcine model of burn wounds. Burns. 2020;46:1632. https://doi.org/10.1016/j.burns.2020.04.004.
19. Coutris N, Gawaziuk JP, Cristall N, Logsetty S. Interrupted nutrition support in patients with burn injuries: a single-centre observational study. Plast Surg. 2019;27:334–9. https://doi.org/10.1177/2292550319880917.
20. Jeschke MG, Finnerty CC, Suman OE, Kulp G, Mlcak RP, Herndon DN. The effect of oxandrolone on the endocrinologic, inflammatory, and hypermetabolic responses during the acute phase postburn. Ann Surg. 2007;246:351–60. https://doi.org/10.1097/SLA.0b013e318146980e.
21. Stone J, Gawaziuk JP, Khan S, Chateau D, Bolton JM, Sareen J, et al. Outcomes in adult survivors of childhood burn injuries as compared with matched controls. J Burn Care Res. 2016;37:e166–73. https://doi.org/10.1097/BCR.0000000000000323.
22. Enns J, Gawaziuk JP, Khan S, Chateau D, Bolton JM, Sareen J, et al. Mental and physical health outcomes in parents of children with burn injuries as compared with matched controls. J Burn Care Res. 2016;37:e18–26. https://doi.org/10.1097/BCR.0000000000000309.
23. Gittings PM, Grisbrook TL, Edgar DW, Wood FM, Wand BM, O'Connell NE. Resistance training for rehabilitation after burn injury: a systematic literature review & meta-analysis. Burns. 2018;44:731–51. https://doi.org/10.1016/j.burns.2017.08.009.
24. Padalko A. Environmental scan of mental health supports across Canadian burn centers: a healthcare providers' perspective. n.d.
25. Padalko AA, Gawaziuk J, Logsetty S. 754 Social determinants associated with Paediatric burn injury: a population based, case-control study. J Burn Care Res. 2020;41:S210–1. https://doi.org/10.1093/jbcr/iraa024.335.
26. Espinoza LF, Friedstat J, Faoro N, Chang PH, McMullen KA, Simko LC, et al. Geographic variation in outcomes after burn injury: a burn model system national database study. Ann Plast Surg. 2020;84:644. https://doi.org/10.1097/SAP.0000000000002287.
27. Carta T, Gawaziuk JP, Cristall N, Forbes L, Logsetty S. Evaluation of a multidisciplinary burn care journal club: lessons learned. Burns. 2018;44:560–5. https://doi.org/10.1016/j.burns.2017.10.017.
28. Corrarino JE, Walsh PJ, Nadel E. Does teaching scald burn prevention to families of young children make a difference? A pilot study. J Pediatr Nurs. 2001;16:256–62. https://doi.org/10.1053/jpdn.2001.25535.
29. Cagle KM, Davis JW, Dominic W, Gonzales W. Results of a focused scald-prevention program. J Burn Care Res. 2006;27:859–63. https://doi.org/10.1097/01.BCR.0000245423.79531.50.

War Zones and Biological Weapons

56

Jason D. Heiner and William Hurley

Abbreviations

HEPA High-efficiency particulate air
PPE Personal protective equipment

War Zones

Introduction to Battlefield Care

War zone trauma providers generally train in civilian and noncombat military settings prior to engaging in battlefield medical care and often have little or no experience in the combat setting prior to their first medical war zone assignment [1, 2]. When not deployed to the combat setting, urban civilian trauma hospitals provide an important environment for training military trauma teams due to the relatively high volume of injured patients at these centers [1–3]. While the dynamics of trauma team care in the war zone and non-war settings share some similarities, notable differences to care within the battlefield exist.

Team Members and Echelons of Battlefield Care

On the battlefield, the individuals composing trauma teams and the specific circumstances in which trauma care is provided can vary considerably. Trauma care occurs along a spectrum from battlefield care at the point of injury while under enemy fire and other combat hazards and with minimal medical resources to larger mobile or fixed structures that resemble more familiar emergency care and resuscitation environments. War zone trauma care in the American military and similar modern military systems utilizes a tiered trauma care and evacuation system to organize and deploy its medical resources (Table 56.1) [4–6]. Advancing capabilities exist upward along the echelons of care. However, with factors including the asymmetric nature of the modern battlefield and availability of rapid casualty transport, the injured may bypass lower echelons for regions of higher care capabilities [4].

The first typical echelon of battlefield care is near the point of injury with trauma care teams often consisting of combat medics or Battalion Aid Station personnel. Care at the second echelon takes place in settings such as the Forward Surgical Team, Mobile Field Surgical Team, and Expeditionary Medical Support Unit where immediate life and limb-saving surgical interventions and stabilization may occur. The third echelon of care occurs in settings such as the Army Combat Hospital, Air Force Theater Hospital, or Naval fleet hospitals—combat trauma casualties may arrive to this level of care from the first or second echelon of care, and from here, may be transferred out of the war zone. These levels of care are connected by medical evacuation services to transport patients efficiently up or between these echelons

Table 56.1 Levels of common warzone patient care settings and typical trauma team member composition [4–6]

Level I/Role 1 (i.e., point of injury)
Combat medic
General physician
Physician assistant
Level II/Role II (i.e., forward surgical team)
Combat medic
Nurse
Surgeon
Anesthesiology provider
Level III/Role III (i.e., combat support hospital)
Combat Medic
Nurse
Physician assistant
Surgeon (including specialists)
Emergency physician
Anesthesiology provider
General physician
Radiologist

J. D. Heiner (✉)
University of Washington, Department of Emergency Medicine, Seattle, WA, USA
e-mail: jheiner@uw.edu

W. Hurley
Olympia Emergency Care Physicians, WA, USA

L. Marshall Gillman, S. Widder (eds.), *Trauma Team Dynamics*, https://doi.org/10.1007/978-3-031-86312-7_56

of care. The varying levels of care allow treatment of minimally injured patients at the lowest tier of care needed to maximally maintain local war fighting strength, while also providing key opportunities to stabilize more critically injured patients prior to their transport out of the war zone.

Members of modern war zone trauma teams can include varying numbers of surgeons and surgical specialists, emergency physicians, combat medics, anesthesiologists, nurses, and additional ancillary providers (Table 56.1) [4–6]. The multidisciplinary physician nature of modern robust military trauma teams provides optimal care to combat casualties and addresses the frequently devastating penetrating, blast, and orthopedic injuries seen on the battlefield. Radiologists may aid in the triage of imaging studies for trauma patients and report immediate results to trauma team leaders. Many additional providers assist in patient care at the higher echelons to include blood bank, pharmacy, laboratory services, and operating room personnel. In multi-casualty and mass-casualty incidents, the trauma team members vary based on number of casualties and the priority and nature of their injuries.

Casualty Care Team Preparation

War zone casualties can include soldiers, adult civilians, children, and enemy combatants and often arrive with little warning, in critical condition, and in multi-casualty or mass-casualty numbers. Team preparedness to ensure effective communication, identified leadership, role clarity, situational awareness, and action anticipation is imperative. The ability of the individual and the trauma teams to function in a predictable manner to dynamic situations is key to care in the combat setting. Team training prior to combat deployment, ongoing training in the war zone, and consistent debriefing is vital to optimizing battlefield care.

Pre-deployment simulation-based training has positively affected trauma team performance in areas such as modern battlefield injury care, individual performance awareness, and team performance during mass-casualty incidents [3, 7–9]. This simulation training may employ a variable of training tools such as high-fidelity mannequins, perfused cadavers, and in situ positioning of field care elements or entire facilities [3, 7–9]. Importantly, pre-deployment training can identify critical areas of needed improvement in trauma team performance such as communication lapses, inappropriate trauma triaging, delays to lifesaving procedures, and failure to recognize hazards such as unexploded ordnance. Often, medical specialists are assigned to differing echelons of care in part due to the specialty expertise they deliver; at times, their specialty background may be less complementary to the battlefield and reveal opportunities to provide additional team and setting training. In the war zone, ongoing team exercises and simulation-based training can be an effective tool to maintain and improve trauma team performance and may be particularly valuable to orient new members to the deployed trauma team. Team exercises can target critical events, complement debriefing tools, and can include all aspects of patient care from initial triage through evacuation to higher levels of care.

Care of the trauma patient can be stressful for care team members in any setting. The consistent high acuity and devastating nature of battlefield casualties within unfamiliar surroundings combined with a setting typically removed from a medical provider's usual personal and professional support can add additional emotional burden. Medical providers in combat settings are at risk of developing syndromes such as post-traumatic stress disorder and should be offered interventions such as critical incident debriefing. Regular debriefing of trauma care as well as critical incident debriefing of particularly stressful events may optimize team and individual performance, enhance individual coping, nurture team communication, and prevent stress reactions or identify individuals in need of more mental health resources.

Biological Weapons

Introduction to Biological Weapons

Biological warfare agents are unconventional weapons considered to be a modern threat in military and civilian settings. Although a natural event, the recent medical, social, and economic disruption produced by the COVID-19 pandemic demonstrates the potential immense impact of the release of an effective infectious biological warfare agent [10]. Such weapons are relatively inefficient on the modern battlefield but are weapons that can be obtained with relative ease and produced with relatively low cost and technology [11]. These factors, coupled with their profound psychosocial impacts, make biological weapons attractive as agents of terrorism and crime. Several unique factors make biological weapons problematic for the trauma team. These include challenges to timely recognition and identification of the agent, the need for protection of trauma team members, control of spread to team members and the community, and recognition of the profound physical and psychological impacts on team members caring for victims of biological weapons. Recognizing and preparing for these unique challenges can promote optimal care of patients and enhance the performance of the trauma team.

Biological Warfare Historical Considerations

Historically, disease has produced greater numbers of casualties in the battlefield when compared to injury. The exploitation of disease as a weapon dates to medieval times and has been used with varying success by the Romans, the United States Calvary, the Japanese, and the Soviets [12]. The use of ricin for assassination and the mailing of anthrax spores demonstrate a recent use of biological weapons in the United Kingdom and in the United States.

The most concerning potential biological weapons have caused the deadliest plagues and pandemics in history. These include anthrax, cholera, plague, smallpox, hemorrhagic fever viruses, and now COVID-19 (SARS-COV2). Victims exposed to biological weapons may require isolation, decontamination, and novel therapies to prevent the further spread of these agents to communities and healthcare providers as secondary casualties [9, 13]. Care of the trauma patient in the setting of biological weapon exposure will be challenged by the physiological impacts of the agent on the patient, as well as the reduction of available resources through diversion to the care of other victims. There will be increased workload and stress in team members through the need to consider their own risks of exposure and the need to work in personal protective equipment (PPE). These challenges may be mitigated by planning, preparation, and training of the trauma team for the care of victims of biological weapons as well as for the care of victims of the next pandemic.

Diversity of Biological Weapons

Agents used as biological weapons in warfare, terrorism, and crime are generally infectious and often living particles or the toxic products of living organisms [9, 11, 13]. The United States Centers for Disease Control and Prevention has categorized biological agents into three categories, with Category A listing the agents of highest priority and risk of use as a weapon [14]. These bacterial, viral, and toxin agents are found in nature and can be most efficiently weaponized as an aerosol (Table 56.2). Bacterial organisms include anthrax, cholera, and plague. Viral agents include smallpox and viral hemorrhagic fevers. Weaponized toxins include ricin and botulism.

Medical Management of Biological Weapon Victims

The recent principles of care for patients with suspected COVID-19 infection provide a useful framework for the care of victims of biological weapons [15, 16]. These include:

1. Personal protection of team members while performing initial assessment, stabilization, and management of the patient.
2. Rapid identification of suspected infection or toxicity.
3. Maintenance of heightened personal protection until the risk of secondary transmission can be eliminated through appropriate decontamination or ruling-out of the suspected agent.
4. Simultaneous care of traumatic injuries as well as illness and injury produced by the biological weapon.

Identification of Bioweapons

Biological weapons may remain unnoticed for days or weeks after exposure due to delayed onset of illness, making identi-

Table 56.2 Selected biological warfare agents, likely mode of delivery, and chosen physiologic effects [9, 11, 13, 14]

Biological agent	Delivery mode	Physiological effect
Bacterial		
Anthrax (*Bacillus anthracis* spores)	Aerosol release Food and water contamination	Pulmonary, gastrointestinal, cutaneous
Brucellosis (*Brucella* bacteria)	Aerosol release	Bone and joint, pulmonary, genitourinary
Plague (*Yersinia pestis* bacteria)	Aerosol release	Pulmonary, hematologic
Cholera (*Vibrio cholerae* bacteria)	Aerosol release Food and water contamination	Gastrointestinal
Viral		
Smallpox (variola major or minor virus)	Aerosol release	Skin, pulmonary, hematologic, neurologic
Viral hemorrhagic fevers (i.e., Ebola)	Aerosol release	Skin, hematologic, neurologic
Toxin		
Clostridium Botulinum toxin	Aerosol release Food and water contamination	Neurologic, gastrointestinal
Ricin	Aerosol release Food and water contamination	Pulmonary, gastrointestinal
Trichothecene Mycotoxin	Aerosol release Food and water contamination	Hematologic, neurologic, pulmonary, Gastrointestinal

fication and control difficult immediately after exposure [9, 13]. The initial suspicion of exposure to a biological weapon occurs through the recognition of a unique pattern of disease in multiple victims [14]. To recognize such a pattern, team members require briefing and familiarization regarding illness patterns and exposure suspicion. This is a critical time for the team to establish and maintain situation awareness, as well as to cross-monitor team members to ensure they maintain awareness and safety. The importance of informed pattern recognition was exemplified by care team members recognizing the unique pattern of hemorrhagic mediastinitis in anthrax victims and the recent recognition of a novel progressive respiratory and inflammatory illness in victims of COVID-19 [17]. Initial suspicions can then be confirmed (or eliminated) through specific testing for the suspected agent.

Victims of biological weapons and the "worried well" may overwhelm healthcare resources [9, 13]. In general, healthcare facilities and their providers are thought to be poorly prepared for these unexpected events that could quickly deplete available protective supplies, treatments, available hospital beds, and other resources [9]. Members of the trauma team must be prepared and supported to treat both contaminated and uncontaminated patients, prioritize trauma care and medical care for biological weapon victims, and efficiently deliver care while protecting other patients, themselves, and other team members from secondary exposure.

Unique to the recent COVID-19 pandemic was an early reduction in the use of Emergency Departments in the United States during the pandemic [18]. This likely came from an informed public recognizing that resources were limited by the need to care for COVID-19 patients, as well as recognizing their personal risk of acquiring the disease through travel and at the healthcare facility. This recent experience demonstrates a public health opportunity to control access and match resources to needs in similar events (such as a biological weapons event) through consistent, trusted, and timely public health messaging.

Victim Decontamination and Isolation

Individuals exposed to a biological weapon may be prevented from becoming ill through early decontamination. Delays in symptom onset and agent identification may make decontamination impossible. Isolation of victims may then be required to prevent the agent from infecting other patients, members of the community, and care team members [9, 13].

The discovery of unidentified contaminates or suspected persistent aerosolized agents on victims (such as toxins or anthrax spores) provides an opportunity for decontamination [9]. For most agents, removal of clothing and washing of the patient with soap and water to remove further biological contaminates is adequate [9]. Decontamination can proceed alongside initial care if providers are appropriately protected. Wounds can be irrigated with copious clean or sterile water to remove the agent and assist in the removal of contaminated foreign bodies [9]. Patient decontamination should not interfere with more immediate lifesaving treatments and may be performed in parallel with other medical and surgical interventions [9, 13]. Patient decontamination increases the work burden and potentially reduces the performance of the trauma team. Trauma team training with explicit inclusion of decontamination scenarios is critical to preparing team members for additional communication requirements, role clarity, and exceptional situational awareness that will be needed in these crisis-rich events.

Personal Protective Equipment

Care of the trauma patient with exposure to a biological weapon is complicated by the need to prevent further exposure and disease. There is limited data or consensus to firmly guide recommendations, but if the biologic agent is identified, specific precautions should be instituted (Table 56.3) [9]. When biological weapon use is suspected but not yet identified, personal protective equipment (PPE) with a non-encapsulated chemical-resistant suit, gloves, boots, and a full-face organic vapor/HEPA (high-efficiency particulate air) filter cartridge mask has been recommended [9].

Personal protective equipment creates barriers to patient care through limiting the maximum duration of work, increasing heat stress, reducing visibility from fogging of eyewear and face shields, and impeding fine motor and palpation skills from glove use. Several distant past studies have been equivocal on the impact of these challenges while more recent studies during the COVID-19 pandemic demonstrated reduced voiced communication and increased isolation from the patient and other team members when wearing protective equipment [19]. These findings underscore the importance of training and practice for healthcare providers in the donning and doffing of PPE, work while in PPE, and challenges to team performance while wearing PPE.

Specific Biological Weapons

Anthrax

The spores of the bacterium *Bacillus anthracis* are commonly found in soil and when activated can produce cutaneous, gastrointestinal, inhalational, and injection-related infections in humans [20]. Most severe is inhalational anthrax, characterized by meningitis and hemorrhagic mediastinitis that occur about a week after inhalation of anthrax

Table 56.3 Suggested precautions and personal protective equipment (PPE) against selected agents of biological warfare [9]

Precautions and PPE	Biological agent
Universal/standard precautions Includes gloves, masks, gown, eye protection, and frequent hand washing	Anthrax Cholera Clostridium Botulinum toxin Ricin Trichothecene mycotoxin
Contact precautions Universal/standard precautions *plus* Patients isolation in a standard room	Brucellosis
Droplet precautions Universal/standard precautions *plus* Contact precautions *plus* N-95 or better respirator *plus* Mask worn by patient	Plague
Airborne precautions Universal/standard precautions *plus* Patient isolation in a negative pressure room *plus* N-95 or better respirator *plus* Mask worn by patient	Smallpox Viral hemorrhagic fevers

spores. Treatment with antibiotics, antitoxin, and intensive supportive care can improve the survival from inhalational anthrax from about 15% to 55% [21]. As with most bacterial infections, secondary spread to care team members does not occur from inhalational anthrax, making the need for specific personal protective equipment (PPE) unnecessary.

Hemorrhagic Fevers (Ebola and Marburg Viruses)

Exposure to a hemorrhagic fever virus produces an abrupt viral syndrome (fever, headache, and myalgia) after an incubation period of about 6–10 days. This is followed by nausea, vomiting, abdominal pain, diarrhea, profound fluid losses, chest pain, cough, and pharyngitis, then a maculopapular rash, and finally hemorrhagic manifestations (petechiae, ecchymoses, and bleeding) as the disease progresses. Intensive supportive care, fluid replacement, antiviral agents, and antitoxins can improve survival from about 10% to over 60% [22]. As with many viral agents, secondary infection of family members and caregivers is common and demands the meticulous use of isolation and personal protective equipment (PPE) to avoid exposure to aerosolized viruses, infected fomites, and infectious body fluids.

Botulism Toxin

Ingestion or inhalation of botulism toxin produces a progressive descending paralysis. Cranial nerve involvement (drooping eyelids, weak jaw clench, difficulty swallowing or speaking) is followed by upper and lower body weakness and respiratory failure from muscle paralysis. Treatment is intensive supportive care and antitoxin administration. Key to the management of botulism is early administration of antitoxin that stops the progression of paralysis but does not reverse it [23]. Once established, paralysis from botulism toxin commonly lasts for weeks or months due to the permanent blockage of neurotramsmitter release at nerve terminals, making prolonged ventilation and intensive care necessary. As with most toxin exposures, decontamination of a victim of botulism toxin exposure may be needed if the agent was aerosolized and liquid remains on the body. Soap and water are effective for decontamination. Otherwise, care team members are of no significant risk of secondary exposure and no specific PPE use is recommended for their protection.

Impact on Trauma Team Members

Easily overlooked are the psychological effects for both the community and the providers involved in a biological weapon attack. It has been well documented that mass population scale attacks cause many non-injured patients to seek care at the emergency department. Some of these patients have stress reactions, while others have psychosomatic complaints mimicking the effects of the biological weapon. Further complicating such scenarios is the psychological toll these events could have on the providers who must deal with unfamiliar protocols, rare disease processes, large number of concerned but well patients, and facing the personal risk of possible exposure to a biologic agent during an immensely unfamiliar and potentially tragic event [24]. Hospitals and trauma team leaders are wise to have well-defined and practiced protocols in place to manage large numbers of unexposed patients and to provide rapid psychological support for trauma team members during a suspected attack with a biological weapon.

Conclusion

Treatment of the trauma patient in unique settings such as the battlefield or with the addition of exceptional hazards such as biological weapons present challenges to trauma team performance. Patient care in war zones is challenged by limited resources, threats of combat, and variable team member composition. Biological weapons can have a myriad of physiologic effects on the patient, and necessary medical precautions and decontamination events can impair the delivery of typical individual and team care. Targeted trauma team and individual preparation can optimize the delivery of patient care in these exceptional settings.

Key Points

- The application of specific teamwork skills in assuring team member fitness to work, cross-monitoring of team members, mutual support, and regular debriefing will be needed to ensure optimal team performance in the unique environments of the battlefield and in caring for victims of biological weapons.
- The COVID-19 pandemic provided a model to demonstrate the profound impacts of an effective biological weapon and present the opportunity to plan, prepare, and mitigate such impacts in the future.
- Team training and practice in identification of victims of biological weapons, decontamination, personal protective equipment use, and novel therapies are needed to mitigate the impacts of biological weapons on the community, care facilities, and trauma team.

References

1. Dubose J, Rodriguez C, Martin M, Nunez T, Dorlac W, King D, et al. Preparing the surgeon for war: present practices of US, UK, and Canadian militaries and future directions for the US military. J Trauma Acute Care Surg. 2012;73:S423–30.
2. Schmied Blackman V, Torres T, Stakley JA, Raiciulescu S, Garcia E, Ross JL, Polk TM, Stotts NA. Quantifying clinical opportunities at the Navy Trauma Training Center. Mil Med. 2021;186(Suppl 1):40–8.
3. Valdiri LA, Andrews-Arce VE, Seery JM. Training forward surgical teams for deployment: the US Army Trauma Training Center. Crit Care Nurs. 2015;35(2):e11–7.
4. Clarke JE, Davis PR. Medical evacuation and triage of combat casualties in Helmand Province, Afghanistan: October 2010–April 2011. Mil Med. 2012;177(11):1261–6.
5. Schoenfeld AJ. The combat experience of military surgical assets in Iraq and Afghanistan: a historical review. Am J Surg. 2012;204:377–83.
6. Beckett A, Pelletier P, Mamczak C, Benfield R, Elster E. Multidisciplinary trauma team care in Kandahar, Afghanistan: current injury patterns and care practices. Injury. 2012;43:2072–7.
7. Schulman CI, Garcia GD, Wyckoff MM, Duncan RC, Withum KF, Graygo J. Mobile learning module improves knowledge of medical shock for forward surgical team members. Mil Med. 2012;177:1316–21.
8. Kim M, Torrie I, Poisson R, Withers N, Bjarnason S, Da Luz LT, Pannell D, Beckett A, Tien HC. The value of live tissue training for combat casualty care: a survey of Canadian combat medics with battlefield experience in Afghanistan. Mil Med. 2017;182(9):e1834–40.
9. Multiservice tactics, techniques, and procedures for treatment of biological warfare agent casualties. Army Techniques Publication; 2013. Report No: 4-02.84.
10. Sarkodie SA, Owusu PA. Global assessment of environment, health and economic impact of the novel coronavirus (COVID-19). Environ Dev Sustain. 2020;5:1–11.
11. Jansen HJ, Breeveld FJ, Stijnis C, Grobusch MP. Biological warfare, bioterrorism, and biocrime. Clin Microbiol Infect. 2014;20(6):488–96.
12. Barras V, Greub G. History of biological warfare and bioterrorism. Clin Microbiol Infect. 2014;20(6):497–502.
13. Eachempati SR, Flomenbaum N, Barie PS. Biological warfare: current concerns for the health care provider. J Trauma. 2002;52:179–86.
14. Bioterrorism agents/diseases. https://emergency.cdc.gov/agent/agentlist-category.asp. Accessed 30 Dec 2020.
15. Sawhney C, Singh Y, Jain K, Sawhney R, Trikha A. Trauma care and COVID-19 pandemic. J Anaesthesiol Clin Pharmacol. 2020;36(Suppl 1):S115–20.
16. Coimbra R, Edwards S, Kurihara H, Bass GA, Balogh ZJ, Tilsed J, Faccincani R, Carlucci M, Martínez Casas I, Gaarder C, Tabuenca A, Coimbra BC, Marzi I. European Society of Trauma and Emergency Surgery (ESTES) recommendations for trauma and emergency surgery preparation during times of COVID-19 infection. Eur J Trauma Emerg Surg. 2020;46:505.
17. Lippi G, Sanchis-Gomar F, Henry BM. COVID-19: unravelling the clinical progression of nature's virtually perfect biological weapon. Ann Transl Med. 2020;8(11):693.
18. Boserup B, McKenney M, Elkbuli A. The impact of the COVID-19 pandemic on emergency department visits and patient safety in the United States. Am J Emerg Med. 2020;38(9):1732–6.
19. Leibner ES, Stokes S, Ahmad D, Legome E. Emergency department COVID management policies: one institution's experience and lessons learned. Emerg Med Pract. 2020;22(5 Suppl):1.
20. Zasada AA. Injectional anthrax in human: a new face of the old disease. Adv Clin Exp Med. 2018;27(4):553–8.
21. Anthrax information for healthcare professionals. https://www.cdc.gov/anthrax/healthcare/index.html. Accessed 30 Dec 2020.
22. Jacob ST, Crozier I, Fischer WA 2nd, Hewlett A, Kraft CS, Vega MA, Soka MJ, Wahl V, Griffiths A, Bollinger L, Kuhn JH. Ebola virus disease. Nat Rev Dis Primers. 2020;6(1):13.
23. Chalk CH, Benstead TJ, Pound JD, Keezer MR. Medical treatment for botulism. Cochrane Database Syst Rev. 2019;4(4):CD008123.
24. Luan R, Pu W, Dai L, Yang R, Wang P. Comparison of psychological stress levels and associated factors among healthcare workers, frontline workers, and the general public during the novel coronavirus pandemic. Front Psych. 2020;11:583971.

57 Nuclear Injuries

Mansoor Ali Khan and Heidi L. Frankel

Introduction

Trauma care can be challenging in the best of environments. However, in certain circumstances the environment can contribute to the severity of injuries or even cause unique and characteristic injury patterns. Herein we will discuss fallout from nuclear disasters or nuclear weapons.

Historical Background

Survivors of the atomic bombing of Hiroshima and Nagasaki in 1945 provide the basis for much of the available literature on the effects of radiation. The Atomic Bomb Casualty Commission (ABCC) was established in 1947 to study the late effects of radiation [1]. There were more than 100,000 documented fatalities as a direct result of radiation exposure [2] following the bombing.

The Chernobyl disaster resulted in 31 immediate fatalities from acute radiation sickness and approximately 6000 deaths from cancers due to radiation exposure. Almost 4000 square kilometers of land is now uninhabited with 120 villages and two major cities left to decay with over 100,000 losing their homes [3].

Information on early internal radiation doses in Fukushima after the nuclear power plant accident on March 11, 2011, is quite limited due to initial organizational difficulties, high background radiation, and contamination of radiation measuring devices [4]. With regard to healthcare infrastructure, the biggest lesson learned was the impact of evacuating healthcare facilities within the emergency planning zones. The vast majority of able-bodied populace evacuated themselves in private or public transportation. There was no medical support provided during transportation of residents to hospitals and care homes. This resulted in deaths directly attributable to lack of healthcare provision during evacuation, whereas, at this point no life has been lost as a result of radiation, although the long-term effects are still unknown as elevated levels of radiation are still being detected 3 years later [5].

Physics of Weaponry

The most feared and deadly environmental hazards that exist today are nuclear. These include both conventional fission or fusion devices and unconventional weapons known as "dirty bombs."

Fission employs high-density elements, with a heavy unstable nucleus, that subsequently splits into two or more lighter nuclei releasing a vast quantity of energy. The most commonly used substances to bring about nuclear reactions are the isotopes of Uranium and Plutonium, which undergo fission readily. The first uranium-based weapons used were "Little Boy" and "Fat Man," used to bomb Hiroshima and Nagasaki at the climax of the First World War.

Fusion, on the other hand, can be described as the combining of light nuclei to form a heavier nucleus-bearing product, the same process that powers stars. It can be seen as the reverse of fission, but still with the production of vast amounts of thermal energy and radiation. Practically, nuclear power plants and weapons are the only existent environmental hazards. Nuclear reactor incidents require special consideration due to the variety of radioactive material released; radioiodine (I^{131}) can travel over long distances.

Dirty bombs, also referred to as Radiological Dispersion Devices (RDD), are munitions that cause a purposeful dissemination of radioactive material without nuclear detonation. The purpose of the weapon is to contaminate the area around the conventional explosion with radioactive material.

M. A. Khan · H. L. Frankel (✉)
St Mary's Hospital, Imperial College Healthcare NHS Trust, London, UK

Keck University Hospital, University of Southern California, Los Angeles, CA, USA
e-mail: manskhan@doctors.org.uk

L. Marshall Gillman, S. Widder (eds.), *Trauma Team Dynamics*, https://doi.org/10.1007/978-3-031-86312-7_57

With thermonuclear weapons, the three main methods of injury from a nuclear explosion result from the initial blast, thermal effects, and ionizing radiation:

- *Initial blast* injuries result from the shearing forces between differing tissue planes, causing severe internal tissue disruption. Individuals near the blast epicenter will suffer instant vaporization, whereas the casualties on the peripheries will suffer varying degrees of internal injuries. Petechial hemorrhages within organs are difficult to diagnose; the mainstays are CT/MRI scanning or postmortem findings. The major problem arises not from diagnosing the injury, but once diagnosed, very few therapeutic measures to save life can be administered. Matters are further complicated when debris is carried in the blast wave; the arising result will cause blunt and penetrating injury to occur. In these situations one can only carry out the usual life support measures.
- *Thermal effects*—The rapidly expanding fireball that develops into the infamous "mushroom cloud" has an initial temperature of many millions of degrees Centigrade. As it expands at a rate of over 100 m/s, it rapidly cools to only a few thousand degrees Centigrade. The thermal radiation emitted can cause severe burns many kilometers away.
- *Radiation*—The types of radiation are important due to the fact that they affect cellular function in differing ways. Alpha (ά) particles are essentially the nucleus of helium atoms. These have a limited airborne range of a few centimeters and are easily absorbed by paper. However, due to their relatively high atomic mass, they cause the most structural cellular damage. Beta (β) particles, ideally described as free-floating electrons, have a range of a few meters and are stopped by a thin sheet of aluminum. These have an atomic mass of 1/1850 of a neutron/proton, and therefore, are less destructive compared to alpha particles. Finally, gamma (γ) radiation is electromagnetic waves, which can only be stopped by concrete or lead; this allows for deeper penetration of the human body and subsequent internal irradiation (Fig. 57.1).

The scale used for quantitative measurement of radiation is known as the Gray (Gy) scale. The cellular effects of radiation are similar for different kinds and doses of ionizing radiation. Cell death is readily observed by light microscopy, with nuclear and cytoplasmic deformational changes. The type and severity of the injury is dependent on the dose of radiation received. A useful indicator of this is the Median Lethal Dose (LD50 2.5–5 Gy), which is the dose that is lethal to 50% of a given population.

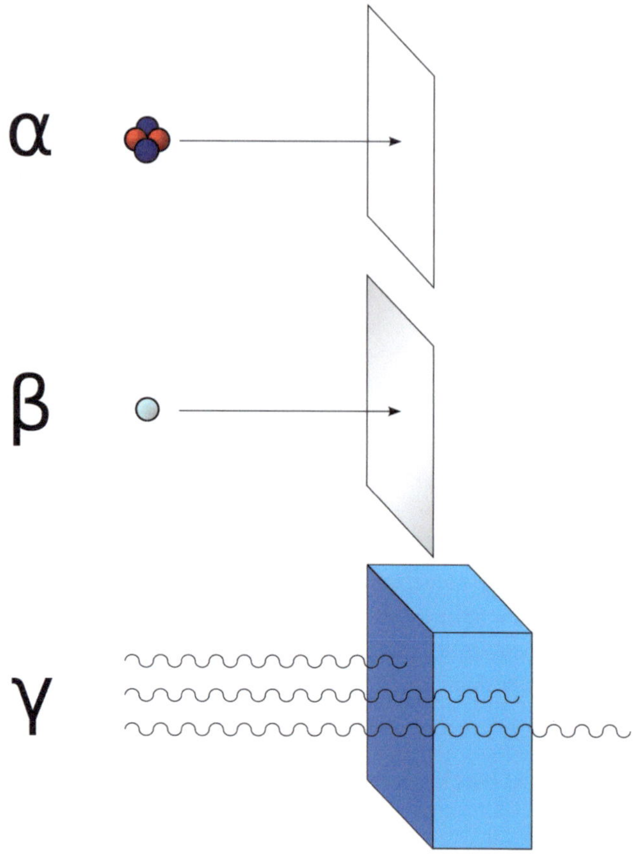

Fig. 57.1 Particle penetration *Alpha radiation*—readily stopped by a sheet of paper *Beta radiation*—is stopped by an aluminum plate *Gamma radiation* is eventually absorbed as it penetrates a dense material. Lead is good at absorbing gamma radiation, due to its density. (Permission is granted to copy, distribute and/or modify this document under the terms of the GNU Free Documentation License, Version 1.2 or any later version published by the Free Software Foundation; with no Invariant Sections, no Front-Cover Texts, and no Back-Cover Texts. A copy of the license is included in the section entitled GNU Free Documentation License)

Medical Management of Nuclear Device-Related Injuries: Scene Considerations

There are two ways in which an individual may be exposed to radiation: *external radiation hazard* and *internal radiation hazard*.

- *External radiation hazard* is received when the radioactive material is external to the body. Emitted radiation travels through space and irradiates the body; however, the radioactive material remains external to the body. Therefore, if one moves away from the source of radiation, the amount of radiation the body is receiving decreases.

- *Internal radiation hazard*, or radioactive contamination as it is often referred to, arises from radioactive material entering the body. The three main routes of entering the body are inhalation, ingestion, and injection. Once inside the body, the radiation from the contamination irradiates the internal organs. Internal problems vary with the type of radiation that is emitted. If a substance is undergoing alpha decay in the gut, then areas of close contact are being exposed to high-energy radiation that will result in immediate cell death. The half-life of the radioactive substance is extremely important, as some isotopes may linger in the body from a time frame of hours to years [6].

The major difference between the two types of radiation hazard is that in one circumstance, getting a distance away from it can considerably reduce one's radiation dose. With radioactive contamination, the fact that the source is internal, distance from the source would make no difference. To prevent ingestion/inhalation, no eating/drinking or smoking should be allowed until after an individual has left the area and has been decontaminated.

Protective equipment, protocols, and procedures should be used for emergency services personnel to eliminate/minimize radioactive contamination. Personal protective equipment provides a physical barrier that allows respiratory protection, and protective clothing that prevents skin contamination. The emergency planning zone for a nuclear reactor incident involves two zones:

- Plume exposure pathway emergency planning zone (within a 10 mile radius)
- Ingestion exposure pathway emergency planning zone (within a 50 mile radius)

Transportation

It is imperative that life-saving tasks be undertaken before moving the casualty. Once completed, then transportation of these casualties can be divided into two groups: those without radiation exposure and those with radiation exposure. Patients without exposure to radiation require no special transport consideration. Those exposed to radiation require removal of contaminated external clothing and covering with two large sheets. Care must be taken to decontaminate the evacuation vehicle.

An initial response team will usually evacuate the casualty to the initial treatment area where the medical team will be given a status on the type of radiation level of contamination [7]. The casualty is then taken through a decontamination procedure in a "dirty area," removing all garments and being cleansed with copious amounts of water.

Once this has been achieved, the casualty is then rechecked for radiation. If contaminants still exist, the casualty is further washed with copious amounts of water and a detergent, and the process is repeated. If radiation-free, the individual is then taken to the "clean area" where he/she can undergo further medical treatment.

Treatment should be extremely limited. For example, intravenous cannulation may introduce radioactive products into the general circulation; intubation may cause radioactive substances to be forced into the upper airways and lung parenchymal tissues. The inhalation of these substances will cause substantial internal radiation, as it is extremely difficult to remove once inhaled.

Ideally, this process must be carried out for all casualties. However, as one can appreciate, if a nuclear device were to be detonated in a large populace, then carrying out the above required decontamination would rapidly use up all available medical resources and present a massive challenge to the command and control structure, especially with regard to who to prioritize for medical treatment.

The sheer power of the initial blast wave is enough to vaporize majority of structures around the detonation zone.

Hospital Care

Initial management of a casualty, as with any medical problem, is the most important phase. However, this is not as simple as it seems. The priority for the individual is for decontamination and administration of potassium iodide—to reduce the uptake of I^{131}. This is one of the many daughter products of nuclear fission of Plutonium and will help reduce the risk of developing thyroid neoplasms.

It is difficult to ascertain what dose of radiation an individual has been exposed to. The diagnosis of radiation sickness is based primarily upon the clinical picture presented by the patient, as radiation dosimetry is unreliable, and also varies based on the organ system primarily affected. Individuals may not realize that they have been exposed to radiation, especially if it is due to fallout.

In order to measure the amount of radiation received, one must obtain samples of sputum, nasal swabs, and urinalysis to check for the amount of radioactive contaminants. Whole body radioactive imaging is also available, but this proves to be time consuming.

A relatively simple test to establish the severity of radiation exposure can be obtained by measuring lymphocytes in the blood [8]. An initial sample must be immediately taken within the first 24 h followed by additional samples. A useful rule of thumb is, if lymphocytes have decreased by 50% and are less than $1000/mm^3$, then the patient has received significant radiation exposure.

Injuries sustained due to the blast wave are directly proportional to the magnitude of the blast. In the majority of cases, the shearing forces between the tissue planes are severe enough to irreparably damage organs/organ systems. Individuals, for example, with blast lung have a very poor chance of survival—the only curative process would be a total lung transplant. Even if this was the case, it is highly unlikely that the lungs are the only organs to be damaged. People generally die in blast injuries due to multisystem failure.

The major complicating factor in a blast wave from a nuclear explosion is that it is highly unlikely that overpressures will be the sole contributors to bodily damage. It is almost impossible not to have airborne missiles within the blast wave. Luckily, the majority of missile injuries caused by nuclear weapons will, in general, be low velocity in nature, and severe injuries may be survived since extensive tissue cavitation would not be a factor. However, greater than 90% of people who have sustained penetrating trauma and the majority of individuals having sustained severe blunt trauma will have some form of vascular injury.

Conclusions

Thankfully the use of nuclear weapons and nuclear disasters is exceedingly rare. However, these incidents carry with them unique considerations from a medical treatment, logistical, and organizational point of view, and each jurisdiction should have a plan in place for such circumstances.

Key Points

- Nuclear disasters can present with a spectrum of manifestations, each with its own challenges.
- The key is to evacuate casualties and limit exposure to radiation to both them and relief personnel.
- A command center should be established in a non-contaminated region, to assess the extent of damage and contamination and to implement control and treatment measures.

References

1. Shigematsu I. The 2000 Sievert Lecture—lessons from atomic bomb survivors in Hiroshima and Nagasaki. Health Phys [Historical Article Lectures]. 2000;79(3):234–41.
2. Hall EJ. Lessons we have learned from our children: cancer risks from diagnostic radiology. Pediatr Radiol [Lectures Research Support, US Gov't, PHS]. 2002;32(10):700–6.
3. Sharma PP. Chernobyl & Fukushima: lessons to be learnt. Indian J Surg. 2011;73(3):173–4.
4. Matsuda N, Kumagai A, Ohtsuru A, Morita N, Miura M, Yoshida M, et al. Assessment of internal exposure doses in Fukushima by a whole body counter within one month after the nuclear power plant accident. Radiat Res. 2013;179(6):663–8.
5. Tanigawa K, Hosoi Y, Hirohashi N, Iwasaki Y, Kamiya K. Evacuation from the restricted zone of the damaged Fukushima nuclear power plant: facing with the reality. Resuscitation [Letter]. 2011;82(9):1248.
6. Fischer L, Kimose HH, Spjeldnaes N, Wara P. Late radiation injuries of the small intestine—management and outcome. Acta Chir Scand. 1989;155(1):47–51.
7. Chin FK. Scenario of a dirty bomb in an urban environment and acute management of radiation poisoning and injuries. Singapore Med J. 2007;48(10):950–7.
8. Berger ME, Christensen DM, Lowry PC, Jones OW, Wiley AL. Medical management of radiation injuries: current approaches. Occup Med (Lond) [Research Support, US Gov't, Non-PHS Review]. 2006;56(3):162–72.

Further Reading

Gusev IA, Guskova AK, Mettler FA. Medical management of radiation accidents. 2nd ed. Fig. 3.1:24.

Ionising Radiation Regulations 1999. Health and safety executive. Government of United Kingdom.

North Atlantic Treaty Organisation. Medical effects of ionising radiation on personnel. STANAG 2866.

North Atlantic Treaty Organisation. Medical support operations in an NBC environment. AmedP-7; STANAG 2873.

North Atlantic Treaty Organisation. NATO handbook on the medical aspects of NBC defensive operations. AmedP-6(B).

Radiation (Emergency Preparedness and Public Information) Regulations 2001. Health and safety executive. Government of United Kingdom.

Trauma and Surgical Capabilities for Space Exploration

58

David J. Alexander

Introduction

Surgeries in space have always been a distinct possibility in the space program. Several studies have been performed to quantify the risk of surgical events in spaceflight using analogs. These studies have shown that illnesses and injuries that require major surgery should be rare [1, 2]. If these events do occur, they can have critical impacts to the mission. These include mission aborts and partial or complete return from low Earth orbit. If these events were to occur on an exploration class mission away from low Earth orbit, the consequences could be devastating. Major surgery, if performed, will impact numerous areas of mission planning and performance. Significant amount will need to be invested in crew training and logistics.

Only noninvasive surgical procedures have been performed on humans thus far. The advantage to being in low Earth orbit is that one can stabilize an astronaut and return in an 8–24 h time period. Throughout the construction phases of the International Space Station (ISS), there was an increased risk of trauma, lacerations, crush injuries, and thermal or electrical burns. The careful planning of the individual phases of construction, with crew safety being a principal concern, resulted in no severe injuries occurring. This is not to say there have not been close calls in the history of spaceflight. On the Soviet space program mission Salyut 7, a cosmonaut experienced severe abdominal pain. This was thought to be appendicitis. This later proved more likely an episode of ureterolithiasis. The cosmonaut recovered and did not require early evacuation. An astronaut on ISS Expedition 30/31 also developed abdominal pain, but was determined by ultrasound on orbit not to be a surgical problem. Numerous minor procedures have been performed aboard the ISS. These principally involve minor superficial lacerations that are common. Although falls do not occur in microgravity, the movement of large masses has resulted in pinched fingers. Uneven surfaces due to excessive use or, in rare cases, bad design have also resulted in superficial injuries.

Exploration missions have an increasing risk of injuries. These are missions beyond low Earth orbit and likely to other planets. The crewmembers will be exposed to gravitational forces that increase the risk of injury. Falls are to be considered in the planning of future missions. The risk of orthopedic injuries will increase with deep exploration missions due to the bone and muscle degradation that occurs in microgravity. The deconditioning in the cardiovascular system also jeopardizes the responses a crewmember can recruit to combat traumatic conditions. Exercise countermeasures to counteract these microgravity effects place the individuals at risk for minor or major orthopedic injuries. Surgical conditions such as appendicitis, cholecystitis, and ureterolithiasis can occur randomly and are a risk for surgical intervention. There is also the possibility that a surgical condition could arise from long duration spaceflight that was previously unpredicted. Wound healing is delayed in microgravity conditions and will affect recovery time. It has been also shown that immunosuppression occurs with spaceflight and may complicate postoperative healing.

Exploration missions will necessitate careful design of the surgical systems and crew training. The driving consideration is the autonomy of the system and crewmembers due to long separation from definitive medical facilities. Communication delays compound the issue as ready availability of consultants may not be possible. The surgical equipment manifested will be limited by weight, power, volume, and lighting in the vehicles. Training on the unique surgical equipment for spaceflight will impact the time a crewmember spends pre-mission in preparation for these contingencies. The crew makeup should include a crew medical officer, specifically trained to handle these situations. Even if a physician is placed on the crew, he will have to maintain the skills required to perform surgical procedures.

D. J. Alexander (✉)
Flight Medicine Johnson Space Center, Houston, TX, USA
e-mail: david.j.alexander@nasa.gov

L. Marshall Gillman, S. Widder (eds.), *Trauma Team Dynamics*, https://doi.org/10.1007/978-3-031-86312-7_58

There is also the psychological impact of being confined and the gravity of a fellow member of a close-knit crew requiring surgery.

The effects of solar radiation are a real concern, and much needs to be learned about spaceflight beyond the limits of the Van Allen radiation belts. In the next section, we will explore the physiological challenges of spaceflight. These take a high priority in trauma treatment for any space exploration mission with prolonged journeys in microgravity or total weightless states.

Physiological Challenges in Spaceflight

There are essentially no differences in physiologic responses between microgravity (low Earth orbit and still under the minimal gravitational pull of the Earth) and zero gravity (away from planetary gravitational forces). For this chapter, essentially they will be treated as interchangeable terms. A vast majority of the experience with spaceflight has been in low Earth orbit or the microgravity environment. Astronauts in microgravity have physiological changes that put them at risk for surgical procedures. One of the biggest alterations in space travel is in the cardiovascular system. When the subject arrives in space, there is no longer a gravitational pull that drives the circulatory components toward the feet [3–5]. This results in a shift of fluid from the lower body to the head and torso. Since the cardiovascular system no longer fights gravity for fluid distribution, the stroke volume is decreased 10–20%. The resultant fluid shift initiates a diuresis resulting in a 10–23% volume reduction which is roughly equivalent to a grade one hemorrhage [6–8]. These changes are seen in the first 24 h of spaceflight. There is an initial 17% reduction in plasma volume that is compounded by transiently increased levels of hematocrit. This appears to cause a decrease in erythropoietin secretion causing a reduction in the mass of red blood cells [9]. The net effect is an overall reduction of about 10% in total blood volume upon entry into the microgravity environment. Cardiovascular reserve is definitely reduced, and the sympathetic responses are altered with greater beta-receptor sensitivity. This has the possibility of preventing the required vasoconstriction needed to combat a traumatic or surgically induced insult [3, 10, 11]. This process is actually started if the astronaut is in a prolonged lying position with the legs elevated above the trunk. This triggers the perceived fluid overload by the kidneys and will activate the concomitant diuresis [12].

Evidence exists that raises the issue of impaired wound healing on orbit [13]. Research done on shuttle flights indicated that incisions performed in microgravity had greater inflammatory responses, fibroplasia, and collagen deposition. There was also evidence of reduced stress loading. During the STS-90 shuttle mission, numerous surgical procedures were performed on rodents. Observationally there was no evidence of dehiscence or infection after 48 h. The incisions made in spaceflight appeared to heal well after surgery [13]. Another area of concern is the loss of bone density with weightlessness. No longer is there a static gravitational load on the skeletal structure. The loads normally imparted by running or walking terrestrially are not present. With lack of a straining force, the bone no longer undertakes remodeling and reinforcement [14]. Other factors that compound the effect are loss of direct sunlight with reduction in vitamin D. Also chronically elevated CO_2 leads to acidosis and reabsorption of the bicarbonate in bone [15–17]. The weight-bearing areas of the bone bear the greatest impact. The lumbar vertebrae, pelvis, femoral neck, trochanter, tibia, and calcaneus lose about 1–2% per month. A 6-month mission on board the ISS can result in the loss of 8–12% of bone mass [16]. Individuals display a wide variety in total amount and the sites of bone loss. The supplementation of vitamin D and the use of resistive exercise regimes have definitely made a positive improvement in prevention of bone loss. The demineralization increases the risk of bone fractures on orbit. This also may have an impact on the risk of fracture in travel to distant planets. The likelihood of fracture would increase initially post landing as the astronauts would be required to do work in the new gravitational plane. Terrestrially more than half of trauma cases admitted to hospitals are for long bone trauma [18]. A long-bone fracture on a microgravity mission is potentially disastrous. Experimental bone fractures in microgravity resulted in impaired callus formation and reduced angiogenesis. Bone healing studies of rodents that were placed in orbit on a Russian biosatellite showed decreased osteoblasts, osteoblastic activity, and reduced angiogenesis in the bone [19]. It is unknown at this time if having no static loading will result in malunion. Immobilization would be a simple matter of splinting, but if a traction force is needed, then external fixation would be in order. One advantage to microgravity is that the risk of fat embolization would probably be reduced.

One factor that needs to be accounted for is the immune system and cellular alterations. The cellular immunity seems to be suppressed in microgravity. Consistently neutropenia, lymphocytopenia, and overall diminished white cell populations are seen. On the individual cell level, there are notable decreases in cellular mobility and interleukin production [19]. Also of note is the occurrence of delayed cutaneous hypersensitivity which indicates an alteration of cell-mediated immunity [20]. These alterations in cellular function would have an impact on the initial inflammatory reactions for wound healing. This increases the likelihood of postoperative infections and increases the risk of sepsis. This may also increase the risk of appendicitis, cholecystitis, and other surgical infectious diseases. Add to this the problem of impaired cellular functions is the "contaminated" environment of the space vehicle. A closed environment with little direct sunlight and difficulties in cleaning the environment lead to increases in microorganisms. Observational studies have revealed an increase in the bacterial growth as compared to the terrestrial environment [21]. The bacteria have thicker cell walls to contend with. This adds to the inhibitory and penetration requirements for antibiotics. The bacteria colonies grown from the Apollo-Soyuz mission displayed increased antibiotic resistance as compared to pre- and post-flight colonies [21]. Manifesting antibiotics to combat these consequences would be critical.

There are a large number of issues surrounding surgery in microgravity. These include, but not limited to the following:

1. Providing and maintaining a sterile field.
2. Maintaining hemostasis.
3. Adequate lighting and exposure—if minimally invasive surgery is used, then adequate visualization by cameras and monitors.
4. Intravenous fluid replacement or blood infusion—examining the pros and cons of blood substitutes and onboard IV fluid generation to reduce up mass of the vehicle.
5. Preventing contamination of the surgical field and the spacecraft—the vehicle likely will use a closed-loop system and will recirculate the atmosphere. Also blood and body fluids have corrosive effects on equipment and surfaces.
6. Providing anesthesia and monitoring.
7. Diagnostic imaging and laboratories required for diagnosis.
   (a) Provisions for ultrasound
   (b) Possible use of endoscopic procedures—laparoscopy, thoracoscopy, cystoscopy, colonoscopy, and esophagoscopy
   (c) Miniaturization of CT/MRI scanners
   (d) Miniaturized and multifunctional lab equipment
8. Accounting for microgravity.
   (a) Restraining the patient and operator to prevent free floating
   (b) Restraining equipment and still readily available in the procedure
   (c) Physiology changes in microgravity—increased risk of intracranial hypertension
   (d) Changes in fluid dynamics that affect the behavior of bleeding and drainage
      - Suctioning
      - Drainage systems modification—functions of cutting and needle insertion will need to be combined with drainage.
   (e) Changes in physical landmarks and shifting of internal organs
9. Modifying advanced life support and defibrillation techniques—limited crew size and space will necessitate compression devices. Also defibrillation will need to be isolated from the vehicle to prevent computer and electrical damage.
10. Waste management—this includes temporary storage during the procedure.
    (a) Contaminated waste
    (b) Needle and sharp disposal
11. Postoperative recovery.

These issues will be explored in more depth in the following sections.

Historical Perspective

Much of the experimentation in surgical capabilities has been with the realization that emergent surgical diseases may occur with prolonged zero-gravity travel. The primary concern recently has been a concern of trauma that may occur with the assembly and maintenance of the ISS. In the future, prolonged zero-gravity transits to planetary surfaces will likely increase the risk of traumatic or emergent surgical conditions. Dr. Iaroshenko experimented with rodents at the Russian Space Agency in 1967 [22]. Since that time, there have been numerous efforts to provide the foundation of surgery in space. The US Space Program history has seen advances in medical equipment and procedures. The Mercury and Gemini programs only carried basic diagnostic equipment to measure physiological changes in spaceflight. Monitoring of blood pressure, pulse, and respiration was a normal procedure. The only medical kits were those deemed necessary for an off-nominal landing in an austere environment. The Apollo spacecraft carried only a rudimentary medical kit for simple medical problems. The Skylab missions had a minor surgical kit to close superficial lacerations [23]. The Space Shuttle medical system had the Shuttle Orbiter Medical System (SOMS kit) and was divided into three parts. One part of the medical emergency kit has a stethoscope, a blood pressure cuff, sutures, disposable thermometers, and medicines that could be injected. The second part of the kit contains adhesive tape, gauze bandages, adhesive bandages, and a variety of oral medicines. The third section contained an instrumentation pack, an oxygen-cycled respirator, intravenous fluid, and a defibrillator. Specialized medicines and equipment could also be added, depending on the requirements of the individual mission. The SOMS kit weighed 20 pounds and could be placed in one of the mid-deck lockers. One of the components was a minor surgical kit for laceration closure. This had conventional instruments that were individually wrapped, which made the logistics of wound closure slightly more complicated than a single sterile pack. Local anesthetics were also included. Items also included in the pack were simple closure items, such as sterile strips, Dermabond ampules, and staples. The hardware on the Mir space station was similar to the Space Shuttle medical system. On board the ISS, the medical system is divided up into sub-packs. Of particular note was that the most famous use of the SOMS kit was not in a human laceration repair. On the STS-117 mission, the Space Shuttle Atlantis was damaged during ascent. A corner of the thermal blanket on the port orbital maneuvering system peeled back, leaving a triangular 4-inch × 6-inch gap. The surgical staple gun was used to repair the damage in a spacewalk (Fig. 58.1). It was discovered through testing that the staples could withstand 5000 °F temperatures for a length of time adequate to deorbit the vehicle.

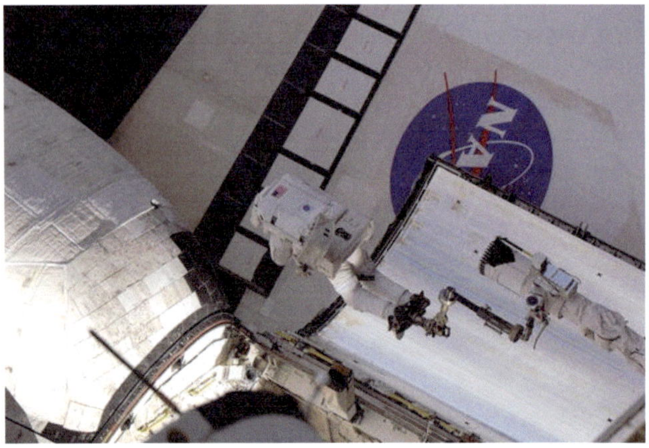

Fig. 58.1 Extravehicular activity during STS-117 to repair the damaged thermal blanket using a surgical staple gun

Parabolic Testing

Numerous procedures were validated in human and animal studies on the microgravity aircraft. The parabolic microgravity program uses an aircraft to simulate low-gravity states induced by parabolic flight. The aircraft pulls up into a 45° nose high attitude and climbs about 5000 ft. At that point, the aircraft pushes the nose over to about 45° nose low (Figs. 58.2 and 58.3). At the top of the parabola, a microgravity state is induced for about 20–30 s. The maneuver is repeated 30–40 times in order to simulate spaceflight conditions for equipment and procedure validation. The problem is that it is only a short duration of time to apply the procedures, but this is the only adequate simulation of the microgravity state available currently. Both the Russian and US space programs have used parabolic flights to evaluate medical procedures and equipment. In 1967, the Russian space program evaluated laparotomies on parabolic flights. The system utilized a transparent surgical canopy with a magnetic instrument holder. It was noticed that the procedures went fairly well. The one complication noted was that arterial bleeding formed droplet streams that spread throughout the containment area decreasing visualization. Bowel evisceration during laparotomy could also obscure the visual field [24]. The US parabolic experimental program found that surgical procedures could be performed with only minor modifications. The requirement for restraining the patient, surgical hardware, and the surgical personnel had to be stringently observed [25]. The patient, even if awake for a minor surgical procedure, must remain restrained. The operating personnel must also be limited in motion from the waist down, but leave the arms and hands free of obstructions.

Bleeding and free blood could be contained with common surgical methods of sponges and suction, but must be addressed immediately [26]. All phases of surgical proce-

Fig. 58.2 NASA parabolic flight profile

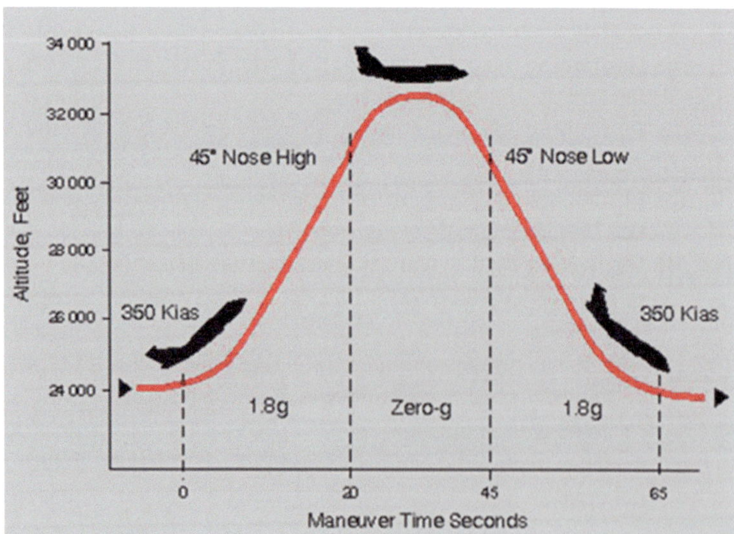

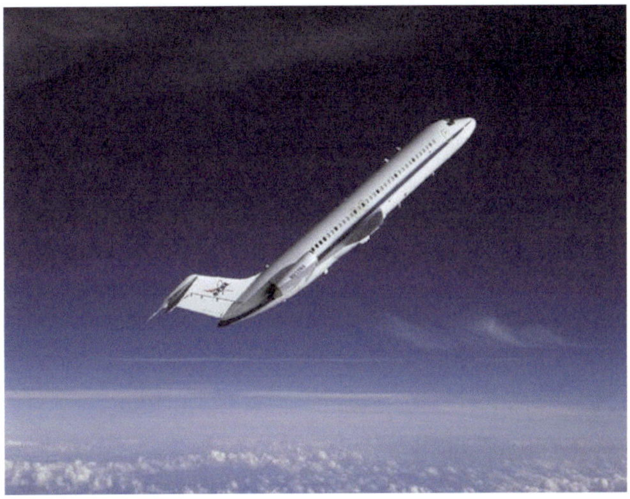

Fig. 58.3 NASA C-9 microgravity aircraft

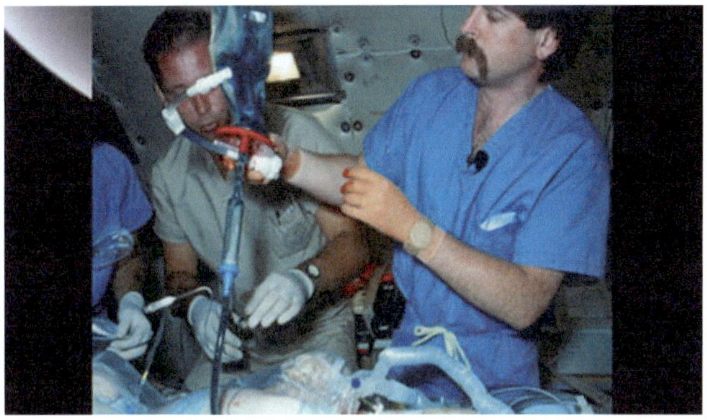

Fig. 58.4 Enclosed surgical field testing on NASA microgravity aircraft

dures have been evaluated. Prepping, draping, equipment prep, and restraining have all been proven in microgravity. Lighting and enclosed environments have also been validated. Again, the emphasis has been on adequate restraint of the equipment. Glove packages must have tape on the backing to secure them, and commercially available surgical drapes with an adhesive band proved to be excellent solutions for microgravity operations. Conventional antiseptics had enough surface tension to remain in place as well [27–29].

It was found that procedure-oriented kits were preferable to individually packaged instruments. Extra packaging became an encumbrance. Standard Velcro, elastic cords, and magnetic surgical tables helped to contain the instruments. Sharp blocks (a block of Styrofoam for sharps), an adhesive pad, and a plastic bag near the surgical table or as a pocket on a gown were used to facilitate rapid trash disposal. Maintaining an organized surgical table and rapid trash disposal are critical in the microgravity arena. This facilitated speeding the procedures and maintaining a good visual field [29]. The ISS uses a floor-level restraint system that was developed from similar devices flown on the Space Shuttle and Russian Mir space station. The CMRS (Crew Medical Restraint System) can act also as a backboard for patient transport if needed. It is easily stored and has built-in belts to restrain patients and operating personnel. There is even a built-in cervical restraint system.

Surgical Field Testing

One of the major impedances to surgical care in microgravity (low Earth orbit) or zero gravity (away from planetary gravitational forces) is the atmospheric contamination of the vehicles' atmosphere with blood or other body fluids. The closed-loop systems could easily be overwhelmed with surgical debris and blood [30]. The spacecraft also presents a hazard to the surgical site. The clean vehicle at launch accumulates dross that increases the risk of contamination of the wound area. Particles tend to be larger and contain dust, food particles, and sloughed skin elements. In a limited space environment, the surgical zone may be in close proximity to the galley or exercise facilities. Also there can be numerous scattered areas or waste disposal. This may aid in surgical trash disposal, but it would also be a potential source of contamination for the procedure. Long-duration spaceflight has shown to produce immunosuppression and altered immune responses [31, 32]. Impaired healing of wounds has also been seen. A system for contaminant containment for the field and prevention of infectious contamination of the surgical site are requisite requirements (Fig. 58.4).

The Russian space community built several enclosed systems and tested them in parabolic flights [24, 32]. In 1978, an inflatable Lexan surgical enclosed bubble was proposed by Mutke [33]. Markham and Rock tested several inflatable enclosures and simulated surgical procedures in parabolic flight [34–36]. These proved to be quite successful at containing floating instruments, solids, and fluids. NASA tested a similar inflatable canopy [32]. Anesthetized animals were used as surgical subjects, and the systems were evaluated for ease of use, portability, and containment. It was noted during these experiments that venous bleeding appeared to be increased. It was surmised to be due to an inability of the venous walls to provide compression in microgravity. Unopposed surface tension caused both arterial and venous areas of bleeding to form large fluid domes [26]. Arterial bleeding was not entrapped by sponges or suction when a large stream of droplets was formed. The overhead canopy placed over the surgical area would be useful in containing uncontrolled bleeding or if copious irrigation was required. Another method of containing contaminants in a surgical field is the use of laminar flow devices. The airflow would direct the fluid or other detritus into a downstream suction collection device. NASA also tested this concept in parabolic flight. Bleeding and debris not restrained by local methods were swept away from the visual field directly over the open wound. Still most bleeding was controlled by surgical sponges, gauze, or suction directly at the site.

Surgical and Advanced Life Support Procedures

NASA conducted numerous parabolic flights to test operative and resuscitative techniques in a microgravity environment. These tests were conducted to see what procedures could be done, how the equipment behaved, and if the procedures could be done with minimal equipment. The crew medical officer (CMO) for each journey may be a non-physician. Cardiopulmonary resuscitation (CPR) was found to be more difficult in lower-gravity environments, but can be accomplished. It was reinforced that restraint of both the subject and the rescuer was critical in most situations. The "handstand" procedure of placing one's feet on the wall opposite to the victim's chest and placing the CMOs hands over his head and on the chest was found to be effective. Also the Heimlich method of standing behind the victim and performing CPR was validated as providing adequate CPR [37–39]. Ventilation support with artificial ventilators was performed, and the parameters were unchanged from the terrestrial environment. Similarly, respiratory mechanics on ventilatory support was not clinically different [40].

ALS (Advanced Life Support) procedures of venous cutdowns, cricothyroidotomies, peritoneal lavages, and chest tube insertions were also evaluated. These proved to be more difficult than in normal gravity. Fluid infusions and drainage systems required modifications to the techniques. Intravenous fluids had to have all the free air removed and required fluid pumps to infuse the fluids. Pressurizing the fluids with external pressure bags did work well. Drainage lines had to be as short as possible and large in diameter to prevent surface tension and capillary action from inhibiting flow. Percutaneous peritoneal lavage was more dangerous. The GI tract is more dilated due to decreased peristalsis in low-gravity environments. This resulted in additional pressure of the bowel on the abdominal wall and increased the risk of perforation. A modification of the technique would be required to increase the air in the abdominal cavity to decrease this likelihood. Another complicating factor was that the increased fluid tension and lack of capillary fluid pull led to decreased lavage fluid drainage. An advantage to this procedure is that it required less training than their open lavage counterpart. Open peritoneal lavage techniques were accomplished, but required more training and the use of surgical canopies.

Chest tube insertion was also performed on the surgical evaluation parabolic flights. The equipment employed incorporated a Heimlich valve and a Sorenson drainage system. This proved to provide adequate drainage and eliminated the risk of contamination from the vehicle environment. Another advantage was that the blood from a hemothorax in this type of system could be used to autotransfuse a trauma victim [41–43]. A percutaneous Seldinger dilatation method proved easy to train, required only a minimal amount of equipment, and did not require a dedicated surgical field. Suture ties around the chest tube site to secure the tube had to perform several functions and were critical in the procedure. Studies have shown that suturing in microgravity is similar but slower than normogravity [44]. They had to retain the tube in position and control fluid and blood leakage. Chest tube drainage generally did not require suction, because the intrathoracic pressure provided the push to the drainage system. The advantage of a chest tube placed in microgravity was that the hemothorax fluid was equally distributed along the chest wall in an adherent sheet rather than pooling in a dependent location. Some loculation did occur though by surface tension, but overall was not as critical as in a one-G environment. The procedure only encompassed about 1 h of ground-based instruction and could possibly be done by computer-based training (CBT). Telemedicine guidance of peritoneal lavage and chest tube insertion could also be done by a remotely located surgeon.

Other surgical procedures have been performed in the simulated microgravity environment. Leg dissection, thoracotomy, laparotomy, and craniotomy were simulated. Specifically craniectomy, C-section, and laminectomy were conducted on the STS-90 Neurolab flight [45]. Other procedures included ureteral stenting, thoracoscopy, and microsurgery [46–48]. The evaluation of surgical skills in these major procedures demonstrates equivocal results. Subjective evaluation suggests that surgical procedural performance decreases when the operator is not acclimated to the microgravity environment which may further lead to task erosion and subsequent tissue injury.

Numerous evaluations of endoscopy and laparoscopy have been performed [45, 47, 49, 50]. The concerns observed during these procedures were the potential for impaired visualization due to lack of bowel retraction from gravity. Also floating debris of blood and detached materials could impede the visual field. The elastic mesenteric tethering of the bowel in position and fluid surface tension caused surgical detritus to adhere to the abdominal wall. Parabolic flights proved insightful with animal subjects used to simulate the human equivalent. The endoscopic tools and procedures proved to be feasible and comparable to the one-G environment. Abdominal laparoscopy has the advantage of providing a natural surgical canopy by the subject's own body.

The weight of the abdominal wall causes the abdominal cavity to form a flattened oval. This oval in microgravity is changed to a more rounded shape. This leads to an increase in the anterior to posterior diameter and increases the visual field. This actually facilitates minimally invasive abdominal procedures. Other advantages of minimally invasive surgeries are preventing contamination of the cabin with biological particulates, preventing abdominal contamination, maintaining thermal regulation, and possible blood collection and autotransfusion [51, 52].

Minimally invasive surgeries (MIS) have several drawbacks. Thoracoscopy presents a different set of problems from laparoscopy. In the microgravity environment, the retraction of the mediastinum by gravity is not present. This causes anatomical obscuration of the visual field. Selective bronchial intubation, pulmonary segmental deflation, and chest insufflation would be required to make a thoracoscopic procedure viable. It is very difficult to establish a pneumoperitoneum without direct visualization of the abdomen and has a high risk of bowel perforation. Minimally invasive surgeries still remain limited in the management of multitrauma cases [53, 54]. There are numerous publications that have raised the question on the use of MIS in critically ill patients [55–57]. This raises questions if an injured astronaut can tolerate the increased intra-abdominal pressures required for MIS [58]. Astronauts have reduced red cell counts and plasma volumes and decreased cardiac output which put the crewmembers at risk for injury and may be compounded with the stresses of laparoscopy.

In any minimally invasive surgical procedure, the CMO would need to have the training, ability, and experience specific to endoscopic procedures in order to perform them. Highly trained surgeons with considerable proficiency would be required to perform these procedures. Also significant deskilling occurs when a surgeon does not continually practice these procedures. It would require a simulated surgical environment to accompany the mission to remain proficient in these skills. Several studies have been undertaken to reduce the required training and skill-level retention to accomplish minimally invasive surgical procedures. Broderick et al. investigated simulating hand-assisted laparoscopy in parabolic flights [51]. Dulchavsky has also proposed the method of using mini-laparoscopes for peritoneal drainage with telemonitoring [47].

New methods and equipment have been developed making space surgery a more viable and easier option. Miniaturization of laparoscopic equipment has made the possibility of these procedures even more viable. Large amounts of supporting equipment are no longer required for most procedures. A portable computer had substituted for large bulky video monitors, and fiber optics can provide adequate lighting and visualization of the field. Stereoscopic three-dimensional displays are coming online that can be incorporated into virtual reality headgear. Abdominal wall lift devices are in development that may eliminate the need for CO_2 or N_2 insufflation [59]. This would allow the abdominal wall to be retracted anteriorly improving the visual field and allow the mesenteric attachments to hold the bowel in place. The change in the abdominal wall shape is different with lift devices than with insufflation. The viscera have a higher propensity to float and obscure the visual field in the intra-abdominal compartment [60]. Controlling hemorrhage is made easier by fibrin glue injectors, laser scalpels, and advanced stapling devices. Tissue sealants and fibrin glues have been compounded into a foam and easily applied. These have been found to be more effective than surgical packing currently in use [61]. A device now is in development that can detect vascular flow prior to cutting and suturing. This uses pulsatile light absorption characteristics of hemoglobin to noninvasively characterize hidden blood vessels. By using a multichannel LED/sensor pair that employs NIR and red light, blood vessels can be detected and vessel size determined. This would help avoid unintended cuts to the vasculature caused by poor visibility in a minimally invasive procedure. Such a device prevents the obscuration of the visual field by streams of blood caused by inadvertent vessel injury [62].

Accessing disease pathology via an intraluminal route is a revolution in medicine. This has been demonstrated in trauma, vascular surgery, and cardiology care. Access to the central circulation also enhances hemodynamic support and measurements and can enhance guided interventional angiographic therapies. It also can provide an extremely efficient method to administer specific pharmacologic treatments. Via central venous access, inotropes and vasopressors can be administered safely. Vasopressors may be required in the treatment of space-adapted physiology. Heparin-bonded extracorporeal circuits are used in multisystem trauma for both rapid rewarming and also facilitating hemodynamic support [63, 64]. Doppler-guided needles are currently available and smart ultrasound-guided "bibs" that use automated algorithms for vascular identification are being developed [65, 66]. In the future, full robotic control may be possible for cannula insertion and diagnostic assessment. This offers some real advantages in deep exploration missions and may reduce the training required for these missions.

Telerobotics and telepresence are offering an increase in precision and the ability to operate from long distances. They offer the capability to enhance the images and dexterity of the individual surgeon. Telemedicine also has the capability to provide consultation and even surgical procedures to be performed from a distance. Investigations have shown that operating across continents and to undersea environments can be accomplished [67, 68]. While these techniques might be practical in low Earth orbit, they would be inhibited by communication delays outside of that realm. A Mars mission could not avail itself of telemedicine. Electronic delays from 8 to 40 min would render this option impossible.

Surgical Procedures in Space

The Space Shuttle Neurolab mission on STS-90 conducted the first surgical procedures on animals in orbit. A leg wound was created and then closed with Dermabond adhesive. Several other procedures were conducted on that mission and provided insight and verified parabolic experiments of surgical procedures in space. The mission confirmed that the procedures were only as difficult as the ones performed on Earth. Spaceflight experience also demonstrated that there were no obvious changes in manual dexterity, proprioception, or fine motor control of the hand. It reinforced the principle that restraint of the operator, patient, and surgical equipment was critical. It took a diligent effort to contain equipment in place and immediately discard any trash. Procedures took longer because of the need to assure restraint of the equipment. It was noticeable that fluids coalesced and surface tension predominated in microgravity. Sponging and suction at the site of bleeding controlled the environment and allowed continued visualization of the field. Scalpels and needles required special care, but that restraint on Styrofoam blocks proved adequate. If not restrained, loose needles needed to be called out and identified immediately in order to prevent accidental punctures.

Diagnostics

The physiological alterations that occur in the spaceflight environment will impact disease presentation, diagnostic evaluation, treatment, and management. Ultrasonography has proved to be the most valuable diagnostic tool in spaceflight. Exams such as the extended focused assessment with sonography for trauma (eFAST) to evaluate the need for emergent surgical intervention have been proven on orbit [69–73]. Ultrasound (US) is dependent on gravity to locate free fluid in the thorax and abdomen. Thus far surface tension has caused these to form on orbit, but may not be counted on in all situations. Ultrasound evaluation has been shown to delineate several conditions, including pneumothoraces and sinus fluid levels [72, 74, 75]. The development of three-dimensional US displays has led to improvements in analysis of injuries in acute abdomens. It can better quantify volumes of fluid when compared to two-dimensional US [76, 77]. US contrast media may also be used to help quantify and follow any hemorrhages in real time [78]. Future developments may include the use of integrated computer programs to help predict the progression of an injury. Hoyt's research predicted survivable outcomes based on terrestrial volumes of hemorrhage to be 2 h if the bleeding was determined to be 25 ml of bleeding per minute. If bleeding exceeded 100 ml/min, a mortal outcome could be expected in 30 min if bleeding was uncontrolled [79]. Programs could be generated based on the physiological changes encountered in spaceflight.

US can also be utilized as an interventional device. It has been utilized for guided percutaneous aspiration of intraperitoneal fluid using a swine model in microgravity [80]. US requires user-dependent skills and requires dedicated training for the onboard operators. Current efforts guide less-experienced users from Mission Control using skilled experts who remotely mentor the onboard astronauts. This will require onboard trained ultrasonographers for deep space missions [81, 82]. NASA scientists have created a research program to facilitate minimally trained crew medical officers to use US autonomously and/or using remote guidance [71, 82]. US offers the greatest potential currently, but miniaturized CT or MRI scanners are also being developed that can be adapted for space travel. These will require specialized operators or automated diagnostic tools for immediate analysis. More than likely images can be transmitted back to consultants for analysis. Thus both diagnostic evaluation and interventional techniques could be performed in microgravity with the use of ultrasound-dependent techniques. A noninvasive way to perform surgery is by focused ultrasound. This can be used to ablate or emulsify soft tissue tumors in the tissues of the abdomen, brain, and heart. It offers a method to also treat benign prostatic hyperplasia and possibly bone cancer. Ultrasonic atomization causes mechanical tissue disruption by boiling histotripsy. Ultrasonic atomization occurs by having an ultrasound wave in liquid encountering an air interface. This interaction ejects small liquid droplets into the air. Boiling histotripsy was developed at the University of Washington that uses high-intensity focused ultrasound (HIFU). This HIFU is then used to fractionate tissue into its submicron components. The HIFU rapidly heats tissue as the transducer focuses to form a millimeter-diameter bubble of boiling material in milliseconds. This fractionates the tissue into its submicron components. This technology offers a method of noninvasive precise tissue atomization and is currently being explored for space usage [83].

Trauma Care in Space

Trauma stabilization and care on long-duration or long-distance mission presents unique difficulties in management. In these situations, the need for rapid evacuation can be a disastrous situation. Physiological alterations of microgravity, diminished immune systems, inexperienced or ill-equipped care providers, limited equipment, and extreme distance can conspire against a reasonable survival in traumatic injuries. The advantage of space exploration is that advanced procedures, training, and advanced technology can be incorporated into the design of these missions. These missions are analogous to rural trauma or trauma in undeveloped countries. Rural trauma in the United States shows that in distant populations, mortality can be up to 50% greater than urban populations. Trauma in rural populations accounts for 60% of deaths in the United States, despite only 20% of the population reside in these areas [84–86].

Crewmembers in orbit are hemodynamically challenged after 72 h in a microgravity environment. They have about a 15% decrease in circulating red blood cells and plasma volume. This is defined as a class I hemorrhage terrestrially. Another factor in space physiology that is unique is the blunting of cardiovascular reflexes. These combined result in a decreased ability for a crewmember in microgravity to respond to blood loss. This can result in a shortened time in which intervention can have the greatest effect. They immediately move into a class II type of hemorrhagic shock. The initial response to trauma must be rapid and consideration to fluid resuscitation must be given priority. As we have seen, ATLS procedures can be readily accomplished in the microgravity environment [40]. Intravenous access has been demonstrated experimentally and aboard the ISS. Securing an airway has also been demonstrated in parabolic flight using endotracheal intubation, laryngeal mask insertion, or surgical tracheostomy. A FAST (focused assessment with sonography for trauma) ultrasound can be utilized to evaluate for traumatic injury as well as confirm the endotracheal tube position [87, 88].

The truncal region requires surgical intervention to control internal bleeding. External pressure is not efficacious to control hemorrhage in this area. Ninety-nine percent of deaths are due to thoracic or abdominal bleeding [89, 90]. Ultrasound has been used to localize intrapleural, intraperitoneal, and retroperitoneal bleeding terrestrially, in parabolic flight and onboard space vehicles. It is as sensitive as terrestrial-based applications [69–73, 91]. Management of these injuries has changed due to rapid diagnostic procedures. No longer is explorative surgery required, and it has given way to observation and repeated scanning techniques. This also implies that surgical or intensive monitoring must be available in case there is recurrent hemorrhage. Observation may also be complicated by and require interventions in the cases of abscesses, pseudoaneurysms, urinomas, or biliomas. Many of these can be treated with percutaneous interventions and have been demonstrated in parabolic as well as actual spaceflights [80, 92]. These conditions still require surgical expertise if severe recurrent hemorrhage occurs. This would require specialized training and physician intervention [3, 93]. In the space environment, it may be better to intervene in a staged fashion rather than going directly to open procedures. In all of these cases, anesthetics would be required. Gaseous anesthetics have innumerable problems in a closed-loop environment. Re-inhalation and intoxication of the ones performing the interventions is a real risk. Also the incorporation of anesthetic decontamination equipment into the environmental control system may be space and cost prohibitive [3]. Intravenous anesthetic techniques are preferable and have been demonstrated in parabolic flights.

Immediate Damage Control Procedures

Severe shock and sepsis may demand an immediate surgical intervention before extensive diagnostics can localize the condition. A group of flight surgeons, trauma surgeons, and biomedical engineers emphasized that a laparotomy may be required to stabilize a patient prior to further procedures or deorbiting to Earth [94]. As discussed in Chaps. 30 and 31, the paradigm of only completing the necessary components via limited procedures is referred to as damage control (DC) surgery. These methods do not require prolonged procedures that tax the patient's physiological reserves. Also these procedures do not require extensive equipment outlays [8, 95]. These procedures are not significantly different from the terrestrial environment. Solid-organ bleeding can be tamponaded with packs around the offending organ. The abdominal wall can be left open for further procedures to follow. An open abdominal wall facilitates converting noncompressible bleeding into compressible visceral bleeding by direct methods. Fibrin glue and tissue sealants can also be used easily in these DC surgeries. These procedures have been demonstrated by physician extenders and non-surgeons [96]. These types of procedures would allow immediate DC surgery to be performed to stabilize the crewmembers' condition. Then planning and further diagnostics can take place with consultation with ground control. Then long-distance training or reviews and simulations can be undertaken to perform a definitive surgical procedure.

Orthopedic injuries lend themselves to damage control procedures. Fixation devices are easy to use and may be the most viable option. Plaster casting requires mixing plaster with water, and this takes up a valuable resource. Fiberglass casting materials produce large amounts of off-gassed products that must be accommodated by the environmental control system. These may not be easily removed. Flexible aluminum splints and elastic bandages can be used on the simpler fractures. Numerous fractures require gravity to heal the break or maintain reduction. Manual traction is difficult to apply in microgravity. Another concern is that bone healing is likely to be delayed in spaceflight [13, 14]. External fixation offers numerous advantages. The techniques for the most part are simple and rapid. They are not physiologically stressing and do not require extensive anesthesia applications. Their application will allow early mobilization, and if placed under tension, they may substitute for gravity and manual traction. US can be used to diagnose and evaluate the reduction [63, 97, 98]. This has been demonstrated in numerous studies [99–101]. The use of US can also be accomplished with external fixation in place.

Addressing these surgical challenges has led to unique solutions that have been incorporated into terrestrial care [102, 103]. Currently, computerized tomography (CT) and magnetic resonance imaging (MRI) are not done in microgravity environments. An MRI is possible as high-power magnets have been incorporated into the ISS particle physics experiments. The AMS-2 superconducting magnet has two coils of niobium-titanium producing a central field of 0.87 teslas. Numerous investigations are undergoing evaluation in the use of advanced US techniques that could be incorporated in the treatment of critically injured patients. These cover a range of subjects from diagnostic studies to addressing the crew training in advanced US techniques [47, 71, 82, 104]. The ISS has a US station aboard to conduct clinical and research efforts in the microgravity environment. The carotid intima-media thickness (CIMT) measurement was developed through a direct venture with NASA. CIMT uses the ArterioVision software initially developed at NASA's Jet Propulsion Lab (JPL). JPL's Image Processing Laboratory is tasked with the processing and interpretation of spacecraft imagery. NASA-invented Video Imaging Communication and Retrieval software has been used to process pictures from numerous space missions, including the Voyagers and Mars Reconnaissance Orbiter. Periodic upgrades of the imaging software have enabled greater accuracy and improved knowledge of our solar system. ArterioVision is incorporated into a standardized US examination of the carotid artery and produces the CIMT [105].

Crew Medical Officers

The CMO (crew medical officer) onboard the shuttle or ISS is not required to be a physician. They undergo 40–60 h of medical training to accomplish specific diagnostic and therapeutic interventions [106]. This includes a broad area of medical subjects, but they do not have the dedicated surgical expertise that a trained physician possesses. A general surgeon with specific training in the unique diagnostic and therapeutic interventions for a long-duration mission would be ideal. Other critical care or emergency physicians would also be excellent candidates. This mission specialist physician would also have other training in psychological support and intervention for a long-duration spaceflight. Their duties would include nonmedical functions in order to equitably distribute the workload of an extended mission. A caveat to this is that the medical specialist would also have the same physiological changes of microgravity and be susceptible to the same risks as the other crewmembers. Another crewmember will need to have some redundancy in capability. Telemedical support is available currently to the ISS, but will be more difficult as the distances grow larger on interplanetary missions. Telemedicine and telerobotics research are constantly ongoing to address many gaps in space medicine care [104]. On these interplanetary missions, acute care will need a large amount of autonomy and a large library of medical information available. Just in time computerized training will need to be available. Also procedural simulation programs can be made available to practice and retain skills. Each mission will have to be scrutinized, and specific requirements and personnel assignments will have to be made with the possibility of a critical medical event likely to occur.

Conclusions

There are numerous advantages of low Earth orbit. In dealing with trauma, having easy communication access to Mission Control and medical consultation resources offers huge potentials. Another advantage is having the option of deorbiting to more dedicated medical facilities. While initiatives to go further than the lunar surface are growing in reality, the option of an immediate return or easy communication with terrestrial resources diminishes with increasing distance. The International Space Station offers unique opportunities to test interventional procedures in order to provide care to traumatized or surgical patients. Landing on other planetary surfaces also increases the risk or trauma due to falls as well as construction injuries as support structures will need to be erected. All of the exploration activities will require dedicated planning to put in place dedicated trauma treatment equipment and personnel. Training will also need to be robust to cover these contingencies. We are explorers and risk takers. In order to minimize the risk, we must plan and test the future capabilities that will extend our reach beyond our terrestrial bonds.

Key Points

- Astronauts in microgravity have a decreased stroke volume, reduced circulating blood volume, suppressed cellular immunity, and impaired wound healing putting them at increased risk from trauma.
- Surgery in space faces many challenges including providing and maintaining a sterile field, maintaining hemostasis, and preventing contamination of both the surgical field and the surrounding environment.
- Imaging in space is also limited and currently relies heavily on ultrasound as the main imaging modality.
- The mission specialist physician on long-duration spaceflights will face multiple challenges including the performance of nonmedical functions in order to equitably distribute the workload, the need for a broad range of medical knowledge, and the ability to retain a specialized surgical skill set with potentially minimal opportunities to practice.

References

1. Wilken DD. Significant medical experiences aboard Polaris submarines: a review of 360 patrols during the period 1963–67, US Naval Submarine Medical Center Report, 560, Groton; 1969.
2. Tansey WA, Wilson JM, Schaefer KE. Analysis of health data from 10 years of Polaris submarine patrols. Undersea Biomed Res. 1979;6(Suppl):S217–46.
3. Kirkpatrick AW, Campbell MR, Novinkov OL, et al. Blunt trauma and operative care in microgravity: a review of microgravity physiology and surgical investigations with implications for critical care and operative treatment in space. J Am Coll Surg. 1997;184:441–53.
4. Kirkpatrick AW, Dulchavsky SA, Boulanger BR, et al. Extraterrestrial resuscitation of hemorrhagic shock: fluids. J Trauma. 2001;50:162–8.
5. Charles JB, Lathers CM. Cardiovascular adaptation to spaceflight. J Clin Pharmacol. 1991;31:1010–23.
6. Leach CS, Inners LD, Charles JB. Changes in total body water during space flight. J Clin Pharmacol. 1991;31:1001–6.
7. McCuaig KE, Houtchens BA. Management of trauma and emergency surgery in space. J Trauma. 1992;33:615–25.
8. Burch JM, Ortiz JB, Richardson J, et al. Abbreviated laparotomy and planned reoperation for critically ill patients. Ann Surg. 1992;215:476–83.
9. Buckey JC. Space physiology, Effect of spaceflight on the cardiovascular system. New York: Oxford University Press; 2006. p. 149–54.
10. Kirkpatrick AW, Campbell MR, Broderick T, et al. Extraterrestrial hemorrhage control: terrestrial developments in technique, technology, and philosophy with applicability to traumatic hemorrhage control during long duration spaceflight. J Am Coll Surg. 2005;200:64–76.
11. Kirkpatrick AW, Ball CG, Campbell M, Williams DR, Parazynski SE, Mattox KL, Broderick TJ. Severe traumatic injury during long duration spaceflight: light years beyond ATLS. J Trauma Manag Outcomes. 2009;3:4.
12. Williams D, Kuipers A, Mukai C, Thirsk R. Acclimation during space flight: effects on human physiology. CMAJ. 2009;180(13):1317–23.
13. Davidson JM, Aquino AM, Woodward SC, et al. Sustained microgravity reduces intrinsic wound healing and growth factor response in the rat. FASEB J. 1999;13:325–9.
14. Nicogossian AE, Sawin CF, Huntoon CL. Overall physiologic response to spaceflight. In: Nicogossian AE, Huntoon CL, Pool SL, editors. Space physiology and medicine. Baltimore: Williams & Wilkins; 1993. p. 213–27.
15. Buckey JC. Bone loss: managing calcium and bone loss in space. In: Barratt MR, Pool SL, editors. Space physiology. New York: Oxford University Press; 2006. p. 5–21.
16. Shackelford LC. Principles of clinical medicine for space flight, Musculoskeletal response to space flight. New York: Springer Science and Business Media; 2008. p. 293–306.
17. Cann C. Response of the skeletal system to spaceflight. In: Churchill SE, editor. Fundamentals of space lifesciences, vol. 1. Malabar: Krieger Publishing Company; 1997. p. 83–103.
18. Tafton PG, McGough RL. Lower extremity fractures and dislocations. In: Moore EE, Feliciano DV, Mattox KL, editors. Trauma. New York: McGraw-Hill; 2004. p. 939–68.
19. Kaplansky A, Durnova G, Burkovskya T, et al. The effect of microgravity o bone fracture healing in rats flown on Cosmos 2044. Physiologist. 1991;34:325–9.
20. Taylor G, Janney R. In vivo testing confirms a blunting of the human cell-mediated immune mechanism during spaceflight. J Leukoc Biol. 1992;48:129–32.
21. Kacena MA, Merrell GA, Manfredi B, et al. Bacterial growth in space flight: logistic growth curve parameters for Escherichia coli and Bacillus subtilis. Appl Microbiol Biotechnol. 1999;51:229–34.
22. Iaroshenko GL, Terent'ev VG, Mokrov MN. Peculiarities of surgical intervention under conditions of weightlessness. Voen Med Zh. 1967;10:69–70.
23. Musgrave S. Surgical aspects of space flight. Surg Annu. 1976;8:1–23.
24. Stazhadze LL, Goncharov IB, Neumyzakin IP, et al. Anaesthesia, surgical aid and resuscitation in manned space missions. Acta Astronaut. 1981;8:1109–13.
25. Campbell MR, Billica RD, Johnston SL. Animal surgery in microgravity. Aviat Space Environ Med. 1993;64:58–62.
26. Campbell MR, Billica RD, Johnston SL. Surgical bleeding in microgravity. Surg Gynecol Obstet. 1993;177:121–5.
27. McCuaig K. Aseptic technique in microgravity. Surg Gynecol Obstet. 1992;175:466–47.
28. McCuaig K. Surgical problems in space: an overview. J Clin Pharmacol. 1994;34:513–7.
29. Campbell MR, Billica RD, Melton S. Surgical instrument restraint in weightlessness. Aviat Space Environ Med. 2001;72:871–6.
30. McCuaig K, Lloyd C, Gosbee J, et al. Simulation of blood flow in microgravity. Am J Surg. 1992;164:114–23.
31. Barratt MR, Pool SL, et al. Chapter 15, Immunolgic concerns. In: Principles of clinical medicine for space flight. Springer Science + Business Media; 2008. p. 307–31.
32. Campbell MR, Billica RD. A review of microgravity surgical investigations. Aviat Space Environ Med. 1992;63(6):52.
33. Mutke HG. Equipment for surgical intervention and childbirth in weightlessness. Aviat Space Environ Med. 1981;8:399–403.
34. Rock J. An expandable surgical chamber for use in a weightless environment. Aviat Space Environ Med. 1984;55:403–4.
35. Markham SM, Rock JA. Deploying and testing an expandable surgical chamber in microgravity. Aviat Space Environ Med. 1989;60:76–9.

36. Markham SM, Rock JA. Microgravity testing of a surgical isolation containment system for space station use. Aviat Space Environ Med. 1991;62:691–3.
37. Bennett TE, Pantalos GM, Sharp MK, Schurfranz T, Everett S, Gillars K, O'Leary S, Lorange R, Woodruff S, Lemon M, Sojka J. Effect of gravitational acceleration on cardiac diastolic function: the hearts in space project, 1985 to 1999. NASA Conference Publication NASA/CP-1999-209476, Daelemans G, Mosier F, editors, p. 97–106; 1999.
38. Jay GD, Lee P, Goldsmith H, Battat J, Maurer J, Suner S. CPR effectiveness in microgravity: comparison of three positions and a mechanical device. Aviat Space Environ Med. 2003;74(11):1183–9.
39. CAPT Zach Perkins, CPR in micro-gravity environments. http://hypospray.thedocnetwork.net/?p=40.
40. Campbell MR, Billica RD, Johnston SL, Muller MS. Performance of advanced trauma life support procedures in microgravity. Aviat Space Environ Med. 2002;73(9):907–12.
41. Schweitzer EJ, Hauer JM, Swan KG, et al. Use of the Heimlich valve in a compact autotransfusion device. J Trauma. 1987;27:537–42.
42. Mattox KL, Walker LE, Beall AC, et al. Blood availability for the trauma patient—Autotransfusion. J Trauma. 1975;15(8):663–9.
43. Rumisek JD. Autotransfusion of shed blood: an untapped battlefield resource. Mil Med. 1982;147:193–6.
44. Kirkpatrick AW, Doarn CR, Campbell MR, Barnes SL, Broderick TJ. Manual suturing quality at acceleration levels equivalent to spaceflight and a lunar base. Aviat Space Environ Med. 2008;79:1065–6.
45. Campbell MR, Williams DR, Buckey JC Jr, Kirkpatrick AW. Animal surgery during spaceflight on the Neurolab Shuttle mission. Aviat Space Environ Med. 2005;76:589–93.
46. Jones JA, Johnston S, Campbell M, Miles B, Billica R. Endoscopic surgery and telemedicine in microgravity: developing contingency procedures for exploratory class spaceflight. Urology. 1999;53:892–7.
47. Campbell MR, Kirkpatrick AW, Billica RD, Johnston SL, Jennings R, Short D, Hamilton D, Dulchavsky SA. Endoscopic surgery in weightlessness: the investigation of basic principles for surgery in space. Surg Endosc. 2001;15:1413–8.
48. Pinsolle V, Martin D, de Coninck L, Techoueyres P, Vaida P. Microsurgery in microgravity is possible. Microsurgery. 2005;25:152–4.
49. Panait L, Merrell RC, Rafiq A, Dudrick SJ, Broderick TJ. Virtual reality laparoscopic skill assessment in microgravity. J Surg Res. 2006;136:198–203.
50. Campbell MR, Billica RD, Jennings R, Johnston S 3rd. Laparoscopic surgery in weightlessness. Surg Endosc. 1996;10:111–7.
51. Broderick TJ, Privitera MB, Parazynski SE, et al. Simulated hand-assisted laparoscopic surgery (HALS) in microgravity. J Laparoendosc Adv Surg Tech A. 2005;15:145–8.
52. Rafiq A, Broderick TJ, Williams DR, et al. Assessment of simulated surgical skills in parabolic flight. Aviat Space Environ Med. 2005;76:385–91.
53. Boffard KD, editor. Manual of definitive surgical trauma care, Minimally invasive surgery in trauma. London: Hodder Headline Group; 2003. p. 172–3.
54. Leppaniemi A, Haapiainen R. Diagnostic laparoscopy in abdominal stab wounds: a prospective, randomized study. J Trauma. 2003;55:636–45.
55. Burch JM, Moore EE, Moore FA, et al. The abdominal compartment syndrome. Surg Clin N Am. 1996;76:833–42.
56. Kirkpatrick AW, Balogh Z, Ball CG, et al. The secondary abdominal compartment syndrome: Iatrogenic or unavoidable? J Am Coll Surg. 2006;202:668–79.
57. Schein M, Wittman DH, Aprahamian CC, et al. The abdominal compartment syndrome: the physiological and clinical consequences of elevated intra-abdominal pressure. J Am Coll Surg. 1995;180:745–52.
58. Kirkpatrick AW, Broderick T, Ball C, et al. Implications regarding the abdominal compartment syndrome in space. ANZ J Surg. 2005;75:A5–A60.
59. Holthausen UH, Nagelschmidt M, Troidl H. CO2 pneumoperitoneum: what we know and what we need to know. World J Surg. 1999;23:794–800.
60. Kirkpatrick AW, Keaney DVM, Kmet L, et al. Intra-abdominal pressure effects on porcine thoracic compliance in weightlessness: implications for physiologic tolerance of laparoscopic surgery in space. Crit Care Med. 2009;37:591–7.
61. Holcomb JB, McClain JM, Pusateri AE, et al. Fibrin sealant foam sprayed directly on liver injuries decreases blood loss in resuscitated rats. J Trauma. 2000;49:246–50.
62. Gunn J, Fehrenbacher P. Northwestern University, Chicago, Illinois presentation at the NASA Human Research Program Investigators' Workshop 2014.
63. Taeger G, Ruchholtz S, Waydas C, et al. Damage control orthopedics in patients with multiple injuries is effective, time saving, and safe. J Trauma. 2005;59:408–15.
64. Perchinsky MJ, Long WB, Hill JG, et al. Extracorporeal cardiopulmonary life support with heparin bonded circuitry in the resuscitation of massively injured trauma patients. Am J Surg. 1995;169:488–91.
65. Vucevic M, Tehan B, Gamlin F, et al. The SMART needle: a new Doppler ultrasound-guided vascular access needle. Anaesthesia. 1994;49:889–91.
66. Yaffe L, Abbott D, Schulte B. Smart aortic arch catheter: moving suspended animation from the laboratory to the field. Crit Care Med. 2004;32:S51–5.
67. Amiko Nevills NEEMO: NASA extreme environment mission operations report; 2006.
68. Marescaux J, Leroy J, Rubino F, et al. Transcontinental robot-assisted remote telesurgery: feasibility and potential applications. Ann Surg. 2002;235:487–92.
69. Kirkpatrick AW, Jones JA, Sargsyan A, Hamilton DR, Melton S, Beck G, Nicolau S, Campbell M, Dulchavsky S. Trauma sonography for use in microgravity. Aviat Space Environ Med. 2007;78:A38–42.
70. Kirkpatrick AW, Hamilton DR, Nicolaou S, Sargsyan AE, Campbell MR, Feiveson A, Dulchavsky SA, Melton S, Beck G, Dawson DL. Focused assessment with sonography for trauma in weightlessness: a feasibility study. J Am Coll Surg. 2003;196:833–44.
71. Sargsyan AE, Hamilton DR, Jones JA, Melton S, Whitson PA, Kirkpatrick AW, Martin D, Dulchavsky SA. FAST at MACH 20: clinical ultrasound aboard the International Space Station. J Trauma. 2005;58:35–9.
72. Hamilton DR, Sargsyan AE, Kirkpatrick AW, Nicolaou S, Campbell M, Dawson DL, Melton SL, Beck G, Guess T, Rasbury J, Dulchavsky SA. Sonographic detection of pneumothorax and hemothorax in microgravity. Aviat Space Environ Med. 2004;75:272–7.
73. Sargsyan AE, Karakitsos D. Ultrasound imaging in space flight. In: Lumb, Karakitsos, editors. Critical care ultrasound. Elsevier; 2014. p. 258–62.
74. Sargsyan AE, Hamilton DR, Nicolaou S, Kirkpatrick AW, Campbell MR, Billica RD, Dawson D, Williams DR, Melton SL, Beck G, Forkheim K, Dulchavsky SA. Ultrasound evaluation of the magnitude of pneumothorax: a new concept. Am Surg. 2001;67:232–5. Discussion pp 235–6
75. Benninger MS, McFarlin K, Hamilton DR, Rubinfeld I, Sargsyan AE, Melton SM, Mohyi M, Dulchavsky SA. Ultrasound evalua-

tion of sinus fluid levels in swine during microgravity conditions. Aviat Space Environ Med. 2009;80:1063–5.
76. Riccabona M, Nelson TR, Pretorius DH. Three-dimensional ultrasound: accuracy of distance and volume measurements. Ultrasound Obstet Gynecol. 1996;7:429–34.
77. Shalev J, Davidi O, Fisch B. Quantitative three-dimensional sonographic assessment of pelvic blood after transvaginal ultrasound-guided oocyte aspiration: factors predicting risk. Ultrasound Obstet Gynecol. 2004;23(2):177–82.
78. Catalano O, Cusati B, Nunziata A, et al. Active abdominal bleeding: contrast-enhanced sonography. Abdom Imaging. 2006;31:9–16.
79. Hoyt DB. A clinical review of bleeding dilemmas in trauma. Semin Hematol. 2004;41:S40–3.
80. Kirkpatrick AW, Nicolaou S, Campbell MR, Sargsyan AE, Dulchavsky SA, Melton S, Beck G, Dawson DL, Billica RD, Johnston SL, Hamilton DR. Percutaneous aspiration of fluid for management of peritonitis in space. Aviat Space Environ Med. 2002;73:925–30.
81. Fincke EM, Padalka G, Lee D, van Holsbeeck M, Sargsyan AE, Hamilton DR, Martin D, Melton SL, McFarlin K, Dulchavsky SA. Evaluation of shoulder integrity in space: first report of musculoskeletal US on the International Space Station. Radiology. 2005;234:319–22.
82. Chiao L, Sharipov S, Sargsyan AE, Melton S, Hamilton DR, McFarlin K, Dulchavsky SA. Ocular examination for trauma; clinical ultrasound aboard the International Space Station. J Trauma. 2005;58:885–9.
83. Simon JC, Sapozhnikov OA, Khokhlova VA, Wang Y-N, Crum LA, Bailey MR, Ultrasonic atomization of tissue: a mechanism for ultrasound-based surgery—presentation at the NASA Human Research Program Investigators' Workshop 2014, NIH grants DK43881, EB007643 and NSBRI through NASA NCC 9–58.
84. Grossman DC, Kim A, MacDonald SC, et al. Urban-rural differences in prehospital care of major trauma. J Trauma. 1997;42:723–9.
85. Mueller BA, Rivara FP, Bergman AB. Urban-rural location and the risk of dying in a pedestrian-vehicle collision. J Trauma. 1988;28:91–4.
86. Sampalis JS, Denis R, Fréchette P, Brown R, Fleiszer D, Mulder D. Direct transport to tertiary trauma centers versus transfer from lower level facilities: impact on mortality and morbidity among patients with major trauma. J Trauma. 1997;43(2):288–95.
87. Chun R, Kirkpatrick AW, Sirois M, et al. Where's the tube? Evaluation of hand-held ultrasound in confirming endotracheal tube placement. Prehosp Disaster Med. 2004;19:366–9.
88. Weaver B, Lyon M, Blaivas M. Confirmation of endotracheal tube placement after intubation using the ultrasound sliding lung sign. Acad Emerg Med. 2006;13:239–44.
89. Martinowitz U, Holcomb JB, Pusateri AE, et al. Intravenous rFVIIa administered for hemorrhage control in hypothermic coagulopathic swine with grade V liver injuries. J Trauma. 2001;50:721–9.
90. Hoyt DB, Bulger EM, Knudson MM, et al. Death in the operating room: an analysis of a multi-center experience. J Trauma. 1994;37:426–32.
91. Melton S, Beck G, Hamilton D, et al. How to test a medical technology for space: trauma sonography in microgravity. McGill J Med. 2001;6:66–73.
92. Demetriades D, Velmahos G. Technology-driven triage of abdominal trauma: the emerging era of nonoperative management. Annu Rev Med. 2003;54:1–15.
93. Hiatt JR, Harrier HD, Koenig BV, et al. Nonoperative management of major blunt liver injury with hemoperitoneum. Arch Surg. 1990;125:101–3.
94. Houtchens B. System for the management of trauma and emergency surgery in space: final report. NASA Johnson Space Center NASA Grant NASW-3744 Houston.
95. Holcomb JB, Helling TS, Hirshberg A. Military, civilian, and rural application of the damage control philosophy. Mil Med. 2001;166:490–3.
96. Tisherman SA, Vandevelde K, Safar P, et al. Future directions for resuscitation research: ultra-advanced life support. Resuscitation. 1997;34:281–93.
97. Harwood PJ, Giannoudis PV, van Griensven M, et al. Alterations in the systemic inflammatory response after early total care and damage control procedures for femoral shaft fracture in severely injured patients. J Trauma. 2005;58:446–54.
98. Scalea TM, Boswell SA, Scott JD, et al. External fixation as a bridge to intramedullary nailing for patients with multiple injuries and with femur fractures: damage control orthopedics. J Trauma. 2000;48:613–23.
99. Dulchavsky SA, Henry SE, Moed BR, et al. Advanced ultrasonic diagnosis of extremity trauma: the FASTER examination. J Trauma. 2002;53:28–32.
100. Kirkpatrick AW, Brown R, Diebel LN, et al. Rapid diagnosis of an ulnar fracture with portable hand-held ultrasound. Mil Med. 2003;168:312–3.
101. Noble VE, Legome E, Marshburn T. Long bone ultrasound: making the diagnosis in remote locations. J Trauma. 2003;54:800.
102. Grigorev AI, Bugrov SA, Bogomolov VV, Egorov AD, Kozlovskaya IB, Pestov ID, Polyakov VV, Tarasov IK. Medicine on Mars. UTMB Center for Aerospace Medicine; 2007.
103. Husted TL, Broderick TJ. NASA Medical results of the MIR year-long mission. Course syllabus: pushing the envelope II. and the emergence of new surgical technologies. J Surg Res. 2006;132:13–6.
104. Foale CM, Kaleri AY, Sargsyan AE, et al. Diagnostic instrumentation aboard ISS; just-in-time training for non-physician crewmembers. Aviat Space Environ Med. 2005;76:594–8.
105. NASA technology helps detect heart disease and strokes. Jet Propulsion Laboratory. California Institute of Technology [Internet] June 6, 2006. http://www.jpl.nasa.gov/news/news.php?release=2007-063.
106. Campbell MR. A review of surgical care in space. J Am Coll Surg. 2002;194:802–12.

Logistical Transformation of Healthcare Systems in the COVID-19 Era

59

Jaffar A. Al-Tawfiq and Ziad A. Memish

Introduction

Pandemics are characterized as being low-chance but high-impact events [1]. In recent years, we have witnessed the emergence of three coronaviruses. These are the Severe Acute Respiratory Syndrome Coronavirus (SARS-CoV) detected in 2002 in Guangdong Province, China [2, 3]. The disease caused 8096 cases and 774 (9.6%) deaths over a four-month period from late 2002 to early 2003 [4]. SARS cases were detected in Vietnam, Hong Kong, Canada, the United States, Ireland, Vietnam, and Singapore [2, 5–12], and all cases were linked to a patient who stayed in Hotel M in Hong Kong [13]. And 10 years later, a novel coronavirus was isolated from a patient in Saudi Arabia [14, 15] which was later named the Middle East Respiratory Syndrome Coronavirus (MERS-CoV) [16].

The third coronavirus is the severe acute respiratory syndrome coronavirus 2 (SARS-CoV-2), which is genetically similar to SARS-CoV [17]. Initial cases were first described in a cluster of patients identified in December 2019 in Wuhan City, China. The initial cases were felt to be secondary to the animal-human interaction, and subsequently, cases were the result of community transmission [17, 18]. After the initial cluster of cases was identified, several studies demonstrated human-to-human transmission of SARS-CoV-2 through either droplets or direct contact [19]. Subsequent cases occurred among travelers from China and those caused local transmission in almost every country around the globe [20, 21].

J. A. Al-Tawfiq
Specialty Internal Medicine and Quality Department, Johns Hopkins Aramco Healthcare, Dhahran, Saudi Arabia

Indiana University School of Medicine, Indiana, IN, USA

Johns Hopkins University School of Medicine, Baltimore, MD, USA
e-mail: jaffar.tawfiq@jhah.com

Z. A. Memish (✉)
King Saud Medical City, Ministry of Health, Riyadh, Saudi Arabia

Al-Faisal University, Riyadh, Saudi Arabia

Hubert Department of Global Health, Rollins School of Public Health, Emory University, Atlanta, GA, USA

The Need for Healthcare Transformation

The need for healthcare transformation is well recognized and emerged from the need to provide adequate and quality healthcare to the patients. In previous studies in the United States and without any stressful pandemics, only 55% (95% CI: 54.3–55.5%) of adult patients received the recommended care they needed [22]. The need for technology to change the healthcare system had been recognized and was put in place to drive such changes. In addition, it was suggested that it is important to improve quality of care, decrease costs, and build strategies across the continuum of care [23]. Of the key components of transformation of healthcare are timing and integral map that brings together the process of integration of various components of behavior, social determinants, culture, and personal domains [24]. There is no better time to drive such transformation than the time of the COVID-19 pandemic [24].

Is COVID-19 an Accelerator of or a Game Changer in Healthcare?

Looking at the changes around the globe and specifically in the healthcare system during the COVID-19, it is thought that COVID-19 was the cause for many of the changes. However, others had thought that COVID-19 is an accelerator of these changes that were to happen regardless of the occurrence of COVID-19. An example of these changes is the use of telemedicine and telehealth (Fig. 59.1).

L. Marshall Gillman, S. Widder (eds.), *Trauma Team Dynamics*, https://doi.org/10.1007/978-3-031-86312-7_59

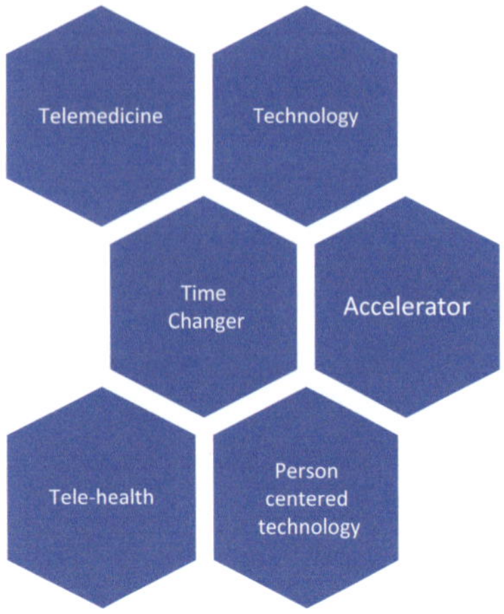

Fig. 59.1 COVID-19 time changer or an accelerator

Pandemic Impact

Previous coronaviruses had caused significant impact on the healthcare systems [25, 26]. In addition, the pandemic has shown many disparities not only in outcome but also in care delivery among affected population [27]. The emergence of COVID-19 pandemic resulted in a global disruption in healthcare infrastructure with significant increase in demand on healthcare to care for the increasing surge of COVID-19 patients and maintaining the needed routine healthcare for non-COVID-19 patients and protecting healthcare workers and other patients [28–30]. There have been multiple interventions to flatten the curve and spare the healthcare system. The lessons we learned from previous pandemics were numerous. However, the current COVID-19 pandemic is of particular importance due to the rapid and persistent increased burden on healthcare organizations and the lack of extra supplies needed to manage it on a global level. All healthcare systems around the globe had to rapidly adopt alternative options for dealing with COVID-19 and non-COVID-19 cases.

The emergence of COVID-19 necessitated the prevention of the spread of infections in healthcare facilities by relying on the United States Centers for Disease Control and Prevention (CDC) strategies of hierarchy of infection prevention and controls [28, 31]. COVID-19 pandemic raised the question about resilience of healthcare systems globally. It is important that we look beyond the current crisis, build on the capacity of healthcare systems to better prepare for future outbreaks and pandemics, identify building blocks of resilient health, and explore ways to build capacity and the ability to maintain healthcare provision for non-COVID-19-related concerns. Many organizations had to also expand the capacity for many activities such as intensive care units, quarantine, isolation, and satellite clinics [32, 33]. Countries around the globe have either used the SARS paradigm or the influenza paradigm in dealing with COVID-19 [34]. The SARS paradigm concentrated on eliminating infections, disease surveillance, redesigning of healthcare facilities, and reducing cross-infection. The influenza paradigm however is based on acceptance that COVID-19 would ultimately spread through the population and that little if any could be done to control the disease [34].

The emergence of COVID-19 tested healthcare organizations for resilience by the ability to absorb the shock of COVID-19, respond effectively, adapt to the shock, change the structure of the organizations, and sustain day-to-day operations. These are the fundamentals of any resilient organization [34]. In order for healthcare organizations to respond to COVID-19 and any future pandemics, they must ensure enough medical supplies, availability of workforce, having additional needed financial support, abilities to deal with non-COVID-19-related issues (e.g., chronic medical conditions, cardiac cases, hemodialysis, and cancer care) [28], and utilizing digital solutions and other innovations to monitor and manage non-COVID-19 and COVID-19 patients.

Empowering Factors for Increasing Organization's Capacity for Improvisation

There is the need to have organizations increase their improvisation through increasing autonomy, more flexibility, fast decision-making, and preserving structure with clear lines of communication and coordination. Rather than materializing "out of thin air," improvisation comes from adjustments and recombination of already existing resources to maintain some structure [35]. For any organization to have a shared understanding, especially of the way to deal with any pandemic, it is important to be fully aware of the interdependence on others, the need to have a holistic awareness of the pandemic and the rapidity of the change, and have excellent communication channels in order to share information in a timely manner [36].

Shortage in Manpower and PPEs/Disinfectant

The emergence of COVID-19 had transformed the healthcare system across the globe [37, 38]. It is noted that there is an international, national, and regional shortage of personal protective equipment [39, 40]. The concern is confounded by the fact that hospital administrators and managers prohibit healthcare workers from discussing these issues openly or raising the flag [41]. In a study from Saudi Arabia, about one-third of respondents to questionnaires reported shortage of PPE [42]. Another factor contributing to the shortage of PPE is inappropriate use and wastage of PPE [43]. This shortage is mainly for single-use PPE which is not designed for reprocessing [44]. Thus, healthcare organizations developed multiple strategies to deal with this shortage including custom-made production and sterilization or high-level disinfection for PPE reprocessing utilizing hydrogen peroxide vapor or ultraviolet C waves [44]. However, manufacturers may not recommend the disinfection or sterilization of respirators [44]. It was also noted that highly energetic ultraviolet germicidal irradiation (UVGI) was effective for the reuse of respirators [45]. Others had used face shields to provide coverage of the respirators and extended the use of such respirators. There was clear disruption of the supply across the globe. China is the supplier of about 50% of surgical masks and the only place that has the capacity of mass production of clinical gowns [46]. On the other hand the United States is the largest market for the use of PPE, and the acute increase in the demand had contributed to the shortage [38]. To address these issues, there is a global need to have extended, reusable, and recyclable PPE [47].

Isolation and Quarantine

The COVID-19 pandemic had caused an urgent demand for isolation rooms to isolate and quarantine individuals who have infection or those who are suspected of being infected for the duration of the incubation period. Quarantine originates from the Latin *quadragina* and the Italian *quaranta* which denotes 40. This refers to the time when sailors had to be managed offshore in their ships for 40 days before being allowed to get into the cities at the time of plague [48]. This practice was used also during the previous coronaviruses outbreaks. During the Severe Acute Respiratory Syndrome Coronavirus (SARS-CoV) outbreak, many governments created quarantine facilities for those needing quarantine such as close contacts and travelers [48]. In addition, during SARS and the Middle East Respiratory Syndrome Coronavirus (MERS-CoV) outbreak, healthcare workers were quarantined after exposure [49, 50]. During COVID-19 pandemic, there had been multiple facilities created around the globe to accommodate especially returning travelers for quarantine [33, 51].

Telehealth and Telemedicine

It is no doubt that the COVID-19 pandemic had changed the way healthcare workers had dealt with long-practiced medical therapies [28] such that patients with acute coronary syndrome were prioritized to receive nonsurgical interventions such as thrombolytic therapy [52]. Telemedicine had become increasingly utilized in many services such as 35% of urologic consultations [53]. Such visits allow healthcare staff to assess the clinical progress of the patients, response to therapy, and adjust or refill medications [28].

Although telemedicine, telehealth, and e-health are used interchangeably, there is a subtle difference between these terms [54–56]. Telehealth encompasses telemedicine and utilizes any telecommunication tools such as texting, messaging, phone calls, e-mails, or other communication portals allowing patient-to-provider communication. On the other hand, telemedicine is a narrower term and refers to the use of videoconferencing and remote patient monitoring. The term e-health is being used to indicate data processing and computer applications. It seems that telemedicine is the most commonly used terminology since the early 1990s, followed by e-health, and the least used terminology is telehealth [54]. Despite the adaptation of telemedicine, there are several challenges that need to be kept in mind. These challenges include availability of infrastructure, access, operational, regulatory, communication, and legislative issues [57]. Of course, telemedicine poses opportunities and has its own challenges that need further evaluation to ensure better utilization [58].

Leadership During the COVID-19 Pandemic

The leadership style and activities during the COVID-19 pandemic had to adapt to making tough decisions without clear and solid data, go beyond the unknown, communicate effectively, integrate different activities and different hospitals, and deal with patient cohorting and staff shortages (Fig. 59.2). The initial events of the COVID-19 pandemic were associated with lots of uncertainties and rapidly changing information. These uncertainties dictate that leaders make decisions with less information and thus these decisions might not be optimal. These uncertainties many times touch the basic needs of individuals to feel safe. Many healthcare workers may act strangely and may not follow appropriate infection control measures due to fear. Leaders need to be equipped to move people from fear to actions to deal with the situation that might be full of emotions and irrational actions. Leaders need to change these situations from fear to positive situations, to practice creative abandonment, and to communicate clear directions, actions, values, and behaviors. This strategy allows actions to be gauged and redirected to the best solution rather than not doing anything. Leaders have to "Be First, Be Right, and Be Credible" in their communications [59]. The communication has to be up, down, and across for effective leadership [60]: upward communication to officials and governmental agencies, communicating down to staff and the community, and communicating across to peers and other organizations [60]. However, such leadership might be further challenged by the need to work from home adding an additional factor and a burden in communication and management [61].

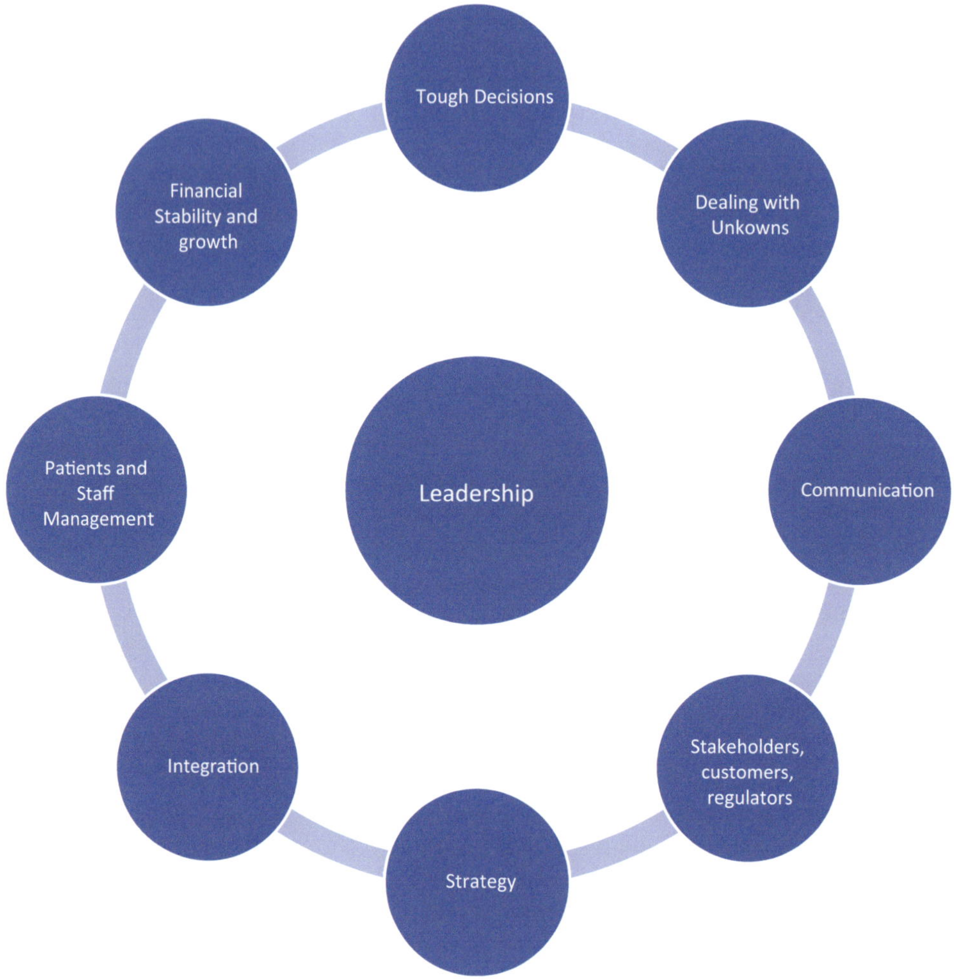

Fig. 59.2 A simplified diagram of different activities leaders of healthcare organizations dealt with during the COVID-19 pandemic

Financial Support

One of the most needed transformations in healthcare is to have financial support for the care of the patients, innovation, maintaining research, and providing care for patients [37]. There were increasing demands on emergency room visits and laboratory tests for COVID-19 with reduction in routine surgical procedures and routine blood tests at the time of the pandemic [62, 63]. The rapid evolution of the pandemic had forced many healthcare organizations around the globe to put and spend extra-financial activities to maintain the needed healthcare. The need to have enhanced partnerships with governmental and private sectors for the development of medications, vaccines, and diagnostic tests is fundamental in the fight against this pandemic [37, 64].

Conclusion

The current COVID-19 pandemic resulted in a major influence on healthcare organizations. This impact had accelerated the transformation of healthcare and impacted the designs of hospitals to manage large influx of patients and care for COVID-19 and non-COVID-19 patients. Healthcare organizations should be in a better position to respond to future challenges and emergencies including pandemics.

Key Points

- Pandemics are characterized as being low-chance but high-impact events.
- The COVID-19 pandemic resulted in a global disruption in healthcare infrastructure.
- The COVID-19 pandemic caused an urgent demand to isolate and quarantine individuals.
- Healthcare transformation is driven by need for quality care.
- Integration of behavior, social determinants, culture, and personal domains is needed for the transformation of healthcare.
- COVID-19 is an accelerator of healthcare transformation including telemedicine, telehealth, and e-health.
- Organizations need more autonomy, flexibility, and fast decision-making.
- Shortage in manpower and PPEs/disinfectant had a significant impact.
- Leadership adapting to tough decisions and uncertainties.
- Financial support is needed for patient care, innovation, and research.

References

1. Lloyd-Smith M. The COVID-19 pandemic: resilient organisational response to a low-chance, high-impact event. BMJ Lead [Internet]. 2020 [cited 2021 Apr 16];4(3):109–12. Available from: http://bmjleader.bmj.com/.
2. Lee N, Hui D, Wu A, Chan P, Cameron P, Joynt GM, et al. A major outbreak of severe acute respiratory syndrome in Hong Kong. N Engl J Med. 2003;348(20):1986–94.
3. Shaw K. The 2003 SARS outbreak and its impact on infection control practices. Public Health [Internet]. 2006 [cited 2018 Feb 3];120(1):8–14. Available from: http://www.ncbi.nlm.nih.gov/pubmed/16297415.
4. Graham RL, Baric RS. Recombination, reservoirs, and the modular spike: mechanisms of coronavirus cross-species transmission. J Virol. 2010;84(7):3134–46.
5. Leung GM, Hedley AJ, Ho L-M, Chau P, Wong IOL, Thach TQ, et al. The epidemiology of severe acute respiratory syndrome in the 2003 Hong Kong epidemic: an analysis of all 1755 patients. Ann Intern Med [Internet]. 2004 [cited 2016 Apr 8];141(9):662–73. Available from: http://www.ncbi.nlm.nih.gov/pubmed/15520422.
6. Tsang KW, Ho PL, Ooi GC, Yee WK, Wang T, Chan-Yeung M, et al. A cluster of cases of severe acute respiratory syndrome in Hong Kong. N Engl J Med. 2003;348(20):1977–85.
7. Poutanen SM, Low DE, Henry B, Finkelstein S, Rose D, Green K, et al. Identification of severe acute respiratory syndrome in Canada. N Engl J Med [Internet]. 2003 [cited 2017 Jan 18];348(20):1995–2005. Available from: http://www.ncbi.nlm.nih.gov/pubmed/12671061.
8. Centers for Disease Control and Prevention (CDC). Outbreak of severe acute respiratory syndrome—worldwide, 2003. MMWR Morb Mortal Wkly Rep [Internet]. 2003 [cited 2019 Oct 12];52(11):226–8. Available from: http://www.ncbi.nlm.nih.gov/pubmed/12665115.
9. Centers for Disease Control and Prevention (CDC). Preliminary clinical description of severe acute respiratory syndrome. MMWR Morb Mortal Wkly Rep [Internet]. 2003 [cited 2019 Oct 12];52(12):255–6. Available from: http://www.ncbi.nlm.nih.gov/pubmed/12680522.
10. Centers for Disease Control and Prevention (CDC). Update: severe acute respiratory syndrome—United States, June 4, 2003. MMWR Morb Mortal Wkly Rep [Internet]. 2003 [cited 2019 Oct 12];52(22):525–6. Available from: http://www.ncbi.nlm.nih.gov/pubmed/12803200.
11. Centers for Disease Control and Prevention (CDC). Severe acute respiratory syndrome (SARS) and coronavirus testing—United States, 2003. MMWR Morb Mortal Wkly Rep [Internet]. 2003 [cited 2019 Oct 12];52(14):297–302. Available from: http://www.ncbi.nlm.nih.gov/pubmed/12731699.
12. Centers for Disease Control and Prevention (CDC). Severe acute respiratory syndrome—Singapore, 2003. MMWR Morb Mortal Wkly Rep [Internet]. 2003 [cited 2019 Oct 12];52(18):405–11. Available from: http://www.ncbi.nlm.nih.gov/pubmed/12807088.
13. Parashar UD, Anderson LJ. Severe acute respiratory syndrome: review and lessons of the 2003 outbreak. Int J Epidemiol [Internet]. 2004 [cited 2019 Oct 12];33(4):628–34. Available from: http://www.ncbi.nlm.nih.gov/pubmed/15155694.
14. Zaki AM, van Boheemen S, Bestebroer TM, Osterhaus ADME, Fouchier RAM. Isolation of a novel coronavirus from a man with pneumonia in Saudi Arabia. N Engl J Med [Internet]. 2012 [cited 2016 Jan 17];367(19):1814–20. Available from: http://www.ncbi.nlm.nih.gov/pubmed/23075143.
15. Corman VM, Eckerle I, Bleicker T, Zaki A, Landt O, Eschbach-Bludau M, et al. Detection of a novel human coronavirus by real-time reverse-transcription polymerase chain reaction. Euro Surveill [Internet]. 2012 [cited 2019 May 10];17(39). Available from: http://www.ncbi.nlm.nih.gov/pubmed/23041020.
16. de Groot RJ, Baker SC, Baric RS, Brown CS, Drosten C, Enjuanes L, et al. Middle East respiratory syndrome coronavirus (MERS-CoV): announcement of the Coronavirus Study Group. J Virol [Internet]. 2013;87(14):7790–2. Available from: https://pmc.ncbi.nlm.nih.gov/articles/PMC3700179/pdf/zjv7790.pdf.
17. Guan W, Ni Z, Hu Y, Liang W, Ou C, He J, et al. Clinical characteristics of coronavirus disease 2019 in China. N Engl J Med. 2020;382(18):1708–20.
18. Zhou F, Yu T, Du R, Fan G, Liu Y, Liu Z, et al. Clinical course and risk factors for mortality of adult inpatients with COVID-19 in Wuhan, China: a retrospective cohort study. Lancet [Internet]. 2020 [cited 2020 Mar 17];6736(20):1–9. Available from: http://www.ncbi.nlm.nih.gov/pubmed/32171076.
19. Lai CC, Shih TP, Ko WC, Tang HJ, Hsueh PR. Severe acute respiratory syndrome coronavirus 2 (SARS-CoV-2) and coronavirus disease-2019 (COVID-19): the epidemic and the challenges. Int J Antimicrob Agents. Elsevier B.V. 2020;55:105924.
20. Zhao D, Yao F, Wang L, Zheng L, Gao Y, Ye J, et al. A comparative study on the clinical features of coronavirus 2019 (COVID-19) pneumonia with other pneumonias. Clin Infect Dis [Internet]. 2020 [cited 2020 May 25];71(15):756–61. Available from: https://pubmed.ncbi.nlm.nih.gov/32161968/?from_single_result=10.1093%2Fcid%2Fciaa247&expanded_search_query=10.1093%2Fcid%2Fciaa247.
21. Peeri NC, Shrestha N, Rahman MS, Zaki R, Tan Z, Bibi S, et al. The SARS, MERS and novel coronavirus (COVID-19) epidemics, the newest and biggest global health threats: what lessons have we learned? Int J Epidemiol. 2020;49(3):717–26.
22. McGlynn EA, Asch SM, Adams J, Keesey J, Hicks J, DeCristofaro A, et al. The quality of health care delivered to adults in the United States. N Engl J Med [Internet]. 2003 [cited 2021 Apr

19];348(26):2635–45. Available from: https://pubmed.ncbi.nlm.nih.gov/12826639/.
23. Jacquin L. A strategic approach to healthcare transformation – PubMed. Heal Financ Manag [Internet]. 2014 [cited 2021 Apr 19];68(4):74–70. Available from: https://pubmed.ncbi.nlm.nih.gov/24757877/.
24. Senzon SA. Five keys to real transformation in health care. J Altern Complement Med [Internet]. 2011 [cited 2021 Apr 19];17(11):1085–9. Available from: https://pubmed.ncbi.nlm.nih.gov/22087617/.
25. Al-Tawfiq JA, Abdrabalnabi R, Taher A, Mathew S, Rahman KA. Infection control influence of Middle East respiratory syndrome coronavirus: a hospital-based analysis. Am J Infect Control [Internet]. 2019 [cited 2019 Jan 3];47(4):431–4. Available from: https://linkinghub.elsevier.com/retrieve/pii/S0196655318309441.
26. Abdullah ASM, Tomlinson B, Thomas GN, Cockram CS. Impacts of SARS on health care systems and strategies for combating future outbreaks of emerging infectious diseases. 2004 [cited 2021 Apr 25]. Available from: https://www.ncbi.nlm.nih.gov/books/NBK92485/.
27. Tirupathi R, Muradova V, Shekhar R, Salim SA, Al-Tawfiq JA, Palabindala V. COVID-19 disparity among racial and ethnic minorities in the US: a cross sectional analysis. Travel Med Infect Dis [Internet]. 2020 [cited 2020 Nov 9];38:101904. Available from: http://www.ncbi.nlm.nih.gov/pubmed/33137491.
28. Al-Tawfiq JA, Al-Yami SS, Rigamonti D. Changes in healthcare managing COVID and non–COVID-19 patients during the pandemic: striking the balance [Internet]. Diagn Microbiol Infect Dis. Elsevier Inc. 2020 [cited 2021 Jan 2];98. Available from: https://pubmed.ncbi.nlm.nih.gov/32891957/.
29. Rosenbaum L. The untold toll — the pandemic's effects on patients without covid-19. N Engl J Med. 2020;382(24):2368–71.
30. Al-Tawfiq JA, Garout MA, Gautret P. Preparing for emerging respiratory pathogens such as SARS-CoV, MERS-CoV, and SARS-CoV-2. Le Infez Med. 2020;28(suppl 1):64–70.
31. de Castro ABB. Hierarchy of controls. [Internet]. Am J Nurs. 2003 [cited 2020 Jul 6];103:104. Available from: https://www.cdc.gov/niosh/topics/hierarchy/default.html.
32. Shoukat A, Wells CR, Langley JM, Singer BH, Galvani AP. Projecting demand for critical care beds during COVID-19 outbreaks in Canada. CMAJ. 2020;192(19):E489–96.
33. Abdulrahman A, AlSabbagh M, AlAwadhi A, Al-Tawfiq JA, Rabaan AA, Atkin S, et al. Quarantining arriving travelers in the era of COVID-19: balancing the risk and benefits a learning experience from Bahrain [Internet]. Trop Dis Travel Med Vaccines. BioMed Central Ltd. 2021 [cited 2021 Mar 22];7. Available from: https://pubmed.ncbi.nlm.nih.gov/33436085/.
34. Union E. The organisation of resilient health and social care following the COVID-19 pandemic. Opinion of the Expert Panel on effective ways of investing in Health (EXPH) [Internet]. 2020 [cited 2021 Apr 9]. Available from: http://ec.europa.eu/dgs/health_food-safety/index_en.htm.
35. WWeick KE. Improvisation as a mindset for organizational analysis. Organ Sci [Internet]. 1998 [cited 2021 Apr 10];9(5):543–55. Available from: https://pubsonline.informs.org/doi/pdf/10.1287/orsc.9.5.543.
36. Bigley GA, Roberts KH. The incident command system: high-reliability organizing for complex and volatile task environments. Acad Manag J [Internet]. 2001 [cited 2021 Apr 10];44(6):1281–99. Available from: https://journals.aom.org/doi/abs/10.5465/3069401.
37. Jazieh AR, Kozlakidis Z. Healthcare transformation in the post-coronavirus pandemic era. Front Med [Internet]. 2020 [cited 2021 Apr 19];7:429. Available from: /pmc/articles/PMC7399067/.
38. Cohen J, van der Meulen Rodgers Y. Contributing factors to personal protective equipment shortages during the COVID-19 pandemic [Internet]. Prev Med. Academic Press Inc. 2020 [cited 2021 Apr 19];141. Available from: https://pmc.ncbi.nlm.nih.gov/articles/PMC7531934/.
39. O'Sullivan ED. PPE guidance for covid-19: be honest about resource shortages [Internet]. BMJ. BMJ Publishing Group. 2020 [cited 2021 Apr 19];369. Available from: https://pubmed.ncbi.nlm.nih.gov/32303504/.
40. Inaba M, Naito H, Sakata T, Nakao A. COVID-19 pandemic and shortage of personal protective equipment in Tokyo clinics. Acute Med Surg [Internet]. 2020 [cited 2021 Apr 19];7(1). Available from: https://pmc.ncbi.nlm.nih.gov/articles/PMC7276792/pdf/AMS2-7-e527.pdf.
41. Mandrola J. COVID-19 and PPE: some of us will die because of the shortage. Recenti Prog Med [Internet]. 2020 [cited 2021 Apr 19];111(4):183. Available from: https://pubmed.ncbi.nlm.nih.gov/32319434/.
42. Aljadeed R, AlRuthia Y, Balkhi B, Sales I, Alwhaibi M, Almohammed O, et al. The impact of COVID-19 on essential medicines and personal protective equipment availability and prices in Saudi Arabia. Healthcare [Internet]. 2021 [cited 2021 Apr 19];9(3):290. Available from: https://pmc.ncbi.nlm.nih.gov/articles/PMC8001971/.
43. Fram DS, Escudero DVDS, Matias LDO, Coelho WEGDS, Antonelli TS, Ferreira DB, et al. Personal protective equipment: shortage or waste? [Internet]. Infect Control Hosp Epidemiol. Cambridge University Press. 2020 [cited 2021 Apr 19]:1. Available from: https://pmc.ncbi.nlm.nih.gov/articles/PMC7399137/pdf/S0899823X20003542a.pdf.
44. Rowan NJ, Laffey JG. Challenges and solutions for addressing critical shortage of supply chain for personal and protective equipment (PPE) arising from Coronavirus disease (COVID19) pandemic – case study from the Republic of Ireland. Sci Total Environ [Internet]. 2020 [cited 2021 Apr 19];725. Available from: https://pubmed.ncbi.nlm.nih.gov/32304970/.
45. Boškoski I, Gallo C, Wallace MB, Costamagna G. COVID-19 pandemic and personal protective equipment shortage: protective efficacy comparing masks and scientific methods for respirator reuse. Gastrointest Endosc [Internet]. 2020 [cited 2021 Apr 19];92(3):519–23. Available from: https://pubmed.ncbi.nlm.nih.gov/32353457/.
46. Burki T. Global shortage of personal protective equipment. Lancet Infect Dis [Internet]. 2020 [cited 2021 Apr 19];20(7):785–6. Available from: https://pmc.ncbi.nlm.nih.gov/articles/PMC7314445/pdf/main.pdf.
47. Dargaville T, Spann K, Celina M. Opinion to address the personal protective equipment shortage in the global community during the COVID-19 outbreak. Polym Degrad Stab [Internet]. 2020 [cited 2021 Apr 19];176. Available from: https://pubmed.ncbi.nlm.nih.gov/32292217/.
48. Centers for Disease Control and Prevention (CDC). Use of quarantine to prevent transmission of severe acute respiratory syndrome-Taiwan, 2003. Morb Mortal Wkly Rep. 2003;52:680–3.
49. [No authors listed]. Will your ED have staff quarantined for SARS? Brace yourself for the worst. ED Manag [Internet]. 2003 [cited 2020 Mar 6];15(5):49–51, suppl 1. Available from: http://www.ncbi.nlm.nih.gov/pubmed/12760151.
50. Saudi Ministry of Health. Middle East respiratory syndrome coronavirus 2018 guidelines for healthcare professionals [Internet]. 2018 [cited 2019 May 23]. Available from: https://www.moh.gov.sa/ccc/healthp/regulations/documents/merscov%20guidelines%20for%20healthcare%20professionals%20-%20may%202018%20-%20v5.1%20%281%29.pdf.
51. Al-Tawfiq JA, Sattar A, Al-Khadra H, Al-Qahtani S, Al-Mulhim M, Al-Omoush O, et al. Incidence of COVID-19 among returning travelers in quarantine facilities: a longitudinal study and lessons learned. Travel Med Infect Dis. 2020;38:101901.

52. Welt FGP, Shah PB, Aronow HD, Bortnick AE, Henry TD, Sherwood MW, et al. Catheterization laboratory considerations during the coronavirus (COVID-19) pandemic: from the ACC's Interventional Council and SCAI. J Am Coll Cardiol. 2020;75(18):2372–5.
53. Borchert A, Baumgarten L, Dalela D, Jamil M, Budzyn J, Kovacevic N, et al. Managing urology consultations during COVID-19 pandemic: application of a structured care pathway. Urology. 2020;141:7.
54. Fatehi F, Wootton R. Telemedicine, telehealth or e-health? A bibliometric analysis of the trends in the use of these terms [Internet]. J Telemed Telecare. 2012 [cited 2021 Apr 17];18:460–4. Available from: https://pubmed.ncbi.nlm.nih.gov/23209265/.
55. Sood S, Mbarika V, Jugoo S, Dookhy R, Doarn CR, Prakash N, et al. What is telemedicine? A collection of 104 peer-reviewed perspectives and theoretical underpinnings. Telemed e-Health [Internet]. 2007 [cited 2021 Apr 17];13(5):573–90. Available from: https://pubmed.ncbi.nlm.nih.gov/17999619/.
56. Oh H, Rizo C, Enkin M, Jadad A. What is eHealth (3): a systematic review of published definitions [Internet]. J Med Internet Res. JMIR Publications Inc. 2005 [cited 2021 Apr 17];7. Available from: https://pubmed.ncbi.nlm.nih.gov/15829471/.
57. Annaswamy TM, Verduzco-Gutierrez M, Frieden L. Telemedicine barriers and challenges for persons with disabilities: COVID-19 and beyond [Internet]. Disabil Health J. Elsevier Inc. 2020 [cited 2021 Apr 17];13. Available from: https://pubmed.ncbi.nlm.nih.gov/32703737/.
58. Blandford A, Wesson J, Amalberti R, AlHazme R, Allwihan R. Opportunities and challenges for telehealth within, and beyond, a pandemic [Internet]. Lancet Glob Health. Elsevier Ltd. 2020 [cited 2021 Apr 17];8:e1364–5. Available from: www.thelancet.com/lancetgh.
59. Remley K. Be first, be right, and be credible: translating lessons from crisis communications [Internet]. J Public Health Manag Pract. Lippincott Williams and Wilkins. 2019 [cited 2021 Apr 16];25:208–9. Available from: https://pubmed.ncbi.nlm.nih.gov/30720596/.
60. Fraser MR. Leading in the COVID-19 crisis: challenges and solutions for state health leaders. J Public Heal Manag Pract [Internet]. 2020 [cited 2021 Apr 16];26(4):380–3. Available from: https://journals.lww.com/10.1097/PHH.0000000000001192.
61. Kirchner K, Ipsen C, Hansen JP. COVID-19 leadership challenges in knowledge work. Knowl Manag Res Pract [Internet]. 2021 [cited 2021 Apr 16]. Available from: https://www.tandfonline.com/doi/abs/10.1080/14778238.2021.1877579.
62. Tartari F, Guglielmo A, Fuligni F, Pileri A. Changes in emergency service access after spread of COVID-19 across Italy [Internet]. J Eur Acad Dermatol Venereol. Blackwell Publishing Ltd. 2020 [cited 2021 Apr 19];34:e350–1. Available from: https://pubmed.ncbi.nlm.nih.gov/32339340/.
63. Hollander JE, Carr BG. Virtually perfect? Telemedicine for covid-19. N Engl J Med [Internet]. 2020 [cited 2021 Apr 19];382(18):1679–81. Available from: https://pubmed.ncbi.nlm.nih.gov/32160451/.
64. Krech R, Kickbusch I, Franz C, Wells N. Banking for health: the role of financial sector actors in investing in global health. BMJ Glob Heal [Internet]. 2018 [cited 2021 Apr 19];3(Suppl 1). Available from: https://pubmed.ncbi.nlm.nih.gov/29736278/.

Trauma in the Setting of a Pandemic

60

Niels D. Martin and Lily Tung

Introduction

Care of trauma patients involves quick decision-making with incomplete information. Occasionally, our ability to care for trauma patients is challenged by pandemics, prompting a need to balance trauma care with preventing a worsening of the pandemic. Defined by Merriam-Webster as "an outbreak of a disease that occurs over a wide geographic area (such as multiple countries or continents) and typically affects a significant proportion of the population," pandemics can affect trauma in unpredictable ways, making preparation for these events difficult. For instance, on March 11, 2020, the World Health Organization declared COVID-19 a global pandemic. During this pandemic, societal lockdowns led to an overall decrease in traumas worldwide; however, some cities witnessed an increase in violent, penetrating traumas [1–12].

Hospitals often have contingency plans or disaster management plans for sudden influxes of patients. When a pandemic is declared, there is a potential need to quickly transition to the mindset of disaster management as a pandemic evolves. The difference between a pandemic and a natural disaster or bioterrorism is that a pandemic has an uncertain endpoint. With a new disease, particularly one on a global scale, there is a constant generation of new information for prevention, diagnosis, and treatment. In spite of the constantly evolving situation and increase in patients secondary to the pandemic, it is still important to try to maintain conventional care for as long as possible before changing to "contingency care" or even "crisis care" under the stress of the pandemic.

In order to best approach adjusting the pandemic response to maintain trauma readiness and the highest possible level of care, there are four categories that are often described in traditional disaster management that must be addressed: staff, stuff, space, and systems [13] (Table 60.1).

N. D. Martin
University of Pennsylvania, Department of Surgery, Philadelphia, PA, USA
e-mail: Niels.Martin@pennmedicine.upenn.edu

L. Tung (✉)
Royal Columbian Hospital, University of British Columbia, Department of Surgery, New Westminster, BC, Canada
e-mail: lily.tung@fraserhealth.ca

L. Marshall Gillman, S. Widder (eds.), *Trauma Team Dynamics*, https://doi.org/10.1007/978-3-031-86312-7_60

Table 60.1 Categories that need to be addressed in a pandemic: staff, stuff, space, and systems

Staff	*Stuff*
Retraining and reassignment of staff	Securing of PPE and supply chains
Modular staffing	Protocols detailing PPE use
Regular monitoring and testing of staff	Judicious use of blood products
Most experienced staff performing high-exposure procedures	
Removal of high-risk staff from direct patient care (older, immunocompromised, students)	
Limit in-person consults	
Monitoring of staff well-being	
Space	*Systems*
Hospital spaces can be reconfigured, repurposed, or reengineered to adapt to new needs (e.g., OR ➔ ICU, clinic ➔ ED)	Guidance from national health authorities and trauma associations
Trauma bay: establish hot/warm/cold zones, limit traffic, prohibit visitors	Regularly scheduled meetings and updates at both regional and hospital levels
OR: minimize staff, environmental contamination, OR time; consider dedicated pandemic ORs and transport routes, recover in OR and not PACU	Updates should be easily accessible online
ICU/floor: cluster work to minimize entry/exit from patient room, organize units by disease status, not service	Retraining of proper PPE use, N95 fittings
Clinic: switch to tele/video conferencing, screen for disease if in-person visit advised	Disaster credentialing and privileging

OR operating room, *ICU* intensive care unit, *ED* emergency department, *PACU* post-anesthetic care unit, *PPE* personal protective equipment

Staff

Management of staff will depend on specifics of the pandemic itself; however, the over-arching focus remains the same—protecting staff while maintaining quality of patient care. As with any new disease, patient care will be constantly evolving as new information becomes available. Until a rapid and accurate diagnostic test is available, all trauma patients need to be presumed positive on arrival. Changes that need to be implemented include retraining and reassignment of staff, modular staffing, establishing protocols for tele-consults, and maintaining staff well-being.

Retraining/Reassignment

A potential bottleneck during a pandemic is a shortage of specialized staff. Specialties most likely to be affected include emergency medicine, intensive care, and infectious disease. In cities where the pandemic results in a rise in trauma, additional support for trauma services may be required. As certain specialties will likely have their practices curtailed or even suspended, these physicians can be retrained and reassigned to assist with clinical coverage as surges occur or when staff become infected and are thus unable to continue to provide patient care. For instance, when elective cases are canceled, general surgeons can be retrained to cover trauma or emergency surgery [1, 13–15]. Given the abbreviated retraining of these physicians, a tiered staffing strategy may be necessary. For example, should a mass casualty occur during the pandemic, one fellowship-trained trauma surgeon may supervise multiple teams each consisting of a general surgeon, resident, and nurse. This allows general surgeons to utilize their transferrable skills to lead trauma resuscitations while having the content expert, the trauma surgeon, use their training and experience to safely run multiple resuscitations at once.

Furthermore, physicians of all specialties should also be updated to become more familiar with treatments or procedures that may become high in demand as a result of the pandemic. For example, during the COVID-19 pandemic, there was an increase in patients requiring intubation, so hospitals expanded their airway teams, developed protocols for proning patients in the intensive care unit (ICU), and implemented tracheostomy guidelines for the COVID-19 positive patients. Similarly, there was a decrease in available ventilators, thus necessitating retraining of staff to understand how to use BIPAP machines as a supportive modality [1]. Finally, if backup staff are limited or have already been exhausted, retired staff can be called upon for clinical duties. This, however, should be a last resort and needs to be balanced with retirees being older and so potentially more susceptible to the pandemic [15].

Modular Staffing

Given the infectious nature of a pandemic, even with proper application of personal protective equipment (PPE), healthcare workers can become infected and unable to work. Besides the aforementioned retraining and reassignment of medical staff, schedules should be revised so that teams work

Table 60.2 Example of modular staffing

	Week 1	Week 2	Week 3	Week 4	Week 5	Week 6
Team 1	Day shift	Night shift	Backup	Day shift	Night shift	Backup
Team 2	Night shift	Backup	Day shift	Night shift	Backup	Day shift
Team 3	Backup	Day shift	Night shift	Backup	Day shift	Night shift

Team 1: physicians A and B, Team 2: physicians C and D, Team 3: physicians E and F. Teams are to remain intact with no exchanging of team members

in isolation from each other to prevent the spread of disease by minimizing in-person physician-to-physician interactions whenever possible [16]. Also, backup teams should be included in the event that a team needs to be isolated. One such method to accomplish this is modular staffing.

Modular staffing involves creating teams of providers such that there are the maximum number of teams with the minimum number of providers needed for patient care per team. The team members do not change to allow for containment of any potential outbreaks, and better contact tracing and quarantining should the need arise [17, 18]. The teams should also be scheduled for shorter shifts with hand-offs being done remotely by phone or video conference [13, 18]. Shorter shifts may be necessary because of the increased risk of burnout from the stress associated with working during a pandemic and work with additional PPE on [13]. An example of a modular staffing schedule is shown in Table 60.2.

Other ways to decrease exposure include having attending physicians only perform high-exposure procedures, particularly in patients who are known to be positive. For example, during the COVID-19 pandemic when aerosolization was a potential mode of transmission, one Philadelphia hospital had only the most experienced person in-house perform intubations, and all intubations were performed in the trauma bay rather than the operating room (OR) in order to further minimize potential exposure [1]. Also, for operative traumas, the operating team should be limited to attending physicians and senior residents. This serves to not only minimize exposure to junior trainees, but it allows for a faster surgery, thus decreasing potential exposure to the entire OR team. Similarly, damage control principles should be utilized to minimize exposure to the entire OR team [19].

Outside the OR, consider having one attending physician cover more than one service while in-house or allowing for attending physicians to take call from home as long as they are within a reasonable distance from the hospital. For example, in a setting where trauma and emergency surgery services are staffed by separate attendings, the decrease in trauma may allow for one in-house attending to cover both services. Alternatively, depending on the local patient population and common injury patterns, the trauma surgeon may take call from home and be called in depending on the severity of the patient's injuries, with an emergency medicine physician or other in-house attending physician available to stabilize and resuscitate until the trauma surgeon's arrival.

Once diagnostic testing is available, consideration must be given for regular diagnostic testing and quarantining of healthcare workers to avoid larger level contamination [20, 21]. This also allows for more rapid containment of an entire team should one member of a team test positive while asymptomatic. Similarly, in order to protect healthcare workers, once vaccinations are available, all healthcare workers should be immunized unless medically contraindicated.

Finally, healthcare workers who are older, immunocompromised, or otherwise more susceptible to the disease may need to be withdrawn from clinical work that requires direct patient contact. Residents should return from satellite sites to their primary institutions to avoid commuting or travel that may contribute to inter-hospital spread. Medical students should be removed from clinical rotations to decrease risk of exposure and conserve PPE [20].

Consultants

Trauma patients are unique in that their injuries may require multiple different consultants. During a pandemic, protocols should be developed to allow for teleconsultations, with clear indications for when in-person consults would be necessary [1]. This would help further decrease potential exposures while still maintaining patient care. Similarly, the number of trauma team members allowed in the radiology suite should be limited to one to two providers to limit the exposure in the often small radiology reading rooms.

Staff Well-Being

The uncertainty and stressors of working in a pandemic can negatively impact healthcare workers' mental health and well-being. Studies have shown that during a pandemic, healthcare workers experience an increased risk of burnout, anxiety, depression, and insomnia [14, 22]. The pandemic's negative impact on healthcare workers can be due to a number of causes such as an increase in stress and fatigue from working with high-risk or positive patients, concern about transmitting the disease to their family or colleagues, the additional PPE required at work, the lack of PPE at work, and the uncertainty of working in the presence of a novel pathogen, especially one with no available treatment [22–24].

Mechanisms need to be put in place to monitor the psychological and emotional well-being of the team. Those who are exposed or test positive will need additional resources and support [18]. For those healthcare workers who choose to isolate themselves from their families to protect them, support for childcare, care of pets, or personal needs may help alleviate some stressors [13, 14]. Additional measures that may benefit the team include well-being sessions, frequent check-ins, and designated areas within the hospital to decompress. Debriefs should also be encouraged to help staff process difficult events or situations [25].

Stuff

Adequate PPE will be necessary to protect staff and avoid further spread of the pandemic. At the same time, careful conservation of PPE may be necessary as supply chains will need to be secured and manufacturers will require time to increase production to meet demands in both healthcare and public sectors. In order to ensure adequate stockpiles or emergency provisions, hospitals may need to reach out to local, provincial, or even federal governments for aid.

Furthermore, protocols may need to be developed to more clearly delineate the use of PPE. This is important particularly at the beginning of a pandemic when information is incomplete and there is increased anxiety among healthcare workers, which could lead to an overestimation of the risk of disease transmission and thus potential overuse of PPE. These concepts are especially important in trauma because of the invasive nature of the initial resuscitation exposing the providers to many patient secretions. For this reason, many trauma centers have staff in full PPE appropriate to the pandemic for every trauma resuscitation.

Finally, there may be potential shortages of blood products during a pandemic due to fear of disease transmission, donation centers being closed, or prospective donors electing to remain at home [18, 19]. As such, transfusions should be given judiciously, conservation methods such as autotransfusion employed, and the public encouraged to continue to donate blood while maintaining the proper precautions.

Space/Structure

Besides staff, space can quickly become a scarce resource during a pandemic. Hospital spaces may need to be reconfigured or repurposed to adapt to new needs. For instance, during the COVID-19 pandemic, engineers were engaged to create temporary negative pressure rooms in trauma bays, and ORs were repurposed to become ICUs. If the region a hospital is in has yet to be fully affected by the pandemic, then simulations to identify potential problems or bottlenecks are recommended so that necessary changes to procedures and protocols can be made and new workflows created and educated [1]. From a trauma perspective, there are four locations that may need to be addressed: trauma bay, OR, ICU, and clinics. Until cleared, trauma patients during a pandemic should be treated as infected in all phases of care.

Trauma Bay

Trauma bays are where the trauma team first encounters the patient. It is where resuscitation and life-saving procedures occur, which necessitates them to be fully equipped and in a space large enough to accommodate the entire trauma team. During a pandemic, trauma bays may need to be modified to better protect both providers and patients, while still maintaining their functionality. If a disease's mode of transmission is airborne, then rapid engagement with hospital engineers may be necessary to create negative pressure rooms in the trauma bay. Alternatively, if time or space does not allow for negative pressure rooms, then physical barriers need to be erected to separate trauma patients and minimize cross-contamination or certain trauma bays need to be designated for disease suspects or positive patients [1]. Regardless of how the space is modified, it needs to be able to continue to accommodate staff, supplies, and PPE [26].

In addition to the aforementioned changes, contamination needs to be minimized by establishing zones within the trauma bay. There should be three zones clearly marked out on the floor with colored tape: hot, warm, and cold zones. Each zone corresponds to the degree of contamination within that zone, with hot being on the patient's side where it is most contaminated (Fig. 60.1). In the warm zone, things are still considered potentially contaminated, but on a lower scale relative to the hot zone. This is where doffing of PPE would occur and where "transfer stations" would be stationed. "Transfer stations" are where supplies from the cold zone are placed for pick up by personnel in the hot zone. Lastly, the cold zone is considered clean and where donning of PPE would occur. All unnecessary equipment and supplies should be removed from the hot zone and placed in the cold zone. Any necessary equipment such as ultrasounds for FAST exams should be covered with a plastic bag similar to the probe covers used during sterile procedures to allow for easier cleaning and decreased contamination. Lead or plexiglass barriers should also be kept in the hot zone for use during X-rays. Equipment bundles for common procedures (chest tubes, thoracotomies, etc.) can be created and passed into the hot zone when required (Table 60.3). The trauma team in the hot zone should include only those who are actively working on the patient. If feasible, the trauma team leader can remain in the cold zone to direct the team to further conserve PPE and minimize exposure. Basic PPE should

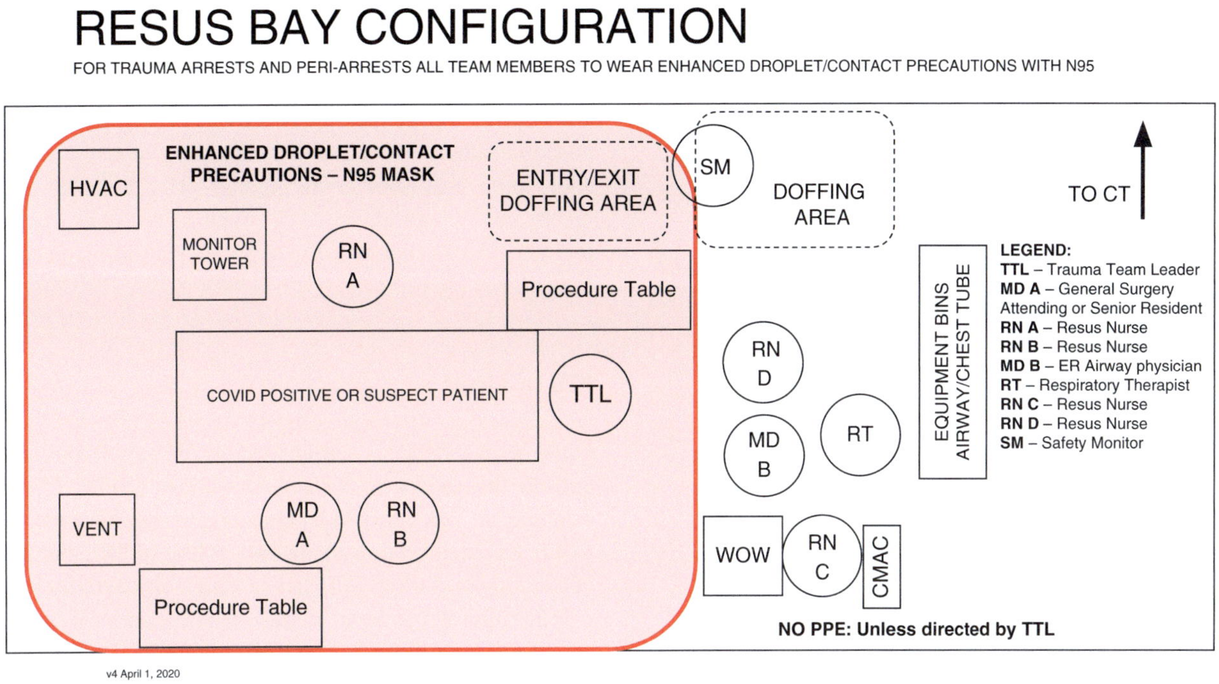

Fig. 60.1 Sample trauma bay layout with hot zone indicated in red

be worn in the warm zone, and additional pandemic-specific PPE is required in the hot zone. The distance between the hot and cold zones should be dictated by how far the pathogen could potentially travel, for example, in COVID-19, it was 6 feet from the patient's head [1, 26].

In order to limit traffic through the trauma bay, clearly designate one entrance and one exit. Only necessary personnel should have access to the trauma bay. Family or visitors should not be allowed in the trauma bay [27]. Consider performing a screening questionnaire and physical exam on arrival of the stable trauma patient. Consider placing a mask on the stable patient to mitigate aerosolization. All suspected cases should have diagnostic tests sent [28]. In the case of an unstable patient or a patient in extremis, omit any screening, assume the patient is positive, and proceed with full pandemic-specific PPE. In situations where the disease can be asymptomatic, there is increasing or high prevalence in the community, or if there are concerns about the hospital reaching capacity, assume all incoming trauma patients are positive [1, 18, 26, 29].

After resuscitation, most trauma patients will ultimately require transport to either imaging, the OR, or be admitted to the hospital. In order to minimize exposure during transport, the shortest possible one-way routes should be delineated beforehand. Not only should transport staff wear PPE, but the patient should as well. Gowns and sheets should either be disposable or placed in clearly marked infectious disease bags. All transport equipment should be disinfected once the patient has been transported to their destination [27]. When possible, consider portable imaging methods such as X-rays or ultrasound, to minimize transport through the hospital [30]. Early trauma patient testing can also de-escalate isolation at an earlier time point and save precious resources.

Operating Room

During a pandemic, resources such as staff and supplies may become severely limited. In such a setting, nonoperative management of trauma should be pursued whenever possible [19, 29, 31]. Goals of management with regard to the OR include minimizing exposure in the OR, environmental contamination, and OR time [16].

Logistical considerations include collaboration with the anesthesia department to establish policies on how to handle positive or presumed positive patients. For example, transport should occur along clearly marked pathways to designated ORs (preferably those closest to the entrance to the OR suites to minimize environmental contamination of entire hallways or OR pods) [32], particularly for patients who are positive or presumed positive. Patients who are not intubated should wear PPE at all times during transport. Stable patients should proceed directly to the ORs without passing through the preoperative area. If space allows, patients should be extubated and recovered in the OR instead of the PACU to minimize contamination to one room [16]. To further minimize exposure, the same transport team should take the patient from the trauma bay to the OR without transfer of

Table 60.3 Sample procedural bundles

Trauma team PPE bundle
6 X Waterproof gowns
6 X N95 masks
6 X Face shields
6 X Facemasks with shield
Chest tube/finger thoracostomy
3 X Chlorhexidine prep sticks (large)
1 x Sterile gown
1 x Medium sheet
2 x Green towels
2 x 5 cc Lidocaine local anesthetic vials
1 x Red 18 gauge blunt needle
1 x 22 Gauge needle
1 x 10 cc syringe
1 x #11 Scalpel blade (disposable)
1 x Chest tube insertion instrument tray
1 X 28Fr chest tube
1 x 0 Prolene suture or 0 silk suture
1 x Gelonet gauze
2 x Trach dressing
1 X ABD pad
1 X Mefix roll
1 X Pleur-evac
Thoracotomy (always handed up with a chest tube tray (above))
1 x Bottle of chlorhexidine
2 x Sterile gowns
1 x Medium sheet
4 x Green towels
1 x #10 Scalpel blade (disposable)
1 x 3–0 Vicryl suture
2 x 4–0 Prolene suture with tapered needles
1 x Skin stapler
1 x Thoracotomy instrument tray
2 x 5 Pack of laparotomy sponges
1 x Yankauer suction and tubing

care between different teams in between. Dedicated donning and doffing areas, similar to the warm zone in the trauma bay, should be located outside the ORs. All necessary PPE should be donned prior to entry into the OR. Additional disinfection measures may be necessary between cases depending on the pandemic disease [18, 19, 33, 34].

During the operation, a runner should be employed so that all staff who are in the OR remain inside until the case is completed [1, 27, 32]. Entry and exit into the OR should be limited [16]. Only equipment or supplies that are required for surgery should be in the OR to minimize waste and cleaning. Suture trees and other general stock should be kept outside of the room to minimize contamination. Preference should be given to instruments or supplies that have disposable alternatives [34]. No personal items should be allowed in the ORs. Disposable scrub caps and shoe covers should be used instead of personal fabric scrub caps [29, 34].

In pandemics in which the disease is airborne, aerosol-generating procedures such as intubation should only be performed in full PPE. Providers should avoid bag valve mask ventilation prior to intubation if possible and consider rapid sequence intubation [19, 27, 32, 34]. Intubation should be done by the most experienced provider using a video laryngoscope rather than direct laryngoscopy, and the endotracheal tube cuff should be inflated prior to commencing mechanical ventilation [34]. Where possible, perform regional blocks instead of general anesthesia, if the procedure allows [32].

ICU or Floor

Once a pandemic is anticipated or declared, policies to enforce the ease of access and correct use of PPE should be established. Work should be clustered to minimize entry and exit from patient rooms to not only conserve PPE, but the act of donning or doffing PPE can be a high-risk activity [6, 26]. If space allows, pandemic disease-positive patients should be separated from those who are negative [13]. In these cases, trauma patients may not be clustered in one unit or floor, and so the trauma team will need to be careful when rounding to not spread the disease within the hospital. If a shortage of ICU beds and ventilators occurs, ORs can be repurposed to become ICUs or PACUs [1, 25].

Clinic

For trauma clinic, most patients can be managed remotely by teleconference or video conference. Infrastructure for this should be deployed widely if not in place already. If a patient needs to be seen in person for follow-up, minimize exposure by limiting the number of staff present and try to coordinate the patient's visit with appointments with other specialties. All patients should be screened for the disease by phone prior to their appointment. They should not come to clinic if they are symptomatic or have recently tested positive for the disease.

Finally, just as ORs can be repurposed to become ICUs, clinics can be repurposed to become temporary emergency rooms in the event of a surge [1].

Systems

Effective communication is key during a pandemic, particularly one involving a new pathogen. The prolonged yet dynamic nature of the event requires constant situational awareness and implementation of effective communication strategies as new information regarding epidemiology, and scientific and clinical data becomes available. Regular updates on important items such as hospital capacity, available resources, prevention strategies, new diagnostic criteria, and potential treatments should be given virtually to minimize potential exposure and conserve PPE [18]. These updates should also be easily accessible online for those unable to attend the virtual meetings.

Below we describe suggestions for what can be done at the country, regional, hospital, and then division level.

Country Level

Regular updates and clear guidance should come from national health authorities such as the Centers for Disease Control and Prevention (United States of America) and Public Health Agency of Canada. In developing nations where resources, even at the national level, are scarce, access to information from other countries will be vital to understanding how to treat patients while protecting healthcare workers.

Regarding treating trauma patients, guidelines should also be sought from national organizations such as the American College of Surgeons Committee on Trauma, Eastern Association for the Surgery of Trauma, and American Association for the Surgery of Trauma.

Regional Level

At the regional level, weekly meetings should occur between trauma medical directors and program managers to discuss census data, facility-level surge activities, resource and PPE availability, any clinical lessons learned, and sharing of newly developed protocols [1]. Establishing a regional triage system, resource allocation, and crisis standards of care while taking into account local and regional resources should be discussed. Crisis standards of care are generally instituted on a regional level, ensuring the community gets equal care at all available centers. Contingency plans for the pandemic's impact on EMS and ability to transfer patients to higher level of care should also be discussed at the regional level. Capacity should be maintained at all level I and II trauma centers. Finally, in the event that the increase in hospitalized patients secondary to the pandemic combined with an increase in trauma patients exceeds the capacity and capabilities of adult hospitals, pediatric hospitals should consider increasing their age limits to accepting young adults [1].

Hospital Level

At the hospital level, a command center should be activated or established. This command center would function 24/7 to manage administrative, clinical, and communication responsibilities such as education and collaboration between different departments, development of protocols, patient flow, and procurement and allocation of resources [13, 18]. Based on factors such as census, resources, and predicted surge activities, elective cases may need to be canceled or limited to those that do not require post-operative admission [34]. Similarly, in-person ambulatory clinics may need to be canceled and transitioned to telehealth in order to minimize traffic and exposure at the hospital, as well as increase available space to be repurposed for other uses [1, 20].

Decisions made at the hospital level should be communicated to departments through regularly scheduled teleconference meetings. Items to discuss at these meetings include community or regional situation, current hospital census, projected number of patients who arrive, and any new policies or protocols or updates to existing ones [18]. Results of the meetings, especially new policies or protocols, should also be easily accessible online to centralize the information and make it available to those unable to attend the meetings.

Education regarding when, how, and how much PPE to use should be available to all healthcare workers [14, 33]. Additional appointments for N95 fittings may be required. This is particularly important at the beginning of the pandemic when anxiety and uncertainty may lead to over-use of PPE and waste [13]. Clear protocols outlining this should be created and distributed.

Given potential staff attrition secondary to the pandemic, disaster credentialing, privileging, degree of supervision needed, clinical scope of practice, and access to electronic medical records should be considered [18].

In order to protect staff and minimize spread of the disease, visitors to the hospital should be limited and hand hygiene encouraged [18].

Division or Trauma Team Level

At the division or trauma team level, hand-overs and morning reports should continue, but with providers participating remotely or from different rooms if possible [25]. Within the same meeting, regular briefings and memos about new policies, protocols, or clinical knowledge on the pandemic should also be given. Similar to a disaster scenario, understanding and establishment of early triage to palliative care for those with severe injuries who are not expected to survive will be important in a resource-scarce environment [18]. As discussed in the staffing section, general surgeons whose elective cases have been canceled can be reassigned to assist with trauma resuscitations or other patient care [1, 13–15]. In short, all efforts should be directed at effective communication while minimizing exposure and maintaining optimal trauma care [18].

Conclusion

Unlike other facets of life, trauma, unfortunately, does not stop with a pandemic. As the COVID-19 pandemic showed, pandemics pose significant challenges to trauma care. Early recognition, flexibility, and communication are key to continuing to provide optimal care for trauma patients. As the pandemic evolves, so must the policies and protocols that have been put in place. Finally, given the potential duration and stress of a pandemic, the well-being of those caring for patients must also be supported.

Key Points

- Maintaining trauma readiness in the setting of a pandemic requires early addressing of each of the four key categories of staff, stuff, space, and systems.
- Staff: to address staff well-being while concurrently maintaining quality of patient care, staff may need to be retrained or reassigned, modular staffing schedules created, and telemedicine considered.
- Stuff: centers need to be prepared for potential supply issues that may affect blood products, PPE, and other supplies.
- Space: hospital spaces may need to be reconfigured or repurposed to adapt to new needs.
- Systems: the prolonged and dynamic nature of a pandemic requires constant situational awareness and effective communication strategies at the hospital, regional, and country levels.

References

1. Qasim Z, Sjoholm LO, Volgraf J, Sailes S, Nance ML, Perks DH, et al. Trauma center activity and surge response during the early phase of the COVID-19 pandemic-the Philadelphia story. J Trauma Acute Care Surg. 2020;89(4):821–8.
2. Yeates EO, Grigorian A, Barrios C, Schellenberg M, Owattanapanich N, Barmparas G, et al. Changes in traumatic mechanisms of injury in Southern California related to COVID-19: penetrating trauma as a second pandemic. J Trauma Acute Care Surg. 2021;90(4):714–21.
3. Chiba H, Lewis M, Benjamin ER, Jakob DA, Liasidis P, Wong MD, et al. "Safer at home": the effect of the covid-19 lockdown on epidemiology, resource utilization and outcomes at a large urban trauma center. J Trauma Acute Care Surg. 2021;90(4):708–13.
4. Kamine TH, Rembisz A, Barron RJ, Baldwin C, Kromer M. Decrease in trauma admissions with COVID-19 pandemic. West J Emerg Med. 2020;21(4):819–22.
5. Fahy S, Moore J, Kelly M, Flannery O, Kenny P. Analysing the variation in volume and nature of trauma presentations during COVID-19 lockdown in Ireland. Bone Jt Open. 2020;1(6):261–6.
6. Forrester JD, Liou R, Knowlton LM, Jou RM, Spain DA. Impact of shelter-in-place order for COVID-19 on trauma activations: Santa Clara County, California, March 2020. Trauma Surg Acute Care Open. 2020;5(1):e000505.
7. Navsaria PH, Nicol AJ, Parry CDH, Matzopoulos R, Maqungo S, Gaudin R. The effect of lockdown on intentional and nonintentional injury during the COVID-19 pandemic in Cape Town, South Africa: a preliminary report. S Afr Med J. 2020;0(0):13183.
8. Harris D, Ellis DY, Gorman D, Foo N, Haustead D. Impact of COVID-19 social restrictions on trauma presentations in South Australia. Emerg Med Australas. 2020;33:152.
9. Jacob S, Mwagiru D, Thakur I, Moghadam A, Oh T, Hsu J. Impact of societal restrictions and lockdown on trauma admissions during the COVID-19 pandemic: a single-centre cross-sectional observational study. ANZ J Surg. 2020;90(11):2227–31.
10. Abdallah HO, Zhao C, Kaufman E, Hatchimonji J, Swendiman RA, Kaplan LJ, et al. Increased firearm injury during the COVID-19 pandemic: a hidden urban burden. J Am Coll Surg. 2021;232(2):159–68 e3.
11. Donnelly MR, Barie PS, Grigorian A, Kuza CM, Schubl S, de Virgilio C, et al. New York state and the nation: trends in firearm purchases and firearm violence during the COVID-19 pandemic. Am Surg. 2020;87:690–7. https://doi.org/10.1177/0003134820954827.
12. DiFazio LT, Curran T, Bilaniuk JW, Adams JM, Durling-Grover R, Kong K, et al. The impact of the COVID-19 pandemic on hospital admissions for trauma and acute care surgery. Am Surg. 2020;86(8):901–3.
13. Faccincani R, Pascucci F, Lennquist S. How to surge to face the SARS-CoV-2 outbreak: lessons learned from Lombardy, Italy. Disaster Med Public Health Prep. 2020;14(5):e39–41.
14. Ellis R, Hay-David AGC, Brennan PA. Operating during the COVID-19 pandemic: how to reduce medical error. Br J Oral Maxillofac Surg. 2020;58(5):577–80.
15. Ehrlich H, McKenney M, Elkbuli A. Strategic planning and recommendations for healthcare workers during the COVID-19 pandemic. Am J Emerg Med. 2020;38(7):1446–7.
16. De Simone B, Chouillard E, Di Saverio S, Pagani L, Sartelli M, Biffl WL, et al. Emergency surgery during the COVID-19 pandemic: what you need to know for practice. Ann R Coll Surg Engl. 2020;102(5):323–32.
17. Nadarajan GD, Omar E, Abella BS, Hoe PS, Do Shin S, Ma MH, et al. A conceptual framework for Emergency department design in a pandemic. Scand J Trauma Resusc Emerg Med. 2020;28(1):118.
18. Maintaining trauma center access and care during the COVID-19 pandemic: guidance document for trauma medical directors American College of Surgeons Committee on Trauma. 2020. Available from: https://www.facs.org/quality-programs/trauma/maintaining-access.
19. Dutton RP, Grissom TE, Herbstreit F. COVID-19 and trauma care: improvise, adapt, and overcome! Anesth Analg. 2020;131(2):323–5.
20. Javor P, Varga E, Fekete K, Toth F, Hartmann P. Novel coronavirus and trauma surgery: successful infection control from a level I trauma centre. Eur J Trauma Emerg Surg. 2020;46(4):737–41.
21. Fransvea P, Sganga G, Cozza V, Di Grezia M, Fico V, Tirelli F, et al. Set up of a dedicated COVID-19 surgical pathway and operating room for surgical emergencies. J Trauma Acute Care Surg. 2020;89(4):e97–e100.
22. Muller AE, Hafstad EV, Himmels JPW, Smedslund G, Flottorp S, Stensland SO, et al. The mental health impact of the covid-19 pandemic on healthcare workers, and interventions to help them: a rapid systematic review. Psychiatry Res. 2020;293:113441.
23. Cabarkapa S, Nadjidai SE, Murgier J, Ng CH. The psychological impact of COVID-19 and other viral epidemics on frontline healthcare workers and ways to address it: a rapid systematic review. Brain Behav Immun Health. 2020;8:100144.
24. Mattila E, Peltokoski J, Neva MH, Kaunonen M, Helminen M, Parkkila AK. COVID-19: anxiety among hospital staff and associated factors. Ann Med. 2021;53(1):237–46.

25. Tahmassebi R, Bates P, Trompeter A, Bhattacharya R, El-Daly I, Jeyaseelan L, et al. Reflections from London's Level-1 Major Trauma Centres during the COVID crisis. Eur J Orthop Surg Traumatol. 2020;30(6):951–4.
26. Livingston DH, Bonne S, Morello C, Fox A. Optimizing the trauma resuscitation bay during the covid-19 pandemic. Trauma Surg Acute Care Open. 2020;5(1):e000488.
27. Chen P, Xiong XH, Chen Y, Wang K, Zhang QT, Zhou W, et al. Perioperative management strategy of severe traumatic brain injury during the outbreak of COVID-19. Chin J Traumatol. 2020;23(4):202–6.
28. Hu P, Jansen JO, Uhlich R, Black J, Pierce V, Hwang J, et al. Early comprehensive testing for COVID-19 is essential to protect trauma centers. J Trauma Acute Care Surg. 2020;89(4):698–702.
29. Gok AFK, Eryilmaz M, Ozmen MM, Alimoglu O, Ertekin C, Kurtoglu MH. Recommendations for trauma and emergency general surgery practice during COVID-19 pandemic. Ulus Travma Acil Cerrahi Derg. 2020;26(3):335–42.
30. Halvachizadeh S, Teuben M, Berk T, Neuhaus V, Pape HC, Pfeifer R. The impact of SARS-CoV-2 (COVID-19) pandemic on trauma bay management and guideline adherence in a European level-one-trauma centre. Int Orthop. 2020;44(9):1621–7.
31. Di Saverio S, Khan M, Pata F, Ietto G, De Simone B, Zani E, et al. Laparoscopy at all costs? Not now during COVID-19 outbreak and not for acute care surgery and emergency colorectal surgery: a practical algorithm from a hub tertiary teaching hospital in Northern Lombardy, Italy. J Trauma Acute Care Surg. 2020;88(6):715–8.
32. Li Y, Zeng L, Li Z, Mao Q, Liu D, Zhang L, et al. Emergency trauma care during the outbreak of corona virus disease 2019 (COVID-19) in China. World J Emerg Surg. 2020;15(1):33.
33. Coccolini F, Perrone G, Chiarugi M, Di Marzo F, Ansaloni L, Scandroglio I, et al. Surgery in COVID-19 patients: operational directives. World J Emerg Surg. 2020;15(1):25.
34. Coimbra R, Edwards S, Kurihara H, Bass GA, Balogh ZJ, Tilsed J, et al. European Society of Trauma and Emergency Surgery (ESTES) recommendations for trauma and emergency surgery preparation during times of COVID-19 infection. Eur J Trauma Emerg Surg. 2020;46(3):505–10.

Part VII

Trauma Team Education

61 Designing a Simulation Curriculum

Jason Park, Reagan L. Robertson, and Ashley S. Vergis

Simulation-based education offers great opportunities for learners in medicine and the health professions. It can be used to teach cognitive or technical skills in a safe environment that is focused on experiential and reflective learning. Too often, however, attention is focused on the simulators themselves and their associated technology. It is important to keep in mind that simulation is an instructional medium, and simulators function only as tools in this context. The focus should not be on the tools, but rather on the educational experience they enable. It is therefore necessary to ensure that simulation is thoughtfully incorporated and appropriately used within an educational curriculum in order to maximize its educational impact.

For the purposes of this chapter on trauma team training, simulation will refer specifically to "simulated clinical immersion" (SCI) [1]. However, many of the curriculum design principles that are discussed can be applied to other simulation modalities as well. SCI involves guided experiences in simulated environments, often with the use of human patient simulators. These experiences are aimed to complement and improve real patient experiences for learners. The distinctive feature of SCI is that the environment reproduces the actual clinical or work environment and directly affects the educational experience. SCI can be used to reproduce the high acuity, dynamic, and often fast-paced environments that characterize the operating room, trauma bay, or emergency department. This simulation modality is an especially valuable method of teaching the non-technical skills involved in trauma team and crisis resource management, including situational awareness, clinical judgment, decision-making, interpersonal behavior and teamwork, and stress management. These skills are essential to competently and efficiently manage trauma situations that present in clinical practice.

Designing an educational curriculum to effectively incorporate simulation can be a daunting task. There are multiple steps that contribute to an effective educational program, and it requires an organized and well-thought-out approach. Many authors have written entire books on curriculum development for medical education, some of which are included in the Refs. [2, 3]. The frameworks described by these authors share common steps or components. With a focus on competencies and educational outcomes, this chapter follows Sherbino and Franks's five-step framework for systematic educational design (Fig. 61.1) [3]. This chapter serves as an overview of the basic steps that are involved in curriculum design, with a focus on how these steps apply to simulation. These steps include the following: (1) conducting a needs assessment, (2) developing learning objectives, (3) selecting and implementing appropriate instructional methods, (4) assessing learning and competence, and (5) evaluating the educational program. Some of these steps are further described in the chapters that follow, including Designing Multidisciplinary Simulation Scenarios (Chap. 62),

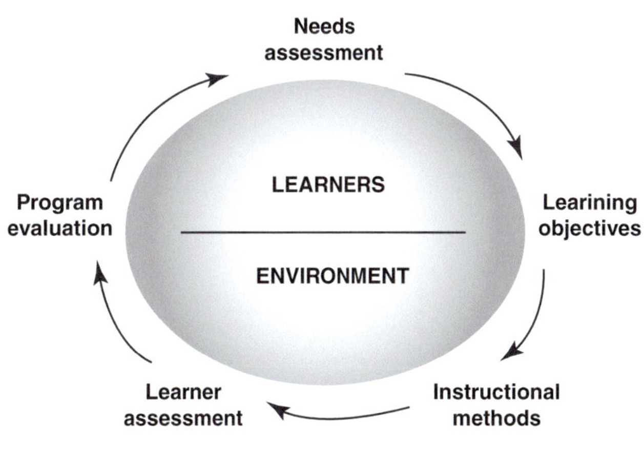

Fig. 61.1 Systematic educational design. (Source: Sherbino and Frank [3]. Reproduced with permission [3])

J. Park
Department of Surgery, University of British Columbia, Vancouver, BC, Canada
e-mail: jpark@sbgh.mb.ca

R. L. Robertson · A. S. Vergis (✉)
Department of Surgery, University of Manitoba, Winnipeg, MB, Canada
e-mail: rrobertson@sbgh.mb.ca; avergis@sbgh.mb.ca

L. Marshall Gillman, S. Widder (eds.), *Trauma Team Dynamics*, https://doi.org/10.1007/978-3-031-86312-7_61

Constructive Debriefing for Trauma Team Education (Chap. 63), and Program Evaluation and Assessment of Learning (Chap. 64).

Needs Assessment

The first step in designing a relevant, comprehensive, and effective educational program is to conduct a needs assessment (NA). This serves as the foundation from which the curriculum structure flows. The curriculum's goals and objectives are written based on the results of the NA. The instructional methods are then chosen to meet these goals and objectives.

NA refers to the systematic process of collecting and analyzing information to define the educational needs of the target group [4]. The NA can target individual learners or entire programs. The main point of the NA is that it makes systematic a process that before was largely based on assumptions. The NA identifies the target group's learning needs, which refers to the gaps between a learner's current and desired ability that can be overcome by a learning activity [5].

Learning needs can be considered from several viewpoints including the learner, educator, institution (including accreditation or licensing bodies, specialty societies, or hospitals), and society [6]. Historically, educators often adopted the idea that they knew best the learner's needs. However, taking the learner's perceived needs into consideration not only addresses gaps that the learners themselves identify but may also increase their engagement in the learning activity. Ultimately, it is necessary to strike a balance that considers the perspectives of learners and educators and also ensures that institutional and societal perspectives are represented.

NAs can be conducted using information from a number of different sources (Table 61.1). Each source has its own complexities, advantages and disadvantages, and resource requirements. Some of the desired information may already be in existence and easily accessible. In other cases, it may have to be acquired, which may add time and costs to the process.

Sources of information that are commonly used for NAs include external sources, internal sources, as well as data generated from questionnaires, surveys, or interviews. These information sources are further described below:

1. *External sources* include literature searches for original studies, reviews, or practice guidelines; published reports or statements from accrediting bodies (e.g., CanMEDS Roles put forth by the Royal College of Physicians and Surgeons of Canada or the core competencies defined by the Accreditation Council for Graduate Medical Education); and the results of accreditation surveys. External sources are often a good starting point because they can be fairly encompassing, yet readily available at a low cost.
2. *Internal sources* refer to data from within the institution that can be used to identify learning needs. These data

Table 61.1 Information sources that can be used for a needs assessment

Method	Description	Strengths	Weaknesses
Questionnaire or survey	Set of written questions or items	Low cost, relatively easy to administer Can assess wide variety of topics and sample a large population Quantitative and/or qualitative data	Skill is required to write questions because the quality of data is dependent on the design and quality of the questions Time and costs of administering, collecting, and analyzing data Responses may be difficult to generalize without an adequate response rate Self-reported data
Individual interviews	Individual face-to-face or telephone interviews	Useful to get in-depth insight into participants' perspectives Can allow for open-ended questions to assess broader range of topics or clarify/elaborate on responses Qualitative data	Resource and time intensive; requires trained interviewers to collect data and often high-level expertise to analyze data Often sample a limited number of participants Self-reported data
Focus group interviews	Group interview, usually 4–10 participants per group	Allows interviewing several participants at a time Many of the same advantages as individual interviews but group interaction can allow participants to express perspectives that they might not express in individual format Qualitative data	Resource and time intensive; requires trained interviewers and often high-level expertise to analyze data Data can sometimes be skewed by participants who dominate the discussion Some participants may be reluctant to disclose information in non-anonymous group settings Self-reported data

(continued)

Table 61.1 (continued)

Method	Description	Strengths	Weaknesses
Internal environmental scans	Examination of data generated within the organization; sources of data can include: Course evaluations Faculty assessments Performance data from previous student cohorts Mortality and morbidity rounds Chart audits	Much of this data has already been collected (with the exception of some chart audits)	Data quality and utility can be variable Data must be re-interpreted and re-purposed Chart audits can sometimes be time-consuming and costly
External environmental scans	Examination of externally generated data; sources of data can include: Accreditation surveys Literature searches Reports or practice guidelines from accrediting bodies or professional organizations	Can provide a starting point for data collection Can be low cost since data is usually already collected and accessible Can identify new topics from outside organizations	May not be applicable at local context Data may have to be re-interpreted and re-purposed
Strategic planning	Activities can include: Review of organization's mission and vision Reviews of survey and interviews, internal and external scan results Brainstorming of participants and stakeholders	Usually involves a range of participants and stakeholders, including learners, teachers, educators, and administrators Allows leadership to develop and prioritize needs Useful for large-scale curriculum development or renewal	Resource and time intensive; requires skilled leadership and facilitation

Adapted from: Ratnapalan et al. [4], Kern et al. [2], and Sherbino and Lockyer [6]

sources include direct observation and faculty assessments, mortality and morbidity rounds, examination results from previous student cohorts, and chart audits. Some of this data may already be available at the institution level, but the quality can be variable and the data usually has to be repurposed and reinterpreted.

3. *Questionnaires, surveys, interviews, or focus groups* can be used to gain insight into the learner's, educator's, and other stakeholders' perspectives. These tools can be used when the available information is insufficient or when there is a need to collect new or more specific information.

The scope of the intended curriculum, including the type, purpose, and available resources, guides the specific information sources selected for use in the NA. In practice, it is best to use these information sources in combination and take into account data from multiple different sources. This approach can enhance the educator's understanding of the target group's learning needs and ensure the curriculum's relevance and comprehensiveness.

Learning Objectives

The next step in designing a curriculum is to transform the learning needs into learning objectives. Learning objectives are clear statements of the intended outcomes of the specific learning activity [7]. They state what the learner will be able to do after the learning activity that they could not do before [8]. Learning objectives are related to learning goals but are more specific. Goals are broader statements about the overall purpose of a curriculum. They are more general and more difficult to measure. In contrast, learning objectives are specific and designed to be more easily measured. Achieving the specific objectives should contribute to achieving the overall goals of the curriculum.

Learning objectives are important for learners and educators in that they set specific expectations for the outcome of the learning activity. The objectives also guide the selection of learning methods and help to prioritize content. Finally, learning objectives enable assessment and program evaluation to demonstrate the effectiveness of the curriculum.

Well-written learning objectives have five elements:

1. A *defined learner*. Objectives should describe "who" they are intended for. This description is especially useful for simulation sessions that involve multiple learners at different levels or from different backgrounds who may have different learning objectives. Furthermore, learning objectives should always be written from the learners' perspective.
2. A *time reference* during which the learning occurs. For example, objectives may apply to a single simulation ses-

Table 61.2 Examples of learning objectives using observable action verbs

"At the end of this simulation session, second-year general surgery residents will identify the causes of hemodynamic instability in patients who sustain blunt abdominal trauma"
"At the end of the simulation course, workshop participants will demonstrate the standard technique for chest compressions"
"At the end of his simulation scenario, trauma team leaders will be able to describe the factors associated with poor compliance with advanced trauma life support guidelines in the resuscitation room"

sion or a series of sessions, or to an entire training program.

3. A *performance description* of what the learner should be able to do. A key point when writing performance descriptors is to use action verbs that identify an observable behavior. Observable action verbs provide clear and more precise guidance for learners than non-observable verbs. They are also easier to assess. Examples of observable action verbs that apply to skills required for trauma team management include "identify," "list," or "demonstrate." In contrast, non-observable verbs, like "appreciate" or "understand," are vague for learners and difficult to measure.
4. The *conditions under which learners will learn*. The educational tools that are provided or can be used are defined.
5. The *criteria for assessing performance*, including the minimal standard for assessing performance.

In some cases, the learning objectives will need to specify each of these elements in detail. In others, some of these elements may be implied. Table 61.2 lists some examples of learning objectives that incorporate these elements. The focus of learning objectives should always be the learners' performance at the end of the learning activity.

Instructional Methods

After establishing objectives, the next step in designing an educational program is to develop content and choose the most appropriate instructional methods to achieve the objectives. Several factors need to be considered when choosing instructional methods for any curriculum. These include the following: (1) the domain of the objectives and competencies of interest, (2) the number of learners, their backgrounds and levels, (3) the learning environment and available resources and expertise, and (4) practical issues associated with implementing an instructional method, such as the time frame.

There are a number of different instructional methods, and some methods are more appropriate for certain objectives than others. Ultimately, it is necessary to select the instructional methods that best achieve the desired learning objectives. To create appropriate training opportunities using simulation, it is necessary to select objectives from your broader needs that can be met using the available simulation technology.

Simulation can be used to teach and assess a range of roles or competencies. It offers the opportunity to bring members of a healthcare team together in a simulated environment, which makes it an ideal platform to teach and assess team processes and outcomes. Consequently, simulation is an especially effective method to teach crisis resource and trauma team management skills like situational awareness, clinical judgment, decision-making, communication, leadership, teamwork, and inter-specialty or inter-professional care. Participants can learn and practice these skills in a structured, safe, and supportive learning environment without compromising the safety of patients. Simulation-based training has been shown to improve crisis management non-technical skills, and quality of care in high acuity situations [9, 10]. The main disadvantage of simulation is that it is only useful for certain types of objectives, so it is crucial to match the learning methods to the type of objectives of interest. Simulation can also be expensive and resource intensive, so it is important to engage leadership early in the curriculum development process to build and maintain support for the program.

Simulation sessions usually have three main parts: (1) a briefing in which the participants get acquainted with the setting, the case, and the available resources, (2) the exposure to a simulated scenario, and (3) the debriefing in which the participants get feedback from the facilitators or preceptors. Because simulation involves active participation from the learner, the learner should have at least some previous experience with the topic. Before any session, the teacher should familiarize him or herself with the characteristics of the learner, their training (specialty or discipline and level of education), and previous experience with the topic in question.

The scenarios used in simulation courses form the core of the educational experience, and their development is discussed in the next chapter. The debriefing session is also an essential part of simulation-based education. The debriefing session gives learners the opportunity to receive feedback and reflect on their performance. The feedback consists of identifying performance gaps, determining the basis of these gaps, and then targeting instruction to close the gaps. It is intended to be constructive and to stimulate reflective practice, focusing on improvement rather than being judgmental or critical.

Simulation for Assessing Learners

An assessment plan for learners is an integral part of a well-developed educational curriculum. Assessment follows the instructional method, which in turn flows from the curriculum's goals and objectives.

Miller previously proposed a framework to assess clinical performance or competence [11]. In his framework, the achievement of competence follows a hierarchical progression from "knows," to "knows how," to "shows how," to "does." Simulation provides a realistic environment where learners must apply and integrate knowledge, skills, and decision-making abilities in real time. By placing learners in this environment, educators can evaluate competency in a way that more closely reflects actual clinical practice compared to other learning methods. In particular, simulation offers educators the opportunity to observe and assess learners' ability to "show how."

Simulation can allow the assessment of multiple skills or roles within a single testing session. Trauma simulation is particularly useful in testing decision-making (medical expert role), teamwork (collaborator role), and communication skills (communicator role). When planning assessments for trauma scenarios, it is not necessary to assess all the roles all the time. It is more appropriate to use specific tools to assess specific objectives for a particular scenario or program. For example, some simulation scenarios may teach medical expertise and communication, and assessment should focus on these roles in these cases. It would be inappropriate to assess roles that did not play a large part of a given scenario.

The choice of assessment tool should match the type and stage of the learning being assessed or taught. In other words, the complexity of the assessment tool should match the complexity of the learning objective. Furthermore, the assessment tools should have evidence to support the reliability and validity of their results. Finally, the assessment needs to be practical to administer with the resources available.

Program Evaluation

Program evaluation refers to a systematic process of reviewing an education program. The most important question when conducting a program evaluation is whether the program achieved its intended goals and objectives. Through this process, educators can decide on whether to continue a program or identify changes that may be needed to improve future programs. Program evaluations also help educators decide whether the program justifies the resources allocated to it.

The program evaluation process has three main components: (1) determining the elements to be evaluated (what to evaluate), (2) selecting the best approach and tools to conduct the evaluation (how to evaluate), and (3) analyzing the data so that decisions can be made about the program. There are several established frameworks for program evaluation that can be applied to simulation-based education, such as the Kirkpatrick Hierarchy (Reaction, Knowledge, Behavior, Results) or CIPP (Context, Input, Process, Product) models [12, 13]. Program evaluations can be based on one or several of the levels or points within these frameworks. The specific tools for evaluation can include questionnaires or semi-structured interviews, structured observations, and examination results. The extent of the evaluation must be consistent with the size of the educational program and the resources available to conduct the evaluation. Last but not least, the intent of the evaluation will determine the types of decisions that can be made on its basis. Program evaluation results are most commonly used for continuous quality improvement.

Summary

Simulation can play an important part of a system aimed at improving performance and enabling high-quality care for trauma patients. However, simulation by itself is merely a means. The success of any simulation activity ultimately depends on how simulation is incorporated and used within a broader educational curriculum.

Designing a comprehensive, cohesive, and effective educational curriculum entails several key steps. Curriculum design usually starts with a needs assessment, which serves as the foundation from which the rest of the curriculum structure flows. The curriculum's goals and learning objectives are developed based on the results of the needs assessment, and instructional methods are then chosen to best meet these goals and objectives. The objectives also facilitate the assessment of learning. Finally, program evaluation should be planned as part of the curriculum design process to evaluate the effectiveness of the curriculum.

Key Points

- The success of any simulation activity ultimately depends on how simulation is incorporated and used within a broader educational curriculum.
- Curriculum design usually starts with a needs assessment, which serves as the foundation from which the rest of the curriculum structure flows.
- The curriculum's goals and learning objectives are developed based on the results of the needs assessment, and instructional methods are then chosen to best meet the goals and objectives.
- Learner assessments and program evaluation should also be planned as part of the curriculum design process to evaluate curriculum's effectiveness.

References

1. Chiniara G, Cole G, Brisbin K, Huffman D, Cragg B, Lamacchia M, et al. Simulation in healthcare: a taxonomy and a conceptual framework for instructional design and media selection. Med Teach. 2013;35:e1380–95.
2. Kern DE, Thomas PA, Hughes MT. Curriculum development for medical education: a six-step approach. 2nd ed. Baltimore: Johns Hopkins University Press; 2009.
3. Sherbino J, Frank JR. Educational design: a CanMEDS guide for the health professions. Ottawa: Royal College of Physicians and Surgeons of Canada; 2011.
4. Ratnapalan S, Hilliard RI. Needs assessment in postgraduate medical education: a review. Med Educ Online. 2002;7:1–8.
5. Jean P, Des Marchais J, Delorme P. Needs assessment. On becoming an educator in the health professions: a systematic approach. Ottawa; 1994.
6. Sherbino J, Lockyer J. Mind the gap: educational needs assessment. In: Sherbino J, Frank JR, editors. Educational design: a CanMEDS guide for the health professions. Ottawa: Royal College of Physicians and Surgeons; 2011.
7. Richardson D, Flynn L. The roadmap: learning objectives. In: Sherbino J, Frank JR, editors. Educational design: a CanMEDS guide for the health professions. Ottawa: Royal College of Physicians and Surgeons; 2011.
8. Amin Z, Eng KH. Basics in medical education. Singapore: World Scientific Publishing Company; 2005.
9. Wayne DB, Didwania A, Feinglass J, Fudala MJ, Barsuk JH, McGaghie WC. Simulation-based education improves quality of care during cardiac arrest team responses at an academic teaching hospital: a case-control study. Chest. 2008;133:56–61.
10. Buljac-Samardzic M, Dekker-van Doorn CM, van Wijngaarden JD, van Wijk KP. Interventions to improve team effectiveness: a systematic review. Health Policy. 2010;94:183–95.
11. Miller GE. The assessment of clinical skills/competence/performance. Acad Med. 1990;65:S63–7.
12. Kirkpatrick DL, Kirkpatrick JD. Evaluating training programs: the four levels. 3rd ed. San Francisco: Berret-Koehler; 2006.
13. Stufflebeam DL. The CIPP model for evaluation. In: Stufflebeam DL, Madaus GF, Kellaghan T, editors. Evaluation in education and human services. New York: Springer; 2002.

Simulation Scenario Design

62

J. Damian Paton-Gay, Peter G. Brindley, and Lawrence Marshall Gillman

The Fundamentals of Scenario Design

In this chapter we will provide a framework for designing simulation scenarios. We will also identify key decision points and pitfalls during the design process. There is much room for creativity in scenario design, but it must rest upon a disciplined adherence to fundamental principles. Deviation from these can result in unwieldy scenarios, unclear learning objectives, inefficiency, confused participants, and frustrated faculty. Careful scenario can mitigate many of the difficulties encountered in debriefing sessions while ensuring a rich learning experience.

A Stepwise Approach to Scenario Design

We will use a series of steps to guide scenario design. They are as follows:

(i) Needs assessment
(ii) Identification of target audience/participants
(iii) Statement of goal
(iv) Creation of objectives
(v) Scenario design
(vi) Running the scenario
(vii) Revising the scenario

J. D. Paton-Gay (✉)
Department of Surgery, University of Alberta, Edmonton, AB, Canada
e-mail: patongay@ualberta.ca

P. G. Brindley
Department of Critical Care Medicine, University of Alberta Hospital, Edmonton, AB, Canada
e-mail: peter.brindley@albertahealthservices.ca

L. Marshall Gillman
Departments of Surgery Section of General Surgery, Internal Medicine Section of Critical Care, University of Manitoba, Winnipeg, MB, Canada
e-mail: lawrence.gillman@umanitoba.ca

It is not critical to adhere only to the order above. A needs assessment is required as a first step, and running and revising the scenario occur once we have done the previous steps; however, as we move through steps ii to v, we often move back and forth steps as logistical limitations or new information come to light that informs earlier steps.

The Importance of Needs Assessment, Goals, and Objectives

Simulation is intuitive as a coaching and educational endeavor. Most of us have experience with simulated training outside of healthcare, such as performing drills during athletic practice, practicing oral presentations in front of friends, or practicing music prior to a recital. There is a risk to that familiarity, however. It can seem that we simply put together a scenario that approximates real life and "voila!" we are practicing. Certainly, some practice will occur when it is run as a simulation event. However, there is a significant risk of merely practicing what we already do, good or bad. In medical simulation, there is also a tendency to increase complexity and stress of simulated cases solely to encourage engagement of participants. Facilitators often feel jubilant watching their participants struggle through difficult cases. *However, key questions to ask are: Did this really accomplish our goal? What was our goal? What were our objectives? Was stress a contributor or a hindrance to learning in this event? Did we learn new skills, hone existing ones or did we practice maladaptive, defensive behaviors?*

Several years ago, leaders in simulation education began using the phrase "It Depends On Your Objectives," shortened to IDOYO. We are not sure who coined the phrase and acronym, but it caught on because of its utility as a response to questions about scenario design. Wondering who your target audience/participants are? IDOYO. Wondering what simulation modality to use? IDOYO. Wondering how much stress/urgency to add? IDOYO. Wondering how much complexity is required? IDOYO.

L. Marshall Gillman, S. Widder (eds.), *Trauma Team Dynamics*, https://doi.org/10.1007/978-3-031-86312-7_62

In short, all of the decisions in scenario design are informed by the *goal and objectives* for the event, and the goal and objectives are informed by a *needs assessment*. Accrediting bodies such as the Royal College of Physicians and Surgeons of Canada provide standards for simulation activities that highlight the importance of high-quality objectives [1].

Needs Assessment

Used to guide an entire curriculum or a single simulation event, the *needs assessment* is exactly how it sounds. It is a determination of why specific practice or an educational event is required. This generally translates easily to a statement of the goal. *Needs* may relate to technical skills (such as performing a procedure), to communication and team function, to system or environmental issues (e.g., identifying latent safety hazards or assessing a new protocol), or to familiarizing participants with the training methods. Below are some examples of needs assessments and goals (Table 62.1):

Objectives

Objectives are clear, concise statements describing the outcome of an educational event. In other words, objectives allow us to answer the question "after this session, how will we know that learning has occurred?" For us to see the effects of an educational event, there must be an identifiable change in participants' behavior. For this reason, objectives are always stated using a verb describing an observable action at the start.

It is critical that objective statements incorporate discrete, identifiable behaviors rather than general terms or descriptions of outcomes [2]. For example, the objective "Use good communication to maximize team efficiency" seems, on the surface, to provide guidance for participants and facilitators. However, "good communication" refers to the outcome we see when specific communication skills are employed. To design and run a scenario that will improve communication, we need to clarify which specific skills are to be practiced. This is similar to a sport coach building a drill to "get the ball out of our zone." This will lead to frustration as the players try, as they do in real games, to create the outcome of clearing the ball out of their own zone without employing specific skills that allow the goal to be realized. The *goal* of the drill is to improve clearance of the zone, while the *objectives* may be to (a) position the offensive players to receive an outgoing pass and (b) use body position by defensive players to create lanes through which the ball can be cleared out of the zone. Below are some examples of objectives for healthcare simulations (Table 62.2).

Tables of objective verbs are widely available. In line with Benjamin Bloom's original work on the topic in 1956, these tables divide objective verbs into domains of knowledge, comprehension, application, analysis, synthesis, and evaluation [3]. An example is available on the Utica University website [4].

Table 62.1 Examples of needs assessments and goals

Needs assessment	Goal of session
Communication errors during resuscitations have led to delays in care	Practice specific communication skills that will minimize errors
During proning of ARDS patients in the ICU, we have had several cases of lines and tubes being dislodged	Practice proning patients while maintaining a high level of situational awareness
A new resuscitation bay is being built, we must determine how it can be best arranged and outfitted prior to completion of the build	Use simulations of resuscitations to guide the organization and building of the new resuscitation bay
Delays in transport of blood products from the blood bank to the operating room have led to delays in care	Determine where delays may be happening by simulating blood ordering, preparation, and transportation
Surgical residents must perform emergency surgical maneuvers quickly and expertly despite seeing very few in real life	Practice high stakes, low frequency surgical maneuvers such as emergency department thoracotomy in a laboratory setting
A needs assessment suggests that simulation will help our emergency department staff manage intubations under airborne precautions, but the staff are unfamiliar with simulation	Familiarize staff with, and demonstrate the feasibility of in situ simulation in our department using straightforward cases and thorough prebriefing before moving on to new skills
Team members have expressed discomfort with having family members present at resuscitations and are unsure of how to incorporate them	Review methods for involving and helping family members through resuscitations, then practice first with lower emotional/psychological realism

Table 62.2 Examples of objectives for healthcare simulation

Goal	Objective(s)
Improve communication in the resuscitation bay	*Target* all communication to a specific audience Employ closed-loop communication
Minimize delays in ordering and transporting blood products during major surgery	*Specify* exactly what blood products are necessary *Delegate* an individual team member to manage ordering blood and communicating with blood bank
Improve team comfort and facility with having family members present at resuscitations	*Position* family members where they are involved, yet safe and not impeding care *Assign* a liaison to the family member *Provide* summaries to family member and liaison while team members are performing tasks
Improve safety of proning ARDS patients in the ICU	*Perform* a time-out prior to proning *Maintain* role clarity by assigning specific roles and responsibilities to each member *Assign* a team leader who will stand back and ensure safety
Familiarize team members with the use of in situ simulation in the emergency department	*Facilitate* an in situ simulation in the emergency department *Coordinate* with triage and charge nurses to ensure real patients are not affected by the event *Coordinate* with ER manager to ensure that staff are available to take part and focus on the event

Choosing a Modality

Once we have determined our goal and objectives for an event and ascertained that simulation is an appropriate teaching method, we must decide on a modality. Combining our objectives with an understanding of the types of realism in simulation typically yields a clear solution for which modality is most important. Thus, we will first explore the types of realism.

Types of Realism in Simulation

Physical Realism

This refers to how closely the physical space, props or trainer/mannequin approximates the real space. In the case of theatre-based simulation, the degree to which the simulation lab approximates a real clinical space is an example of physical realism. For task trainers, such as intubation mannequins, the required physical realism is very high for the area being worked on. In situ simulation provides the benefit of extremely high environmental physical realism. Interestingly, "high fidelity" mannequins are quite limited in terms of physical realism. They have limited movements, use lights to demonstrate cyanosis, and vibrating motors to simulate seizure activity, all of which only loosely approximate actual clinical findings. These limitations are offset by the ability to perform medical procedures, such as defibrillation, intubation, and cardiopulmonary resuscitation on a fairly close physical approximation of an actual patient.

Cognitive Realism

This is the accuracy with which the simulation responds to participants' actions compared with the responses expected in real life. Learners are typically much less tolerant of lapses in cognitive realism than physical realism [5]. This can impair or degrade learner engagement and complicate the debriefing process.

An important consideration when designing scenarios is how time is managed during the simulation. Some medications and actions may take longer in real life to have an effect than the amount of time we have available during the simulation. In these cases, facilitators are sometimes obliged to undermine some realism in the interest of having the case progress. It is important that participants are made aware of this potential during prebriefing as the simulator's responses to their actions may not align with their previous real-life experiences. Another consideration is whether team members will be acting in their usual, real-life roles, or have to assume another professional role during the simulation (which sometimes occurs when there are no team members present from a particular discipline). Participants should almost always act in their own professional roles (maximizing this component of realism) unless the objectives call for something else, for example, developing interprofessional empathy and understanding other team members' roles.

Emotional Realism

This is the degree to which emotional reactions common to real-life scenarios are recreated in the simulation event. There is a very strong temptation for simulation educators and facilitators to maximize emotional realism, particularly stress. However, a robust body of research indicates that this does not yield the best learning and can in fact be highly detrimental. It is critical that facilitators return to the objectives of their scenario and carefully consider the effects of emotional realism before deciding on what level of stress to incorporate. If stress management is a goal of the scenario, then participants must be provided with specific skills for stress management. Participants should be prebriefed on this aspect of the training, and it must be clear what skills they are to employ/practice. If stress management is not a specific goal of the event, then the appropriate level of emotional realism must be sought to maintain engagement while not undermining the educational objectives [6].

Social or Sociological Realism

A recent addition to our framework of realism in situations is social realism, i.e., the degree to which social interactions from real life are recreated in the simulated environment. Social interactions are complex and can shape decisions and actions of team members. These effects may not be accurately recreated in the simulation lab and facilitators should be cognizant of the potential loss of fidelity inherent in simulation. This domain is particularly material to multidisciplinary simulation [7].

Simulation Modalities

A broad range of simulation modalities exists. Scenario designers with access to a simulation lab and "high-fidelity" mannequins will often default to these tools. However, as mentioned above, the key to choosing a modality is to review the goal and objectives of the scenario, and then consider the components of realism that are required to accomplish them. Below is a list of simulation modalities with a brief description of strengths. This list should be viewed as a toolkit from which elements can be chosen, mixed, and matched.

Theatre-Based Simulation

Simulation takes place in a dedicated space, often mixed with other modalities, such as mannequins, task trainers, and standardized patients.

Strengths:

- Does not impact actual patient care areas
- Allows for added audiovisual technology (video debriefing for example)
- Typically has dedicated control rooms and debriefing rooms, simplifying logistics

Weaknesses:

- Impaired physical realism as space often quite different than actual rooms
- Can be expensive
- Sometimes remote from patient care areas, decreasing the number of staff who can participate

In Situ Simulation

Simulation takes place in the actual area used by participants at work. Again, can be mixed with other modalities including task trainers, mannequins, and standardized patients.

Strengths:

- Very high physical realism
- Close to/in actual work area so staff can frequently take part during a break or while others cover their duties
- Allows assessment of team/participant interaction with physical space

Weaknesses:

- Can interrupt actual patient care
- Lack of dedicated debrief space and control room complicates logistics

High-Fidelity Mannequin

Use of mannequins with various levels of functionality has become ubiquitous in medical simulation. When their use aligns with the goals and objectives of a simulation event, mannequins are a valuable tool. A clear understanding of the weaknesses of high-fidelity mannequins also allows us to choose another modality when appropriate.

Strengths:

- Allows painful/dangerous procedures to be performed with actual apparatus
- Approximates the size and positioning of a real patient increasing some elements of physical realism

Weaknesses:

- Some poor elements of physical realism
- Expensive to purchase and maintain
- Require a control computer and human resources to run

Standardized Patient

Having actors perform the role of the patient is a long-standing tradition of medical education both for teaching and assessment [8]. When painful or dangerous procedures are not required for the scenario, standardized patients can sometimes provide the highest form of physical and cognitive realism.

Strengths:

- Can be very high physical, cognitive, and emotional realism.
- Patient is interactive and can adjust to behaviors of team.

Weaknesses:

- Require very specific coaching
- Can be expensive
- Lack of cognitive and physical realism if painful or dangerous procedures are to be performed

Task Trainer

A model of one area of the body is used for practicing specific procedures. These models are built with high physical realism for that procedure while minimizing other domains of realism to allow focus on a specific technical skill.

Strengths:

- Focus on one skill without added cognitive load
- Reusable
- Easily transported

Weaknesses:

- Specific purpose and sometimes awkward to incorporate into larger scenarios
- Can be expensive to purchase, maintain

Tabletop Exercise

The recreation of an event using a white board, chalkboard, computer, or pieces on a table. This allows for simulation of patient movements and resource utilization at the department, institution, or system level.

Strengths:

- Minimal resources required to execute the simulation event
- Can recreate "high-level" view of system

Weaknesses:

- Does not incorporate bedside skills and assessments unless paired with another modality
- May overlook latent safety threats as actual patient movements are not performed

Virtual Reality

Recreation of physical space and events on a virtual platform is rapidly growing as a simulation modality. Medical simulation software is available for consumer virtual reality gaming devices such as the Oculus headset (ref: https://www.oculus.com/experiences/go/878262692296965/). In addition with the development of artificial intelligence, simulated patients are becoming more realistic to interact with.

Strengths:

- Allows recreation of high-stakes events with no risk to participants
- Rapid cycling simulation allows repetitive practice
- Recording allows review of performance in debrief
- Scalable by adding extra participants

Weaknesses:

- Technology is still new and software is under development.
- Technical skills are still not easy to reproduce as most use consumer grade gaming controllers, though this may improve as haptic devices become more readily accessible..
- May overlook safety and system issues in real life if they are not programmed into scenario.

Telephone Simulations

Trauma often involves large distances and low population densities. This means acutely ill patients are routinely transported before definite treatment. Much care is coordinated by telephone, but blind communication skills are rarely deliberately taught. Telephone simulation provides many of the putative benefits of high-fidelity simulation but with little cost [9].

Strengths:

- Very low tech (only requires a telephone connection and separate spaces for facilitator and participant).
- Low cost.
- Wide variety of situations can be simulated (e.g., trauma bay calling up to operating room, or rural physician phoning for advice).
- Can also supplement a mannequin-based simulation.

Blindfolded Simulation

Physician leaders often want to do everything themselves, rather than delegating. Accordingly, they may not communicate what they are doing or why. Equally, nurses and respiratory therapists (RTs) do not always share what they have done, or when they first identified deteriorating vital signs. To mitigate this, simulations can be redone but with the physician-leader blindfolded [10]. This has been shown to immediately improve adherence to CRM principles: physicians elicit more help and confirm that instructions are fulfilled. Interestingly, non-blindfolded team members also perform better: they communicate task completion and volunteer changes in vital signs sooner. This simple intervention also enhances role clarity.

Strengths:

- Immediate improvement in CRM skill use
- Inexpensive

Weaknesses:

- Requires careful prebrief and safe environment.
- Some debriefing time must be used to address the change in realism (it is important to establish that this is a drill/practice and to emphasize which objectives are being highlighted).

Staged Entry Scenarios

Staged entry, where part of the team starts and others arrive later, creates opportunities to practice handover and leadership transition. It also allows team members, who would normally be in a supporting role, to do more of the initial assessment and resuscitation.

Strengths:

- Improved cognitive realism as real-life crises often unfold in the same way
- Emphasizes establishment of role clarity, maintenance of shared mental model

Distance Resuscitations

A unique hybrid of the blindfolded simulations described earlier in the chapter and the staged entry scenarios discussed above. By setting the scenario in a remote center (i.e., staffed by non-physicians), we can provide unique multidisciplinary simulations. For example, non-physician team members can be in one room performing the physical simulation (i.e., hands-on resuscitation), while, in another room, physicians perform telephone simulation (i.e., they direct the resuscitation). Our experience is that these blended scenarios are well received by both the non-physician group (who get to manage the entire resuscitation including procedures) and the physician group (who realize it requires as much "verbal dexterity" as "manual dexterity" to rescue a trauma victim). As outlined above, physicians frequently receive calls from distant centers but rarely practice "over-the-phone" resuscitations (where they cannot see the patient and must learn to rely upon others).

Confederates in Simulation

Although not a "modality" per se, confederates are team members who act as participants during team-based simulations but have knowledge about the case and facilitate the performance of the simulation. Whether or not to use confederates is a very frequent decision confronting simulation facilitators.

Strengths:

- Can add cognitive realism to the case by responding to team members' actions with knowledge about the underlying problem so that the responses are realistic
- Can add emotional, social realism
- Can take the place of participants who cannot attend the event thus allowing participants to remain in their usual professional roles

Weaknesses:

- Can be distracting if their behavior is not aligned with educational objectives (i.e., can help "too much"). Confederates need very specific guidance and prebriefing to avoid this problem.
- Often require payment.
- Can detract from cognitive and social realism as they become more familiar or, sometimes, bored with sequential runs of the scenario.

Creating the Scenario: The Importance of Templates

Once we have decided on a goal, objectives, and modality, we must build a scenario. Again, this requires frequent revisiting of the objectives. Each component of the event (location, modality, prebrief, events, and debrief) must be directed toward achieving our objectives. For this, the use of a template is invaluable. Below is an example of a scenario design template. Under each heading, there is a description of what information should be included.

Summary

In this chapter, we have outlined the key principles and steps to designing simulation scenarios. Creating effective, engaging, and well-organized scenarios takes time and practice. Adhering to the principles above will minimize the number of difficulties you encounter while building and running your simulation educational. Adjusting simulation scenarios based on the experience and feedback from previous runs is critical. Encourage feedback from participants, facilitators, and confederates so that each scenario can be honed with each use.

Key Points

- This chapter explores how to conduct needs assessment and then design and finesse simulations.
- We explore how to develop objectives, write a scenario, and choose the appropriate simulation modality.
- We explore the pros and cons of simulation and how to finesse simulations to ensure they work for various learner groups, and based on feedback.

Simulation Scenario Design Template

Simulation Scenario Design Template

Title of Simulation Scenario:

Designer:

Date:

Goal:

This is a statement of the overall outcome we are seeking from the event.

Target Audience

A list of participants including training level.

Objectives

At the end of this session, participants will: 1. 2. 3. This is a list of specific skills/behaviours that participants will be able to perform.

Summary

This is a summary of the case including description of the patient, mechanism of injury or circumstances of illness, presenting symptoms, expected course.

Patient Details

Further information about the patient including medical and surgical histories, allergies, medications and any other information germane to the scenario.

Location, Equipment

A list of all equipment required

Case Progression

Time / Action	Event / Response

This is a list of time points and/or actions by participants that will elicit specific responses by the simulator (mannequin, equipment, standardized patient or confederates). It should include an end-point at which the scenario will be halted.

Expected Debrief points

This will include the objectives, and any other foreseeable performance gaps or exceptional performances by the team.

Case Stem

This is the basic information that will be given to the participants prior to their entry into the simulation.

Supplemental Materials

ECG's, printouts of labs, ABG's X-ray and CT images Ultrasound images Charting including recent vital signs, medication list.

References

1. CPD accreditation: simulation-based learning activities. Royal College of Physicians and Surgeons of Canada. Available at: http://www.royalcollege.ca/rcsite/cpd/accreditation/cpd-accreditation-simulation-based-learning-activities-e. Accessed 6 May 2023.
2. Sherbino J, Frank JR. Educational design: a CanMEDS guide for the health professions. Ottawa: Royal College of Physicians and Surgeons; 2011.
3. Bloom BS, editor. Taxonomy of educational objectives: the classification of educational goals: handbook I, cognitive domain. New York: David McKay; 1956.
4. Utica University. Available at: https://www.utica.edu/academic/Assessment/new/Blooms%20Taxonomy%20-%20Best.pdf. Accessed 6 May 2023.
5. Smink DS, Yule SJ, Ashley SW. Realism in simulation: how much is enough? JAMA Surg. 2017;152(9):825–6.
6. LeBlanc VR. The effects of acute stress on performance: implications for health professions education. Acad Med. 2009;84(10):S25–33.
7. Armenia S, Thangamathesvaran L, Caine AD, King N, Kunac A, Merchant AM. The role of high-fidelity team-based simulation in acute care settings: a systematic review. Surg J (N Y). 2018;4(3):e136–51.
8. Wilbur K, Elmubark A, Shabana S. Systematic review of standardized patient use in continuing medical education. J Contin Educ Heal Prof. 2018;38(1):3–10.
9. Brindley P. Novel technique for critical care training. Can Med Assoc J. 2007;176(1):68.
10. Brindley PG, Lord J, Hudson D. The blindfolded learner: a simple intervention to improve crisis resource management skills. J Crit Care. 2008;23:253–4.

Constructive Debriefing for Trauma Team Education

63

Adam Cheng, Vincent Grant, and Naminder Sandhu

Introduction

The role of simulation-based education in training trauma teams and educating trauma team members is rapidly expanding [1–3]. As the key educational element of simulation-based education [2, 3], educator-guided debriefings are being increasingly studied and discussed in an effort to improve the effectiveness of the educational intervention. Debriefing, defined as a "facilitated or guided reflection in the cycle of experiential learning," [4] involves an active discourse between the debriefing facilitator and the various participants (e.g., learners), with the purposes of enhancing individual and team-based knowledge, skills, and performance. The over-arching goal of post-event debriefings is to positively influence change in provider behavior, thus leading to improved patient care and outcomes [4–9].

There is an increasing body of literature examining how debriefing should be delivered to enhance educational outcomes from simulation-based education [10–20]. Video-assisted debriefing is often used by facilitators to promote after-action review by highlighting specific behaviors, both positive and negative, and using them as trigger points for discussion [10–13]. While the use of video-assisted debriefing is quite common among resource-rich simulation programs, studies of its use in simulation-based education have demonstrated mostly negligible effects for improving provider skills in a simulated environment [10–13]. The optimal method and context of use for video-assisted debriefing are still yet to be defined. Studies support the application of personalized debriefing (with a facilitator) over the use of multimedia debriefing (with no instructor present) [15, 16] or group-led debriefing (with no facilitator) [17]. Finally, the combination of debriefing with participants viewing expert-modeled performance of desired behaviors has shown promise in improving learner satisfaction, knowledge, and skills [18–20]. These studies help provide some insight into how post-simulation debriefing should ideally be conducted when training trauma teams.

A. Cheng (✉) · V. Grant
Alberta Children's Hospital, Calgary, AB, Canada

Department of Pediatrics, University of Calgary, Calgary, AB, Canada
e-mail: vjgrant@ucalgary.ca

N. Sandhu
Alberta Children's Hospital, Calgary, AB, Canada
e-mail: naminder.sandhu@albertahealthservices.ca

Debriefing Structure and Method

Post-event debriefing, when applied to either simulation-based education or after a real patient case, is most efficiently and effectively performed when conducted in a systematic and structured fashion [6–9]. This section will review the overall structure of a debriefing event and discuss several methods that a facilitator can choose when reviewing the events of the case with the participating trauma teams.

Debriefing Structure

Structuring a post-event debriefing into various phases helps the facilitator manage time and content and also provides participants with a familiar flow when the same structure is consistently used within a single institution or program. The structure of a debriefing may vary depending on the preferences of the facilitator, their training in simulation-based education, and the amount of time available for the debriefing. Some of the potential phases of debriefing include: a reactions phase, a descriptive phase, an analysis phase, and a summary phase (Table 63.1) [4–9] (Walter Eppich, December 18, 2013, re: PEARLS blended method of debriefing, "personal communication").

The reactions phase allows the facilitator to identify the initial thoughts and feelings of the participants, and ultimately, define learning objectives that are most important to the participants [4, 6–9]. In this phase, the facilitator asks

L. Marshall Gillman, S. Widder (eds.), *Trauma Team Dynamics*, https://doi.org/10.1007/978-3-031-86312-7_63

Table 63.1 Debriefing structure

Phase	Description
Reaction	Identify initial thoughts and feelings of participants Define learning objectives that are important to participants Emotional washout, unwrap mental mindset of participants Facilitators track topics and plan how to address them
Description	Serve to establish a shared understanding of the case Solicit a brief summary of the case from a medical point of view and main issues May be abbreviated if team members had clear shared understanding of the underlying diagnosis and key issues
Analysis	Facilitators use various techniques to guide discussion and address learning and performance gaps Integrate selected topics raised by participants Multiple potential approaches Debriefer prompts plus-delta list generation Debriefer gives performance feedback Debriefer facilitates a discussion using advocacy inquiry Close performance gaps through discussion and/or teaching
Summary	Allows learners to state take-home messages and how lessons learned apply to real-life clinical practice Instructor may add final comments to augment essential elements

open-ended questions to provide participants the opportunity to vent their initial emotions related to the simulation, which may be feelings of frustration, fear, angst, confusion, appreciation, or elation over the event that has just taken place. Through this process, participants will also provide valuable information on their initial thoughts around the perceived care of the patient (both positive and negative). This step is vital to unwrapping the mental mindset of the participants (especially the emotional ones). If steps are not taken to allow the team members to share these emotions, they will be less likely to effectively reflect on their previous actions and hence, unable to fully engage in interactive discussion during the remainder of the debriefing. Their initial thoughts are also key indicators of the areas that the participants want to review during the debriefing. Facilitators should carefully track these topics as they arise during the reactions phase and actively plan how and when they will address them during the analysis portion of the debriefing. As specific analysis and discussion of issues do not typically occur during this phase of the debriefing, the facilitator should consider summarizing the issues that have been brought forth by participants before proceeding to the next phase of debriefing.

The key purpose of the descriptive phase is to ensure that all team members have a shared collective understanding of the main details of the case, including the primary diagnosis and main clinical issues (Walter Eppich, December 18, 2013, re: PEARLS blended method of debriefing, "personal communication"). The facilitator typically asks one member of the team to summarize these details briefly in one to two sentences, followed by confirmation from other team members. In some cases, there are differing perspectives of the primary diagnosis or core issues. These should be clarified by the facilitator and/or the group before proceeding with the analysis of specific behaviors. Failure to do so at this point in the debriefing may lead to confusion and/or misperceptions among some or all of the participants, thus increasing the risk of dissatisfaction or disengagement with the simulation debriefing at hand (Walter Eppich, December 18, 2013, re: PEARLS blended method of debriefing, "personal communication").

The bulk of debriefing is performed in the analysis phase [4, 6–9]. During this phase of debriefing, facilitators use various techniques to guide the team members toward identifying both positive and negative actions, as well as better understanding the rationale behind those actions and behaviors. By managing the flow and time available for discussion, the facilitator guides the group through issues that have been brought forth by participants while also covering the predefined learning objectives of the simulation scenario. Through reflective learning and feedback, the facilitator is able to promote the acquisition of new knowledge, skills, and attitudes, with the eventual goal of improving both individual and team performance in real patient care.

Once all of the performance issues have been identified, the final phase of debriefing typically involves a summary phase [4, 6–9] (Walter Eppich, December 18, 2013, re: PEARLS blended method of debriefing, "personal communication"). During this phase, a summary of the key take-home points is either provided directly by the facilitator or brought up and reviewed by the team. This ensures that the main learning points from the case are reinforced, with the hopes of positively influencing change in provider behavior for future trauma cases.

Debriefing Method

Several formats exist allowing the facilitator options when conducting the analysis portion of the debriefing. The method selected by the facilitator is most likely based on various factors: the time allotted for the debriefing event, the rationale evident behind the teams' actions during the scenario or event, the facilitators' comfort with using the selected method, the type of learning objective, and the level of insight/experience of the participants. The methods that will be reviewed here include Advocacy Inquiry (Debriefing with Good Judgement) [6–9], Plus Delta [4, 5], Directive Feedback, and Blended Methods of Debriefing (Walter Eppich, December 18, 2013, re: PEARLS blended method of debriefing, "personal communication").

Advocacy Inquiry

As a debriefing technique, Advocacy Inquiry (AI) attempts to uncover the "frame" or rationale behind a participant's behavior [7–9]. By uncovering the "frame" of an action, the facilitator better understands how to provide feedback for an action. This technique is particularly useful when the rationale behind an action is not clear or immediately apparent (to the facilitator or other team members). AI uses a series of factual statements to uncover the positive and negative performance issues without making assumptions as to the driving rationale behind these actions. The first statement is a clear, concise, and specific observation about an action or behavior that was seen or heard. The second is a short statement of appreciation or concern, reflecting the facilitator's point of view related to the issue at hand. The third statement then asks the individual or team to share their point of view related to the topic at hand (Table 63.2). The responses from team member(s) will then guide further discussion from the team around the topic area, with a goal of consolidating positive performance and/or improving negative performance [7–9]. By promoting reflection on previous actions in this manner, the facilitator can effectively engage learners in discussion and even have insightful teams address performance issues and answer questions on their own. Although AI is a highly powerful method when done appropriately by a skilled facilitator, it often takes much time to practice and master this technique. That being said, facilitators should consider practicing this technique in lower-stakes learning environments before using it in environments where patient and/or learner safety is at higher risk.

Plus-Delta

The plus-delta technique is another established technique where a facilitator guides a team to verbally produce two lists [4–6]. One list is the "plus"; the items that the team felt went particularly well during a case or simulation scenario. The second list is the "delta"; the items that the team felt could be improved upon for future performance. The advantages of this technique are that it is quick to learn and use and rapidly establishes a list of issues to frame further discussion. It is a particularly effective technique when there is very little time for debriefing (Walter Eppich, December 18, 2013, re: PEARLS blended method of debriefing, "personal communication"). Once the list of items is generated, specific issues may still require discussion, or at a minimum, the facilitator should provide some teaching to emphasize key take-home messages. The main disadvantage of the plus-delta method is that unless the individual items are further discussed in a reflective manner, the facilitator runs the risk of making inaccurate assumptions related to the underlying rationale driving specific actions, and subsequently delivering the wrong teaching point (Walter Eppich, December 18, 2013, re: PEARLS blended method of debriefing, "personal communication"). For example, in a trauma resuscitation scenario, a nurse participant may comment that the team struggled executing the severe head injury protocol in a timely fashion. If the instructor makes the wrong assumption and assumes there was a knowledge deficit, and subsequently starts teaching the severe head injury protocol, he/she may be missing out on the other potential causes for this performance deficit (e.g., errors in teamwork and communication).

Directive Feedback

Directive feedback is another technique when the facilitator provides teaching around a specific behavior or action. In its purest form, directive feedback is one directional (i.e., from teacher to learner) and does not involve discussion or reflective learning. This method is most suitable when the time available for debriefing is short, when the rationale behind a specific performance issue is clear and self-evident (to the facilitator and the group), or if the learners are inexperienced and/or have poor insight. This technique is particularly useful for clinical and technical skills, review of established guidelines or algorithms, and positive behaviors that one may want to reinforce. Similar to the plus-delta method, the main disadvantage is that the presumed rationale may be incorrect, with the consequence that the feedback provided targets the wrong objective.

Table 63.2 Advocacy inquiry [7–9]

Step	Possible statements/phrases
Observation	I noticed that…. I saw that…..
Facilitator point of view	At the time I was thinking….. I was wondering…..
Learner point of view	What were your thoughts at the time? How did you see it?

Blended Methods

Experienced facilitators using the techniques described above have discovered that the use of one single debriefing method in isolation may not be optimally effective for all debriefing and learning environments. As such, some experts have advocated for a blended approach to debriefing, while using various methods within a single debriefing event (Walter Eppich, December 18, 2013, re: PEARLS blended method of debriefing, "personal communication"). This allows for some flexibility based on the time allotted to debriefing, while still allowing the facilitator the ability to further uncover the rationale behind certain behaviors when there is uncertainty (Walter Eppich, December 18, 2013, re: PEARLS blended method of debriefing, "personal communication"). The blended approach allows for a more precise match of the specific learning needs of a team with the goals of the educator and should allow for more precise feedback in consolidating positive performance and/or improving negative performance.

Debriefing Real Trauma Teams

Advantages of Post-Trauma Debriefing

Simulation provides fertile grounds for the practice of effective resuscitation of critically ill patients and debriefing-generated learning on team process. Yet despite the growing evidence of the positive role of debriefing after surgical, anesthetic, or critical care-based simulation events [21–28], translating debriefing practice from the simulation setting to real-life events has been a challenge.

The concept of team-based debriefing after stressful events developed out of an intention to integrate profound personal experiences on the personal, emotional, and group levels. Debriefing in healthcare moved into the spotlight in 1983, when Mitchell described a formal technique targeted toward emergency services and disaster response teams which aimed to protect and support the group exposed to a critical incident by minimizing the development of abnormal stress responses [29]. Originating as an early psychological intervention after critical incidents associated with psychological stress and trauma, the intention of debriefing has expanded and evolved with a focus on improvement of team process by way of an educational intervention.

Debriefing is becoming recognized as an increasingly important procedure in medical team training, although the literature on debriefing in-hospital trauma teams is sparse. Anecdotally, healthcare providers perceive a need for debriefing in the acute care setting. Individuals who have attended debriefing often rate the experience as "valuable," "helpful," and as a "morale maintenance" intervention [30, 31]. As a performance enhancement tool, debriefing is beginning to receive significant attention from major international organizations in resuscitation such as the American Heart Association and International Liaison Committee on Resuscitation; in fact, they are endorsing debriefing for events such as cardiac arrest and identifying its impact on future performance and actual patient outcomes as an important area of research [32–35].

Review of Literature

A review of the literature shows that formalized debriefing has not yet become a standard practice in medical settings. In particular, surveys of emergency department staff in various countries have demonstrated a clear lack of formal debriefing practice after resuscitations despite a significant value placed on this process by healthcare providers. For example, pediatric emergency department physicians and nurses in Australia, the UK, and Canada have revealed that post-resuscitative debriefing is an uncommon practice, although most find it helpful in reducing stress, thus identifying a perceived need but lack of a structured debriefing process [36–39].

Despite anecdotal evidence from surveys and short-term observational studies, stronger empirical evidence for the efficacy of debriefing as a stress-reduction intervention is lacking. In the small number of randomized control trials studying debriefing as a stress management intervention in various contexts (including non-medical), early single-session debriefing of individuals exposed to traumatic experiences did not appear to reduce the risk of psychological distress or post-traumatic stress disorder [40]. It is difficult to translate this information to debriefing of trauma teams and does not speak to its efficacy as an educational intervention.

Studies focusing on debriefing benefits for team training are mostly extrapolated from the simulation education literature. Unfortunately, research and theory on debriefing have been spread across diverse disciplines, so it has been difficult to definitively ascertain debriefing effectiveness and how to enhance it. Yet the potential benefit to medical teams such as trauma teams is gradually being established. A meta-analysis from human factors literature done across a diverse body of published and unpublished research on team- and individual-level debriefs suggested that organizations can improve individual and team performance by approximately 20–25% by using properly conducted debriefings [41].

In recent years, attempts at designing and implementing real-time debriefing programs have been made in acute care settings. For one, there is promising literature coming from the management of cardiac arrest in both adult and pediatric settings. Quantitative debriefing targeting pediatric cardiac arrest events has been shown to be feasible and useful for providers [42]. Quantitative debriefing refers to programs building upon classic qualitative debriefing (i.e., facilitated discussions of participant actions and thought processes) by the addition of actual quantitative patient information gathered from bedside CPR recording devices, patient monitors, and resuscitation records. The effect of debriefing techniques on real-life performance and patient outcomes is also fertile territory for translation of current simulation-based knowledge and experience in debriefing. The use of playback of actual resuscitation events with targeted discussion of CPR performance is an effective way of improving rescuer knowledge and team performance in cardiac resuscitation, along with improved patient outcomes [34]. This work has broad applicability for improving trauma teamwork and the potential to improve outcomes from trauma events in general.

The challenge faced in assessing complex clinical team activities such as trauma resuscitation is developing validated metrics to assess competency. In terms of specific trauma team training tools, there is growing experience since the 1980s in performance review using videotapes as a technique to achieve behavioral changes and algorithm compliance, which has revealed some positive results. In fact, in some trauma centers, video analysis has become a standard quality assurance method [43–46]. Video recording trauma resuscitations and regular review have been shown to improve trauma team leadership and the performance of residents in subsequent real-life resuscitations; overall, this method of debriefing seems to lead to reduced time in the emergency department prior to definitive care and improved delivery of key trauma resuscitation interventions. Videotape review based on trauma resuscitation guidelines has also been compared to verbal feedback and has been shown to be more impactful in changing behavior. With such results, there is promising evidence that ongoing videotape review can be an important quality assurance adjunct, as improved algorithm compliance should be associated with improved patient care. Of course, videotaping of patient care requires overcoming substantial obstacles including medico-legal issues, confidentiality, and logistical and resource issues which restrict its use significantly [43–46].

Recommendations

There is growing evidence that supports the use of structured debriefing as an educational strategy to improve clinician knowledge and skill acquisition and implementation of those skills in practice. Debriefing of clinical teams after a life-threatening traumatic emergency can lead to improved processes and patient-focused outcomes. However, the effect of debriefing on long-term patient outcomes is still uncertain. Furthermore, details of the most effective and pragmatic debriefing program for trauma teams are yet to be determined.

Given their potential efficacy and lessons learned from cardiac arrest, trauma videotape review, and simulation literature, debriefing should be a standard part of any team training intervention that incorporates, at minimum, a simulated team experience. In such cases, to promote alignment, the debriefing should involve the full team, focus on team improvements, and assess effectiveness with team-level performance measures.

Key Points

- Debriefing is an important component of simulation-based trauma team education.
- Post-event debriefing is most effective when conducted in a structured fashion.
- The method of debriefing should be tailored to the learning environment and context.
- Debriefing teams after real trauma events have the potential to improve clinical outcomes in the future.

References

1. Cook DA, Hatala R, Brydges R, Zendejas B, Szostek JH, Wang AT, et al. Technology enhanced simulation for health professions education: a systematic review and meta-analysis. JAMA. 2011;3306:978–88.
2. Issenberg SB, McGaghie WC, Petrusa ER, Gordon DL, Scalese RJ. Features and uses of high-fidelity medical simulations that lead to effective learning: a BEME systematic review. Med Teach. 2005;27:10–28.
3. McGaghie WC, Issenberg SB, Petrusa ER, Scalese RJ. A critical review of simulation-based medical education research: 2003–2009. Med Educ. 2010;44:50–63.
4. Fanning RM, Gaba DM. The role of debriefing in simulation-based learning. Simul Healthc. 2007;2:115–25.
5. Raemer D, Anderson M, Cheng A, Fanning R, Nadkarni V, Savoldelli G. Research regarding debriefing as part of the learning process. Simul Healthc. 2011;6:S52–7.
6. Arafeh JM, Hansen SS, Nichols A. Debriefing in simulated-based learning: facilitating a reflective discussion. J Perinat Neonat Nurs. 2010;24:302–9.
7. Rudolph JW, Simon R, Raemer D, Eppich WJ. Debriefing as formative assessment: closing performance gaps in medical education. Acad Emerg Med. 2008;15:1–7.
8. Rudolph JW, Simon R, Rivard P, Dufresne RL, Raemer DB. Debriefing with good judgment: combining rigorous feedback with genuine inquiry. Anesth Clin. 2007;25:361–76.
9. Rudolph JW, Simon R, Dufresne RL, Raemer DB. There's no such thing as a "non-judgmental" debriefing: a theory and method for debriefing with good judgment. Simul Healthc. 2006;1:49–55.
10. Savoldelli GL, Naik VN, Park J, Joo HS, Chow R, Hamstra SJ. Value of debriefing during simulated crisis management: oral versus video-assisted oral feedback. Anesthesiology. 2006;105:279–85.
11. Grant JS, Moss J, Epps C, Watts P. Using video-facilitated feedback to improve student performance following high-fidelity simulation. Clin Sim Nurs. 2010;6:e177–84.
12. Byrne AJ, Sellen AJ, Jones JG, Aitkenhead AR, Hussain S, Gilder F, et al. Effect of videotape feedback on anaesthetists' performance

while managing simulated anaesthetic crises: a multicenter study. Anaesthesia. 2002;57:169–82.
13. Sawyer T, Sierocka-Castaneda A, Chan D, Berg B, Lustik M, Thompson M. The effectiveness of video-assisted debriefing versus oral debriefing alone at improving neonatal resuscitation performance: a randomized trial. Simul Healthc. 2012;7:213–21.
14. Van Heukelom JN, Begaz T, Treat R. Comparison of postsimulation debriefing versus in-simulation debriefing in medical simulation. Simul Healthc. 2010;5:91–7.
15. Xeroulis GJ, Park J, Moulton CA, Reznick RK, LeBlanc V, Dubrowski A. Teaching suturing and knot-typing skills to medical students: a randomized controlled study comparing computer-based video instruction and (concurrent and summary) expert feedback. Surgery. 2007;141:442–9.
16. Welke TM, LeBlanc VR, Savoldelli GL, Joo HS, Chandra DB, Crabtree NA, et al. Personalized oral debriefing versus standardized multimedia instruction after patient crisis simulation. Anesth Analg. 2009;109:183–9.
17. Boet S, Bould D, Bruppacher HR, Desjardins F, Chandra DB, Naik VN. Looking in the mirror: self-debriefing versus instructor debriefing for simulated crises. Crit Care Med. 2011;39:1377–81.
18. LeFlore JL, Anderson M, Michael JL, Engle WD, Anderson J. Comparison of self-directed learning versus instructor-modeled learning during a simulated clinical experience. Simul Healthc. 2007;2:170–7.
19. LeFlore JL, Anderson M. Effectiveness of 2 methods to teach and evaluate new content to neonatal transport personnel using high-fidelity simulation. J Perinat Neonat Nurs. 2008;22:319–28.
20. LeFlore JL, Anderson M. Alternative educational models for interdisciplinary student teams. Simul Healthc. 2009;4:135–42.
21. Gururaja RP, Yang T, Paige JT, Chauvin SW. Examining the effectiveness of debriefing at the point of care in simulation-based operating room team training. In: Henriksen K, Battles JB, Keyes MA, Grady ML, editors. Advances in patient safety: new directions and alternative approaches – vol. 3: performance and tools. Rockville: Agency for Healthcare Research and Quality; 2008.
22. Papaspyros SC, Javangula KC, Adluri RK, O'Regan DJ. Briefing and debriefing in the cardiac operating room. Analysis of impact on theatre team attitude and patient safety. Interact Cardiovasc Thorac Surg. 2010;10(1):43–7.
23. Clay AS, Que L, Petrusa ER, Sebastian M, Govert J. Debriefing in the intensive care unit: a feedback tool to facilitate bedside teaching. Crit Care Med. 2007;35(3):738–54.
24. Morgan PJ, Tarshis J, LeBlanc V, Cleave-Hogg D, DeSousa S, Haley MF, et al. Efficacy of high-fidelity simulation debriefing on the performance of practicing anaesthetists in simulated scenarios. Br J Anaesth. 2009;103(4):531–7.
25. Tan H. Debriefing after critical incidents for anaesthetic trainees. Anaesth Intensive Care. 2005;33:768–72.
26. Dine CJ, Gersh RE, Leary M, Riegel BJ, Bellini LM, Abella BS. Improving cardiopulmonary resuscitation quality and resuscitation training by combining audiovisual feedback and debriefing. Crit Care Med. 2008;36(10):2817–22.
27. Ahmed M, Sevdalis N, Paige J, Paragi-Gururaja R, Nestel D, Arora S. Identifying best practice guidelines for debriefing in surgery: a tri-continental study. Am J Surg. 2012;203(4):523–9.
28. Arora S, Ahmed M, Paige J, Nestel D, Runnacles J, Hull L, et al. Objective structured assessment of debriefing: bringing science to the art of debriefing in surgery. Ann Surg. 2012. https://doi.org/10.1097/SLA.0b013e3182610c91. Publication before print.
29. Mitchell J. When disaster strikes: the critical incident stress debriefing process. J Emerg Med Serv. 1983;8:36–9.
30. Tuckey MR. Issues in the debriefing debate for the emergency services: moving research outcomes forward. Clin Psychol Sci Pract. 2007;14(2):106–16.
31. Devilly GJ, Cotton P. Psychological debriefing and the workplace: defining a concept, controversies and guidelines for intervention. Aust Psychol. 2003;38:144–50.
32. Soar J, Monsieurs KG, Ballance JH, Barelli A, Biarent D, Greif R, et al. European Resuscitation Council Guidelines for Resuscitation 2010 Section 9. Principles of education in resuscitation. Resuscitation. 2010;81:1434–44.
33. Weng TI, Huang CH, Ma MH, Chang WT, Liu SC, Wang TD, et al. Improving the rate of return of spontaneous circulation for out-of-hospital cardiac arrests with a formal, structured emergency resuscitation team. Resuscitation. 2004;60:137–42.
34. Edelson DP, Litzinger B, Arora V, Walsh D, Kim S, Lauderdale DS, et al. Improving in-hospital cardiac arrest process and outcomes with performance debriefing. Arch Intern Med. 2008;168(10):1063–9.
35. Bhanji F, Mancini ME, Sinz E, Rodgers DL, McNeil MA, Hoadley TA, et al. American Heart Association guidelines for cardiopulmonary resuscitation and emergency cardiovascular care science. Part 16: education, implementation, and teams. Circulation. 2010;2010:S920–33.
36. Theophilos T, Magyar J, Babl FE. Debriefing critical incidents in the paediatric emergency department: current practice and perceived needs in Australia and New Zealand. Emerg Med Aust. 2009;21:479–83.
37. Ireland S, Gilchrist J, Maconochie I. Debriefing after failed paediatric resuscitation: a survey of current UK practice. Emerg Med J. 2008;25:328–30.
38. Burns C, Harm NJ. Emergency nurses' perceptions of critical incidents and stress debriefing. J Emerg Nurs. 1993;19(5):431–6.
39. Sandhu N, Eppich W, Mikrogianakis A, Grant V, Robinson T, Cheng A. Postresuscitation debriefing in the pediatric emergency department: a national needs assessment. Can J Emerg Med. 2013;15(0):1–10.
40. Rose S, Bisson J, Churchill R, Wessely S. Psychological debriefing for preventing post traumatic stress disorder (PTSD). Cochrane Database Syst Rev. 2002;2(2):CD000560.
41. Tannenbaum SI, Cerasoli CP. Do team and individual debriefs enhance performance? A meta-analysis. Hum Factors. 2013;55(1):231–45.
42. Zebuhr C, Sutton RM, Morrison W, Niles D, Boyle L, Nishisaki A, et al. Evaluation of quantitative debriefing after pediatric cardiac arrest. Resuscitation. 2012;83(9):1124–8.
43. Hoyt DB, Shackford SR, Fridland PH, Mackersie RC, Hansbrough JF, Wachtel TL, et al. Video recording trauma resuscitations: an effective teaching technique. J Trauma Acute Care Surg. 1988;28(4):435–40.
44. Scherer LA, Chang MC, Meredith JW, Battistella FD. Videotape review leads to rapid and sustained learning. Am J Surg. 2003;185(6):516–20.
45. Townsend RN, Clark R, Ramenofsky ML, Diamond DL. ATLS-based videotape trauma resuscitation review: education and outcome. J Trauma Acute Care Surg. 1993;34(1):133–8.
46. Santora TA, Trooskin SZ, Blank CA, Clarke JR, Schinco MA. Video assessment of trauma response: adherence to ATLS protocols. Am J Emerg Med. 1996;14(6):564–9.

64 Program Evaluation and Assessment of Learning

Vicki R. LeBlanc and Walter Tavares

The use of simulation modalities for health professions education is both resource and time intensive. As such, there is an expectation to demonstrate that the program offered had the desired outcome, in terms of participant experiences, impact on learning or behavior of the participants, as well as in terms of desired institutional or patient-related outcomes. The goal of this chapter is to present a brief overview of program evaluation (outcomes-based and process-based). It will conclude with a more focused discussion of the assessment of learners, as this is a common foci of interest, not only for program evaluation but also for those interested in using simulation to determine their learners' level of abilities.

Program Evaluation

Because simulation-based education is time and resource intensive, there is often the need to demonstrate that the resources and time allotted to simulation-based courses or program are effective in meeting the desired learning objectives. Program evaluation is the systematic investigation of a program's worth [1]. It is the process of determining whether the program or course that has been designed works (or not) and whether (and how) it needs to be modified or improved. Program evaluation is the systematic collection, analysis, and use of information to answer questions about projects, policies, and programs, particularly about their effectiveness and efficiency.

V. R. LeBlanc (✉)
Wilson Centre, Washington, DC, USA

Department of Innovation in Medical Education, Faculty of Medicine, University of Ottawa, Ottawa, ON, Canada
e-mail: vleblan3@uottawa.ca

W. Tavares
Wilson Centre, Washington, DC, USA

McMaster University, Hamilton, ON, Canada

School of Community and Health Studies, Centennial College, Toronto, ON, Canada
e-mail: walter.tavares@utoronto.ca

There are several foci for program evaluation, including but not limited to:

- Assessment of the program's cost and efficiency
- Assessment of program design
- Assessment of the program's outcome (i.e., what it has actually achieved)
- Assessment of the program's impact on learning
- Assessment of how the program is being implemented (i.e., is it being implemented according to plan?)

The two main approaches to program evaluation are outcomes-based evaluation and process-based evaluations. Program evaluation is often conceptualized as occurring at the end of the program (outcome-based), to determine whether the desired outcomes came to be. However, program evaluation can occur at several stages of a program (process-based), with the goal of determining how a program was implemented, as well as how and why it did—or did not—work as intended [2].

Outcomes-Based Program Evaluation

Outcomes-based program evaluation is aimed at answering the question of whether the program brings about the desired outcomes, generally defined by the course and learning objectives [2]. This is the type of program evaluation that is most familiar to health professions educators. There are several models to guide outcomes-based program evaluation that have been used related to health professions education.

The Kirkpatrick framework involves four levels designed as a sequence of ways to evaluate programs [3]. The four levels of the Kirkpatrick framework are as follows:

Learner reactions: How the participants thought and felt about the program.

Learning: The increase in knowledge and/or skill, or the changes in attitudes that occurred as a result of the program.

L. Marshall Gillman, S. Widder (eds.), *Trauma Team Dynamics*, https://doi.org/10.1007/978-3-031-86312-7_64

Behavior: The transfer of the knowledge, skills, or attitudes to the work or clinical setting.

Results: The tangible results of the program in terms of costs, quality, or efficiency.

A similar framework, specifically applied to health professions, was proposed by Miller [4]. It is similar to the Kirkpatrick framework, in that there are several levels of assessment of skills and performance. The four levels of the Miller framework are as follows:

Knows (Knowledge): Whether the student's knowledge has increased. This is considered the foundation of clinical skills, but is not sufficient to demonstrate changes in clinical skills and performance itself. It is generally measured with written exams.

Knows how (Competence): Whether a student can apply the knowledge learned. This is generally assessed using tests involving clinical problem solving.

Shows how (Performance): Whether the student can demonstrate a change in clinical skills and performance. This is generally assessed with behavioral examinations such as OSCEs and simulation modalities.

Does (Action): Whether the learner's clinical skills and knowledge are improved during daily patient care. This is generally assessed with direct observation in real clinical contexts during patient care.

Program Evaluation Designs

In addition to determining the level of outcomes at which they are going to evaluate their program, educators also need to determine the design by which they will assess if desired improvement of knowledge, skills, performance, or patient care has occurred.

The most straightforward method for conducting a program evaluation is to measure the impact of the program on the desired outcome measures after the program has been delivered. The limitation of this type of measure is that it does not provide any information regarding a learner's level of knowledge or performance before the course. As such, this approach does not allow the educator to determine whether a learner's current level of performance or knowledge is due to the program itself, due to baseline levels before the course, or other factors that occurred in parallel to the course.

One way to determine whether improvements occurred through the program is to use a pre-post design, where the outcome of interest is measured before the program, and then once again after the completion of the program. While this design allows educators to determine whether knowledge or skills improved from the baseline, it does not eliminate the possibility that the improvements were due to other factors that occurred in parallel to the program or due to increase in performance merely due to repeated testing.

The next level of program evaluation design is to have an experimental design, with pre-course and post-course assessments, and a comparison group that is identical to the learners in the program, but does not receive the program. This design is considered a superior one for program evaluation, as it allows educators to separate out the influence of baseline ability and parallel events from those of the program itself. However, the limitation of this type of design is that it is resource and time intensive, and may create ethical concerns if the learners in the control group are withheld a particular learning opportunity. This last concern can be overcome with a cross-over design, in which the students in the control group are offered the learning intervention after the post-course measures have been obtained.

In designing their outcomes-based program evaluation, educators are often challenged by the difficulties in obtaining outcome measures at the level of "behavior" or "does," as well as with creating rigorous experimental designs. One question often asked is how strong is the need to prove that a program delivers the desired outcomes. In the case of a program that is already supported and established, in which other educators have shown that it works, it is generally acceptable to focus on learner feedback, pre- and post-course knowledge and skills assessments, mostly as a form of continuous monitoring of the quality of a program. If a program is novel, and potentially contested and challenged, educators will need to focus on behavioral or patient outcomes data and will need to move toward a true experimental design with pre- and post-course measures and a comparison group. If one objective is to publish the results of the program evaluation in a peer-reviewed journal, the standards for publication have been consistently increasing over the years. A design with a control group or comparison training method, with validated measures of performance, is generally required for publication in peer-reviewed journals targeted to health professions educators.

Process-Based Program Evaluation

Process-based program evaluation, in addition to assessing the measurable outcomes of a program, is also geared to fully understanding how a program was implemented as well as how and why the program did or did not have the desired outcomes [5]. This type of program evaluation looks beyond what a program is supposed to do, to evaluate how a program is being implemented and to determine whether the components critical to the success of the program are—or have been—implemented [2].

It is an ongoing process in which multiple measures are used to evaluate how the program is being developed and delivered:

- How was the intervention developed, delivered, and received?
- Are target populations being reached?
- Are people receiving the intended program?
- Are instructors, facilitators, and technicians adequately prepared?
- What are the barriers to and facilitators of the development and delivery of the program?

In process-oriented program evaluation, the evaluator is not just interested in the outcomes of a program, but also in developing an understanding of the perspectives, experiences, and expectations of all stakeholders, in order to determine whether the program was delivered in the manner it was intended.

The methodologies used in process-oriented outcome measures include both quantitative and qualitative methods. They can include, among others, structured observations, questionnaires, semi-structured interviews, focus groups, logs of meetings and program preparations, and analysis of course documents.

One model that can guide process-based program evaluation is the CIPP model, which looks at Context, Input, Process, and Product [1]. Depending on the point at which the CIPP model is applied during program evaluation, it allows for formative questions at the beginning of the program, as well as a guide for evaluating the program's process and input throughout and at the end of the program:

- Context: What needs to be done? Were important needs addressed?
- Input: How should it be done? Was a defensible design employed?
- Process: Is it being done? Was the design well executed?
- Product: Is it succeeding? Did the effort succeed?

Assessment of Learning

Program evaluation may take on many forms; however, a common approach is to evaluate the impact a program has on learners. As an outcome measure, this may include the achievement of competencies, successful attainment of objectives, or changes in behavior. In each of these outcomes, there is a requirement to engage learners in a process of assessment at one of the levels of the Miller or Kirkpatrick framework discussed earlier in this chapter. As with any outcome measures, those engaging in the *assessment of learning* must ensure (at a minimum) that the process demonstrates evidence of both reliability and validity. A comprehensive review of all stimulus and response formats (e.g., written, oral, computer-based simulations) is beyond the scope of this chapter. Therefore, we focus here on the complex process of performance-based assessments, specifically as it relates to the direct observation, by one or more raters, of trainee performance in a simulation or work-based setting.

The assessment of clinical performance is a complex process, involving broadly, four phases including (a) a stimulus, (b) learner behaviors, (c) direct observation by a rater/assessor, and (d) rating or judgment transferred to a rating tool. The stimulus generally involves the development of a clinical challenge intended to elicit or expose a learner's ability as they relate to predetermined objectives or competencies. The learner then exhibits behaviors in response to the clinical challenge and a rater observes the performance, making reference to some performance expectations or standards along the way. This is then all transformed into some form of categorical judgment or rating regarding the candidate's ability and used to inform decisions regarding the learner's degree of competence, achievement of competencies, or objectives. Importantly, with the exception of phase 2 (learner behaviors) assessment developers have control of these facets, and the decisions and/or processes that assessment developers put in place have implications for both reliability and validity.

Reliability

Reliability serves as a type of quality index in assessments and refers to the ability to *consistently differentiate* between candidates [6, 7], with both consistency and differentiation being equally important. Consistency suggests that scores on a performance assessment would be relatively similar between raters (inter-rater reliability) within raters (intra-rater reliability), if tested a second time (test-retest reliability), across different stations (inter-station reliability), etc. On the other hand, differentiation suggests the assessment process is designed such that differences between candidates (if present) can be detected.

Reliability provides an indication of the ability to achieve this consistent differentiation but also an indication regarding the amount of error associated with the process [7, 8]. Error is present when a score is generated that is different than the "true" score. Error can be systematic (e.g., a rater is excessively or inappropriately stringent and scores are subsequently lower than the "true" score) or random (i.e., unpredictable). There is always a degree of measurement error associated with rater-based assessments and ideally, those sources are identified and then mitigated where possible. Strategies to maximize reliability therefore involve both improving differentiation and minimizing error.

The question thus remains; how does one meaningfully maximize the ability to differentiate between candidates and minimize error? First, with regard to maximizing differentiation (i.e., the range of scores obtained in the assessment process), case development, the number of cases included, and the rating tools used are all strategies that can be applied (just to name a few). Individual case development and the collection of cases used should ensure students are adequately challenged such that they are neither too difficult nor too simple. Rating scales with too few discrimination points (e.g., a dichotomous done/not done rating tool) may not allow for the necessary differentiation to support reliable assessments.

A second strategy to improve reliability involves minimizing the amount or degree of error associated with the process. Previous research exploring sources of error in performance-based assessments typically finds *context specificity* as the greatest source of error [9–13]. Context specificity refers to the counterintuitive finding that a candidate's performance in one case is a poor predictor of performance in another. For example, a candidate's clinical performance when presented with a patient experiencing an asthmatic exacerbation would not necessarily be predictive of performance when presented with a patient suffering from hemorrhagic shock. These findings suggest that in order to achieve the reliability expected of high stakes assessments, a number of cases (or samples) should be used. As the number of cases increases, the effect of context specificity (a significant source of error) is minimized and the closer one is to determining the individual's true performance ability [14]. Other sources of error (e.g., raters, rating tools) should also be considered and mitigated as much as possible, in order to further minimize error and improve reliability associated with performance-based exams.

Validity

Validity refers to the degree of confidence one has in the inferences drawn based on the scores generated by an assessment process [15–17]. That is, validity refers to the plausibility, accuracy, or appropriateness of a proposed interpretation (e.g., degree of competence), proposed use (e.g., certification vs. remediation), or use of test scores (e.g., advancement) and not the test itself. Validity refers to the degree to which the interpretation, for example, is supported by evidence [16, 18–20]. There are numerous implications associated with this conceptualization of validity. To begin with, validity is never actually achieved and there are different levels or degrees of evidence; some stronger than others. For example, demonstrating that a 5 station performance exam is perceived by experts, candidates, and stakeholders to be a suitable measure of clinical performance (referred to as face validity) is a much weaker argument or source of evidence than having evidence of predictive validity in which performance on the 5 station exam actually predicts performance in future clinical settings (an admittedly difficult form of evidence to achieve) [21]. The stronger the arguments (i.e., empirical evidence in support of the interpretations) the more one can have confidence in and defend decisions made based on scores generated from an assessment process.

Unfortunately, there are many threats to validity [9]. Broadly, these include poor reliability (discussed previously), lack of authenticity, under- or over-construct representation, and/or construct irrelevant variance [22]. These threats may be present in the stimuli (i.e., the clinical cases the candidates are presented with) or the response format (i.e., the rating tool used and/or raters themselves) [22, 23]. When one or more of these threats are present and/or not reasonably mitigated, the extrapolations that one makes from the assessment context to future clinical contexts are weakened.

Focusing first on authenticity, where possible, the assessment format (i.e., stimuli) should match or align with the settings with which inferences and generalizations are eventually to be made [24]. Extrapolations from assessment contexts to future clinical contexts require less of a leap when the two settings are closely matched. For example, providing a multiple choice exam when the goal is to make inferences regarding a person's intravenous insertion skills is an inappropriate stimulus because it lacks authenticity and thus validity associated with the assessment process is threatened. Therefore making inferences regarding intravenous skills based on scores generated on the written exam is difficult. However, using a highly realistic task trainer is far more authentic and therefore likely to be a stronger argument because it is a closer approximation to the future performance setting. Extending the example further, integrating the procedural skill into the broader context of assessment, prioritization, clinical reasoning, communication, and resource considerations, offers additional authenticity. Finally, using a real patient in a real clinical environment with real contextual forces would require even less of a leap when extrapolating from assessment contexts to future clinical performance contexts. Therefore, when assessment at the "does" level (obviously the most authentic stimulus) is not feasible, simulations designed to replicate physical, conceptual, and emotional realism should be employed to maximize validity [24]. This extends to ensuring cases involve full clinical encounters consistent with the health profession, as opposed to fragmented decontextualized skills (arguably less authentic).

A second and third threat to validity involves construct under- and over-representation [16]. In the context of the cases used (and assuming a performance examination at the "shows how" or "does" level), construct under-representation refers to under-sampling of the domain of possible encounters. Hypothetically speaking, if there are 100 different skills or patient types in the domain of possible encounters, and the sampling strategy only includes 10 of each, the risk of construct underrepresentation is higher than if 20 of each were included. Of course, not all elements of the construct can be included in a given assessment process. Therefore, one must apply a reasonable sampling strategy using a structured blueprint and appropriate framework. Construct over-representation would essentially be the opposite (albeit less common of a problem). That is, including content in a performance-based assessment that was not representative of trauma care. One final threat that can be assigned to either under- or over-construct representation is in the representativeness of the sample. This refers to the degree to which the cases selected for an assessment process, for example, represent the frequency of actual clinical encounters. This has significant implications for making predictions regarding future clinical performance. This is often addressed using a matrix of frequency and importance for a domain of possible encounters. Decisions need to be made regarding the distribution of cases across these two domains in addition to the sampling strategy issues described above.

Closely related is the concept of construct irrelevant variance, which refers to any systematic sources of error [8]. Construct over-representation, for example, may be considered a type of construct irrelevant variance. Other sources may include flawed cases, poor rating scales, inappropriate rating items, various forms of rater biases (e.g., leniency and stringency, or restriction of range), inadequate sampling, and poor case difficulty (either too easy or too difficult) [23]. Any of these may artificially lower or elevate scores (causing scores to inappropriately deviate from the "true score") thereby threatening validity claims.

With regard to the response format (i.e., direct observation measurement tools), both construct representation and construct irrelevant variance are applicable here as well. For instance, when developing or using a checklist or global rating scale, if the measurement tool does not adequately represent the construct by either missing important items or dimensions, or including items or dimensions that should not be included, then both construct under- and over-representation are possible. The measurement tools/response format used should demonstrate evidence of reliability and validity on their own but also in the context in which they are used to avoid threats to validity.

Summary

Simulation-based education requires significant time and resources. As such, educators are often required to provide evidence that the program accomplishes the desired goals and that the performance measures obtained in this format are valid and reliable. In this light, the current chapter provided an overview of two related concepts. Program evaluation is conducted to determine whether a program led to the desired outcomes (outcomes-based evaluation) and to determine how a program was implanted (process-based evaluation). In a related goal, assessment of learning is conducted to determine a learner's level of knowledge or ability, and requires attention to ensuring the reliability and validity of the measures used.

Key Notes

- It is important for educators to provide evidence that simulation programs accomplish the desired goals and that assessments made in the simulation context are sound.
- Program evaluation is used to determine whether a program led to the desired outcomes (outcomes-based), as well as how a program was implemented (process-based).
- Educators engaging in the assessment of learning must ensure that the process demonstrates evidence of both reliability and validity.

References

1. Singh MD. Evaluation framework for nursing education programs: application of the CIPP model. Int J Nurs Educ Scholarsh. 2005;1(1):13.
2. Haji F, Morin MP, Parker K. Rethinking programme evaluation in health professions education: beyond 'did it work?'. Med Educ. 2013;47(4):342–51.
3. Kirkpatrick DL. Evaluation. In: Craig RL, editor. Training and development handbook. New York: McGraw-Hill; 1976. p. 301–19.
4. Miller G. The assessment of clinical skills/competence/performance. Acad Med. 1990;65(9):S63.
5. Saunders RP, Evans MH, Joshi P. Developing a process-evaluation plan for assessing health promotion program implementation: a how-to guide. Health Promot Pract. 2005;6(2):134–47.
6. Eva K. Assessment strategies in medical education. In: Salerno-Kennedy R, O'Flynn S, editors. Medical education: state of the art. New York: Nova Science Publishers; 2010. p. 93–106.
7. Downing S. Reliability: on the reproducibility of assessment data. Med Educ. 2004;38(9):1006–12.
8. Haladyna TM, Downing S. Construct-irrelevant variance in high-stakes testing. Educ Meas Issues Pract. 2004;23(1):17–27.
9. Eva KW. On the generality of specificity. Med Educ. 2003;37(7):587–8.
10. Eva KW, Neville AJ, Norman GR. Exploring the etiology of content specificity: factors influencing analogic transfer and problem solving. Acad Med. 1998;73(10):S1.
11. van der Vleuten CP, Schuwirth LW, Scheele F, Driessen EW, Hodges B. The assessment of professional competence: building blocks for theory development. Best Pract Res Clin Obstet Gynaecol. 2010;24:703.
12. van der Vleuten C, Swanson D. Assessment of clinical skills with standardized patients: state of the art. Teach Learn Med. 1990;2(2):58–76.

13. Newble D, Swanson D. Psychometric characteristics of the objective structured clinical examination. Med Educ. 1988;22(4):325–34.
14. Downing S, Yudkowsky R. Assessment in health professions education. New York: Routledge; 2009.
15. Kane M. Validation. In: Educational measurement, vol. 4. Westport: American Council on Education/Praeger; 2006. p. 17–64.
16. Downing S. Validity: on the meaningful interpretation of assessment data. Med Educ. 2003;37(9):830–7.
17. Schuwirth LW, van der Vleuten CP. Programmatic assessment and Kane's validity perspective. Med Educ. 2012;46(1):38–48.
18. Kane M. Current concerns in validity theory. J Educ Meas. 2001;38(4):319–42.
19. Kane M. Validating score interpretations and uses. Lang Test. 2012;29(1):3–17.
20. Kane M. An argument-based approach to validity. Psychol Bull. 1992;112(3):527.
21. Tavares W, LeBlanc VR, Mausz J, Sun V, Eva KW. Simulation based assessment of paramedics and performance in real clinical contexts. Prehosp Emerg Care. 2013;18:116.
22. Downing S, Haladyna T. Validity threats: overcoming interference with proposed interpretations of assessment data. Med Educ. 2004;38(3):327–33.
23. Downing S. Threats to the validity of clinical teaching assessments: what about rater error? Med Educ. 2005;39(4):353–5.
24. Hodges B, Hanson M, McNaughton N, Regehr G, University of Toronto Psychiatric Skills Assessment Project. Creating, monitoring, and improving a psychiatry OSCE: a guide for faculty. Acad Psychiatry. 2002;26(3):134.

65 Teaching Technical and Procedural Skills

Garrett G. R. J. Johnson and Ashley S. Vergis

Introduction

Healthcare providers who care for trauma patients must be fluent in a variety of clinical procedures. Previous chapters have examined the role of training and simulation for non-technical skills such as communication, teamwork, and management of stress and physical resources. However, just as importantly, trauma providers must also be expert technicians. Procedures vary widely in complexity, from the very simple (proper placement of blood pressure cuff and oxygen saturation monitor) to the more complex (emergency resuscitative thoracotomy). In order to perform those skills in a trauma setting, they must first be learned and retained beyond the period of initial practice, and then recalled and executed appropriately in the requisite clinical setting. To ensure the technical competency of future generations, capable trauma providers must regularly teach these skills to their more junior peers. However, for reasons we will explore in this chapter, technical expertise unfortunately does not necessarily ensure teaching proficiency. Therefore, the efficacy of procedural skills teaching is highly variable in clinical practice [1].

Procedural Skills Learning

Traditional methods for technical skills instruction in medicine can be ascribed to Halsted's original surgical residency training program where medical students and residents were taught surgical skills according to an apprenticeship model. According to this approach, students were expected to learn both the technical and nontechnical aspects required of their profession through sheer exposure and repetition. Trainees assumed that because they were learning from an expert, they too would attain expertise eventually. There was little focus on the quality of the instruction that was taking place, or the "trainers" themselves. Rather, the onus was on the trainees to learn what they could, or else move on to alternate pursuits [2]. While this method has been used to train surgeons in complex technical and procedural skills for over a century, it is no longer viewed as appropriate. In a modern medical training environment, which is resource-intensive and in high-demand, skilled providers must be trained effectively in a reasonable timeframe. More efficient, and thoughtful training is required to optimize the learning environment so that medical trainees can attain the requisite skills with less wasted time [3].

Learning Competence

One major limitation of the historical apprenticeship approach is a flawed premise upon which it is based—that expert proceduralists are also expert teachers. Rather, expertise in procedural instruction has little to do with procedural proficiency [1]. That is not to say that novices can train other novices in procedures as well as experts can. Rather, technical expertise is likely required but is not sufficient to ensure expert teaching. This phenomenon can be partly explained according to Peyton's learning cycle theory [4]. According to this theory, learners move through a variety of stages before attaining procedural competency. Initially, novices, by definition, are not competent at the procedure at hand, and due to lack of exposure may not necessarily be aware of this reality. This initial stage is termed *unconsciously incompetent.* As learners gain exposure to the procedure/task at hand, they become more aware of their skill deficit, and progress to *consciously incompetent.* As they gain more experience, and learn the steps of the procedure through expert instruction, they may become *consciously competent*. Finally, experts

G. G. R. J. Johnson
Department of Surgery, and Clinician Investigator Program, University of Manitoba, Winnipeg, MB, Canada
e-mail: umjoh529@myumanitoba.ca

A. S. Vergis (✉)
Department of Surgery, University of Manitoba, Winnipeg, MB, Canada
e-mail: avergis@sbgh.mb.ca

L. Marshall Gillman, S. Widder (eds.), *Trauma Team Dynamics*, https://doi.org/10.1007/978-3-031-86312-7_65

Table 65.1 Key aspects of adult learning theory for teaching technical skills

1. Adults retain skills better by doing rather than by watching
2. Adults learn better when content is immediately relevant (i.e., to their clinical practice)
3. Adult learners have surprisingly short attention spans and need to be actively engaged
4. Clear goals and objectives are important
5. Feedback is essential
6. Adults need opportunities for reflection

Adapted from: Hamdorf and Davies [6]

attain a level of *unconscious competence*, where through repeated exposure, they have a high degree of pattern recognition and muscle memory so that they may no longer consciously appreciate the intricacies of the task at hand. The challenge for the teacher when providing good procedural instruction is to remain mindful of these stages and to make explicit to the learner those factors that may have become implicit to the instructor. Importantly, experts may revert into a state of unconscious incompetence in the long term if they fall out of practice (i.e., become rusty), or do not stay up to date with the latest advances.

Adult Learning

Another important factor to consider when training medical professionals in technical procedures is the concept of adult learning theory. Adult learning theory has multiple components, and entire textbooks have been written about the topic and on how adults learn differently from children [5]. While interesting, not all these factors are necessarily important to consider when determining how best to provide technical procedural instruction to trauma care providers. According to Hamdorf et al., the most important features for successful adult learning of clinical skills include clear goal setting, identifying relevance to clinical practice, and providing the opportunity for reflection [6]. Other important aspects of adult learning for teaching procedural skills are listed in Table 65.1. These factors are important to remember when applying the tips to enhance teaching technical and procedural skills below.

Components of Skill Learning

The methods used to teach technical skills (e.g., endotracheal intubation, intravenous line insertion, or tube thoracostomy) differ from those used to teach medical content (e.g., how to read an ECG or the differential diagnosis for abdominal pain). Therefore, a skill is a useful exercise to define. According to Burgess et al., a skill [7]:

1. Is learned, not innate
2. Can be divided into discrete steps
3. Requires practice to improve
4. Has a specific and measurable goal or outcome

According to this definition, a technical skill could be taught in isolation from the clinical context. However, teachers should recognize the relevance of established learning domains for skills acquisition. Bloom's taxonomy provides a useful framework that may help classify some of the factors influencing technical skills development for trainees. Bloom's taxonomy has three overarching domains [8].

The Cognitive Domain

The cognitive domain focuses on the knowledge required for skills learning (Fig. 65.1). These levels were originally developed as a stepwise progression, with the lower rungs representing simple functions such as pure recall (i.e., list the indications for tube thoracostomy) required to achieve before higher functions such as comprehension, application analysis, synthesis, and evaluation, could be accomplished [8]. More contemporary editions of this taxonomy now represent each sub-domain as more parallel processes rather than a strict stepwise progression [9]. The constructs within the cognitive domains have been used to design educational objectives and curricula for various surgical procedures. The constructs within the cognitive domain may be applied to trauma procedures according to the following examples: *remember* relevant definitions, anatomy, and clinical criteria; *understand* the pathophysiology and etiology of a given condition; *apply* knowledge to diagnose and propose management; *analyze* knowledge such as the value of further diagnostic tests; *evaluate* alternative treatment options in complex situations; and *create new knowledge* by investigating innovative techniques/solutions [10]. Instructors should consider these complex cognitive processes involved in learning procedural skills.

The Affective Domain

The affective domain involves the emotional response and desire for satisfaction in good performance of a skill and an appreciation of its clinical significance (e.g., a lifesaving

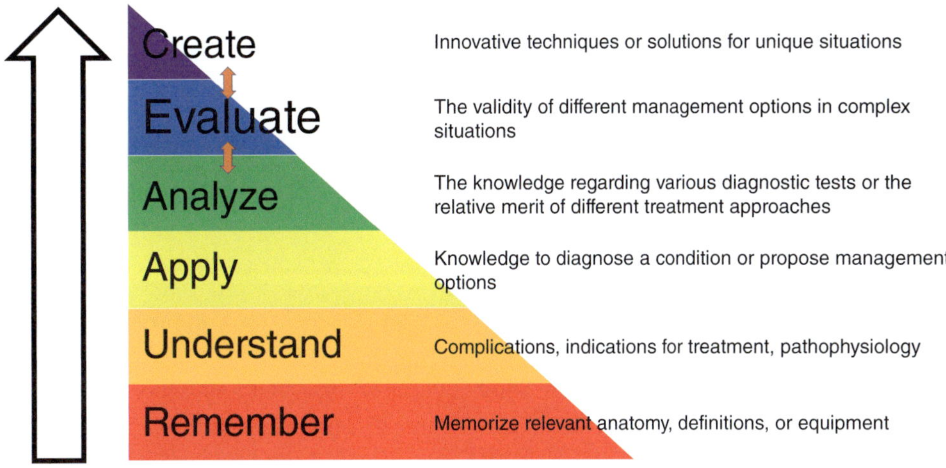

Fig. 65.1 The cognitive domain according to Bloom's taxonomy with teaching points applicable to trauma procedure skills development. (Adapted from Krathwohl [9])

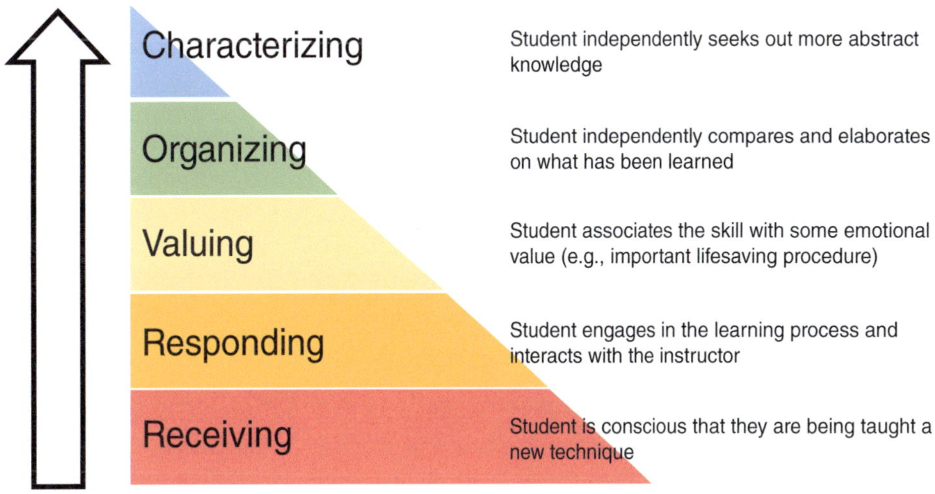

Fig. 65.2 Taxonomy of the affective domain. (Adapted from Krathwohl et al. [11])

tube thoracostomy). A major part of this affective process is the motivation from the teacher (extrinsic motivation) as a positive role model. This motivation, which is initially extrinsic, becomes intrinsic when the student learns to internally value the skill and no longer requires extrinsic motivation from the teacher. The process begins with *receiving* when, at the appropriate moment, the student consciously notes the concept being taught and follows this with a positive *response*. This leads to embracing the concept with emotional *value*, followed by internalization and permanent change in the student's reaction to the concept or skill being taught (Fig. 65.2) [11]. A key element of this process is the recognition of "the teachable moment" when the student is most eager to observe and be receptive to the teacher's efforts. The effective teacher creates a receptive positive environment as a role model and stimulator of intrinsic motivation. This self-motivation then leads to development of the higher levels of the affective domain: *organizing* where the student considers different values and ideas, and *characterization* where the student seeks to build more abstract knowledge related to the task. This progression along the affective domain is not accomplished by command, rather it is stimulated by a highly motivated, sensitive teacher, acting as a role model.

Included in this domain is the concept of a "safe learning environment," where students feel secure to ask questions, take risks, and make mistakes. The safe learning environment is an essential location for the acquisition of new procedural skills [12]. However, as discussed in Chap. 13, after initial skills competency is achieved, the application of external stressors enhances memory consolidation [13] and can help learners develop strategies to deal with stressors inherent to the clinical environment that might otherwise impair effective performance in practice [14].

The Psychomotor Domain

The psychomotor domain focuses on the necessary neuromuscular and motor coordination aspects of acquiring a technical skill. Bloom's original taxonomy had no subcategories for this domain. Subsequently, multiple frameworks

Table 65.2 Five-step approach to skills teaching

1. Overview	Learner can describe why the procedure is needed and how to use it in clinical care—provides motivation to learn/practice
2. Demonstration	Instructor demonstrates the skill at normal speed and without commentary
3. Deconstruction	Instructor breaks skill down into simple steps and demonstrates while describing each step
4. Comprehension	Instructor demonstrates the skill while being "talked through" the steps by the learner
5. Performance	Student demonstrates the skill, while describing each step

Adapted from: George and Doto [18]

under this domain have been proposed [15–17]. Table 65.2 lists one application of the psychomotor domain which was used as a theoretical basis for a popular method of technical skills instruction in healthcare [4, 18]. The application of this method will be discussed in the following section.

All three domains of Bloom's taxonomy complement each other in the acquisition of technical skills. For instance, the cognitive aspects allow understanding of the anatomy, physiology, and indications for performing the skill; the psychomotor aspect focuses on the physical details of accomplishing the skill and performing it proficiently; while the affective component stimulates intrinsic motivation and emphasizes the value of the skill in the clinical management of a patient. As opposed to mere physical acquisition of a skill, the other domains lead to more complete learning. While this may not necessarily make a procedure easier to master, a student that is sensitized to a skill's clinical significance through the cognitive and affective domains may be more likely to expend the effort and energy required for mastery. We implore the reader to consider their own teachers who have had the greatest impact on their own clinical skills development. They were not necessarily the most technically skilled surgeons or clinicians that they can identify. Rather, they were excellent teachers because they were inspiring, made challenging concepts seem easy, or made uninteresting topics appear relevant and exciting. When focusing on procedural skills education, it may seem simpler to ignore concepts outside of the psychomotor domain. However, we argue those additional components (e.g., indications, risks, benefits, documentation, communication, and psychoemotional interactions between the patient, and providers) should be addressed for their important cognitive and affective influence.

Techniques for Teaching Procedures

Since Bloom's original taxonomy for learning, multiple frameworks have been developed in order to expand upon Bloom's psychomotor domain [15–17]. We have curated some of the more useful techniques that have demonstrated effectiveness in the literature for enhanced procedural skills instruction in healthcare and can be applied for teaching useful skills required in trauma resuscitation.

Five Steps for Technical Skills Teaching

Skills are more easily taught when broken down into small, discrete steps. One popular method for teaching using this principle is George and Doto's five-step approach (Table 65.2). According to this framework, the learner has an opportunity to observe the skill performed competently, can recite the component steps, and then ultimately perform the skill under supervision. Steps that are performed incorrectly can be recognized and repeated before proceeding to the next [18]. This instructional method is relatively intuitive and may occur naturally to some. However, one common pitfall is the tendency for teachers to talk themselves through the initial demonstration, which robs the learner from seeing an expert demonstration unimpeded [6]. Peyton's four-step approach, another popular teaching method in the literature, is identical to the five-step method, but skips the "overview" step [4]. We prefer the five-step model, as in the overview phase the learner establishes the knowledge relating to the importance of the skill in clinical practice. This provides context and motivation to help with learning according to the cognitive and affective domains of Bloom's taxonomy.

These four- and five-step methods work particularly well for simple procedures (with less than seven steps), which can be easily maintained in working memory [7]. Owing to the simplicity and effectiveness of the five-step method, it has been adopted into the Advanced Trauma Life support teaching program [19]. However, as procedures become lengthier and more complex, the efficacy of the four- and five-step methods is less clear [20].

Cognitive task analysis (CTA) is a method used to enhance division of technical procedures into parts. CTA was developed by the United States military, and uses a panel of experts to identify the key components of a procedure. An example of the major steps for a cricothyroidotomy task generated through CTA is shown in Fig. 65.3. In addition to the major steps of the procedure, during CTA the cognitive processes behind each step are also identified, including key decision points, technical tips, potential pitfalls, solutions, observable trainee behaviors, and even simulator fidelity issues [21, 22]. For example, during cricothyroidotomy, for the "palpate for landmarks" step, Cannon-Bowers et al. describe a procedural cue as the tactile feedback from the depression over the cricothyroid membrane. Potential pit-

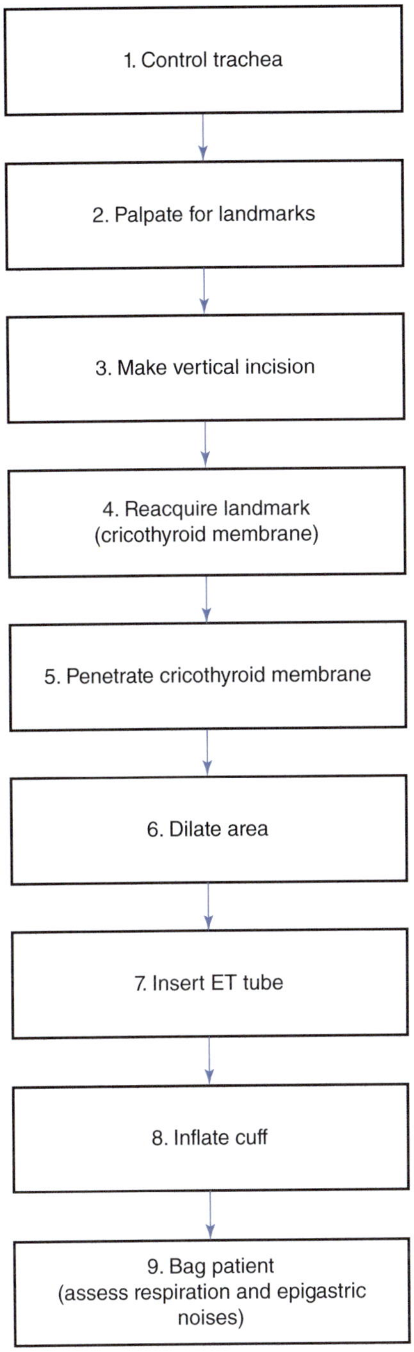

Fig. 65.3 Major task list for open cricothyrotomy procedure generated through cognitive task analysis of nine military trauma personnel. (Adapted from Cannon-Bowers et al. [21])

falls during this step may include insufficient grip on the trachea, misinterpreting anatomical landmarks, or using two hands to palpate. Solutions include grasping the trachea firmly between thumb and middle finger and leaving the index finger free to palpate. Objective observable trainee behaviors include forming the grip as described, and palpation for the anatomical landmarks using the index finger with a vertical trachea orientation [21]. This information is then used as part of procedural instruction, rather than to have expert instructors provide procedural steps on an ad hoc basis. Procedural instruction using CTA is more efficient and effective than conventional training, and has been applied by the United States military for teaching trauma medical personnel for decades [21, 22].

Feedback

The provision of specific, immediate, and constructive feedback is perhaps the most important component of successful procedural skills teaching. By following the structured approach to teaching above, learners can see the skill being performed with excellent technique first, before attempting it for themselves. However, immediate feedback and therefore error correction prevents the unfortunate circumstance from occurring where the skill is initially practiced incorrectly, thereby reinforcing unconscious incompetence, which can be difficult to remedy [23].

During procedural instruction, the optimal timing of feedback is debated [24, 25]. Some suggest it should be withheld until the conclusion of the skill session in order to allow the learner to practice while focusing on each element of the skill, without excessive verbal information [26]. Allowing the opportunity for learners to self-correct during the procedure without excessive input from the instructor, can help develop valuable problem-solving skills. This delayed feedback is termed *summary feedback*. This summary feedback should be given immediately after the procedure ends so that errors in performance can be corrected in a timely fashion [25]. Summary feedback can be used during low-risk procedures or during simulation, where there is no risk of patient harm. However, when teaching procedures on live patients, which is often necessary for complex surgical operations, then *concurrent feedback* (throughout the procedure) is often necessary so as to prevent inadvertent injury [27].

Ideally, feedback is a two-way process involving dialogue between instructor and student. Prior to beginning a procedural instruction session, the trainee and teacher should establish clearly stated learning objectives, based upon the student's past training experience. For a review of the components of learning objectives, see Chap. 58. In brief, these objectives should be viewed as a contract between student and teacher in which the gap between present skills and those to be learned is filled. The student must understand what needs to be achieved, by what timeframe, how this will be achieved, and by what metric these skills will be measured. In this way, they are best prepared to pursue these changes as outlined and guided by the instructor [28]. A participant-driven method of feedback is also helpful to ensure the trainee has an opportunity for self-reflection. An example of this method is asking the participant what they felt went well

Table 65.3 Six-step approach to skill teaching incorporating simulation and practice

1. Learn	Knowledge acquisition
2. See	Observation of the procedure
3. Practice	Deliberate practice using simulation
4. Prove	Competency is assessed
5. Do	The procedure is performed on a patient, with direct supervision until the learner is entrusted to perform the procedure independently
6. Maintain	Continued clinical practice, supplemented by simulation-based training

Adapted from: Sawyer et al. [35]

and what could be improved, prior to telling them the instructor's perspective [29].

The "Feedback Sandwich" model is another popular method. In this model the instructor begins with identifying and complimenting the student's good performance followed by discussion of deficiencies. Feedback should end on a positive, supportive but balanced note with defined plans for further development of the skills emphasizing the concept that expertise comes with continued practice and develops over years. Limitations of the feedback sandwich model are that if not used skillfully, it can appear patronizing. Furthermore, the emphasis of feedback should be on areas for improvement. Trainees may find this critical "middle" element of the feedback sandwich too subtle, resulting in them failing to reflect on what needs to change [30].

Assessment of Competency

An essential element of trainee development interconnected with constructive feedback is the concept of assessment. Compared to feedback, competency assessments aim to evaluate whether the trainee can safely perform the procedure as part of their clinical role. Using simulation to assess learners is discussed in Chaps. 64, 66. Miller's pyramid provides a hierarchy of four steps for evaluation of clinical procedures: knows, knows how, shows how, and does. The base of the pyramid assesses knowledge, whereas the point of the pyramid evaluates actual performance in clinical practice [31]. Historically, competency assessments have taken the form of a high-stakes examination at the end of the expected training process. However, recognizing the importance of repeated evaluations of consistent performance, modern medical training programs have been increasingly blending feedback with formal assessments [32]. Examples include the recent integration of daily entrustable professional activity (EPA) evaluations into surgical and medical residency programs in Canada [33].

Deliberate Practice

Most procedural skills required in the care of trauma patients are impossible to master in a single session. Therefore, after initial learning, trainees must practice in order to enhance their skills and prevent natural skill decay. As instructors, we have a finite ability to influence the private study habits of our students. However, we can position them for success by imparting certain practice habits that are associated with high degrees of success. In medicine, sports, and the arts, those that attain high levels of skill use deliberate practice. Deliberate practice is characterized by continual reflection on performance and focused practice to enhance areas of weakness [34]. Instructors can foster those positive practice traits by providing both opportunities for practice (i.e., in clinical practice or in simulation) and for reflection (i.e., participant-driven feedback above). Instructors can also help identify areas for weakness and opportunities for improvement through constructive feedback. A modification to the five-step teaching model emphasizing the importance of deliberate practice for skills acquisition and maintenance is listed in Table 65.3 [35].

Future Directions

Importantly, while constructive feedback and deliberate practice are repeatedly identified as essential to ensuring skills development, they are also limited resources in the modern healthcare education environment. Dedicated practice for complex skills requires significant time investment. Many procedural skills can only be practiced in the hospital or clinical setting, which effectively means only during working hours. In the past two decades, residency training programs have had their working duty hours limited. That factor, combined with increased public scrutiny further, limits our ability to provide opportunities for dedicated practice in the workplace. Procedural task simulators have been used as one solution and have demonstrated significant efficacy for training a variety of simple and complex medical procedures. However, high-quality simulators with evidence of efficacy do not exist for all medical procedures and are an active area of research [36]. Procedural task simulators can also be costly, so they too are often limited to the workplace. Therefore, methods to enhance trainee practice at home in their spare time is another evolving area. Serious gaming, or gamification, the process of turning procedural performance in simulation into a skill-based competition, has shown promise to increase self-guided after-hours practice [37]. Similarly, procedural task simulators have been combined with videogames, in order to stimulate trainee interest and encourage practice during leisure time [38, 39]. As the number of procedural and surgical techniques continues to expand, the demands for efficient and effective trauma skills training will too. Techniques to supplement training, such as home simulators and more efficient instructional methods, will continue to become more important.

Key Points

- An apprenticeship model is not efficient enough in the modern procedural training environment. Structured learning programs are required.
- When teaching procedural skills, remember the importance of clear goal setting, identifying relevance to clinical practice, and providing the opportunity for reflection.
- The teacher has likely achieved task-related unconscious competence and therefore must be mindful of the procedural steps and instructional method.
- A five-step approach for skill teaching ensures that learners develop an appropriate level of awareness before attempting a skill.
- Expert learners employ deliberate practice.
- Deliberate practice is characterized by continual reflection on performance and focused practice to enhance areas of weakness.
- Appropriate feedback is crucial for successfully teaching technical skills.

References

1. Wall D, McAleer S. Teaching the consultant teachers: identifying the core content. Med Educ. 2000;34(2):131–8.
2. Cameron JL. William Stewart Halsted: our surgical heritage. Ann Surg. 1997;225(5):445–58.
3. Nataraja RM, Webb N, Lopez P-J. Simulation in paediatric urology and surgery. Part 1: an overview of educational theory. J Pediatr Urol. 2018;14(2):120–4.
4. Peyton JWR. The learning cycle. In: Teaching & learning in medical practice. 1st ed. Rickmansworth: ManticCore Europe Ltd; 1999. p. 13–9.
5. Bierema LL. Adult learning theories and practices. In: Fedeli M, Bierema LL, editors. Connecting adult learning and knowledge management: strategies for learning and change in higher education and organizations, Knowledge management and organizational learning. Cham: Springer International Publishing; 2019. p. 3–25. Available from: https://doi.org/10.1007/978-3-030-29872-2_1.
6. Hamdorf JM, Davies R. Teaching a clinical skill. In: Manual of simulation in healthcare. 2nd ed. Oxford: Oxford University Press; 2015. Available from: http://oxfordmedicine.com/view/10.1093/med/9780198717621.001.0001/med-9780198717621-chapter-6.
7. Burgess A, van Diggele C, Roberts C, Mellis C. Tips for teaching procedural skills. BMC Med Educ. 2020;20(2):458.
8. Bloom BS, Krathwohl DR, Masia BB. Taxonomy of educational objectives: the classification of educational goals. Longmans, Green; 1956. Available from: https://books.google.ca/books?id=rJNqAAAAMAAJ.
9. Krathwohl DR. A revision of Bloom's taxonomy: an overview. Theory Pract. 2002;41(4):212–8.
10. Tuma F, Nassar AK. Applying Bloom's taxonomy in clinical surgery: practical examples. Ann Med Surg. 2021;69:102656.
11. Krathwohl DR, Masia BB, Bloom BS. Affective domain: the classification of educational goals. London: Longman Schools Division; 1965.
12. Yanofsky SD, Nyquist JG. Using the affective domain to enhance teaching of the ACGME competencies in anesthesiology training. J Educ Perioper Med. 2014;12(1):E055.
13. Bong CL, Fraser K, Oriot D. Cognitive load and stress in simulation. In: Grant VJ, Cheng A, editors. Comprehensive healthcare simulation pediatric, vol. 1. 1st ed. Cham: Springer; 2016. p. 3–18.
14. Zakay D, Wooler S. Time pressure, training and decision effectiveness. Ergonomics. 1984;27(3):273–84.
15. Harrow AJ. A taxonomy of the psychomotor domain: a guide for developing behavorial objectives. New York: David McKay Co.; 1972. 190 p.
16. Dave RH. Psychomotor levels. In: Developing and writing educational objectives. Tucson: Educational Innovators Press; 1970. p. 20–1.
17. Simpson EJ. The classification of educational objectives, psychomotor domain [Internet]. 1966 [cited 2021 Dec 21]. Available from: https://eric.ed.gov/?id=ED010368.
18. George JH, Doto FX. A simple five-step method for teaching clinical skills. Fam Med. 2001;33(8):577–8.
19. American College of Surgeons Committee on Trauma. ATLS advanced trauma life support: instructor course manual. 10th ed. Chicago: American College of Surgeons; 2018.
20. Giacomino K, Caliesch R, Sattelmayer KM. The effectiveness of the Peyton's 4-step teaching approach on skill acquisition of procedures in health professions education: a systematic review and meta-analysis with integrated meta-regression. PeerJ. 2020;8:e10129.
21. Cannon-Bowers J, Bowers C, Stout R, Ricci K, Hildabrand A. Using cognitive task analysis to develop simulation-based training for medical tasks. Mil Med. 2013;178(10 Suppl):15–21.
22. Edwards TC, Coombs AW, Szyszka B, Logishetty K, Cobb JP. Cognitive task analysis-based training in surgery: a meta-analysis. BJS Open. 2021;5(6):zrab122.
23. Hattie J, Timperley H. The power of feedback. Rev Educ Res. 2007;77(1):81–112.
24. Al Fayyadh MJ, Hassan RA, Tran ZK, Kempenich JW, Bunegin L, Dent DL, et al. Immediate auditory feedback is superior to other types of feedback for basic surgical skills acquisition. J Surg Educ. 2017;74(6):e55–61.
25. Xeroulis GJ, Park J, Moulton C-A, Reznick RK, LeBlanc V, Dubrowski A. Teaching suturing and knot-tying skills to medical students: a randomized controlled study comparing computer-based video instruction and (concurrent and summary) expert feedback. Surgery. 2007;141(4):442–9.
26. Salmoni AW, Schmidt RA, Walter CB. Knowledge of results and motor learning: a review and critical reappraisal. Psychol Bull. 1984;95(3):355–86.
27. Nazari T, Bogomolova K, Ridderbos M, Dankbaar MEW, van Merriënboer JJG, Lange JF, et al. Global versus task-specific postoperative feedback in surgical procedure learning. Surgery. 2021;170(1):81–7.
28. Richardson D, Flynn L. The roadmap: learning objectives. In: Educational design: a CanMEDS guide for the health professions. Ottawa: Royal College of Physicians and Surgeons; 2011.
29. Pendleton D. The consultation: an approach to learning and teaching. Oxford/New York: Oxford University Press; 1984.

30. James IA. The rightful demise of the Sh*t Sandwich: providing effective feedback. Behav Cogn Psychother. 2015;43(6):759–66.
31. Miller GE. The assessment of clinical skills/competence/performance. Acad Med. 1990;65(9 Suppl):S63–7.
32. Ten Cate O. Entrustability of professional activities and competency-based training. Med Educ. 2005;39(12):1176–7.
33. CBD Program Evaluation Operations Team. Competence by design (CBD) implementation pulse check. The Royal College of Physicians and Surgeons of Canada; 2020. Available from: https://www.royalcollege.ca/rcsite/cbd/competence-by-design-cbd-e.
34. Ericsson KA. Deliberate practice and the acquisition and maintenance of expert performance in medicine and related domains. Acad Med. 2004;79(10 Suppl):S70–81.
35. Sawyer T, White M, Zaveri P, Chang T, Ades A, French H, et al. Learn, see, practice, prove, do, maintain: an evidence-based pedagogical framework for procedural skill training in medicine. Acad Med. 2015;90(8):1025–33.
36. Borgersen NJ, Naur TMH, Sørensen SMD, Bjerrum F, Konge L, Subhi Y, et al. Gathering validity evidence for surgical simulation: a systematic review. Ann Surg. 2018;267(6):1063–8.
37. Gentry SV, Gauthier A, Ehrstrom BL, Wortley D, Lilienthal A, Car LT, et al. Serious gaming and gamification education in health professions: systematic review. J Med Internet Res. 2019;21(3):e12994.
38. Jalink MB, Goris J, Heineman E, Pierie JPEN, ten Cate Hoedemaker HO. Construct and concurrent validity of a Nintendo Wii video game made for training basic laparoscopic skills. Surg Endosc. 2013;28(2):537–42.
39. Johnson G, Vergis A, Unger B, Park J, Gillman L. Design and validity evidence for a unique endoscopy simulator using a commercial video game. Cureus. 2021;13(9):e18379.

Competency-Based Education

66

Brett Mador

Introduction

Competency-based education (CBE) represents the most significant paradigm shift in medical education since the aftermath of the Flexner report over 100 years ago [1, 2]. While still in its early stages of implementation, CBE has gained a foothold in many countries with the aim of avoiding pitfalls of traditional training models and producing healthcare professionals that are well-rounded and fully competent to meet the needs of target populations. CBE has been adapted to multiple areas of healthcare and is immediately applicable to trauma team training.

History

In the late twentieth century, the traditional, process and time-based training curriculum for healthcare practitioners was brought into question. One of the main driving forces behind this was the patient safety movement [3, 4], which had the twinned effects of limiting trainee work-hours and clinical responsibilities [5, 6], while also elevating the expected standards of medical graduates. The result was an uneven bar of competence, and a highly variable quality of new graduates across training programs [7]. This imbalance has been further compounded by an ever-increasing amount of required knowledge and skills related to ongoing intellectual and technological advances in health care. The described concerns were met by many in medical education as a crisis of training, and after much discourse and deliberation, and based on the central premise of ensuring high patient care standards and transparency, a transition to a competency-based model of training was endorsed [8, 9].

This education crisis was arguably even more pronounced in regard to trauma care. Developed countries have witnessed a measurable decline in major trauma cases, due to a combination of factors including motor vehicle safety and prevention campaigns [10, 11]. At the same time, trauma care underwent a paradigm shift of its own, away from invasive diagnostic procedures and frequent operative intervention, and toward noninvasive diagnostic procedures and nonoperative management of many traumatic injuries [12]. Specifically, diagnostic peritoneal lavage has been largely supplanted by bedside point-of-care ultrasound, and nonoperative management of blunt spleen and liver injuries has become the standard of care. Admittedly, the main quantitative and volume-related issues relate more to surgical management of trauma [13, 14]. However, the loss of technical experience in vivo has effects on the trauma team as a whole, and expectations for performance in cases of severe trauma (i.e., resuscitative thoracotomy) remain high. Combined with the more generalized issues mentioned previously, and an overreliance on simulation and ex vivo training to supplement existing education opportunities, a modern crisis in trauma care training has been described [15, 16].

The competency-based model (or outcomes-based model) was adapted from vocational fields and introduced theoretically to the medical field in the 1970s and 1980s, before being formally introduced into medical education practice in the 1990s [1, 17]. Further adaptation and ideas have been developed over the ensuing decades, in order to adequately apply the principles to medical education. The foundation of this transition began with the development and implementation of various competency frameworks such as the Outcome Project in the United States [8], the Scottish Doctor in the United Kingdom [18], and CanMEDS in Canada [19]. These frameworks attempted to distill down the key attributes of an ideal physician, going beyond medical expertise to encompass additional faculties. The CanMEDS framework includes medical expert, communicator, collaborator, health advocate, leader, scholar, and professional as its competency domains [19], whereas the ACGME core competencies include practice-based learning and improvement, patient care and procedural skills, systems-based practice, medical

B. Mador (✉)
Department of Surgery, University of Alberta, Edmonton, AB, Canada

L. Marshall Gillman, S. Widder (eds.), *Trauma Team Dynamics*, https://doi.org/10.1007/978-3-031-86312-7_66

Table 66.1 Comparison of competency-based and traditional time-based curricula

Competency-based curriculum	Traditional time-based curriculum
Focus on competencies (what the learner does in practice)	Focus on time spent and acquired knowledge (what the learner knows)
Competencies determined based on societal needs	Knowledge/time required based on historical standards
Assessment based on observable abilities	Assessment based on knowledge-based objectives
Primary mode of assessment is multiple workplace-based performance evaluations	Primary mode of assessment is summative examinations
Assessment for learning: assessment used primarily to promote learning	*Assessment of learning*: assessment used primarily to gauge learning progress
Learner centered	Teacher centered
Time-flexible; emphasis on individual sequential progression	Time-based; emphasis on quantitative experience
Criterion-referenced standards	Norm-referenced standards

knowledge, interpersonal and communication skills, and professionalism [8]. These and other core competencies were then adapted to formal curricula. CBE curricula have now been deployed in multiple countries [20], and spanning all disciplines of medicine. Given the relatively new introduction of the model, data specific to medical education is still being collected, and unforeseen advantages and disadvantages are actively being reported and considered [21, 22].

CBE can be envisioned and delivered in a myriad of different ways, although it generally follows a few guiding principles which include: an outcomes-based focus, emphasis on specific observable abilities, time flexibility, learner centeredness [23], and a robust system of assessment [24]. While a pure CBE model requires all of these components, it is also possible, and perhaps preferable, to apply some combination of CBE and traditional principles in practice [25]. A comparison of CBE and traditional curricula is shown in Table 66.1.

Outcomes-Based

Traditional medical curricula often focus on the curricula itself; the content and required training experiences that most closely resemble current medical practice, and from this derive a set of learning objectives and assessment methods. Further, traditional curricula utilize a prespecified time-period over which training is required, based largely on historical standards. An outcomes-based curriculum takes a different approach. It begins, instead, with the target patient population and its specific needs, both current and projected. Needs-based information is used to develop a very specific set of outcomes or competencies for trainees. It is this set of requirements that then determines the curriculum, including assessment and program evaluation. An outcomes-based approach differs from the traditional model in that the focus shifts away from process-related factors, such as how curricula will be delivered, what teaching methods will be employed, and how long training will take.

Within a CBE model, objectives of training should be organized as specific, assessable criteria that are required by all trainees in order to provide a minimum standard of care to a specific patient population. These criteria are generally referred to as "competencies" within such a framework. The crucial difference between a competency and an objective is that a competency must be specific, comprehensive, measurable, and directly related to work-based activities [26]. Further, judgment of these competencies should be criterion-referenced, or based on a very specific standard of care, as opposed to norm-referenced, or compared to peers [24]. Each should be considered, and designed, with the knowledge, skills, and abilities (outcomes) of a competent physician in mind. It is crucial that these competencies, and the methods by which they will be achieved and assessed, be transparent to all parties.

Focus on Observable Abilities

Traditional curricula place an unbalanced emphasis on knowledge, at the expense of skills and attitudes (i.e., competencies). More specifically, traditional objectives, which often feature excessively long lists of knowledge-based objectives, may not translate into a trainee's ability to perform very specific, workplace-oriented tasks [23]. For example, knowledge of how a trauma resuscitation should occur, while easy to test, does not guarantee an individual's ability to perform all the requisite tasks and demonstrate the appropriate attitudes required for competent performance. CBE tends to favor a more complete, varied list of competencies that are more functionally relevant and readily observable.

The focus shifts from knowledge, to the application of knowledge and/or skills in the appropriate context where they can be observed and assessed. Miller's pyramid of assessment (Fig. 66.1) exhibits this well, and aiming for a higher level of assessment, specifically "does" as opposed to "knows," assures a more accurate assessment of true performance compared to traditional models of medical education [27]. This connects directly to another key pillar of effective CBE, which is a robust system of assessment.

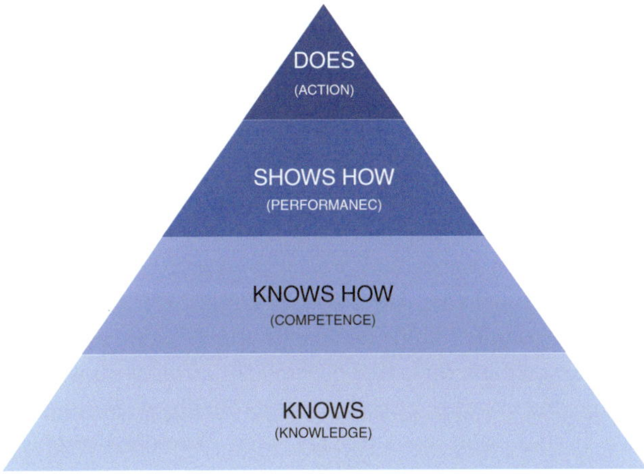

Fig. 66.1 Miller's pyramid of assessment. (Reproduced with permission from Miller [27])

Robust System of Assessment

Perhaps the most crucial practical aspect of effective CBE implementation is a robust system of learner assessment [24]. Given the previously mentioned focus on outcomes and abilities, a more detailed and thorough system is required than the traditional final evaluations and knowledge-based examinations. Assessment within the workplace is particularly nuanced, given the problems inherent to differing contexts and case specificity [28]. Workplace-based assessment is therefore a crucial component of CBE and requires multiple assessments by multiple raters to achieve reliable determinations of competency in a given area [24].

This increased volume of assessments, in turn, makes each assessment lower stakes; it becomes increasingly unlikely that a single assessment can independently result in a "pass" or "fail." Generally, these frequent workplace-based assessments are considered more formative (for development) than summative (for final evaluation), though elements of both concepts are present, as each assessment will contribute to eventual promotion decisions. This highlights the idea of *assessment for learning*, or the idea that assessments, and resultant feedback provided, may actually be more effective as tools to promote learning, as opposed to purely reporting what has already been learned [24]. For example, a CBE observation that a trainee did poorly with closed-loop communication during a trauma resuscitation, when shared directly with the trainee in a timely and constructive manner, may lead to significant improvement in future performance. In contrast, the traditional notion was that an assessment simply served to show the trainee's deficiencies and prevent progression until achieved (*assessment of learning*).

Along these lines, the nature of feedback and coaching that is provided to trainees should be optimized in a CBE model. As opposed to traditional models, where feedback would be provided in a more summative manner at the end of a course or rotation, CBE models typically favor regular feedback that can be applied to ongoing trainee improvement. Ideally, this feedback should be specific, timely, constructive, and focused on behaviors [29]. Principles of coaching have often been borrowed from other fields, such as sports and music, for this purpose as well. CBE favors a positive teacher-learner relationship, with frequent observations and associated feedback with the goal of continuous trainee improvement. This process of expertise development is further supported by the theory of deliberate practice, which relies on regular and valid assessments and feedback to optimize progression [30].

Time Flexibility

Traditional training specifically prescribes the amount of time, or number of cases, required by a trainee to achieve competence in a given subject. A simple example is the fixed length of a trauma simulation course, or the prescribed time spent on a trauma or emergency medicine rotation. Unfortunately, these prescribed time frames have changed little despite the major constraints on medical training previously described. Furthermore, trainees learn at different rates, both based on personal aptitude and the specific context. A trauma service experience during a busy summer month could have very different learning opportunities compared to a slower winter rotation. All of these factors question the adequacy of time-based training. CBE allows for flexibility of timing that can be adjusted to a given learner, allowing them to achieve competence without the constraints of time-based curricula [22]. More specifically, CBE focuses on individual learner progression through defined, sequential milestones.

Not surprisingly, in postgraduate residency training settings, true time-flexibility has been particularly difficult to achieve [22, 31]. There are multiple contributing factors, including service-based requirements of many medical learners, and logistical difficulties in programs that are training multiple learners simultaneously. Despite these difficulties, even relative time-flexibility, and the concept that learners achieve competence at different rates, is a key principle of CBE [23].

Learner-Centric

The last key principle of CBE is a shift from teacher to learner-centered curricula. Given the previously described tenets, specifically outcome-based and time-flexibility, it serves that the curriculum would be more focused on the learner, and their specific needs to achieve competence, than on the teacher's goals or ideas. Traditionally curricula have been designed, at least partly, around teacher-developed curricula and their chosen instructional methods. However, the needs of the learner and their quest for individual competence are given more emphasis in the CBE model. The learner is able to use the competencies, as well as milestones which provide a described pathway to competence, to self-direct their learning. This takes shape primarily in targeting specific short-term goals and choosing workplace-based assessments to complement these goals. The focus of the teacher is more focused on guiding the learner on their individual journey toward competency than it is on specifically prescribing all steps in the process.

Application to Trauma Team Training

To date, CBE has been primarily applied at the post-graduate training level for medical doctors. However, the principles described can, and have been, applied to many other areas of health professional training [32, 33], and can be specifically applied to trauma care and trauma team training for all trauma care practitioners. In fact, CBE has been identified as a key area in the redesign of trauma care curricula to address the increased needs and difficulties previously described [34].

Given the reduction in overall trauma volume, procedural trauma cases, and trainee work-hours and responsibilities, CBE provides an important avenue by which to ensure the competence of graduating trainees when it comes to trauma care. The use of high-fidelity simulation to help achieve these goals, including assessment of requisite abilities, also contributes significantly to improving trauma training [35]. Video reviews have been utilized to facilitate teaching and fit well into CBE by providing another opportunity for more in-depth observation, as well as learner self-reflection [36]. Given the current state of trauma training, it behooves all curriculum planners to seriously consider CBE principles when designing training opportunities of all types.

While it is certainly possible to develop entire CBE curricula for trauma training, it is more feasible to apply specific principles or hybrid approaches. The simplest method is to introduce competency-based assessment tools to existing curricula, as described in the next section. Specifically, to introduce new assessment tools aimed to measure competence in specific abilities, with the goal of developing learner expertise in a given workplace-based activity. These units of competence are often referred to as entrustable professional activities, or EPAs. EPAs are particularly useful for providing a bridge between the competencies that a trainee is required to possess, and the actual application of knowledge, skills, and attitudes that they exhibit on a regular basis [37]. These units tend to encompass a variety of specific milestones and competencies and are considered a surrogate for practice-based performance.

Workplace-Based Assessment

As described elsewhere in this book, trauma team training is a crucial yet elaborate and previously undervalued aspect of effective trauma care. Developing competence and expertise in such a complex field can benefit greatly from workplace-based assessment tools that provide a scaffold with which to prompt and organize effective learner feedback. Fortunately, several such tools have already been developed, typically adapted from preexisting tools from other fields. The most well-studied and validated of these is the Trauma Non-Technical Skills Scale, or T-NOTECHS [38]. This scale was borrowed from the aviation industry and initially adapted for use in the operating room before being further modified for use with trauma resuscitation teams. The scale utilizes five essential behavior domains rated on a 5-point Likert scale: leadership, cooperation and resource management, communication and interaction, assessment and decision-making, and situation awareness/coping with stress [38]. The formal tool is shown in Fig. 66.2. Behavioral anchors are provided to assist with accurate and reliable assessment. Statistical analysis shows good reliability and correlation of higher scores with improved performance. Many similar tools have been developed and validated, both specific to trauma, such as the Trauma Team Performance Observation Tool (TPOT) [39], and more general crew resource management tools, such as the Mayo High Performance Teamwork Scale [36] and the Ottawa Crisis Resource Management Global Rating Scale (Ottawa GRS) [40].

Competency-based assessment tools provide a new avenue by which to train and assess trauma teams and their members. They provide relevance and utility as both a formative and summative training tool and can be applied both as an interim assessment to improve future performance and as an end-of-training assessment to judge readiness for in situ trauma resuscitation. Given the complexity of trauma team training, including team composition and patient/situation context, having a validated tool to assist in team development is essential. Course directors and curriculum planners are strongly encouraged to consider adopting these types of tools into their curricula. They also serve a role in programmatic evaluation, providing a validated tool with which to measure learner progression during a program of training. Notably, the utilization of technology, including mobile applications, for the use of these assessment tools can improve uptake and efficiency [41].

Tools have also been developed to facilitate more specific roles and responsibilities within the trauma team. Gregg et al. developed a tool specifically designed to assess

TRAUMA NOTECHS

Leadership

5	4	3	2	1
Clearly defined team leader. Good time management, all tasks completed, non-hierarchical		Individual defined, but some tasks not completed.		Indentify of team leader not clear

Cooperation and Resource Management

5	4	3	2	1
All team members clearly fill a role and perform all designated tasks		Identity of all members not clear, some do not perform assigned tasks		Unable to discern role identity of team members

Communication and Interaction

5	4	3	2	1
Clear communication with Team Leadr as a hub, relayed to scribe		Communication not always through Team Leader, or not relayed rapidly to scribe		Unorganized or incoherent communication on many different levels

Assessment and Decision Making

5	4	3	2	1
Orderly and completed 1° (ABCDE) and 2° surveys Plan communicated team.		Assessment somewhat out of order, all major tasks complete		1° and 2° surveys disorderly and/or incomplete. Plan not clear.

Situation Awareness / Coping with Stress

5	4	3	2	1
Untoward findings and distractions did not upset systematic and orderly flow. Team is calm and plans ahead.		Untoward findings caused disruption but did not preclude task completion.		Untoward findings or interruptions completely upset orderly assessment and task completion Not anitcipatory.

Fig. 66.2 Trauma NOTECHS. (Reproduced with permission from Steinemann et al. [38])

the performance of the trauma team leader [42]. More general leadership tools, such as the modified Campbell Leadership Descriptor tool, have also been effectively used to measure trauma team leadership [43]. Given the elaborate nature of this role, including both clinical acumen and nontechnical skills, this can be incredibly difficult to assess holistically. These tools provide a comprehensive method to do so, either in real-time or utilizing video recordings, and either in situ or using simulation. By utilizing CBE principles, and providing multiple assessments with appropriate feedback over time in a learner-centered fashion, one can greatly facilitate learner progression in ways that were previously much more nebulous.

Technical skills crucial to trauma team functioning can similarly be assessed using existing workplace-based assessment tools. These tools have been previously validated and are useful for evaluation of skills in areas such as endotracheal intubation [44], point-of-care ultrasound [45], chest tube insertion [46], and central venous access [47]. These tools are immediately amenable for integration into existing trauma courses, formal rotations, simulation exercises, and in situ trauma care. Again, the tools are especially helpful for fostering appropriate and effective feedback to assist in training progression, while also maintaining a role in more summative assessment of competence.

Case Examples

To better understand the relevance and impact of CBE in trauma training, it is helpful to consider specific examples for context, specifically course-based and rotation-based learner settings.

Advanced Trauma Life Support (ATLS) is a course that is well-known to most readers and has integrated certain components of CBE over its numerous iterations [48]. The general organization of ATLS maintains a more traditional curriculum, composed of a specified number of interactive and skills-based sessions delivered over a fixed period of time. However, the curriculum has for some time also included "optional" sessions (i.e., ocular trauma) that can be utilized depending on learner needs. Furthermore, the most recent 10th edition has improved the flexibility of course delivery by allowing a hybrid flipped classroom approach, which can be optioned depending on learner preferences. However, the most notable competency-based aspect of the course has been the final learner assessment. To successfully complete the course, participants are required to demonstrate their learned abilities in simulated moulage scenarios which are assessed using a standardized, criterion-referenced form. This is fairly unique to courses of this type, but this concept is outcomes-based and focused on observable abilities, aligning well with CBE by ensuring competence within a specific context for all graduates of the course.

Potential future CBE-related adaptations of ATLS could include introducing additional competency-based assessments to other aspects of the course such as small group sessions. For example, integrating a specific competency-based assessment tool for tube thoracostomy and cricothyrotomy, ideally supported through a smartphone application. It could also use these formative assessments to offer additional learning opportunities and time-flexibility to participants that require it. While admittedly resource-intensive and logistically challenging, these modifications would be advantageous to the learner by improving learner-centeredness and flexibility.

Another relevant and common example is that of a postgraduate rotation on a trauma service. Several key changes can be introduced to transform a standard rotation to a competency-based format. One such consideration is to convert the traditional, comprehensive list of specialty-determined objectives into a more compact list of easily observable EPAs. An example EPA, such as "lead a trauma resuscitation," would incorporate multiple overlapping competencies such as leadership, knowledge/expertise, and collaboration. Each competency would also encompass multiple traditional objectives such as "selects appropriate resuscitation fluids" and "differentiates the causes of shock." These EPAs can be observed directly in the workplace or in simulation, and utilize pre-selected, validated assessment forms to provide both formative feedback and summative evaluation. These assessment forms can also be split among multiple learners to improve efficiency of team-based learning (i.e., tube thoracostomy for the junior resident, trauma team leader for the senior resident). The individual learner will have access to their collated assessments throughout the rotation, in order to understand areas of competence and deficiency and therefore self-direct future learning on the rotation. As discussed previously, transitioning from the ingrained time-based format of these rotations is a challenging aspect of CBE implementation [22]. Given the difficulties of eliminating postgraduate service requirements, programs may instead consider adding additional clinical opportunities such as call shifts, drop-in clinics, or dedicated simulations in areas of identified deficiency. Together, these strategies emphasize the interrelated core principles of CBE, aimed at providing improved learning opportunities along with more objective evidence of learner development.

Conclusion

Competency-based education is considered the biggest paradigm shift in medical education in the last 100 years [1]. While the theoretical model presents significant challenges to implementation, it is much more feasible to consider the core principles and apply them as necessary to existing or redeveloped curricula and courses. Specifically, applying existing workplace-based assessment tools that are designed to measure observed learner competence within a flexible and learner-centered environment. These tools have previously been developed for, tested, and applied to the areas of trauma team performance, trauma team leadership, and various technical skills essential to trauma team functioning. Taken together, integration of CBE principles into trauma team training offers a unique opportunity to improve overall competence in an observable, measurable fashion, and with anticipated positive impact on downstream patient outcomes.

Key Points

- Competency-based education is the most significant paradigm shift in medical education in a century.
- Core principles include an outcomes-based approach, an emphasis on trainee abilities, a robust system of assessment, time flexibility, and learner-centeredness.
- Several validated workplace-based assessment tools exist for use in trauma team training and can greatly impact learner development.

References

1. Carraccio C, Wolfsthal SD, Englander R, Ferentz K, Martin C. Shifting paradigms: from Flexner to competencies. Acad Med. 2002;77(5):361–7.
2. Flexner A. Medical education in the United States and Canada. Washington, DC: Science and Health Publications, Inc.; 1910.
3. Holzman IR, Barnett SH. The Bell Commission: ethical implications for the training of physicians. Mt Sinai J Med. 2000;67(2):136–9.
4. Kohn LT, Corrigan JM, Donaldson MS, editors. To err is human: building a safer health care system. Washington, DC: National Academies Press; 1999.
5. Byrnes MC, Narciso VC, Brantley L, et al. Impact of resident work-hour restrictions on trauma care. Am J Surg. 2006;191(3):338–43.
6. Philibert I, Friedmann P, Williams WT, for the members of the ACGME Work Group on Resident Duty Hours. New require-

ments for resident duty hours. JAMA J Am Med Assoc. 2002;288(9):1112–4.
7. Asch DA, Nicholson S, Srinivas SK, Herrin J, Epstein AJ. How do you deliver a good obstetrician? Outcome-based evaluation of medical education. Acad Med. 2014;89(1):24–6.
8. Swing SR. The ACGME outcome project: retrospective and prospective. Med Teach. 2007;29(7):648–54.
9. Frenk J, Chen L, Bhutta ZA, Cohen J, Crisp N, Evans T, Fineberg H, Garcia P, Ke Y, Kelley P, Kistnasamy B. Health professionals for a new century: transforming education to strengthen health systems in an interdependent world. Lancet. 2010;376(9756):1923–58.
10. Bolen JR, Sleet DA, Chorba T, Brewer R, Dellinger A, Wallace LJ, Johnson VR. Overview of efforts to prevent motor vehicle-related injury. In: Prevention of motor vehicle-related injuries: a compendium of articles from the Morbidity and Mortality Weekly Report 1985–1996. Atlanta: CDC; 1997. p. 36–52.
11. Cothren CC, Moore EE, Hedegaard HB, Meng K. Epidemiology of urban trauma deaths: a comprehensive reassessment 10 years later. World J Surg. 2007;31(7):1507–11.
12. Lukan JK, Carrillo EH, Franklin GA, et al. Impact of recent trends of noninvasive trauma evaluation and nonoperative management in surgical resident education. J Trauma Acute Care Surg. 2001;50(6):1015–9.
13. Barmparas G, Navsaria PH, Dhillon NK, Edu S, Margulies DR, Ley EJ, Gewertz BL, Nicol AJ. The gap in operative exposure in trauma surgery: quantifying the benefits of an international rotation. Surg Open Sci. 2020;2(1):46–50.
14. Engels PT, Versolatto A, Shi Q, Coates A, Rice TJ. Cause for concern: resident experience in operative trauma during general surgery residency at a Canadian centre. Can Med Educ J. 2020;11(6):e54.
15. Engels PT, Bradley NL, Ball CG. The current state of resident trauma training: are we losing a generation? Can J Surg. 2018;61(3):14417.
16. Strumwasser A, Grabo D, Inaba K, Matsushima K, Clark D, Benjamin E, Lam L, Demetriades D. Is your graduating general surgery resident qualified to take trauma call? A 15-year appraisal of the changes in general surgery education for trauma. J Trauma Acute Care Surg. 2017;82(3):470–80.
17. McGaghie WC, Miller GE, Sajid AW, Telder TV. Competency-based curriculum development in medical education. An introduction. Public Health Papers No. 68. Geneva: WHO; 1978.
18. Simpson JG, Furnace J, Crosby J, Cumming AD, Evans PA, Friedman Ben David M, Harden RM, Lloyd D, McKenzie H, McLaughlan JC, et al. The Scottish doctor – learning outcomes for the medical undergraduate in Scotland: a foundation for competent and reflective practitioners. Med Teach. 2002;24(2):136–43.
19. Frank JR. The CanMEDS 2005 physician competency framework: better standards, better physicians, better care. Ottawa: Royal College of Physicians and Surgeons of Canada; 2005.
20. Graham IS, Gleason AJ, Keogh GW, Paltridge D, Rogers IR, Walton M, De Paola C, Singh J, McGrath BP. Australian curriculum framework for junior doctors. Med J Aust. 2007;186(S7):S14–9.
21. Hall AK, Rich J, Dagnone JD, Weersink K, Caudle J, Sherbino J, Frank JR, Bandiera G, Van Melle E. It's a marathon, not a sprint: rapid evaluation of competency-based medical education program implementation. Acad Med. 2020;95(5):786–93.
22. Nousiainen MT, Mironova P, Hynes M, Glover Takahashi S, Reznick R, Kraemer W, Alman B, Ferguson P, CBC Planning Committee. Eight-year outcomes of a competency-based residency training program in orthopedic surgery. Med Teach. 2018;40(10):1042–54.
23. Frank JR, Snell LS, Cate OT, Holmboe ES, Carraccio C, Swing SR, Harris P, Glasgow NJ, Campbell C, Dath D, Harden RM. Competency-based medical education: theory to practice. Med Teach. 2010;32(8):638–45.
24. Holmboe ES, Sherbino J, Long DM, Swing SR, Frank JR, International CBME Collaborators. The role of assessment in competency-based medical education. Med Teach. 2010;32(8):676–82.
25. Harris KA, Frank JR. Competence by design: reshaping Canadian medical education. Ottawa: Royal College of Physicians and Surgeons of Canada; 2014.
26. Ten Cate O. Entrustability of professional activities and competency-based training. Med Educ. 2005;39:1176–7.
27. Miller GE. The assessment of clinical skills/competence/performance. Acad Med. 1990;65(9):S63–7.
28. Norman G, Bordage G, Page G, Keane D. How specific is case specificity? Med Educ. 2006;40(7):618–23.
29. Jug R, Jiang XS, Bean SM. Giving and receiving effective feedback: a review article and how-to guide. Arch Pathol Lab Med. 2019;143(2):244–50.
30. Ericsson KA. An expert-performance perspective of research on medical expertise: the study of clinical performance. Med Educ. 2007;41(12):1124–30.
31. Van Rossum TR, Scheele F, Sluiter HE, Bosman PJ, Rijksen L, Heyligers IC. Flexible competency based medical education: more time efficient, higher costs. Med Teach. 2018;40(3):315–7.
32. Gravina EW. Competency-based education and its effect on nursing education: a literature review. Teach Learn Nurs. 2017;12(2):117–21.
33. Mejicano GC, Bumsted TN. Describing the journey and lessons learned implementing a competency-based, time-variable undergraduate medical education curriculum. Acad Med. 2018;93(3):S42–8.
34. Mador B, Kim M, White J, Harris I, Tekian A. Development of a novel conceptual framework for curriculum design in Canadian postgraduate trauma training. Can Med Educ J. 2020;11(1):e62.
35. Gjeraa K, Møller TP, Østergaard D. Efficacy of simulation-based trauma team training of non-technical skills. A systematic review. Acta Anaesthesiol Scand. 2014;58(7):775–87.
36. Hamilton NA, Kieninger AN, Woodhouse J, Freeman BD, Murray D, Klingensmith ME. Video review using a reliable evaluation metric improves team function in high-fidelity simulated trauma resuscitation. J Surg Educ. 2012;69(3):428–31.
37. ten Cate O, Scheele F. Competency-based postgraduate training: can we bridge the gap between theory and clinical practice? Acad Med. 2007;82(6):542–7.
38. Steinemann S, Berg B, DiTullio A, Skinner A, Terada K, Anzelon K, Ho HC. Assessing teamwork in the trauma bay: introduction of a modified "NOTECHS" scale for trauma. Am J Surg. 2012;203(1):69–75.
39. Capella J, Smith S, Philp A, Putnam T, Gilbert C, Fry W, Harvey E, Wright A, Henderson K, Baker D, Ranson S. Teamwork training improves the clinical care of trauma patients. J Surg Educ. 2010;67(6):439–43.
40. Kim J, Neilipovitz D, Cardinal P, Chiu M, Clinch J. A pilot study using high-fidelity simulation to formally evaluate performance in the resuscitation of critically ill patients: the University of Ottawa Critical Care Medicine, High-Fidelity Simulation, and Crisis Resource Management I Study. Crit Care Med. 2006;34(8):2167–74.
41. Lockyer J, Carraccio C, Chan MK, Hart D, Smee S, Touchie C, Holmboe ES, Frank JR, ICBME Collaborators. Core principles of assessment in competency-based medical education. Med Teach. 2017;39(6):609–16.
42. Gregg SC, Heffernan DS, Connolly MD, Stephen AH, Leuckel SN, Harrington DT, Machan JT, Adams CA Jr, Cioffi WG. Teaching leadership in trauma resuscitation: immediate feedback from a real-time, competency-based evaluation tool shows long-term improvement in resident performance. J Trauma Acute Care Surg. 2016;81(4):729–34.
43. Sakran JV, Finneman B, Maxwell C, Sonnad SS, Sarani B, Pascual J, Kim P, Schwab CW, Sims C. Trauma leadership: does perception drive reality? J Surg Educ. 2012;69(2):236–40.

44. Ryason A, Petrusa ER, Kruger U, Xia Z, Wong VT, Jones DB, De S, Jones SB. Development of an endotracheal intubation formative assessment tool. J Educ Perioper Med. 2020;22(1):e635.
45. Ziesmann MT, Park J, Unger BJ, Kirkpatrick AW, Vergis A, Logsetty S, Pham C, Kirschner D, Gillman LM. Validation of the quality of ultrasound imaging and competence (QUICk) score as an objective assessment tool for the FAST examination. J Trauma Acute Care Surg. 2015;78(5):1008–13.
46. Ghazali A, Léger A, Petitpas F, Guéchi Y, Boureau-Voultoury A, Oriot D. Development and validation of a performance assessment scale for chest tube insertion in traumatic pneumothorax. J Pulm Respir Med. 2016;6(346):2.
47. Huang GC, Newman LR, Schwartzstein RM, Clardy PF, Feller-Kopman D, Irish JT, Smith CC. Procedural competence in internal medicine residents: validity of a central venous catheter insertion assessment instrument. Acad Med. 2009;84(8):1127–34.
48. American College of Surgeons Committee on Trauma. Advanced Trauma Life Support® (ATLS®): student course manual. 10th ed. Chicago: American College of Surgeons; 2018.

Simulation Center Design, Development, and Management

67

Susan Carter and Tariq Al Shanteer

Introduction

The demand for healthcare simulation has become increasingly prevalent in all aspects of the medical arena, including education, the hospital setting, specialty credentialing, and licensing or board certification. Though simulated events are well integrated into most trauma training offerings, comprehensive simulation centers are becoming more interprofessional and offer a new level of complexity not seen before. When designing a simulation center, there are a myriad of factors that come into play and each location has its own needs and own special interest groups. This chapter serves to be thought-provoking, whether in stimulating creativity with existing equipment and existing personnel or developing a stand-alone simulation center with a massive budget. This discussion will hopefully offer some ideas and concepts specific to the task at hand.

Learning Styles

The simulation center leader must recognize current trends in education and adapt to an ever-rapidly-changing landscape. Demand for smaller class sizes, remote and modular classes, larger training spaces, and increased class frequency are examples of recent medical simulation tendencies. Increasing numbers of educational offerings are remote, virtual, hybridized classrooms, flipped classrooms, and asynchronous learning—all of which are here to stay in some aspect or another. Therefore, it may be beneficial to embrace the future of distance learning and enjoy certain benefits such as maximizing faculty interaction and conserving expenses. For example, widely broadcasting a case scenario vignette using one set-up prevents the necessity for repetitively setting up and breaking down the scenario and offering the same vignette repeatedly to small groups. Fortunately, the move toward hands-on and observational learning appeals to different learner types for knowledge acquisition. It has been suggested that experiential learning, also known as simulation-based education (SBE), may increase retention versus traditional assigned reading or lectures. Many students are participatory and visual learners but adding sound to vignettes creates a realistic environment and appeals to auditory learners. This is certainly beneficial in trauma simulations, as desensitization to loud noises and numerous distractions has been proven to improve decision-making and procedural skills [1].

Attention to multisensory experience is increasingly important. "To excel in this environment as a surgical simulation leader requires unique knowledge, skills, and abilities that are different from those used in traditional clinically based education" [2].

Observational Learning

Observational or Social Learning is a teaching method where the learner watches others practice this behavior or skill, relying predominantly on the sense of sight and hearing. Albert Bandura in his social learning theory has emphasized that four conditions were necessary for any form of observing and modeling a teaching method: attention, retention, reproduction, and motivation [3]. A person starts from his first moment to learn about the manner of witnessing the behavior and actions of others and applying them in his life as a basic instinct for learning, such as a child watching his parent's behavior, and the acquisition of language and other basic skills. The observational learning theory applies in the field of healthcare and medical education in which the learner watches a set of both non-sensory and sensory skills prac-

S. Carter (✉)
Rocky Vista University, Englewood, CO, USA

Colorado Children's Hospital, Aurora, CO, USA
e-mail: SCarter@rvu.edu

T. Al Shanteer
Colorado Children's Hospital, Aurora, CO, USA
e-mail: tariq.alshanteer@childrenscolorado.org

L. Marshall Gillman, S. Widder (eds.), *Trauma Team Dynamics*, https://doi.org/10.1007/978-3-031-86312-7_67

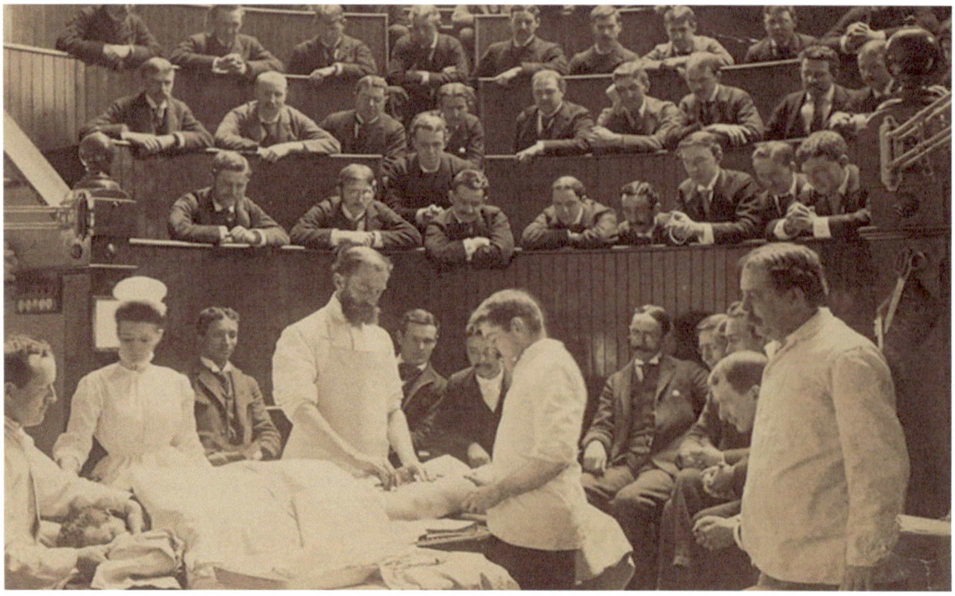

Fig. 67.1 Boston City Hospital operating theater, circa 1890. A. H. Folsom

ticed in front of him by the seasoned professional to learn the correct way to perform this skill by viewing and memorizing. Traditionally, this method is considered the first step in teaching health practitioners, with the basic cognitive acquisition and skills in dealing with various pathologies through observation and preservation. This is accomplished by live viewing or using modern communication technology and available media resources. Teaching halls, auditoriums, and skill labs are fully equipped with this technology (Fig. 67.1).

Transition to Experiential Learning

Reflective observation plus concrete learning completes the first two stages of the Experiential Learning Theory, described by Kolb in 1984 [4].

After these stages have been grasped, the final two phases in Kolb's theory follow. They are abstract conceptualization and active experimentation, which transform the experience. Space for observational learning is a needed consideration in design of a simulation center, but the major emphasis becomes in creating an arena for experiential learning, where students will participate directly in doing the task themselves. Learning by doing.

> Ensuring the safe, effective management of patients requires efficient processes of care within a smoothly operating system in which highly reliable teams of talented, skilled health care providers are able to use the vast array of high-technology resources and intensive care techniques available. Simulation can play a unique role in exploring and improving the complex perioperative system by proactively identifying latent safety threats and mitigating their damage to ensure that all those who work in this critical health care environment can provide optimal levels of patient care. [5]

Administrative Support

One of the major driving factors of simulation center design is prioritization by upper management and administration. If the governing body of an institution is enthusiastic about cutting-edge technology, simulation modalities will certainly be involved. When introducing the simulation center concept, it is important to present an organized approach with definite goals, strategic plan, and budget. Numerous basic business plans for 3- and 5-year projections are widely available and can be utilized as a template for the specific project at hand [6]. Creating a video or PowerPoint presentation of state-of-the-art simulation in trauma training is an effective tool to create interest and increase participation for an upcoming simulation center. Even if the project is small, utilizing current space that is re-purposed, having administration support the idea is crucial. Concepts of growth, quality of education, and enhanced patient safety will serve an institution well. Several templates exist for creating a strategic plan with short- and long-term goals and can help one navigate this process. Involving local trauma team members and their institutions can help drive this process. Input from hospital administration, emergency medicine staff, and faculty, operating room, recovery room, local fire and rescue, swat, police, ambulance, and transport are essential. Tying the strategic plan to university goals, course objectives, institutional learning objectives, and credentialing criteria will be most cohesive in the long run. A return on investment (ROI) is often queried, so an answer should be prepared in advance.

Assessing Needs

Comprehensive due diligence, including identifying healthcare and service program gaps in the community, guides programmatic decisions. Engaging internal and external stakeholders through surveys or personal discussions is essential for the simulation program's success. Leadership buy-in from the initial stage of development is critical, as it lays the groundwork for a cohesive and committed effort throughout the planning, project, and operational phases. For instance, if local first responders are expected to conduct simulated training events at the facility, including an ambulance ramp and/or entrance becomes a key consideration. Resources mapping further supports the alignment of services, reducing competition and fostering a collaborative community environment.

Shared Resources

It is often easier to start small and grow gradually and incrementally so that the existing culture can keep pace with new technology and techniques. Involvement in successful simulated events can be initiated by learning from local healthcare entities that commonly utilize hands-on training, such as those who instruct Advanced Cardiovascular Life Support (ACLS), Advanced Trauma Life Support (ATLS), and stage Mass Casualty Incidents (MCIs). It may be advantageous and cost-effective to "piggyback" onto these established simulation exercises in the local community, for example, local fire and rescue service providers, who are well-versed in simulation and task training. Reciprocating by providing volunteers for role-playing, set-up, or clean-up is usually appreciated by all involved. These relationships are crucial in the trauma team setting and offer a cohesive front as a multi-team simulation event. Creating a simulation center advisory board can include representatives from these community entities to brainstorm and develop new simulation events. Also, if expenses are shared and funds are used frugally, a financial drain on the system is prevented. Simulation education will expand rapidly when working with these experienced and collegial resources.

> Recommendations were provided on topics such as building a simulation team, preparing for accreditation requirements, what to ask for during early stages of development, identifying tools and resources needed to meet educational goals, expanding surgical simulation programming, and building educational curricula. [2]

Timeline Development

A timeline is important for any project design. Remodeling or converting existing space versus new construction must be carefully considered. Repair or modification of current equipment versus acquisition of new simulation devices may take many months. Development of existing instructors and staff versus hiring and training new employees is a significant undertaking. All these tasks initially seem daunting. Six months is a reasonable period to convert a space and operate as a designated simulation center, whereas 2 years may be more realistic regarding major remodeling or de novo construction. Supply chain problems or personnel shortages may thwart even the best-laid plans, so a time "cushion" may be warranted in your region. It also may take 3–5 years to convert a culture of traditional education to one adopting newer models of learning techniques. A well-thought-out plan can be updated and modified at any time but will save much time and expense in the long run.

Accreditation Considerations

If repurposing within an existing building, meeting early with representatives from the grounds or facilities department and a local contractor may provide valuable input and ideas regarding the location of present water lines, electricity, structural support, etc. Once a rough floorplan is created, specialists, including a structural engineer and architect, can then be called in to start finalizing blueprints. Recognition of accreditation requirements may factor in at this point, as governing bodies may have different minimal square footage requirements and recommendations. As part of the accreditation process, for example, the American College of Surgeons (ACS) requires 800 contiguous square feet to meet criteria as a focused Accredited Educational Institute (AEI), while 1200 contiguous square feet plus 4000 square feet of additional space is required to gain the comprehensive Accredited Educational Institution status [7]. The Society for Simulation in Healthcare (SSH) has several options for accreditations, and standards note that the size of the simulation center is important. The SSH Accreditation Standards, under Section 3b of Resource Management—"The Simulation Program has appropriate physical space for simulation activities to support the mission and/or vision of the Program" [8]—offer a detailed narrative description of the facilities employed by the program for simulation activities as outlined by Al-Elq (2010) [9]. This should be accompanied by comprehensive floor plans, blueprints, and photographs of the utilized facilities.

Systems Integration: Internal

One of the key considerations during the design process is system integration. Simulation is an effective part of the education process if it is a part of the existing curriculum rather than a standalone training. Interweaving simulation structure into the organizational hierarchy is important, creating a network and communication paths to other departments in the institution. This includes positioning the simulation classrooms as part of the organization's assets and integrating existing technology into technical departments in your organization, such as the Facility department, Informational Technology, and Biomedical. Another factor is human integration involving facility members as part of the simulation-based curriculum and encouraging them to utilize evolving technology (simulation modalities) in their learning process. Staff development assistance could be offered with fully simulation-based teaching and training.

Systems Integration: External

Pathways and communication also need to be created for relevant external entities. The design of a simulation program must also consider these vital programs and systems and integrate them to be successful for all parties. With increasing implementation of infrastructure for telehealth and telemedicine, opportunities exist for triage algorithms and "dashboard" applications to provide up-to-the-minute communication from the field and during transportation to the emergency center that are ultimately in the victim/patient's best interest. There are numerous components and multiple roles involved when one considers field triage, patient stabilization, transport, hand-offs, emergency and operative care, administration, facility, communication, and follow-up, to name a few important programs outside of the institution.

Low-Fidelity Simulation

Low-fidelity simulation is a popular topic; numerous "Do-It-Yourself" articles and videos abound. Minding cost efficiency by inadvertently reallocating funds from other departments can create future animosity toward the simulation center, so one must be wary and meticulous during budgeting processes. Using existing or expired materials, as well as commonly found materials, plus some ingenuity, can engage learners and greatly benefit the program without significant capital expenditure. For instance, running a trauma code can be done with as few as three vignettes, encompassing a skill session and debrief. This exercise can include fundamentals of the FAST (Focused Assessment with Sonography for Trauma) exam, relevant surface anatomy for central line insertion, chest tube insertion, running a team trauma code, and multiple trauma management as described by David Farley and his creative team [10].

Competency Assessments

Numerous licensing bodies employ simulation-based assessments to evaluate whether students possess the requisite clinical competencies for professional practice [11]. Students interview, examine, and treat an actor or standardized patient. Both verbal and nonverbal cues are assessed. The move to virtual OSCEs (Objective Structured Clinical Examination) evaluates nonverbal cues more complicated but can be adapted to allow these examinations to continue. This is the bulk of activity in many healthcare simulation centers, so adaptation to virtual may be considered. These summative examinations have been used by the National Assessment Collaboration (NAC) Examination and the Medical Council of Canada Qualifying Examination (MCCQE) Part II, and by the United States Medical Licensing Examination (USMLE) Step I. In 2021, the United States Medical Licensing Examination (USMLE) discontinued the clinical skills test portion of Step II Board examinations. In the press release, the USMLE and cosponsor of the Federation of State Medical Boards (FSMB) stated that OSCEs have been utilized with minimal change in healthcare for decades for many healthcare programs. Technological advances have produced a trend of incorporating Virtual Reality modules with interactive holographic patients in addition to standardized patient encounters and other testing modalities. These modules may offer more objectivity in grading and may decrease some expenses associated with live actor sessions. They also allow for repetition and rote practice before encounters with a live actor. If competency assessment and licensure exams are to be a large focus within a center, considerations must include ensuring adequate numbers of exam rooms are available for one or more streams of students, observation stations with one-way mirrors, flow of both students and standardized patients through the center, video recording, announcement, and timing technology to facilitate exam and access to computers for pre- and post-station probes. Besides the contracted labor costs, a significant hardware and subscription software budget must also be allotted.

Budgetary Concerns

When preparing a budget for a simulation center, costs are often categorized into personnel, capital expenditures, and operational budget, which includes maintenance and licenses. Capital expenditures will have a ceiling determined by the institution and necessitate a rationale for the purchase. Maintenance includes repairs, warranties, disposables, and items used in less than a year. Subscription costs encompass Learning Management Systems (LMS) software from vendors that run standardized patient programs, video capture technology, and virtual/augmented reality modules purchased yearly. Simulation technology is rapidly evolving and thus simulators, which are costly purchases, may have a limited lifespan. Leasing opportunities are increasingly available and may help convert capital purchases into more manageable and predictable operating costs; multi-year option and finance department may find depreciation schedule useful.

Incorporating both static and flexible budgeting approaches is critical in the operational budget planning process. A static budget sets a fixed financial plan for essential resources, while a flexible budget allows for adjustment in response to evolving needs or technological advancement [12].

This dual approach ensures that the simulation center can maintain high operating standards and adapt to changes without compromising financial stability. A comprehensive capital plan that includes timely upgrades and simulator replacement is also vital to the center's long-term success.

Immersive Realism

Total immersion is a technique utilized in simulated events. If numerous senses are utilized in the experience, the learner feels like they are in the scene, not just observing. A well-known example is a room converted to an ambulance interior, mimicking transport of a patient. Murals or wallpaper and decals are effective ways to create realism in a given space, without creating clutter or safety hazards. Noise amplification can add to realism with sirens and alarms. Olfactory sense stimulation works well in certain settings such as smoke or rotten garbage. Taste, though not often considered, may be indirectly perceived with salt water during a sea rescue scenario for example. Other effects easily accomplished are crowd noise, flashing lights, and intermittent darkness. Very hot or very cold environments can be implemented without much difficulty depending upon the current environment. More complex simulations have been done performing an operation onboard a pitching naval vessel, and in the weightlessness of space [13]. The more realistic the environment, the more immersed learners feel. While generally resulting in increased learner satisfaction it remains unclear how much and which of these potentially costly additions improve learning and have more concrete outcomes. For instance, simple task trainers have been shown to be equivalent to more complex laparoscopic simulators [14]. Cost and benefit must be carefully balanced when considering costly purchases, and more robust studies of these novel simulation technologies are required [15].

Multi-Use Rooms

Consideration of utilizing one room for multiple functions can be cost effective and space efficient. A standard size for a clinic examination room is often 3 m by 3 m, or ~9.3 sq m (10 × 10 ft, 100 sq ft). If multiple learners are expected, such as in team training, 4.5 × 5 m, 22.5 sq m (14 × 16 ft, 224 sq ft) is preferable. Although variable, the average inpatient room size in the United States increased from 22.3 sq m (240 sq ft) in 2002 to 29.7 sq m (320 sq ft) in 2012, according to [16]. Recommended Emergency Room Trauma Bay space is close to the same size, averaging between 225 and 300 sq ft. Two adjoining examination rooms with a collapsible wall in between allow the two smaller rooms to be opened into one larger room now utilized as an Operating Room or Trauma Bay, for example. The examination rooms are traditionally utilized for Standardized Patients, the interior of an ambulance cabin, task training events, and simulating the home environment. When opened, the larger rooms can also be used to simulate Post-Anesthesia Care Units, Intensive Care Units, and Preoperative Preparation areas. They can also accommodate team training where multiple specialties and programs are represented. A larger space for team debriefing is necessary, which is often accomplished immediately after a simulated event. Traffic flow must be considered, so formal debriefing or a quick "hot wash" is not occurring in a hallway or area setting up for the next scenario. Similarly, square footage of hallways must accommodate groups of people moving gurneys around corners and through doorways.

Class A—150 sq ft minimum clear floor area, 12-foot minimum clear dimension, 3′-6″ clearance at both sides, the foot, and the head of the operating table

Class B—250 sq ft minimum clear floor area, 15-foot minimum clear dimension, 3′-6″ clearance at both sides, the foot, and the head of the operating table

Class C—400 sq ft minimum clear floor area, 18-foot minimum clear dimension, 4′-0″ clearance at both sides, the foot, and the head of the operating table

Floor Plans of Simulation Centers—Examples (Figs. 67.2, 67.3, 67.4, and 67.5)

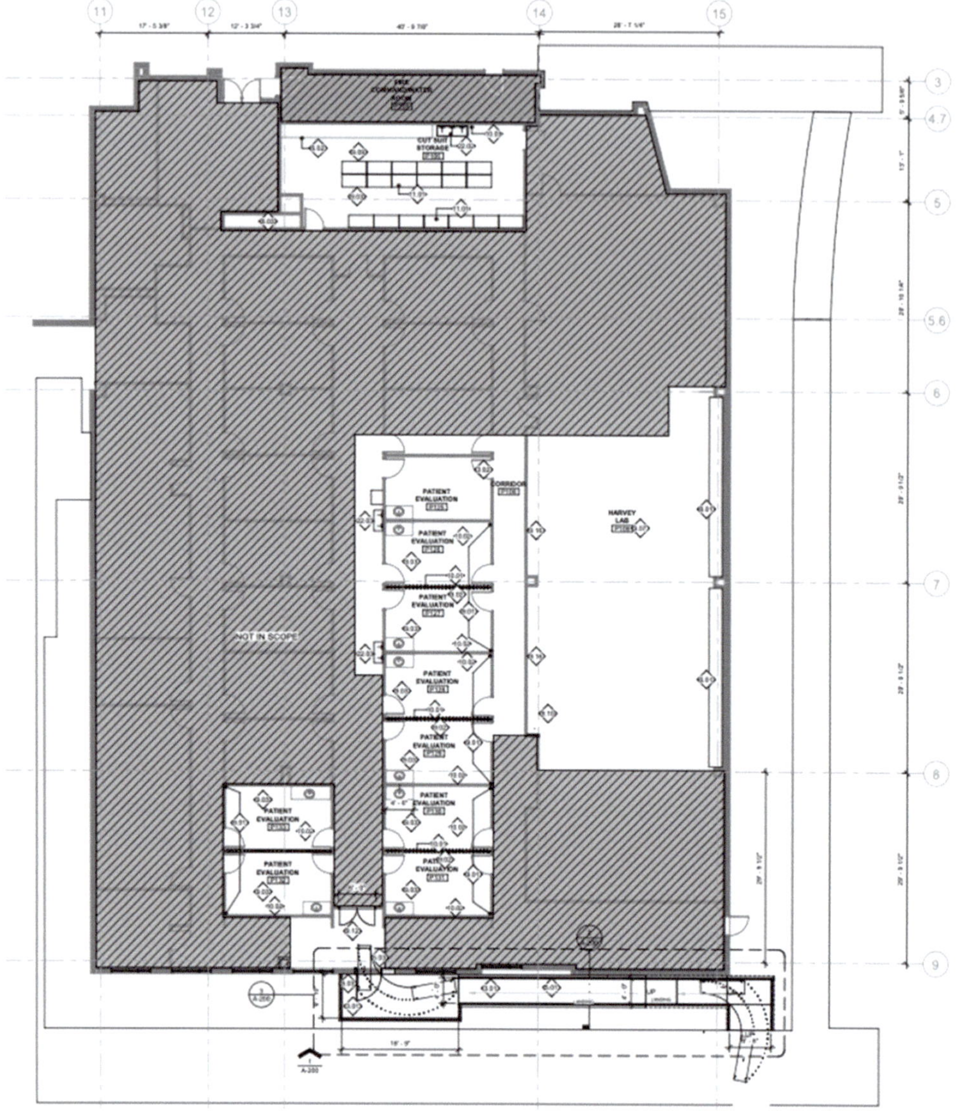

Fig. 67.2 Floorplan A

Fig. 67.3 Floorplan B

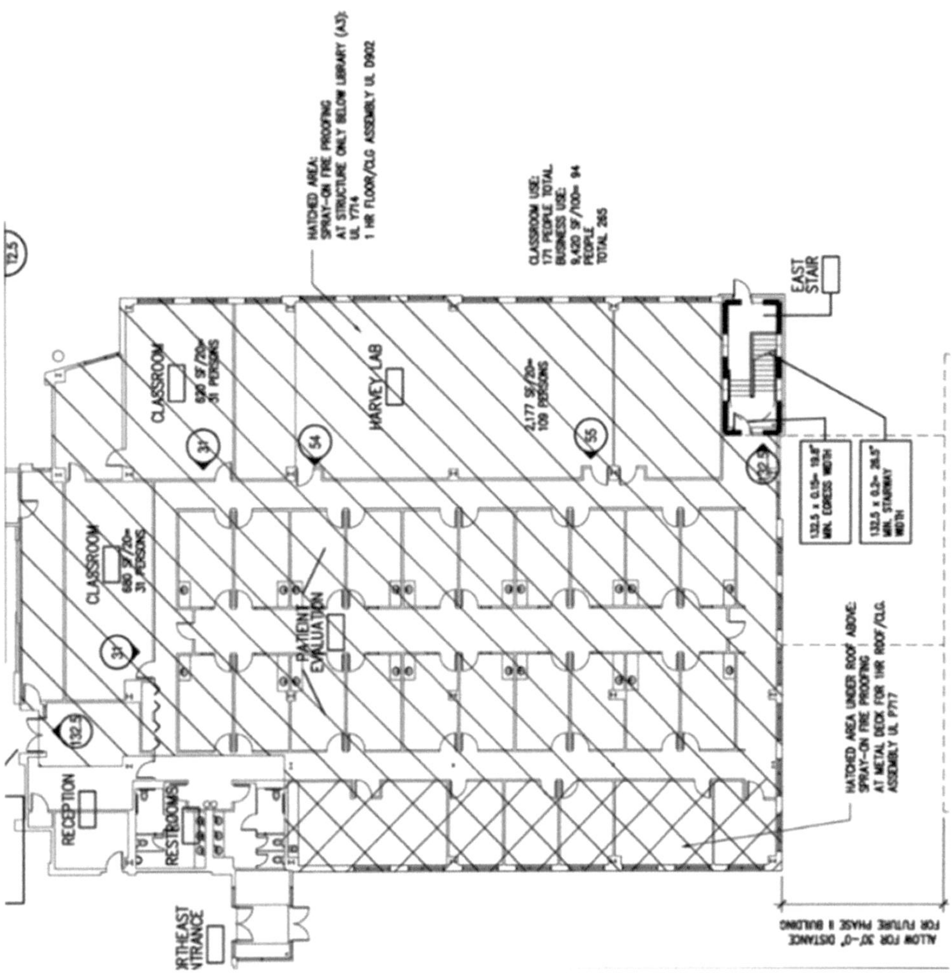

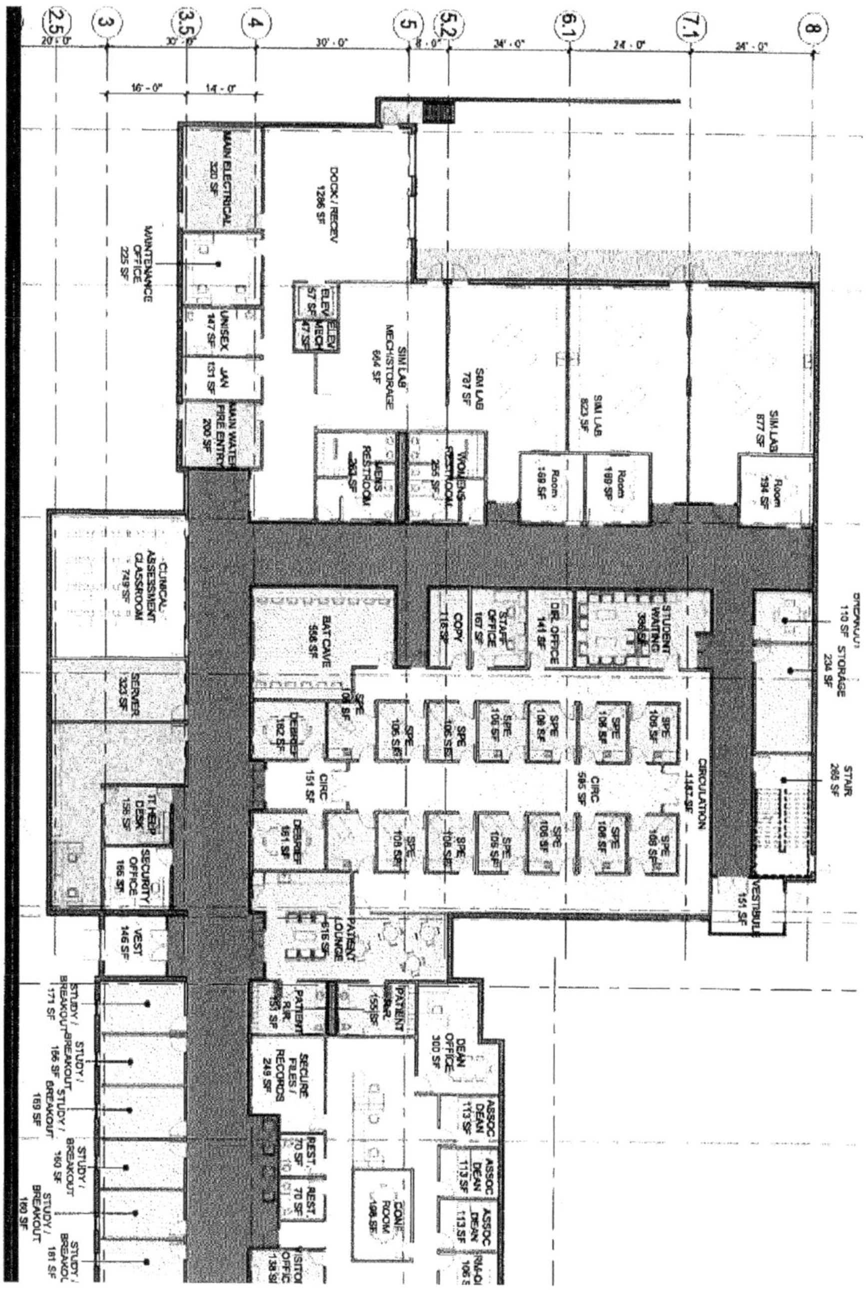

Fig. 67.4 Floorplan C

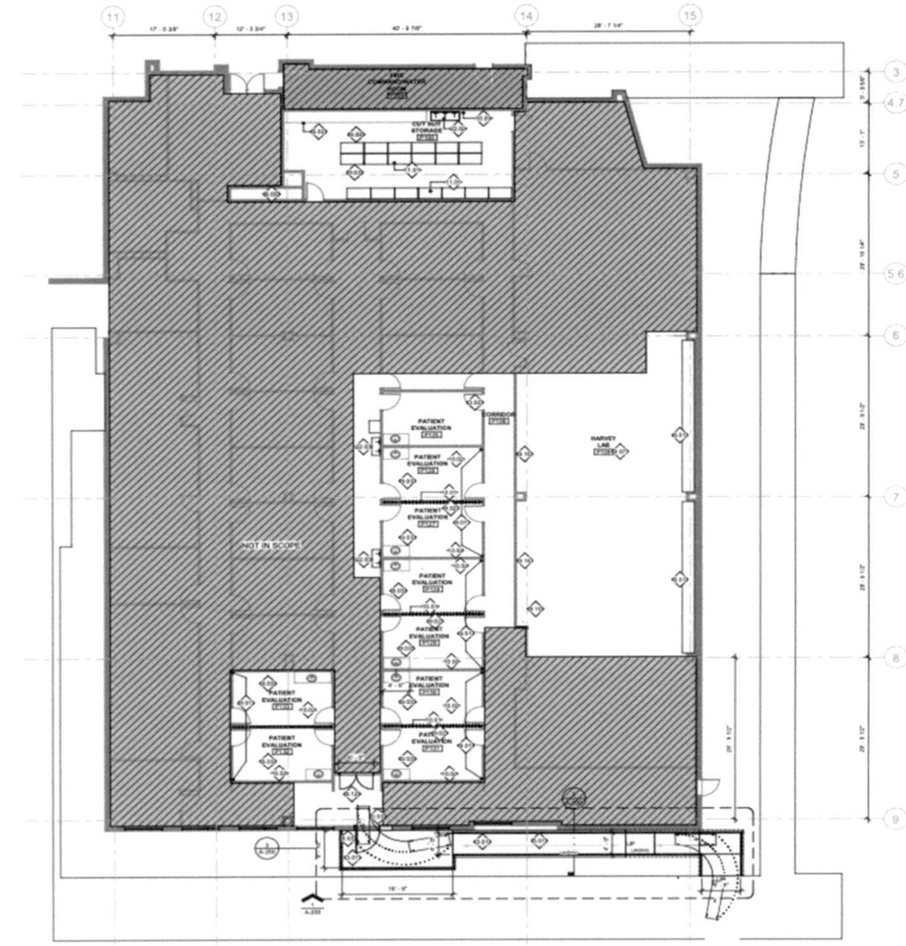

Fig. 67.5 Floorplan D

Interactive Learning Stations

Individual spaces are becoming more common as the move from traditional auditoriums continues. Instead of occupying an auditorium seat amongst many others, a personal area equipped with necessary technology may be considered. The user station may include a recliner with 3-D goggles and headphones, a convertible standing desk for a laptop, a background with green screen capabilities, dimmable lighting, a student storage cubby, and pop-up partitions to accommodate individual versus team activities. Outdoor spaces can also be equipped with mobile learning stations if needed.

Gathering Areas

The lobby of a simulation center serves as a crucial space for learners' check-in, staging, and security management. Additionally, the inclusion of a lounge or gathering area is highly recommended. This space provides a place for participants to take breaks and decompress after intense training sessions and serves as a welcoming area for visitors touring the center. Strategically positioning the lounge near restroom facilities enhances its convenience and functionality, further supporting the center's operations.

Audiovisual Considerations

Audiovisual systems and recording technologies have become indispensable in the design process of a simulation center, regardless of the nature of training or training modality used. The healthcare simulation manufacturing companies compete to provide multiple solutions that suit the needs of each center in terms of space, budget, and the availability of infrastructure to accommodate them.

A low-cost camera can be used as a minimal-budget solution to document and record simulated events. It can be an IP-based camera or a direct-wired solution where data is stored on a computer hard drive or network drive. Low-cost multi-room configurations or a mobile solution can be considered adequate and serve for in situ training if necessary.

An expansion plan must be drawn out when purchasing an AV system and considered from the early stages of design. Mapping the location of cameras and their number in proportion to the size of the room, lighting, and the location of windows, entry, and exit doors can influence the success of video recordings. Several views with different cameras are helpful, especially positioned directly overhead when procedures are being taught and broadcast. Mobile or wearable webcams can be facile in the field, but stability is preferred when intricacy is increased. Sound is often crucial, muffling insulation is carried out in the construction stages, as well as appropriate server locations and ventilation. A separate diagram for the audiovisual system, including the network wires, audio mixer system, speakers, laptops, control rooms, and debriefing areas, should be created by specialists in this field.

Several ways to record and document cases/courses have been developed in simulation. These are important parts of the proper evaluation of students, instructors, and staff and an efficient way of logging hours of utilization. Tracking hours, numbers, types of learner feedback of both learners and instructors, and accomplished goals for the events are a significant part of the accreditation process. An annual report from all users will significantly aid in coalescing data from numerous sources, especially if accreditation cycles are reported every 3–5 years.

Documentation can be performed using a direct paper form, especially when participants are remote, or technology is not feasible in the environment. Alternatively, electronic entries can be utilized for documentation and feedback, with many template options from several vendors. The budget must be considered for hardware, software subscription, and maintenance plus upgrades of these tracking systems.

It is essential to establish a specific policy governing the recording section, which includes obtaining informed consent from participants. This policy should align with the institutions' guidelines on the duration for which recorded videos are stored on servers or in the cloud and must comply with federal governmental regulations, such as Health Insurance Portability and Accountability Act (HIPPA) and (Family Educational Rights and Privacy Act (FERPA).

Observation

Incident records and bookmark events can be directly witnessed by the observer as part of the simulation event or witnessed invisibly in the control station. Visibility may be accomplished by a one-way mirror to control station design or through a high-resolution camera (Pan-tilt-zoom or PTZ), allowing the observer to judge and evaluate remotely with a clear picture of participants. For a makeshift "operatorium," choir bleachers or stepstools can be set up around the OR table for better viewing if numerous learners are participating.

Accessibility

When designing a simulation center, consider that the space mimics what would be seen in any actual health facility, inside and out. For example, the nursing station is an integral part of an ICU (Intensive Care Unit) and should be centrally located. The same reasoning applies to the core design, including entrances, exits, waiting rooms, pathways for emergency vehicles and hand-offs, handrails for stairs, wheelchair lanes, electric doors, tactile tiles for outer and inner hallways, gurney turning space, large debriefing room, supply rooms, organized storage space, a pharmacy area, laboratory and preparatory space, and visible signage. The external space should accommodate parking, ambulance, and fire truck maneuverability (covered, if possible, with vestibule), large doors, external cameras, adjacent Emergency Room/Trauma Bay access, and

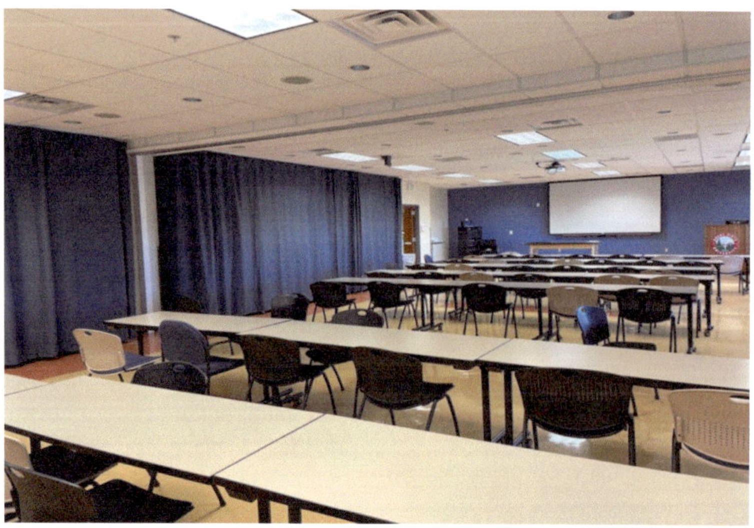

Fig. 67.6 Class room—with lateral storage spaces, concealed by curtains

a nearby lounge for first responders. Valuable free space such as a greenbelt, field, or park can provide excellent "field" simulated mass casualty events.

Control Center

The control center is the "brain" of the simulation center, as it enables the controller (Educator, Sim Tech, Faculty Member, etc.) to watch events, record incidents, and control the different computerized simulation modalities. It also serves to communicate with participants. Chaperoning is also possible via the Control Center.

It is necessary to consider several important factors in the design process of the control center, as multiple rooms can be connected if the area is large and multiple technologies have been implemented. Two control centers can be considered if a categorized floor or specialized wing is available. Consideration of the control center includes the following:

1. Cloud vs. Hardwired
2. Audio visual Requirements
3. Servers
4. Data Management
5. Technology Specialist Space

Storage Space

A quintessential problem in every simulation center is adequate storage space. Organization of equipment, whether by a function or specialty, allows users to locate and replace items easily. Cluttering of simulation equipment in hallways and thoroughfares prevents realistic transportation of victims or patients from area to area, as would be seen in a normal trauma situation. Fire codes may be violated as well. Adjustable shelving housing clear tubs with labeled lids can identify stored equipment, such as disposables, surgical instruments, and airway management tools. If shelving is in a shared space, obscuring curtains can provide a professional appearance when the equipment is not in use, yet they provide easy accessibility when needed. Electronic high-fidelity manikins are often best left on their respective beds or gurneys so they can be transported easily from space to space as needed (Fig. 67.6). As with other sensitive equipment, damage can result from constant jostling. Retention of traveling cases or shipping boxes is another consideration, depending on how often the simulation devices are transported to other locales. Flattening cardboard boxes used for shipping can be done and placed in a central location at the institution or discarded. Travel cases can protect equipment during transport but can be tedious to open and reassemble task trainers if utilized on a day-to-day basis (Fig. 67.7).

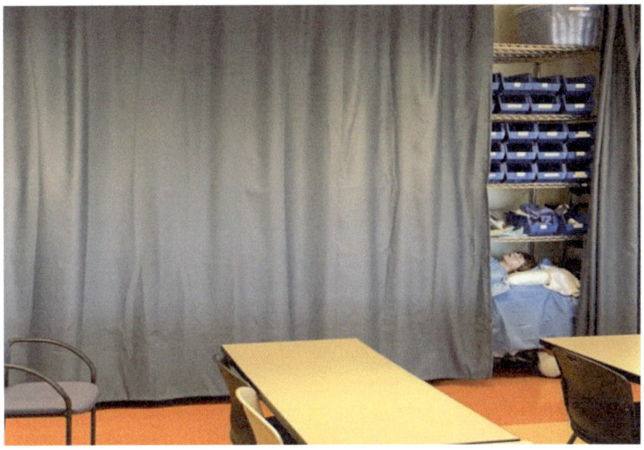

Fig. 67.7 Extensive storage on shelves behind curtains

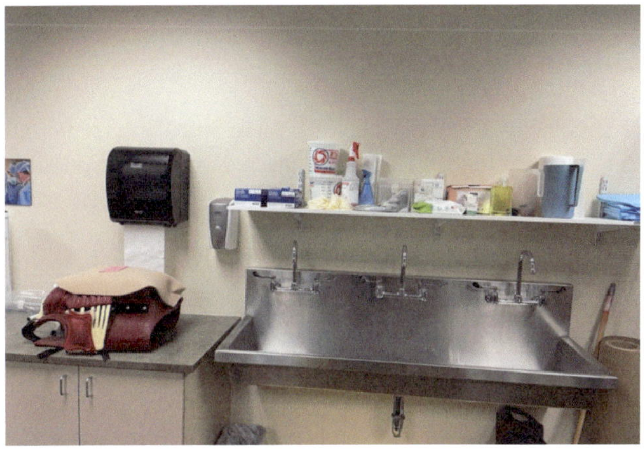

Fig. 67.8 Prep. room with large sink

Preparation Area

A large room complete with counters and sinks and space for manikins on gurneys or multiple task trainers to cohabitate is necessary for a simulation center. Moulage of actors and manikins will occur here, with accessible and adjacent storage of costumes, makeup, artificial blood, tubing, batteries for replacement, etc. Appropriate cleaning supplies in this area are clearly labeled to indicate which cleaning product is acceptable and which training tool is needed to avoid costly errors (Fig. 67.8).

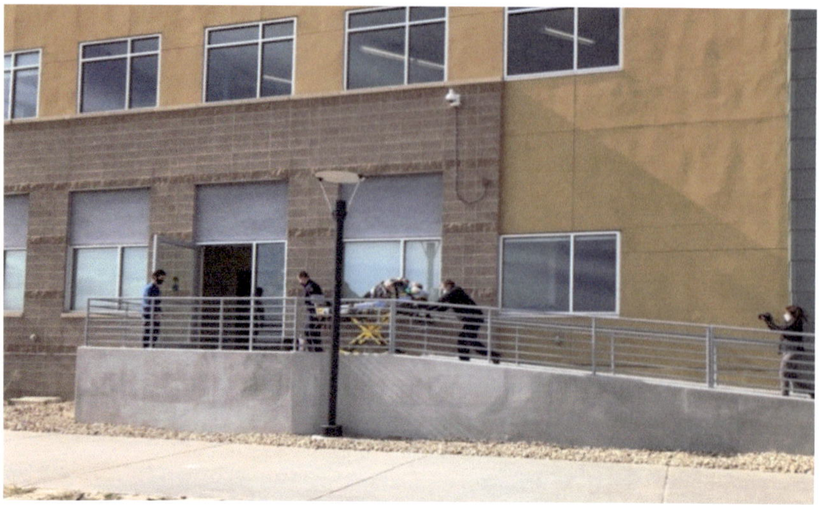

Fig. 67.9 First responders transport during mass casualty training

Entrances and Exits

If simulating a Trauma Center, a large ambulance ramp and entryway are preferable, with a covered vestibule if possible. Care should be taken regarding appearance and signage, so the public does not confuse simulated emergency services with the real thing. This area facilitates hand-off practice from the field to the hospital. If space is available in an adjacent parking lot or green area, appropriate personnel can also practice crowd control. Hospital Staff and Administration are heavily involved in full-blown scenarios and will be engaged with entrance control. Regarding exits from the simulation center, private or separate exits for students after summative exercises and live actor standardized patient encounters will be needed (Fig. 67.9).

Development of Extracurricular Activities

Student engagement in the simulation center is beneficial. Developing a student simulation interest group or club within the institution has several advantages. Involving existing clubs that use simulation for demonstrations, guest lecturers, and other special events will engage numerous students. Creating a Simulation Competition with critical thinking manikin case scenario and a virtual reality interactive patient module competition can incentivize students to participate and embrace simulation technology. Student Affairs or the Marketing Department can be involved and sometimes offer financial incentives to the students. Perpetual plaques can be displayed at the institution, giving the competitors a sense of pride, or prizes won will be satisfying to those learners involved. Developing an interest in simulation may introduce students to career opportunities, advanced electives, or fellowships.

Scholarly Activity

Each simulated event can provide an opportunity for student involvement by authoring an account of the occurrence, analyzing the success and limitations of the event, or measuring the impact on SBE. Even the uninitiated student can create a summary of the event for an internal newsletter or public coverage of the simulation. This can increase awareness of simulation modalities to other students, institutional staff, faculty, and community members. Abstracts and poster presentations can often be accomplished with minimal mentoring and guidance, with numerous opportunities to present at simulation conferences and meetings.

Research

With guidance from research and statistics departments and the Institutional Review Board (IRB), students can be actively involved in simulation research projects. Often simulation projects preclude concern with healthcare privacy issues when live subjects are not utilized. In addition, research in medical simulation can be accomplished when clinical access is limited, and at all stages of learning. Numerous opportunities for publications are present, as simulation-related journals have become more prevalent in the past few years. For example, subtle aspects of modification of simulation equipment, variation of roles, scenario setup specifics, and learner perceptions can be explored, as simulation is a relatively new research area in the healthcare arena over the past few decades.

Reflection

Journaling and reflective writing can also prove useful in simulation-based education. Gibbs's six-stage cycle of reflection is a theory used to incorporate this practice during debriefing [17]. Many learners find reflective writing valuable and may enjoy rereading their perceptions years later.

Individualized Remediation

Simulation provides a unique opportunity to help struggling students. Providing a virtual reality case module or a manikin case scenario that can be mentored by a senior level student, resident, or attending can provide enormous opportunity for growth and clarification of the areas in which the student was previously confounded. The unique environment of simulation may be less threatening than the real live events, and opportunities to pause, discuss, and reflect on each facet of the desired skill set and care have high value. This endeavor is clearly labor intensive and depends on faculty or instructors available to accomplish these sessions.

Multisensory Reality

The importance of creating a realistic environment has been mentioned previously in regard to stimulating the senses including creating sight, audio, olfactory, and lighting manipulations in scenarios when possible. Specific to the trauma team, the hostile environment simulation should also be considered as many first responders and frontline healthcare workers carry out their respective duties in harsh or threatening conditions (Figs. 67.10 and 67.11).

According to Tactical Emergency Casualty Care (TECC) Guidelines for First Care Providers June 2016, relevant definitions include the following:

First Care Provider (FCP)—Empowered and trained community members who can serve a critical role during the initial moments after complex and dynamic disasters. These FCPs often have immediate access to severely injured victims and can provide time-sensitive, life-saving interventions; the FCP is the first link in the trauma chain of survival.

First Responder—Responding law enforcement, fire, and EMS personnel.

Direct Threat Care (Hot Zone)—describes actions taken in response to a casualty where the external, on- going threat to life is as dangerous, or more dangerous, than the injury sustained. Essentially, care is provided to the injured in

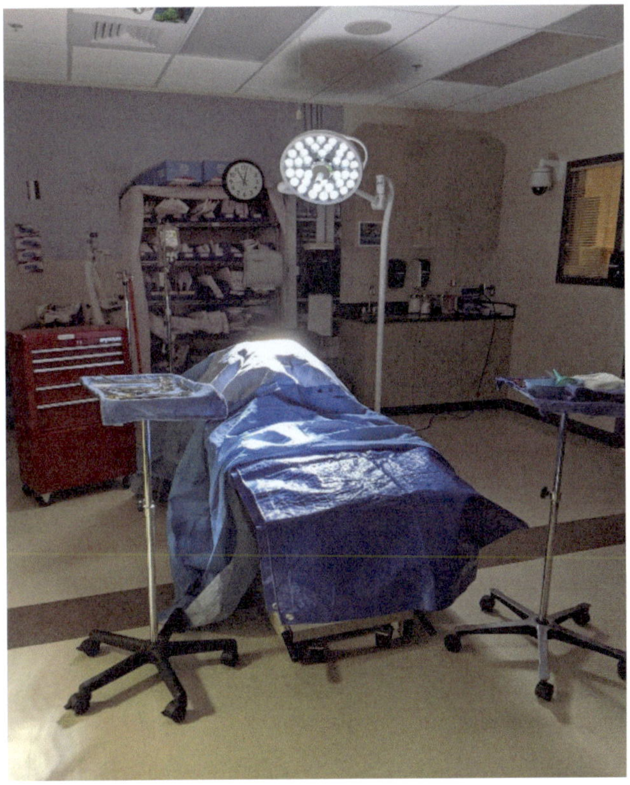

Fig. 67.10 Simulated OR setup

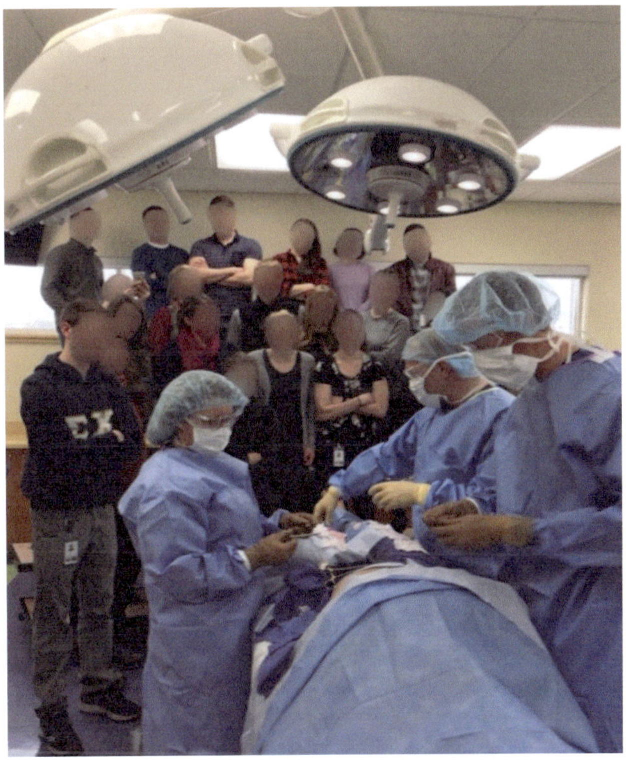

Fig. 67.11 "Operatorium" using choir bleachers to improve visibility

any area where there is a direct and immediate threat of additional external injury to the First Care Provider or the patient. This threat includes, but is not limited to gunfire, a potential building collapse, fire, secondary explosive devices, etc.

Indirect Threat Care (Warm Zone)—Care provided once the first care provider and injured person(s) are no longer under an immediate threat of additional injury, but there remains the possibility of additional unknown or unmitigated threats; for example, in an area of the building where active shooting/violence is no longer occurring or once the patient has been moved to an area of higher security with cover and/or concealment (e.g. casualty collection point (CCP) or barricaded room).

Environments may include cold, fire or smoke, water, noxious chemicals, motion, and gravity [18].

Advanced Simulation Events

In addition to hostile environments, other advanced scenarios most likely will be undertaken as the simulation center matures. Examples include Crisis Team Training, Biopreparedness, large-scale Mass Casualty Incidents, Disaster Training, High Acuity-Low incidence events, ICU Patient Management, Multiple Organ Failure cases, and Complex Surgeries for Multiple Trauma victims. These may require specialized task trainers and equipment, skilled simulation personnel, proficient simulation technology operators, significant event preparation, and experienced organizers of these types of events to interact with many programs and volunteers, depending on the scale of the event.

Simulation Center Management

After garnering administration support and creating and governance board, the organizational structure should be delineated. This will require frequent updates as the simulation center expands and roles are reassigned and may require updates at frequent intervals. The simulation entity may be classified and reclassified as a center, an office, an institute, or a department. Existing institutional organizational charts will be helpful as a template, and guidance can be obtained from Administration and Human Resources regarding job descriptions and the nature of direct and indirect reporting structure. If the institution is affiliated with the military, management of the center may be affected directly or tangentially.

Governance/Advisory Board

As mentioned previously, albeit briefly, a simulation center needs governance in the form of an advisory board or committee to assist in the center's administration. Members may include representatives from administration, active internal programs, external affiliates (EMT, Paramedic, SWAT, Fire and Rescue, Police Force), a community member, local hospital trauma personnel, institution simulation staff, alumni/graduate medical education, and a marketing liaison. This body can help prepare a Mission Statement and Goals and work cooperatively for community outreach and multi-team simulation events. An agenda is helpful and allows each member to prepare a report on their activities and concerns. Likewise, the minutes of the meeting provide history and communication when members are unable to attend. Requirements for monthly or quarterly meetings may be a part of an accreditation, which should be appropriately honored.

Conclusion

The information relayed in this chapter stems from our combined experience after designing healthcare spaces and simulation centers over several years. We have recently focused on establishing simulation centers that serve trauma, first responder, and surgical staff, with aligned skills. Many experts in the medical design arena may offer sage advice and innovative solutions to your specific application.

Numerous factors will be at play in designing your simulation facility, including time frame, targeted learners, the extent of administrative support, and available budget. In addition, the technical readiness of the lead operators and the availability of space is paramount.

During the recent pandemic and the subsequent changes in techniques necessary for the educational process, simulation center design has changed accordingly. Attention must be given to more hybridized and remote learning, with high expectations when hands-on events do occur. Some examples of distance learning trends include teaching anatomy through dimensional programs with 3D goggles worn by the students for dissection while an instructor remotely explains through stereoscopic three-dimensionality, and the student practices skills through a mobile kit.

Simulation technology continues to develop rapidly, and it is exciting to be a part of new modalities that speak to different learner types than ever before. It is an honor to be able to play a small part in developing quality healthcare professionals to serve the sick and wounded for years to come.

Key Points, Development of Simulation Center

- Appeal of a Simulation Program
- Support and Governance
- Internal and External Integration
- Timeline and Accreditation Considerations
- Budget and Resources
- Learner Assessment and Evaluations
- Technology Concerns
- Layout and Design
- Scholarly Activities

References

1. Aebersold M. Simulation-based learning: no longer a novelty in undergraduate education. Online J Issues Nurs. 2018;23. https://ojin.nursingworld.org/MainMenuCategories/ANAMarketplace/ANAPeriodicals/OJIN/TableofContents/Vol-23-2018/No2-May-2018/Articles-Previous-Topics/Simulation-Based-Learning-Undergraduate-Education.html.
2. Gardner A, Ritter E, Dunkin B, Smink D, Lau J, Paige J, Phitayakorn R, Acton R, Stefanidis D, Gee D. Leaders by example: best practices and advice on establishing a state-of-the art surgical simulation center that optimizes available resources. Am J Surg. 2018;215(2):259–65. https://doi.org/10.1016/j.amjsurg.2017.11.007.
3. Stone SM. Observational learning | Psychology, behavior & cognitive processes. Encyclopedia Britannica. 1 Aug 2016. https://www.britannica.com/science/observational-learning.
4. Levine AI, DeMaria S Jr, Schwartz AD, Sim AJ. The comprehensive textbook of healthcare simulation. Springer eBooks; 2013. https://doi.org/10.1007/978-1-4614-5993-4.
5. Gardner AK, Johnston M, Korndorffer JR, Haque I, Paige JT. Using simulation to improve systems-based practices. Jt Comm J Qual Patient Saf. 2017;43(9):484–91. https://doi.org/10.1016/j.jcjq.2017.05.006.
6. Khan M, Sasso RA. Obtaining Medical Simulation Center accreditation. StatPearls – NCBI Bookshelf; 2022. https://www.ncbi.nlm.nih.gov/books/NBK554424/.
7. ACS. Accreditation standards and criteria. n.d. https://www.facs.org/for-medical-professionals/education/programs/accredited-education-institutes/accreditation-standards-and-criteria/.
8. SSIH. Full accreditation. n.d. https://www.ssih.org/Credentialing/Accreditation/Full-Accreditation.
9. Al-Elq A. Simulation-based medical teaching and learning. J Fam Community Med. 2010;17(1):35. https://doi.org/10.4103/1319-1683.68787.
10. Jackson JJ, Mabry CD, Savarise MT, Senkowski CK. Effectively using E/M codes for trauma care. Bull Am Coll Surg. 2013;98(6):56–65. https://pubmed.ncbi.nlm.nih.gov/23789201
11. Gillette, C. Improving Pharmacy Student Communication Outcomes Using Standardized Patients. American Journal of Pharmaceutical Education 2017;81(6) Article 110, p 1–6. https://www.ajpe.org/article/S0002-9459(23)02413-0/pdf
12. Reiter KL, Song PH. Gapenski's healthcare finance: an introduction to accounting and financial management. 7th ed. Health Administration Press; 2021. https://openlibrary.telkomuniversity.ac.id/home/catalog/id/167289/slug/gapenski-s-healthcare-finance-an-introduction-to-accounting-and-financial-management-7-e-.html
13. Hoang TN, LaPorta AJ, Malone JD, Champagne R, Lavell K, De La Rosa GM, Gaul L, Dukovich M. Hyper-realistic and immersive surgical simulation training environment will improve team performance. Trauma Surg Acute Care Open. 2020;5(1):e000393. https://doi.org/10.1136/tsaco-2019-000393.
14. Steigerwald SN, Park J, Hardy KM, Gillman LM, Vergis AS. Does laparoscopic simulation predict intraoperative performance? A comparison between the Fundamentals of Laparoscopic Surgery and LapVR evaluation metrics. Am J Surg. 2015;209(1):34–9. https://doi.org/10.1016/j.amjsurg.2014.08.031.
15. Johnson GG, Brindley PG, Gillman LM. Fidelity in surgical simulation: further lessons from the S.T.A.R.T.T. course. Can J Surg. 2020;63(2):E161–6. https://doi.org/10.1503/cjs.017818.
16. cheresearch.org. n.d. https://cheresearch.org/.
17. Husebø SE, O'Regan S, Nestel D. Reflective practice and its role in simulation. Clin Simul Nurs. 2015;11(8):368–75. https://doi.org/10.1016/j.ecns.2015.04.005.
18. Tactical Emergency Casualty Care (TECC) Guidelines. Tactical Emergency Casualty Care (TECC) guidelines for first care providers. 2016. https://www.c-tecc.org/images/TECC-Guidelines-for-First-Care-Providers-June-2016.pdf.

The Story of "Hyper-Realism": From Hollywood to the Bedside

68

Kit Lavell and Lawrence Marshall Gillman

Facing the tyrannies of time and trauma, a third-year surgical resident has mere minutes to save the life of a victim of a motorcycle accident. Swiftly performing an emergency open surgery splenectomy, the resident's attention turns to the hilum, where he identifies the splenic artery and veins, and dissects, but too close to the pancreas and clips its tail. The attending allows the resident to make this critical mistake. Why? Because the attending can stop the process, pause the vital signs, and take a timeout for a teaching moment. The patient is not human. The resident is operating on the world's only hyper-realistic open surgery simulator.

This scene has a Hollywood connection. But the connection is not from a television medical drama. While it *is* a simulation, it is not done for a camera. The anatomy, the tissues, vessels, and organs don't just look real they feel real to the surgeons. They dissect, clamp, ligate, cut, and suture realistically.

A year after 9/11, in the middle of San Diego, the regional headquarters of the Drug Enforcement Headquarters quietly opened. DEA (Drug Enforcement Administration) agents had just occupied the new building when gunfire erupted on the mesa about 70 feet above them. Weapons drawn, agents scurried up the hillside, only to confront actors in middle-eastern garb brandishing AK-47 assault rifles. Only the agents had real weapons and real bullets, so a standoff quickly turned into inquisitive bemusement, and eventually into a conversation with Stu Segall, a Hollywood producer.

In 1991, Stu came to San Diego planning to film a TV series. Having spent years in Los Angeles as a TV producer, he wanted to find a location for "Silk Stalkings," a new detective TV series fictionally set in Palm Beach Florida. Eleven years later and after shooting 1000 hours of prime-time TV series, movies of the week, and features, Stu's business took a nose dive. The events of September 11, 2001, pushed action-oriented entertainment into hiatus because of audience sensitivities to violence. Stu Segall Productions operated 10 sound stages on 20 acres and most were not being used a year later, but they were not empty. Talking with the DEA agents, Stu offered them the use of his sound stages for training. Filled with elaborate sets depicting residential, commercial, and industrial interiors, the agents saw a unique contrast to the bare warehouses in which they trained, where yellow tape on the floors simulated walls, doors, and windows.

Sweaty and tired, but excited, the agents emerged from the sound stages shaking their heads. Stu asked them if he could make the sets better for their use. They laughed, but appreciatively. Stu however had ideas. While he has no military or law enforcement background, he thinks like a "bad guy," with years of creatively conveying this kind of action onto small and big screens. So the first thing he did was create complications to "mess with their minds." DEA and other local law enforcement officers (LEO) trained in "room clearing" exercises in this new environment. Stu would "reverse-hang" doors, so instead of opening expectedly 90° into the side wall of an interior room, for example, a door would open 180° into the opening wall. This would take the LEO unexpectedly out of their comfort zone. Stu would also change the configuration of the rooms between training days, and sometimes between training exercises. What everyone noticed was that the "unexpected" kept them guessing. This was more like the "real world" instead of an unchallenging training exercise.

Richard Carmona, MD, FACS, MPH, Surgeon General of the United States under President George W. Bush visited Stu not long after this. Stu told Dr. Carmona that he wanted to give back to the law enforcement and military communities and thought his facilities would make a unique training environment. Dr. Carmona told Stu that there was not much money in this endeavor and that the most he could expect

K. Lavell
Strategic Operations, Inc., San Diego, CA, USA
e-mail: kit@e-stops.com

L. Marshall Gillman (✉)
Departments of Surgery Section of General Surgery, Internal Medicine Section of Critical Care, University of Manitoba, Winnipeg, MB, Canada
e-mail: Lawrence.Gillman@umanitoba.ca

L. Marshall Gillman, S. Widder (eds.), *Trauma Team Dynamics*, https://doi.org/10.1007/978-3-031-86312-7_68

was hats and T-shirts, pointing to the ones behind Stu's desk. The Department of Homeland Security had not yet become a Cabinet-level department and federal, state, and local governments were just beginning to meet the challenge of this new threat. There did not appear to be much of a business model for what Stu wanted to do, but he was game for volunteering his facilities.

A mutual friend of Stu's and mine, a reserve marine colonel and publisher of the *San Diego Business Journal* introduced us, with the thought that I might help create a business. A dozen years before I sold an engineering and construction business I had started from scratch. Between that time and meeting Stu I did some consulting, but mostly I was writing for magazines, newspapers, a book, and some screenplays. And I was intrigued by what Stu was trying to do.

As a Naval Aviator, I flew 243 combat missions in Vietnam. I spent the better part of a year in the Mekong Delta flying close air support for Navy SEALs, riverine forces, and Army advisors and infantry before flying A-4 Skyhawk jets. I had been a military and civilian flight instructor, witnessed the growth of flight simulators, and was keenly interested in training of all types. My stepfather had retired as a cop. I remember talking to him about job-related stress. While visiting my home in California, he died from a heart attack just weeks after retiring in Chicago. My wife, an RN, tried unsuccessfully to resuscitate him before I got home from flying as a Navy flight instructor. The shock from this caused me to reflect for years on how to reduce stress in occupations like policing and military aviation. I studied aviation safety at the Naval Postgraduate (NPG) School in Monterey California and investigated aircraft accidents as a collateral duty as an aviator. This groundbreaking interdisciplinary program at NPG examined how stress, both material and psychological, contributes to failure. The effects of stress intrigued me.

After leaving the Navy and working on a master's degree, I became an executive with the City of San Diego in the late 1970s. This was a time when urban crime rates were rising. Officer-involved shootings led to lawsuits against cities across the nation. Courts ruled that a city's defense of law enforcement officers' training adequacy could not rely solely on marksmanship at a static live-fire range. Training had to be "realistic," conducted in conditions found in the real world, and incorporating "judgmental" shoot-no-shoot scenarios. I left the City to start my own company in 1981, but my interest in training under conditions of stress stayed with me.

Years later I was introduced to the writings of Bruce Siddle who is the managing partner of Human Factor Research Group, an organization that provides consulting, training, and services to educators, emergency medical providers, law enforcement, and military personnel. Bruce is a pioneer in the study of survival stress and how it impacts the performance of law enforcement officers and military personnel including combat aviators. His important research into how the Sympathetic Nervous System affects perceptual and cognitive processing, motor performance and memory, has been introduced into performance-based training for law enforcement and, military, including special operations and combat aviation.[1]

Twenty-plus years later, Stu Segall and I hit it off immediately. I joined the new Strategic Operations (STOPS) as Executive Vice President, wrote a business plan, helped create a training model, and marketed our unique training to law enforcement and especially the military. The wars in Afghanistan and Iraq left our nation inadequately prepared to train for asymmetric warfare. As a nation, we were still training to fight the Soviets in Eastern Europe. Government leaders spoke of the need for a "Revolution in Military Training." I had written a six-part feature series on the subject for the Sunday editions of the Insight section of the San Diego Union-Tribune, the last part of which appeared on the Sunday before the invasion of Iraq began. The editors and I planned this series several months before, to end on a date that I predicted would be the start of the war. I missed it by a few days.

Five months before "Operation Iraqi Freedom," we were preparing to introduce a unique military training experience at STOPS. We created a Military Operation on Urban Terrain (MOUT), jargon for a replica of an urban environment, in this case a town on the "back lot" of the TV/Movie Studio that could be re-configured to look like any geographic area of the world.

In addition to the realistic sets, we used role players who had immigrated to the United States. San Diego has one of the largest Middle Eastern immigrant populations. Hundreds were on the casting rolls of Stu Segall Productions as "background actors" (extras). They would convey the culture and language to the scenarios. With realistic scripts, sets, props, wardrobe, makeup, and pyrotechnic special effects, one could see the effect on a trainee who was immersed in one of these scenarios. In the movie business, there is a phrase: "the willing suspense of disbelief." When the lights go down in a theater and the movie starts, you willingly suspend your disbelief that you are not on the Titanic in 1912 or are not on the planet Avatar—if it is done well. We have all seen movies where you are transported into disbelief when it is not done well. It is much easier to manipulate the sights and the sounds in a two-dimensional (and sometimes 3-D) moving picture to create this "disbelief" than it is to accomplish it in the real world. Why? It is much more difficult because training scenarios are more complex, the audience (trainee) is interacting with the environment and actors, whose actions may be unpredictable, and the special effects are closer (with safety now becoming a factor). No one had done this kind of

[1] Sharpening the Warriors Edge: The Psychology & Science of Training, PPCT Research Publications, 1995.

military training before. When we first started this type of training you could see in the eyes and in the actions of the participants that they were so immersed in the scenarios that they "thought" it was real. I coined the phrase hyper-realistic to describe it. We trademarked it as Hyper-Realistic® and defined it as "such a high degree of fidelity in the replication of real-world conditions in a training environment that participants so willingly suspend disbelief that they become totally immersed and eventually stress inoculated in a way that can be quantifiably and qualitatively verified."

Calling it "stress inoculation" initially met with skepticism. Nineteen years later, and 46 peer-reviewed scientific papers about what we do, corroborate early anecdotal evidence that hyper-realistic immersion training produces a stress inoculation effect and that repetitive training in controlled, stressful situations enables people to lower their stress levels from the detrimental range to a more beneficial one, in a measurable way. (This is discussed below.)

The Fig. 68.1 flow chart illustrates how Strategic Operations transform ordinary tactical training scenarios into hyper-realistic training scenarios. Strategic Operations uses all the techniques of the theater, TV, and film industry—the "magic of Hollywood"—to enhance live training in a way that is unique in the training world. (See the lower "lane" in the flow chart.) However, employing Hollywood techniques is not enough. Two additional ingredients are necessary. The first is an understanding of and expertise in, military tactics, techniques, and procedures. (See the middle "lane" in the flow chart.) And most importantly, add to this mix all the proprietary techniques, methods, procedures, and ideas that enable the effects to be not only extremely realistic, but dynamic, interactive, and repeatable. Large numbers of military can experience combat conditions in a training environment that truly reflects real-world conditions but in a safe, controlled, duplicable, dynamic setting.

The original footprint of the TV/Movie Studio was 20 acres. The training area included a MOUT facility that could be configured as a village representing various third-world geographies. Additional features include a 4-story Close Quarters Battle (CQB) tactical training building, a rappel/fast rope tower with a helicopter on a lift that goes up to 60 feet, a merchant ship simulator, a Navy DDG simulator, an Emergency Room, two Operating Rooms, helicopter fuselages, classrooms, a bunk house for 45, and an armory. Under a Cooperative Research and Development Agreement (CRADA) with Naval Medical Center San Diego, an MV-22 Osprey (without wings or engines) is used for medical research at Strategic Operations.

It has long been known that larger numbers of casualties occur within the first several combat missions. Fear of the unknown, lack of adequate preparation, and the unexpected account for these statistics. By bringing modern technology and proven techniques of the movie industry together to faithfully replicate real combat in training scenarios, military participants are in effect experiencing those first combat missions in a safe, fully immersive hyper-realistic environment where they can make their mistakes without real-world casualties. The result is a better-prepared warfighter, validated by recent scientific evidence, and thus lives saved. A Defense Science Board study[2] found about 50% of all casualties in war occur in the first several significant exposures to combat. After these, the rate drops to less than 6%. Facing hyper-realistic RPGs, (rocket propelled grenades), IEDs (improvised explosive device) insurgents, battlefield effects, and horrific medical trauma in a training environment created by STOPS allows warfighters to hone their skills in a controlled setting rather than in the real world, and in turn, this helps save lives. This is the value of hyper-realistic training (see Fig. 68.2).

STOPS has helped develop and facilitate a wide spectrum of medical courses using the Cut Suit that range from Tactical Combat Casualty Care (TCCC) for Medics and Corpsmen at Point of Injury (POI) care under fire, transitioning to tactical field care and then to more definitive care, to advanced courses for medical providers, including surgeons and other operating room professionals. Again, the advantage of STOPS training is that it allows/requires the provider to interact with a live human model. The patients' pain, emotional well-being, and full injury profile are now part of a complete training regimen that creates a training standard found nowhere else.

In addition to military training, STOPS is an Authorized Training Facility for the National Association of EMTs (NAEMT Training Center No. 6653) and can deliver the entire menu of NAEMT nationally certified programs. STOPS is also an official training site and presenter for the California Commission on Peace Officers Standards & Training (POST Presenter No. 1102) and is capable of submitting curriculums for POST accreditation.

By 2021 STOPS has provided training support to more than a million military and civilian first responders. STOPS Tactical Training Canada provides support to UK forces training at the British Army Training Unit Suffield in Alberta. From 2004 to 2010 STOPS was designated as an Alternative Training Venue (ATV), an official pre-deployment training facility for the Marine Corps, the only civilian facility so designated. Whole battalions trained at STOPS prior to being sent overseas.

In late 2006, Lieutenant General James Mattis, then commanding general of I Marine Expeditionary Force asked STOPS to convert an abandoned 32,000 square foot tomato processing plant on Camp Pendleton California into an "infantry training simulator," officially designated as the

[2]Report of the Defense Science Board Task Force on Training Superiority and Training Surprise: https://www.cl.cam.ac.uk/~rja14/shb08/chatham3.pdf, January 2001.

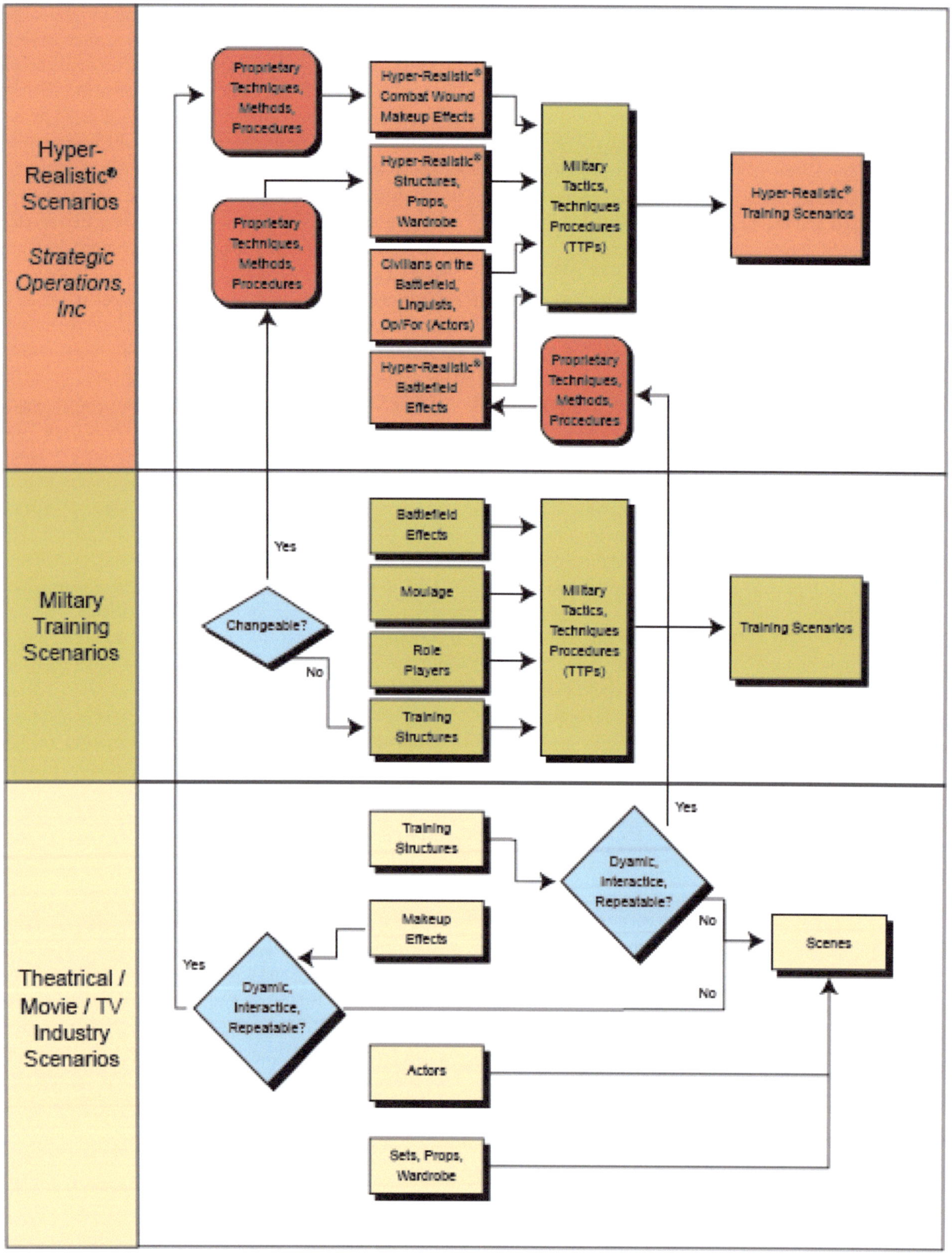

Fig. 68.1 Strategic operations

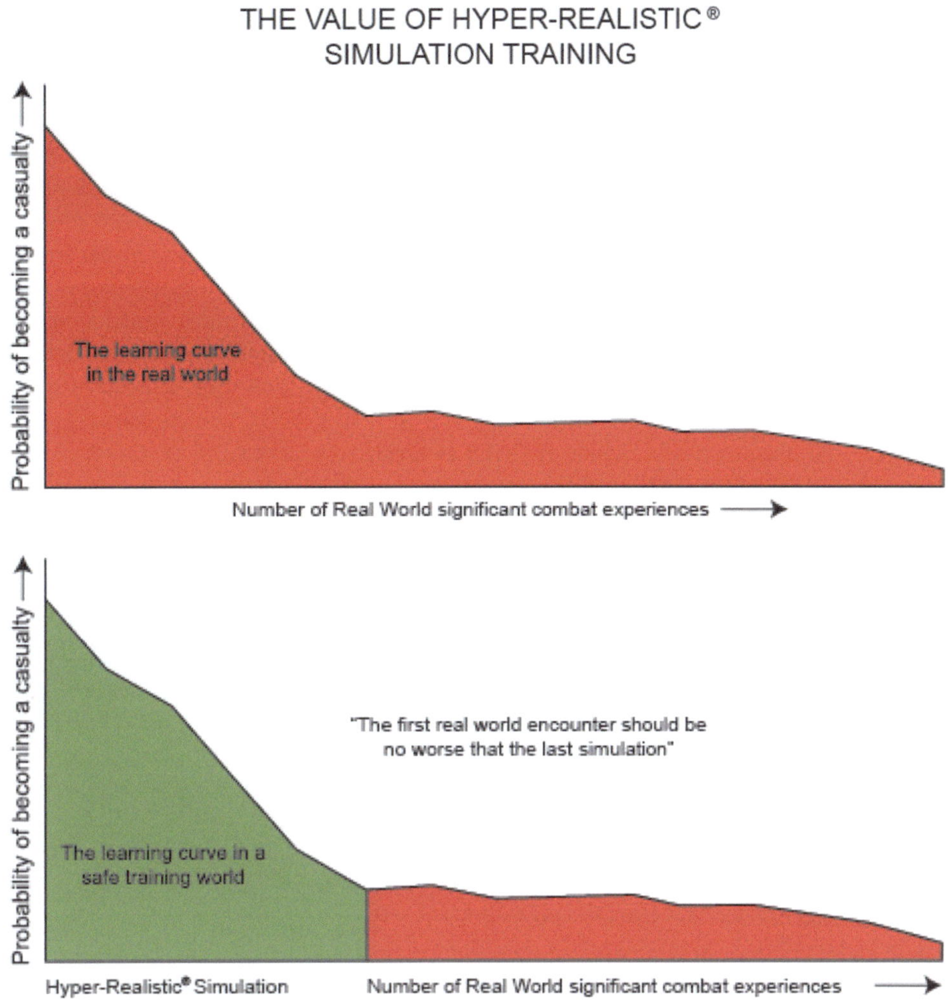

Fig. 68.2 Hyper-realistic simulation training

Infantry Immersion Trainer (IIT). Aviators have multi-million-dollar flight simulators but the Infantry that has sustained more than 85% of the casualties in Iraq and Afghanistan has no such simulators. STOPS created movie-set-like villages inside the building with pyrotechnics and other special effects. Designed for squads of 13 marines to perform urban patrolling and to interact with indigenous populations, cameras record scenarios for after-action playback and debriefing. For a time STOPS provided role players pyrotechnic and medical special effects training support. In 2007, as marines trained in the IIT, a researcher from the US Naval Health Research Center evaluated marines training in the IIT for stress reactivity, mitigation, and inoculation. Preliminary results in this study found the "acute stress response to the IIT training is substantial." Salivary hormone levels indicated that this type of "training provided a stress inoculation effect."[3]

This was the beginning of 46 scientific papers about how this type of training produces a stress inoculation effect in trainees in different types of scenarios, ranging from LEO and military tactical training to mass casualties training to surgical team training to damage control training in high sea states to zero-gravity environments.[4]

At the request of Captain Greg Bowman, MD, US Navy (Ret.) of first Medical Battalion, STOPS simulated in 2010 a number of the most horrific wounds that Captain Bowman treated in Iraq for a medical training exercise at MCB Camp Pendleton. In order to more comprehensively simulate these wounds on a live actor, the idea was born for the Cut Suit human-worn simulator; the most realistic way to simulate the look, feel, and smell effects of severe traumatic events on a live human while concurrently allowing corpsmen, medics, combat lifesavers, Soldiers, Sailors, Marines, Airmen, doctors, and civilian first responders to safely perform real

[3]"Stress Reactions and Mitigation in Immersive Training," 31 March 2009, Paul Miller, MD, MS.

[4]The reader can find a list of these papers at the bottom of the homepage of Strategic Operations: https://www.strategic-operations.com/v/vsp-files/downloadables/Articles_and_Abstracts_26_February_2021.pdf.

procedures on this person. As a result of a 2012 study for the Naval Health Research Center (NHRC)[5] STOPS was invited to bid on a Navy research contract. In August 2013, STOPS was competitively awarded a multi-year contract to support the Simulated Ambulant Lab Technology II (SALT II) Program.

Anthony J. LaPorta (Col. USA, ret.), MD, FACS, Professor of Surgery at Rocky Vista University (RVU) and head of the military track, approached me at the Special Operations Medical Association (SOMA) annual meeting in December 2011 with a request to develop the Cut Suit into a surgical trainer and a curriculum for RVU. By May 2012, the first surgical Cut Suit was used in a weeklong Intensive Surgical and Trauma Skills Course (ISTSC) at RVU, followed by ISTSC 2 at RVU in 2013. Beginning in 2014 STOPS has hosted the ISTSC at its facilities every year until the Ninth Annual course in 2020 was cancelled because of COVID-19. It has been rescheduled for June 2021. Other medical schools have joined ISTSC and efforts are underway to expand the curriculum nationwide. Second-year medical students enrolled in the military track as *Health Professions Scholarship Program (HPSP)* students stay at the STOPS bunkhouse and immerse themselves in scenarios 18 hours a day from point of injury through emergency room to operating room. They work with real first responders in point of injury scenarios ranging from overturned cars, high-rise fires, and industrial accidents to military simulations including IEDs and RPGs. The students work in the emergency room and participate in more than 40 operations during the 5-day course. As part of an ongoing study, salivary hormone samples are taken from student volunteers throughout the week and analyzed. Papers have been published about how this course better prepares these students academically.

RVU credits its partnership with STOPS and its incorporation of the Cut Suit into its curriculum with helping RVU become a distinguished medical school in the few short years it has been in existence. The RVU Surgical Simulation Center that uses the Cut Suit and STOPS technology has been accredited by the American College of Surgeons (ACS) and is the only osteopathic medical school and one of only two medical schools in the Mountain West Region to receive this distinction. The American College of Surgeons (ACS) has called RVU's use of the Cut Suit a "best practice."

In cooperation with Tuan Hoang, MD, FACS, Captain USN (Ret.) STOPS, helped develop the Shipboard Surgical Trauma Training (S2T2) Curriculum, originally a 6-day (now 5-day) training course for Navy Fleet Surgical Teams (FST) with hyper-realistic scenarios featuring Surgical Cut Suits. The training is designed to immerse the team in a hyper-realistic combat environment with complex, challenging combat casualty care scenarios, requiring the team to work on cohesion, asset management, communication, and other team dynamics to take care of the overwhelming crises. The Defense Health Board report to the Secretary of Defense in October 2018 recommended that all DOD (Department of Defense) surgical training adopt this course.[6]

STOPS partnered with Naval Medical Center San Diego to complete a 2-year Joint Program Committee (JPC)-1 grant titled "Determining the Use of a Hyper-Realistic® and Immersive Simulation Training Environment to Illustrate Improved Team Performance across the Continuum of Care." The team conducted five 6-day Navy FST and one Army FST training exercises based on the S2T2 Curriculum with extensive salivary biometric and R-to-R micro variability of heart rate data gathered along with other objective and subjective data which were reported in peer-reviewed papers.

Ten trauma surgeons from Canada and the United States performed emergency surgery in a weightless environment in a first-of-its-kind proof-of-concept experiment. This was damage control surgery in the ultimate austere environment. A specially equipped Falcon 20 jet (a "vomit comet") from the Flight Research Laboratory (FRL) at the National Research Council (NRC), the Government of Canada's premier research and technology organization, entered parabolic flight maneuvers, each of which produced 30–40 seconds of weightlessness to simulate zero-g. While weightless the surgeons performed a laparotomy on the Cut Suit. The surgeons wore sensors monitoring their physiology, cameras inside the aircraft recorded images, and onboard electronics recorded g-forces, acceleration, flight data, blood loss, and time to complete the task of stopping the bleeding. Bleeding to death is the most preventable cause of post-traumatic death worldwide. While many of these deaths can be prevented with relatively basic surgical interventions, they remain lethal when no facilities or skills exist to perform basic damage control surgery. This experiment in parabolic flight has implications for terrestrial applications from battlefield to rural to wilderness areas.

To determine the effects of high sea states on Navy surgical teams performing surgery on ships, STOPS created a Cut Suit system like the one used in the zero-g study. Hundreds of simulated surgeries were performed in a land-based simulator with six degrees of motion, simulating high sea states, and then on a Navy ship at sea for 3 weeks.

Numerous studies report that the quality of open surgical education has deteriorated for a variety of factors, including the demise of the Halstead paradigm of residency structure, effectively ending the "see one, do one, teach one" era of

[5]"Hyper-Realistic® Immersive Corpsman Training Process Evaluation Survey Results," Booz Allen Hamilton (BAH), 30 November 2012.

[6]Low-Volume High-Risk Surgical Procedures: Surgical Volume and Its Relationship to Patient Safety and Quality of Care Second Report, May 20, 2019. https://www.health.mil/About-MHS/OASDHA/Defense-Health-Agency/Defense-Health-Board/Reports.

surgery training on a live human due to patient safety and its ethical and legal issues. Additionally, here is what retired surgeon Joan F. Tryzelaar, MD, FACS, FACCP, says:

- "The 80-hour workweek has effectively taken 6 months to 1 year of in-hospital time out of residency.
- "50% of the graduates had not performed even half of 121 'essential operations' (2005 data).
- "Only 6–14% of the resident's total working time during a 5-year training program is spent in the Operating Room learning those essential operations.
- "30% of (graduates accepted into fellowship programs) were not prepared for operative cases and nearly two thirds could not work unsupervised for a significant period of time (Based on a survey of program directors): '… Residents have markedly decreased experience with open surgery because of the conversion of open surgery to laparoscopic surgery. The problem here is that the complex open operations that were previously done by general surgical residents have not been replaced by comparable laparoscopic operations of equal complexity…'
- "Fellowship/subspecialty training increased from 30% to more than 80%, in part from a feeling of inadequacy to pursue a more broad-based practice.
- "Burnout is common among American surgeons (35%) and is the single greatest predictor of surgeons' satisfaction with career and specialty choice.
- "General surgeons have decreased as a proportion of the total U.S. surgical workforce.
- "35% of general surgeons are >55 years old and capable of 'open' procedures. In contrast, many younger surgeons are not, and will replace only a portion of their older colleagues when they retire…
- "Fewer general surgeons will be available to treat an increasing demand for their services.
- "Surgical graduates are unable to perform a broad range of open and laparoscopic operations competently, as a consequence of inadequate exposure during their residency training.
- "Trauma and emergency surgery often requires the knowledge and ability to perform an *open* procedure, a skill that will be less and less available.
- "In 2006, 30% (925) of the 3,107 US counties lacked a single surgeon and nearly 9.5 million Americans lived in those counties."[7]

The Defense Science Board's "Low-Volume High-Risk Surgical Procedures: Surgical Volume and Its Relationship to Patient Safety and Quality of Care Second Report," cited above, states,

Establishing a cohesive team dynamic is critical prior to entering a combat zone. Although not recognized as an ACS-approved simulation course, the S2T2 aligns with some of the best practices identified by the ACS-AEI, including its ability to develop customized simulation environments. The highlight of the course is its use of realistic trauma training scenarios that place students in a high-anxiety training "bubble" and a state of suspended disbelief. The immersed simulation training progresses in intensity and complexity throughout the week-long program to create a "crawl, walk, run" approach to learning. This Hyper-Realistic™ field-based casualty scenario replicates battlefield conditions for point-of injury scenarios, Role 2 (resuscitative and surgical care), and en route care mock-ups.[8]

For decades, the aviation industry has embraced, adopted, and advanced simulation as an integral part of training and education. Accident rates have decreased immensely as safety has resulted from simulation. From Level D Full Flight Simulators (FFS) to Crew Resource Management (CRM) to checklists, the aviation industry has much to demonstrate to medical training and education.

If an image of fighter pilots in aerial combat training—integrating flight simulators and aircraft—comes to mind, the analogy is correct: there needs to be a "Top Gun" for surgical training. Surgery and a simulation environment should be so realistic that a medical student's *first* surgical experience on a human should be with no less confidence than the *last* surgery on an open surgery simulator. Since the end of the "see one, do one, teach one" era (the "Halstead method"), physicians in training have had significantly less hands-on experience in which they have been allowed to make decisions and be responsible for the consequences of those decisions. Success is often born of failure. But being allowed to make mistakes—to fail—is no longer permissible in surgical education, for obvious and good reasons: patient safety. But it has unintended consequences, as discussed above.

Interestingly, the US military over the last few decades developed a system of training that recognized that only by being allowed to make mistakes—and learn from them—could true learning be achieved. The military created Combat Training Centers (CTCs) at Fort Irwin, California, and Fort Polk, Louisiana, for ground combat training (the Top Gun school for aviators serves the same purpose) based on five principles: (1) provide a realistic setting; (2) allow trainees to fail; (3) face a credible opponent; (4) objective assessment of

[7] "Surgical Competence, a Crisis in US Health Care?" http://www.cardiachealth.org/, posted on February 20, 2014 – 12:45 pm.

[8] Low-Volume High-Risk Surgical Procedures: Surgical Volume and Its Relationship to Patient Safety and Quality of Care Second Report, May 20, 2019. https://www.health.mil/About-MHS/OASDHA/Defense-Health-Agency/Defense-Health-Board/Reports. Appendix E, p. 77.

performance; and (5) trainees are given a chance to remediate mistakes. While these principles may seem simple, and maybe even obvious, the CTC training system incorporating them sets the US military apart from *all* other militaries in the world.

Figure 68.3 shows how and why these five principles should be incorporated into immersive, Hyper-Realistic® surgical simulations using the Cut Suit and Advanced Surgical Simulation Packages (ASSP).

The Cut Suit coupled with the ASSP is the only open surgery simulator that is Hyper-Realistic®, repairable and thus cost-effective, the subject of numerous peer-reviewed scientific papers, and is part of curricula for medical students, surgical residents, and military and civilian surgeons.

Designed by surgeons, for surgeons, to teach surgeons, abdominal and thoracic ASSPs drop into the patented Cut Suit surgical simulator. Several surgeons consulted in the design of the Cut Suit/ASSP system, led by Reginald Franciose, MD, FACS. From the start, Dr. Franciose designed into the ASSP the pitfalls and the complications that could be encountered in each procedure. ASSPs replicate various trauma and pathology scenarios, so realistic that participants willingly suspend disbelief that they are not working on a real person. Unlike performing surgery on a real person, "time out" can be taken for instruction and education, and then restarted. Mistakes could be made and taken to a point where true learning of how to recover from the mistake can be experienced, safely. The system could be paused, reset, started over, and stopped to be analyzed and reviewed for lessons learned.

Since the end of the "see one, do one, teach one" era of the Halstead method, physicians in training have had significantly less hands-on experience in which they have been allowed to make decisions and be responsible for the consequences of those decisions. The Cut Suit and ASSP allows for that experience. Besides improving individual surgical skills and decision-making, the Cut Suit simulator enhances surgical team training just as flight simulators enhance Crew Resource Management in the airline industry.

Hopefully, in the coming years, surgical residents will receive as much practice with open surgical procedures as older generations did—and even much more—using Hyper-Realistic® surgical simulation. And surgeons in rural and wilderness areas who occasionally encounter high-risk, low-volume trauma can better prepare themselves and regularly hone their skills using these kinds of simulations. Hopefully, many lives will be saved.

	Military Combat Training Centers (CTC)	Hyper-Realistic® Surgical Simulations
Realistic Setting	Unique training environment. Units do not come to the CTC to do what they are capable of doing at home station. The CTC'c advantages in training high-intensity warfare over vast maneuver space and translated to real world distances with multiple towns, villages, caves, and urban live-fire venues. Hyper-Realistic® simulations including battlefield and medical special effects. Scenarios are created where the outcome is not assured and that promote initiative-oriented warfighting skills. Mastery of fundamentals is stressed for both individuals and collective (team) tasks. The CTC is hard, and in many ways, more difficult than actual combat. The first combat mission should be no worse than the last simulation. Make your mistakes here, do the "dying" here.	Unique training environment (simulation operating room). Surgeons and their teams come here to do what they cannot do in a real operation room: practice on "humans" (Hyper-Realistic® "Cut Suits"). Scenarios are created where the outcome is not assured and that promote initiative-oriented surgical skills. Mastery of fundamentals is stressed, for both individual and collective (team) tasks. The surgical simulations are hard, and in many ways more difficult than actual surgery. Complications and resulting stress levels can be ramped up, mistakes can be allowed, then reversed, and simulations can be reset, over and over. The first surgery should be no worse that the last simulation. Make your mistakes here, do the "dying" here.
Allowed to Fail	Stressing units to their organizational limits. Units learn best when pushed to the threshold of failure, and allowed to fail. The CTC continues to push units to their limits, continuously raising the threat, modifying conditions, and maintaining standards of performance to expose weaknesses in key systems and functions. The CTC should be hard-in many ways more difficult than actual combat.	Stressing surgical teams to their organizational limits. Individuals and teams learn best when pushed to the thresholds of failure, and allowed to fail. Hyper-Realistic® Surgical Simulations pushes individuals and teams to their limits, continuously raising the threat, modifying conditions, and maintaining standards of performance to expose weaknesses in key systems and functions. Surgical simulations should be hard-in many ways more difficult than actual surgery.
Credible Opponent	Provide a freethinking, capabilities-based, opposing force (OPFOR) with and equal chance to win. The training unit must be allowed to fail.	Surgeons and teams face credible, complicated, interactive crises (pathologies and trauma) with an equal chance to win. Surgeons and teams must be allowed to fail.
Objective Assessment	Unblinking feedback. The CTC prides itself on providing brutally honest and irrefutable feedback on unit performance while providing a forum that encourages candid discussion and self-analysis by the unit. Subjective assessment is significantly enhanced with instrumentation, including position location of individuals, weapons, and weapons' effects, as well as video, all of which can be used for after-action review (AAR).	Unblinking feedback. Hyper-Realistic® Surgical Simulations provide brutally honest and irrefutable feedback on individual and team performance while providing a forum that encourages candid discussion and self-analysis by the individual and team. Subjective assessment is significantly enhanced by instrumentation, including position location of individuals, instruments, and organs within the Cut Suit, as well as video, all of which can be used for after-action review (AAR).
Chance to Remediate.	Dedicate a portion of the exercise to retraining those tasks which the commander deems essential for their unit to increase proficiency. (Retraining is not an indication of failure)	With Hyper-Realistic® Surgical Simulations, remediation can occur immediately, or following an after-action review. (retraining is not an indication of failure.)

Fig. 68.3 Cut Suit and advanced surgical simulation packages (ASSP) principals

Index

L. Marshall Gillman, S. Widder (eds.), *Trauma Team Dynamics*, https://doi.org/10.1007/978-3-031-86312-7

D

E

MIX
Papier aus verantwortungsvollen Quellen
Paper from responsible sources
FSC® C105338

If you have any concerns about our products,
you can contact us on
ProductSafety@springernature.com

In case Publisher is established outside the EU,
the EU authorized representative is:
Springer Nature Customer Service Center GmbH
Europaplatz 3, 69115 Heidelberg, Germany

Printed by Libri Plureos GmbH
in Hamburg, Germany